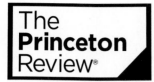
The
Princeton
Review®

The Princeton Review

MCAT® PREP

2021-2022

The Staff of The Princeton Review

Penguin
Random
House

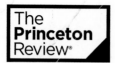

The Princeton Review
110 East 42nd St, 7th Floor
New York, NY 10017
E-mail: editorialsupport@review.com

Published in the United States by Penguin Random House LLC, New York, and in Canada by Random House of Canada, a division of Penguin Random House Ltd., Toronto.

Terms of Service: The Princeton Review Online Companion Tools ["Student Tools"] for the Cracking book series and MCAT Review series are available for only the two most recent editions of that book. Student Tools may be activated only once per eligible book purchased. Activation of Student Tools more than once per book is in direct violation of these Terms of Service and may result in discontinuation of access to Student Tools Services.

ISBN: 978-0-525-57041-7
ISSN 2693-2016

The MCAT is a registered trademark of the Association of American Medical Colleges.

The Princeton Review is not affiliated with Princeton University.

Editor: Selena Coppock
Production Artist: Jason Ullmeyer
Production Editors: Liz Dacey, Sarah Litt

Printed in China

10 9 8 7 6 5 4 3 2 1

Editorial

Rob Franek, Editor-in-Chief
David Soto, Director of Content Development
Stephen Koch, Student Survey Manager
Deborah Weber, Director of Production
Gabriel Berlin, Production Design Manager
Selena Coppock, Managing Editor
Aaron Riccio, Senior Editor
Meave Shelton, Senior Editor
Chris Chimera, Editor
Anna Goodlett, Editor
Eleanor Green, Editor
Orion McBean, Editor
Patricia Murphy, Editorial Assistant

Penguin Random House Publishing Group

Tom Russell, VP, Publisher
Alison Stoltzfus, Publishing Director
Amanda Yee, Associate Managing Editor
Ellen Reed, Production Manager
Suzanne Lee, Designer

CONTRIBUTORS

TPR MCAT Biology and Biochemistry Development Team:
Jessica Adams, Ph.D.
Britney McMurren, B.H.Sc., M.Sc.
Judene Wright, M.S., M.A.Ed., Senior Editor, Lead Developer
Sarah Woodruff, B.S., B.A., Lead Developer

TPR MCAT CARS Development Team:
Gina Granter, M.A.
Christopher Hinkle, Th.D.
Jennifer S. Wooddell, Senior Editor, Lead Developer

TPR MCAT General Chemistry Development Team:
Bethany Blackwell, M.S., Senior Editor, Lead Developer
William Ewing, Ph.D.
Chris Fortenbach, B.S.

Edited for Production by:
Judene Wright, M.S., M.A.Ed.
    National Content Director, MCAT Program,
    The Princeton Review

TPR MCAT Organic Chemistry Development Team:
Bethany Blackwell, M.S.
William Ewing, Ph.D.
Brandon Kelley, Ph.D.
Jason Osman, Ph.D., Senior Editor, Lead Developer

TPR MCAT Physics Development Team:
Jon Fowler, M.A., Senior Editor
Tomislav Kurtovic, M.A.

TPR MCAT Psychology and Sociology Development Team:
Matthew Dempsey, Ph.D., Senior Editor, Lead Developer
Kevin Keogh
Anthony Krupp, Ph.D.
Tomislav Kurtovic, M.A.

The Princeton Review would like to thank the following people for their contributions to this book :
Elizabeth Aamot (Fatith), Rizwan Ahmad, M.A., Kashif Anwar, M.D., M.M.S., Farhad Aziz, B.S., John Bahling, M.D.,
Gary Bedford, Kendra Bowman, Ph.D., Kristen Brunson, Ph.D., Jessica Burstrem, M.A., Brian Butts, B.S., B.A., Argun Can,
Phil Carpenter, Ph.D., Erika C. Castro, B.A., Brian Cato, Khawar Chaudry, B.S., Nita Chauhan, H.BSc, MSc, Dan Cho, M.P.H.,
Maria S. Chushak, M.S., Alix Claps, M.A., Doug Couchman, Cynthia Cowan, B.A., Glenn E. Croston, Ph.D., Sara Daniel, B.S.,
Douglas S. Daniels, Ph.D., Nathan Deal, M.D., Guenevieve O. del Mundo, B.A., B.S., C.C.S., Ian Denham, B.Sc., B.Ed.,
Joshua Dilworth, M.D., Ph.D., Annie Dude, Amanda Edward, H.BSc., H.BEd., Cory Eicher, B.A., Rob Fong, M.D., Ph.D.,
Chris Fortenbach, B.S., Michelle E. Fox, B.S., Kirsten Frank, Ph.D., (James) Ben Gill, Jacqueline R. Giordano, Carlos Guzman,
Corinne Harol, Alison Howard, James Hudson, M.A., Isabel L. Jackson, B.S., Adam Johnson, Nadia Johnson, M.A., M.S.,
Ryan Katchky, Jason N. Kennedy, M.S., Erik Kildebeck, Omair Adil Khan, Paul Kugelmass, George Kyriazis, Ph.D.,
Ali Landreau, B.A., Steven A. Leduc, M.S., Ben Lee, Jay Lee, Heather Liwanag, Ph.D., Brendan Lloyd, B.Sc., M.Sc.,
Stefan Loren, Ph.D., Travis Mackoy, B.S., Rohit Madani, B.S., Neil Maluste, B.S., Joey Mancuso, M.S., D.O.,
Chris Manuel, M.P.H., Ashley Manzoor, Ph.D., Janet Marshall, Ph.D., Douglas K. McLemore, B.S., Evan Martow, BMSc,
Mike Matera, B.A., Jennifer A. McDevitt, M.A., Marion-Vincent L. Mempin, B.S., Donna Memran, Ashleigh Menhadji,
Al Mercado, Brian Mikolasko, M.D., M.BA, Katherine Miller, Ph.D., Abhisehk Mohapatra, B.A., Katherine Montgomery,
Christopher Moriates, M.D., Paola A. Munoz, M.A., Stephen L. Nelson, Jr., Ph.D., Tenaya Newkirk, Ph.D., Don Osborne,
Daniel J. Pallin, M.D., Gina Passante, Rupal Patel, B.S., Vivek Patel, Tyler Peikes, Chris Pentzell, M.S., Bikem Ayse Polat,
Mary Qiu, Chris Rabbat, Ph.D., Steven Rines, Ph.D., Ina C. Roy, M.D., M.S., Jayson Sack, M.D., M.S., Karen Salazar, Ph.D.,
Will Sanderson, Jeanine Seitz-Partridge, M.S., Maryam Shambayati, M.S., Sina Shahbaz, B.S., Shalom Shapiro,
Mark Shew, H.BSc., Carolyn J. Shiau, M.D., Gillian Shiau, M.D., Oktay Shuminov, B.S., Andrew D. Snyder, M.D., Angela Song,
Kate Speiker, Teri Stewart, B.S.E., David Stoll, Dylan Sweeney, Preston Swirnoff, Ph.D., M.S., Jonathan Swirsky,
Felicia Tam, Ph.D., Jenkang Tao, B.S., B.A., Neil Thornton, Lara Tubelle de Gonzales, Rhead Uddin, Danish Vaiyani,
Christopher Volpe, Ph.D., Betsy Walli, M.S., Ph.D., Jia Wang, Tom Watts, B.A., David Weiskopf, M.A., Barry Weliver,
Chelsea K. Wise, M.S., Hesham Zakaria.

Periodic Table of the Elements

1 H 1.0																	2 He 4.0
3 Li 6.9	4 Be 9.0											5 B 10.8	6 C 12.0	7 N 14.0	8 O 16.0	9 F 19.0	10 Ne 20.2
11 Na 23.0	12 Mg 24.3											13 Al 27.0	14 Si 28.1	15 P 31.0	16 S 32.1	17 Cl 35.5	18 Ar 39.9
19 K 39.1	20 Ca 40.1	21 Sc 45.0	22 Ti 47.9	23 V 50.9	24 Cr 52.0	25 Mn 54.9	26 Fe 55.8	27 Co 58.9	28 Ni 58.7	29 Cu 63.5	30 Zn 65.4	31 Ga 69.7	32 Ge 72.6	33 As 74.9	34 Se 79.0	35 Br 79.9	36 Kr 83.8
37 Rb 85.5	38 Sr 87.6	39 Y 88.9	40 Zr 91.2	41 Nb 92.9	42 Mo 95.9	43 Tc (98)	44 Ru 101.1	45 Rh 102.9	46 Pd 106.4	47 Ag 107.9	48 Cd 112.4	49 In 114.8	50 Sn 118.7	51 Sb 121.8	52 Te 127.6	53 I 126.9	54 Xe 131.3
55 Cs 132.9	56 Ba 137.3	57 *La 138.9	72 Hf 178.5	73 Ta 180.9	74 W 183.9	75 Re 186.2	76 Os 190.2	77 Ir 192.2	78 Pt 195.1	79 Au 197.0	80 Hg 200.6	81 Tl 204.4	82 Pb 207.2	83 Bi 209.0	84 Po (209)	85 At (210)	86 Rn (222)
87 Fr (223)	88 Ra 226.0	89 †Ac 227.0	104 Rf (261)	105 Db (262)	106 Sg (266)	107 Bh (264)	108 Hs (277)	109 Mt (268)	110 Ds (281)	111 Rg (272)	112 Cn (285)	113 Uut (286)	114 Fl (289)	115 Uup (288)	116 Lv (293)	117 Uus (294)	118 Uuo (294)

*Lanthanide Series:

58 Ce 140.1	59 Pr 140.9	60 Nd 144.2	61 Pm (145)	62 Sm 150.4	63 Eu 152.0	64 Gd 157.3	65 Tb 158.9	66 Dy 162.5	67 Ho 164.9	68 Er 167.3	69 Tm 168.9	70 Yb 173.0	71 Lu 175.0
90 Th 232.0	91 Pa (231)	92 U 238.0	93 Np (237)	94 Pu (244)	95 Am (243)	96 Cm (247)	97 Bk (247)	98 Cf (251)	99 Es (252)	100 Fm (257)	101 Md (258)	102 No (259)	103 Lr (260)

†Actinide Series:

TABLE OF CONTENTS

PART 1: MCAT OVERVIEW

CHAPTER 1: MCAT BASICS 3

CHAPTER 2: OVERVIEW AND STRATEGY OF THE SCIENCE SECTIONS 13

CHAPTER 3: STRESS MANAGEMENT, STUDY SCHEDULES, AND FINAL PREPARATION 25

CHAPTER 4: MCAT STATISTICS 33

CHAPTER 5: LAB TECHNIQUES 47

PART 2: MCAT BIOCHEMISTRY

CHAPTER 6: BIOCHEMISTRY BASICS 105

CHAPTER 7: AMINO ACIDS AND PROTEINS 111

CHAPTER 8: CARBOHYDRATES AND CARBOHYDRATE METABOLISM 137

CHAPTER 9: LIPIDS 159

CHAPTER 10: NUCLEIC ACIDS 177

PART 3: MCAT BIOLOGY

CHAPTER 11: MOLECULAR BIOLOGY 193

CHAPTER 12: MICROBIOLOGY 235

CHAPTER 13: EUKARYOTIC CELLS 259

CHAPTER 14: GENETICS AND EVOLUTION 297

CHAPTER 15: THE NERVOUS AND ENDOCRINE SYSTEMS 329

CHAPTER 16: THE CIRCULATORY, RESPIRATORY, LYMPHATIC, AND IMMUNE SYSTEMS 369

CHAPTER 17: THE EXCRETORY AND DIGESTIVE SYSTEMS 407

CHAPTER 18: THE MUSCULOSKELETAL SYSTEM AND SKIN 435

CHAPTER 19: THE REPRODUCTIVE SYSTEMS 455

PART 4: MCAT PSYCHOLOGY AND SOCIOLOGY

CHAPTER 20: RESEARCH METHODS 481

CHAPTER 21: SOCIAL STRUCTURE, GROUP IDENTITY, AND SELF IDENTITY 497

CHAPTER 22: PERSONALITY, MOTIVATION, ATTITUDES, AND PSYCHOLOGICAL DISORDERS 535

CHAPTER 23: LEARNING, MEMORY, AND BEHAVIOR 551

CHAPTER 24: INTERACTING WITH THE ENVIRONMENT 567

PART 5: MCAT GENERAL CHEMISTRY

CHAPTER 25: CHEMISTRY FUNDAMENTALS 589

CHAPTER 26: ATOMIC AND MOLECULAR STRUCTURE AND PROPERTIES 603

CHAPTER 27: THERMODYNAMICS 647

CHAPTER 28: PHASES AND GASES 663

CHAPTER 29: KINETICS 683

CHAPTER 30: EQUILIBRIUM 693

CHAPTER 31: ACIDS AND BASES 709

CHAPTER 32: ELECTROCHEMISTRY 731

PART 6: MCAT ORGANIC CHEMISTRY

CHAPTER 33: ORGANIC CHEMISTRY FUNDAMENTALS 747

CHAPTER 34: STRUCTURE AND STABILITY 757

CHAPTER 35: ORGANIC CHEMISTRY REACTIONS: NUCLEOPHILIC SUBSTITUTION AND ADDITION.... 803

CHAPTER 36: BIOLOGICALLY IMPORTANT MOLECULES 835

PART 7: MCAT PHYSICS

CHAPTER 37: KINEMATICS AND DYNAMICS 863

CHAPTER 38: WORK AND ENERGY 919

CHAPTER 39: THERMODYNAMICS 945

CHAPTER 40: FLUIDS AND ELASTICITY OF SOLIDS 961

CHAPTER 41: ELECTROSTATICS, ELECTRICITY, AND MAGNETISM 991

CHAPTER 42: OSCILLATIONS, WAVES, AND SOUND 1083

CHAPTER 43: LIGHT, OPTICS, AND QUANTUM PHYSICS 1113

PART 8: MCAT CRITICAL ANALYSIS AND REASONING SKILLS

CHAPTER 44: INTRODUCTION TO MCAT CRITICAL ANALYSIS AND REASONING SKILLS 1143

CHAPTER 45: CARS: ACTIVE READING 1173

CHAPTER 46: CARS QUESTION TYPES AND STRATEGIES 1201

CHAPTER 47: CARS: THE PROCESS OF ELIMINATION (POE) AND ATTRACTORS 1237

CHAPTER 48: CARS SECTION-WIDE STRATEGY 1255

PASSAGE PERMISSIONS INFORMATION 1290

INDEX 1291

16-PAGE TEAR OUT SUMMARY SECTION 1311

Get More (Free) Content
at **PrincetonReview.com/prep**

As easy as **1·2·3**

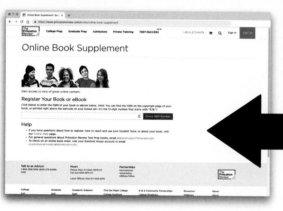

1 Go to PrincetonReview.com/prep and enter the following ISBN for your book:
9780525570417

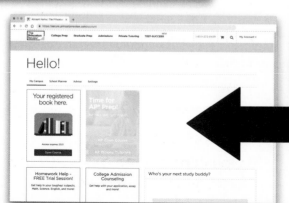

2 Answer a few simple questions to set up an exclusive Princeton Review account. *(If you already have one, you can just log in.)*

3 Enjoy access to your **FREE** content!

Once you've registered, you can...

- Take **4** full-length practice MCAT exams

- Find useful information about taking the MCAT and applying to medical school

- Check to see if there have been any corrections or updates to this edition

- Get our take on any recent or pending updates to the MCAT

Need to report a potential **content** issue?

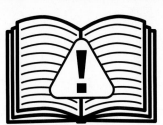

Contact **EditorialSupport@review.com** and include:

- full title of the book
- ISBN
- page number

Need to report a **technical** issue?

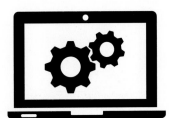

Contact **TPRStudentTech@review.com** and provide:

- your full name
- email address used to register the book
- full book title and ISBN
- Operating system (Mac/PC) and browser (Firefox, Safari, etc.)

Part 1

MCAT Overview

Chapter 1
MCAT Basics

SO YOU WANT TO BE A DOCTOR

So...you want to be a doctor. If you're like most premeds, you've wanted to be a doctor since you were pretty young. When people asked you what you wanted to be when you grew up, you always answered "a doctor." You had toy medical kits, bandaged up your dog or cat, and played "hospital." You probably read your parents' home medical guides for fun.

When you got to high school you took honors and AP classes. You studied hard, got straight As (or at least really good grades!), and participated in extracurricular activities so you could get into a good college. And you succeeded!

At college you knew exactly what to do. You took your classes seriously, studied hard, and got a great GPA. You talked to your professors and hung out at office hours to get good letters of recommendation. You were a member of the pre-med society on campus, volunteered at hospitals, and shadowed doctors. All that's left to do now is get a good MCAT score.

Just the MCAT.

Just the most confidence-shattering, most demoralizing, longest, most brutal entrance exam for any graduate program. At about 7.5 hours (including breaks), the MCAT tops the list...even the closest runners up, the LSAT and GMAT, are only about 4 hours long. The MCAT tests significant science content knowledge along with the ability to think quickly, reason logically, and read comprehensively, all under the pressure of a timed exam.

The path to a good MCAT score is not as easy to see as the path to a good GPA or the path to a good letter of recommendation. The MCAT is less about what you know, and more about how to apply what you know...and how to apply it quickly to new situations. Because the path might not be so clear, you might be worried. That's why you picked up this book.

We promise to demystify the MCAT for you, with clear descriptions of the different sections, how the test is scored, and what the test experience is like. We will help you understand general test-taking techniques as well as provide you with specific techniques for each section. We will review the science content you need to know as well as give you strategies for the Critical Analysis and Reasoning Skills (CARS) section. We'll show you the path to a good MCAT score and help you walk the path.

After all...you want to be a doctor. And we want you to succeed.

WHAT IS THE MCAT...REALLY?

Most test-takers approach the MCAT as though it were a typical college science test, one in which facts and knowledge simply need to be regurgitated in order to do well. They study for the MCAT the same way they did for their college tests, by memorizing facts and details, formulas and equations. And when they get to the MCAT they are surprised...and disappointed.

It's a myth that the MCAT is purely a content-knowledge test. If medical school admission committees want to see what you know, all they have to do is look at your transcripts. What they really want to see, though, is how you *think*. Especially, how you think under pressure. And *that's* what your MCAT score will tell them.

The MCAT is really a test of your ability to apply basic knowledge to different, possibly new, situations. It's a test of your ability to reason out and evaluate arguments. Do you still need to know your science content? Absolutely. But not at the level that most test-takers think they need to know it. Furthermore, your science knowledge won't help you on the Critical Analysis and Reasoning Skills (CARS) section. So how do you study for a test like this?

You study for the science sections by reviewing the basics and then applying them to MCAT practice questions. You study for the CARS section by learning how to adapt your existing reading and analytical skills to the nature of the test.

The book you are holding will review all the relevant MCAT content you will need for the test, and a little bit more. It includes hundreds of questions designed to make you think about the material in a deeper way, along with full explanations to clarify the logical thought process needed to get to the answer. It also comes with access to four full-length online practice exams to further hone your skills: see below.

GO ONLINE!

In addition to the review material you'll find in this book, there is a wealth of practice content available online at **PrincetonReview.com/prep.** There you'll find the following:

- 4 full-length practice MCATs with complete answers and explanations
- useful information about taking the MCAT and applying to medical school

To register your book, go to **PrincetonReview.com/prep.** You'll see a welcome page where you can register your book by its ISBN number (found on the back cover above the barcode). Set up an account using this number and your email address. Then you can access all of your online content.

MCAT NUTS AND BOLTS

Overview

The MCAT is a computer-based test (CBT) that is *not* adaptive. Adaptive tests base your next question on whether or not you've answered the current question correctly. The MCAT is *linear*, or *fixed-form*, meaning that the questions are in a predetermined order and do not change based on your answers. However, there are many versions of the test, so that on a given test day, different people will see different versions. The following table highlights the features of the MCAT exam.

Registration	Online via www.aamc.org. Begins as early as six months prior to test date; available up until week of test (subject to seat availability).
Testing Centers	Administered at small, secure, climate-controlled computer testing rooms.
Security	Photo ID with signature, electronic fingerprint, electronic signature verification, assigned seat.
Proctoring	None. Test administrator checks examinee in and assigns seat at computer. All testing instructions are given on the computer.
Frequency of Test	Many times per year distributed over January, April, May, June, July, August, and September.
Format	Exclusively computer-based. NOT an adaptive test.
Length of Test Day	7.5 hours
Breaks	Optional 10-minute breaks between sections, with a 30-minute break for lunch.
Section Names	1. Chemical and Physical Foundations of Biological Systems (Chem/Phys) 2. Critical Analysis and Reasoning Skills (CARS) 3. Biological and Biochemical Foundations of Living Systems (Bio/Biochem) 4. Psychological, Social, and Biological Foundations of Behavior (Psych/Soc)
Number of Questions and Timing	59 Chem/Phys questions, 95 minutes 53 CARS questions, 90 minutes 59 Bio/Biochem questions, 95 minutes 59 Psych/Soc questions, 95 minutes
Scoring	Test is scaled. Several forms per administration.
Allowed/ Not allowed	No timers/watches. Noise reduction headphones available. Noteboard booklet and wet-erase marker given at start of test and taken at end of test. Locker or secure area provided for personal items.
Results: Timing and Delivery	Approximately 30 days. Electronic scores only, available online through AAMC login. Examinees can print official score reports.
Maximum Number of Retakes	The test can be taken a maximum of three times in one year, four times over two years, and seven times over the lifetime of the examinee. An examinee can be registered for only one date at a time.

Registration

Registration for the exam is completed online at https://students-residents.aamc.org/applying-medical-school/article/2015-mcat-registration-fees/. The AAMC opens registration for a given test date at least two months in advance of the date, often earlier. It's a good idea to register well in advance of your desired test date to make sure that you get a seat.

Sections

There are four sections on the MCAT exam: Chemical and Physical Foundations of Biological Systems (Chem/Phys), Critical Analysis and Reasoning Skills (CARS), Biological and Biochemical Foundations of Living Systems (Bio/Biochem), and Psychological, Social, and Biological Foundations of Behavior (Psych/Soc). All sections consist of multiple-choice questions.

Section	Concepts Tested	Number of Questions and Timing
Chemical and Physical Foundations of Biological Systems	Basic concepts in chemical and physical sciences, scientific inquiry, reasoning, research and statistics skills	59 questions in 95 minutes
Critical Analysis and Reasoning Skills	Critical analysis of information drawn from a wide range of social science and humanities disciplines	53 questions in 90 minutes
Biological and Biochemical Foundations of Living Systems	Basic concepts in biology and biochemistry, scientific inquiry, reasoning, research and statistics skills	59 questions in 95 minutes
Psychological, Social, and Biological Foundations of Behavior	Basic concepts in psychology, sociology, and biology, research methods and statistics	59 questions in 95 minutes

Most questions on the MCAT (44 in the science sections, all 53 in the CARS section) are passage-based. The science sections have 10 passages with 4–6 questions per passage and 15 freestanding questions (more on that below). The CARS section has 9 passages with 5–7 questions per passage. A passage consists of a few paragraphs of information on which several following questions are based. In the science sections, passages often include equations or reactions, tables, graphs, figures, and experiments to analyze. CARS passages come from literature in social sciences, humanities, ethics, philosophy, cultural studies, and population health, and they do not test content knowledge in any way.

Some questions in the science sections are *freestanding questions* (FSQs). These questions are independent of any passage information. These questions appear in several groups of about four to five questions, and are interspersed throughout the passages. About 1/4 (15 of 59) of the questions in the sciences sections are freestanding, and the remainder are passage-based.

Each section on the MCAT is separated by either a 10-minute break or a 30-minute lunch break.

Section	Time
Test Center Check-In	Variable, can take up to 40 minutes if center is busy.
Tutorial	10 minutes
Chemical and Physical Foundations of Biological Systems	95 minutes
Break	10 minutes
Critical Analysis and Reasoning Skills	90 minutes
Lunch Break	30 minutes
Biological and Biochemical Foundations of Living Systems	95 minutes
Break	10 minutes
Psychological, Social, and Biological Foundations of Behavior	95 minutes
Void Option	5 minutes
Survey	5 minutes

The survey includes questions about your satisfaction with the overall MCAT experience, including registration, check-in, et cetera, as well as questions about how you prepared for the test.

Scoring

The MCAT is a scaled exam, meaning that your raw score will be converted into a scaled score that takes into account the difficulty of the questions. There is no guessing penalty. All sections are scored from 118–132, with a total scaled score range of 472–528. Because different versions of the test have varying levels of difficulty, the scale will be different from one exam to the next. Thus, there is no "magic number" of questions to get right in order to get a particular score. Plus, some of the questions on the test are considered "experimental" and do not count toward your score; they are just there to be evaluated for possible future inclusion in a test.

At the end of the test (after you complete the Psychological, Social, and Biological Foundations of Behavior section), you will be asked to choose one of the following two options: "I wish to have my MCAT exam scored" or "I wish to VOID my MCAT exam." You have five minutes to make a decision, and if you do not select one of the options in that time, the test will automatically be scored. If you choose the VOID option, your test will not be scored (you will not now, or ever, get a numerical score for this test), medical schools will not know you took the test, and no refunds will be granted. You cannot "unvoid" your scores at a later time.

So, what's a good score? The AAMC is centering the scale at 500 (i.e., 500 will be the 50th percentile) and recommends that application committees consider applicants near the center of the range. To be on the safe side, aim for a total score of 506–508. And remember that if your GPA is on the low side, you'll need higher MCAT scores to compensate, and if you have a strong GPA, you can get away with lower MCAT scores. But the reality is that your chances of acceptance depend on a lot more than just your MCAT scores. It's a combination of your GPA, your MCAT scores, your undergraduate coursework, letters of recommendation, experience related to the medical field (such as volunteer work or research), extracurricular activities, your personal statement, etc. Medical schools are looking for a complete package, not just good scores and a good GPA.

GENERAL LAYOUT, TEST TOOLS, AND PACING

Layout of the Test

In each section of the test, the computer screen is divided vertically, with the passage on the left and the range of questions for that passage indicated above (e.g., "Passage 1 Questions 1–5"). The scroll bar for the passage text appears in the middle of the screen. Each question appears on the right, and you need to click "Next" to move to each subsequent question.

In the science sections, the freestanding questions are found in groups of 4–5, interspersed with the passages. The screen is still divided vertically; on the left is the statement "Questions [X–XX] do not refer to a passage and are independent of each other" and each question appears on the right as described above.

CBT Tools

There are a number of tools available on the test, including highlighting, strike-outs, the Flag for Review button, the Navigation and Review Screen buttons, the Periodic Table button, and of course, the noteboard booklet. All tools are available with both mouse control (buttons to click) or keyboard commands (Alt + a letter). As everyone has different preferences, you should practice with both types of tools (mouse and keyboard) to see which is more comfortable for you personally. The following is a brief description of each tool.

1) **Highlighting:** This is done in the passage text (including table entries and some equations, but excluding figures and molecular structures), in the question stems, and in the answer choices (including Roman numerals). Select the words you wish to highlight (left-click and drag the cursor across the words), and in the upper left corner click the "Highlight" button to highlight the selected text yellow. Alternatively, press "Alt+H" to highlight the words. Highlighting can be removed by selecting the words again and in the upper left corner clicking the down arrow next to "Highlight." This will expand to show the "Remove Highlight" option; clicking this will remove the highlighting. Removing highlighting via the keyboard is cumbersome and is not recommended.

2) **Strike-outs:** This can be done on the answer choices, including Roman numeral statements, by selecting the text you want to strike out (left-click and drag the cursor across the text), then clicking the "Strikethrough" button in the upper left corner. Alternatively, press "Alt+S" to strikeout the words. The strike-out can be removed by repeating these actions. Figures or molecular structures cannot be struck out, however, the letter answer choice of those structures can.

3) **Flag for Review button:** This is available for each question and is found in the upper right corner. This allows you to flag the question as one you would like to review later if time permits. When clicked, the flag icon turns yellow. Click again to remove the flag. Alternatively, press "Alt+F."

4) **Navigation button:** This is found near the bottom of the screen and is only available on your first pass through the section. Clicking this button brings up a navigation table listing all questions and their statuses (unseen, incomplete, complete, flagged for review). You can also press "Alt+N" to bring up the screen. The questions can be sorted by their statuses, and clicking a question number takes you immediately to that question. Once you have reached the end of the section and viewed the Review screen (described below), the Navigation screen is no longer available.

5) **Review Screen button:** This button is found near the bottom of the screen after your first pass through the section, and when clicked, brings up a new screen showing all questions and their statuses (either incomplete, unseen, or flagged for review). Questions that are complete are assigned no additional status. You can then choose one of three options by clicking with the mouse or with keyboard shortcuts: Review All (Alt+A), Review Incomplete (Alt+I), or Review Flagged (Alt+R); alternatively, you can click a question number to go directly back to that question. You can also end the section from this screen.

6) **Periodic Table button:** Clicking this button will open a periodic table (or press "Alt+T"). Note that the periodic table is large, covering most of the screen. However, this window can be resized to see the questions and a portion of the periodic table at the same time. The table text will not decrease, but scroll bars will appear on the window so you can center the section of the table of interest in the window.

7) **Noteboard Booklet (Scratch Paper):** At the start of the test, you will be given a spiral-bound set of four laminated 8.5"×14" sheets of paper and a wet-erase black marker to use as scratch paper. You can request a clean noteboard booklet at any time during the test; your original booklet will be collected. The noteboard is only useful if it is kept organized; do not give in to the tendency to write on the first available open space! Good organization will be very helpful when/if you wish to review a question. Indicate the passage number, the range of questions for that passage, and a topic in a box near the top of your scratch work, and indicate the question you are working on in a circle to the left of the notes for that question. Draw a line under your scratch work when you change passages to keep the work separate. Do not erase or scribble over any previous work. If you do not think it is correct, draw one line through the work and start again. You may have already done some useful work without realizing it.

Pacing

Since the MCAT is a timed test, you must keep an eye on the timer and adjust your pacing as necessary. It would be terrible to run out of time at the end only to discover that the last few questions could have been easily answered in just a few seconds each.

In the science sections you will have about one minute and thirty-five seconds (1:35) per question, and in the CARS section you will have about one minute and forty seconds per question (1:40).

Section	# of Questions in passage	Approximate time (including reading the passage)
Chem/Phys, Bio/Biochem, and Psych/Soc	4	6.5 minutes
	5	8 minutes
	6	9.5 minutes
CARS	5	8.5 minutes
	6	10 minutes
	7	11.5 minutes

When starting a passage in the science sections, make note of how much time you will allot for it and the starting time on the timer. Jot down on your noteboard what the timer should say at the end of the passage. Then just keep an eye on it as you work through the questions. If you are near the end of the time for that passage, guess on any remaining questions, make some notes on your noteboard, Flag the questions, and move on. Come back to those questions if you have time.

For the CARS section, keep in mind that many people will maximize their score by *not* trying to complete every question or every passage in the section. A good strategy for test takers who cannot achieve a high level of accuracy on all nine passages is to randomly guess on at least one passage in the section and spend your time getting a high percentage of the other questions right. To complete all nine CARS passages, you have about ten minutes per passage. To complete eight of the nine, you have about 11 minutes per passage.

TESTING TIPS

Before Test Day

- Take a trip to the test center a day or two before your actual test date so that you can easily find the building and room on test day. This will also allow you to gauge traffic and see if you need money for parking or anything like that. Knowing this type of information ahead of time will greatly reduce your stress on the day of your test.
- Don't do any heavy studying the day before the test. Try to get a good amount of sleep during the nights leading up to the test.
- Eat well. Try to avoid excessive caffeine and sugar. Ideally, in the weeks leading up to the actual test you should experiment a little bit with foods and practice tests to see which foods give you the most endurance. Aim for steady blood sugar levels during the test: sports drinks, peanut-butter crackers, trail mix, etc. make good snacks for your breaks and lunch.

General Test Day Info and Tips

- On the day of the test, arrive at the test center at least a half hour prior to the start time of your test.
- Examinees will be checked in to the center in the order in which they arrive.
- You will be assigned a locker or secure area in which to put your personal items. Textbooks and study notes are not allowed, so there is no need to bring them with you to the test center.
- Your ID will be checked, your palm vein will be scanned, and you will be asked to sign in.
- You will be given your noteboard booklet and wet-erase marker, and the test center administrator will take you to the computer on which you will complete the test. You may not choose a computer; you must use the computer assigned to you.
- Nothing is allowed at the computer station except your photo ID, your locker key (if provided), and a factory sealed packet of ear plugs; you cannot even bring your watch.
- If you choose to leave the testing room at the breaks, you will have your palm vein scanned again, and you will have to sign in and out.
- You are allowed to access the items in your locker, except for notes and cell phones. (Check your test center's policy on cell phones ahead of time; some centers do not even allow them to be kept in your locker.)
- Don't forget to bring the snack foods and lunch you experimented with in your practice tests.
- At the end of the test, the test administrator will collect your noteboard.
- Definitely take the breaks! Get up and walk around. It's a good way to clear your head between sections and get the blood (and oxygen!) flowing to your brain.
- Ask for a clean noteboard at the breaks if you use up all the space, or if you just want a fresh one for the next section.

Chapter 2
Overview and Strategy
of the Science Sections

This chapter is designed to present you with an overview of the types of passages and questions that will appear in the science sections of the MCAT and to give you some general strategies for dealing with them. An overview of CARS passages and questions, along with strategies for that section, appear in the CARS section of this book.

2.1 SCIENCE SECTIONS OVERVIEW

There are three science sections on the MCAT.

- Chemical and Physical Foundations of Biological Systems
- Biological and Biochemical Foundations of Living Systems
- Psychological, Social, and Biological Foundations of Behavior

The Chemical and Physical Foundations of Biological Systems section (Chem/Phys) is the first section on the test. It includes questions from General Chemistry (about 35%), Physics (about 25%), Organic Chemistry (about 15%), and Biochemistry (about 25%). Further, the questions often test chemical and physical concepts within a biological setting: for example, pressure and fluid flow in blood vessels. A solid grasp of math fundamentals is required (arithmetic, algebra, graphs, trigonometry, vectors, proportions, and logarithms); however, there are no calculus-based questions.

The Biological and Biochemical Foundations of Living Systems section (Bio/Biochem) is the third section on the test. Approximately 65% of the questions in this section come from biology, approximately 25% come from biochemistry, and approximately 10% come from Organic and General Chemistry. Math calculations are needed for certain subtopics (like genetics probability questions), but are generally not required on this section of the test; however, a basic understanding of statistics as used in biological research is helpful.

The Psychological, Social, and Biological Foundations of Behavior section (Psych/Soc) is the fourth and final section on the test. About 65% of the questions will be drawn from Psychology (and about 5% of these will be biologically-based), about 30% from Sociology, and about 5% from Biology. As with the Bio/Biochem section, calculations are generally not required, however, a basic understanding of statistics as used in research is helpful.

Most of the questions in the science sections (44 of the 59) are passage-based, and each section has ten passages. Passages consist of a few paragraphs of information and include equations, reactions, graphs, figures, tables, experiments, and data. Four to six questions will be associated with each passage.

The remaining 25% of the questions (15 of 59) in each science section are freestanding questions (FSQs). These questions appear in approximately four groups interspersed between the passages. Each group contains four to five questions.

95 minutes are allotted to each of the science sections. This breaks down to approximately one minute and 35 seconds per question.

2.2 PASSAGES VS. FSQS: WHAT TO START WITH

Passages vs. FSQs in the Science Sections: What to Start With

Since the questions are displayed on separate screens, it is awkward and time consuming to click through all of the questions up front to find the FSQs. Therefore, go through the section on a first pass and decide whether to do the passage now or to save it for later, basing your decision on the passage text and the first question. Tackle the FSQs as you come upon them. More details are below.

Here is an outline of the procedure:

1) For each passage, write a heading on your noteboard with the passage number, the general topic, and its range of questions (e.g., "Passage 1, Q 1–5, thermodynamics" or "Passage 2, Q 6–9, enzymes"). The passage numbers do not currently appear in the Navigation or Review screens, thus having the question numbers on your noteboard will allow you to move through the section more efficiently.

2) Skim the text and decide if you want to do the passage now or later. If a passage is a "Now," complete it before moving on to the next passage (also see "Attacking the Questions" below). If it is a "Later" passage, first write "SKIPPED" in block letters under the passage heading on your noteboard and leave room for your work when you come back to complete that passage. (Note that the specific passages you skip will be unique to you; in the Bio/Biochem section, you might choose to do all Biology passages first, then come back for Biochemistry. Or in Chem/Phys you might choose to skip experiment-based or analytical passages…know ahead of time what type of passage you are going to skip and follow your plan.)

3) If you have skipped a passage, click on the "Navigation" button at the bottom to get to the Navigation screen. Click on the first question of the next passage; you'll be able to identify it because you know the range of questions from the passage you just skipped. This will take you to the next passage, where you will repeat steps 1–3.

4) Once you have completed your first pass through the section, go to the Review screen and click the first question for the first passage you skipped. Answer the questions and continue going back to the Review screen and repeating this procedure for other passages you have skipped.

Attacking the Questions

As you work through the questions, if you encounter a particularly lengthy question, or a question that requires a lot of analysis, you may choose to skip it. This is a wise strategy because it ensures you will tackle all the easier questions first, the ones you are more likely to get right. If you choose to skip the question (or if you attempt it but get stuck), write down the question number and the word "SKIP" on your noteboard and move on to the next question. At the end of the passage, click "Previous" to move back through the set of questions and complete any that you skipped over the first time through. Make sure that you have filled in an answer for every question.

2.3 SCIENCE PASSAGE TYPES

The passages in the science sections fall into one of three main categories: Information and/or Situation Presentation, Experiment/Research Presentation, or Persuasive Reasoning.

Information and/or Situation Presentation

These passages either present straightforward scientific information or they describe a particular event or occurrence. Generally, questions associated with these passages test basic science facts or ask you to predict outcomes given new variables or new information. Here is an example of an Information/Situation Presentation passage:

Figure 1 shows a portion of the inner mechanism of a typical home smoke detector. It consists of a pair of capacitor plates which are charged by a 9-volt battery (not shown). The capacitor plates (electrodes) are connected to a sensor device, D; the resistor, R, denotes the internal resistance of the sensor. Normally, air acts as an insulator and no current would flow in the circuit shown. However, inside the smoke detector is a small sample of an artificially produced radioactive element, americium-241, which decays primarily by emitting alpha particles, with a half-life of approximately 430 years. The daughter nucleus of the decay has a half-life in excess of two million years and therefore poses virtually no biohazard.

The decay products (alpha particles and gamma rays) from the 241Am sample ionize air molecules between the plates and thus provide a conducting pathway which allows current to flow in the circuit shown in Figure 1. A steady-state current is quickly established and remains as long as the battery continues to maintain a 9-volt potential difference between its terminals. However, if smoke particles enter the space between the capacitor plates and thereby interrupt the flow, the current is reduced, and the sensor responds to this change by triggering the alarm. (Furthermore, as the battery starts to "die out," the resulting drop in current is also detected to alert the homeowner to replace the battery.)

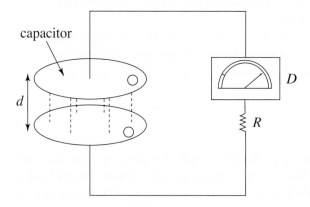

capacitor

d

D

R

Figure 1 Smoke detector mechanism

$$C = \varepsilon_0 \frac{A}{d}$$

Equation 1

where ε_0 is the universal permittivity constant, equal to 8.85×10^{-12} C^2/(N·m^2). Since the area A of each capacitor plate in the smoke detector is 20 cm^2 and the plates are separated by a distance d of 5 mm, the capacitance is 3.5×10^{-12} F = 3.5 pF.

Experiment/Research Presentation

These passages present the details of experiments and research procedures. They often include data tables and graphs. Generally, questions associated with these passages ask you to interpret data, draw conclusions, and make inferences. Here is an example of an Experiment/Research Presentation passage:

The development of sexual characteristics depends upon various factors, the most important of which are hormonal control, environmental stimuli, and the genetic makeup of the individual. The hormones that contribute to the development include the steroid hormones estrogen, progesterone, and testosterone, as well as the pituitary hormones FSH (follicle-stimulating hormone) and LH (luteinizing hormone).

To study the mechanism by which estrogen exerts its effects, a researcher performed the following experiments using cell culture assays.

Experiment 1:

Human embryonic placental mesenchyme (HEPM) cells were grown for 48 hours in Dulbecco's Modified Eagle Medium (DMEM), with media change every 12 hours. Upon confluent growth, cells were exposed to a 10 mg per mL solution of green fluorescent-labeled estrogen for 1 hour. Cells were rinsed with DMEM and observed under confocal fluorescent microscopy.

Experiment 2:

HEPM cells were grown to confluence as in Experiment 1. Cells were exposed to Pesticide A for 1 hour, followed by the 10 mg/mL solution of labeled estrogen, rinsed as in Experiment 1, and observed under confocal fluorescent microscopy.

Experiment 3:

Experiment 1 was repeated with Chinese Hamster Ovary (CHO) cells instead of HEPM cells.

Experiment 4:

CHO cells injected with cytoplasmic extracts of HEPM cells were grown to confluence, exposed to the 10 mg/mL solution of labeled estrogen for 1 hour, and observed under confocal fluorescent microscopy.

The results of these experiments are given in Table 1.

Experiment	Media	Cytoplasm	Nucleus
1	+	+	+
2	+	+	+
3	+	+	+
4	+	+	+

Table 1 Detection of Estrogen (+ indicates presence of Estrogen)

After observing the cells in each experiment, the researcher bathed the cells in a solution containing 10 mg per mL of a red fluorescent probe that binds specifically to the estrogen receptor only when its active site is occupied. After 1 hour, the cells were rinsed with DMEM and observed under confocal fluorescent microscopy. The results are presented in Table 2. The researcher also repeated Experiment 2 using Pesticide B, an estrogen analog, instead of Pesticide A. Results from other researchers had shown that Pesticide B binds to the active site of the cytosolic estrogen receptor (with an affinity 10,000 times greater than that of estrogen) and causes increased transcription of mRNA.

Experiment	Media	Cytoplasm	Nucleus	Estrogen effects observed?
1	G only	G and R	G and R	Yes
2	G only	G only	G only	No
3	G only	G only	G only	No
4	G only	G and R	G and R	Yes

Table 2 Observed Fluorescence and Estrogen Effects (G = green, R = red)

Based on these results, the researcher determined that estrogen had no effect when not bound to a cytosolic, estrogen-specific receptor.

Persuasive Reasoning

2.3

These passages typically present a scientific phenomenon along with a hypothesis that explains the phenomenon, and may include counter-arguments as well. Questions associated with these passages ask you to evaluate the hypothesis or arguments. Persuasive Reasoning passages in the science sections of the MCAT tend to be less common than Information Presentation or Experiment-based passages. Here is an example of a Persuasive Reasoning passage:

Two theoretical chemists attempted to explain the observed trends of acidity by applying two interpretations of molecular orbital theory. Consider the pK_a values of some common acids listed along with the conjugate base:

acid	pK_a	conjugate base
H_2SO_4	< 0	HSO_4^-
H_2CrO_4	5.0	$HCrO_4^-$
H_2PO_4	2.1	$H_2PO_4^-$
HF	3.9	F^-
HOCl	7.8	ClO^-
HCN	9.5	CN^-
HIO_3	1.2	IO_3^-

Recall that acids with a $pK_a < 0$ are called strong acids, and those with a $pK_a > 0$ are called weak acids. The arguments of the chemists are given below.

Chemist #1:

"The acidity of a compound is proportional to the polarization of the H—X bond, where X is some nonmetal element. Complex acids, such as H_2SO_4, $HClO_4$, and HNO_3 are strong acids because the H—O bonding electrons are strongly drawn towards the oxygen. It is generally true that a covalent bond weakens as its polarization increases. Therefore, one can conclude that the strength of an acid is proportional to the number of electronegative atoms in that acid."

Chemist #2:

"The acidity of a compound is proportional to the number of stable resonance structures of that acid's conjugate base. H_2SO_4, $HClO_4$, and HNO_3 are all strong acids because their respective conjugate bases exhibit a high degree of resonance stabilization."

A Note about Psych/Soc Passages

Passages in the Psychology and Sociology section of the MCAT tend to be a blend of Information and Experiment Presentation passages. They often present data from recent research studies. For example, consider the following Psych/Soc passage:

Psychotic disorders—most notably schizophrenia and bipolar disorder with psychotic features—affect approximately 2% of Americans. These disorders are extremely manageable with psychotropic medications—to relieve symptoms such as hallucinations and delusions—and behavioral therapy, such as social skills training and hygiene maintenance.

However, individuals with psychotic disorders have the lowest level of medication compliance, as compared to individuals with mood or anxiety disorders. Antipsychotic medications can have extremely negative side effects, including uncontrollable twitching of the face or limbs, blurred vision, and weight gain, among others. They also must be taken frequently, and at high doses, in order to be effective. While relatively little is known about the reasons for noncompliance, studies do suggest that in schizophrenia, age of schizophrenia diagnosis and medication compliance is positively correlated. Evidence also suggests that medication noncompliance is disproportionally prevalent in individuals of a low socioeconomic status (SES) due to issues such as homelessness, lack of insurance benefits, and lack of familial or social support.

Researchers were interested to see how drug education might affect compliance or noncompliance with psychotropic medications based on patient socioeconomic status. In a study of 1200 mentally ill individuals in the Los Angeles metro area, researchers measured baseline psychotropic medication compliance, then provided patients with a free educational seminar on drug therapy, and then measured psychotropic medication compliance six months later. The one-day, 8-hour seminar included information on positive effects of psychotropic medication, side effects of psychotropic medication, psychotropic medication interactions with other substances such as alcohol and non-prescribed drugs, and information on accessing Medicare benefits. Compliance was measured by number of doses of prescribed psychotropic medication that the patients took in a week, over the course of 12 weeks, as compared to the number of doctor-recommended doses per week. Compliance was measured using a self-report questionnaire.

Results indicated that post-seminar, mentally ill patients from middle or upper class backgrounds (Upper and Middle SES) were significantly more compliant with their psychotropic medication regimens than prior to the seminar. However, no significant differences were found in patients at or below the poverty level (Lower SES). Table 1 displays psychotropic medication compliance by SES and disorder.

Disorder	SES	Pre-Seminar Compliance	Post-Seminar Compliance
Bipolar I	Upper	60%	73%
	Middle	57%	61%
	Lower	25%	27%
Schizophrenia	Upper	53%	65%
	Middle	51%	62%
	Lower	22%	26%

Table 1 Psychotropic Medication Compliance by Socioeconomic Status (SES) and Disorder

2.3

MAPPING A PASSAGE

"Mapping a passage" refers to the combination of skimming, on-screen highlighting, and noteboard notes that you take while working through a passage.

Reading the Passage

"Reading" in the sense that we commonly use the word is seldom the best way to read MCAT passages. A kind of "informed skimming" is usually the best strategy. A quick scan of the passage, including reading the first sentence, should be enough to tell you its topic and type, and it will help you decide whether to do it now or postpone it until you've tackled easier passages. Once you decide to do a passage, try not to get bogged down reading all the little details. Generally, you should read for location of information, without doing too much heavy analysis of data or experiments at this time. You can always come back and ponder them further if you are asked a question about them.

Highlighting

Resist the temptation to highlight everything! (Everyone has done this: you're reading a science textbook with a highlighter, and then look back and realize that the whole page is yellow!) Restrict your highlighting to a few things:

- the main theme of a paragraph
- an unusual or unfamiliar term that is defined specifically for that passage (e.g., something that is italicized)
- statements that either support the main theme or contradict the main theme
- list topics
- equations
- relationships (for example, one thing increases while another decreases)

The Noteboard Booklet

Keep your noteboard organized! Resist the temptation to write on any blank space.

1) Label your noteboard with the passage number, range of questions, and topic for that passage (for example, "P2, Q5–9, enzymes")
2) For each paragraph, note P1, P2, etc. on the noteboard and jot down a few notes about that paragraph.
3) Jot down any important conclusions you come to as you skim the passage and/or answer the questions.
4) For physics passages only: write down any given equations and leave some space to work with them. Also, redraw any simple diagrams and label any values given (note that some values might be found in the text around the diagram). In some cases, you may need to manipulate the figures to answer questions, and you can't do this with figures on the computer screen. For passages that don't include many diagrams or equations, write down any equations and basic ideas you recall about the passage topic. For example, in a passage about perfectly inelastic collisions, you might write down $\mathbf{p} = m\mathbf{v}$, and "momentum conserved, KE not."
5) As you tackle the questions, label each question and its work (if needed) on the noteboard.

2.4 SCIENCE QUESTION TYPES

Question in the science sections are generally one of three main types: Memory, Explicit, or Implicit.

Memory Questions

These questions can be answered directly from prior knowledge, with no need to reference the passage or question text. Memory questions represent approximately 25% of the science questions on the MCAT. Usually, Memory questions are found as FSQs, but they can also be tucked into a passage. Here's an example of a Memory question:

> Which of the following acetylating conditions will convert diethylamine into an amide at the fastest rate?
>
> A) Acetic acid / HCl
> B) Acetic anhydride
> C) Acetyl chloride
> D) Ethyl acetate

If you find that you are missing a fair number of Memory questions, it is a sure sign that you don't know the science content well enough. Go back and review.

Explicit Questions

Explicit questions can be answered primarily with information from the passage, along with prior knowledge. They may require data retrieval, graph analysis, or making a simple connection. Explicit questions make up approximately 35–40% of the science questions on the MCAT; here's an example (taken from the Information/Situation Presentation passage above):

> The sensor device D shown in Figure 1 performs its function by acting as:
>
> A) an ohmmeter.
> B) a voltmeter.
> C) a potentiometer.
> D) an ammeter.

If you find that you are missing Explicit questions, practice your passage mapping. Make sure you aren't missing the critical items in the passage that lead you to the right answer. Slow down a little; take an extra 15–30 seconds per passage to read or think about it more carefully.

Implicit Questions

These questions require you to take information from the passage, combine it with your prior knowledge, apply it to a new situation, and come to some logical conclusion. They typically require more complex connections than do Explicit questions, and they may also require data retrieval, graph analysis, etc. Implicit questions usually require a solid understanding of the passage information. They make up approximately 35–40% of the science questions on the MCAT; here's an example (taken from the Experiment/Research Presentation passage above):

If Experiment 2 were repeated, but this time exposing the cells first to Pesticide A and then to Pesticide B before exposing them to the green fluorescent-labeled estrogen and the red fluorescent probe, which of the following statements will most likely be true?

A) Pesticide A and Pesticide B bind to the same site on the estrogen receptor.
B) Estrogen effects would be observed.
C) Only green fluorescence would be observed.
D) Both green and red fluorescence would be observed.

Here's another example of an Implicit Question taken from the Psych/Soc passage above:

Suppose the experiment described in the passage were repeated, but instead of testing how drug education affects compliance, researchers measured how incentives affect compliance in low SES schizophrenics. The low SES schizophrenia group was broken into two groups. Group A received an incentive every time they took their medication for seven consecutive days, while Group B received an incentive every two weeks, regardless of compliance level. Based on operant conditioning principles, what results should the researchers see?

A) No difference in compliance levels from the first study.
B) Group A's compliance should be higher than Group B's compliance.
C) Group B's compliance should be higher than Group A's compliance.
D) Both groups should demonstrate increased compliance from the first study but it is impossible to tell which group's compliance is expected to be higher.

If you find that you are missing a lot of Implicit questions, make sure first of all that you are using POE aggressively. Second, go back and review the explanations for the correct answer, and figure out where your logic went awry. Did you miss an important fact in the passage? Did you forget the relevant science content? Did you miss a connection to the data? Did you follow the logical train of thought to the right answer? Once you figure out where you made your mistake, you will know how to correct it.

Science Question Strategies

1) Remember that the potential content in the science sections is vast, so don't panic if something seems completely unfamiliar. Understand the basic content well, find the basics in the unfamiliar topic, and apply them to the question.

2) Process of Elimination is paramount! The Strikethrough button allows you to eliminate answer choices; this will improve your chances of guessing the correct answer if you are unable to narrow it down to one choice.

3) Answer the straightforward questions first (typically the memory questions). Leave questions that require analysis of experiments and graphs for later. Take the test in the order YOU want. Make sure to use your noteboard to indicate questions you have skipped.

4) Make sure that the answer you choose actually answers the question, and isn't just a true statement.

5) Try to avoid answer choices with extreme words such as "always," "never," etc. In the sciences, there is almost always an exception and answers are rarely black-and-white.

6) I-II-III questions: Whenever possible, start by evaluating the Roman numeral item that shows up in exactly two answer choices. This will allow you to quickly eliminate two wrong answer choices regardless of whether the item is true or false. Typically then, you will only have to assess one of the other Roman numeral items to determine the correct answer. Always work between the I-II-III statements and the answer choices. Once an item is found to be true (or false), strike out answer choices which do not contain (or do contain) that item number. Make sure to strike out the actual Roman numeral item as well, and highlight those items that are true.

7) LEAST/EXCEPT/NOT questions: Don't get tricked by these questions that ask you to pick the answer that doesn't fit (the incorrect or false statement). It's often good to use your noteboard and write a T or F next to answer choices A–D. The one that stands out as different is the correct answer!

8) 2 × 2 style questions: These questions require you to know two pieces of information to get the correct answer, and are easily identified by their answer choices, which commonly take the form A because X, B because X, A because Y, B because Y. Tackle one piece of information at a time, which should allow you to quickly eliminate two answer choices.

9) Ranking questions: When asked to rank items, look for an extreme—either the greatest or the smallest item—and eliminate answer choices that do not have that item shown at the correct end of the ranking. This is often enough to eliminate one to three answer choices. Based on the remaining choices, look for the other extreme at the other end of the ranking and use POE again. If you're not sure where to begin your analysis, looking at the answer choices may help you narrow down your options for one of the extreme values.

10) If you read a question and do not know how to answer it, look to the passage for help. It is likely that the passage contains information pertinent to answering the question, either within the text or in the form of experimental data.

11) If a question requires a lengthy calculation, mark it and return to it later, particularly if you are slow with arithmetic or dimensional analysis.

12) Don't leave any question blank. There is no guessing penalty on the MCAT.

2.4

2.5 SUMMARY OF THE APPROACH TO SCIENCE PASSAGES AND QUESTIONS

How to Map the Passage and Use the Noteboard Booklet

1) The passage should not be read like textbook material, with the intent of learning something from every sentence (science majors especially will be tempted to read this way). Passages should be read to get a feel for the type of questions that will follow, and to get a general idea of the location of information within the passage.

2) Highlighting—Use this tool sparingly, or you will end up with a passage that is completely covered in yellow highlighter! Highlighting in a science passage should be used to draw attention to a few words that demonstrate one of the following:
   - the main theme of a paragraph
   - an unusual or unfamiliar term that is defined specifically for that passage (e.g., something that is italicized)
   - statements that either support the main theme or counteract the main theme
   - list topics (see below)

3) Pay brief attention to equations, figures, and experiments, noting only what information they deal with. Do not spend a lot of time analyzing at this point. For physics passages, jot down the equations in a row with room to work beneath them. Copy simple figures to which you can add force or kinematics vectors, simplified circuit diagrams, or other details that allow you to see directly what's happening. Physics generally involves the most noteboard work of all the sciences.

4) For each passage, start by noting the passage number, the general topic, and the range of questions on your noteboard. You can then work between your noteboard and the Review screen to easily get to the questions you want to.

5) For each paragraph, note "P1," "P2," etc. on the noteboard and jot down a few notes about that paragraph. Try to translate science jargon into your own words using everyday language. Especially note down simple relationships (for example, the relationship between two variables).

6) Lists—Whenever a list appears in paragraph form, jot down on the noteboard the paragraph and the general topic of the list. It will make returning to the passage more efficient and help to organize your thoughts.

7) The noteboard will only be useful if it is kept organized! Make sure that your notes for each passage are clearly delineated and marked with the passage number and question range. This will allow you to easily read your notes when you come back to review a Flagged question. Resist the temptation to write in the first available blank space as this makes it much more difficult to refer back to your work.

Chapter 3
Stress Management, Study Schedules, and Final Preparation

Mental Preparation

Managing your psychological state is just as important to your score as studying content and learning techniques. Here are some suggestions to help you get the most out of your preparation, and to maximize your performance on test day.

3.1 REDUCING ANXIETY

Most students feel some level of stress before and during an important exam. A certain level of anxiety, while uncomfortable, is beneficial: it sharpens your attention, keeps you alert, and intensifies your focus. However, if you find that your stress and anxiety get out of control to the point where your performance suffers, there are ways to manage it and reduce it to a reasonable level. You will find that some of these techniques work better for you than others. Try them all out, settle on some that work for you (or come up with your own), and then use them consistently up to and on the day of the test.

Use Positive Reinforcement

- When we place high demands on ourselves, it's easy to fall into negative thinking at moments of frustration. You may find yourself thinking self-critical thoughts while studying or doing a practice test. Do "How could I miss that question!", "I'm so stupid!", or "I'm never going to get this!" sound familiar?

- Recognize these responses for what they are: a reaction from stress, not a representation of reality. Find words and phrases to replace the negative thoughts, such as "I know I'm smart, I'm working hard, and it will all pay off in the end." It may sound goofy, but it works.

Practice Creative Visualization

- Creative visualization, if practiced over time, can offer significant long-term anxiety reduction. Lie on the floor (at home, not during the test!) on your back, with your arms and legs stretched out. Adjust your position until you feel comfortable and relaxed. Then close your eyes and picture the most wonderful, relaxing place you have ever visited or would like to visit, or a situation that makes you feel safe and at peace. It may be a tropical island, a quiet forest, a deserted beach, or a gathering at home with friends and family. See your surroundings clearly, smell the air, hear the birds, or picture the faces of the people who make you happy. When you are ready to stop, picture the most relaxing part of the scene one last time. Count to three slowly, then open your eyes. If you practice this regularly for a few weeks, especially at times when you feel tense, you should begin to feel less anxious. Then, if you do find yourself becoming anxious during the test, breathe deeply and imagine yourself back in that peaceful place. You will find yourself relaxing quickly, because you're trained yourself to respond that way.

- While thinking about the aftermath of the test, it is helpful to focus on positive outcomes, imagining success. Who will be the first person you tell about your MCAT score? How will that person react to the good news? Imagine the look on your parent's face, the hugs you will get, and the feeling of accomplishment you will have, as you share news of your score. Thinking of these things as part of your goal, rather than simply focusing on the numerical score you want to achieve, can help you feel more motivated.

Use Music

Many people use music to control and manage anxiety, and just to feel better overall. If you are a music person, create a playlist with a set of songs you can listen to whenever you find yourself feeling negative or non-productive emotions, be it anxiety and fear, or fatigue and lethargy.

Have a Plan

In the table below, describe any symptoms of anxiety you may have experienced when taking a practice test or doing homework and the method or methods you use (or will use in the future) to help manage it.

Symptoms	Management Methods

3.2   MAXIMIZING YOUR PRODUCTIVITY

Preparing to take the MCAT is a rigorous process that requires many hours of work spread over a significant amount of time. Don't burn yourself out by trying to cram hundreds of hours of work into just a few weeks, or by studying 20 hours a day for several months.

Anxiety comes in part from feeling as if you are unable to control a situation. Just as a clear pacing strategy will help you to work more methodically and stay calm during the MCAT, pacing yourself in your preparation will help you feel more in control, ensure that you get through the work that needs to be done, and allow you to relax and spend time with friends and family (and therefore maintain your sanity). If you set a reasonable schedule and stick to it, you will walk into the MCAT mentally and physically healthy, with the confidence that comes from knowing that you have done everything you need to do.

Prepare for Actual Test Conditions

- **Build up your stamina.**
  It is difficult to maintain concentration over many hours under normal circumstances, let alone under stressful conditions. Prepare for test day by working passages over longer and longer periods with shorter and shorter breaks, until you can comfortably concentrate for a few hours at a time.

- **Take as many full practice tests as possible.**
  Experience builds confidence. Once you have practiced doing several passages at a stretch, take on doing more and more practice tests. Complete full tests in one sitting, taking the breaks between sections. Don't have any food or water during the test except at the breaks. If you get cold or hot, don't put on or take off clothing except at the breaks. That is, take your practice tests under the same conditions as the real MCAT. On test day, you can walk in to the testing center knowing that you know how to do this—this is just one more test in a long line of tests you've already completed.

- **Practice dealing with distraction.**
  Do passages or practice tests under less-than-ideal conditions. Go to a coffee house, or an area of the library where people are moving around. Practice tuning out your surroundings while you work.

Set a Schedule

- Consider how many hours of MCAT preparation you should do in a week and create a daily schedule of the hours of the day you will dedicate to it. Be practical in your estimation of hours: you may feel like you should be studying all the time but you likely have other responsibilities and commitments, plus you need time to eat, rest, exercise, and unwind.

- You may only be able to manage two hours of MCAT prep if you have a heavy day with classes, work, or other commitments—set your schedule accordingly. And, if you can manage it, having one day a week that is completely, or at least significantly, free of MCAT study can be restorative (and help you to get even more out of the other six days of the week). A great benefit of creating a schedule to manage your time is that when you are not scheduled to study, you don't have to feel guilty about not studying!

- Your schedule should be personalized based on when you tend to wake, eat, sleep, and on your own individual activities. Do make sure to adjust your sleep and study schedule to correspond to the time of day you are taking the MCAT, at least in the last few weeks before your test.

- On the following page are two sample schedules. Both are for days when you don't have to go to class or work: the first is for a day dedicated to reading and passage drills, and the second is for days on which you are taking full practice tests. Both entail 8–9 hour prep days. Notice how much time is left to do other things.

Construct your own agenda for the weeks or months remaining before the MCAT, using these sample schedules as guidelines.

Sample Schedule: No Full Practice Test

6:30A.M.–8:00A.M.: Wake up, breakfast, quick morning walk/run or workout, shower

8:00A.M.–11:30A.M.: MCAT prep (this could be half a practice test, practice questions and passages, test review, or some chapter reading for various subjects)

11:30A.M.–1:00P.M.: Lunch and leisure time (read a magazine, check social media news, meet with a friend, dance to your favorite song)

1:00P.M.–4:00P.M.: MCAT prep

4:00P.M.–5:00P.M.: Snack, stretch, unwind

5:00P.M.–7:00P.M.: MCAT prep

7:00P.M.–10:30P.M.: Dinner and leisure time

10:30P.M.–11:00P.M.: Go to bed

Sample Schedule: Full Practice Test

6:30A.M.–7:30A.M.: Wake up, breakfast, quick morning walk/run or workout, shower

7:30A.M.–9:00A.M.: Warm up for the test (do a few practice questions and passages to get your mind going)

9:00A.M.–4:30P.M.: Full practice MCAT (including break times)

4:30P.M.–6:00P.M.: Dinner/snack, relax

6:00P.M.–8:00P.M.: Test review (always review your performance as soon as possible; review CARS on the same day as the test so that you can remember your thought process during the test)

8:00P.M.–10:30P.M.: Relax, do whatever else needs to be done
10:30P.M.–11:00P.M.: Go to bed

3.3 PREPARING FOR THE DAY OF THE TEST

There are a variety of things you can do in the time remaining to make the day of the MCAT as comfortable and familiar as possible.

- Make peace with your anxiety. Everyone experiences it, including the highest scorers. Feel free to be nervous on test day and the several days (or weeks) before. Even if you don't sleep well the night before the test, you'll be fine. Nervousness can be a good thing; adrenaline intensifies your ability to concentrate intensely.

- Let go of the need to be perfect. You don't need to complete every question, or get every question that you complete correct, to get a high score.

- This is not the time to quit smoking (do that *after* the MCAT) or give up caffeine, but take care of your health. Keep eating well and exercising up until the test date. And don't turn to drugs or alcohol for stress management, and definitely don't start experimenting with black-market ADHD drugs! Maintain a habit of 7–8 hours of sleep (per night, not per week).

- Get up roughly at the same time each morning as you will on test day, and go to bed at the same time that you will the night before the test. If you are in the habit of staying up until 2 A.M., but need to go to bed at 10 P.M. in order to get a reasonable amount of sleep the night before the test, you won't be able to magically change your sleeping habits at the last minute. Get into a good sleep schedule at least the week or two before the test, and you will thank yourself on test day!

- Whenever possible, practice at the same time of day as the real test.

- Make a plan for getting to your testing site, and practice it. What time will you get up? What will you eat? What route will you take to the test site? Make sure that you plan to leave in plenty of time to get there a little early. Travel to the site at the same time as you will on the day of the test to see how long it takes you.

- Visualize success. Elite athletes, before each competition, visualize themselves going through each step of a successful performance. This both calms their nerves and focuses them on the task at hand. Remember a time in which you worked through a passage or set of passages with good results, and mentally run through the steps you took. Recall the sense of control and confidence you have when you stay calm and focused, use the techniques you've learned, and take charge of the material. If you begin to feel stress or anxiety, close your eyes and remember that feeling.

- Your main job in the last week before the exam is to keep yourself relaxed and focused. Don't burn yourself out at the end. Taper off the hours you spend per day on homework as you approach the test day. Continue to practice your stress reduction techniques. Make time for some enjoyable activities.

- The day before the test, at most do some basic review; in fact, feel free to take the day off from the MCAT altogether! Try to do some light exercise (don't overdo it), eat well, watch a funny movie, and get to bed at your regular set time.

- Plan to reward yourself after the test. Make plans with friends of family to do something that you like to do. You deserve a reward!

3.4 MAXIMIZING YOUR PERFORMANCE ON TEST DAY

Before the Test

- Don't rush. Make sure that you set your alarm—or better still, alarms!—to ensure that you have time to eat a good breakfast, take a shower, and do what you need to do before you leave the house. Most importantly, NO CRAMMING! Aside from doing a quick warm-up (see below), don't open your MCAT books on the day of the test, and don't bring any books or notes with you to the test center.

- Warm up before the test. Get your mind working in the right direction before you leave home. That could mean just reading through some MCAT-like material, or doing a passage or two (best to redo passages you have already done) untimed. You are not trying to learn anything new; you just want to get your mind into "MCAT mode."

- Use music to set a good tone. Have a playlist selected ahead of time. As you get ready to leave the house, or as you make your way to the testing center, use music to either calm down or rev up.

- While waiting to be seated, if other test takers are gathered together talking frantically about their fears or, on the other hand, about their superior preparation, step away. Don't let anyone make you nervous or negatively influence your calm, confident state of mind.

- During the test, follow the strategy that you have outlined for yourself. Work calmly and methodically. Do not rethink your strategy or your career choice at this point!

- **Take a breath.**
  The more tense we get, the more shallow our breathing becomes. Lack of oxygen can then contribute to your anxiety in a feedback loop. Stop this process the minute you realize that your muscles are tightening or your focus is fading. Sit back in your chair and take three deep breaths. Take your eyes off the screen for 10–15 seconds, and move your arms and shoulders around to release the muscles. Don't force yourself onward to the next question if you realize that you're not working at your peak. Rather than wasting a big chunk of time getting questions wrong because you can't think straight, take a few seconds to relax and regroup, and make the most of the rest of your time.

- **Take the breaks you are given.**
  The MCAT is designed to give you a feeling of burnout. The test makers give you as little help as possible during your test day, so use what they give you! Just as you should use the annotation tools provided, such as highlighting and strikeout, you must also take advantage of the breaks you are offered. Use them for the basics (eating, using the restroom) but also to clear your mind, breathe deeply, get your eyes away from the screen, and shift gears for the next session.

- **Don't obsess about time.**
  Of course you are going to check the timer while you work, but checking the time constantly will distract you and make things more stressful. Doing lots of practice tests will help you develop a sense of timing while you work, so you know how long you take to read passages and get through questions. Only check the clock between passages or if you are stuck on a question and feel the need to move on; otherwise, immerse yourself in the task of working passages and attacking questions efficiently and effectively.

- Don't wait until the actual test to follow these guidelines. Implement them during every practice test. If you train yourself to manage your mental state during your preparation, your training will kick in automatically during the real test, allowing you to get the most out of all that hard work you have invested and maximize your score.

Chapter 4
MCAT Statistics

4.1 BASIC RESEARCH METHODS AND STATISTICS

The MCAT tests your knowledge of basic research methods and statistical concepts within the context of science passages and questions, particularly in the social and behavioral sciences section. The MCAT will not test your knowledge about statistics explicitly, per se, but will test whether you are able to apply statistical concepts and an understanding of research methodology while answering content-related questions. Application questions might include the following:

- graphical analysis and interpretation
- determining whether results are supported by data presented in figures
- demonstrating an understanding of basic statistics and research methods
- interpreting data presented in graphs, figures, and tables
- drawing conclusions about data and methodology

What Is Statistics?

Statistics is a tool that organizes data. Statistics are often employed to organize data sets and present data in a logical manner such that it can be analyzed and conclusions can be drawn. Data often include numerical information collected through research. The different types of statistical data that you might encounter on the MCAT are described in this section.

Descriptive Statistics

Descriptive statistics quantitatively describe a population or set of data; in behavioral fields, descriptive statistics will often provide information about the data involved in the study, such as number of subjects (or sample size), proportion of subjects of each sex, average age (or weight, or height, or IQ...whatever is relevant to the study) of the sample, etc. Descriptive statistics include **measures of central tendency** (such as mean, median, mode) and **measures of variability** (such as range and standard deviation).

4.2 MEASURES OF CENTRAL TENDENCY

Measures of central tendency summarize or describe the entire set of data in some meaningful way.

Mean

The mean is the average of the sample. The average is derived from adding all of the individual components and dividing by the number of components. The mean is not necessarily a number provided in the sample. You should be able to recognize what the mean of a given data set is and be able to calculate it.

Example Mean Question:

Subject	Starting Weight (in pounds)	Final Weight (in pounds)
Subject 1	184	176
Subject 2	200	190
Subject 3	221	225
Subject 4	235	208
Subject 5	244	225

Table 1 Starting and Final Weights for Study Subjects

What is the average amount of weight lost in pounds for all five subjects whose data is represented in Table 1, rounded to the nearest pound?

Solution:

In order to answer this question, you must first calculate how much weight each subject lost, and then divide by the number of subjects (in this case, five).

Subject	Starting Weight (in pounds)	Final Weight (in pounds)	Weight Lost (in pounds)
Subject 1	184	176	8
Subject 2	200	190	10
Subject 3	221	225	–4*
Subject 4	235	208	27
Subject 5	244	225	19

Subject 3 gained 4 pounds

Total weight lost is 60 pounds (remember to subtract 4 pounds for Subject 3, not add), divided by 5 subjects is 12 pounds. The average weight lost is **12 pounds**.

Note: The mean can be both useful and deceptive. Using the example above, what sort of conclusions could be drawn from the fact that the subjects lost an average of 12 pounds? One might conclude that the subjects were successful at losing weight. However, the mean does not reflect the fact that one of the participants, Subject 3, actually gained weight. Nor does it reflect that one the participants, Subject 4, was very successful, losing over twice the mean. Consider another example: If ten people are in a room together and all of them earn salaries at or below minimum wage, but one of them is a billionaire, the mean salary for the ten people might make it seem like they were all quite wealthy. Therefore, use caution when making assumptions about a data set when given just the mean.

Median

The median is the middle number in a data set. The median is determined by putting the numbers in consecutive order and finding the middle number. If there is an odd number of numbers, there will be a single number that is the median. If there is an even number of numbers, the median is determined by averaging the two middle numbers. Therefore, the median is not necessarily one of the numbers in the data set. You should be able to recognize what the median of a given data set is and be able to calculate it.

Example Median Question:

Subject	Height (in inches)
Subject 1	67
Subject 2	61
Subject 3	72
Subject 4	70
Subject 5	66
Subject 6	68

Table 2   Height of Study Subjects

Is Subject 6 taller than the median for all subjects whose height is displayed in Table 2?

Solution:

In order to determine the median height for all six subjects, their heights must first be organized in ascending order: 61, 66, 67, 68, 70, 72. The middle two numbers are 67 and 68; when averaged, this produces a median of **67.5 inches**. Subject 6 is taller than the median.

Note: The median can be useful in gauging the midpoint of the data, but it will not necessarily tell you much about the **outliers** (a numerical observation that is far removed from the rest of the observations). Using the example where nine people earn salaries at or below minimum wage and the tenth is a billionaire, the median will give you a pretty good idea about the income for most of the people in the room, but it will not indicate that one person makes much more than the rest. Therefore, also use caution when making assumptions about a data set when given just the median.

Mode

The mode is the most frequently recurring number in the data set. If there are no numbers that occur more than once, there is no mode. If there are multiple numbers that occur most frequently, each of those numbers is a mode. The mode must be one of the numbers in the sample, and modes are never averaged. You should be able to recognize what the mode of a given data set.

Example Mode Question:
   In the following set of test scores, what is the mode?

   Test Scores: 32, 65, 66, 67, 68, 68, 69, 70, 71, 72, 73, 75, 75, 75, 75, 78, 82

Solution:
   The most frequently recurring number in the set above is **75**.

Note: Like the mean and median, the mode is only useful in describing some types of data sets. Mode is particularly useful for scores (such as test scores). For example, looking at the test scores above, the mean is 69.5 and the median is 71. Using all three measures you could conclude that while the mean was low, most of the students in the class scored above the mean, and the most common score was 75. There was one very low score that brought down the mean, but there were no very high scores.

4.3   MEASURES OF VARIABILITY

Knowing information about the central tendency of a data set can be useful, but it is also useful to know something about the variation in the data set. In other words, how similar or diverse are the data?

Range

The range is the difference between the smallest and largest number in a sample. You should be able to recognize what the range of a given data set is and be able to calculate it.

Example Range Question:
   In the following set of values, what is the range? Values: –5, 8, 11, –1, 0, 4, 14

Solution:
   The smallest value in the set above is –5, and the largest is 14. The difference between these two is the range, which is **19**.

Note: The range only provides limited information about a data set, however. Returning to the example of the ten people in a room, the range of incomes might be 3 billion dollars, but that provides relatively little information about the individual salaries of the people in the room. Knowing just the range does not tell us that the majority of the people in the room all have salaries around minimum wage.

Standard Deviation

The standard deviation is more useful than the range for calculating how much the data vary. It can determine if numbers are packed together or dispersed because it is a measure of how much each individual number differs from the mean. The best way to understand standard deviation is to consider a normal distribution (also called a bell-shaped curve). You will not need to calculate standard deviation, but you should understand what it is and should be able to make assumptions and draw conclusions from standard deviation data.

Normal Distributions

A normal distribution is a very important class of statistical distributions for the study of human behavior, because many psychological, social, and biological variables are normally distributed. Large sets of data (such as heights, weights, test scores, IQ) often form a symmetrical, bell-shaped distribution when graphed by frequency (number of instances). For example, if you took the individual weights of all 25-year-old males in America and plotted weight on the x-axis and frequency on the y-axis, the results will be normally distributed.

Standard Deviation

Standard deviation describes the degree of variation from the mean. A low standard deviation reflects that data points are all similar and close to the mean, while a high standard deviation reflects that the data are more spread out. For the purposes of the MCAT, you should be familiar with a normal distribution (or bell-shaped curve) and should be able to determine what a standard deviation means for a set of data. You will not be expected to calculate the standard deviation. Figure 1 demonstrates the relationship between a normal distribution and standard deviation.

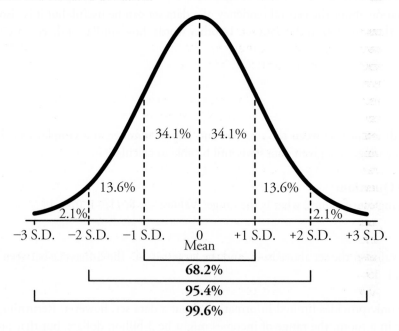

Figure 1   Normal Distribution and Standard Deviation Rules

All normal distributions have the following properties:

- 34.1% of the data will fall within one standard deviation above or below the mean, thus 68.2% of the data will fall within one standard deviation of the mean
- 13.6% of the data will fall between one and two standard deviations above or below the mean, thus 95.4% of the data will fall within two standard deviations of the mean
- 2.1% of the data will fall between two and three standard deviations above or below the mean, thus 99.6% of the data will fall within three standard deviations of the mean
- 0.2% of the data will fall beyond three standard deviations above or below the mean, thus 0.4% of the data will fall beyond three standard deviations of the mean

So for a normal distribution, almost all of the data lie within **3 standard deviations** of the mean.

Example Standard Deviation Question:

Suppose that 1,000 subjects participate in a study on reaction time. The reaction times of the subjects are normally distributed with a mean of 1.3 seconds and a standard deviation of 0.2 seconds. How many subjects had a reaction time between 1.1 and 1.5 seconds? How many participants had reaction times slower than 1.9 seconds? A reaction time of 0.9 seconds is within how many standard deviations of the mean?

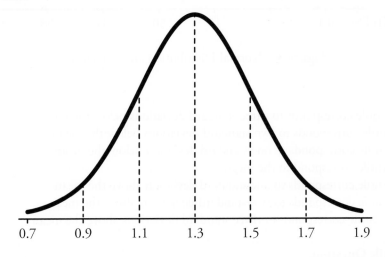

Figure 2   Subjects' Reaction Time

Solution:

Subjects' reaction times would produce a normal distribution like the one above. Reaction times within 1.1 and 1.5 seconds would include all of the data within one standard deviation of the mean (or, in other words, one standard deviation above and below the mean). 68.2% of the data fall within one standard deviation of the mean (34.1% above and 34.1% below), so **682** subjects have a reaction time between 1.1 and 1.5 seconds.

0.2% of the data will fall above 3 standard deviations of the mean, so only **2** subjects will have a reaction time slower than 1.9 seconds.

A reaction time of 0.9 seconds is **two standard deviations below the mean**.

4.3

Percentile

Percentiles are often used when reporting data from normal distributions. Percentiles represent the area under the normal curve, increasing from left to right. A percentile indicates the value or score below which the rest of the data falls. For example, a score in the 75th percentile is higher than 75% of the rest of the scores. Each standard deviation represents a fixed percentile as follows:

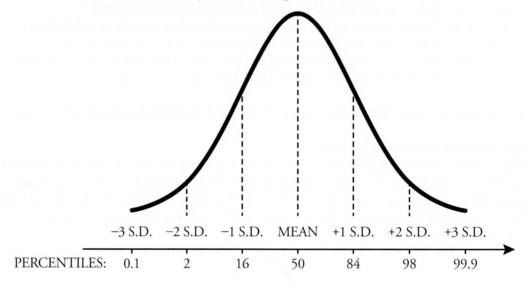

Figure 3 Normal Distribution and Percentiles

- 0.1th percentile corresponds to three standard deviations below the mean
- 2nd percentile corresponds to two standard deviations below the mean
- 16th percentile corresponds to one standard deviation below the mean
- 50th percentile correspond to the mean
- 84th percentile corresponds to one standard deviation above the mean
- 98th percentile corresponds to two standard deviations above the mean
- 99.9th percentile corresponds to three standard deviations above the mean

Example Percentile Question:

If the scores for an exam are normally distributed, the mean is 20 and the standard deviation is 6, a score of 14 would be what percentile? What score would correspond to the 99.9th percentile?

Solution:

A score of 14 would be one standard deviation below the mean, which corresponds to the **16th percentile**. The 99.9th percentile is three standard deviations above the mean, which would correspond to a score of **38**.

4.4 INFERENTIAL STATISTICS

Beyond merely describing the data, inferential statistics also allows inferences or assumptions to be made about data. Using inferential statistics, such as a regression coefficient or a *t*-test, you can draw conclusions about the population you are studying. Inferential statistics starts with a hypothesis and checks to see if the data prove or disprove that hypothesis. You will not be expected to calculate any of the following statistical measures on the MCAT, but you will be expected to recognize these statistical analyses and apply information about these various measures.

Variables

Variables are the things that statistics is designed to test; more specifically, statistics measures whether or not a change in the independent variable has an effect on the dependent variable. An **independent variable** is the variable that is manipulated to determine what effect it will have on the dependent variable. A **dependent variable** is a function of the independent variable, as the independent variable changes, so does the dependent variable. Typically, the independent variable is the one *manipulated* by the scientist in an experiment and the dependent variable is the one *measured* by the scientist. Common independent variables in behavioral sciences include: age, sex, race, socioeconomic status, and other group characteristics. Standardized measures and scores are also common independent variables. Dependent variables could be any number of things, such as test scores, behaviors, symptoms, etc.

Example Variable Question:

Two scientists want to measure the impact of caffeine consumption on fine motor performance. Therefore, they devise an experiment where a treatment group receives 50 mg of caffeine (in the form of a sugar-free beverage) 20 minutes before performing a standardized motor skills test, and the control group receives a non-caffeinated sugar-free beverage 20 minutes before performing a standardized motor skills test. What is the independent variable in this example? What is the dependent variable?

Solution:

The independent variable is caffeine because the researchers are attempting to determine the impact of this variable on another, the dependent variable (which in this example is performance on the standardized motor skills test).

Sample Size

Sample size refers to the number of observations or individuals measured. Simply enough, if an experiment involves 100 people, the sample size is 100. Sample size is typically denoted with: N (the total number of subjects in the sample being studied) or n (the total number of subjects in a subgroup of the sample being studied). While larger sample sizes always confer increased accuracy, in practicality, particularly for behavioral research where it is likely impossible to test *all* of the people in the country who are clinically depressed, the sample size used in a study is typically determined based on convenience, expense, and the need to have sufficient **statistical power** (which is essentially the likelihood that you have enough subjects to accurately prove the hypothesis is true within an acceptable margin of error). Bigger sample sizes are always better; the larger the sample size, the more likely that you can draw accurate inferences about the population from which the sample was drawn.

Random Samples

Since it is often not possible to test everyone in the population, it is crucial to select a random sample from the larger population in order to conduct research. A **random sample** is a subset of individuals from within a statistical population that can be used to estimate characteristics of the whole population. A population can be defined as including all of the people with a given condition or characteristic that you wish to study. Except under the rarest of circumstances, it will not be possible to study everyone with a given characteristic or condition, so a subset of the population is selected. If the subset is not selected randomly, then this non-randomness might unintentionally skew the results (which is called **sampling bias**). A classic example of this occurred during the 1948 Presidential Election in the United States: a survey was conducted by randomly calling households and asking people who they were planning to vote for, Harry Truman or Thomas Dewey. Based on this phone survey, Dewey was projected to win, but Truman actually did. What could have possibly gone wrong? Well it turns out that in 1948 having a phone was not such a common thing; in fact, only wealthier households were likely to have a telephone. So the "random" selection of telephone numbers was in fact not a representative random sample of the U.S. population, because many people (of whom a large proportion were clearly voting for Truman) did not have telephone numbers. For the purposes of the MCAT, you should be able to identify the following types of sampling biases:

- The bias of selection from a **specific real area** occurs when people are selected in a physical space. For example, if you wanted to survey college students on whether or not they like their football team, you could stand on the quad and survey the first 100 people that walk by. However, this is not a completely random sample, because people who don't have class that day at that time are unlikely to be represented in the sample.
- **Self-selection bias** occurs when the people being studied have some control over whether or not to participate. A participant's decision to participate may affect the results. For example, an Internet survey might only elicit responses from people who are highly opinionated and motivated to complete the survey.
- **Pre-screening or advertising bias** occurs often in medical research; how volunteers are screened or where advertising is placed might skew the sample. For example, if a researcher wanted to prove that a certain treatment helps with smoking cessation, the mere act of advertising for people who "want to quit smoking" could provide only a sample of people who are highly motivated to quit and would be likely to quit without the treatment.
- **Healthy user bias** occurs when the study population is likely healthier than the general population. For example, recruiting subjects from the gym might not be the most representative group.

t-test and p-values

The *t*-test is probably one of the most common tests in the social sciences, because it can be used to calculate whether the means of two groups are significantly different from each other, statistically. For example, if you have a control group and a treatment group both take a standardized test, the means of the two groups can be compared statistically. Furthermore, *t*-tests are also often used to calculate the difference between a pre-treatment measure and a post-treatment measure for the same group. For example, you could have a group of subjects take a survey before and after some sort of treatment, and statistically compare the means of the two tests.

The *t*-test is most often applied to data sets that are normally distributed. You will not be required to know how to perform a *t*-test, but you will need to understand what **significance** is. For the purposes of most experiments, two samples are considered to be significantly different if the *p*-value is below ± 0.05 (the *p*-value can be found using a table of values from the *t*-test). If two data sets are determined to be statistically significantly different (the *p*-value is below ± 0.05), then it can be concluded with 95% confidence that the two sets of data are actually different, instead of containing data that could be from the same data set.

Again, understanding how *p*-values are calculated and mathematically how *t*-tests are done is not important here. Instead, it's important that you understand how these values are used to interpret data.

Let's work through an example to demonstrate how common statistics are used in science. A researcher has sections of two different types of skin cancers from human patients. She stains them for the protein CD31, which is a marker of endothelial cells. She then takes digital pictures of the immunofluorescent sections, and she counts how many blood vessels are present in each picture. She takes five pictures of each slide:

Slide A	Slide B
10	3
8	2
7	4
8	4
11	4

a) What is the mean, median, and mode for each dataset?
b) The standard error of group A is 0.735, and the standard error for group B is 0.400. What does this tell you about the data?
c) The researcher conducts a two-sided *t*-test and gets a *p*-value of 2.66×10^{-3}, and then she performs a one-sided *t*-test and gets a *p*-value of 1.33×10^{-3}. What does this tell you?
d) What assumptions are made about the data in performing these tests?
e) What could the researcher do to increase her confidence in the results?

Solutions:

a) The means are:

$$Mean_{Group\ A} : \frac{10 + 8 + 7 + 8 + 11}{5} : 8.8$$

$$Mean_{Group\ B} : \frac{3 + 2 + 4 + 4 + 5}{5} : 3.4$$

Remember, the median is the middle number, so it's best to put the data in order first:

Slide A	Slide B
7	2
8	3
8	4
10	4
11	4

The median of group A is 8, and the median of group B is 4.

The mode is the most frequent value. For group A, this is 8. For group B, the mode is 4.

b) Standard error is the standard deviation divided by the square root of the sample size. The sample size is 5 for both group A and group B, because five pictures were taken for each slide. Since the standard error of group A is larger than that of group B, and since the two groups have the same sample size, the standard deviation of group A must also be larger than that of group B. Note that this may or may not be the case if the sample sizes were different. A larger standard deviation means the data is more variable, so you can conclude that the data from group A has a larger spread than the data from group B.

c) Since both p-values are less than 0.05, they are both significant. The two-sided t-test result tells you the two datasets have significantly different means. The one-sided t-test tells you group A has a significantly larger mean than group B.

d) As with most datasets, the researcher is assuming the data fits a normal distribution, and that her sample size is large enough to be meaningful.

e) More data allows for more confident conclusions. The researcher could therefore take more pictures from each slide, to increase the sample size.

Correlation

Correlation expresses a relationship between two sets of data using a single number, the correlation coefficient (if represented at all, the correlation coefficients will usually be represented as R or r). This value measures the direction and magnitude of linear association between these two variables. A correlation coefficient can have a maximum value of 1 and a minimum value of –1. A **positive correlation** (meaning a coefficient greater than 0) indicates a *positive* association between the two variables; that is, when one variable increases, the other also tends to increase as well (similarly, as one variable decreases, the other tends to decrease). A **negative correlation** (meaning a coefficient that is less than 0) indicates a negative association between the two variables; that is, when one increases, the other tends to decrease (or vice versa). A correlation coefficient of exactly 0 indicates that there is no linear relationship between the two variables.

Example Correlation Question:

Psychologists studied 500 male infants from birth to age 16. Infants were measured on "agreeableness" at age one using a standardized questionnaire given to the parents (with scores ranging from 0 to 5). As the infants aged, the psychologists would collect standard measures of behavior problems (including cheating, fighting, getting put in detention, and later delinquency, smoking, and drug use) every two years. Overall behavior problems were summed. The psychologists found a correlation between agreeableness and later behavior problems of –0.6 (Figure 4). What does a higher "agreeableness" score correlate to? An "agreeableness" score of 4.0 corresponds to roughly how many accumulated behavior problems by age 16? What conclusions can we draw about the causes of behavior problems?

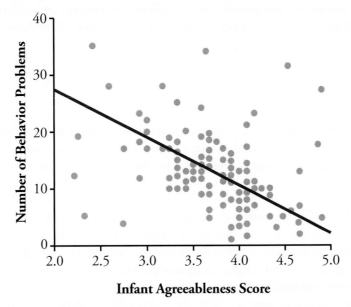

Figure 4   Correlation Between Infant Agreeableness and Later Behavior Problems ($R = -0.6$)

Solution:

Because the two variables are inversely correlated, as scores for "agreeableness" increase, behavioral problems decrease (this is also demonstrated by Figure 4).

An "agreeableness" score of 4.0 corresponds to approximately 10 accumulated behavior problems by age 16; note that correlations are not best used to make assumptions about people's behavior like this in behavioral psychology and medicine, though they may be used to make generalizations.

Note: We can draw no conclusions about behavioral problems based on a correlation! A very important concept in statistics is that **correlation does not imply causation**. A famous example is this one: In New York City, the murder rate is directly correlated to the sale of ice cream (as ice cream sales increase, so do murders). Does this mean that buying ice cream somehow causes murders? Of course not! When two variables are correlated (especially two variables that are as complex as measures of human behavior), there are always a number of other factors that could be influencing either one. In the ice cream/murder example, a logical third factor might be temperature; as the temperature rises, more crimes are committed, but people also tend to eat more cold food, like ice cream.

Reliability

Reliability is the degree to which a specific assessment tool produces stable, consistent, and replicable results. The two types of reliability you should be able to recognize on the exam are test-retest reliability and inter-rater reliability.

- **Test-retest reliability** is a measure of the reliability of an assessment tool in obtaining similar scores over time. In other words, if the same person takes the assessment five times, their scores should be roughly equal, not wildly different.
- **Inter-rater reliability** is a measure of the degree to which two different researchers or raters agree in their assessment. For example, if two different researchers are collecting observational data, their judgments of the same person should be similar, not wildly different.

Validity

Generally, **validity** refers to how well an experiment measures what it is trying to measure. There are three important types of validity: internal, external, and construct. For the purposes of the MCAT, you should know what each type of validity is, and should be able to recognize threats to internal and external validity.

1) **Internal validity** refers to whether the results of the study properly demonstrate a causal relationship between the two variables tested. Highly controlled experiments (with random selection, random assignment to either the control or experimental groups, reliable instruments, reliable processes, and safeguards against confounding factors) may be the only way to truly establish internal validity. **Confounding factors** are hidden variables (those not directly tested for) that correlate in some way with the independent or dependent variable and have some sort of impact on the results.

2) **External validity** refers to whether the results of the study can be generalized to other situations and other people. Generalizability is limited to the independent variable, so the following must be controlled for in order to protect the external validity:
   - sample must be completely random (any of the sampling errors discussed above will threated external validity)
   - all situational variables (treatment conditions, timing, location, administration, investigator, etc.) must be tightly controlled
   - cause and effect relationships may not be generalizable to other settings, situations, groups, or people, etc.

3) **Construct validity** is used to determine whether a tool is measuring what it is intended to measure; for example, does a survey ask questions clearly? Are the questions getting at the intended construct? Are the correct multiple choices present? Et cetera.

Chapter 5
Lab Techniques

5.1 SEPARATIONS

Extractions

One of the more useful techniques in experimental organic chemistry is solvent extraction. Complex mixtures of organic compounds can be separated using careful choice of solvents based on the differential solubilities of the various components of the mixture. We'll see that the acid/base properties of organic molecules play an important role in the extraction process.

Extraction allows us to separate one substance from a mixture of substances by adding a solvent in which the compound of interest is highly soluble. The solution containing the compound of interest is shaken with a second solvent (completely immiscible with the first) in an apparatus called a separatory funnel. The solvents are allowed to separate into two distinct phases, and the compound of interest will distribute itself between the two phases based upon its solubility in each of the individual solvents. This is called a **liquid-liquid extraction**.

Solubility largely depends on two things: the polarity of the solute and the polarity of the solvent. When it comes to solubility, *like dissolves like*. Polar molecules are soluble in polar solvents, and nonpolar molecules are soluble in nonpolar solvents. For example, water is a polar solvent and hydrocarbons are nonpolar molecules. Hydrocarbons will therefore have very low solubility in water. The simplest liquid-liquid extraction is accomplished when an organic compound is extracted with water. A simple water extraction can remove substances that are highly polar or charged, including inorganic salts, strong acids and bases, and polar, low molecular weight compounds (less than five carbons) such as alcohols, amines, and carboxylic acids.

A second class of organic extraction involves the use of acidic or basic water solutions. Organic compounds that are basic (e.g., amines) can be extracted from mixtures of organic compounds upon treatment with dilute acid, usually HCl. This treatment will protonate the basic functional group, forming a positively charged ion. The resulting cationic salts of these basic compounds are usually freely soluble in aqueous solution and can be removed from the organic compounds that remain dissolved in the organic phase.

On the other hand, extraction with a dilute weak base—typically sodium bicarbonate ($NaHCO_3$)—results in converting carboxylic acids into their corresponding anionic salts. These anionic salts are generally soluble in aqueous solution and can be removed from the organic compounds that remain dissolved in the organic phase. Dilute sodium hydroxide could also be used for this kind of extraction, but it is basic enough to also convert phenols into their corresponding anionic salts. When phenols are present in a mixture of organic compounds and need to be removed, a dilute sodium hydroxide solution will succeed in converting phenols into their corresponding anionic salts. The anionic salts of the phenols are generally soluble in the aqueous phase and can therefore be removed from the organic phase. Note that NaOH will also extract carboxylic acids, but that $NaHCO_3$ cannot extract phenols.

As an example, let's step through an extraction that will separate four organic compounds from one another: *para*-cresol, benzoic acid, aniline, and naphthalene, all of which are dissolved in diethyl ether.

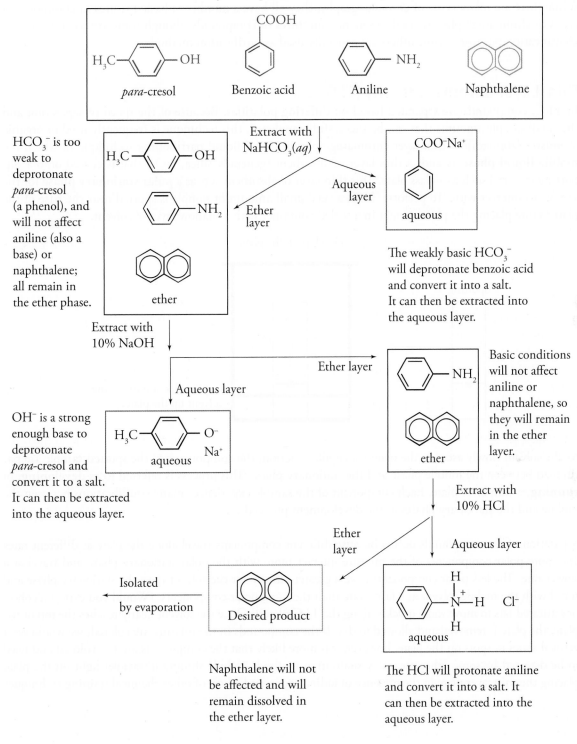

All four components dissolved in diethyl ether

COOH — Benzoic acid
H_3C—⟨⟩—OH — *para*-cresol
—NH_2 — Aniline
Naphthalene

Extract with NaHCO$_3$(*aq*)

HCO$_3^-$ is too weak to deprotonate *para*-cresol (a phenol), and will not affect aniline (also a base) or naphthalene; all remain in the ether phase.

ether

COO$^-$Na$^+$
aqueous

The weakly basic HCO$_3^-$ will deprotonate benzoic acid and convert it into a salt. It can then be extracted into the aqueous layer.

Aqueous layer

Ether layer

Extract with 10% NaOH

Ether layer

Aqueous layer

OH$^-$ is a strong enough base to deprotonate *para*-cresol and convert it to a salt. It can then be extracted into the aqueous layer.

H_3C—⟨⟩—O$^-$ Na$^+$
aqueous

Basic conditions will not affect aniline or naphthalene, so they will remain in the ether layer.

—NH_2

ether

Extract with 10% HCl

Ether layer

Aqueous layer

Isolated by evaporation

Desired product

Naphthalene will not be affected and will remain dissolved in the ether layer.

N$^+$—H with H's, Cl$^-$
aqueous

The HCl will protonate aniline and convert it into a salt. It can then be extracted into the aqueous layer.

Chromatography

While there are many types of chromatography, they all have a number of basic features in common. All types of chromatography are used to separate mixtures of compounds, though some are used mostly for identification purposes, while others are generally used as purification methods.

Thin-Layer Chromatography (TLC)

In TLC, compounds are separated based on differing polarities. Because of the speed of separation and the small sample amounts that can be successfully analyzed, this technique is frequently used in organic chemistry laboratories. Thin-layer chromatography is a solid-liquid partitioning technique in which the **mobile liquid phase** ascends a thin layer of absorbent (generally silica, SiO_2) that is coated onto a supporting material such as a glass plate. This thin layer of absorbent acts as a **polar stationary phase** for the sample to interact with. To perform TLC, a very small amount of sample is spotted near the base of the plate before placing the plate upright in a sealed container with a shallow layer of solvent.

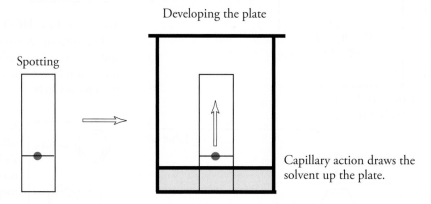

Developing the plate

Spotting

Capillary action draws the solvent up the plate.

As the solvent slowly ascends the plate via capillary action, the components of the spotted sample are partitioned between the mobile phase and the stationary phase. This process is referred to as **developing**, or **running**, a thin layer plate. Each component of the sample experiences many equilibrations between the mobile and the stationary phases as the development proceeds.

Separation of the compounds occurs because different components travel along the plate at different rates. The more polar components of the mixture interact more with the polar stationary phase and travel at a slower rate. The less polar components have a greater affinity for the solvent than the stationary phase and travel with the mobile solvent at a faster rate than the more polar components. [Would you expect alcohols or saturated fats to move more quickly along the TLC plate?[1]] Once the solvent nearly reaches the top of the plate, the plate is removed and allowed to dry. If the compounds in the mixture are colored, we would see a vertical series of spots on the plate; however, it is more likely that the components are not colored and need to be detected by some other means. Visualization methods include shining ultraviolet light on the plate, placing the thin layer plate in the presence of iodine vapor, and a host of other chemical staining techniques.

---

[1]   Since the alcohols are more polar than the saturated fats, the alcohols would interact more strongly with the silica gel coating the plate. The nonpolar saturated fats would interact more strongly with the solvent, and would travel more quickly along the plate.

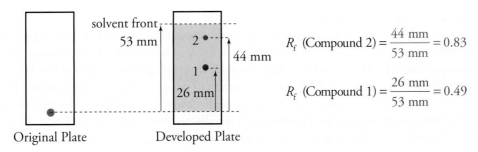

$$R_f \text{ (Compound 2)} = \frac{44 \text{ mm}}{53 \text{ mm}} = 0.83$$

$$R_f \text{ (Compound 1)} = \frac{26 \text{ mm}}{53 \text{ mm}} = 0.49$$

(Note that the R_f is always positive and never greater than 1.)

Once the separated components have been visualized, R_f values can be computed. This "ratio to front" value (R_f) is simply the distance traveled by an individual component divided by the distance traveled by the solvent front.

Example 5-1:

A TLC plate was spotted with an unknown mixture of amino acids along with three known amino acids: phenylalanine (R_f 0.62), lysine (R_f 0.12), and valine (R_f 0.44). The developed plate displayed spots with the following R_f values: 0.12, 0.55, 0.62. What can be concluded about the composition of the unknown mixture of amino acids?

Solution:

R_f values of two of the three spots observed for the unknown mixture of amino acids in the developed plate correspond to R_f values of lysine (0.12) and phenylalanine (0.62). However, the R_f value of the third spot observed for the mixture (0.55) differs from that observed for valine (0.44). We conclude that the unknown mixture of amino acids contains phenylalanine and lysine but not valine. The identity of the third component of the mixture remains unknown.

Example 5-2:

A TLC plate coated with silica gel was spotted with a mixture of benzoic acid, benzyl alcohol, and benzyl benzoate. Subsequently, the plate was eluted with a moderately polar organic solvent. Spots on the developed plate displayed R_f values of 0.11, 0.32, 0.72. To which compound does each of the three spots correspond?

Solution:

Silica gel is a highly polar stationary phase; hence, more polar solutes will have greater affinity for the stationary phase and are expected to display small R_f values. In contrast, less polar solutes will display greater affinity for the solvent and thus are expected to display larger R_f values. Note that as polarity increases R_f value decreases, in the order ester (benzyl benzoate), alcohol (benzyl alcohol), carboxylic acid (benzoic acid). We therefore can assign the three spots as follows: benzoic acid (R_f 0.11), benzyl alcohol (R_f 0.32), and benzyl benzoate (R_f 0.72).

Column (Flash) Chromatography

While TLC is a good technique for separating very small amounts of material, it's not a good technique for isolating bulk compounds. A common technique known as column or flash chromatography employs the same principles behind TLC toward just such a goal. A chromatography column is filled with silica gel (predominantly SiO_2, as in the TLC plate), which is saturated with a chosen organic solvent. The mixture of compounds to be separated is then added to the top and allowed to travel down through the silica. The flow of solvent (along with the separated compounds) is collected from the bottom. Just as in TLC, polar compounds will spend more time adsorbed on the polar solid phase, and as such travel more slowly down the column than nonpolar compounds. Therefore, compounds can be expected to leave the column, and be collected, in order of polarity (least polar to most polar).

Column Chromatography

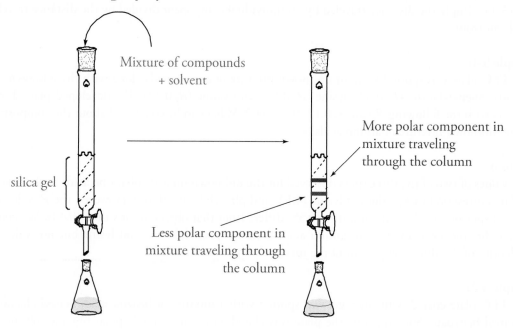

Ion Exchange Chromatography

In applications where the materials to be separated have varying charge states, ion exchange chromatography may be employed. This method, again involving passing a mobile liquid phase containing the analyte through a column packed with a solid stationary phase, utilizes a polymeric resin functionalized with either positive or negatively charged moieties on the polymer surface.

The schematic below depicts the passage of an analyte containing both positively and negatively charged ionic species, as well as neutral molecules, through a pore of an ion exchange resin. The particular stationary phase resin depicted below is functionalized with anionic sulfonate groups, initially coordinated to sodium cations.

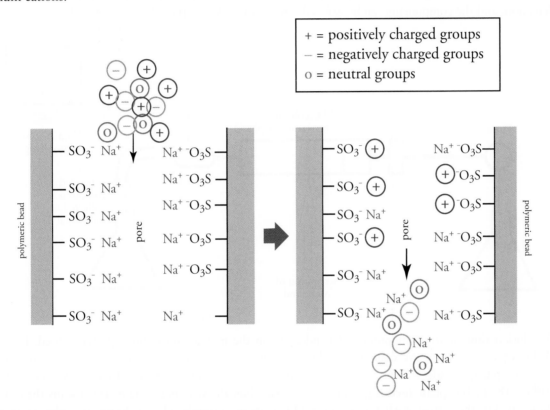

As the analyte passes through the resin, positively charged groups displace sodium ions and coordinate to the anionic functionalities tethered to the polymer surface. While these groups are retained, and their progress through the column retarded, the negatively charged groups and neutral species quickly pass through the material and are eluted first. Once all the negatively charged and neutral species have been eluted, the column can be treated with a concentrated sodium-containing solution to displace all adsorbed positively charged species.

Ion exchange chromatography is frequently used in the separation of mixtures of proteins. At any given pH, proteins within a mixture may exist in a variety of charge states. If such a mixture is passed through a cation exchange resin (one functionalized with negatively charged groups and cationic substances as shown in the figure above), those proteins with pI values greater than the pH of the mobile phase will be positively charged and elute slowly compared to those with pI values below the solution pH. If the same mixture at the same pH were passed through an anion exchange resin, the opposite would be true, and proteins with pI values above the pH of the solution will elute first. If the pI values of the proteins to be separated are known, the pH of the mobile phase may be buffered to a specific pH, thereby ensuring different charge states and hence good separation.

High Performance Liquid Chromatography (HPLC)

HPLC uses the same principles as all chromatographic separation techniques, and it takes advantage of the differing affinities of various compounds for either a stationary phase or a mobile phase. However, because the mobile phase is forced through the stationary phase at very high pressures, both the speed and efficiency of the separation is increased, making this technique an improvement over column chromatography.

The basic configuration of an HPLC system is shown in the figure below. The pumping unit is where pressurization of the mobile phase first occurs. The sample to be separated is solubilized and injected by syringe, then the mobile phase carries the sample to the column. The sample is separated into its constituent components, which are detected and analyzed as they exit the column. The eluent is collected after detection, and the components can be isolated after evaporation of the solvent, if desired.

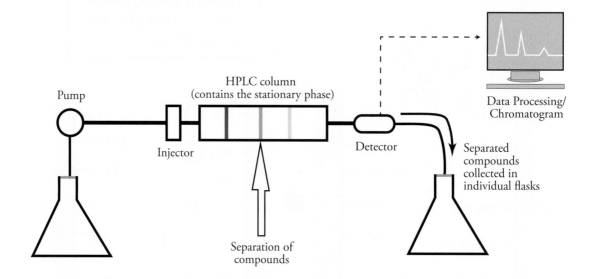

The elution time of any compound is dependent upon the mobile and stationary phases used. For most HPLC separations of organic compounds, the stationary phase is a silica gel that has been bonded to a nonpolar group (e.g., octadecylsilane), creating a relatively *nonpolar* stationary phase. This is called reverse phase HPLC. The mobile phase used is generally *more polar* than the stationary phase. This means the order of elution will be the reverse of what occurs on a TLC plate or in simple column chromatography. More polar compounds elute first in HPLC, as they have a high affinity for the mobile phase. The less polar compounds are slowed by their interactions with the nonpolar stationary phase, and therefore elute last.

Size Exclusion Chromatography

Size exclusion chromatography is a technique used to separate bulk materials based on molecular size. Much like flash chromatography, the materials to be separated are dissolved in solvent, loaded onto a column packed with a stationary phase, and allowed to travel to the bottom of the column where they are collected.

In contrast to flash chromatography, which uses a polar silicate stationary phase, the stationary phase employed in size exclusion chromatography most often consists of chemically inert, porous polymer beads. The sizes of the pores in the bead are carefully controlled to allow permeation of small molecules in the eluent, while excluding larger ones. A schematic for the beads and the paths taken by large and small molecules is depicted below.

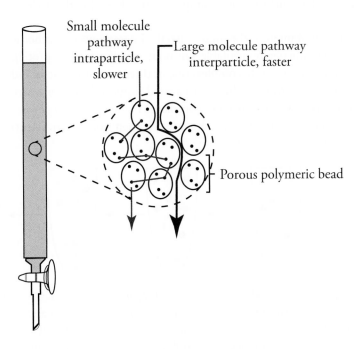

The exclusion of large molecules from the pore volume creates a more direct path down the column for large species than the more complicated intraparticle pathway taken by compounds small enough to permeate the beads. The overall result is the quick elution of large molecules and longer retention of smaller species.

Size exclusion chromatography is frequently used for the separation of large polymers from small oligomeric fragments, or the separation of full proteins from smaller peptide chains. The lack of chemical interaction between the mobile and stationary phases results in relatively speedy elution (compared to chromatography on silica) and minimal loss of material on the column. However, though materials of very different sizes are easily separated, the technique is not particularly effective at separating different compounds of similar sizes.

- Would an amino acid such as glycine or a triglyceride elute more rapidly from the column during size exclusion chromatography?[2]

---

[2] Since the amino acid is much smaller than the triglyceride, it would enter the pores of the stationary phase beads more easily. The triglyceride would be excluded from the pores, and take a more direct path through the column, thus eluting more rapidly than the amino acid.

Affinity Chromatography

Affinity chromatography is most commonly used to purify proteins or nucleic acids from complex biochemical mixtures like cell lysates, growth media, or blood, rather than a reaction mixture. It is based on highly specific interactions between macromolecules. As a result of this specific binding, the target molecule is trapped on the stationary phase, which is then washed to remove the unwanted components of the mixture. The target protein is then released (or eluted) off the solid phase in a highly purified state.

In large-scale work, the stationary phase is a column packed with a solid resin, and the sample is poured through the column. In smaller scale experiments, the solid phase can be mixed in a small tube with the sample to allow interaction with the components of the mixture. The sample is then centrifuged (spun at high speeds) so the heavy solid resin settles to the bottom of the tube. Since the protein of interest is bound to the solid resin, the liquid (or supernatant) is simply decanted, leaving the desired compound behind.

In order to isolate a protein of interest, the highly specific interactions of antibodies can be used, as shown in the figure below. A commercially available antibody specific for the protein is added to the lysate sample. To isolate the antigen-antibody complex, one of three common microbe-derived proteins (Protein A, Protein G, or Protein L) is covalently linked to a solid support. These proteins are useful because they bind mammalian antibodies, so upon mixing, complexes made of *Protein of Interest – Antibody – Protein A/G/L – Solid Support Bead* form in solution. The target is then isolated after centrifuging the sample and decanting the supernatant.

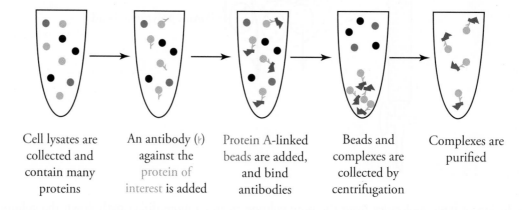

Figure 1 Purifying a Protein of Interest using an Antibody and Protein A-linked Beads

Instead of centrifugation, magnetic beads can be used as the solid phase, as shown on the next page. The beads are isolated from the solution by using a magnet to hold them (bound to the protein of interest) against the sides of the tube, while the solution containing any undesired compounds is decanted. Then the desired compound can be released from the beads in a pure state.

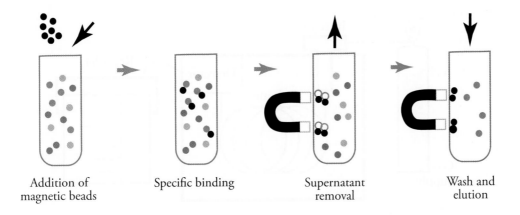

Figure 2 Using Magnetic Beads as the Solid Phase in Affinity Chromatography

Not all proteins of interest have a commercial antibody available. In this case, researchers can use an **affinity tag.** Using recombinant technology (described later in this chapter), a small molecular tag is added to the N-terminus or the C-terminus of the protein. DNA sequences coding for affinity tags are well known, and these can be subcloned into a plasmid with the gene of interest. Affinity-tagged proteins can be produced in large amounts in laboratory bacteria, and the cell lysate collected is rich in tagged protein.

There are many types of affinity tags, and they are generally small enough that they don't interfere with protein folding or function. One class of commonly used affinity tags are the His tags (made of 6–10 histidine amino acids), which bind ions such as nickel. When a cell lysate is applied to a column packed with nickel-based resin, the His-tagged proteins bind to the resin. This is done under high pH conditions, and the His-tagged protein can be eluted off the solid phase using lower pH conditions.

Gas Chromatography

Gas chromatography (GC) is a form of column chromatography in which the partitioning of the components to be separated takes place between a **mobile gas phase** and a **stationary liquid phase**. This partitioning, or separation, between mixtures of compounds occurs based on their *different volatilities*. In a typical gas chromatograph, a sample is loaded into a syringe and injected into the device through a rubber septum. The sample is then vaporized by a heater in the injection port and carried along by a stream of inert gas (typically helium). The vaporized sample is quickly moved by the inert gas stream into a column composed of particles that are coated with a liquid absorbent.

As the components of the mixture pass through the column, they interact differently with the absorbant based on their relative volatilities. Each component of the mixture is subjected to many gas-liquid partitioning processes which separates the individual components. The less volatile components will spend more time dissolved in the liquid stationary phase than the more volatile component that will be carried along by the carrier gas at a faster rate. It is this equilibrium between the component (the absorbed liquid phase and the carrier gas mobile phase) that results in the separation of the mixture. If the interactions of the substrates with the column are similar (this is usually the case with most GC columns), the more volatile components emerge from the column first, while the less volatile components emerge from the column later.

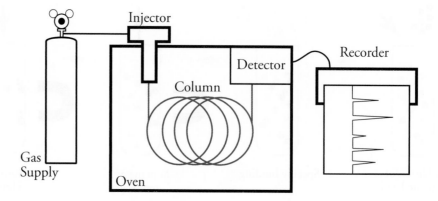

As each component exits the column, it is burned, and the resulting ions are detected by an electrical detector that generates a signal that is recorded by a chart recorder. The chart recorder printout enables us to determine the number of components and their relative amounts.

Distillations

Distillation is the process of raising the temperature of a liquid until it can overcome the intermolecular forces that hold it together in the liquid phase. The vapor is then condensed back to the liquid phase and subsequently collected in another container.

Simple Distillation

A simple distillation is performed when trace impurities need to be removed from a relatively pure compound, or when a mixture of compounds with significantly different boiling points needs to be separated. For example, an appropriate use of a simple distillation would be to purify fresh drinking water away from a salt water solution. The more volatile water can be boiled away, then condensed and collected, leaving behind the nonvolatile salts.

Fractional Distillation

Fractional distillation is a different type of distillation process that is used when the difference in boiling points of the components in the liquid mixture is not large. A fractional distillation column is packed with an appropriate material, such as glass beads or a stainless steel sponge. The packing of the column results in the liquid mixture being subjected to many vaporization-condensation cycles as it moves up the column toward the condenser. As the cycles progress, the composition of the vapor gradually becomes enriched in the lower boiling component. Near the top of the column, nearly pure vapor reaches the condenser and condenses back to the liquid phase where it is subsequently collected in a receiving flask.

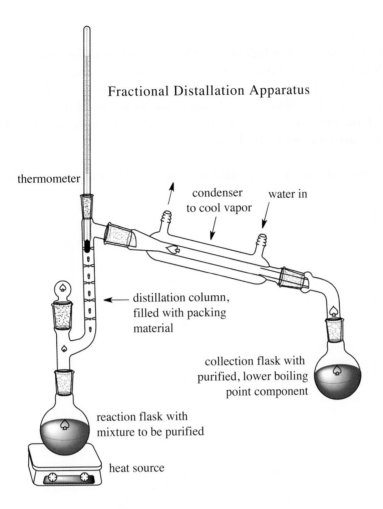

Fractional Distallation Apparatus

thermometer

condenser
to cool vapor

water in

distillation column,
filled with packing
material

collection flask with
purified, lower boiling
point component

reaction flask with
mixture to be purified

heat source

5.2 SPECTROSCOPY

Most types of spectroscopy that we will discuss are examples of absorption spectroscopy. A short explanation of the molecular events involved in absorption spectroscopy will help you remember the details of IR and NMR spectroscopy. Molecules normally exist in their lowest energy form, called their **ground state**. When a molecule is exposed to light, it *may* absorb a photon, provided that the energy of this photon matches the energy between two of the fixed electronic energy levels of the molecule. When this happens, the molecule is said to be in an **excited state**. Molecules tend to prefer their ground state to an excited state, but in order for them to return to their ground state, they must lose the energy they have gained. This loss of energy can occur by the emission of heat, or less commonly, light. In absorption spectroscopy, scientists induce the absorption of energy by a sample of molecules by exposing the sample to various forms of light, thereby exciting molecules to a higher energy state. They then measure the energy released as the molecules relax back to their ground state. This measured energy can reveal structural features of the molecules in the sample.

There are many different forms of light, as displayed in the electromagnetic spectrum. In principle, any of these forms of light could be used to do absorption spectroscopy on molecules, and, in fact, many are! The different forms of light induce different transitions in ground state molecules to different excited states of the molecules and allow for the acquisition of different structural information about the molecules.

Mass Spectrometry

Mass spectrometry is a very useful technique that allows researchers to determine the mass of compounds in a sample. Within the mass spectrometer, molecules are ionized in a high vacuum, usually by bombarding them with high energy electrons. Once ionized, compounds enter a region of the spectrometer where they are acted on by a magnetic field. This field causes the flight path of the charged species to alter, and the degree to which the path is changed is determined by the mass of the ion. This difference is detected and translated into a mass readout in the detector.

A schematic of a portion of the mass spectrum for *n*-nonane (MW = 128 g/mol) follows:

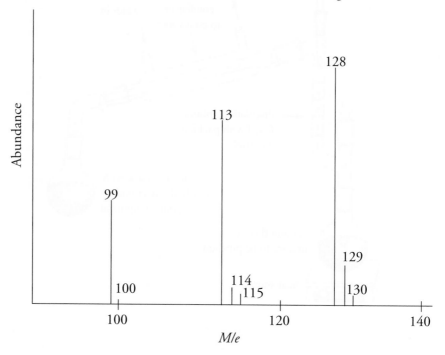

The *M/e* label on the *x*-axis represents the ratio of mass (*M*) to charge (*e*). In most cases *e* = +1, so peaks can simply be viewed as molecular mass. The *y*-axis represents the relative abundance of each species of a particular mass detected in the sample. Masses, though generally not labeled as such, are measured in amu.

Two aspects of the above spectrum may be puzzling: 1) if the molecular weight of nonane is 128 g/mol, why are there peaks greater than this value, and 2) why are there significant peaks in the sample with masses lower than 128?

Remember, atoms can come in a number of different isotopes. For example, the most prevalent mass of hydrogen in nature is 1, but deuterium has an extra neutron and weighs 2 (natural abundance = .015%). Likewise, the most abundant isotope of carbon is ^{12}C, but ^{13}C exists as 1.1% of all carbon atoms. So, the small peaks with masses larger than the main peak represent molecules that have one or more of these less abundant isotopes.

The masses lower than 128 in the above scan represent the masses of molecular fragments. The high energy beam of electrons used to ionize molecules in the mass spectrometer can cause the molecule to break into smaller parts. The figure on the next page shows where *n*-nonane might have been broken to produce peaks with the masses found above. The outer, curved brackets represent a fragment which has lost the terminal CH_3 group and hence is 15 less than the peak at 128. The inner, square brackets show a fragment weighing 99, having lost CH_2CH_3.

Particular atoms present in a molecule may give characteristic peaks in their mass spectra thanks to isotopic ratios. The two most important are Br and Cl. Bromine naturally occurs in two isotopes (79 and 81) of nearly identical natural abundance. This means that any mass spectrum involving a brominated compound will have two major peaks, nearly equal in height, 2 amu apart. Chlorine also occurs as two main isotopes: 35 (75% natural abundance) and 37 (25% natural abundance). Mass spectra for chlorinated molecules will have a peak 2 amu heavier than the main peak and about one-third its height.

Ultraviolet/Visible (UV/Vis) Spectroscopy

UV/Vis spectroscopy is a type of absorption spectroscopy used in organic chemistry. It is very similar to IR (which we'll discuss next), but instead focuses on the slightly shorter, more energetic wavelengths of radiation in the ultraviolet and visible area of the spectrum. The wavelengths in the UV and visible ranges of the electromagnetic spectrum are strong enough to induce electronic excitation, promoting ground state valence electrons into excited states.

In general, UV/Vis spectroscopy is used with two kinds of molecules. It is very useful in monitoring complexes of transition metals. The easy promotion of electrons from ground to excited states in the closely spaced *d*-orbitals of many transition metals gives them their bright color (by absorbing wavelengths in the visible region), and since many of these promotions involve energies in the UV range, these promotions allow study of these species.

More importantly in organic chemistry, UV/Vis spectroscopy is used to study highly conjugated organic systems. Molecular orbital theory tells us that when molecules have conjugated π-systems, orbitals form many bonding, non-bonding, and anti-bonding orbitals. These orbitals can be reasonably close together in energy, and in fact, close enough to allow promotion of electrons between electronic states through absorption of ultraviolet, or even visible photons. The wavelength of maximum absorption for any compound is directly related to the extent of conjugation in the molecule. The more extensive the conjugated system is, the longer the wavelength of maximum absorption will be. To illustrate this relationship, let's look at a series of polycyclic aromatic hydrocarbons in Table 1 on the next page.

		λ_{max}	absorbs	appears
Anthracene		363 nm	UV	white
Tetracene		475 nm	blue	orange
Pentacene		595 nm	yellow/orange	blue/violet

Table 1   UV/Vis Spectroscopic Data for Select Polycyclic Aromatic Hydrocarbons

With the addition of each aromatic ring, the conjugated system grows longer and the wavelength of maximum absorption increases. Since each λ_{max} corresponds to a particular color of light, a simple color wheel can be used to predict the color the compound will appear. As a general rule, the color a compound maximally absorbs is complementary to the color it will appear to our eyes. For a compound that absorbs only ultraviolet radiation, ALL of the visible wavelengths will be reflected and thus the compound will appear white or colorless. However, a compound that absorbs blue light will appear to us as orange, since blue and orange are complementary colors on opposites sides of the color wheel.

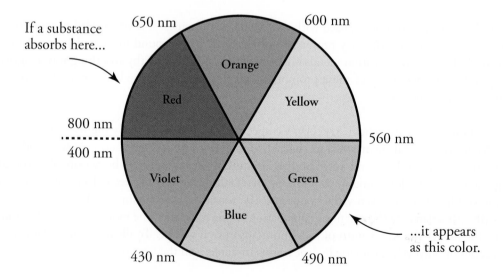

Infrared (IR) Spectroscopy

Electromagnetic radiation in the infrared (IR) range λ = 2.5 to 20 μm has the proper energy to cause bonds in organic molecules to become vibrationally excited. When a sample of an organic compound is irradiated with infrared radiation in the region between 2.5 and 20 μm, its covalent bonds will begin to *vibrate at distinct energy levels* (wavelengths, frequencies) within this region. These wavelengths correspond to frequencies in the range of 1.5×10^{13} Hz to 1.2×10^{14} Hz. In IR spectroscopy, vibrational frequencies are more commonly given in terms of the **wavenumber**. Wavenumber ($\overline{v}$) is simply the reciprocal of wavelength:

$$\overline{v} = \frac{1}{\lambda} = \frac{1}{c}v$$

and is therefore directly proportional to both the frequency (since $\lambda v = c = 3 \times 10^{10}$ cm/sec) and the energy of the radiation (since $E = hv$). That is, the higher the wavenumber, the higher the frequency and the greater the energy. Wavenumbers are usually expressed in *reciprocal centimeters*, cm^{-1}, and MCAT IR spectra will typically cover the range from 4,000 to 1,000 cm^{-1}.

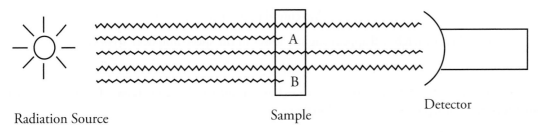

Radiation Source   Sample   Detector

When a bond absorbs IR radiation of a specific frequency, that frequency is not recorded by the detector and is thus seen as a peak in the IR spectrum (since low transmittance corresponds, naturally, to absorbance):

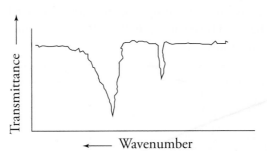

Important Stretching Frequencies

In order to do well on the MCAT, it is important that you know the stretching frequencies of the common functional groups. The most important ones are listed below.

The Double Bond Stretches

We'll begin by examining the carbonyl, or C=O, stretch. The carbonyl stretch is centered around 1,700 cm^{-1} and is very **strong** and very **intense**. *Strength* is reflected in the percent absorbance (or transmittance). *Intensity* is reflected in the sharpness or distinctiveness ("V" shape) of the spike appearing on the spectrum.

The carbonyl stretch is one of the most important absorptions, and you should commit its location to memory. In any spectrum, always look for this stretch first. If it is *not* present, you can eliminate a wide range of compounds that contain a carbonyl group, including aldehydes, ketones, carboxylic acids, acid chlorides, esters, amides, and anhydrides. On the other hand, if the carbonyl stretch *is* present, you know that one of the carbonyl-containing functional groups is indeed present.

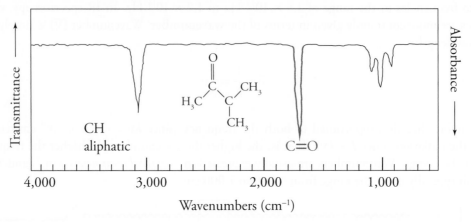

The C=C double bond stretch will appear slightly lower in the spectrum, near 1650 cm^{-1}.

The Triple Bond Stretch
The next stretch to consider is the triple bond. This is an easy one because few molecules possess these functional groups.

The O—H Stretch
Next we come to the hydroxyl stretch. *The O—H stretch is strong and very broad.* **Strength** is reflected as the degree of absorption a peak displays in the spectrum. **Broadness** is reflected as a wide "U"-shaped appearance on the absorption spectrum, as opposed to a "V," or spiked shape. The broadness is due to hydrogen bonding. Like the carbonyl stretch that occurs at 1,700 cm^{-1}, one should always look for the O—H stretch at 3,600–3,200 cm^{-1}. Amines also have stretches in this region, although they vary in intensity.

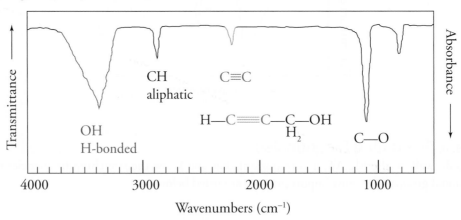

The C—H Stretches

Finally we come to the C—H stretching region (3,300–2,850 cm^{-1}). Since the vast majority of organic compounds contain C—H bonds, you will almost always see absorbances in this region. Note that aliphatic C—H bonds stretch at wavenumbers a little less than 3,000 cm^{-1}, and aromatic C—H bonds stretch at wavenumbers slightly greater than 3,000 cm^{-1}.

Summary of Relevant Infrared (IR) Stretching Frequencies

Bond	Frequency (Wavenumber) Range (cm^{-1})	Intensity
C=O	1735–1680	strong
C=C	1680–1620	variable
C≡C	2260–2100	variable
C≡N	2260–2220	variable
C—H	3300–2700	variable
N—H	3150–2500	moderate
O—H	3650–3200	broad

Example 5-3:

IR spectra, labeled A, B, and C, are obtained for three isomeric C_4H_8O compounds: 2-butanone, 3-buten-2-ol, and cyclobutanol. Characteristic features of their respective IR spectra are described below. Which isomer corresponds to each spectrum?

IR spectrum A: 3600–3200 cm^{-1} and 1620–1680 cm^{-1}
IR spectrum B: 3600–3200 cm^{-1}
IR spectrum C: 1720–1700 cm^{-1}

Solution:

Spectrum A displays absorptions in the regions 3600–3200 cm^{-1} (O—H stretching vibration) and 1620–1680 cm^{-1} (C=C stretching vibration). The absence of absorption in the region 1720–1700 cm^{-1} indicates that this compound does not contain a C=O group. Thus, Spectrum A is assigned to 3-buten-2-ol.

Spectrum B displays an intense absorption signal in the region 3600–3200 cm^{-1}. The lack of absorption in the regions 1720–1700 cm^{-1} and 1620–1680 cm^{-1} indicates the absence of C=O and C=C groups, respectively. Accordingly, Spectrum B can be assigned to cyclobutanol.

Spectrum C displays intense absorption in the regions 1720–1700 cm^{-1} (C=O stretching vibration) but does not contain absorption in the regions 3600–3200 cm^{-1} and 1620–1680 cm^{-1}. Among the three compounds of interest only 2-butanone is consistent with the IR spectral information.

^{1}H Nuclear Magnetic Resonance (NMR) Spectroscopy

^{1}H NMR spectroscopy, commonly called proton NMR, is the third type of absorption spectroscopy that we will consider. In all types of NMR spectroscopy, light from the radio frequency range of the electromagnetic spectrum is used to induce energy absorptions. The interpretation of ^{1}H NMR spectral data is important for the MCAT, but the theory underlying NMR spectroscopy is beyond the scope of the exam. Here, we'll only cover the interpretation of ^{1}H NMR spectra.

Four essential features of a molecule can be deduced from its ^{1}H NMR spectrum, and while we'll review all four, it is most important for the MCAT to focus on the first two. First, the number of sets of peaks in the spectrum indicates the number of chemically nonequivalent sets of protons in the molecule. Second, the splitting pattern of each set of peaks indicates how many protons are interacting with the protons in that set. Third, the mathematical integration of the sets of peaks indicates the relative numbers of protons in each set. Fourth, the chemical shift values of those sets of peaks gives information about the environment of the protons in that set. These four key features of ^{1}H NMR spectroscopy are explained in the next four sections.

Chemically Equivalent Hydrogens

Determining which hydrogens, or protons, are **equivalent** in an organic molecule is the first important skill to master with respect to NMR spectroscopy. Equivalent hydrogens in a molecule are those that have *identical electronic environments*. Such hydrogens have identical locations in the ^{1}H NMR spectrum, and are therefore represented by the same signal, or resonance. Nonequivalent hydrogens will have different locations in the ^{1}H NMR spectrum and be represented by different signals. One must be able to determine which hydrogens (or, usually, groups of hydrogens) are equivalent to which other groups, so that you can predict how many distinct NMR signals there will be in any ^{1}H NMR spectrum. Hydrogens are considered equivalent if they can be interchanged by a free rotation or a symmetry operation (mirror plane or rotational axis). Check yourself on the following examples:

Splitting

The second aspect of NMR spectroscopy that you should be familiar with is the **spin-spin splitting phenomenon**. This occurs when nonequivalent hydrogens interact with each other. This interaction exists because the magnetic field felt by a proton is influenced by surrounding protons. This effect tends to fall off with distance, but it can often extend over two adjacent carbons. Nearby protons that are nonequivalent to the proton in question will cause a splitting in the observed ^1H NMR signal. The degree of splitting depends on the number of adjacent hydrogens, and a signal will be split into $n + 1$ lines, where n is the number of nonequivalent, neighboring (interacting) protons. The important information one must determine is how a proton or a group of chemically equivalent protons will be split by their hydrogen neighbors.

This is best demonstrated by an example:

Three distinct types of hydrogens:
  3 H_a hydrogens
  2 H_b hydrogens
  2 H_c hydrogens

H_a signal split into **three** peaks due to the two neighboring, but different, H_b atoms.

H_b signal split into **six** peaks due to the five neighboring, but different, H_a and H_c atoms.

H_c signal split into **three** peaks due to the two neighboring, but different, H_b atoms.

Note that, for MCAT purposes, the H_a and H_c protons neighboring H_b do not have to be equivalent in order to add them together to get $n = 5$.

$n + 1$ RULE

n = Number of neighboring nonequivalent hydrogens	Splitting ($n + 1$)
0	1—Singlet
1	2—Doublet
2	3—Triplet
3	4—Quartet
4	5—Quintet (or multiplet)
5	6—Sextet (or multiplet)

Consider the NMR spectrum of CH_3CH_2I:

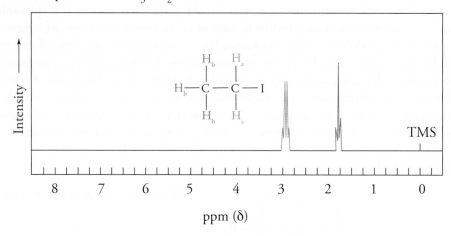

The α-hydrogens have three neighboring hydrogens and are therefore split into a quartet, according to the $n + 1$ rule. The β-hydrogens are split into a triplet because they have two neighboring hydrogens.

Integration

The third important piece of information obtained from the ^1H NMR spectrum of a molecule is the mathematical integration. As the NMR instrument obtains a spectrum of the sample, it performs a mathematical calculation, called an **integration**, thereby measuring the area under each absorption peak (resonance). The calculated area under each peak is proportional to the relative number of protons giving rise to each peak. Thus, the integration indicates the relative number of protons in each set in the molecule.

The Chemical Shift

The fourth and final aspect of an NMR spectrum is the **chemical shift**, which indicates the location of the resonance (set of peaks) in the ^1H NMR spectrum. Differences in the chemical shift values for different sets of protons in a molecule are the result of the differing electronic environments that different sets of protons experience. The magnetic field created by electrons near a proton will **shield** the nucleus from the applied magnetic field created by the instrument, shifting the resonance **upfield**. The more a proton is **deshielded** (i.e., the more distorted away from the atom the electron cloud is), the further **downfield** (to the left) in an NMR spectrum it will appear. For example, a set of protons *near* an electronegative group is said to be deshielded and will appear downfield (to the left) in the ^1H NMR spectrum, relative to a set of protons that are farther away from the electronegative group, which is more shielded and appears more upfield (to the right) in the ^1H NMR spectrum.

downfield   upfield

⟵   ⟶

more deshielded   less deshielded

We will now briefly examine the factors involved in proton deshielding.

Electronegativity Effects on Chemical Shift Values

If an electronegative atom is in close proximity to a proton, it will decrease the electron density near the proton and thereby deshield it. This will result in a *down*field shift in the chemical shift value. Examples:

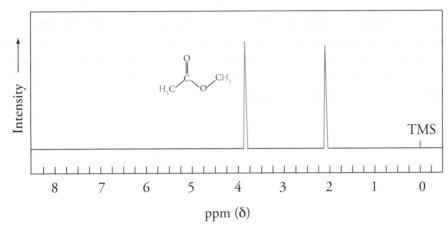

$\delta = 0.26$ ppm $\delta = 3.06$ ppm $\delta = 3.25$ ppm

The spectrum of methyl acetate below shows how the two electronegative groups in the molecule (the O of the ester and the carbonyl) contribute to shifting both methyl signals downfield.

Hybridization Effects on Chemical Shift Values

The **hybridization effect** occurs as a result of the varying bond characteristics of carbon atoms *connected* to the hydrogens. The greater the *s*-orbital character of a C—H bond, the less electron density on the hydrogen. Thus, when considering the hybridization effect alone, the greater the *s*-orbital character, the more deshielded the set of protons is, which will result in a downfield shift for the peak corresponding to that set of protons.

Hybridization effects alone would indicate the alkyne proton to be more deshielded than the alkene proton. However, due to a more complicated physical phenomenon, which is beyond the scope of the MCAT, this turns out not to be the case. To simplify for the MCAT, two other very characteristic chemical shifts you should be familiar with are that of the aromatic protons (δ = 6.5–8 ppm) and alkene protons (δ = 5–6 ppm).

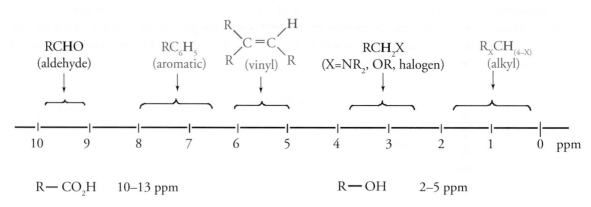

δ = 1 ppm   δ = 2 ppm   δ = 6.5–8 ppm   δ = 6 ppm

Acidity and Hydrogen Bonding Effects on Chemical Shift Values

Protons that are attached to **heteroatoms** (oxygen and nitrogen, for example) are quite deshielded. Acidic protons on a carboxylic acid are an extreme example of a very large downfield shift. You should also be aware that the chemical shifts of alcohol protons are quite variable depending upon the particular compound, but they are in the range of δ = 2–5 ppm.

H_3C—OH

δ = 2–5 ppm

δ = 10–13 ppm

As with IR stretching frequencies, memorizing some commonly encountered ^1H NMR chemical shift values will be helpful. Below is a correlation chart for some common chemical shifts, the most important of which are in red:

| RCHO (aldehyde) | RC_6H_5 (aromatic) | $R_2C=CR_2$ H (vinyl) | RCH_2X (X=NR₂, OR, halogen) | $R_XCH_{(4-X)}$ (alkyl) |

10   9   8   7   6   5   4   3   2   1   0   ppm

R—CO_2H 10–13 ppm   R—OH   2–5 ppm

Example 5-4:

The ^1H NMR spectrum of which of the following three compounds contains one singlet (3H) and one triplet (2H)?

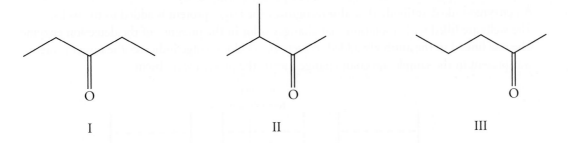

I II III

A) II only
B) III only
C) I and II only
D) II and III only

Solution:

According to the splitting shown below, only structure III contains a combination of a singlet and a triplet. Therefore, choice B is correct.

I II III

5.3 ENZYME-LINKED IMMUNO-SORBENT ASSAY (ELISA)

As the name suggests, an ELISA is a biochemical technique that utilizes antigen-antibody interactions ("immuno-sorbency") to determine the presence of either

- antigens (like proteins or cytokines), or
- specific immunoglobulins (antibodies)

in a sample (such as cells recovered from a tumor biopsy or a patient's serum). The steps on the next page describe the basic protocol when testing for the presence of a specific antigen.

Step 1: The experimental wells are coated with antibodies that are specific for the target antigen.

Step 2: A sample of serum or cell extract is added to the wells.

Step 3: The antibodies immobilize the antigen by binding to it (if it is present in the sample).

Step 4: Any unbound proteins remaining in the sample are washed away.

Step 5: An enzyme-linked antibody that also recognizes the target protein is added to the wells.

Step 6: The wells are filled with a solution that changes color in the presence of the detection enzyme (the one linked to the antibody added in Step 5). A color change indicates the target protein was present in the sample; no color change means the protein was absent.

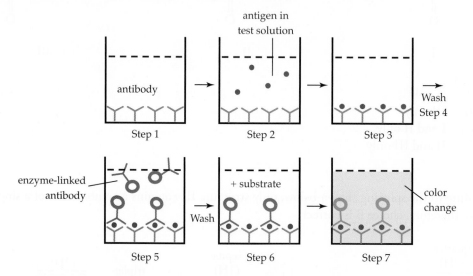

Figure 3   Testing for the Presence of Antigen

When testing for the presence of a specific antibody in a sample, the *antigen* (for which the antibody is specific) is first allowed to adhere directly to the wells. The sample is added as above, and then mixed with enzyme-linked antibodies.

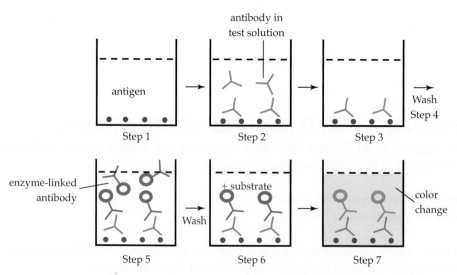

Figure 4   Testing for the Presence of Antibody

ELISA can be used to screen patients for viral infections. For example, serum from a patient suspected to be infected with HIV is loaded into wells that are coated with HIV coat proteins. If the serum contains anti-HIV antibodies (indicating infection), the antibodies will adhere to the proteins on the wells, bind enzyme-linked antibodies, and effect a color change.

- A patient presents with a sore throat and is swabbed to test for the presence of *Streptococcus*. The rapid, in-office test needs to be a version of which type of ELISA in order to detect the presence of the bacteria?[3]

5.4 RADIOIMMUNOASSAY (RIA)

RIAs are similar to ELISAs but use radiolabeled antibodies rather than enzyme-linked antibodies. Thus, the presence of target proteins or antibodies is assayed by measuring the amount of radioactivity instead of a color change. RIAs are more extensively used in the medical field to measure the relative amounts of hormones or drugs in patients' sera.

Step 1: A known amount of radiolabeled antigen (for example, insulin that was synthesized with ^{125}I-labeled tyrosines) is incubated with a known amount of antibody that is specific to the antigen.

Step 2: The insulin:antibody complexes are isolated.

Step 3: The total amount of radioactivity is measured.

Step 4: Unlabeled insulin (also called *cold insulin*) is mixed into the solution in increasing amounts. The cold insulin competes with the labeled insulin (*hot insulin*) for the antibody. As more cold insulin is added, less total radioactivity is recovered and measured. This competition assay helps formulate a standard curve (see below).

Step 5: Steps 1–3 are repeated using patient serum instead of the cold insulin. The standard curve is used to extrapolate the amount of insulin that is circulating in a patient's serum.

---

[3] Since the test is being done for the presence of the bacterium (and thus for bacterial antigen), the "sandwich" style of ELISA in Figure 3 would be utilized. Depending on how long the person had been sick, testing for the antigen would be more effective as the patient's body may not yet be producing antibodies.

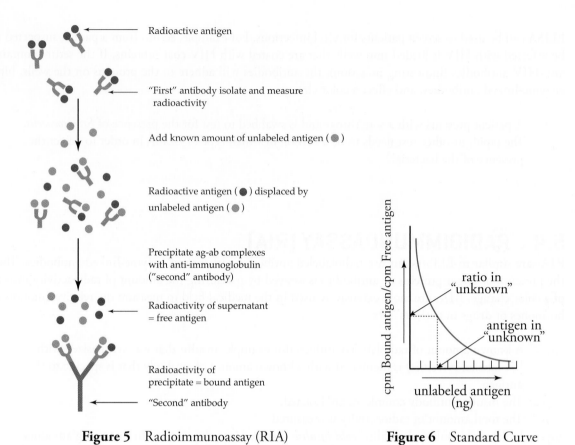

Figure 5 Radioimmunoassay (RIA)

Figure 6 Standard Curve

5.5 ELECTROPHORESIS

Electrophoresis is a means of separating things by size (for example, nucleic acids or proteins) or by charge (for example, proteins or individual amino acids). A "gel" is made out of either acrylamide or agarose, by solubilizing the acrylamide or agarose, pouring it into a rectangular mold, and then allowing it to cool and solidify. Acrylamide and agarose form "nets" as they solidify; the more acrylamide or agarose used in the initial solution, the smaller the pores in the nets.

The mold used to pour the gel creates wells in the gel into which samples can be loaded. An electrical current is applied such that the end of the gel with the wells is negatively charged and the opposite end is positively charged. This causes the samples to migrate toward the positive pole, according to size; smaller things migrate faster (because they fit more easily through the pores of the gel), and larger things migrate more slowly.

For example, here are the steps for separating DNA fragments by size:

Step 1: Isolate the sample DNA from cells.

Step 2: Expose the DNA to enzymes called **restriction endonucleases** (see Section 5.7), which cleave the strands of DNA into smaller fragments of varying size. This may not be necessary in some cases.

Step 3: Add a loading dye to the DNA sample. This makes the sample visible as it is being loaded into the gel. Loading dye also contains a chemical to help inhibit DNA degradation. Finally, glycerol in the loading dye makes the sample more dense than the surrounding buffer, which means the DNA sample sinks to the bottom of the gel wells.

Step 4: Load the mixture of fragments into the gel wells, and apply the electrical current (this is called "running a gel"). Each strand of DNA (negatively charged!) migrates toward the positive end of the gel, but the smaller fragments migrate more quickly, and thus are found farther from the wells at any point in the experiment. You run the samples alongside a "standard" lane, which contains fragments of known size (this help identify the size of the unknowns).

Step 5: Visualize the bands of DNA in the gel. This is done using a dye that binds to nucleic acids and fluoresces when exposed to UV light. This dye is typically added to the gel when it is being made, but can also be applied after the gel is run. The size of each DNA band can be approximated by comparing it to the ladder.

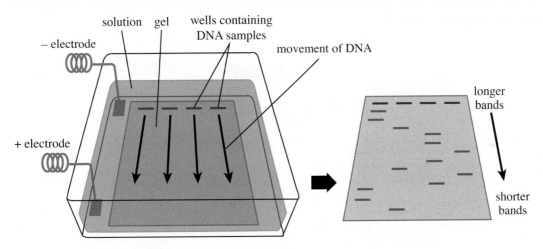

Figure 7   Agarose Gel Electrophoresis of DNA

- If the current was run through the gel indefinitely, what would happen to the loaded sample?[4]

In addition to determining their sizes, fragments of DNA (or RNA) in an electrophoresed gel can be transferred to a more solid and stable membrane in a process called "blotting." There are several types of blots used in biology laboratories.

---

[4]   Eventually, the sample would be pushed off the far edge of the gel and would end up being lost in the solution. The current drives the movement and the edge of the gel does not provide a barrier.

5.6 BLOTTING

Simply put, blotting is the transfer of DNA or proteins from an electrophoresis gel to a nitrocellulose or PVDF membrane. Once transferred, further experiments can be run to isolate or detect a particular nucleic acid fragment or protein (called "probing"). Blotting is classified by the type of molecule being probed.

Southern Blotting

Southern blotting allows you detect the presence of specific sequences within a heterogeneous sample of DNA. This process also allows you to isolate and purify target sequences of DNA for further study.

Step 1: Separate the DNA fragments on an electrophoresis gel.

Step 2: Transfer the fragments to a nitrocellulose membrane.

Step 3: The filter is "probed" for the target DNA sequence. Hybridization probes are short, single-stranded sequences of nucleic acid (usually DNA) that have two important features:
- they are complementary to (and thus will base-pair with) a portion of the target DNA sequence, and
- they are constructed with radiolabeled nucleotides, which allows the visualization of the target sequence with special film.

Probes are often engineered to complement mutations or certain gene rearrangements, making Southern blotting a useful diagnostic tool.

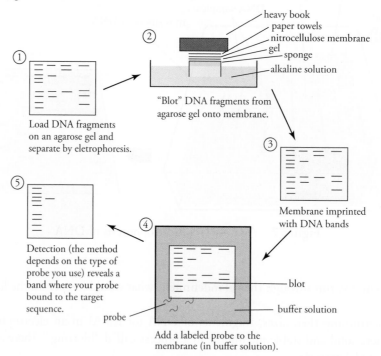

Northern Blotting

Northern blotting is almost identical to Southern blotting, except that RNA is separated via gel electrophoresis instead of DNA. The rest of the process is the same; once the RNA has been separated on a gel, it is transferred to a nitrocellulose membrane and detected via radiolabeled nucleic acid probe. This technique allows you to determine whether specific gene products (normal or pathologic) are being expressed (if their mRNA is present in a cell, they are probably being translated to protein).

Western Blotting

Western blotting allows you to detect the presence of certain proteins within a sample and also serves as a diagnostic tool. You are able to determine, for example, whether cancer cells express certain tumor-promoting growth receptors on their surface. Here are the steps:

Step 1: Cells are collected and solubilized in detergent to release their cytoplasmic contents.

Step 2: Cell lysates, which contain hundreds of different proteins, are denatured (meaning they lose their secondary and tertiary structures). Lysates and a ladder are loaded onto a gel. Similar to nucleic acid gel electrophoresis, a ladder is used so protein size can be compared to a standard.

Step 3: An electric current is applied. Because of the detergent used, the proteins are all negatively charged. They therefore migrate toward the positive electrode, with the smaller proteins migrating the farthest from the wells.

Step 4: The separated proteins from the gel are transferred to a nitrocellulose or PVDF membrane.

Step 5: The membrane is probed for the target protein. Probing for proteins in Western blotting differs from probing in Southern or Northern blotting in that antibodies are used as the probes rather than nucleic acids. This is similar to the technique in ELISA; a primary antibody is used first, which will recognize only the target protein via its antigen-binding portions. Then an enzyme-linked secondary antibody is used that recognizes the constant region of the primary antibody. The enzyme on the secondary antibody will fluoresce when a detection substrate is added, and this light can be photographed with special film. The target protein will show up as a band with an intensity that is proportional to the abundance of the protein in the sample.

- Why do the proteins need to be denatured as part of preparing a Western blot?[5]

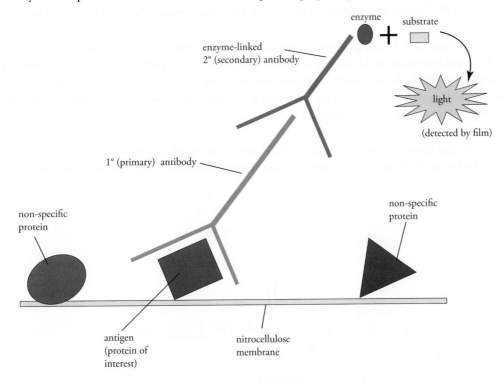

Figure 8 Western Blotting Detection

---

[5] Breaking down the levels of protein structure beyond primary ensures the exposure of binding sites; this allows the protein to be probed as thoroughly as possible.

Eastern Blotting

Several variations of Eastern blotting have been reported, but these tests are not commonly used in molecular biology labs. Eastern blots are used to analyze post-translational modification of peptides, such as the addition of lipids or carbohydrates. The details of this protocol depend on the specifics of the experiment.

5.7   RECOMBINANT DNA

In the past twenty years, a major change has occurred in biology that has allowed it to not only describe the mechanisms of life, but also to manipulate living organisms. The cloning and sequencing of genes, production of recombinant DNA, and the subsequent production of recombinant proteins for use as therapeutic agents in medicine have now become commonplace procedures. A **recombinant protein** is one which has been obtained by transcribing and translating a novel combination of DNA (**recombinant DNA**) from different organisms. For example, the gene for human insulin can be placed in a bacterial **plasmid** (described below). Bacteria with the plasmid will then produce insulin that can be used to treat diabetes. To a large extent these advances are due to the development of new technologies for the handling of DNA, such as the discovery of restriction endonucleases that cleave particular DNA sequences.

Restriction endonucleases are bacterial enzymes that recognize specific sequences of DNA and cut the double-stranded molecule in two pieces. A **nuclease** is an enzyme that cuts nucleic acids. An **endonuclease** cuts in the middle of a DNA chain (contrast with **exonucleases**, which nibble nucleotides from the ends of DNA chains). They are isolated from bacteria and used in the lab. Their natural role in the bacterium is to destroy viral DNA which gets injected into the cell; thus, they *restrict* the reproduction of hostile viruses.

Restriction enzymes have found great use in molecular biology, where they have permitted manipulation of genes to create recombinant DNA. For example, in Figure 9, the cutting-specificity of a restriction enzyme known as *Eco*RI is shown (other restriction enzymes cut at different sequences). The free ends of the DNA molecule that were complementary are known as **sticky ends** since they are able to base pair with other DNA molecules with similar sequences.

- If a circular plasmid containing three *Eco*RI sites is digested to completion, how many pieces will be formed? Would this number be the same or different if the sequence was linear?[6]

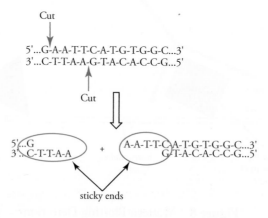

Figure 9   Restriction Digestion of DNA by *Eco*RI

---

[6] The fully digested circular plasmid would generate three pieces. The fully digested linear sequence would generate four pieces.

When a fragment of double-stranded DNA is created by cutting with a restriction endonuclease, it can be inserted into DNA from any source that was also digested by the same restriction endonuclease. For example, *Eco*RI-generated DNA fragments from a human can be isolated, mixed with *Eco*RI-digested DNA from a bacterial plasmid, then joined by the enzyme DNA ligase. Hybrid DNA produced in this fashion is referred to as recombinant DNA.

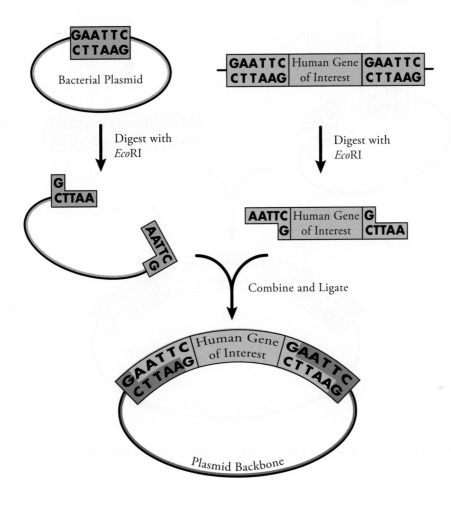

5.7

Figure 10   Cloning DNA Using a Sticky-End Restriction Enzyme

Some restriction enzymes generate DNA with blunt ends rather than sticky ends. That is, the 3' and 5' ends at the cut site are even, with no overhanging bases. Ligating blunt ends together is less specific, and restriction sites may or may not be retained. If the same blunt-cutting restriction enzyme is used on both pieces of DNA, the restriction site will be maintained after ligation. If, however, different blunt-cutting enzymes are used, the products can be ligated together but neither restriction site will be maintained. In Figure 11, a bacterial plasmid was digested with the restriction enzyme SmaI (which is a blunt cutter and recognizes the restriction site CCCGGG). A human gene of interest was digested with the restriction enzyme EcoRV (which is a blunt cutter and recognizes the sequence GATATC). Because both enzymes generate blunt ends, these products can be ligated together. However, the recombinant DNA has lost the restriction sites for both enzymes. The DNA that remains is a combination of the two blunt sites (CCCATC and GATGGG), and cannot be digested with either SmaI or EcoRV.

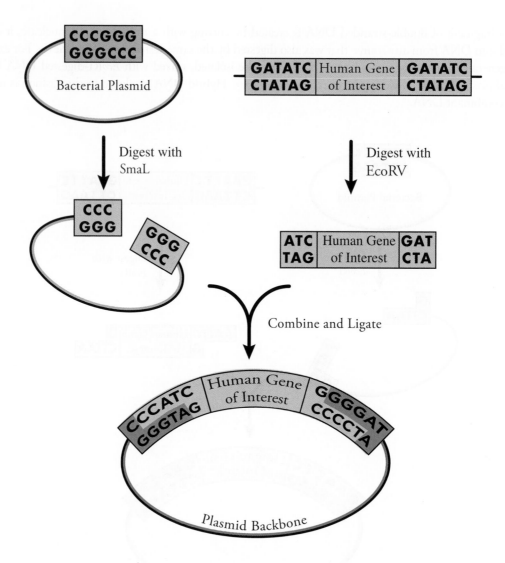

Figure 11   Cloning DNA Using Two Blunt-End Restriction Enzymes

Plasmids

Plasmids are small circular ds-DNA molecules found in bacteria that are capable of autonomous replication (replication that is independent of chromosome replication). Plasmids have been manipulated by recombinant techniques to propagate and express foreign genes in bacteria. Plasmid replication still requires an origin of replication (ORI); in addition to an ORI, they also contain a multiple cloning site, which has restriction sites for dozens of restriction enzymes. This means the plasmid can be digested and any desired sequence with complementary ends can be ligated into the plasmid. Second, plasmids have a drug resistance gene, which helps select and isolate bacteria possessing the plasmid from other bacteria. Lastly, a prokaryotic promoter and start site allow the bacteria to express an inserted gene.

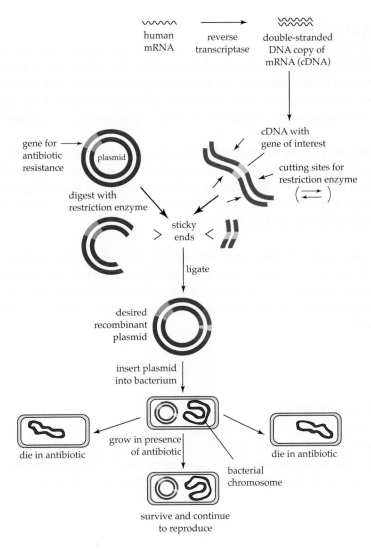

Figure 12   Expression of a Human Gene in Bacteria

Bacterial Transformation

Plasmids can be reintroduced into bacterial cells via transformation, however, only a very small percentage of bacteria are naturally willing to accept pieces of DNA floating around in their environment. More often, the bacteria (or other cell types) must be coaxed to take up the plasmid by heat shocking or electroporation.

Once inside, the plasmid will be exposed to the host's replication and transcription machinery. Newly synthesized mRNA can then access host ribosomes, which translate the encoded protein; on completion of translation, the cells are lysed to release the protein.

Complementary DNA

Many applications of DNA technology involve expressing eukaryotic genes in prokaryotic cells such as *E. coli*. This is conceptually simple: all you have to do is get eukaryotic DNA into a plasmid and get the plasmid into a bacterium, and the bacterium should express the gene. However, prokaryotes lack the equipment necessary for splicing out introns, and many eukaryotic genes are extremely long, making them hard to work with. One way to overcome these obstacles is to work with eukaryotic complementary DNA.

Complementary DNA (or cDNA) is produced from fully spliced eukaryotic mRNA using reverse transcriptase. This enzyme reads an RNA template and builds complementary DNA. cDNAs carry the complete coding sequences for genes, but lack introns (and thus are smaller than the genomic sequence of the gene). Once a cDNA is ligated into a bacterial plasmid and bacteria are transformed with this plasmid, they can produce the protein encoded by the cDNA.

cDNA libraries are also commonly generated. This is where each of the thousands of mRNAs being generated by a given cell type or tissue are converted into cDNAs. Each cDNA is then cloned into a plasmid. This generates thousands of plasmids (the library), with each one containing one cDNA molecule. cDNA libraries can be compared across tissue types of a certain organism (brain versus liver for example) to study tissue-specific gene expression.

5.7

Artificial Chromosomes

Plasmids can only carry inserts up to a certain size. If large inserts are required, artificial chromosomes can be used. Bacterial artificial chromosomes (BACs) typically carry inserts of 100 to 350 kilobase pairs (kb), while yeast artificial chromosomes (YACs) can carry inserts between 100 and 3000 kb. In other words, BACs can easily carry up to 350,000 base pairs of DNA, and YACs can contain up to 3 million base pair inserts!

Eukaryotic Plasmids

Eukaryotic plasmids also exist. They require many of the same components as bacterial plasmids. Eukaryotes use different selection agents, usually either puromycin or neomycin. They also require different promoters in expression plasmids, as well as a poly-adenylation signal downstream of the inserted gene, to terminate transcription.

Eukaryotic plasmids can be introduced into mammalian host cells via transfection. Similar to transformation, there are several experimental options for transfection. Cells can be chemically transfected, usually using calcium phosphate precipitates, or plasmid packaging in liposomes. These lipid vesicles mask the plasmid, but deliver it to the interior of the cell by fusing with the plasma membrane. Non-chemical options for transfection include electroporation, optical transfection with lasers, or shooting the DNA coupled to a gold nanoparticle into a cell nucleus using a gene gun.

Viruses can also deliver DNA into eukaryotic cells, a process called viral transduction. Transduced cells can express genes carried by the viral vector.

5.8   POLYMERASE CHAIN REACTION

Polymerase chain reaction (PCR) is a very quick and inexpensive method for detecting and amplifying specific DNA sequences, screening hereditary and infectious diseases, cloning genes, and fingerprinting DNA. Designed to generate myriad copies of a single template sequence, PCR allows the amplification and subsequent analysis of very small samples of DNA.

Let's say that PCR is to be used to determine whether a certain viral gene has been integrated within a bacterial host genome. A nuclear extract of the bacteria is obtained. Then primers are carefully constructed that will help locate the viral gene (if it is present within the host). Primers are engineered DNA oligonucleotides (~15 bases of single stranded DNA) that will recognize and base pair with specific DNA sequences; in this example, the primers will each recognize a 15-base stretch of the viral gene. Two primers, which will flank a total of ~10 kb of DNA, are used. The "forward primer" will recognize a 15-base stretch at the 3' end of the antisense strand, and the "reverse primer" will recognize a 15-base stretch at the 3' end of the sense strand. When base-paired to their respective gene sequences, the primers will bookend (on opposite sides) the intervening target gene segment.

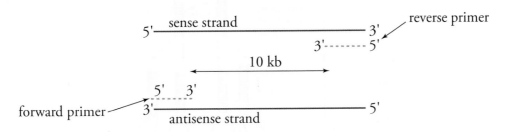

Figure 13   PCR Primers

The primers have free 3' hydroxyl groups, to which dNTPs can be added in a 5' to 3' direction. This will allow the elongation of complementary strands of DNA. The bacterial DNA is mixed with multiple copies of the forward and reverse primers, lots of dNTP bases, a heat-sensitive DNA polymerase, and ions into a buffer. The mixture is then placed into a PCR machine, which will carry out three basic steps:

Step 1:   Initialization. The sample is heated to ~95°C. Heating the sample "melts" the hydrogen bonds that hold the ds-DNA together and, thus, creates single-stranded DNA.

Step 2:   Annealing. The sample is cooled to ~55°C. At this temperature, the primers base-pair with the template strands.

Step 3:   Elongation. The sample is heated to ~72°C. Using the primers as starting points, the heat-sensitive DNA polymerase (usually *Taq* polymerase isolated from algae that thrive in hot springs) elongates strands of DNA that are complementary to each of the template strands. Each strand is polymerized in the 5' to 3' direction. Any mismatched primers will dissociate from the template strands and will not be extended (this helps ensure the purity of the PCR product). Longer DNA targets take longer to synthesize, so the length of the elongation step depends on the length of the product DNA.

- In Step 1, why is the temperature limited to ~95°C? [7]

---

[7]   The temperature needs to be high enough to break the hydrogen bonds between the strands of DNA, but if the temperature is too high, the strands of DNA can denature entirely and the sequence is lost. The balance in PCR is achieving a high enough temperature to separate the strands without destroying them.

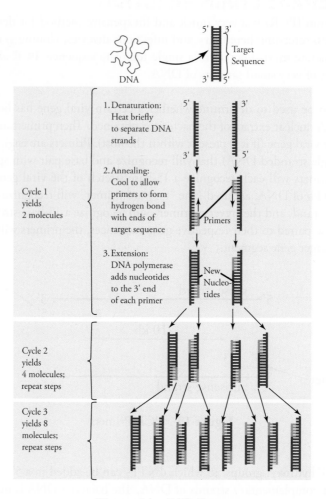

Figure 14 PCR Steps

Each cycle of three steps takes between 0.5 and 5 minutes, depending on the length of the target DNA product (and subsequent length of the elongation step). Because two new complementary strands are synthesized for each template strand in the sample, the PCR product grows at an exponential rate, yielding over a billion copies in just 30 cycles. The sample of DNA is separated via electrophoresis and stained to visualize the products, including the amplified viral gene segment (if present).

Reverse Transcriptase-Polymerase Chain Reaction (RT-PCR)

This is an extension of classic PCR and is used to detect the relative expression of specific gene products. While RT-PCR does not measure the actual expression or abundance of proteins, the technique provides a gauge of gene transcription by measuring the relative amount of target mRNAs. To conduct an RT-PCR experiment, all of the mRNAs from within a cell population are first isolated, then converted into complementary DNA (cDNA) using the enzyme reverse transcriptase. This "library" of cDNAs is then subjected to PCR, using primers specific for a certain gene of interest. If the gene was actively transcribed at the time of harvest, its mRNA will have yielded a cDNA, which will be amplified by the PCR reaction and visualized on a gel.

Quantitative Polymerase Chain Reaction (qPCR)

In quantitative PCR (qPCR, also called real-time PCR), the PCR product is both detected and quantified, as either an absolute number of copies or as a relative amount normalized to a control. The amplified DNA is detected in "real time," as the reaction progresses. The detection process can either use a dye that is fluorescent and binds DNA, or a fluorescent oligonucleotide probe which hybridizes to the sequence of interest. qPCR can be performed on either DNA or cDNA templates, meaning it can give information on the presence and abundance of a particular DNA sequence in samples (if DNA is the template), or on gene expression (if the template is cDNA).

5.9 DNA SEQUENCING AND GENOMICS

DNA sequencing is a method by which scientists can determine gene sequences. This provides the basis for investigating the genetics of health and disease. Knowing gene sequences is also a critical component of other experimental techniques, for example, when constructing primers for PCR reactions.

The most widely used DNA sequencing method (the Sanger technique) hinges on a simple yet important structural characteristic of DNA molecules. The ringed ribose of a dNTP has a hydroxyl group at the 3' carbon. This 3' carbon hydroxyl group serves as the binding site for another dNTP; without it dNTPs could not be linked together, and DNA synthesis would not be possible. The Sanger technique utilizes a modified dNTP, which lacks the 3' carbon hydroxyl group. These dideoxynucleotide triphosphates (ddNTPs) can be incorporated normally into a growing DNA molecule, however, because they lack the 3' carbon hydroxyl group, no further bases can be added to them and they terminate strand elongation at the point of their insertion. The basic protocol is as follows:

Step 1: Obtain a sample of DNA to sequence.

Step 2: Denature the DNA into single strands.

Step 3: Mix the sample of DNA with radiolabeled primers, DNA polymerase, and a mixture of dCTP, dTTP, dGTP, dATP, and ddATP (with the dideoxy form making up 1 percent of the adenine base population). This step of the assay will yield a population of newly synthesized DNA fragments, varying in length, each complementary to the template strand and covalently bonded to a radiolabeled primer at the 5' end (this will aid in the detection of the newly synthesized fragments later). The variety in length of the fragments results from the random insertion of a ddATP into the growing chain.

Step 4: Conduct three more separate reactions as in the previous step, using each of the three other bases in dideoxy form (ddCTP, ddGTP, and ddTTP).

Step 5: Separate the fragments via gel electrophoresis, running each reaction from Steps 3 and 4 in a separate lane.

Step 6: Transfer the fragments to a membrane, and visualize them with radio-sensitive film.

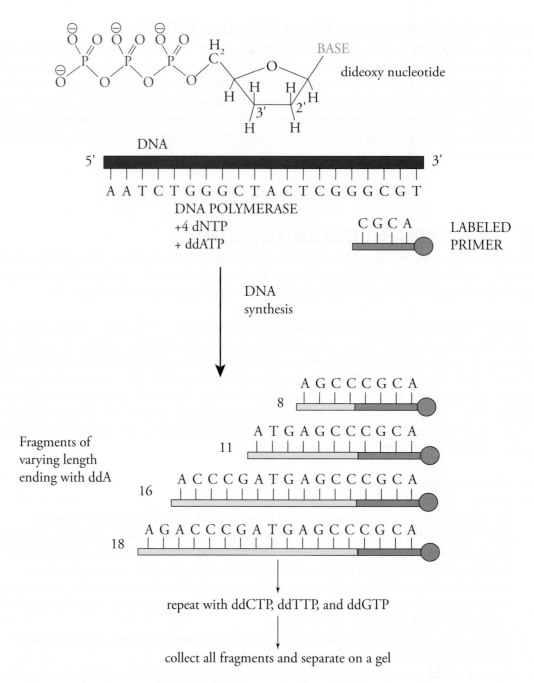

Figure 15 DNA Sequencing Reactions

The smallest fragment (that is, the fragment that migrates the farthest from the well) is a primer with only a single ddNTP attached to it. The lane it ran in corresponds to the first base incorporated into the strand and, thus, the first base of the sequence of the complementary strand. The second smallest fragment is a primer with two bases attached; this fragment ran in the lane corresponding to the base at the second position in the complementary strand (see Figure 16). Reading the membrane from bottom (farthest from the wells) to top (closest to the wells) indicates the sequence (in the 5' to 3' direction) of the complementary strand. Remembering the simple rules of base-pairing (A:T and C:G), you can easily extrapolate the sequence of the template strand.

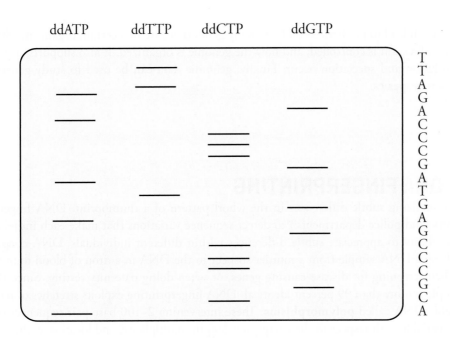

DNA sequence can be read from bottom of gel up

Figure 16 DNA Sequencing Gel

Genomics

The genome of the bacterium *Haemophilus influenzae* was the first to be sequenced and published in 1995. Since then, the genomes of hundreds of organisms have been sequenced and published, including humans and model organisms commonly used in biology laboratories (for example, *E. coli*, *D. melanogaster*, etc.). Researchers and clinicians have recently started sequencing the genome of many cancers, which allows comparative studies between different types and subtypes of cancer, as well as a better understanding of how the cancer genome is different from a normal one.

Genomic sequencing is generally done in two ways, which can be complementary. The first strategy is to generate a genetic linkage map, with several hundred markers per chromosome. This map is then refined to a physical map by preparing YAC or BAC libraries containing large chromosomal fragments. The library is put in order, then gradually cloned into libraries containing smaller and smaller fragments. Each of these small fragments are eventually sequenced and assembled into an overall sequence.

The second strategy is a whole-genome shotgun approach, where chromosomes are cut into small fragments, which are cloned and sequenced. This strategy skips generating maps, and because of this, requires much more extensive analysis of sequencing data by computers in order to align fragments.

Genomic data can lead to predictions on how many genes there are in a certain organism, where they are located, how expression is controlled, and how the genome is organized. It also supports larger questions, like how evolution and speciation occur. Finally, genomic data can be used to study genetic variation within and across species.

5.10 DNA FINGERPRINTING

Much like visualizing subtle differences in the whorl pattern of a thumbprint, DNA fingerprinting allows scientists (and police departments!) to detect sequence variations that make each individual's DNA unique. The ability to appreciate subtle differences within different individuals' DNA comes in handy when matching a DNA sample from a murder suspect to the DNA in a drop of blood found at a crime scene, or when screening for disease-causing genes, or when doing paternity testing. Since the DNA of any two people is more than 99 percent identical, DNA fingerprinting exploits stretches of repetitive and highly variable DNA called **polymorphisms**. These intervening 2–100 base-pair sequences of DNA are structurally variable with respect to their sequence, length, multiplicity, and location within the genome. Two of the several methods of fingerprinting are described below, **restriction fragment length polymorphism** (RFLP) analysis and **short tandem repeat** (STR) analysis.

Restriction Fragment Length Polymorphism (RFLP) Analysis

Step 1: This method uses restriction endonucleases to cut 10–100 base-pair stretches of polymorphic DNA (called minisatellites) into small fragments. Because of the size variations inherent in this DNA, the resulting DNA fragments (now referred to as RFLPs) also vary in size, and are unique to an individual.

Step 2: The RFLPs are separated via gel electrophoresis and transferred to a membrane. Southern blotting techniques are used to analyze the sample. The membrane is probed with radio-labeled DNA oligonucleotides that base-pair with specific RFLP sequences, and the membrane is visualized with special film. Polymorphic DNA, even though recovered from the same chromosomal region, will yield unique band distributions for each person. When RFLPs are recovered from DNA sequences within genes, mutations can be detected. For example, sickle cell disease is caused by a single base substitution in the beta chain of hemoglobin. The substituted valine at the sixth position (normally, glutamic acid is present) will introduce a novel restriction site within the gene. When cut with restriction endonucleases, the point mutation generates a different sized RFLP (when compared to the normal gene cut with the same enzymes) and will yield an anomalous banding pattern.

Short Tandem Repeat (STR) Analysis

Step 1: This method uses PCR to amplify 5–10 base-pair stretches of highly polymorphic and repetitive DNA located within noncoding (introns) regions of the genome. These STRs vary with respect to the sequence and number of repeats found at each locus. To profile an individual, a sample of DNA is obtained and the polymorphic DNA is amplified with PCR.

Step 2: The amplified STRs are separated via electrophoresis and analyzed with Southern blotting.

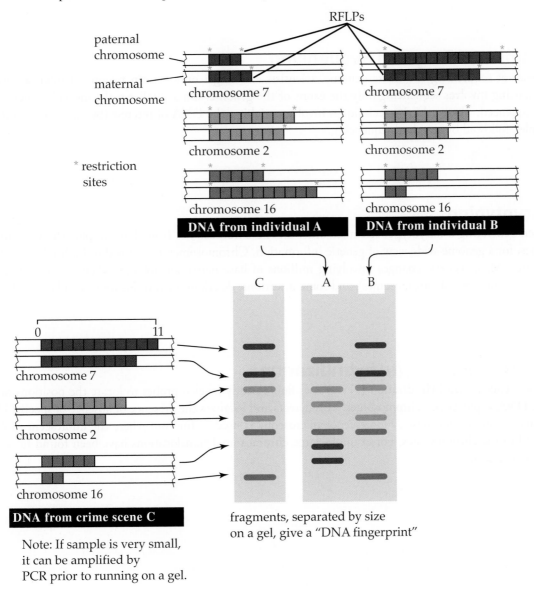

Figure 17   RFLP Analysis

5.11 ADDITIONAL METHODS TO STUDY THE GENOME

Genomic sequencing is the ultimate study of the genome. However, it is very costly and takes a long time. Depending on the experiment, one of the following methods may be better suited to answering a biological question.

Exome and Targeted Sequencing

Instead of sequencing the entire genome, scientists can target only certain regions of interest. Exome sequencing involves sequencing only the exons of the genome. On a smaller scale, individual genes can be sequenced. These selective techniques involve enriching the DNA of interest (by amplification for example), followed by standard sequencing.

Karyotyping

When generating a karyotype, scientists order all the chromosomes from 1 to 22 plus the sex chromosomes, for a genome-wide view of genetic information. Chromosomes are stained to highlight structural features. Major genetic changes (involving millions of base pairs), aneuploidy (when a cell contains an abnormal number of chromosomes), and some insertions, deletions, or translocations can be revealed.

5.11

Fluorescence *in situ* hybridization

Fluorescence *in situ* hybridization (FISH) uses fluorescently labeled probes to locate the positions of specific DNA sequences on chromosomes. This detects and localizes the presence or absence of specific DNA sequences on chromosomes. Fluorescence microscopy is used to find out where the fluorescent probe is bound to the chromosomes. For example, large chromosomal translocations have been found in several types of cancer.

5.12 ANALYZING GENE EXPRESSION

Many of the techniques discussed above give information about gene expression. For example, RT-PCR and qPCR give information on which genes are being transcribed in a given cell population. Western blot analysis can directly test protein expression, and it is limited only by the amount of starting lysate and the availability of antibodies specific for the protein being studied. Additional methods have been developed to study gene expression. Each of these techniques can be used to study a certain gene and gather information about its expression and function, or to study certain cells and gain information on which genes they are expressing and how they grow and survive.

In situ Hybridization

In situ hybridization (ISH) can be used to determine expression of a gene of interest in a tissue, or in an embryo. A very thin slice (or "section") of a tissue sample is mounted onto a microscope slide. The tissue is fixed to keep transcripts in place, and then permeabilized to open the cell membrane. A labeled probe, which is specific for the transcript of interest, is added to the section and binds to the transcript being studied. An enzyme-linked antibody is added and binds to the probe. When a substrate for the enzyme is added, the target transcript-probe-antibody complex is detected. In this way, it can be determined when and where transcripts are expressed on a multicellular level.

Immunohistochemistry

This technique is similar to ISH, but is specific for proteins instead of nucleic acids. As such, it gives a direct report on protein expression in a tissue. Immunohistochemistry (IHC) requires an antibody against a known protein. This antibody is recognized by a secondary antibody, which is either linked to an enzyme or a fluorescent molecule. IHC is commonly used in the clinic. For example, breast cancer biopsies from women are stained for the estrogen receptor (ER), the progesterone receptor (PR) and a plasma membrane receptor called HER2. Breast tumors are then classified as ER$^+$ or ER$^-$, PR$^+$ or PR$^-$, and HER2$^+$ or HER2$^-$. These classifications affect which therapy the patient is given.

Flow Cytometry

Flow cytometry again uses many of the same principles already discussed. Here, single cells (either from lab culture or tissue samples) are stained for certain protein markers using specific antibodies. The antibodies are then linked to a fluorescent tag. Next, the labeled cells are suspended in a fluid stream and passed through a beam of light. Light detectors are found on the other side of, and perpendicular to, the laser. As the labeled cells pass through the light, the beam scatters and the fluorescent tag(s) on the cells can emit light. This combination of scattered and emitted light is measured to give information on cell size, and how many cells in the sample express each of the markers that were labeled. Flow cytometers can have over a dozen different light channels, so many labeled antibodies can be added to one experimental sample. In addition to being analyzed, cells can also be sorted as they go through the machine (a technique called fluorescence-activated cell sorting, or FACS). In this way, a heterogeneous mixture of cells can be sorted based on expression of markers.

5.12

5.13   DETERMINING GENE FUNCTION

Genomic sequencing has revealed thousands of genes with unknown function. There are many ways to discover the function of these genes.

Evolutionary Comparisons

Gene sequences can be compared to all other organisms sequenced. If a human gene of unknown function has much of its sequence in common with a fission yeast protein phosphatase, researchers will test if the unknown human gene may code for a phosphatase.

Protein Domains

Protein domains are conserved patterns in protein sequence and structure. These domains are typically between 25 and 500 amino acids in length and contribute to protein function. Some domains repeat in tandem and others are found in single copies. For example, zinc fingers are small protein domains that are DNA-binding and commonly found in transcription factors. Pleckstrin homology (PH) domains are approximately 120 amino acids long and function in lipid binding, which targets proteins to appropriate cellular compartments. As such, PH domains occur in a wide range of proteins involved in signaling pathways. Thousands of protein domains have been experimentally determined, and the presence of certain domains can shed light on protein function.

Protein Interactions

Knowing which proteins bind to a protein of interest can shed light on protein function, especially since many proteins function in complexes and pathways. Immunoprecipitations are commonly used to find protein-binding partners. In this experiment, cell lysates are collected (as described above) and incubated with an antibody specific for the protein of interest. A complex forms, including the protein of interest, its binding partners, and an antibody. An antibody binding protein covalently linked to a microscopic bead is added next. The bead can be pulled out of solution (or precipitated) by simple centrifugation (spinning the tube at high speeds). This collects bead complexes at the bottom of the tube. These complexes are then washed and purified from the lysate solution. Proteins that don't bind to the protein of interest are lost. Precipitated proteins can then be identified by Western blot analysis (if you have an idea of what proteins you're looking for), or mass spectrometry (if you have no idea what will be there). Data from these experiments can generate network maps, where protein interactions are used to elucidate functional maps of how proteins are working together in a cell.

Cellular Expression

Subcellular location can give information on protein function. To determine the subcellular location of a protein of interest, the gene for this protein can be attached to a reporter system to see where it is expressed. For example, the gene of interest can be cloned into an expression vector and linked to a fluorescent tag such as GFP (green fluorescent protein). This effectively tags the protein with a fluorescent molecule, meaning cellular location can be determined using a fluorescent microscope. In Figure 18 below, the first cell (A) is expressing the GFP-tagged protein of interest on the plasma membrane, the second cell (B) expresses it in the cytoplasm, while the last cell (C) expresses it in the nucleus. In this experiment, the nucleus is also stained with a fluorescent dye called DAPI (which shows up blue under the fluorescent microscope). Since the nucleus of cell C has both blue DAPI and green protein, it shows up as a teal circle.

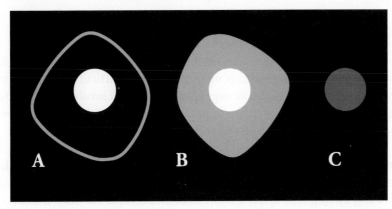

Figure 18   Using GFP-Tagged Proteins to Determine Subcellular Protein Expression

Altering Expression

Altering gene expression can also be used to help determine gene function. Gene expression can be inhibited or increased, and the subsequent phenotype can shed light on protein function.

Gene expression can be knocked down via RNA interference (or RNAi), which uses microRNA (miRNA) or small interfering RNA (siRNA). These short RNA molecules can bind to mRNAs and decrease their activity, often by promoting degradation of the mRNA transcript. Synthetic RNA has been used in both cell culture and in living organisms as a way to decrease protein expression.

- Why would the cell's response to siRNA binding to mRNA transcripts be to trigger degradation of the transcript?[8]

The opposite experiment can also be done, where a protein of interest is over-expressed in a biological system. This can be achieved by attaching the gene of interest to a strong promoter, which will induce high levels of transcription, and therefore gene expression. This genetic construct can be on an expression plasmid, or it can be recombined into the genome. These "knock-in" systems can also be made by

---

[8]   A form of double-stranded RNA is being created, which is not a normal form of nucleotide arrangement in cells. Double-stranded RNA can compose certain viral genomes, and these could be dangerous to the cell; thus, a cell is going to view dsRNA as a foreign construct and degrade it.

increasing gene copy number or increasing transcript stability (usually by decreasing transcript degradation). No matter how it is done, the cellular and biochemical effects of over-expressing a gene of interest can be investigated.

In vitro mutagenesis is when a gene is cloned, specifically mutated, then returned to a cell. Mutations can alter, destroy, or enhance gene function. These mutated genes can even be put into early multicellular embryos, to study the role of a protein in development and whole-organism function.

5.14 PROTEIN QUANTIFICATION

A good understanding of genomics has led to the field of **proteomics**, the systematic and large-scale study of protein structure and function. This is usually done in a particular context, such as in a certain biochemical pathway, organelle, cell, tissue, or organism. Often, this involves quantitative analysis of proteins. This means measuring amounts of different proteins from a functional standpoint, looking at how the amount, state, or location of a protein changes. Here are some examples:

- It's been hypothesized that a particular protein under study functions in G_1 of the cell cycle, but not the other phases. A biochemist tags the protein with a fluorescent molecule, and he observes live and cycling cells under a fluorescent microscope. He finds that the cells have high levels of fluorescence in G_1, but very low levels of fluorescence in the other cell phases. This suggests the protein under study is expressed at high levels in G_1, then is degraded at the beginning of S phase.
- A biochemist is studying the function of an unknown protein, which has been shown to have important functions when a specific transcription factor is mutated. The biochemist obtains two cell lines. One has a mutation in the transcription factor and the other doesn't. She generates lysate samples from the two cell lines and examines the two lysate samples, looking specifically at the protein of interest. She finds it is not phosphorylated in the cell line without the transcription factor mutation, but it is phosphorylated in the cell line with the mutation.

5.14

Many different techniques can help with studying proteins quantitatively. Some of these look at proteins in a cell, either alive (FACS, labeling a protein and looking and subcellular location) or not (immunohistochemistry, flow cytometry). Others measure proteins harvested from a cell (ELISA, Western blotting, immunoprecipitation). These techniques were discussed earlier.

It's common for proteins to be grown in a biological system, then extracted and studied. Often, protein levels in lysates or purified samples must be quantified before an experiment can be started. For example, before performing a Western blot, biochemists typically measure protein concentrations in each sample being studied, to make sure the same amount of lysate is loaded into each well of the gel.

The most commonly used quantification method is Bradford Quantification, using UV-Vis spectrophotometers designed for biochemical analysis. This method uses a Bradford reagent containing a blue pigment called Coomassie blue. When proteins bind the pigment, it shifts the absorption peak of the sample. Absorption is measured at 600 nm. This technique is very simple and has good sensitivity.

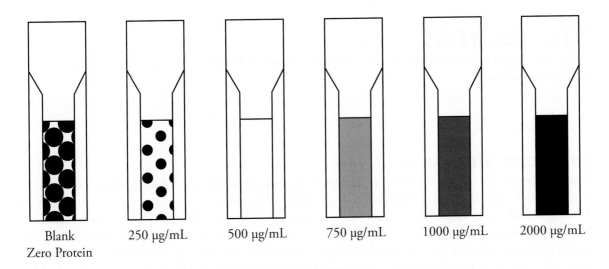

Figure 19   Bradford Quantification of Proteins

To perform quantification, first, the negative control sample is put in the spectrophotometer, to set the zero value. Next, the samples with known concentration are applied, and the spectrophotometer generates a concentration curve. This relates absorbance of the sample with protein concentration. A new curve should be made every time proteins are being quantified. Next, the samples are put in the machine one by one. The spectrophotometer applies light in the visible and adjacent (near-UV and near-infrared) ranges. Absorbance is determined and compared to the calibration curve, and the machine usually reports both the absorbance and the subsequent protein concentration.

AFFINITY CHROMATOGRAPHY

Affinity chromatography is used to separate biochemical mixtures, and it is based on highly specific interactions between macromolecules. While affinity chromatography is most commonly used to purify proteins, it can also be used on other macromolecules (such as nucleic acids). It uses many of the same principles described above: you start with a heterogeneous mixture of molecules (such as cell lysate, growth media or blood). To isolate a protein of interest, you can either use an antibody or tag the protein with an affinity tag (for example, His-tagged proteins can be purified with nickel-based resins and slightly basic conditions; the bound proteins are eluted by adding imidazole or by lowering the pH). The target molecule is trapped on a stationary phase due to specific binding, and the stationary phase is washed to increase purity. The target protein is then released (or eluted) off the solid phase, in a highly purified state. For more detail, see Section 5.1, Affinity Chromatography.

5.14

5.15   STEM CELLS

Stem cells are undifferentiated cells that can differentiate to become other cell types. Stem cells self-replicate by mitosis.

Embryonic Stem Cells

Embryonic stem cells (ESCs) are found in the inner cell mass of the blastocyst and are the only stem cells in humans which are pluripotent. Pluripotent cells are able to differentiate into any of the three germ layers (endoderm, mesoderm, or ectoderm), and they can generate all of the over 220 cells types in the human body. ESCs can replicate indefinitely. While ESCs are the only known pluripotent cells, it's possible that other pluripotent stem cells exist in adults and have not yet been found. In addition, it's possible that multipotent stem cells could de-differentiate into a pluripotent state, but this has not yet been demonstrated in the lab.

Adult Stem Cells

Adult stem cells are found in various tissues, and they function in tissue repair and regeneration. They are multipotent, meaning they can produce many cell types. Adult stem cells are usually tissue-specific, and they differentiate into slightly more differentiated progenitor cells, before completely differentiating.

Applications of Stem Cells

Stem cells have many important uses in biology. First, therapy using ESCs could revolutionize regenerative medicine and alleviate human suffering. Many diseases could be treated using pluripotent cells, such as blood and immune system genetic disorders, many cancers, spinal cord injuries, Parkinson's disease, juvenile diabetes, and blindness. The basic idea behind these stem cell therapies is to manipulate ESCs to become other cells for use in treatment. For example, ESCs induced to become oligodendrocytes have been used to treat patients with spinal cord injuries.

Many ESCs used in the lab come from embryos that were created for *in vitro* fertilization, but then not required. Because generating human ESC lines requires destroying the blastocyst, work on human ESCs is controversial. In addition to ethical concerns, there are additional risks of host-graft rejection and formation of tumors from therapeutic ESCs.

Second, ESCs from model organisms (such as mice and rats) can be isolated and manipulated in the lab. These targeted ESCs can then be aggregated with a normal morula or injected into a normal blastocyst. The morula or blastocyst is then injected into the uterus of a pseudopregnant female animal, which carries the embryos to term. Pseudopregnant mice are produced by mating fertile females with vasectomized males.

A few weeks later, chimeric pups are born, which are a mix of targeted stem cells and normal stem cells. Usually animals with different coat colors are used in these experiments. For example, the ESCs used for targeting in the lab could be from a brown mouse, while the normal donor morula or blastocyst could come from an albino strain. Chimeric pups typically have a mix of white and brown fur and are screened

5.15

to find "founder" animals where the germ line was derived from the targeted ESCs. In this way, new transgenic lines can be generated and used for study. For example, a knock-in mouse could be made which over-expresses a gene of interest. Models are often made using tissue-specific promoters, so studies can be done on certain tissues without affecting all cells in the animal.

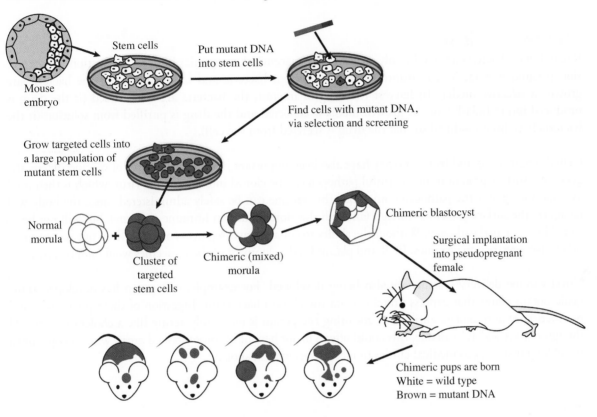

Figure 20   Gene Targeting to Generate Transgenic Mice

Because of the ethical implications of working with human ESCs, there has been a lot of excitement over induced pluripotent stem cells (iPS cells). These cells are made from adult somatic cells by inducing expression of certain genes, usually transcription factors. Induced expression of these proteins causes the somatic cells to re-gain pluripotency, a characteristic which only ESCs have. iPS cells have many other characteristics in common with ESCs, including morphology and replicative ability. Despite the initial excitement however, iPS cells have not yet replaced ESCs because they are potentially tumorigenic and have low replication rates.

5.15

5.16   PRACTICAL APPLICATIONS OF DNA TECHNOLOGY

Pharmaceuticals

Recombinant bacteria are commonly used by pharmaceutical companies in drug production. An expression plasmid is made and transformed into competent bacteria and large cultures of the bacteria are grown in selective media. To harvest the drug of interest, the bacteria are either lysed (if the drug is produced intracellularly), or the growth media is collected and the drug is purified from solution (if the bacteria have been modified so that the drug is secreted from the cell).

Genetic engineering and biotechnology have also been important in the development of vaccines. Here, the gene for a surface protein from a harmful pathogen can be cloned into a harmless virus, which is then used as a vaccine against the pathogenic microbe. This vaccine can be safely administered, since the body will recognize the surface protein as foreign (and will therefore mount an immune response), but will not be infected by the actual pathogen. Without the ability to cut and paste segments of DNA from one source to another (using restriction enzymes, PCR and plasmids), development of these vaccines would not be possible.

Novel vaccine delivery systems are also being developed. For example, one group has developed transgenic potato plants that express proteins from the cholera bacterium. Ingestion of these potatoes causes production of anti-cholera antibodies, meaning the potato is effectively acting like a cholera vaccine. Although not yet widely available, this could offer a major benefit to impoverished areas, where people must travel long distances to medical clinics to receive vaccination shots.

Industry

Genetically modified bacteria are also used to produce enzymes required for food processing. For example, the gene for chymosin has been cloned into both prokaryotic and eukaryotic expression plasmids, and bacteria or yeast containing these plasmids produce large amounts of the enzyme chymosin. This enzyme is then purified and used to clot milk in cheese production.

Transgenic cows are being generated to produce milk that has the same characteristics as human breast milk. (A transgenic organism is one that carries a foreign gene that has been deliberately inserted into its genome.) Additional transgenic animals are being made to produce useful substances (such as goats that excrete silk proteins in their milk or pigs that produce omega-3 fatty acids).

Both bacteria and plants (such as algae, corn and poplars) have been genetically modified for use in biofuel production. Biofuel is derived from living organisms and contains energy from geologically recent carbon fixation. Bioethanol (made from carbohydrates via fermentation) and biodiesel (made from animal and plant fats) are common examples of biofuel.

5.16

Agriculture

DNA technology has had a great impact on the science of agriculture. Scientists have been able to transfer genes to plants in order to optimize crop yield. For example, some plants express a transgenic enzyme that is harmful to pests, which decreases the need for pesticide use. Others express enzymes making them resistant to diseases or herbicides.

Transgenic plants that are capable of nitrogen fixation are also in production. Some plants, such as legumes, can fix their own nitrogen. Scientists have identified genes involved in this process and are working to develop transgenic corn and rice strains also capable of nitrogen fixation. Success in this project would mean a decrease in global fertilizer use, which could have a beneficial impact on the environment.

Food has also been modified to increase shelf life and nutritional value. For example, tomatoes have been altered to stay firm during ripening. This means green tomatoes can be picked and transported to grocery shelves without going soft. Golden rice, which contains beta-carotene, has been developed to combat vitamin A deficiency. New rice strains with higher iron content are also being developed.

DNA technology has also been applied to agriculture biotechnology in the form of animal husbandry. DNA fingerprinting has been applied to certain endangered animals (such as the Puerto Rican parrot, orangutans and some species of African livestock). This allows scientists to identify individual animals, verify their pedigree and ancestors, and track both desirable and undesirable traits. Animals can be registered and mating pairs can be tracked to make sure the population maintains enough variation to be viable and that deleterious traits are not passed on to offspring. This is especially important for species that have a small population. These biotechnology based breeding programs have also been applied to common agriculture livestock species such as cattle and horses.

Environmental Applications

Bacteria are being engineered to express genes that will help cope with some environmental problems. For example, genetically engineered bacteria have been made to help with sewage treatment and to degrade harmful compounds. Some bacteria have been made to extract heavy metals from the environment. These metals are then incorporated into different compounds that can be isolated and used to extract the metal. This means bacteria could play a role in the future of both the clean-up of toxic mining waste and the actual mining process.

Phosphorus water pollution promotes algae growth. Genetically modified pigs, which produce the enzyme phytase in their saliva, are able to break down indigestible phosphorus. These pigs may help reduce water pollution, as their manure contains about half the amount of phosphorus as normal pigs.

5.16

Gene Therapy

Gene therapy is when a genetic disorder is treated by introducing a gene into a cell. This is often to correct or supplement a defective gene. Gene therapy uses genetically modified viruses to deliver genes to somatic human cells. Ideally, the targeted gene will be incorporated into the genome of the cell, but this doesn't always occur. This means treatment efficacy can gradually decrease over time, and repeated treatments may be necessary.

Gene therapy-based treatments for sickle cell anemia, Parkinson's disease, cystic fibrosis, cancer, HIV, diabetes, muscular dystrophy, and heart disease are currently being developed. While the theory behind this technology is not new, it has been difficult to optimize gene therapy in practice. Because of this, gene therapy is not in widespread practice, but it shows promise as a future treatment. Gene therapy of the germ line is also possible in theory, but because of ethical controversy, has not been well developed.

There are some problems associated with gene therapy. Because a foreign particle is being introduced, there is a chance the immune system will respond, and this can reduce treatment efficacy. Current gene therapies are limited to one or two genes, while many disorders are caused by many genes. Finally, there is a small chance of tumor development if the therapy DNA integrates into the genome incorrectly.

Genetic Testing

Biotechnology has also been crucial in developing DNA-based tests. You already learned how RFLP and STR analysis can be used in forensics (to compare crime scene samples to suspects for example): to establish relationships between people or to study the evolutionary relationship between two species. Genetic testing is another application of these tests. Genetic testing can be done before birth (to look for diseases like hemophilia, cystic fibrosis, and Duchene muscular dystrophy) or after birth (to test for mutations that may lead to increased disease risk).

5.17 SAFETY AND ETHICS OF DNA TECHNOLOGY

Regulatory agencies and governments have started implementing regulations on how biotechnology can be used in industry, medicine, and agriculture. These agencies focus on assessing risk, public education, and mandating policies to protect both scientists and the public. However, with a hot topic like biotechnology, there will always be opponents. Serious considerations of risk and implications are important to mitigate any potential downsides to new technology.

Criticisms of genetically modified crops have received widespread news coverage. Opponents argue introduction of transgenic crops into ecosystems could cause unpredictable results. For example, if pesticide resistance is somehow transferred to the pest, this could cause widespread ecological problems. Biotechnology could therefore inadvertently generate new and hazardous pathogens. Opponents also point out that eating transgenic crops may not be safe, and some critics argue that they're not necessary to solve food availability issues. While there is little data supporting the hypothesis that transgenic foodstuffs are dangerous, it is important to consider that this may be the case.

Concerns over gene therapy are also common. Some are worried about the long-term implications of introducing a foreign gene into a human being. Germ line gene therapy is highly controversial, as development of this technology could lead to eugenics: a deliberate effort to control the genetic makeup of human populations. Some see germ line gene therapy as interfering with evolution. Since genetic variation is important for species survival, some argue that gene therapy is a way of decreasing alleles in a population. While this might seem like a good idea, it is possible that alleles that have a disadvantage in one situation might prove to be advantageous in another situation. If gene targeting or eugenics causes this allele to be

5.17

lost, the species could suffer. A common example of an allele with multiple effects is the sickle cell allele. In the homozygous form, this allele causes sickle cell disease. However, in the heterozygous form, this allele provides some protection against malaria. What looks like a "bad allele" from one perspective, can actually be a good thing in other situations.

Working with any animal in a laboratory setting raises ethical issues. Agencies have been appointed to ensure lab animals have a good quality of life, are treated humanely, and are used in justified and important experiments. A rigorous peer-reviewed process (usually overseen by veterinarians) ensures researchers justify the use for each and every experimental animal. Despite these attempts, additional concerns exist. For example, in generating experimental animals, many labs also generate normal animals, which are sacrificed simply because they don't have the correct genotype. Also, transgenic animals typically suffer from decreased fertility and may be susceptible to conditions and diseases besides those they are bred to develop and model. Again, close monitoring of animal facilities, usually in conjunction with both local and federal regulations, ensures researchers are acting in a responsible and ethical manner when working with transgenic animals.

5.17

Part 2

MCAT Biochemistry

Chapter 6
Biochemistry
Basics

6.1 THERMODYNAMICS

Thermodynamics is the study of the energetics of chemical reactions. There are two relevant forms of energy in chemistry: heat energy (movement of molecules) and potential energy (energy stored in chemical bonds). [What is the most important potential energy storage molecule in all cells?[1]]

A practical way to discuss thermodynamics is the mathematical notion of **free energy** (**Gibbs free energy**), defined by Josiah Gibbs as follows:[2]

$$\textbf{Eq. 1} \quad \Delta G = \Delta H - T\Delta S$$

T denotes temperature, H denotes **enthalpy**, and S denotes **entropy** (a measure of disorder).

ΔG increases with increasing ΔH (bond energy) and decreases with increasing entropy.

- The Second Law of Thermodynamics states that disorder tends to increase. Consider, then, the mathematical definition of ΔG above. Which reaction will be less favorable: one with a decrease in free energy ($\Delta G < 0$) or one with an increase in free energy ($\Delta G > 0$)?[3]

The change in the Gibbs free energy of a reaction determines whether the reaction is favorable (**spontaneous**, ΔG negative) or unfavorable (**nonspontaneous**, ΔG positive). In terms of the generic reaction

$$A + B \rightarrow C + D$$

the Gibbs free energy change determines whether the reactants (denoted A and B) will stay as they are or be converted to products (C and D).

Spontaneous reactions, ones that occur without a net addition of energy, have $\Delta G < 0$. They occur with energy to spare. Reactions with a negative ΔG are **exergonic** (energy *exits* the system); reactions with a positive ΔG are **endergonic**. Endergonic reactions only occur if energy is added. In the lab, energy is added in the form of heat; in the body, endergonic reactions are driven by reaction coupling to exergonic reactions (more on this later). Reactions with a negative ΔH are called **exothermic** and liberate heat. Most metabolic reactions are exothermic (which is how homeothermic organisms such as mammals maintain a constant body temperature). Reactions with a positive ΔH require an input of heat and are referred to as **endothermic**.

The signs of thermodynamic quantities are assigned from the point of view of *the system*, not the surroundings or the universe. Thus, a negative ΔG means that the system goes to a lower free energy state, and a system will always move in the direction of the lowest free energy.

---

[1] ATP, which stores energy in the ester bonds between its phosphate groups.

[2] As in ΔS, the Greek letter Δ (delta) indicates "the change in." For example, $\Delta G_{rxn} = G_{products} - G_{reactants}$.

[3] Unfavorable reactions have $\Delta G > 0$. We can deduce this from the second law and Equation 1 because the second law states that decreasing entropy is unfavorable, and the equation has ΔG directly related to $-T\Delta S$.

If ΔG is equal to 0, then the reaction is said to be at equilibrium. **Equilibrium** is defined as the point where the rate of reaction in one direction equals the rate of reaction in the other. At equilibrium, there is constant product and reactant turnover as reactants form products and vice versa, but overall concentrations stay the same. Theoretically (given enough time), all reactant/product systems will eventually reach this point.

While all reactions will eventually reach an equilibrium, we can disturb this balance with the addition or removal of a reactant or product, and the reaction will proceed in the direction necessary to re-establish equilibrium. (The shift to restore equilibrium is a demonstration of Le Châtelier's principle.) Using this principle, a reaction which favors reactants at equilibrium can be driven to generate additional products (such strategies are employed frequently in cellular respiration).

- Which direction, forward or backward, will be favored in a reaction if $\Delta G = 0$?[4]
- Radiolabeled chemicals are often used to trace constituents in biochemical reactions. The following reaction with $\Delta G = 0$ is in aqueous solution:

$$A \rightleftharpoons B + C, \quad K_{eq} = \frac{[B][C]}{[A]}$$

A small amount of radiolabeled C is added to the solution. After a period of time, where will the radiolabel most likely be found: in A, in C, or in both?[5]

Thermodynamics vs. Reaction Rates

The term *spontaneous* is used to describe a reaction system with $\Delta G < 0$. This can be misleading, since the common usage of the word *spontaneous* has a connotation of *rapid rate*; this is not what spontaneous means in the context of chemical reactions. For example, many reactions have a negative ΔG, indicating that they are "spontaneous" from a thermodynamic point of view, but they do not necessarily occur at a significant rate. Spontaneous means that a reaction may proceed without additional energy input, *but it says nothing about the rate of reaction.*

Thermodynamics will tell you where a system starts and finishes but nothing about the path traveled to get there. The difference in free energy in a reaction is only a function of the nature of the reactants and products. Thus, ΔG does not depend on the pathway a reaction takes or the rate of reaction; it is only a measurement of the difference in free energy between reactants and products.

- How does the ΔG for a reaction burning (oxidizing) sugar in a furnace compare to the ΔG when sugar is broken down (oxidized) in a human?[6]

---

[4] If ΔG is 0, then neither the forward nor the reverse reaction is favored. Understand and memorize the following: When $\Delta G = 0$, you are at equilibrium; forward reaction equals back reaction, and the net concentrations of reactants and products do not change.

[5] The reaction is in dynamic equilibrium where reactions are occurring in both directions, but at an equal rate. Because $\Delta G = 0$, we know that the forward reaction and the reverse reaction proceed at equal rates, even though we don't know the actual value. Therefore, after a period of time, the radiolabel will be present in both A and C.

[6] The ΔG is the same in both cases. ΔG does not depend on the pathway, only on the different energies of the reactants and products.

6.2 KINETICS AND ACTIVATION ENERGY (E_A)

The reason some spontaneous (that is, *thermodynamically favorable*) reactions proceed very slowly or not at all is that a large amount of energy is required to get them going. For example, the burning of wood is spontaneous, but you can stare at a log all day and it won't burn. Some energy (heat) must be provided to kick-start the process.

The study of reaction rates is called **chemical kinetics**. All reactions proceed through a transient intermediate that is unstable and takes a great deal of energy to produce. The energy required to produce the transient intermediate is called the **activation energy** (E_a). This is the barrier that prevents many reactions from proceeding even though the ΔG for the reaction may be negative. The match you use to light your fireplace provides the activation energy for the reaction known as burning. It is the activation energy barrier that determines the kinetics of a reaction. [How would the rate of a spontaneous reaction be affected if the activation energy were lowered?[7]]

A **catalyst** lowers the E_a of a reaction *without changing the ΔG*. The catalyst lowers the E_a by *stabilizing the transition state*, making its existence less thermodynamically unfavorable. The second important characteristic of a catalyst is that it is not consumed in the reaction; it is *regenerated* with each reaction cycle.

The traditional way to represent a reaction system like this is using a *reaction coordinate* graph, as shown in Figure 1. This is just a way to look at the energy of the reaction system as compared to the three possible states of the system: 1) reactants, 2) [TS]‡, and 3) products. The *x*-axis plots the physical progress of the reaction system (the "reaction coordinate"), and the *y*-axis plots free energy.

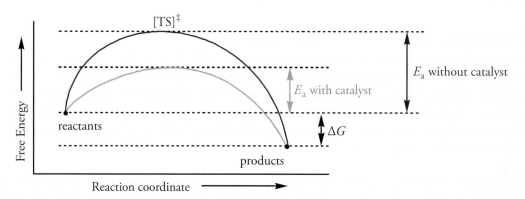

Figure 1   The Reaction Coordinate Graph

Enzymes are catalysts. They increase the rate of a reaction by lowering the reaction's activation energy, but they *do not affect ΔG* between reactants and products. As catalysts, enzymes have a kinetic role, *not* a thermodynamic one. [Will an enzyme alter the concentration of product at equilibrium?[8]] Enzymes may alter the rate of a reaction enormously: a reaction that would take a hundred years to reach equilibrium without an enzyme may occur in just seconds with an enzyme. More information about enzymes can be found in Chapters 7, 9, and 10.

---

[7]   The rate would be increased, since lowering E_a is tantamount to reducing the energy required to achieve the transition state. The more transition state intermediates that are formed, the greater the amount of product produced, that is, the more rapid the rate of reaction.

[8]   No. It will only affect the rate at which the reactants and products reach equilibrium.

6.3   OXIDATION AND REDUCTION

Energy Metabolism and the Definitions of Oxidation and Reduction

Where does the energy in foods come from? How do we make use of this energy? Why do we breathe? The answers begin with **photosynthesis**, the process by which plants store energy from the Sun in the bond energy of carbohydrates. Plants are **photoautotrophs** because they use energy from light ("photo") to make their own ("auto") food. We are **chemoheterotrophs**, because we use the energy of chemicals ("chemo") produced by other ("hetero") living things, namely plants and other animals. Plants and animals store chemical energy in reduced molecules such as carbohydrates and fats. These reduced molecules are oxidized to produce CO_2 and ATP. The energy of ATP is used in turn to drive the energetically unfavorable reactions of the cell. That's the basic energetics of life; all the rest is detail.

In essence, the production and utilization of energy boil down to a series of oxidation/reduction reactions. **Oxidation** is a chemical term meaning the loss of electrons. **Reduction** means the opposite, the gain of electrons. Molecules can gain or lose electrons depending on the other atoms that they are bound to. There are three common ways to identify oxidation/reduction reactions on the MCAT, and it is important for you to know them:

Recognizing Oxidation Reactions:
1) gain of oxygen atoms
2) loss of hydrogen atoms
3) loss of electrons

Recognizing Reduction Reactions (just the opposite):
1) loss of oxygen atoms
2) gain of hydrogen atoms
3) gain of electrons

Though you should memorize this, it is not a subject worthy of philosophizing. If you can answer questions like the following, you're set: Is changing CH_3CH_3 to $H_2C=CH_2$ an oxidation, a reduction, or neither?[9] What about changing Fe^{3+} to Fe^{2+}?[10] What about this: $O_2 \rightarrow H_2O$?[11] You can also identify oxidation/reduction reactions visually by looking at the structure of the molecules. Is the formation of a disulfide bond (Figure 2) an oxidation or a reduction reaction?[12]

---

[9] It's an oxidation, because hydrogens have been removed.

[10] It's a reduction, because an electron has been added.

[11] It's a reduction, because hydrogens have been added to the oxygen molecule.

[12] It's an oxidation, because hydrogens have been removed.

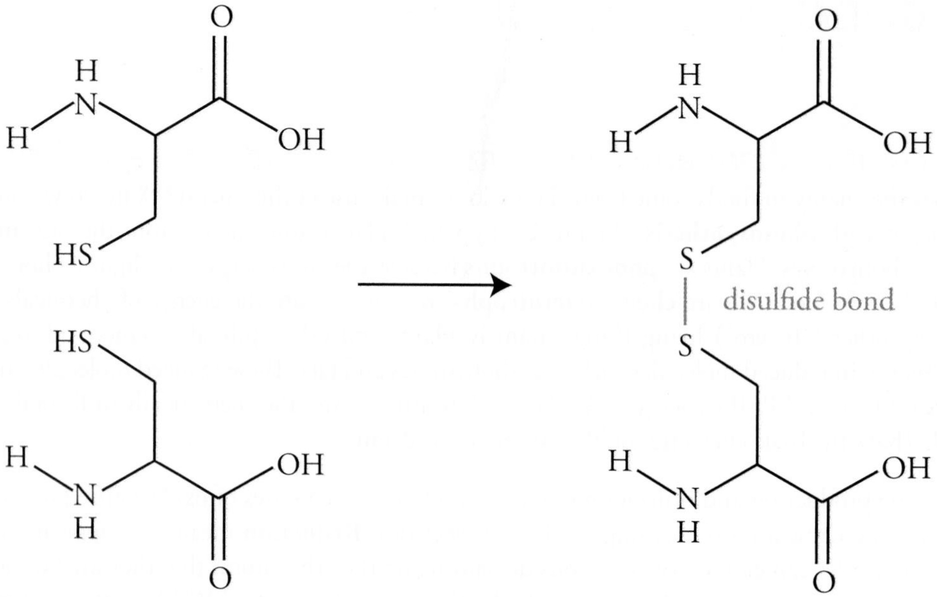

Figure 2 Formation of a Disulfide Bond

Here is one other important fact about oxidation and reduction: when one atom gets reduced, another one *must* be oxidized; hence the term ***redox pair***. As you study the process of glucose oxidation, you will see that each time an oxidation reaction occurs, a reduction reaction occurs too.

Catabolism is the process of breaking down molecules. The opposite is **anabolism**, which is "building-up" metabolism.[13] For example, the way we extract energy from glucose is by **oxidative catabolism**. We break down the glucose by oxidizing it. The stoichiometry of glucose oxidation looks like this:

$$C_6H_{12}O_6 + 6\,O_2 \rightarrow 6\,CO_2 + 6\,H_2O$$

- In the reaction above, what is being oxidized? What is being reduced?[14]

As we oxidize foods, we release the stored energy plants got from the Sun. But we don't make use of that energy right away. Instead, we store it in the form of ATP. Alternatively, we can use the energy in ATP to generate storage molecules such as glycogen and fatty acids. Fatty acids are generated by successive reductions of a carbon chain, thus anabolic processes are generally reductive. More details on redox reactions can be found in the General Chemistry section of this book.

---

[13] The mnemonics are *cata* = breakdown, as in catastrophe, and *ana* = buildup, sounds like "add-a." (Think of anabolic steroids, which weight-lifters use to bulk up.)

[14] The carbons in the sugar are oxidized (to CO_2), and oxygen is reduced (to H_2O).

Chapter 7
Amino Acids and Proteins

7.1 AMINO ACIDS

Proteins are biological macromolecules that act as enzymes, hormones, receptors, channels, transporters, antibodies, and support structures inside and outside cells. Proteins are composed of twenty different amino acids linked together in polymers. The composition and sequence of amino acids in the polypeptide chain is what makes each protein unique and able to fulfill its special role in the cell. Here, we will start with amino acids, the building blocks of proteins, and work our way up to three-dimensional protein structure and function.

Amino Acid Structure and Nomenclature

Understanding the structure of amino acids is key to understanding both their chemistry and the chemistry of proteins. The generic formula for all twenty amino acids is shown below.

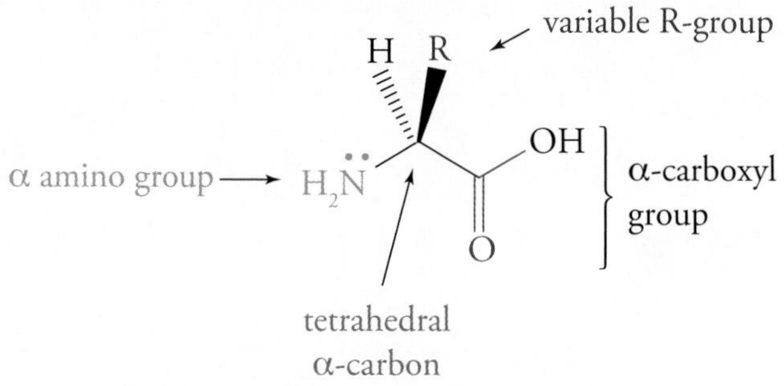

Figure 1   Generic Amino Acid Structure

All twenty amino acids share the same nitrogen-carbon-carbon backbone. The unique feature of each amino acid is its **side chain** (variable R-group), which gives it the physical and chemical properties that distinguish it from the other nineteen.

Classification of Amino Acids

Each of the twenty amino acids is unique because of its side chain, but many of them are similar in their chemical properties. You should be very familiar with the side chains, and it is important to understand the chemical properties that characterize them, such as their varying *shape, ability to hydrogen bond, and ability to act as acids or bases (which determines their charge at physiological pH).*

As you study the 20 amino acids, do so by organizing them into four broad categories: ACIDIC, BASIC, NONPOLAR, and POLAR amino acids. Each amino acid has a three-letter abbreviation and a one-letter abbreviation, which are both important to know for the MCAT.

Acidic Amino Acids

Aspartic acid and glutamic acid are the only amino acids with carboxylic acid functional groups ($pK_a \approx 4$) in their side chains, thereby making the side chains acidic. Thus, there are three functional groups in these amino acids that may act as acids—the two backbone groups and the R-group. You may hear the terms aspart*ate* and glutam*ate*—these simply refer to the anionic (deprotonated) form of each molecule, which is how these amino acids are observed at physiological pH.

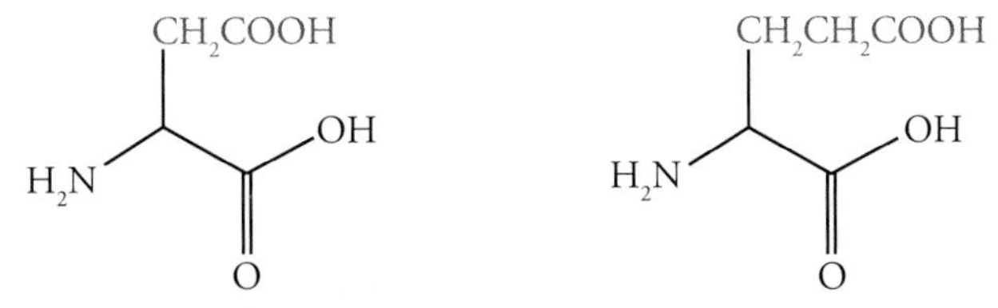

ASPARTIC ACID Asp **D**   GLUTAMIC ACID Glu **E**

Figure 2 Acidic Amino Acids

Basic Amino Acids

Lysine, arginine, and histidine have basic R-group side chains. The pK_a values for the side chains in these amino acids are 10 for Lys, 12 for Arg, and 6.5 for His. Both Lys and Arg are cationic (protonated) at physiological pH, but histidine is unique in having a side chain with a pK_a close to physiological pH. At pH 7.4, histidine may be either protonated or deprotonated—we put it in the basic category, but it often acts as an acid too. This makes it a readily available proton acceptor or donor, explaining its prevalence at protein active sites. A mnemonic is "His goes both ways." This contrasts with amino acids containing –COOH or $–NH_2$ side chains, which are *always* anionic ($RCOO^-$) or cationic (RNH_3^+) at physiological pH. [By the way, *histamine* is a small molecule that has to do with allergic responses, itching, inflammation, and other processes. (You've heard of antihistamine drugs, for example.) It is not an amino acid; don't confuse it with *histidine*.]

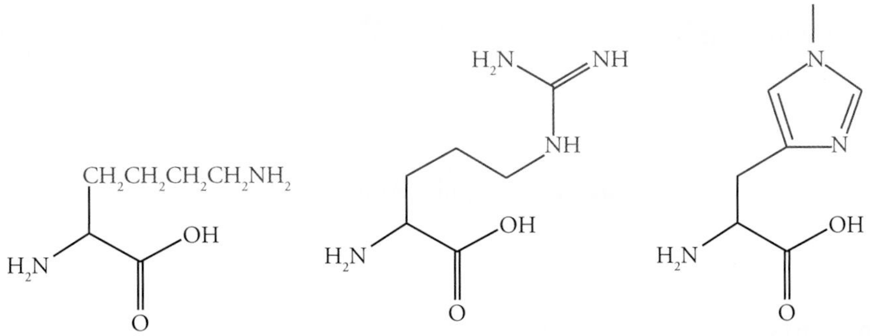

LYSINE Lys **K**   ARGININE Arg **R**   HISTIDINE His **H**

Figure 3 Basic Amino Acids

Hydrophobic (Nonpolar) Amino Acids

Hydrophobic amino acids have either aliphatic (alkyl) or aromatic side chains. Amino acids with aliphatic side chains include glycine, alanine, valine, leucine, and isoleucine. Amino acids with aromatic side chains include phenylalanine, tryptophan, and tyrosine (though the latter is a polar amino acid). Hydrophobic residues tend to associate with each other rather than with water, and therefore are found on the interior of folded globular proteins, away from water. The larger the hydrophobic group, the greater the hydrophobic force repelling it from water.

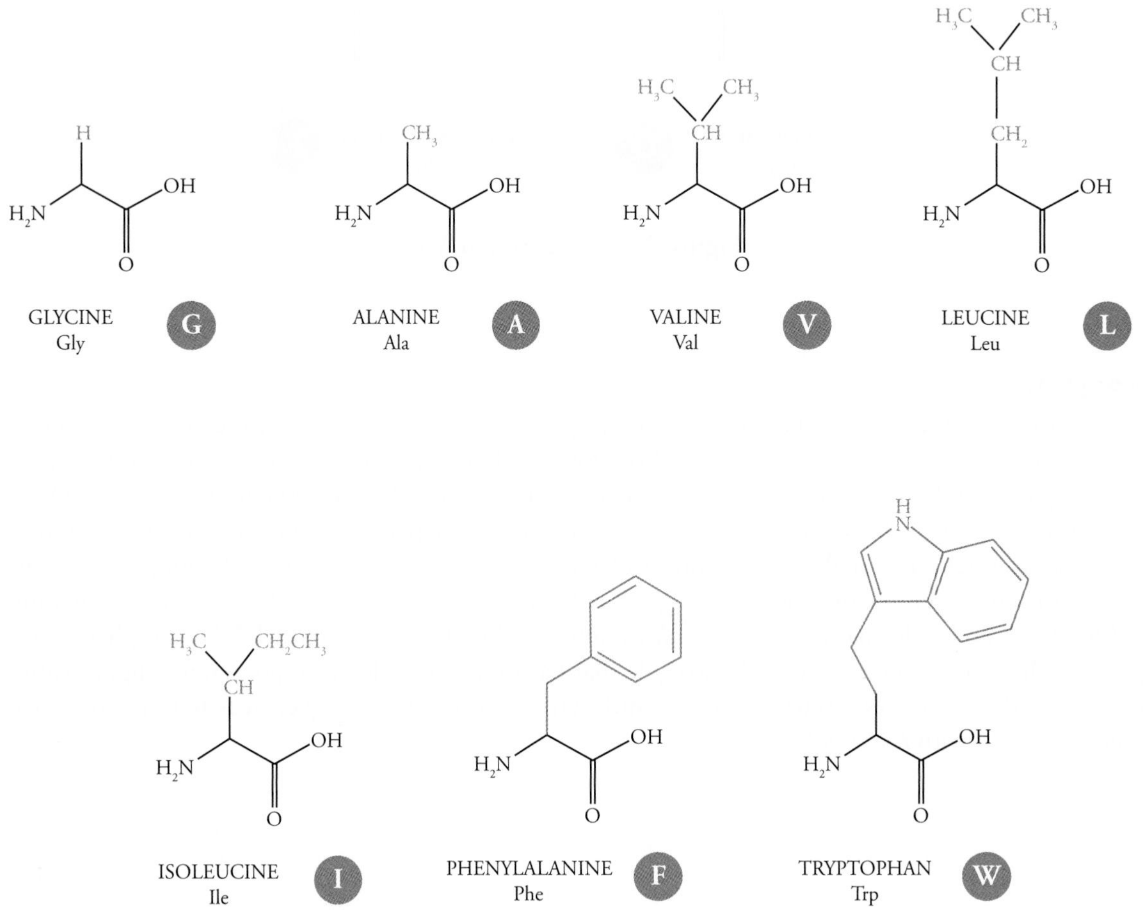

GLYCINE Gly **G**   ALANINE Ala **A**   VALINE Val **V**   LEUCINE Leu **L**

ISOLEUCINE Ile **I**   PHENYLALANINE Phe **F**   TRYPTOPHAN Trp **W**

Figure 4   Nonpolar Amino Acids

Polar Amino Acids

These amino acids are characterized by an R-group that is polar enough to form hydrogen bonds with water but that does not act as an acid or base. This means they are hydrophilic and will interact with water whenever possible. The hydroxyl groups of serine, threonine, and tyrosine residues are often modified by the attachment of a phosphate group by a regulatory enzyme called a kinase. The result is a change in structure due to the very hydrophilic phosphate group. This modification is an important means of regulating protein activity. This category also includes the amide derivatives of aspartic acid and glutamic acid, which are named asparagine and glutamine, respectively.

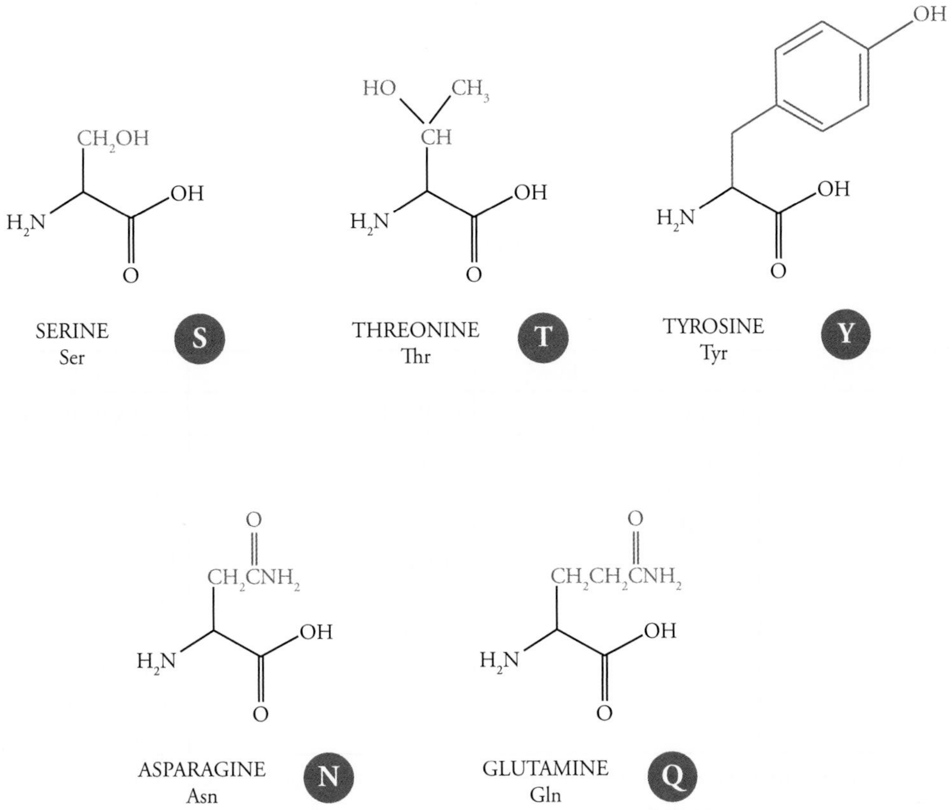

Figure 5   Polar Amino Acids

Sulfur-Containing Amino Acids

Amino acids with sulfur-containing side chains include cysteine and methionine. Cysteine, which contains a thiol (also called a sulfhydryl—like an alcohol that has an S atom instead of an O atom), is fairly polar, and methionine, which contains a thioether (like an ether that has an S atom instead of an O atom), is fairly nonpolar.

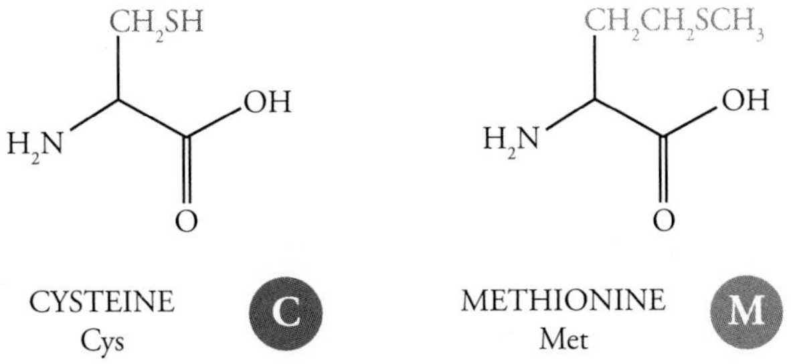

Figure 6   Sulfur-Containing Amino Acids

Proline

Proline is unique among the amino acids in that its amino group is covalently bound to its nonpolar side chain, creating a secondary α-amino group and a distinctive ring structure. This unique feature of proline has important consequences for protein folding (see Section 7.3).

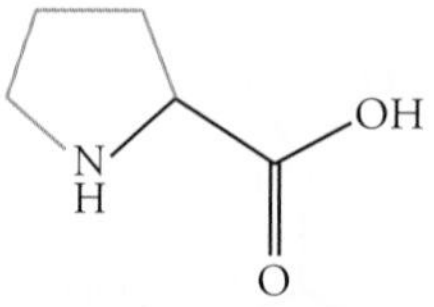

PROLINE
Pro

Hydrophilic			Hydrophobic
ACIDIC	BASIC	POLAR	NONPOLAR
Aspartic acid	Lysine*	Serine	Glycine
Glutamic acid	Arginine	Cysteine	Alanine
	Histidine*	Tyrosine	Valine*
		Threonine*	Leucine*
		Asparagine	Isoleucine*
		Glutamine	Phenylalanine*
			Tryptophan*
			Methionine*
			Proline
*Denotes one of the **nine essential** amino acids, those that cannot be synthesized by adult humans and must be obtained from the diet.			

Table 1   Summary Table of Amino Acids

- Which of the following amino acids is most likely to be found on the interior of a protein at pH 7.0?[1]
   - A) Tyrosine
   - B) Valine
   - C) Arginine
   - D) Glutamic acid

---

[1]   Valine (choice B) is a hydrophobic residue and is thus the most likely to be found on the interior of the proteins. Tyrosine, arginine, and glutamic acid are all hydrophilic, and are more likely to be found on the exterior of a protein.

7.2 AMINO ACID REACTIVITY

Since amino acids are composed of an acidic group (the carboxylic acid) and a basic group (the amine), we must be sure to understand the acid/base chemistry of amino acids.

Reviewing the Fundamentals of Acid/Base Chemistry

Amino acids are **amphoteric**, which means that amino acids can act as acids or bases. This should make sense since an amino acid contains the acidic carboxylic acid group and the basic amino group. The details of amino acid reactivity is discussed in detail in the Organic Chemistry section of this book.

7.3 PROTEIN STRUCTURE

There are two common types of covalent bonds between amino acids in proteins: the **peptide bonds** that link amino acids together into polypeptide chains and **disulfide bridges** between cysteine R-groups.

The Peptide Bond

Polypeptides are formed by linking amino acids together in peptide bonds. A peptide bond is formed between the carboxyl group of one amino acid and the α-amino group of another amino acid with the loss of water. The figure below shows the formation of a dipeptide from the amino acids glycine and alanine.

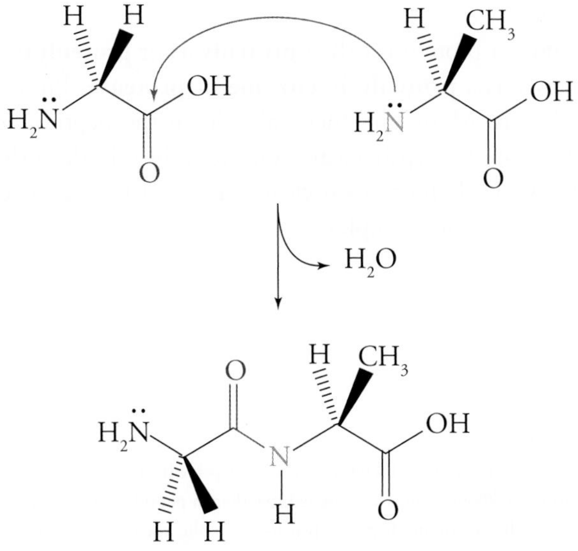

Figure 7   Peptide Bond (Amide Bond) Formation

In a polypeptide chain, the N–C–C–N–C–C pattern formed from the amino acids is known as the **backbone** of the polypeptide. An individual amino acid is termed a **residue** when it is part of a polypeptide chain. The amino terminus is the first end made during polypeptide synthesis, and the carboxy terminus is made last. Hence, by convention, the amino-terminal residue is also always written first.

- In the oligopeptide Phe-Glu-Gly-Ser-Ala, state the number of acid and base functional groups, which residue has a free α-amino group, and which residue has a free α-carboxyl group. (Refer to the beginning of the chapter for structures.)[2]
- How many unique dipeptides (made from linking two amino acids) can be synthesized using only alanine and glycine residues?[3]
- Thermodynamics states that free energy must decrease for a reaction to proceed spontaneously and that such a reaction will spontaneously move toward equilibrium. The diagram below shows the free energy changes during peptide bond formation. At equilibrium, which is thermodynamically favored: the dipeptide or the individual amino acids?[4]

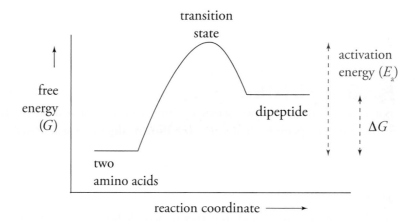

- In that case, how are peptide bonds formed and maintained inside cells?[5]

Hydrolysis of a protein by another protein is called **proteolysis** or **proteolytic cleavage**, and the protein that does the cutting is known as a **proteolytic enzyme** or **protease**. Proteolytic cleavage is a specific means of cleaving peptide bonds. Many enzymes only cleave the peptide bond adjacent to a specific amino acid. For example, the protease trypsin cleaves on the carboxyl side of the positively charged (basic) residues arginine and lysine, while chymotrypsin cleaves adjacent to large hydrophobic residues such as phenylalanine. (Do *not* memorize these examples.)

---

[2] As stated above, the amino end is always written first. Therefore, the oligopeptide begins with an exposed Phe amino group and ends with an exposed Ala carboxyl; all the other backbone groups are hitched together in peptide bonds. Out of all the R-groups, there is only one acidic or basic functional group, the acidic glutamate R-group. This R-group plus the two terminal backbone groups gives a total of three acid/base functional groups.

[3] Four (Gly-Gly, Ala-Ala, Gly-Ala, Ala-Gly). Note that Ala-Gly and Gly-Ala are not identical peptides. In Ala-Gly, the N-terminus is Gly and the C-terminus is Ala. In Gly-Ala, the N-terminus is Gly and the C-terminus is Ala.

[4] The dipeptide has a higher free energy, so its existence is less favorable. In other words, existence of the chain is less favorable than existence of the isolated amino acids.

[5] During protein synthesis, stored energy is used to force peptide bonds to form. Once the bond is formed, even though its destruction is thermodynamically favorable, it remains stable because the activation energy for the hydrolysis reaction is so high. In other words, hydrolysis is thermodynamically favorable but kinetically slow.

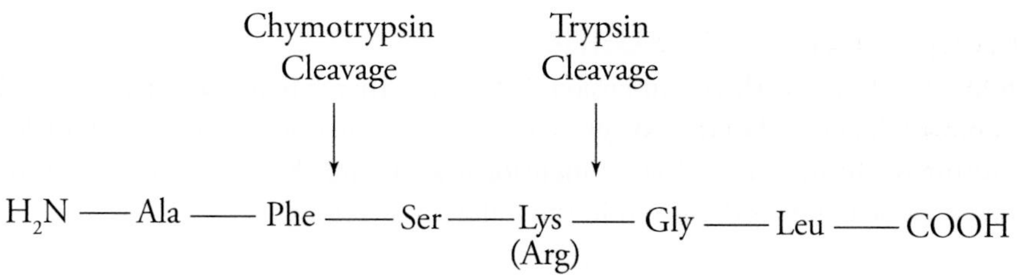

$$H_2N \longrightarrow Ala \longrightarrow Phe \longrightarrow Ser \longrightarrow \underset{(Arg)}{Lys} \longrightarrow Gly \longrightarrow Leu \longrightarrow COOH$$

Chymotrypsin Cleavage ↓   Trypsin Cleavage ↓

Figure 8   Specificity of Protease Cleavage

- Based on the above, if the following peptide is cleaved by trypsin, which amino acids will be on the new N-termini and how many fragments will result: AGRQKFYFK?[6]

The Disulfide Bond

Cysteine is an amino acid with a reactive thiol (sulfhydryl, SH) in its side chain. The thiol of one cysteine can react with the thiol of another cysteine to produce a covalent sulfur-sulfur bond known as a disulfide bond, as illustrated below. The cysteines forming a disulfide bond may be located in the same or different polypeptide chain(s). The disulfide bridge plays an important role in stabilizing tertiary protein structure; this will be discussed in the section on protein folding. Once a cysteine residue becomes disulfide-bonded to another cysteine residue, it is called *cystine* instead of cysteine.

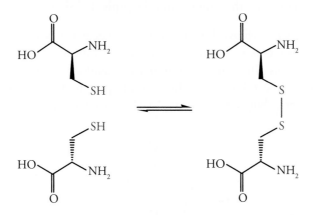

Figure 9   Formation of the Disulfide Bond

- Which is more oxidized, the sulfur in *cysteine* or the sulfur in *cystine*?[7]
- The inside of cells is known as a reducing environment because cells possess antioxidants (chemicals that prevent oxidation reactions). Where would disulfide bridges be more likely to be found, in extracellular proteins, under oxidizing conditions, or in the interior of cells, in a reducing environment?[8]

---

[6] Trypsin will cleave on the carboxyl side of the positively-charged amino acid residues Arg (R) and Lys (K). There will be three fragments after trypsin cleavage: AGR (Ala-Gly-Arg), QK (Glu-Lys), and FYFK (Phe-Tyr-Phe-Lys), with the N-terminal amino acids being alanine, glutamine, and phenylalanine.

[7] In forming cystine from two cysteine residues, hydrogen atoms are removed (an oxidation reaction), indicating that the sulfur in cystine is more oxidized.

[8] In a reducing environment, the S-S group is reduced to two SH groups. Disulfide bridges are found only in extracellular polypeptides, where they will not be reduced. Examples of protein complexes held together by disulfide bridges include antibodies and the hormone insulin.

Protein Structure in Three Dimensions

Each protein folds into a unique three-dimensional structure that is required for that protein to function properly. Improperly folded, or **denatured**, proteins are non-functional. There are four levels of protein folding that contribute to their final three-dimensional structure. Each level of structure is dependent upon a particular type of bond, as discussed in the following sections.

Denaturation is an important concept. It refers to the disruption of a protein's shape without breaking peptide bonds. Proteins are denatured by *urea* (which disrupts hydrogen bonding interactions), by *extremes of pH*, by extremes of *temperature*, and by *changes in salt concentration (tonicity)*.

Primary (1°) Structure: The Amino Acid Sequence

The simplest level of protein structure is the order of amino acids bonded to each other in the polypeptide chain. This linear ordering of amino acid residues is known as primary structure. **Primary structure** is the same as **sequence**. The bond that determines 1° structure is the peptide bond, simply because this is the bond that links one amino acid to the next in a polypeptide.

Secondary (2°) Structure: Hydrogen Bonds Between Backbone Groups

Secondary structure refers to the initial folding of a polypeptide chain into shapes stabilized by hydrogen bonds between backbone NH and CO groups. Certain motifs of secondary structure are found in most proteins. The two most common are the α-**helix** and the β-**pleated sheet**.

All α-helices have the same well-defined dimensions that are depicted below with the R-groups omitted for clarity. The α-helices of proteins are always right-handed, 5 angstroms in width, with each subsequent amino acid rising 1.5 angstroms. There are 3.6 amino acid residues per turn with the α-carboxyl oxygen of one amino acid residue hydrogen-bonded to the α-amino proton of an amino acid three residues away. (*Don't* memorize these numbers, but *do* try to visualize what they mean.)

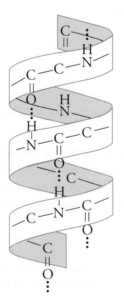

Figure 10   An α-Helix

The unique side chain of proline causes two problems in polypeptide chains:

1. The formation of a peptide bond with proline (shown below) eliminates the only hydrogen atom on the nitrogen atom of proline. The absence of the N-H bond disrupts the backbone hydrogen bonding in the polypeptide chain.
2. The unique structure of proline forces it to kink the polypeptide chain.

For both reasons, proline residues never appear within the α-helix.

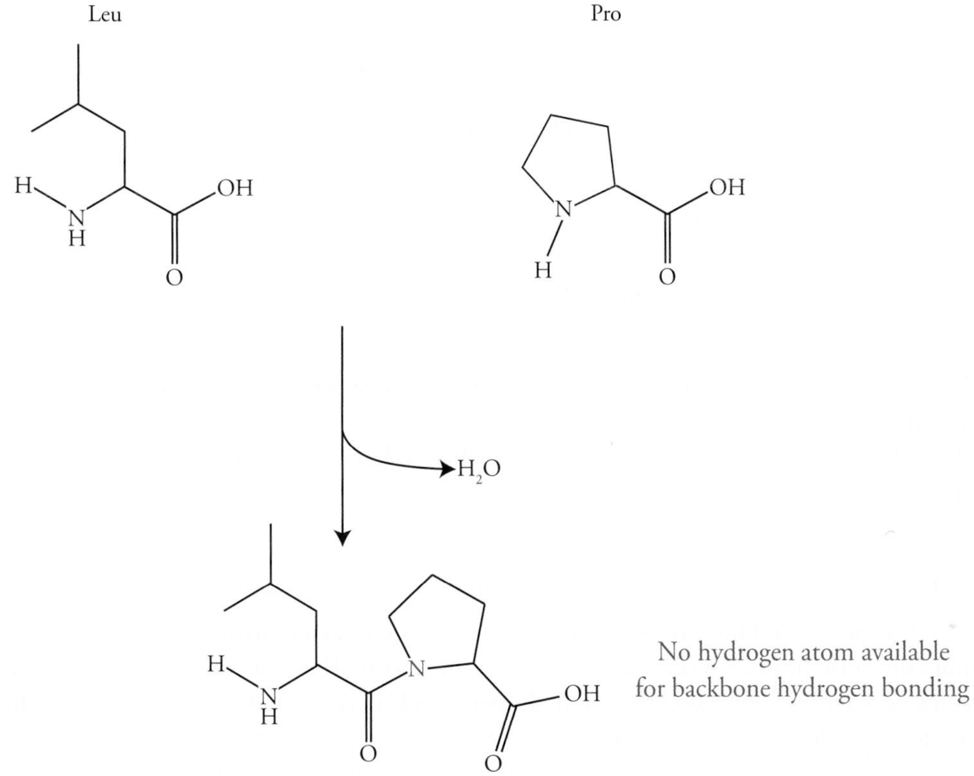

No hydrogen atom available for backbone hydrogen bonding

Figure 11   Proline

Proteins such as hormone receptors and ion channels are often found with α-helical transmembrane regions integrated into the hydrophobic membranes of cells. The α-helix is a favorable structure for a hydrophobic transmembrane region because all polar NH and CO groups in the backbone are hydrogen-bonded to each other on the inside of the helix, and thus don't interact with the hydrophobic membrane interior. α-Helical regions that span membranes also have hydrophobic R-groups, which radiate out from the helix, interacting with the hydrophobic interior of the membrane.

β-Pleated sheets are also stabilized by hydrogen bonding between NH and CO groups in the polypeptide backbone. In β-sheets, however, hydrogen bonding occurs between residues distant from each other in the chain or even on separate polypeptide chains. Also, the backbone of a β-sheet is extended, rather than coiled, with side groups directed above and below the plane of the β-sheet. There are two types of β-sheets, one with adjacent polypeptide strands running in the *same* direction (**parallel** β-pleated sheet) and another in which the polypeptide strands run in *opposite* directions (**antiparallel** β-pleated sheet).

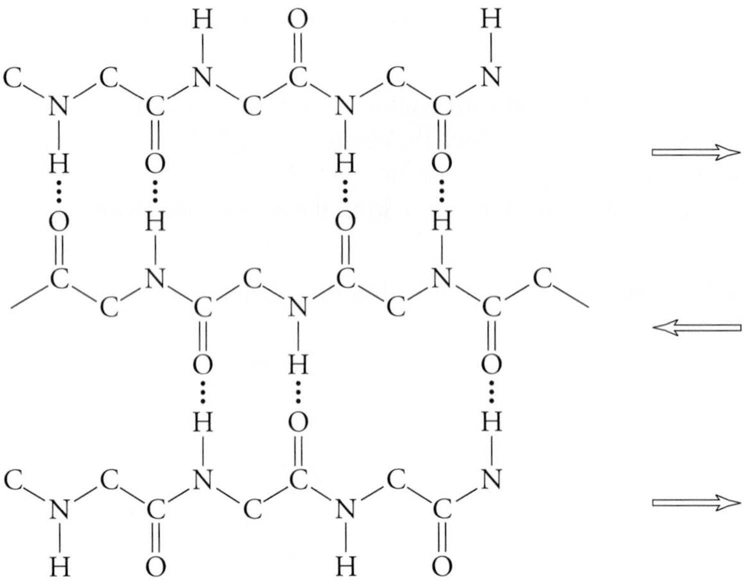

Figure 12 A β-Pleated Sheet

- If a single polypeptide folds once and forms a β-pleated sheet with itself, would this be a parallel or antiparallel β-pleated sheet?[9]
- What effect would a molecule that disrupts hydrogen bonding, such as urea, have on protein structure?[10]

Tertiary (3°) Structure: Hydrophobic/Hydrophilic Interactions

The next level of protein folding, tertiary structure, concerns interactions between amino acid residues located more distantly from each other in the polypeptide chain. These interactions may include **van der Waals forces** between nonpolar side chains, hydrogen bonds between polar side chains, disulfide bonds between cysteine residues, and electrostatic interactions between acidic and basic side chains. The folding of secondary structures such as α-helices into higher order tertiary structures is driven by interactions of R-groups with each other and with the solvent (water). Hydrophobic R-groups tend to fold into the interior of the protein, away from the solvent, and hydrophilic R-groups tend to be exposed to water on the surface of the protein (shown for the generic globular protein). This is called the **hydrophobic effect.**

---

[9] It would be antiparallel because one participant in the β-pleated sheet would have a C to N direction, while the other would be running N to C.

[10] Putting a protein in a urea solution will disrupt H-bonding, thus disrupting secondary structure (and possibly tertiary and quaternary) by unfolding α-helices and β-sheets. It would not affect primary structure, which depends on the much more stable peptide bond. Disruption of 2°, 3°, or 4° structure without breaking peptide bonds is *denaturation*.

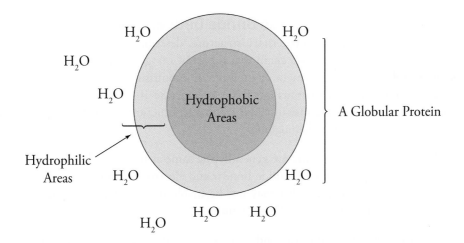

Figure 13   Folding of a Globular Protein in Aqueous Solution

Under the right conditions, the forces driving hydrophobic avoidance of water and hydrogen bonding will fold a polypeptide spontaneously into the correct conformation, the lowest energy conformation. In a classic experiment by Christian Anfinsen and coworkers, the effect of a denaturing agent (urea) and a reducing agent (β-mercaptoethanol) on the folding of a protein called ribonuclease were examined. In the following questions, you will reenact their thought processes. Try to answer the questions before reading the footnotes.

- Ribonuclease has eight cysteines that form four disulfides bonds. What effect would a reducing agent have on its tertiary structure?[11]
- If the disulfides serve only to lock into place a tertiary protein structure that forms first on its own, then what effect would the reducing agent have on correct protein folding?[12]
- Would a protein end up folded normally if you (1) first put it in a reducing environment, (2) then denatured it by adding urea, (3) next removed the reducing agent, allowing disulfide bridges to reform, and (4) finally removed the denaturing agent?[13]
- What if you did the same experiment but in this order: 1, 2, 4, 3?[14]
- Which of the following may be considered an example of tertiary protein structure?[15]
  - I. van der Waals interactions between two Phe R-groups located far apart on a polypeptide
  - II. Hydrogen bonds between backbone amino and carboxyl groups
  - III. Covalent disulfide bonds between cysteine residues located far apart on a polypeptide

---

[11] The disulfide bridges would be broken. Tertiary structure would be less stable.

[12] The shape should not be disrupted if breaking disulfides is the only disturbance. It's just that the shape would be less sturdy—like a concrete wall without the rebar.

[13] No. If you allow disulfide bridges to form while the protein is still denatured, it will become locked into an abnormal shape.

[14] You should end up with the correct structure. In step one, you break the reinforcing disulfide bridges. In step two, you denature the protein completely by disrupting H-bonds. In step four, you allow the H-bonds to reform; as stated in the text, normally the correct tertiary structure will form spontaneously if you leave the polypeptide alone. In step three, you reform the disulfide bridges, thus locking the structure into its correct form.

[15] This is a simple question provided to clarify the classification of the disulfide bridge. **Item I** is a good example of 3° structure. Item II describes 2°, not 3°, structure. **Item III** describes the disulfide bond, which is another example of tertiary structure.

Quaternary (4°) Structure: Various Bonds Between Separate Chains

The highest level of protein structure, quaternary structure, describes interactions between polypeptide subunits. A **subunit** is a single polypeptide chain that is part of a large complex containing many subunits (a **multisubunit complex**). The arrangement of subunits in a multisubunit complex is what we mean by quaternary structure. For example, mammalian RNA polymerase II contains twelve different subunits. The interactions between subunits are instrumental in protein function, as in the cooperative binding of oxygen by each of the four subunits of hemoglobin.

The forces stabilizing quaternary structure are generally the same as those involved in tertiary structure—van der Waals forces, hydrogen bonds, disulfide bonds, and electrostatic interactions. It is key to understand, however, that there is one bond that may not be involved in quaternary structure—the peptide bond—because this bond defines sequence (1° structure).

- What is the difference between a disulfide bridge involved in quaternary structure and one involved in tertiary structure?[16]

7.4 PROTEINS AS ENZYMES

Enzymes are biological catalysts. They increase the rate of a reaction by lowering the reaction's activation energy, but they *do not affect* ΔG between reactants and products. As catalysts, enzymes have a kinetic role, *not* a thermodynamic one. Enzymes may alter the rate of a reaction enormously: a reaction that would take a hundred years to reach equilibrium without an enzyme may occur in just seconds with an enzyme.

Given that thousands of enzymes have been discovered, scientists frequently classify them based upon reaction type. On the following page, Table 2 lists several examples but note that enzymes cannot control the direction in which a reaction proceeds; it is common to see enzymes in a given class function in reverse.

---

[16] Quaternary disulfides are bonds that form between distinct subunits of a protein. Tertiary disulfides are bonds that form between residues in the same polypeptide and can be part of creating one small protein (with no other subunits), or creating one subunit of a larger protein.

Enzyme Class	Reaction
Hydrolase	hydrolyzes chemical bonds (includes ATPases, proteases, and others)
Isomerase	rearranges bonds within a molecule to form an isomer
Ligase	forms a chemical bond (for example, DNA ligase)
Lyase	breaks chemical bonds by means other than oxidation or hydrolysis (for example, pyruvate decarboxylase)
Kinase	transfers a phosphate group to a molecule from a high energy carrier, such as ATP (for example, phosphofructokinase [PFK])
Oxidoreductase	runs redox reactions (includes oxidases, reductases, dehydrogenases, and others)
Polymerase	polymerization (for example, addition of nucleotides to the leading strand of DNA by DNA polymerase III)
Phosphatase	removes a phosphate group from a molecule
Phosphorylase	transfers a phosphate group to a molecule from inorganic phosphate (for example, glycogen phosphorylase)
Protease	hydrolyzyes peptide bonds (for example, trypsin, chymotrypsin, pepsin, et cetera)

Table 2 Enzyme Classes

ATP as an Energy Source: Reaction Coupling

Enzymes increase the rate of reactions that have a negative ΔG. These reactions would occur on their own without an enzyme (they are spontaneous) but far more slowly than with one. However, there are many reactions in the body that occur which have a positive ΔG. The biosynthesis of macromolecules such as DNA and protein is not spontaneous ($\Delta G > 0$), but clearly these reactions *do* take place (or we wouldn't be here). How can this be? Thermodynamically unfavorable reactions in the cell can be driven forward by **reaction coupling**. In reaction coupling, one very favorable reaction is used to drive an unfavorable one. This is possible because *free energy changes are additive*. [What is the favorable reaction that the cell can use to drive unfavorable reactions?[17]] In the cell, ΔG is for the hydrolysis of one phosphate group from ATP, about −12 kcal/mol, so it is a very favorable reaction.

How does ATP hydrolysis drive unfavorable reactions? There are many ways. One example is by causing a conformational change in a protein; in this way ATP hydrolysis can be used to power energy-costly events like transmembrane transport. Another example is by transfer of a phosphate group from ATP to a substrate. Take the unfavorable reaction A + B → C. Let's say that Reactant A must proceed through an intermediate, APO_4^{2-} in order to participate. Let's say $\Delta G = +7$ kcal/mol for the overall reaction. What if the two partial reactions have ΔGs as follows:

$$A + PO_4^{2-} \rightarrow APO_4^{2-} \qquad \Delta G = \quad +2 \text{ kcal/mol}$$

$$\underline{APO_4^{2-} + B \rightarrow C + PO_4^{2-} \qquad \Delta G = \quad +5 \text{ kcal/mol}}$$

$$\textit{Total} \quad \Delta G = \quad +7 \text{ kcal/mol}$$

---

[17] ATP hydrolysis!

These reactions will not proceed, because the overall ΔG will be +7 kcal/mol. What will be the *overall* ΔG if we *couple* the reaction A + B → C to the hydrolysis of one ATP? All we have to do is add up all the ΔG values, as follows:

$$\text{ATP} \rightarrow \text{ADP} + \text{PO}_4^{2-} \qquad \Delta G = \quad -12 \text{ kcal/mol}$$

$$\text{A} + \text{PO}_4^{2-} \rightarrow \text{APO}_4^{2-} \qquad \Delta G = \quad +2 \text{ kcal/mol}$$

$$\underline{\text{APO}_4^{2-} + \text{B} \rightarrow \text{C} + \text{PO}_4^{2-} \qquad \Delta G = \quad +5 \text{ kcal/mol}}$$

$$\textit{Total} \quad \Delta G = \quad -5 \text{ kcal/mol}$$

Now the overall reaction, shown below, is thermodynamically favorable. We have *coupled* the unfavorable reaction A + B → C to the highly favorable hydrolysis of ATP:

$$\text{A} + \text{B} + \text{ATP} \rightarrow \text{C} + \text{ADP} + \text{PO}_4^{2-} \quad \Delta G = -5 \text{ kcal/mol}$$

Note that we first stated that the enzyme has only a kinetic role (influencing rate only), not a thermodynamic one (determining favorability). Then we went on to discuss reaction coupling, which allows enzymes to promote otherwise unfavorable reactions. There is no contradiction, however. The only difference is viewing reactions in an isolated manner or in the complex series of linked reactions more commonly found in the body. The same rule applies in either case: ΔG must be negative for either a single reaction or a series of linked reactions to occur spontaneously. In summary:

- One reaction in a test tube: the enzyme is a catalyst with a kinetic role only. It influences the rate of the reaction, but not the outcome.
- Many "real life" reactions in the cell: enzyme controls outcomes by selectively promoting unfavorable reactions via reaction coupling.

7.5 ENZYME STRUCTURE AND FUNCTION

Most enzymes are proteins that must fold into specific three-dimensional structures to act as catalysts. (Some enzymes are RNA or contain RNA sequences with catalytic activity. For a discussion on biologically important molecules, such as proteins, carbohydrates, lipids, and nucleic acids, see Chapter 35 and Section 35.2.) An enzyme may consist of a single polypeptide chain or several polypeptide subunits held together via the protein's quaternary structure. The reason for the importance of folding in enzyme function is the proper formation of the **active site**, the region in an enzyme's three-dimensional structure that is directly involved in catalysis. [What shape are enzymes more likely to have: fibrous/elongated or globular/spherical?[18]] The reactants in an enzyme-catalyzed reaction are called **substrates**. (Products have no special name; they're just "products.") What is the role of the active site, that is, how do enzymes work? The **active site model**, commonly referred to as the "lock and key hypothesis," states that the substrate and active site are perfectly complementary. This differs from the **induced fit model** which asserts that the substrate and active site differ slightly in structure and that the binding of the substrate induces a conformational change in the enzyme. The induced fit model has gained greater acceptance in recent years, but regardless of the model, enzymes accelerate the rate of a given reaction by helping to *stabilize the transition state*. This lowers the activation energy barrier between reactants and products.

- Is it possible that amino acids located far apart from each other in the primary protein sequence may play a role in the formation of the same active site?[19]
- If, during an enzyme-catalyzed reaction, an intermediate forms in which the substrate is covalently linked to the enzyme via a serine residue, can this occur at any serine residue or must it occur at a specific serine residue?[20]
- Consider the reaction $A \rightleftharpoons B$, which has the following equilibrium constant: $K_{eq} = [B]_{eq}/[A]_{eq} = 1000$. If pure B is put into solution in the presence of an enzyme that catalyzes the reaction between A and B, which one of the following will be true?[21]
  A) All the B will be converted into A, until there is 1,000 times more A than B.
  B) All of the B will remain as B, since B is favored at equilibrium.
  C) The enzyme will have no effect, since enzymes act on the transition state and there is no transition state present.
  D) The reaction that produces A will predominate until $\Delta G = 0$.

The active site for enzymes is generally highly specific in its substrate recognition, including stereospecificity (the ability to distinguish between stereoisomers). For example, enzymes which catalyze reactions involving amino acids are specific for D or L amino acids, and enzymes catalyzing reactions involving monosaccharides may distinguish between stereoisomers as well.

Given the importance of the active site, it becomes clear that small alterations in its structure can drastically alter enzymatic activity. Therefore, both temperature and pH play a critical role in enzymatic function. As

---

[18] Globular. Structural proteins such as collagen tend to be fibrous, but proteins that act as catalysts tend to be roughly spherical to form an active site in a cleft in the sphere.

[19] Yes, the amino acids at the active site may be distant from each other in a polypeptide's primary sequence but be near each other in the final folded protein. This is why protein folding is crucial for enzyme function.

[20] It must occur at a particular serine residue which sticks out into the active site.

[21] If only B exists in solution, then the back-reaction producing A will predominate until equilibrium is reached ($\Delta G = 0$), regardless of the presence or absence of enzyme (choice **D** is correct, and choice B is wrong). According to the K_{eq} given, at equilibrium there will be 1000 times more B than A, not the other way around (choice A is wrong). Note that enzymes do not act on the transition state; they act to produce the transition state (choice C is wrong).

temperature increases, the thermal motion of the peptide and surrounding solution destabilize its structure. If the temperature rises sufficiently, the protein denatures and loses its orderly structure. The pH of the surrounding medium also impacts protein stability; several amino acids possess ionizable –R groups that change charge depending on pH. This can decrease the affinity of a substrate for the active site and, if the pH deviates sufficiently, the protein can denature.

- The transition state intermediate for a reaction possesses a transient negative charge. The active site for an enzyme catalyzing this reaction contains a His residue to stabilize the intermediate. If the His residue at the active site is replaced by a glutamate which is negatively charged at pH 7.0, what effect will this have on the reaction, assuming that the reactants are present in excess compared to the enzyme?[22]

  A) The repulsion caused by the negative charge in the glutamate at the altered active site will increase the activation energy and make the reaction proceed more slowly than it would in solution without enzyme.

  B) The rate of catalysis will be unaffected, but the equilibrium ratio of products and reactants will change, favoring reactants.

  C) The transition state intermediate will not be stabilized as effectively by the altered enzyme, lowering the rate relative to the rate with catalysis by the normal enzyme.

  D) The rate of catalysis will decrease, and the equilibrium constant will change.

Enzymatic function can also depend upon the association of additional molecules. **Cofactors**, which are metal ions or small molecules (not themselves a protein), are required for activity in many enzymes. In fact, the majority of the vitamins in our diet serve as precursors for cofactors (for example, niacin [B3] is ultimately transformed into NAD^+). When a cofactor is an organic molecule, it is referred to as a **coenzyme**; these often bind to the substrate during the catalyzed reaction. One prime example of a coenzyme, which we will focus on later in the chapter, is coenzyme A (CoA).

---

[22] Beware of long, complex-sounding questions! They may not be as bad as they look; for instance, the phrase "assuming that the reactants are present in excess compared to the enzyme" adds nothing to the substance of this question. If His (which is positive or neutral at pH 7) is replaced by Glu (negatively charged at pH 7), this could decrease the effectiveness of—or destroy altogether—the active site of the enzyme. This means the transition state would not be effectively stabilized, and the rate of the reaction would simply reduce to that of the uncatalyzed reaction (choice **C** is correct). The rate would not proceed more slowly than the uncatalyzed reaction (that is, "in solution without enzyme," choice A is wrong), and remember that enzymes do not alter reaction equilibria (K_{eq} will be unaffected; choices B and D are wrong).

7.6 REGULATION OF ENZYME ACTIVITY

Metabolic pathways in the cell are not all continually on, but must be tightly regulated to maintain health. For example, if glycogen synthesis and breakdown occur in the same cell at the same time, a great deal of energy will be wasted without accomplishing anything. Therefore, the activity of key enzymes in metabolic pathways is usually regulated in one or more of the following ways:

1) **Covalent modification.** Proteins can have several different groups covalently attached to them, and this can regulate their activity, lifespan in the cell, and/or cellular location. The addition of a phosphoryl group from a molecule of ATP by a protein **kinase** to the hydroxyl of serine, threonine, or tyrosine residues is the most common example. Phosphorylation of these different sites on an enzyme can either activate or inactivate the enzyme. Protein **phosphorylases**, also phosphorylate proteins, use free-floating inorganic phosphate (P_i) in the cell instead of ATP. Protein phosphorylation can be reversed by protein **phosphatases**.

2) **Proteolytic cleavage.** Many enzymes (and other proteins) are synthesized in inactive forms (zymogens) that are activated by cleavage by a protease.

3) **Association with other polypeptides.** Some enzymes have catalytic activity in one polypeptide subunit that is regulated by association with a separate regulatory subunit. For example, there are some proteins that demonstrate continuous rapid catalysis if their regulatory subunit is removed; this is known as **constitutive activity** (*constitutive* means continuous or unregulated). There are other proteins that require association with another peptide in order to function. Still, other proteins can bind many regulatory subunits. There are numerous examples of this in the cell, and many of them have diverse and complex regulatory mechanisms that all revolve around the theme of "associations with other polypeptides can affect enzyme activity."

4) **Allosteric regulation.** The modification of active-site activity through interactions of molecules with other specific sites on the enzyme (called **allosteric sites**). Let's look at this in a little more detail.

Allosteric Regulation

If the cell is to make use of the enzyme as a biochemical switch, there must be a way to turn the enzyme *on* or *off*. One mechanism of regulation is the binding of small molecules to particular sites on an enzyme that are distinct from the active site; this is allosteric regulation. The binding of the allosteric regulator to the allosteric site is generally noncovalent and reversible. When bound, the allosteric regulator can alter the conformation of the enzyme to increase or decrease catalysis, even though it may be bound to the enzyme at a site distant from the active site or even on a separate polypeptide.

Feedback Inhibition

Enzymes usually act as part of pathways, not alone. Rather than regulate every enzyme in a pathway, usually there are one or two key enzymes that are regulated, such as the enzyme that catalyzes the first irreversible step in a pathway. The easiest way to explain this is with an example. Three enzymes (E1, E2, and E3) catalyze the three steps required to convert Substrate A to Product D. When plenty of D is around, it would be logical to shut off E1 so that excess B, C, and D are not made. This would conserve A and would also conserve energy. Commonly, an end-product such as D will shut off an enzyme early in the pathway, such as E1. This is called **negative feedback**, or **feedback inhibition**.

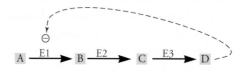

Figure 14   Feedback Inhibition

There are examples of positive feedback ("feedback *stimulation*"), but negative feedback is by far the most common example of feedback regulation. On the other hand, *feedforward stimulation* is common. This involves the stimulation of an enzyme by its substrate, or by a molecule used in the synthesis of the substrate. For example, in Figure 14, A might stimulate E3. This makes sense because when lots of A is around, we want the pathway for utilization of A to be active.

Allosteric regulation can be quite complex. It is possible for more than one small molecule to be capable of binding to an allosteric site. For example, imagine a reaction pathway from A through Z, where each step (A → B, B → C, etc.) is catalyzed by an enzyme. Let's say that an allosteric enzyme called E15 catalyzes the reaction O → P. It would be possible for A to allosterically activate E15 (feedforward stimulation) and for Z to allosterically inhibit E15 (feedback inhibition). This may sound complex, but it's quite logical. What it means is that when lots of A is around, E15 will be stimulated to use the molecules made from A (B, C, D, etc.) to make P, which could then be used to make Q, R, S, etc., all the way up to Z. On the other hand, if a lot of excess Z built up, it would inhibit E15, thereby conserving the supply of A, B, C, etc. and preventing more build-up of Z, Y, X, etc. Hence, in addition to acting as switches, enzymes act as *valves*, because they regulate the flow of substrates into products.

7.7 BASIC ENZYME KINETICS

Enzyme kinetics is the study of the rate of formation of products from substrates in the presence of an enzyme. The **reaction rate** (V, for velocity) is the amount of product formed per unit time, in moles per second (mol/s). It depends on the concentration of substrate, [S], and enzyme.[23] If there is only a little substrate, then the rate V is directly proportional to the amount of substrate added: double the amount of substrate and the reaction rate doubles, triple the substrate and the rate triples, and so forth. But eventually there is so much substrate that the active sites of the enzymes are occupied much of the time, and adding more substrate doesn't increase the reaction rate as much, that is, the slope of the V vs. [S] curve decreases. Finally, there is so much substrate that every active site is continuously occupied, and adding more substrate doesn't increase the reaction rate at all. At this point, the enzyme is said to be **saturated**. The reaction rate when the enzyme is saturated is denoted $\boldsymbol{V_{max}}$; see Figure 15. This is a property of each enzyme at a particular concentration of enzyme. You can look it up in a book for the common ones. [If an enzyme in a solution is acting at V_{max}, and the substrate concentration is doubled, how would the reaction rate be altered?[24]]

Another commonly used parameter on these enzyme kinetics graphs is the Michaelis constant K_m. K_m is the substrate concentration at which the reaction velocity is half its maximum. To find K_m on the enzyme kinetics graph, mark the V_{max} on the y-axis, then divide this distance in half to find $V_{max}/2$. K_m is found by drawing a horizontal line from $V_{max}/2$ to the curve, and then a vertical line down to the x-axis. K_m is unique for each enzyme-substrate pair and gives information on the affinity of the enzyme for its substrate. If an enzyme-substrate pair has a low K_m, it means that not very much substrate is required to get the reaction rate to half the maximum rate; thus the enzyme has a high affinity for this particular substrate.

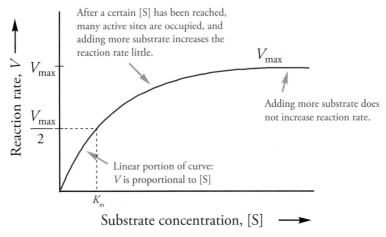

Figure 15   Saturation Kinetics

---

[23] Usually the concentration of enzyme is kept fixed, and [S] is taken as the only independent variable (the one the rate depends on). This is applicable to biological systems, where substrate concentrations change much more than enzyme concentrations.

[24] If the enzyme is acting at V_{max}, it is saturated with substrate; adding more substrate will not increase the reaction rate; the rate is still V_{max}.

Cooperativity

Many multi-subunit enzymes do not behave in the simple kinetic manner described above. In such enzymes, the binding of substrate to one subunit modulates the affinity of other subunits for substrate. Such enzymes are said to bind substrate *cooperatively*. There are two types of cooperativity: positive and negative. In positive cooperativity, the binding of a substrate to one subunit increases the affinity of the other subunits for substrate. The conformation of the enzyme prior to substrate binding, with low substrate affinity, is sometimes termed "tense," and the conformation of enzyme with increased affinity is termed "relaxed" (Figure 16). Negative cooperativity (which is less important for the MCAT) is the opposite: the binding of a substrate to one subunit reduces the affinity of the other subunits for substrate. Cooperative enzymes must have more than one active site. They are usually multisubunit complexes, composed of more than one protein chain held together in a quaternary structure. They may also be a single-subunit enzyme with two or more active sites.

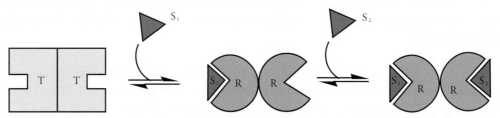

Figure 16   Enzyme Cooperativity

A sigmoidal curve results from cooperative binding. In Figure 17 below, the flat part at the bottom left (Region 1) is explained by the notion that at low [S] the enzyme complex has a low affinity for substrate (is in the tense state), and adding more substrate increases the rate little. The steep part in the middle of the curve (Region 2) represents the range of substrate concentrations where adding substrate greatly increases the reaction rate, because the enzyme complex is in the relaxed state. [What does Region 3 represent?[25]]

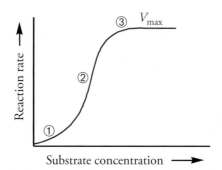

Figure 17   Sigmoidal Kinetics of Cooperativity

Cooperativity does not apply just to catalytic enzymes. For example, hemoglobin (Hb) is a protein complex made of four polypeptide subunits, each of which contains a heme prosthetic group with a single O_2-binding site. (So one Hb has four hemes and four binding sites.) Hb is a carrier (of oxygen), not a catalyst of any reaction (not an enzyme). It exhibits cooperative O_2 binding. This is why the Hb-O_2 dissociation curve is sigmoidal. [What is the relationship between allosteric binding and cooperative binding?[26]]

---

[25] Saturation, just as in the case of a noncooperative enzyme.

[26] Cooperativity is a special kind of allosteric interaction. One active site acts like an allosteric regulatory site for the other active sites. Secondly, cooperative enzyme complexes are often allosterically regulated also. Hb is an excellent example. Not only does O_2 binding to one subunit increase the other subunits' affinities, but also several other molecules can bind to various sites to change the affinity of the complex. For example, CO_2 stabilizes tense Hb, causing each of the four binding sites to have a lower affinity for oxygen. As a result, in the presence of CO_2, Hb tends to give up whatever O_2 it has bound. The most important thing to remember, though, is that the binding in cooperativity takes place at the active site, while the binding in allosteric regulation takes place at "other sites."

Inhibition of Enzyme Activity

Enzyme inhibitors can reduce enzyme activity by a few different mechanisms, including **competitive inhibition**, **noncompetitive inhibition**, **uncompetitive inhibition**, and **mixed-type inhibition**. **Competitive inhibitors** are molecules that *compete* with substrate for binding at the active site. [You can predict that structurally, competitive inhibitors resemble what?[27]] The key thing to remember about competitive inhibitors is that their inhibition can be overcome by adding more substrate; if the substrate concentration is high enough, the substrate can *outcompete* the inhibitor. Hence, V_{max} is not affected. You can get to the same V_{max}, but it takes more substrate (see Figure 18). Therefore, the K_m of the reaction to which a competitive inhibitor has been added is increased compared to the K_m of the uninhibited reaction. [If an enzyme has a reaction rate of 1 μmole/min at a substrate concentration of 50 μM and a rate of 10 μmole/min at a substrate concentration of 100 μM, does this indicate the presence of a competitive inhibitor?[28]]

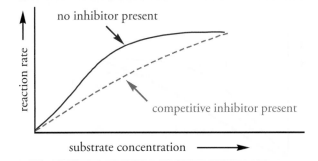

Figure 18   Competitive Inhibition

Noncompetitive inhibitors bind at an allosteric site, not at the active site. No matter how much substrate you add, the inhibitor will not be displaced from its site of action (see Figure 19). Hence, noncompetitive inhibition *does* diminish V_{max}. Remember that V_{max} is always calculated at the same enzyme concentration, since adding more enzyme will increase the measured V_{max}. Addition of a noncompetitive inhibitor changes the V_{max} and $V_{max}/2$ of the reaction, but typically does not alter K_m. This is because the substrate can still bind to the active site, but the inhibitor prevents the catalytic activity of the enzyme.

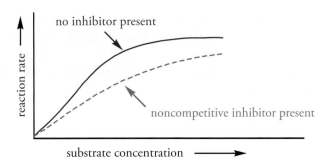

Figure 19   Noncompetitive Inhibition

---

[27]   Structurally, competitive inhibitors must at least resemble the substrate; however, the most effective competitive inhibitors resemble the transition state which the active site normally stabilizes.

[28]   No. The rate increase is greater than linear, indicating that the effect is caused by cooperativity.

- Carbon dioxide is an allosteric inhibitor of hemoglobin. It dissociates easily when Hb passes through the lungs, where the CO_2 can be exhaled. Carbon *mon*oxide, on the other hand, binds at the oxygen-binding site with an affinity 300 times greater than oxygen; it can be displaced by oxygen, but only when there is much more O_2 than CO in the environment. Which of the following is/are correct?[29]

> I. Carbon monoxide is an irreversible inhibitor.
> II. CO_2 is a reversible inhibitor.
> III. CO_2 is a noncompetitive inhibitor.

- In the figure below, the kinetics of an enzyme are plotted. In each case, an inhibitor may be present or absent. Which of the following statements is most likely true?[30]

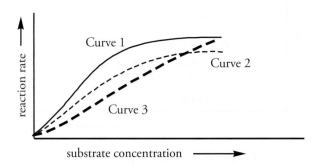

A) The enzyme is uninhibited in Curve 3.
B) Curve 1 represents noncompetitive inhibition of the enzyme.
C) The V_{max} values of Curve 2 and Curve 3 are the same.
D) Curve 3 represents competitive inhibition of the enzyme, and the enzyme is uninhibited in Curve 1.

If an inhibitor is only able to bind to the enzyme-substrate complex (that is, it cannot bind before the substrate has bound), it is referred to as an **uncompetitive inhibitor**. This effectively decreases V_{max} by limiting the amount of available enzyme-substrate complex which can be converted to product. By sequestering enzyme bound to substrate, this increases the apparent affinity of the enzyme for the substrate as it cannot readily dissociate (decreasing K_m).

---

[29] Item I: False. The question states that CO can be displaced by oxygen. **Item II: True.** The question states that it dissociates easily. **Item III: True.** The question states it binds allosterically, which means "at another site" (not the active site).

[30] Since Curve 3 and Curve 1 have the same V_{max}, but Curve 3 has a reduced rate of product formation, it suggests that Curve 3 represents competitive inhibition of the enzyme in Curve 1 (choice **D** is correct). If Curve 3 represented an uninhibited enzyme, it would have no other curves above it (choice A is wrong), and in no case would an inhibitor have a higher V_{max} than an uninhibited reaction (choice B is wrong). Lastly, it can be seen on the graph that Curve 2 has a reduced V_{max} compared to Curve 3 (choice C is wrong).

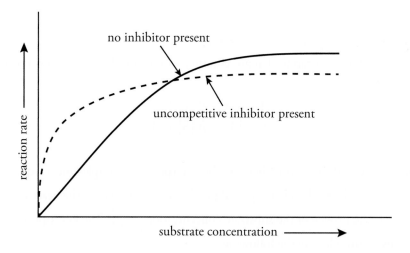

Figure 20   Uncompetitive Inhibition

Mixed-type inhibition occurs when an inhibitor can bind to either the unoccupied enzyme or the enzyme-substrate complex. If the enzyme has greater affinity for the inhibitor in its free form, the enzyme will have a lower affinity for the substrate similar to competitive inhibition (K_m increases). If the enzyme-substrate complex has greater affinity for the inhibitor, the enzyme will have an apparently greater affinity (K_m decreases) for the substrate similar to what we saw in uncompetitive inhibition. On the rare occasion where it displays equal affinity in both forms, it would actually be a noncompetitive inhibitor (many textbooks list noncompetitive inhibition as an example of mixed-type inhibition). In each of these situations, the inhibitor binds to an allosteric site and additional substrate cannot overcome inhibition (V_{max} decreases).

Inhibition Type	$V_{max,\,app}$	$K_{m,\,app}$
Competitive	V_{max}	↑
Noncompetitive	↓	no change
Uncompetitive	↓	↓
Mixed-type	↓	varies

Table 3   Changes in the Apparent V_{max} and K_m in Response to Various Types of Inhibition

7.8 LINEWEAVER-BURK PLOT

The Lineweaver-Burk plot is a graphical representation of enzyme kinetics using the Lineweaver-Burk Equation:

$$\frac{1}{V} = \left(\frac{K_m}{V_{max}}\right)\left(\frac{1}{[S]}\right) + \frac{1}{V_{max}}$$

The equation may appear intimidating but can be interpreted a simple linear equation of the form: $y = mx + b$. The graph is called a double reciprocal plot because the y-axis is the inverse of the reaction rate $\left(\frac{1}{V}\right)$ and the x-axis is the inverse of the substrate concentration $\left(\frac{1}{[S]}\right)$. The key aspects you need to know about the Lineweaver-Burk plot are the following:

1) The slope of the graph is $\dfrac{K_m}{V_{max}}$.

2) The y-intercept of the graph is $\dfrac{1}{V_{max}}$.

3) The x-intercept of the graph is $\dfrac{-1}{K_m}$.

Recall that increasing the substrate concentration ([S]) increases the reaction rate V up to a point. An increase in substrate concentration, however, is a *decrease* in the inverse of the substrate concentration $\left(\frac{1}{[S]}\right)$. Thus, an interesting aspect of the Lineweaver-Burk plot is that an increase in substrate concentration means a decrease in the value along the x-axis. Similarly, an increase in the reaction rate V is a *decrease* in the inverse of the reaction rate $\left(\frac{1}{V}\right)$. Thus, as the reaction rate increases, the value along the y-axis decreases.

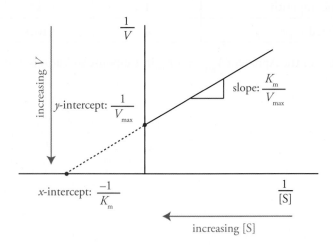

Figure 21   Lineweaver-Burk Plot

- How would the Lineweaver-Burk plot change when a uncompetitive inhibitor is added?[31]

---

[31] An uncompetitive inhibitor decreases the K_m (so the x-intercept shifted to the left) and decreases the V_{max} (so the y-intercept is shifted upward). The new line is parallel to the graph of the uninhibited enzyme.

Chapter 8
Carbohydrates and Carbohydrate Metabolism

8.1   MONOSACCHARIDES AND DISACCHARIDES

A single carbohydrate molecule is called a **monosaccharide** (meaning "single sweet unit"), also known as a **simple sugar**. Monosaccharides have the general chemical formula $C_nH_{2n}O_n$.

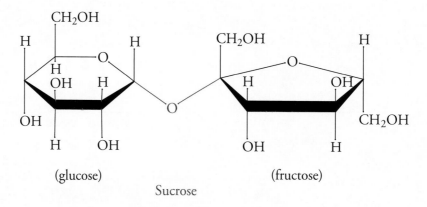

Fructose   Glucose   Ribose

Figure 1   Some Metabolically Important Monosaccharides

Two monosaccharides bonded together form a **disaccharide**, a few form an oligosaccharide, and many form a polysaccharide. The bond between two sugar molecules is called a **glycosidic linkage**. This is a covalent bond, formed in a dehydration reaction that requires enzymatic catalysis.

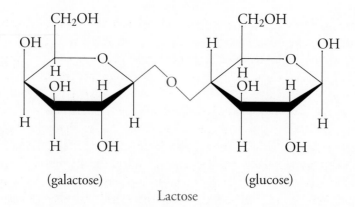

Figure 2   Disaccharides and the α- or β-Glycosidic Bond

Glycosidic linkages are named according to which carbon in each sugar comprises the linkage. The configuration (α or β) of the linkage is also specified. For example, lactose (milk sugar) is a disaccharide joined in a galactose-β-1,4-glucose linkage (above). Sucrose (table sugar) is also shown above, with a glucose unit and a fructose unit.

- Does sucrose contain an α- or β-glycosidic linkage?[1]

Some common disaccharides you might see on the MCAT are sucrose (Glc-α-1,2-Fru), lactose (Gal-β-1,4-Glc), maltose (Glc-α-1,4-Glc), and cellobiose (Glc-β-1,4-Glc). However, you should NOT try to memorize these linkages.

8.2 POLYSACCHARIDES

Polymers (polysaccharides) made from the common disaccharides listed above form important biological macromolecules. Glycogen serves as an energy storage carbohydrate in animals and is composed of thousands of glucose units joined in α-1,4 linkages; α-1,6 branches are also present. Starch is the same as glycogen (except that the branches are a little different), and it serves the same purpose in plants. Cellulose is a polymer of cellobiose, but note that cellobiose does not exist freely in nature. It exists only in its polymerized, cellulose form. The β-glycosidic bonds allow the polymer to assume a long, straight, fibrous shape. Wood and cotton are made of cellulose.

Hydrolysis of Glycosidic Linkages

The hydrolysis of polysaccharides into monosaccharides is favored thermodynamically. Hydrolysis is essential in order for these sugars to enter metabolic pathways (e.g., glycolysis) and be used for energy by the cell. However, this hydrolysis does not occur at a significant rate without enzymatic catalysis. Different enzymes catalyze the hydrolysis of different linkages. The enzymes are named for the sugar they hydrolyze. For example, the enzyme that catalyzes the hydrolysis of maltose into two glucose monosaccharides is called **maltase**. Each enzyme is highly specific for its linkage.

This specificity is a great example of the significance of stereochemistry. Consider cellulose. A cotton T-shirt is pure sugar. The only reason we can't digest it is that mammalian enzymes generally can't break down the β-glycosidic linkages found in cellulose. Cellulose is actually the energy source in grass and hay. Cows are mammals, and all mammals lack the enzymes necessary for cellulose breakdown. To live on grass, cows depend on bacteria that live in an extra stomach called a rumen to digest cellulose for them. If you're really on the ball, you're next question is: Humans are mammals, so how can we digest lactose, which has a β linkage? The answer is that we have a specific enzyme, **lactase**, which can digest lactose. This is an exception to the rule that mammalian enzymes cannot hydrolyze β-glycosidic linkages. People without lactase are **lactose malabsorbers**, and any lactose they eat ends up in the colon. There it may cause gas and diarrhea, if certain bacteria are present; people with this problem are said to be **lactose intolerant**. People produce lactase as children so that they can digest mother's milk, but most adults naturally stop making this enzyme, and thus become lactose malabsorbers and sometimes intolerant.

---

[1] The oxygen on the anomeric carbon of glucose is pointing down, which means the linkage is α-1,2. So, sucrose is Glc-α-1,2-Fru.

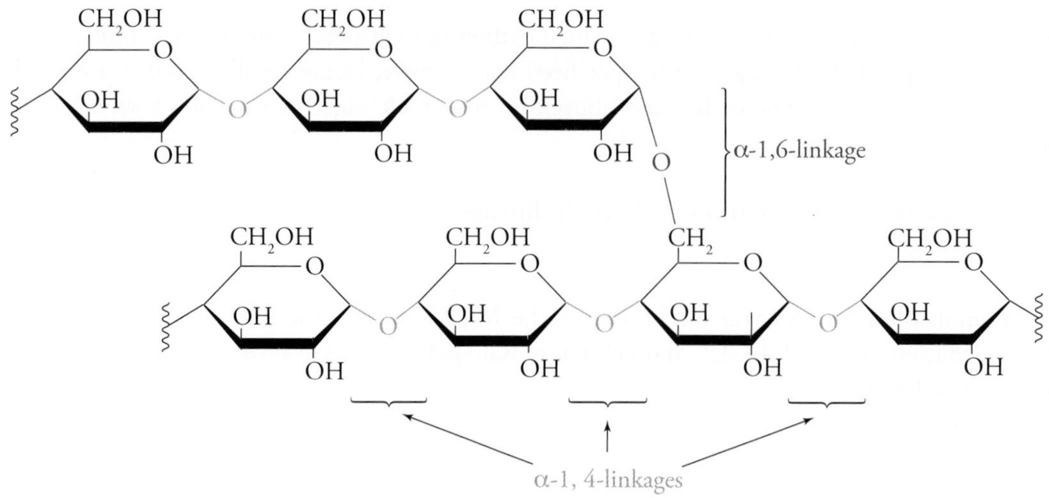

Figure 3 The Polysaccharide Glycogen

- Which requires net energy input: polysaccharide synthesis or hydrolysis?[2]
- If the activation energy of polysaccharide hydrolysis were so low that no enzyme was required for the reaction to occur, would this make polysaccharides better for energy storage?[3]

8.3 INTRODUCTION TO CELLULAR RESPIRATION

When glucose is oxidized to release energy, very little ATP is generated directly. Instead, the oxidation of glucose is accompanied by the reduction of high-energy electron carriers, nicotinamide adenine dinucleotide (**NAD**[+]) and flavin adenine dinucleotide (**FAD**). Each of these carriers accept high-energy electrons during redox reactions (forming **NADH** and **FADH₂**) and are later oxidized when they deliver the electrons to the electron transport chain. This generates the proton gradient that is used to generate ATP. Both of these carriers can serve as enzymatic cofactors and fulfill diverse roles in biological processes. For instance, NAD[+] is required for activation of adenylate cyclase by cholera toxin, and FAD can associate with a protein to become a **flavoprotein**. Dozens of flavoproteins have been characterized and are commonly involved in redox reactions (for example, amino acid metabolism).

Glucose is oxidized to produce CO_2 and ATP in a four-step process: glycolysis, the pyruvate dehydrogenase complex (PDC), the Krebs cycle, and electron transport/oxidative phosphorylation. The first stage is **glycolysis** ("glucose splitting"). Here glucose is partially oxidized while it is split in half, into two identical **pyruvic acid** molecules. [How many carbon atoms does pyruvic acid have?[4]] Glycolysis produces a small quantity of ATP and a small quantity of NADH. Glycolysis occurs in the cytoplasm and does not require oxygen.

In the second stage (the **pyruvate dehydrogenase complex**), the pyruvate produced in glycolysis is decarboxylated to form an acetyl group. The acetyl group is then attached to **coenzyme A**, a carrier that can transfer the acetyl group into the Krebs cycle. A small amount of NADH is produced.

---

2 Because hydrolysis of polysaccharides is thermodynamically favored, energy input is required to drive the reaction toward polysaccharide synthesis.

3 No, because then polysaccharides would hydrolyze spontaneously (they'd be unstable). The high activation energy of polysaccharide hydrolysis allows us to use enzymes as gatekeepers—when we need energy from glucose, we open the gate of glycogen hydrolysis.

4 The text states that glucose is split in half in the formation of pyruvate. Since glucose has six carbons, pyruvate must have three.

In the third stage, the Krebs cycle (also known as the tricarboxylic acid cycle (TCA cycle) or the citric acid cycle), the acetyl group from the PDC is added to oxaloacetate to form citric acid. The citric acid is then decarboxylated and isomerized to regenerate the original oxaloacetate. A modest amount of ATP, a large amount of NADH, and a small amount of $FADH_2$ are produced. Note that although the PDC and the Krebs cycle can only occur when oxygen is available to the cell, *neither uses oxygen directly*. Rather, oxygen is necessary for stage four, in which NADH and $FADH_2$ generated throughout cellular respiration are reconverted into NAD^+ and FAD. The PDC and the Krebs cycle occur in the innermost compartment of the mitochondria: the **matrix**.

In stage four of energy harvesting, **electron transport/oxidative phosphorylation**, the high-energy electrons carried by NADH and $FADH_2$ are oxidized by the **electron transport chain** in the inner mitochondrial membrane. The reduced electron carriers dump their electrons at the beginning of the chain, and oxygen is reduced to H_2O at the end. (The word *oxidative* in "oxidative phosphorylation" refers to the use of oxygen to oxidize the reduced electron carriers NADH and $FADH_2$.) The electron energy liberated by the transport chain is used to pump protons out of the innermost compartment of the mitochondrion. The protons are allowed to flow back into the mitochondrion, and the energy of this proton flow is used to produce the high-energy triphosphate group in ATP.

Glycolysis

Glycolysis is an extremely old pathway, having evolved several billion years ago. It is the universal first step in glucose metabolism, the extraction of energy from carbohydrates. All cells from *all domains* (a domain is the highest taxonomic category) possess the enzymes of this pathway. In glycolysis, a glucose molecule is oxidized and split into two pyruvate molecules, producing a net surplus of 2 ATP (from ADP + P_i) and producing 2 NADH (from NAD^+ + H^+):

$$\text{Glucose} + 2\text{ ADP} + 2\text{ P}_i + 2\text{ NAD}^+ \rightarrow 2\text{ Pyruvate} + 2\text{ ATP} + 2\text{ NADH} + 2\text{ H}_2\text{O} + 2\text{ H}^+$$

Of course, it's not quite that simple. Glycolysis involves several reactions, each of which is catalyzed by a different enzyme (see Figure 4). The general strategy is to first phosphorylate glucose on both ends and then split it into two 3-carbon units which can go on to the PDC and Krebs cycle. In the first step of glycolysis, a phosphate is taken from ATP and used to phosphorylate glucose, producing glucose 6-phosphate (G6P). This is isomerized to fructose 6-phosphate (F6P), which is then phosphorylated on carbon #1 (with the phosphate again taken from ATP) to produce fructose-1,6-bisphosphate (F1,6bP). This is split into two 3-carbon units that are oxidized to pyruvate, producing 2 ATP and 1 NADH per pyruvate, or 4 ATP and 2 NADH per glucose (since we get two 3-carbon units from each glucose). Don't forget that *each* glucose gives rise to *two* 3-carbon units which pass through the second part of glycolysis and into the Krebs cycle.

- An extract of yeast contains all of the enzymes required for glycolysis, ADP, P_i, Mg^{2+}, NAD^+ and glucose, but when these are all combined, none of the glucose is consumed. Provided that there are no enzyme inhibitors present, why doesn't the reaction proceed?[5]

---

[5] Although glycolysis results in a net ATP production, ATP is initially required to drive the reaction forward in the phosphorylation of glucose to glucose-6-phosphate and the phosphorylation of fructose-6-phosphate to fructose-1,6-bisphosphate. Without ATP to "prime the pump," there is no way to start the pathway. In case you're wondering about the Mg^{2+}, it's necessary for all reactions involving ATP.

Hexokinase catalyzes the first step in glycolysis, the phosphorylation of glucose to G6P. G6P feedback-inhibits hexokinase.

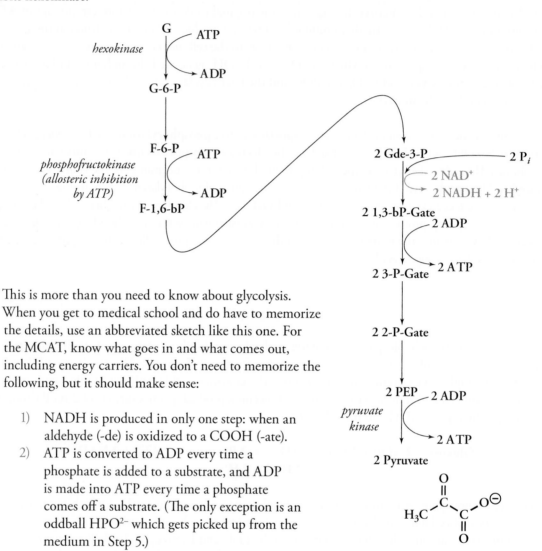

Figure 4 The 9 Reactions (Steps) of Glycolysis

This is more than you need to know about glycolysis. When you get to medical school and do have to memorize the details, use an abbreviated sketch like this one. For the MCAT, know what goes in and what comes out, including energy carriers. You don't need to memorize the following, but it should make sense:

1) NADH is produced in only one step: when an aldehyde (-de) is oxidized to a COOH (-ate).

2) ATP is converted to ADP every time a phosphate is added to a substrate, and ADP is made into ATP every time a phosphate comes off a substrate. (The only exception is an oddball HPO^{2-} which gets picked up from the medium in Step 5.)

Phosphofructokinase (PFK) catalyzes the third step: the transfer of a phosphate group from ATP to fructose-6-phosphate to form fructose-1,6-bisphosphate (F1,6bP). This is an important step because the reaction catalyzed by PFK is thermodynamically very favorable (like burning wood: $\Delta G \ll 0$), so it's practically irreversible. Also, G6P can be shunted to various pathways, but F1,6bP can only react in glycolysis. So once you light the PFK fire, you're committed to glycolysis. Hence, PFK is the key biochemical valve controlling the flow of substrate to product in glycolysis, and the conversion of F6P to F1,6bP is known as a **committed step**. In the remainder of glycolysis, F1,6bP is split into two 3-carbon molecules that are converted to pyruvate, with the production of NADH and ATP. Very favorable steps in enzymatic pathways (those with a large negative ΔG) are practically irreversible (because the back-reaction is so unfavorable). These reactions are the ones that are usually subject to allosteric regulation. Another generalization about what steps get regulated is this: early steps in a long pathway tend to be regulated. This makes sense; if you're going from A to Z, it's more practical to regulate the A → B reaction than the W → X one.

For example, the enzyme PFK is a key regulatory point in glycolysis. PFK is allosterically regulated by ATP. [What effect would you think a high concentration of ATP would have on PFK activity?[6]]

Two molecules of NAD^+ are reduced in glycolysis per glucose catabolized, forming 2 NADH. As discussed above, NADH is an electron carrier, a molecule that is responsible for shuttling energy in the form of **reducing power** (that is, reduction potential). Remember, these high energy electron carriers are not used directly as an energy source but are used later to generate ATP through electron transport and oxidative phosphorylation.

Fermentation

Under **aerobic** conditions (that is, in the presence of oxygen), the pyruvate produced in glycolysis enters the PDC and Krebs cycle to be oxidized completely to CO_2. The NADH produced in glycolysis and the PDC, as well as NADH and $FADH_2$ produced in the Krebs cycle, are all reoxidized in electron transport, where O_2 is the final electron acceptor. In **anaerobic** conditions (without oxygen), electron transport cannot function, and the limited supply of NAD^+ becomes entirely converted to NADH. [What effect would a limited supply of NAD^+ have on glycolysis?[7]]

Fermentation has evolved to regenerate NAD^+ in anaerobic conditions, thereby allowing glycolysis to continue in the absence of oxygen. Fermentation uses pyruvate as the acceptor of the high energy electrons from NADH (see Figure 5). Two examples of this process are (1) the reduction of pyruvate to ethanol (yeast do this in the making of beer, wine, etc.), and (2) the reduction of pyruvate to lactate in human muscle cells.

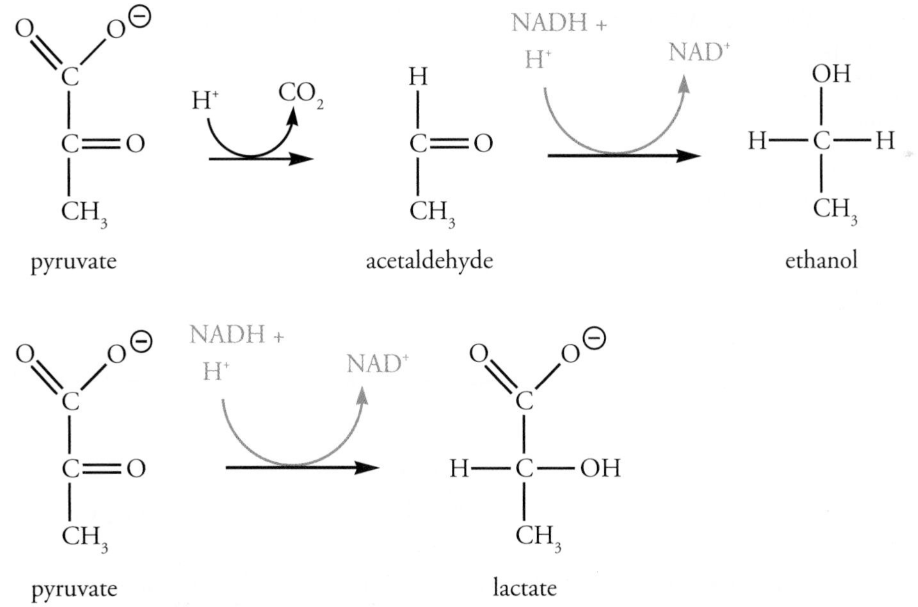

Figure 5   Anaerobic Pathways for Regeneration of NAD^+ from NADH

---

[6]   When energy (ATP) is abundant, the cell should slow glycolysis. High concentrations of ATP inhibit PFK activity by binding to an allosteric regulatory site. It is interesting to note that since ATP is a reactant in the reaction catalyzed by PFK, you would expect a high concentration of ATP to increase the rate of the reaction (Le Châtelier's principle). However, the inhibitory allosteric effects of ATP on PFK outweigh this thermodynamic consideration. So lowering the concentration of ATP will increase the reaction rate, even though ATP is a reactant. Of course, if the ATP level went too low, the reaction could not proceed at all.

[7]   If NAD^+ has all been converted to NADH, then the step in glycolysis that produces NADH (catalyzed by glyceraldehyde 3-phosphate dehydrogenase) cannot occur because it requires NAD^+ as a substrate. Thus, a lack of NAD^+ will *inhibit* glycolysis.

The NAD$^+$ produced by reducing pyruvate anaerobically is available for re-use in the glycolytic pathway, so more ATP can be produced. There is a limit to the use of anaerobic glycolysis as an energy source, however. The ethanol or lactate that is produced builds up, having no other use in the cell, and acts as a poison at high concentrations. Wine yeast die when the ethanol concentration reaches about 12 percent, and lactic acid is damaging at high concentrations in our tissues as well.

The Pyruvate Dehydrogenase Complex

The pyruvate produced in glycolysis in the cytoplasm is transported into the mitochondrial matrix, where it will be entirely oxidized to CO_2. Pyruvate does not enter the Krebs cycle directly, however. First it is oxidatively decarboxylated by the pyruvate dehydrogenase complex (PDC; Figure 6). **Oxidative decarboxylation** is a reaction repeated again in the Krebs cycle, in which a molecule is oxidized to release CO_2 and produce NADH. [In oxidative decarboxylation, pyruvate is changed from a 3-carbon molecule to a __, while __ is given off and __ is produced.[8]] The PDC changes pyruvate into an activated acetyl unit. An acetyl unit is [$(CH_3)(O=C-)$], and *activated* means the acetyl is not floating around freely but rather is attached to a carrier, namely **coenzyme A.** This coenzyme is basically a long handle with a sulfur at the end, abbreviated CoA-SH. It is used in many reaction systems to pass acetyl units around (for example, fatty acid and cholesterol synthesis and degradation). When loaded with an acetyl unit, CoA-SH is abbreviated acetyl-CoA. The bond between sulfur and the acetyl group is high energy, making it easy for acetyl-CoA to transfer the acetyl fragment into the Krebs cycle for further oxidation. Regulation of the PDC is crucial. [AMP (adenosine monophosphate) is a low-energy molecule produced by the hydrolysis of ATP during metabolism. [What effect would you predict a high level of AMP to have on the activity of pyruvate dehydrogenase?[9]]

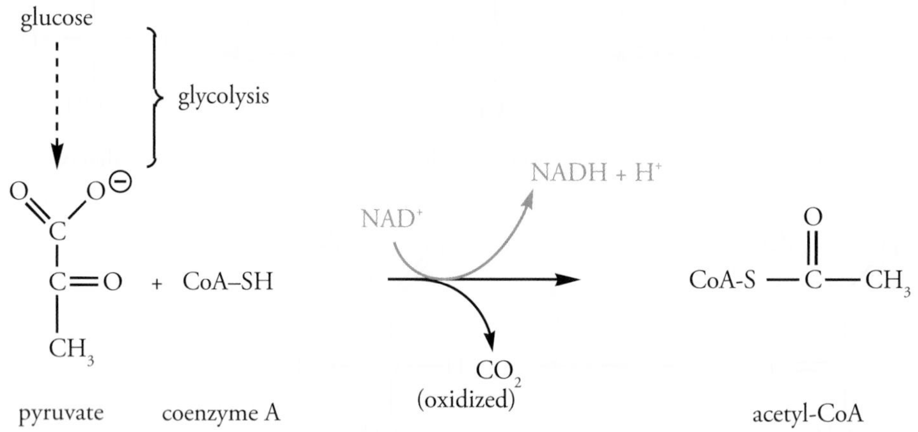

Figure 6   Oxidation of Pyruvate by Pyruvate Dehydrogenase

---

[8] Pyruvate is converted to a 2-carbon molecule, CO_2 is given off, and NADH is made from NAD$^+$. You can figure all of this out based on your knowledge of oxidative decarboxylation. Also, note the name of the enzyme, "dehydrogenase." To remove a hydrogen (*dehydrogenate*) is to oxidize. So the name of the enzyme also tells us that pyruvate is oxidized.

[9] A high ratio of AMP or ADP to ATP is described as low-energy charge. A low-energy charge will stimulate the PDC, increasing the rate of entry of pyruvate into the Krebs cycle.

The Krebs Cycle

The **Krebs cycle** is a group of reactions which take the 2-carbon acetyl unit from acetyl-CoA, combine it with oxaloacetate, and release two CO_2 molecules. NADH and $FADH_2$ are generated in the process. The figure below shows an overview of the process; note that many of the names are not necessary to know and have intentionally been left out.

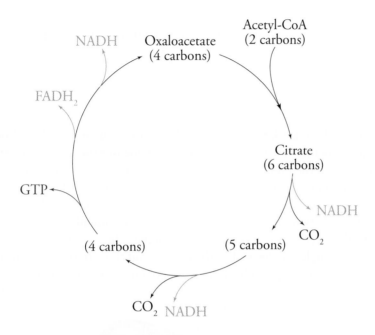

Figure 7   Overview of the Krebs Cycle

These reduced electron carriers (NADH and $FADH_2$) go on to generate ATP in electron transport and oxidative phosphorylation. Two other names for the Krebs cycle are the **tricarboxylic acid cycle** (**TCA cycle**) and the **citric acid cycle**. Citrate is the first intermediate produced in the cycle, as soon as the acetyl unit is supplied. Citrate possesses three carboxylic acid functional groups, hence the term "tricarboxylic acid." Note that a molecule with three carboxylic acids is ready to be oxidatively decarboxylated. We will now break the multistep cycle down into three general stages.

Krebs Stage 1: The two carbons in the acetate fragment of acetyl-CoA are condensed with the 4-carbon compound **oxaloacetate** (OAA; the name is worth remembering), producing **citrate.**

Krebs Stage 2: Citrate is further oxidized to release CO_2 and to produce NADH from NAD^+ with each oxidative decarboxylation. Citrate is first isomerized to form isocitrate, which is then oxidatively decarboxylated to yield the 5-carbon compound α-ketoglutarate, one carbon dioxide, and one NADH. Then α-ketoglutarate is oxidatively decarboxylated to produce succinyl-CoA (four carbons), releasing another CO_2 and producing another NADH.

Krebs Stage 3: OAA is regenerated so that the cycle can continue. In the process, reducing power is stored in 1 NADH and 1 $FADH_2$, and a high-energy phosphate bond is produced directly as GTP. Here GTP plays the role normally reserved for ATP. This GTP will eventually transfer its high-energy phosphate bond to ADP, converting it into ATP. $FADH_2$ is similar to NADH, but ultimately results in the production of less ATP.

8.3

To review, the oxidation of glucose has so far created:

1) 2 ATP and 2 NADH per glucose molecule in glycolysis
2) Pyruvate Dehydrogenase: 2 NADH per glucose (one per pyruvate)
3) Krebs cycle: 6 NADH, 2 $FADH_2$, and 2 GTP per glucose

Thus, most of the energy of glucose is not extracted directly as ATP (or GTP) but in high-energy electron carriers.

Compartmentalization of Glucose Catabolism in Eukaryotes: The Mitochondria

To understand oxidative phosphorylation, you must know the structure of the mitochondrion (Figure 8). The mitochondrion contains two membranes, an **outer membrane** and an **inner membrane**, each composed of a lipid bilayer. The outer membrane is smooth and contains large pores formed by **porin** proteins. The inner membrane is impermeable, even to very small items like H^+, and is densely folded into structures termed **cristae**. The cristae extend into the **matrix**, which is the innermost space of the mitochondrion. The space between the two membranes, the **intermembrane space**, is continuous with the cytoplasm due to the large pores in the outer membrane. The enzymes of the Krebs cycle and the pyruvate dehydrogenase complex are located in the matrix, and those of the electron transport chain and ATP synthase involved in oxidative phosphorylation are bound to the inner mitochondrial membrane.

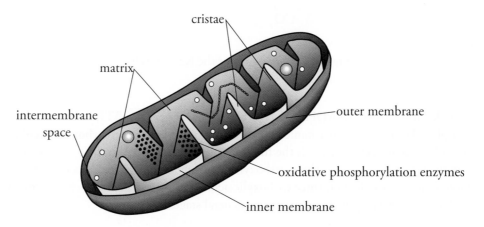

Figure 8 The Mitochondrion

The two goals of electron transport/oxidative phosphorylation are to:

1) reoxidize all the electron carriers reduced in glycolysis, PDC, and the Krebs cycle, and
2) store energy in the form of ATP in the process.

Where are all the reduced electron carriers located? Per each glucose catabolized, two NADH are created by glycolysis in the cytoplasm; the electrons from these NADH will have to be transported into the mitochondria before they can be passed along the electron transport chain. All the other NADHs and $FADH_2$s were produced inside the mitochondrial matrix, so they are in the right place to donate electrons to the electron transport chain.

The situation in prokaryotes is a bit different: all of the reduced electron carriers are located in the cytoplasm. In fact, everything is located in the cytoplasm, since there are *no membrane-bound organelles at all* in prokaryotes (no mitochondria, no nucleus, no lysosomes—everything just floats around in the cytoplasm). Since they have no mitochondria, can bacteria perform oxidative phosphorylation? *Yes, they can!* The way the process works is that a proton gradient must be created and then used to power ATP synthesis by the membrane-bound **ATP synthase**. So all that's required is a membrane impermeable to protons. Eukaryotes use the inner mitochondrial membrane; bacteria just use their cell membrane. The end result of this difference is that when eukaryotes perform aerobic respiration, they have to shuttle the electrons from cytosolic NADH into the mitochondrial matrix (at the cost of some energy) but bacteria do not. So, all things considered, prokaryotes get two more high-energy phosphate bonds from aerobic respiration than eukaryotes do (this will be discussed in more detail in just a bit). From this point forward, we will discuss the eukaryotic system. Remember that it's the same in prokaryotes except that they do it on the cell membrane instead of on the inner mitochondrial membrane (since they have no mitochondria!).

Electron Transport and Oxidative Phosphorylation

Oxidative phosphorylation is the oxidation of the high-energy electron carriers NADH and $FADH_2$ coupled to the phosphorylation of ADP to produce ATP. The energy released through oxidation of NADH and $FADH_2$ by the electron transport chain is used to pump protons out of the mitochondrial matrix. This proton gradient is the source of energy used to drive the phosphorylation of ADP to ATP. The **electron-transport chain** is a group of five electron carriers (Figure 9). Each member of the chain reduces the next member down the line. All five are named for their redox roles. Three of them are large protein complexes found embedded in the inner mitochondrial membrane. They are classified as **cytochromes** due to the presence of a heme group, a porphyrin ring containing a tightly-bound iron atom. The other two members of the electron transport chain are small mobile electron carriers. The chain is organized so that the first large carrier receives electrons (reducing power) from NADH; the NADH is thus oxidized to NAD^+. Hence, the first large carrier in the e^- transport chain ("A" in the figure) is called **NADH dehydrogenase**. It passes its electrons to one of the small carriers in the transport chain, called **ubiquinone**, also known as **coenzyme Q**. NADH dehydrogenase is also known as **coenzyme Q reductase**.

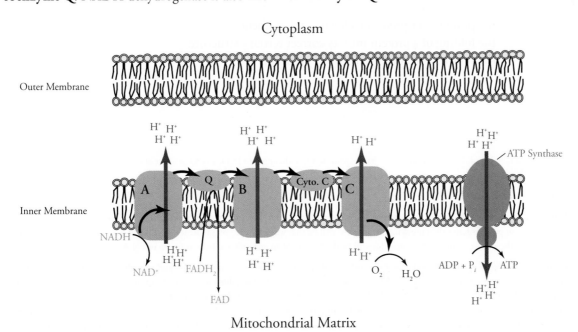

Figure 9 The Electron Transport Chain

Ubiquinone then passes its electrons to the second large membrane-bound complex in the chain ("B"), known as **cytochrome C reductase**. From this name, you can guess what the next carrier in the chain is called; it is **cytochrome C**, a small hydrophilic protein bound loosely to the inner mitochondrial membrane. The last member of the electron transport chain ("C") is simply called **cytochrome C oxidase**. [What accepts electrons from cytochrome C oxidase?[10]]

Each of the three large membrane-bound proteins in the electron transport chain pumps protons across the inner mitochondrial membrane every time electrons flow past. Protons are pumped out of the matrix, into the intermembrane space. The inner mitochondrial membrane is highly impermeable to protons. As a result, the electron transport chain creates a large proton gradient, with the pH being much __[11] (higher/lower) inside the matrix than in the rest of the cell.

What does this have to do with ATP synthesis? Well, there is one more very important protein embedded in the inner mitochondrial membrane: **ATP synthase**. It is a large protein complex which contains a proton channel that spans the inner membrane. The passage of protons from the intermembrane space through the ATP synthase channel causes it to synthesize ATP from ADP + P_i. Thus, ATP production is dependent on a **proton gradient**. The overall process of electron transport and ATP production is said to be *coupled* by the proton gradient. Together, electron transport and ATP production are known as **oxidative phosphorylation**. Make sure you understand these questions:

- Dinitrophenol (DNP) is an uncoupler: It destroys the proton gradient by allowing protons to flow into the matrix. Which one of the following processes does it inhibit first?[12]
  A) Pyruvate decarboxylation by the PDC
  B) The TCA cycle
  C) Electron transport
  D) Muscular contraction

- Which one of the following processes has a negative ΔG under normal aerobic conditions in the cell?[13]
  A) ATP synthesis
  B) The pumping of protons to form a pH gradient
  C) The folding of a protein into its correct tertiary structure
  D) The synthesis of acetyl-CoA from pyruvate

---

[10] If it's the last member of the chain, it must pass its electrons to O_2, reducing it to H_2O, an end product of electron transport. This is the only reason we breathe and the only reason we evolved with lungs, RBCs, etc.

[11] higher (remember, high pH = low $[H^+]$)

[12] If the proton gradient is destroyed, the processes in A, B, and C will continue unabated, because NADH will be reoxidized to NAD^+ at a normal rate, or perhaps faster than normal. The problem will be that without a proton gradient no ATP will get made from all this glucose breakdown. The answer is choice **D** because this will be the first problem encountered from running out of ATP.

[13] Choices A, B, and D are all thermodynamically unfavorable processes that have a positive ΔG and must be driven forward by coupling to thermodynamically favorable processes. ATP synthesis is coupled to the favorable movement of protons down a gradient, pumping of protons against their gradient is coupled to the favorable movement of electrons down the electron transport chain, and the synthesis of acetyl-CoA from pyruvate is coupled to the favorable loss of carbon as carbon dioxide. However, folding of a protein into its correct tertiary structure is thermodynamically favorable and will occur spontaneously without any external energy input; it would have a negative ΔG.

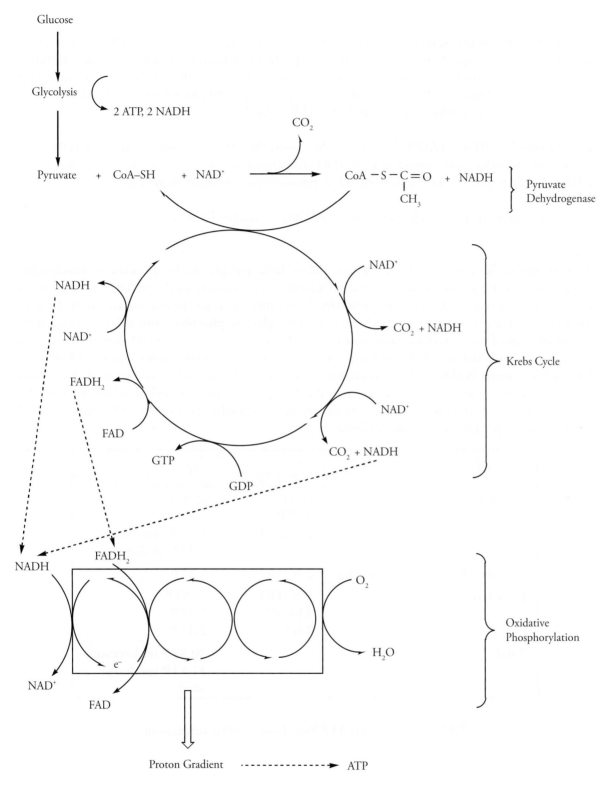

Figure 10   Cellular Respiration

Energetics of Glucose Catabolism

How is electron transport quantitatively connected to ATP synthesis? For every NADH that is oxidized to NAD$^+$, the three large electron transport proteins pump about ten protons across the inner mitochondrial membrane, into the intermembrane space. The "cost" of ATP synthesis is about four protons per molecule of ATP. Since NADH is responsible for the pumping of 10 protons, each molecule of NADH provides the energy to produce approximately 2.5 ATP molecules.

Even though NADH and FADH$_2$ have similar functions, their fates are a little different. FADH$_2$ gives its electrons to ubiquinone instead of to NADH dehydrogenase. By bypassing the first proton pump, FADH$_2$ is only responsible for the pumping of six protons across the inner membrane.

- How many ATP are made every time an FADH$_2$ is reoxidized to FAD?[14]

As mentioned earlier, the PDC, the Krebs cycle and oxidative phosphorylation all occur in mitochondria in eukaryotes, while glycolysis occurs in the cytoplasm. The electrons from the NADH generated in glycolysis must be transported into the mitochondria before they can enter the electron transport chain. In most cells, they are transported by a pathway termed the **glycerol phosphate shuttle**. This shuttle delivers the electrons directly to ubiquinone (just like FADH$_2$ does), bypassing NADH dehydrogenase, and results in the production of only 1.5 molecules of ATP per cytosolic NADH, rather than the 2.5 normally formed from matrix NADH.[15] Bacteria, because they lack cellular organelles, do not need to transport cytosolic electrons across any membranes; hence the discrepancy in the table below in how much ATP is yielded from each NADH from glycolysis in eukaryotes compared to prokaryotes. All values in the following table are per glucose molecule catabolized.

Process	Molecules Formed/Used	ATP Equivalents
Glycolysis	−2 ATP 4 ATP 2 NADH	−2 ATP 4 ATP 3 ATP (eukaryotes) 5 ATP (prokaryotes)
Pyruvate Dehydrogenase Complex	2 NADH	5 ATP
Krebs Cycle	6 NADH 2 FADH$_2$ 2 GTP	15 ATP 3 ATP 2 ATP
Total		**30 ATP (eukaryotes)** **32 ATP (prokaryotes)**

Table 1   Theoretical ATP Yield from Cellular Respiration

---

[14] Only 1.5 ATP are made as a result of the reoxidation of FADH$_2$. Six protons divided by four protons per ATP equals 1.5 ATP.

[15] Some high energy-requiring tissues (such as liver and cardiac muscle cells) utilize a different shuttle (the malate-aspartate shuttle) to bring the electrons to NADH hydrogenase, thus getting the full 2.5 ATP from those electrons. But this is the exception, and generally the MCAT does not test exceptions.

Notes:

1) These numbers are an estimate of the theoretical maximum amount of ATP that can be produced from a single molecule of glucose. As the proton gradient is used to transport other molecules into or out of the matrix, the actual yield may differ depending on the number of protons (that is, the gradient) available for ATP synthesis.

2) These numbers reflect the most recent understanding of ATP synthesis, and as such, may not appear in some textbooks that still cling to the previously established counts of 36 ATP per glucose in eukaryotes and 38 ATP per glucose in prokaryotes.

8.4 GLUCONEOGENESIS

Gluconeogenesis occurs when dietary sources of glucose are unavailable and when the liver has depleted its stores of glycogen and glucose (more on glycogen metabolism in a bit). This process occurs primarily in the liver (and to a lesser extent in the kidneys), and it involves converting non-carbohydrate precursor molecules (such as lactate, pyruvate, Krebs cycle intermediates, and the carbon skeletons of most amino acids) into intermediates of the above pathways where they ultimately become glucose. Gluconeogenesis is an 11-step pathway that uses many of the same enzymes as glycolysis. In simplified terms, it can be thought of as "glycolysis-in-reverse," where those enzymes catalyzing the irreversible reactions (hexokinase, phosphofructokinase, and pyruvate kinase) have been replaced.

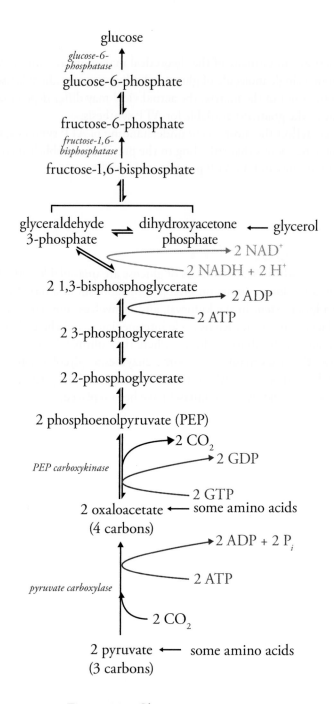

Figure 11   Gluconeogenesis

In Figure 11, starting from the bottom and working towards the top (i.e., starting with pyruvate), the first reaction of gluconeogenesis adds CO_2 to pyruvate, converting it to oxaloacetate. This step requires ATP hydrolysis and is run by the enzyme **pyruvate carboxylase**. In the very next step, oxaloacetate is decarboxylated and phosphorylated to form phosphoenolpyruvate (PEP); this step is run by **phosphoenolpyruvate carboxykinase (PEPCK)**. While this might seem odd (add CO_2 to then remove CO_2), oxidative decarboxylation is a favorable process, and it is often used to drive less favorable reactions. This same process is used in fatty acid synthesis as well.

The next several steps are run by the same enzymes as in glycolysis (PEP to fructose-1,6-bisphosphate). However, the phosphorylation of fructose-6-P to form fructose-1,6-bisP in glycolysis is essentially irreversible ($\Delta G \ll 0$), so it will require an enzyme other than PFK to reverse it. **Fructose-1,6-bisphosphatase** catalyzes the removal of a phosphate group from fru-1,6-bisP to form fru-6-P. This is then isomerized to glu-6-P and dephosphorylated by the final enzyme, **glucose-6-phosphatase** (as with fru-1,6-bisP, the reaction to form glucose-6-P in glycolysis is irreversible; therefore, its dephosphorylation must be run by an enzyme other than hexokinase). Furthermore, the dephosphorylation of glu-6-P is required in order for glucose to be released from liver cells into the bloodstream. Phosphorylated glucose is charged and cannot cross the cell membrane. This "newly-made" glucose can now travel to other cells in the body so that they can take it up and use it for energy.

Altogether then, gluconeogenesis requires six high-energy phosphate bonds (four ATP and two GTP) and two reduced electron carriers (two NADH).

- As discussed previously, glycolysis is a thermodynamically favorable process with an overall $\Delta G < 0$. Since gluconeogenesis primarily reverses the steps of glycolysis, what allows it to also be thermodynamically favorable?[16]

Note that while the majority of the intermediates discussed in cellular respiration can take part in gluconeogenesis, acetyl-CoA cannot. This helps explain why free fatty acids cannot be converted to glucose during periods of starvation, while the glycerol backbone of a triglyceride can.

8.5   REGULATION OF GLYCOLYSIS AND GLUCONEOGENESIS

Pathways that serve opposing roles (e.g., glycolysis and gluconeogenesis) must be tightly regulated to prevent the net loss of energy due to **futile cycling** (running both pathways at the same time). Therefore, **reciprocal control** in response to current cellular needs is critical. In reciprocal control, the same molecule regulates two enzymes in opposite ways.

As we already know, glycolysis and gluconeogenesis utilize many of the same enzymes. Attempts to regulate any one of these would fail to isolate a single pathway, so regulation must focus on those enzymes catalyzing irreversible reactions. Two such heavily-regulated enzymes are **phosphofructokinase (PFK)** and **fructose-1,6-bisphosphatase (F-1,6-BPase)**. These enzymes serve opposing roles in glycolysis and gluconeogenesis, respectively. Both enzymes are allosterically regulated by glycolytic intermediates that activate one enzyme while inhibiting the other. For instance, in energy-starved states, elevated cellular AMP levels activate PFK while inhibiting F-1,6-BPase, resulting in enhanced glycolysis activity and a suppression of gluconeogenesis.

---

[16] There are three major steps in glycolysis with a $\Delta G < 0$ (the other steps have a ΔG close to 0). In gluconeogenesis, these same steps would have a $\Delta G > 0$. However, they are made thermodynamically favorable ($\Delta G < 0$) by coupling the reactions to the hydrolysis of the high energy phosphate bonds of GTP and ATP ($\Delta G \ll 0$).

Another metabolic intermediate that exerts reciprocal control on these two enzymes is **fructose-2,6-bisphosphate (F-2,6-BP)**. Its intracellular concentration is set by a single large protein that functions as two separate enzymes: one that synthesizes F-2,6-BP and one that breaks it down. **Insulin** and **glucagon** help control the concentration of intracellular F-2,6-BP by regulating the activity of this large protein. Note that F-2,6-BP stimulates PFK (thus stimulating glycolysis) and inhibits fructose-1,6-bisphosphatase (thus inhibiting gluconeogenesis). To better illustrate how this works, let us consider an example. When blood glucose levels are high, insulin is released from the pancreas. Insulin stimulates the formation of F-2,6-BP, leading to the stimulation of PFK and activation of the glycolytic pathway. Simultaneously, the F-2,6-BP inhibits fructose-1,6-bisphosphatase, turning off gluconeogenesis so that these opposing pathways do not run at the same time. The reverse situation occurs when blood glucose levels are low; under these conditions, glucagon (also released from the pancreas) triggers the breakdown of F-2,6-BP. The drop in F-2,6-BP levels stops the stimulation of PFK, thus inhibiting glycolysis, and stops the inhibition of fructose-1,6-bisphosphatase, thus stimulating gluconeogenesis.

- Following a high carb meal, the blood concentration of insulin _____ and glucagon _____.[17]

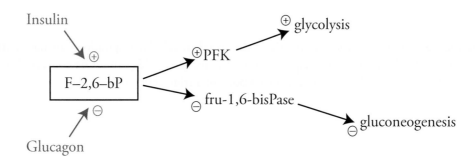

Figure 12 Hormonal Regulation of Glycolysis and Gluconeogenesis

Overview

In order to meet the varied metabolic demands of the cell, many additional forms of regulation occur beyond the limited examples outlined here. The following general principles, however, allow for reasonable predictions of the activity of a given pathway in response to cellular conditions:

1) In a pathway, those enzymes which catalyze irreversible (that is, exergonic) reactions are frequently sites of regulation.
2) Increased concentrations of intermediates in a pathway generally serve to decrease the activity of that pathway (for example, citrate decreases the activity of PFK in glycolysis).
3) Each pathway responds to the energy state of the cell. Cellular respiration is stimulated by energy deficits (for example, high ADP:ATP or NAD^+:NADH ratios) and inhibited by energy surpluses (for example, high ATP:ADP or NADH:NAD^+ ratios).

---

[17] Following a high-carb meal, the blood concentration of insulin increases and glucagon decreases. If you have a lot of carbs in your blood, you don't need to make any more!

The table below outlines some of the regulatory steps described in this chapter.

Pathway	Enzyme	Positive Regulators	Negative Regulators
Glycolysis	Phosphofructokinase	Fructose-2,6-bisphosphate	ATP
		AMP	
Gluconeogenesis	Fructose-1,6-bisphosphatase	ATP	Fructose-2,6-bisphosphate
			AMP

Table 2 Summary of Metabolic Regulation

8.6 GLYCOGEN METABOLISM

Glycogen is a polymer of glucose that is found in muscle and liver cells, and it is the main form of carbohydrate storage in animals. Glycogenesis, the formation of glycogen, starts with glucose-6-phosphate. The molecule is isomerized in a reversible reaction to glucose-1-phosphate by the enzyme phosphoglucomutase. Glu-1-P is activated with UTP to form UDP-glucose, which is added to the growing glycogen polymer by glycogen synthase.

Glycogenolysis starts with the phosphorylation and removal of one glucose unit at the end of the polymer, producing glucose-1-P. This is isomerized to glu-6-P, which can then reenter the glycolytic pathway. As in gluconeogenesis, in order to release the glucose into the bloodstream it must be dephosphorylated with glucose-6-phosphatase.

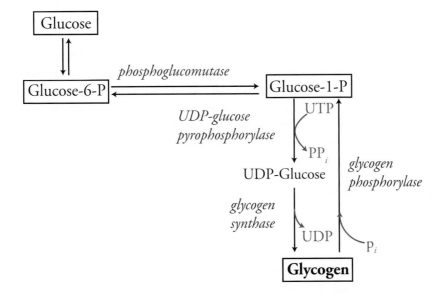

Figure 13 Glycogen Metabolism

Glycogenesis and glycogenolysis occur in both the liver and in skeletal muscle. Liver glycogen is broken down to maintain blood glucose levels during fasting states, while skeletal muscle glycogen is broken down to supply the skeletal muscle with glucose during exercise. Thus, skeletal muscle lacks glucose-6-phosphatase; the absence of this enzyme keeps the glucose phosphorylated and unable to leave the muscle cell.

Glycogenesis and glycogenolysis are opposing processes, controlled by the hormones that regulate blood sugar levels and energy. Insulin, released when blood glucose is high, stimulates glycogenesis. At first this seems paradoxical, as insulin was discussed above as a positive regulator of glycolysis (i.e., glucose breakdown), and it is not immediately apparent why breakdown and storage would be stimulated by the same hormone. However, it makes sense when you consider that it's unnecessary for all of the food just consumed to be immediately turned into energy, just as you don't necessarily need to spend your entire paycheck the moment you get it. You might spend some and put the rest in the bank. So insulin stimulates glycolysis (spending some of your paycheck) as well as glycogenesis (putting the rest in the bank).

Glycogenolysis occurs in response to glucagon, when blood sugar levels are low. It results in glucose being released from the liver into the blood where it can then be taken up by cells and enter glycolysis.

- Patients with Von Gierke's disease have a deficiency in the enzyme glucose-6-phosphatase. What would you expect these patients' blood glucagon and insulin levels to be?[18]

8.7 PENTOSE PHOSPHATE PATHWAY

The **pentose phosphate pathway** (PPP, also known as the hexose monophosphate shunt) diverts glucose-6-phosphate from glycolysis in order to form NADPH, ribose-5-phosphate, and glycolytic intermediates. This cytoplasmic pathway is composed of an irreversible oxidative phase followed by a non-oxidative phase consisting of a series of reversible reactions. NADPH and ribose-5-P are made in the oxidative phase, while the glycolytic intermediates are formed in the non-oxidative phase.

NADPH, although sharing much of its structure with NADH, has a different cellular role and serves as an important reducing agent in many anabolic processes (most notably, fatty acid synthesis). It also aids in the neutralization of reactive oxygen species. Ribose-5-P is used to synthesize nucleotides, while the other carbohydrate intermediates can be returned to glycolysis. Therefore, the "shunt" part of hexose monophosphate shunt...glucose can be shunted out of glycolysis to generate NADPH and ribose-5-P when necessary, and the glycolytic intermediates shunted back in.

- In order for NADPH to be an effective reducing agent, should the ratio of NADPH to $NADP^+$ in the cell be high or low?[19]

---

[18] Without glucose-6-phosphatase, patients with von Gierke's disease are unable to produce free glucose from glycogen (and gluconeogenesis). As a result, these patients would have low blood-glucose levels, leading to chronically high levels of glucagon and low levels of insulin.

[19] A reducing agent is a substance that causes other molecules to be reduced (and is itself oxidized). As NADPH is the reduced form of $NADP^+$, you would want a high NADPH to $NADP^+$ ratio. This would favor the oxidation of NADPH in order for other molecules to be reduced.

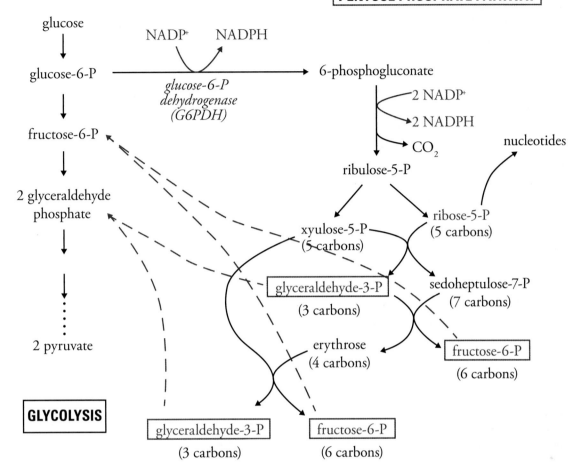

Figure 14   Pentose Phosphate Pathway

The first enzyme in the PPP, **glucose-6-phosphate dehydrogenase (G6PDH)**, is the primary point of regulation. Its product, NADPH, acts via negative feedback to inhibit G6PDH. The two successive oxidations in this part of the pathway (thus the name "oxidative phase") generate 2 NADPH. A deficiency of this enzyme (which is a common heritable disease) limits the ability of red blood cells to eliminate reactive oxygen species; this can lead to cell death and potential renal and hepatic complications.

Chapter 9
Lipids

9.1 INTRODUCTION TO LIPIDS

Lipids are oily or fatty substances that play three primary physiological roles, summarized here and discussed below.

1) In adipose cells, triglycerides (fats) store energy.
2) In cellular membranes, phospholipids constitute a barrier between intracellular and extracellular environments.
3) Cholesterol is a special lipid that serves as the building block for the hydrophobic steroid hormones.

The cardinal characteristic of the lipid is its **hydrophobicity**. *Hydrophobic* means "water-fearing." It is important to understand the significance of this. Since water is very polar, polar substances dissolve well in water; these are known as "water-loving," or **hydrophilic** substances. Carbon-carbon bonds and carbon-hydrogen bonds are nonpolar. Hence, substances that contain only carbon and hydrogen will not dissolve well in water. Some examples: Table sugar dissolves well in water, but cooking oil floats in a layer above water or forms many tiny oil droplets when mixed with water. Cotton T-shirts become wet when exposed to water because they are made of glucose polymerized into cellulose, but a nylon jacket does not become wet because it is composed of atoms covalently bound together in a nonpolar fashion.

Fatty Acid Structure

Fatty acids are composed of long unsubstituted alkanes that end in a carboxylic acid. The chain is typically 14 to 18 carbons long, and because they are synthesized two carbons at a time from acetate, predominantly *even-numbered* fatty acids are made in human cells. A fatty acid with no carbon-carbon double bonds is said to be **saturated** with hydrogen because every carbon atom in the chain is covalently bound to the maximum of hydrogens. **Unsaturated** fatty acids have one or more double bonds in the tail. These double bonds are almost always (Z) (or *cis*).

Saturated fatty acid

Unsaturated fatty acid

- Compared to a saturated fat, would it take more or less energy to change the state of an unsaturated fat from solid to liquid?[1]
- If fatty acids are mixed into water, how are they likely to associate with each other?[2]

---

[1] The presence of cis double bonds in unsaturated fats causes them to pack together less tightly than saturated fats, which have a more regular carbon chain structure. The result is that it takes less energy to change the state of an unsaturated fat from solid to liquid than it does to change a saturated fat.

[2] The long hydrophobic chains will interact with each other to minimize contact with water, exposing the charged carboxyl group to the aqueous environment.

Figure 1 illustrates how free fatty acids interact in an aqueous solution; they form a structure called a **micelle**. The force that drives the tails into the center of the micelle is called the **hydrophobic interaction**. The hydrophobic interaction is a complex phenomenon. In general, it results from the fact that water molecules must form an orderly **solvation shell** around each hydrophobic substance. The reason is that H_2O has a dipole that "likes" to be able to share its charges with other polar molecules. A solvation shell allows for the most water-water interaction and the least water-lipid interaction. In the case of the fatty acid micelle, water forms a shell around the spherical micelle with the result being that water interacts with polar carboxylic acid head groups while hydrophobic lipid tails hide inside the sphere.

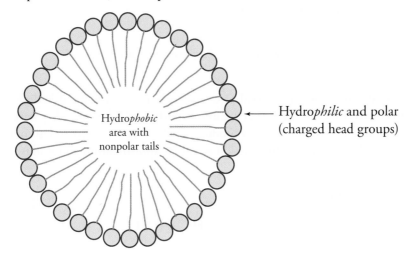

Figure 1   A Fatty Acid Micelle

- How does soap help to remove grease from your hands?[3]

9.2   TRIACYLGLYCEROLS (TG)

The storage form of the fatty acid is fat. The technical name for fat is **triacylglycerol** or **triglyceride** (see Figure 2 on the next page). The triglyceride is composed of three fatty acids esterified to a glycerol molecule. Glycerol is a three-carbon triol with the formula $HOCH_2–CHOH–CH_2OH$. As you can see, it has three hydroxyl groups that can be esterified to fatty acids. It is necessary to store fatty acids in the relatively inert form of fat because free fatty acids are reactive chemicals.

---

[3]   Grease is hydrophobic. It does not wash off easily in water because it is not soluble in water. Scrubbing your hands with soap causes micelles to form around the grease particles.

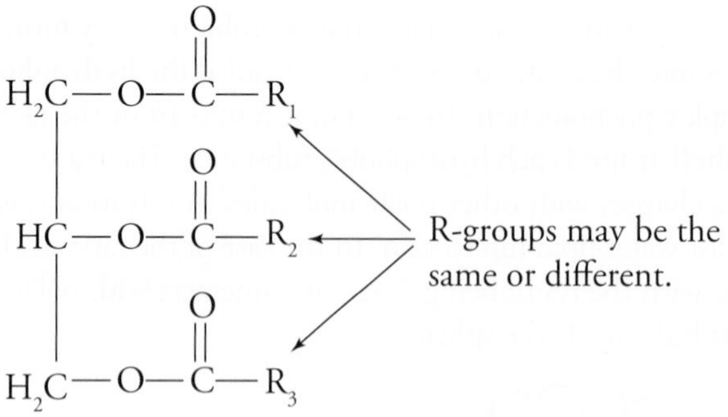

9.2

Figure 2   A Triglyceride (Fat)

The triacylglycerol undergoes reactions typical of esters, such as base-catalyzed hydrolysis. Soaps are the sodium salts of fatty acids (RCOO–Na⁺). They are **amphipathic**, which means they have both hydrophilic and hydrophobic regions. Soap is economically produced by base-catalyzed hydrolysis of triglycerides from animal fat into fatty acid salts (soaps). This reaction is called **saponification** and is illustrated below.

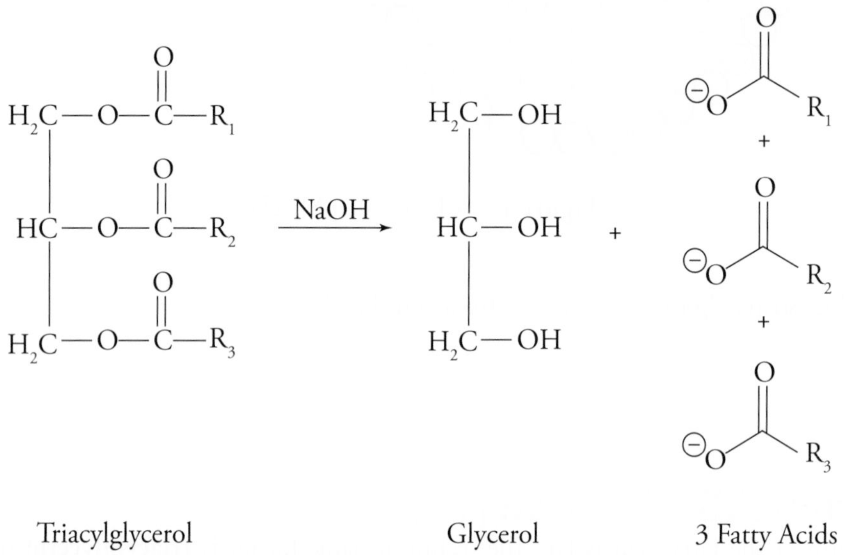

Figure 3   Saponification

Lipases are enzymes that hydrolyze fats. Triacylglycerols are stored in fat cells as an energy source. Fats are more efficient energy storage molecules than carbohydrates for two reasons: packing and energy content.

1)   **Packing:** Their hydrophobicity allows fats to pack together much more closely than carbohydrates. Carbohydrates carry a great amount of water-of-solvation (water molecules hydrogen-bonded to their hydroxyl groups). In other words, the amount of carbon per unit area or unit weight is much greater in a fat droplet than in dissolved sugar. If we could store sugars in a dry powdery form in our bodies, this problem would be obviated.

2)   **Energy content:** All packing considerations aside, fat molecules store much more energy than carbohydrates. In other words, regardless of what you dissolve it in, a fat has more energy carbon-for-carbon than a carbohydrate. The reason is that fats are much more reduced.

Remember that energy metabolism begins with the oxidation of foodstuffs to release energy. Since carbohydrates are more oxidized to start with, oxidizing them releases less energy. Animals use fat to store most of their energy, storing only a small amount as carbohydrates (glycogen). Plants such as potatoes commonly store a large percentage of their energy as carbohydrates (starch).

9.3 PHOSPHOLIPIDS AND LIPID BILAYER MEMBRANES

Membrane lipids are **phospholipids** (also called phosphatides) derived from diacylglycerol phosphate or DG-P. Often the phosphate group has even bigger polar molecules attached to it, such as choline (phosphatidylcholine), ethanolamine (phosphatidylethanolamine), and inositol (phosphatidylinositol).

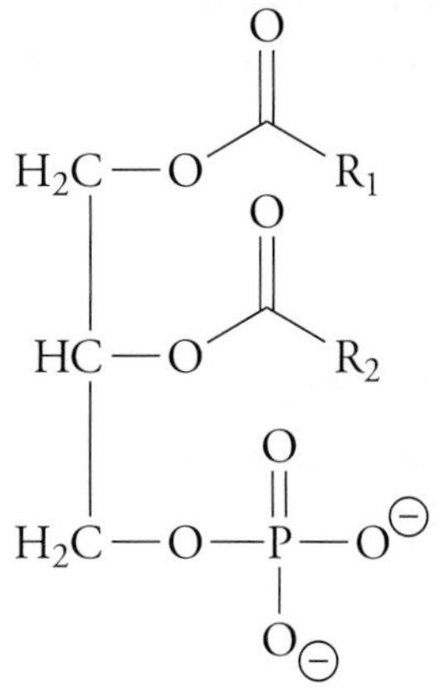

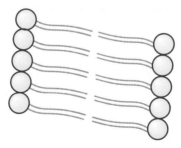

Figure 4   A Phosphoglyceride (Diacylglycerol Phosphate, or DG-P)

We saw above how fatty acids spontaneously form micelles. Phospholipids also minimize their interactions with water by forming an orderly structure—in this case, it is a **lipid bilayer** (Figure 5). Hydrophobic interactions drive the formation of the bilayer, and once formed, it is stabilized by van der Waals forces between the long tails.

Figure 5   A Small Section of a Lipid Bilayer Membrane

- Would a saturated or an unsaturated fatty acid residue have more van der Waals interactions with neighboring alkyl chains in a bilayer membrane?[4]

---

[4]   The bent shape of the unsaturated fatty acid means that it doesn't fit in as well and has less contact with neighboring groups to form van der Waals interactions. Phospholipids composed of saturated fatty acids make the membrane less fluid.

A more precise way to give the answer to the question on the previous page is to say that double bonds (unsaturation) in phospholipid fatty acids *tend to increase membrane fluidity*. Unsaturation prevents the membrane from solidifying by disrupting the orderly packing of the hydrophobic lipid tails. The right amount of fluidity is essential for function. Decreasing the *length* of fatty acid tails also increases fluidity. The steroid **cholesterol** (discussed a bit later) is a third important modulator of membrane fluidity. At low temperatures, it increases fluidity in the same way as kinks in fatty acid tails; hence, it is known as *membrane antifreeze*. At high temperatures, however, cholesterol attenuates (reduces) membrane fluidity. Don't ponder this paradox too long; just remember that cholesterol keeps fluidity at an *optimum level*. Remember, the structural determinants of membrane fluidity are: degree of saturation, tail length, and amount of cholesterol.

The lipid bilayer acts like a barrier surrounding the cell in the sense that it separates the interior of the cell from the exterior. However, the cell membrane is much more complex than a simple barrier; it is a dynamic structure that regulates what comes into and goes out of the cell and transmits extracellular signals to the interior of the cell. More information about the plasma membrane can be found in the Biology section of this book.

9.4 TERPENES AND STEROIDS

A terpene is a member of a broad class of compounds built from isoprene units (C_5H_8) with a general formula $(C_5H_8)_n$.

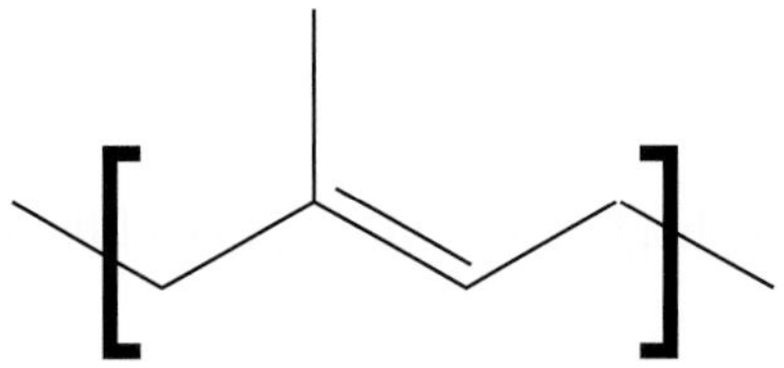

Figure 6 Isoprene Unit

Terpenes may be linear or cyclic, and they are classified by the number of isoprene units they contain. For example, monoterpenes consist of two isoprene units, sesquiterpenes consist of three, and diterpenes contain four.

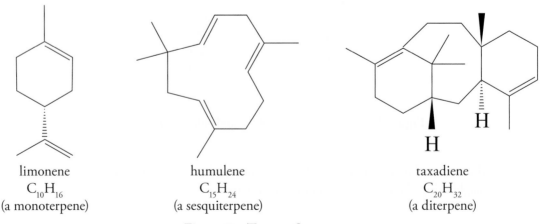

limonene
$C_{10}H_{16}$
(a monoterpene)

humulene
$C_{15}H_{24}$
(a sesquiterpene)

taxadiene
$C_{20}H_{32}$
(a diterpene)

Figure 7 Terpene Structures

Squalene is a triterpene (made of six isoprene units), and it is a particularly important compound, as it is biosynthetically utilized in the manufacture of steroids. Squalene is also a component of earwax.

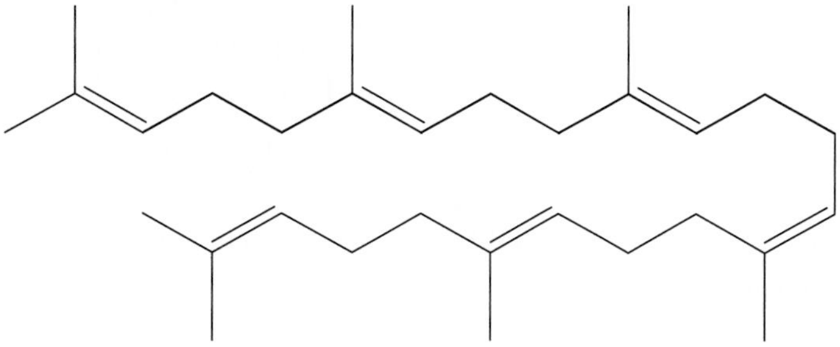

Figure 8 Squalene

Whereas a terpene is formally a simple hydrocarbon, there are a number of natural and synthetically derived species that are built from an isoprene skeleton and functionalized with other elements (O, N, S, etc.). These functionalized-terpenes are known as *terpenoids*. Vitamin A ($C_{20}H_{30}O$) is an example of a terpenoid.

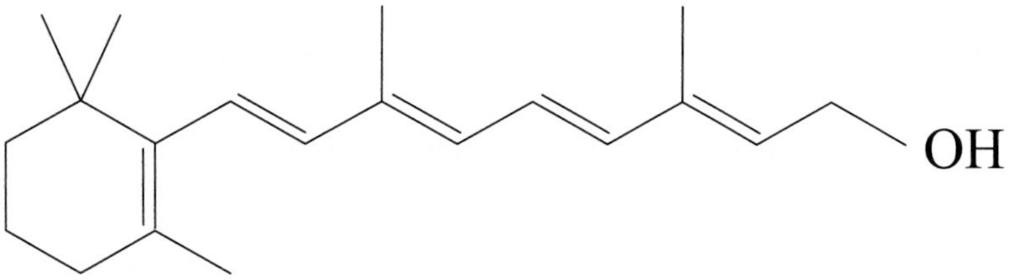

Figure 9 Vitamin A

Steroids

Steroids are included here because of their hydrophobicity, and, hence, similarity to fats. Their structure is otherwise unique. All steroids have the basic tetracyclic ring system (Figure 10 on the next page), based on the structure of **cholesterol**.

As discussed earlier, the steroid cholesterol is an important component of the lipid bilayer. It is both obtained from the diet and synthesized in the liver. It is carried in the blood packaged with fats and proteins into **lipoproteins**. One type of lipoprotein has been implicated as the cause of atherosclerotic vascular disease, which refers to the build-up of cholesterol "plaques" on the inside of blood vessels.

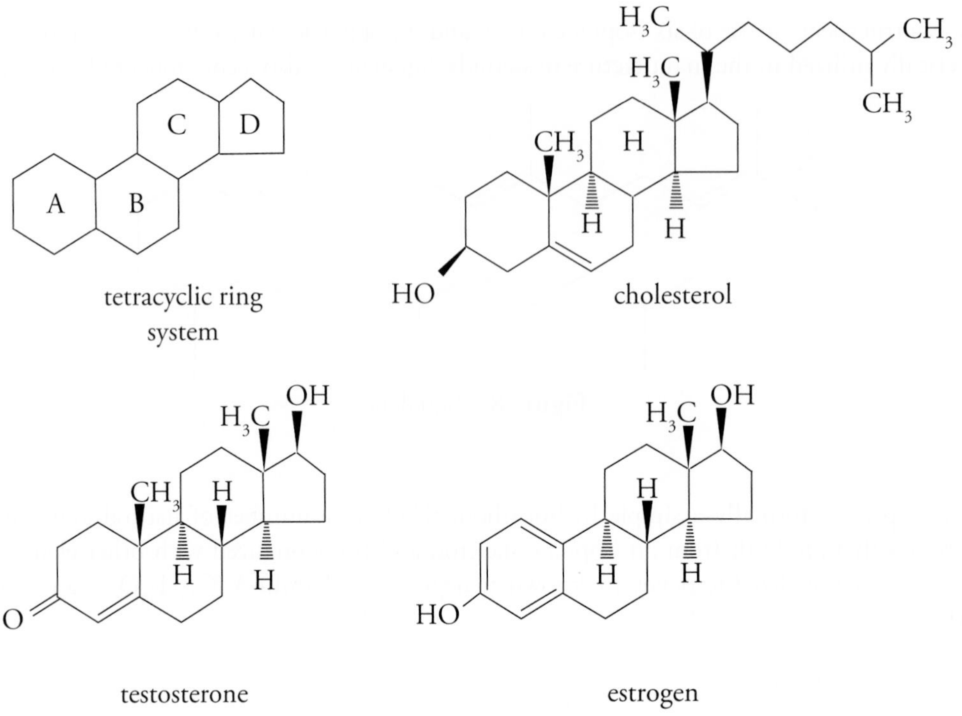

Figure 10 Cholesterol-Derived Hormones

Steroid hormones are made from cholesterol. Two examples are **testosterone** (an androgen or male sex hormone) and **estradiol** (an estrogen or female sex hormone). There are no receptors for steroid hormones on the surface of cells; because steroids are highly hydrophobic, they can diffuse right through the lipid bilayer membrane into the cytoplasm. The receptors for steroid hormones are located within cells rather than on the cell surface. This is an important point! You must be aware of the contrast between *peptide* hormones, such as insulin, which exert their effects by binding to receptors at the cell-surface, and *steroid* hormones, such as estrogen, which diffuse into cells to find their receptors.

9.5 OTHER LIPIDS

Beyond fatty acids, triglycerides, phospholipids, terpenes, cholesterol, and steroids, there are a few other lipids with which you should be familiar for the MCAT.

Sphingolipids

Sphingolipids are structured in a similar manner as phospholipids, except that the backbone is sphingosine instead of glycerol. The only significant sphingolipid in humans is sphingomyelin, an important component of the myelin sheath around neurons.

sphingosine

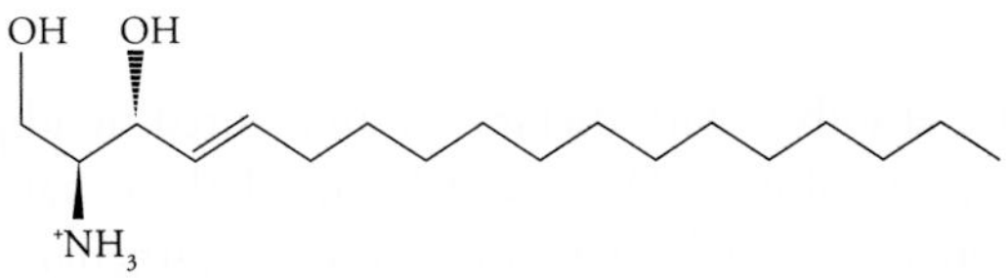

a ceramide

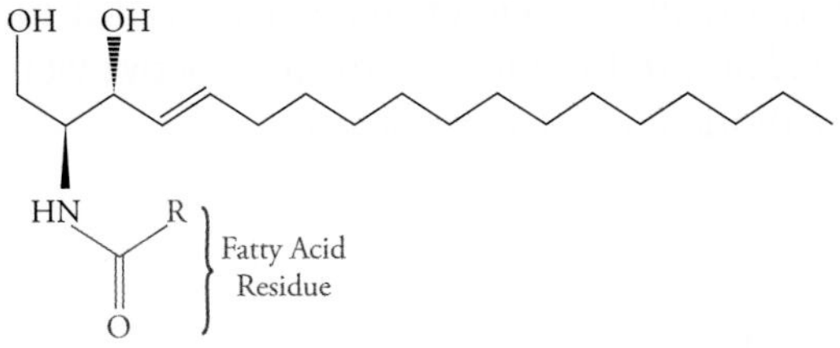

Fatty Acid
Residue

Phosphocholine
group

a sphingomyelin
(phosphatidylcholine)

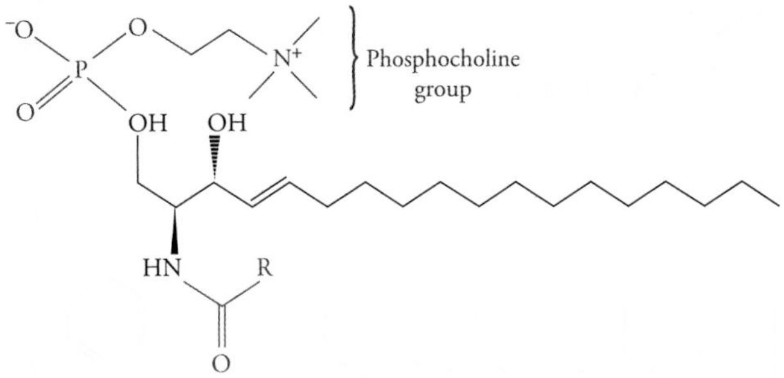

Phosphoethanolamine
group

a sphingomyelin
(phosphatidylethanolamine)

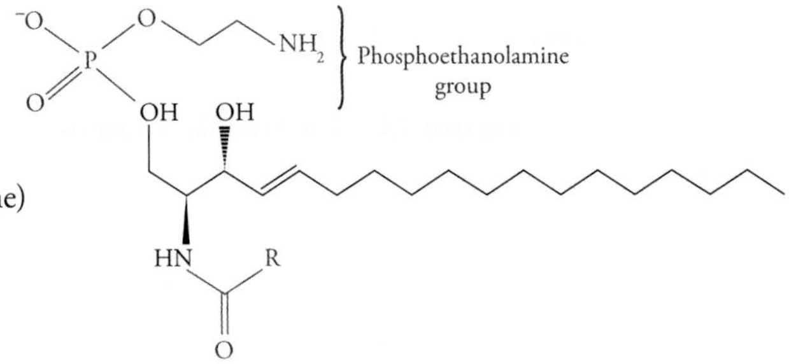

Figure 11 Sphingolipids

Waxes

Waxes are long-chain fats esterified to long-chain alcohols. They are extremely hydrophobic and often form waterproof barriers, most notably in plants. Animals also use waxes to form a protective barrier (e.g., earwax).

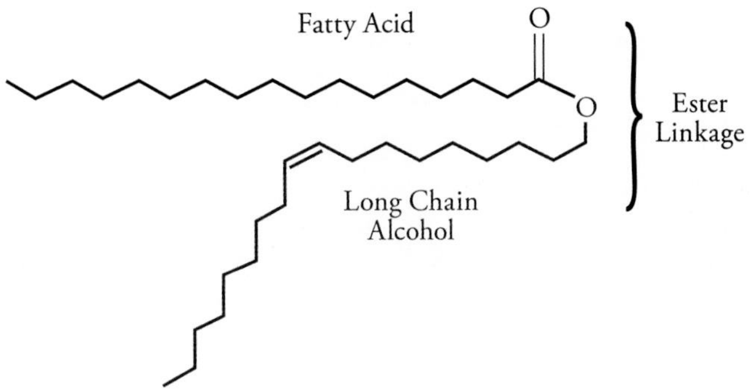

Fatty Acid

Ester
Linkage

Long Chain
Alcohol

Figure 12 Wax

Fat-Soluble Vitamins

Fat-soluble vitamins are absorbed with dietary fat and stored in adipose tissue and in the liver. The four fat-soluble vitamins are vitamins A, D, E, and K; all of them have ring structures. Vitamin A is a terpenoid (mentioned earlier) essential for vision, growth, epithelial maintenance, and immune function. Vitamin D is derived from cholesterol (it is a steroid) important in regulating blood levels of calcium and phosphate. Vitamin E is actually a group of compounds, called **tocopherols** (methylated phenols), that are important as antioxidants. α-Tocopherol is the most active vitamin E. Vitamin K serves as an important coenzyme in the activation of clotting proteins.

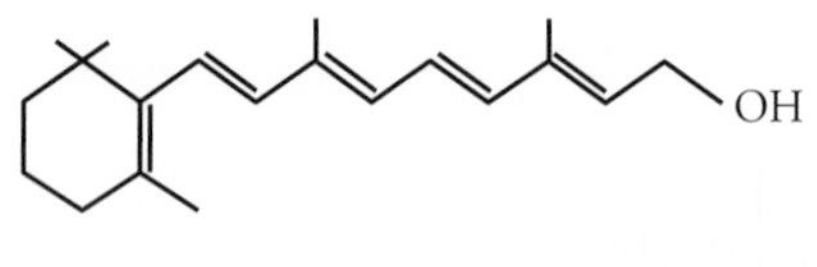

Vitamin A

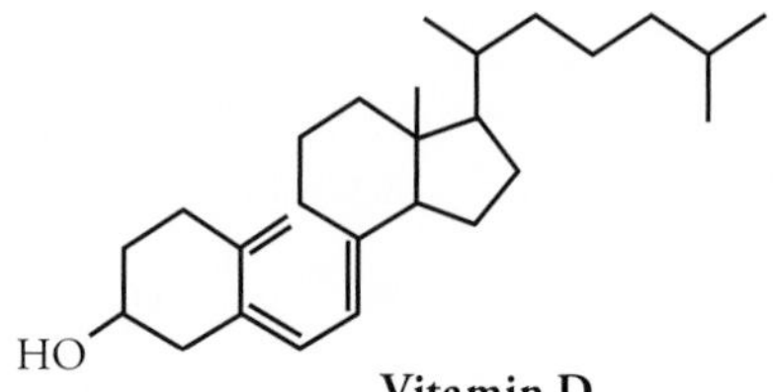

Vitamin D_3

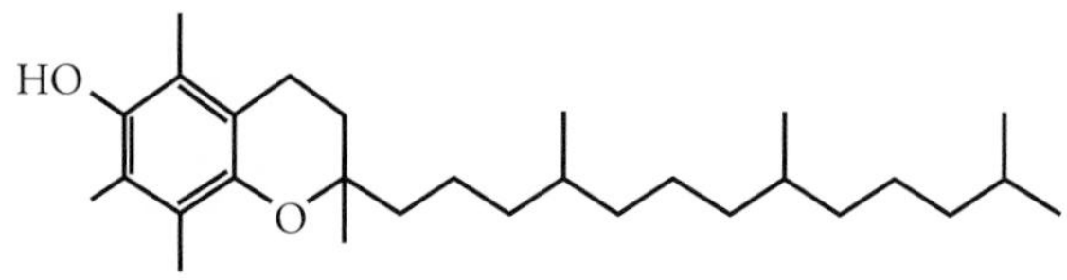

Vitamin E

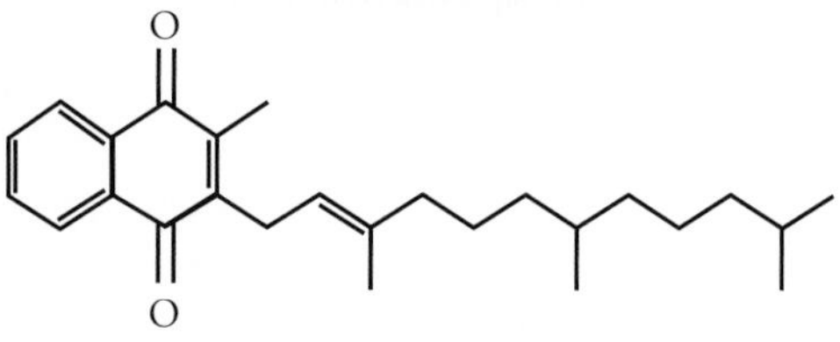

Vitamin K_1

Figure 13 Fat-Soluble Vitamins

Prostaglandins

Prostaglandins belong to a group of molecules known as eicosanoids, derived from 20-carbon fatty acids (the prefix *eicosa* means "20"). They have vastly different roles in different tissues, depending on the receptor to which they bind. Their roles include regulating smooth muscle contraction in the intestines and uterus, regulating blood vessel diameter, maintaining gastric integrity (by decreasing acid secretion and increasing mucus secretion), among others. They all have the same general structure, including a five-membered ring. See Figure 14.

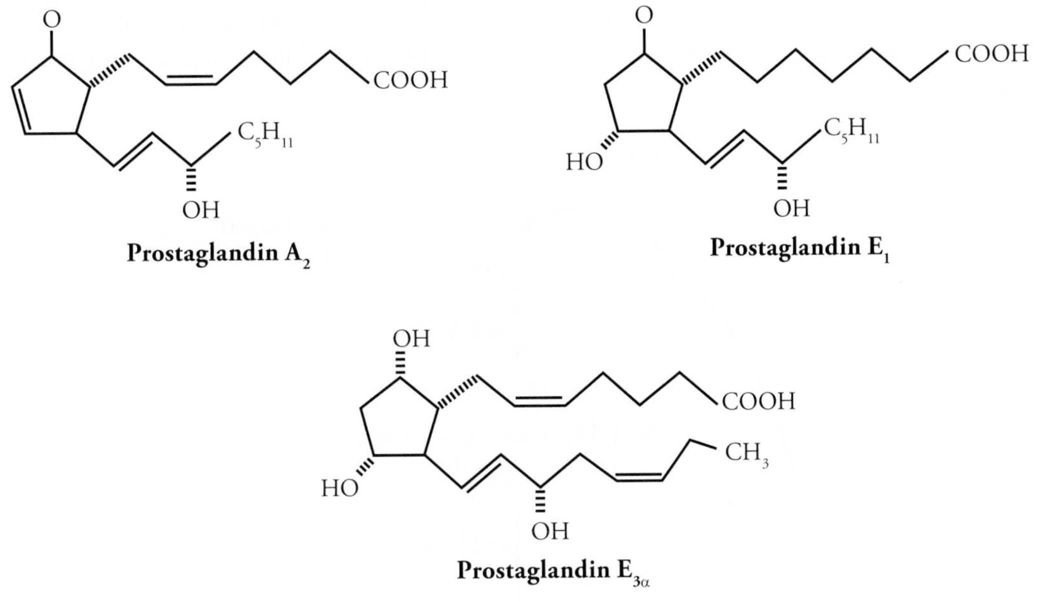

Prostaglandin A$_2$

Prostaglandin E$_1$

Prostaglandin E$_{3\alpha}$

Figure 14   Prostaglandins

9.6   FATTY ACID METABOLISM

Fatty Acid Oxidation

Following the initial steps in fat digestion, **chylomicrons** composed of fat and lipoprotein are transported via the lymphatic system and blood stream to the liver, heart, lungs, and other organs. This dietary fat, or triacylglycerol, is hydrolyzed to liberate free fatty acids which can then undergo β-**oxidation**. This process begins at the outer mitochondrial membrane with the activation of the fatty acid. This reaction, catalyzed by **acyl-CoA synthetase,** requires the investment of two ATP equivalents to generate a fatty acyl-CoA which is then transported into the mitochondrion.

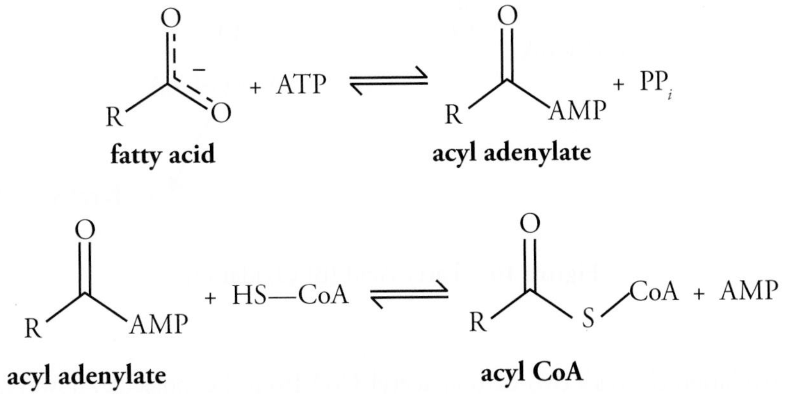

Figure 15   Fatty Acid Activation

Once in the matrix, the fatty acyl-CoA undergoes a repeated series of four reactions which cleave the bond between the alpha and beta carbons to liberate an acetyl-CoA in addition to generating one FADH$_2$ and NADH.

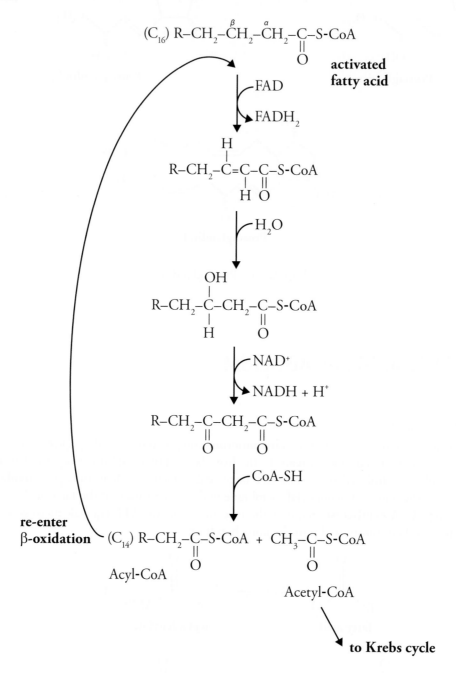

Figure 16 Fatty Acid (β) Oxidation

Each round of β-oxidation cleaves a two-carbon acetyl-CoA from the molecule; however, the final round cleaves a four-carbon fatty acyl-CoA to generate two acetyl-CoA. For instance, the complete β-oxidation of lauric acid (a twelve-carbon saturated fatty acid) involves the following: an investment of two ATP equivalents to convert it to a fatty acyl-CoA and then *five* rounds of β-oxidation. This generates five FADH$_2$, five NADH, and *six* acetyl-CoA which can then enter the Krebs cycle. When these six acetyl-CoA go through the Krebs cycle, they will generate an additional 18 NADH, 6 FADH$_2$, and 6 GTP. We then have a grand total of eleven FADH$_2$ (five from β-oxidation and six from the Krebs cycle), 23 NADH (five from β-oxidation and 18 from the Krebs cycle), and six ATP equivalents (from the Krebs cycle). After the electron transport chain (and subtracting the two ATP equivalents required at the beginning of β-oxidation), we obtain 78 ATP from lauric acid.

Ketogenesis

During periods of starvation, glycogen stores become exhausted and blood glucose falls significantly. To help supply the central nervous system with energy when glucose is in short supply, the liver generates **ketone bodies** via a process in the mitochondrial matrix known as **ketogenesis**. The ketone bodies are generated from acetyl-CoA and include acetone, acetoacetate, and β-hydroxybutyrate. These molecules can cross the blood-brain barrier and be converted back to acetyl-CoA once they arrive at their target organ; the acetyl-CoA can then enter the Krebs cycle (see Figure 17).

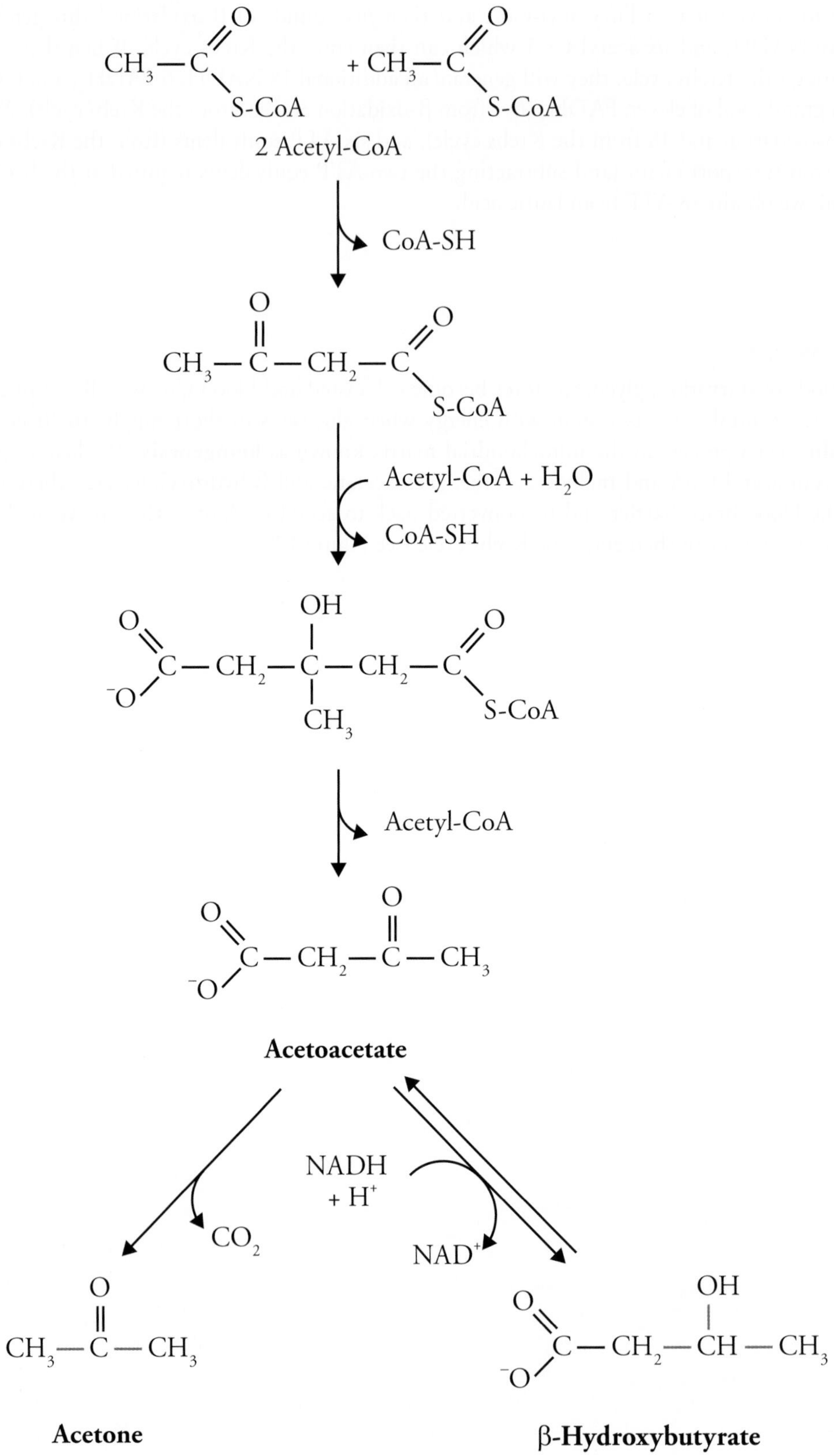

9.6

$$CH_3 - \overset{\overset{\displaystyle O}{\|}}{C} - \text{S-CoA} \quad + \quad CH_3 - \overset{\overset{\displaystyle O}{\|}}{C} - \text{S-CoA}$$

2 Acetyl-CoA

↓ CoA-SH

$$CH_3 - \overset{\overset{\displaystyle O}{\|}}{C} - CH_2 - \overset{\overset{\displaystyle O}{\|}}{C} - \text{S-CoA}$$

↓ Acetyl-CoA + H_2O

CoA-SH

$$^-O - \overset{\overset{\displaystyle O}{\|}}{C} - CH_2 - \overset{\overset{\displaystyle OH}{|}}{\underset{\underset{\displaystyle CH_3}{|}}{C}} - CH_2 - \overset{\overset{\displaystyle O}{\|}}{C} - \text{S-CoA}$$

↓ Acetyl-CoA

$$^-O - \overset{\overset{\displaystyle O}{\|}}{C} - CH_2 - \overset{\overset{\displaystyle O}{\|}}{C} - CH_3$$

Acetoacetate

NADH + H⁺   NAD⁺

CO₂

$$CH_3 - \overset{\overset{\displaystyle O}{\|}}{C} - CH_3$$

Acetone

$$^-O - \overset{\overset{\displaystyle O}{\|}}{C} - CH_2 - \overset{\overset{\displaystyle OH}{|}}{CH} - CH_3$$

β-Hydroxybutyrate

Figure 17   Ketogenesis

In some circumstances, ketogenesis can take place when adequate glucose is present in the blood but cannot enter the cell. This can occur, for example, when a patient suffering from type I diabetes does not receive an insulin injection for a prolonged period of time. Without insulin, glucose cannot enter cells in order to be used for energy, and the patient relies exclusively on fatty acid oxidation for the acetyl-CoA to turn the Krebs cycle. However, because the levels of acetyl-CoA are so high, many of them get converted into ketone bodies. Ketone bodies are acidic, and this can result in diabetic ketoacidosis, which is a potentially life-threatening condition.

Fatty Acid Synthesis

The *de novo* synthesis of fatty acids is reminiscent of β-oxidation with several notable exceptions. While fatty acid catabolism occurs in the mitochondrial matrix, anabolism takes place in the cytoplasm. This compartmentalization allows for easier regulation, since the enzymes required for synthesis and break-down are separated. Much as β-oxidation involved the removal of two-carbon subunits from a fatty acid chain, the synthesis of a fatty acid involves the repeated addition of two-carbon subunits. Rather than building the nascent fatty acid directly with acetyl-CoA, acetyl-CoA is first activated in a carboxylation reaction. The activation is the committed step in fatty acid synthesis and requires the investment of ATP; it is facilitated by **acetyl-CoA carboxylase** to generate **malonyl-CoA**.

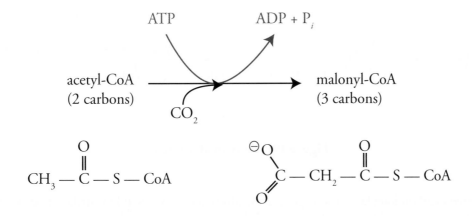

Figure 18   Synthesis of Malonyl-CoA

Fatty acid synthase is a large enzyme with multiple catalytic domains. Acetyl-CoA first binds to a domain known as the **acyl carrier protein (ACP)**. It is then shifted to another domain on the enzyme with a cysteine residue, and malonyl-CoA binds to the ACP. The acetyl group condenses with the malonyl group as the malonyl is decarboxylated. (Recall that the successive addition, then removal of CO_2 can drive unfavorable reactions; this same process occurs in gluconeogenesis with the carboxylation of pyruvate to oxaloacetate, and the subsequent decarboxylation of oxaloacetate to PEP.) The ACP domain now holds a four-carbon unit, which undergoes two reductions. This process requires the reducing power of NADPH, which is generally obtained from the pentose phosphate pathway (see Chapter 8). The saturated four-carbon acyl unit is shifted to the domain with the cysteine residue, and another malonyl-CoA binds to the ACP. The process then repeats: the four-carbon unit condenses with malonyl as CO_2 is lost, two successive reductions occur, and the now six-carbon chain is shifted to the cysteine residue.

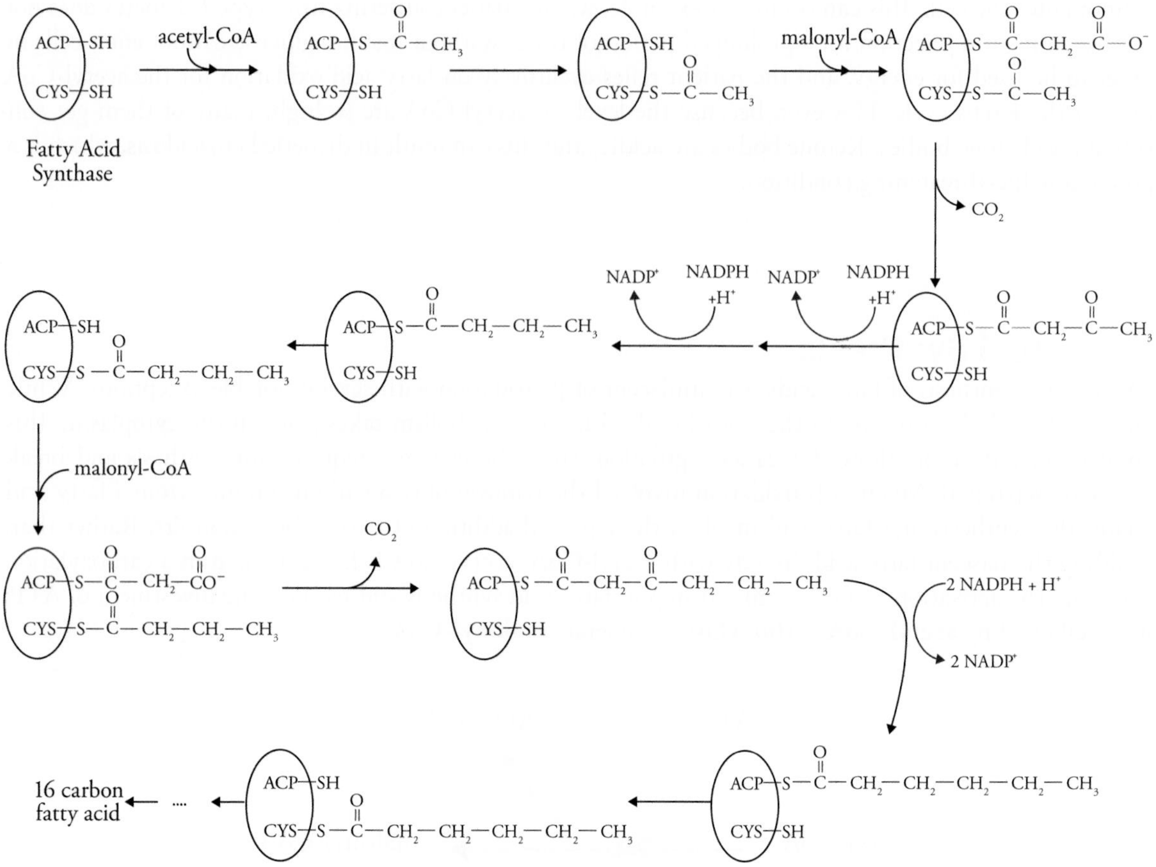

Figure 19 Fatty Acid Synthesis

Once a sixteen-carbon long fatty acid is generated, additional enzymes aid in further modification of the fatty acid (e.g., addition of functional groups and elongation). Note that this process requires no template (nor does glycogen or amino acid synthesis), which means that nothing is "read" to generate the products. This differs from the template-based syntheses of polypeptides (mRNA is "read" to generate an amino acid sequence) and nucleic acids (DNA is "read" to generate DNA during replication and RNA during transcription).

9.7   AMINO ACID CATABOLISM AND METABOLIC SUMMARY

We discussed amino acid structure and protein structure and function in Chapter 7, but we haven't yet really touched on the idea of proteins as fuel. Proteins in cells are constantly being made, kept for a certain period of time (minutes to weeks), and then degraded back into amino acids. In addition, humans absorb amino acids from dietary proteins. These free amino acids can be catabolized via several pathways. They can be taken up by cells and used to make cellular proteins. The amino group can be removed and either used to synthesize nitrogenous compounds, such as nucleotide bases, or it can be converted into urea for excretion. The remaining carbon skeleton (also called an α-keto acid) can either be broken down into water and CO_2, or it can be converted to glucose (glucogenic amino acids) or acetyl-CoA (ketogenic amino acids).

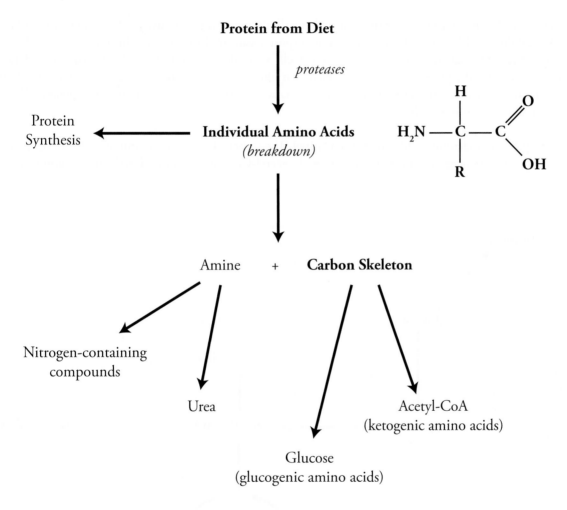

Figure 20   Protein Breakdown

Metabolism Summary

Generally speaking, cells prefer to use carbohydrates as fuel. When blood sugar is high, cells will take up glucose and make ATP via glycolysis. Liver and muscle cells will also store glucose as glycogen (glycogenesis), and the liver can also take some of the acetyl-CoA generated by the pyruvate dehydrogenase complex to make fatty acids (fatty acid synthesis). These are converted into triglycerides and stored in adipose tissue. These pathways are shown in black in Figure 21.

When blood sugar levels fall (starved state), the liver will break down the stored glycogen (glycogenolysis) and release glucose into the bloodstream. It will also begin the process of gluconeogenesis to synthesize "new" glucose that can also be released into the bloodstream. This glucose can be taken up by other body cells and used in glycolysis to generate ATP. These pathways are show in gray in the diagram below.

If the starved state continues past the point where all glycogen stores are used (12–24 hours), then fatty acid breakdown will occur. Triglycerides from adipose tissue are broken down into free fatty acids and glycerol that are released into the bloodstream. Cells will take up the fatty acids and run β-oxidation. The liver can use the glycerol to generate glucose in gluconeogenesis. Some of the acetyl-CoA made in β-oxidation is used to turn the Krebs cycle, and some is converted into ketone bodies (ketogenesis). These pathways are shown in gray below.

Finally, proteins and amino acids can be used as fuel. The carbon skeleton of the amino acids can be used in gluconeogenesis (glucogenic amino acids) or to make acetyl-CoA and ketone bodies (ketogenic amino acids).

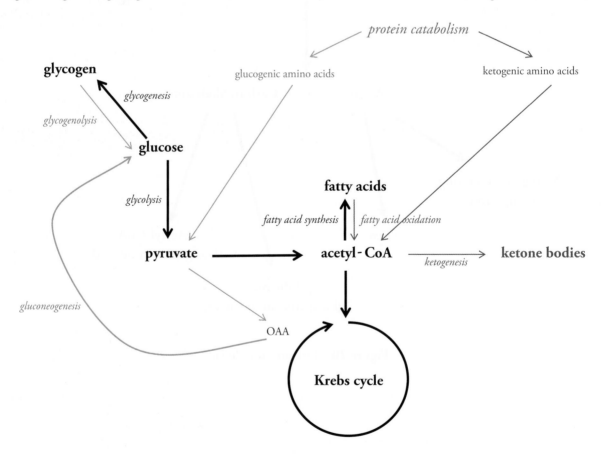

Figure 21   Summary of Metabolism

Chapter 10
Nucleic Acids

10.1 PHOSPHORUS-CONTAINING COMPOUNDS

Phosphoric acid is an *inorganic* acid (it does not contain carbon) with the potential to donate three protons. The K_as for the three acid dissociation equilibria are 2.1, 7.2, and 12.4. Therefore, at physiological pH, phosphoric acid is significantly dissociated, existing largely in anionic form. The most common species (approximately 60% in extracellular fluid) is hydrogen phosphate (HPO_4^{-2}), and the second most common (approximately 40%) is dihydrogen phosphate ($H_2PO_4^-$).

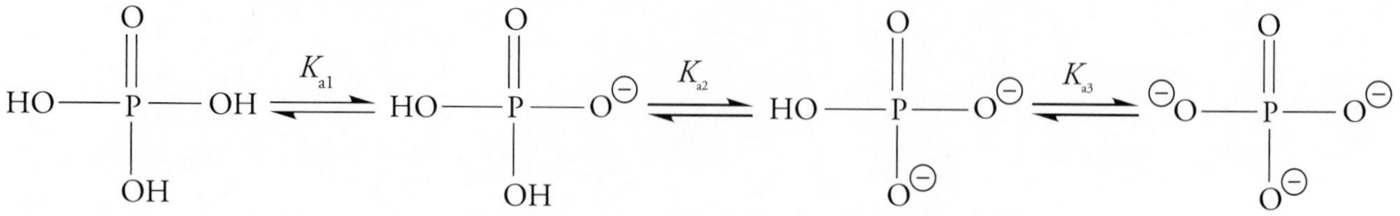

Figure 1 Phosphoric Acid Dissociation

Phosphate is also known as orthophosphate. Two orthophosphates bound together via an **anhydride linkage** form **pyrophosphate**. The P–O–P bond in pyrophosphate is an example of a **high-energy phosphate bond**. This name is derived from the fact that the hydrolysis of pyrophosphate is thermodynamically extremely favorable. The $\Delta G°$ for the hydrolysis of pyrophosphate is about –7 kcal/mol. This means that it is a very favorable reaction. The actual ΔG in the cell is about –12 kcal/mol, which is even more favorable. How is this possible?[1]

There are three reasons that phosphate anhydride bonds store so much energy:

1) When phosphates are linked together, their negative charges repel each other strongly.
2) Orthophosphate has more resonance forms and thus a lower free energy than linked phosphates.
3) Orthophosphate has a more favorable interaction with the biological solvent (water) than linked phosphates.

The details are not crucial. What is essential is that you fix the image in your mind of linked phosphates acting like compressed springs, just waiting to fly open and provide energy for an enzyme to catalyze a reaction.

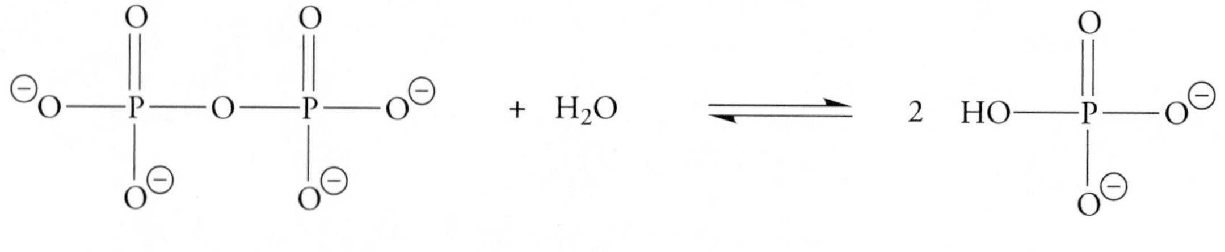

Figure 2 The Hydrolysis of Pyrophosphate

---

[1] Remember that $\Delta G°$ is the free energy change at standard conditions. The concentrations of reactants and products inside the cell are not at standard conditions. In fact, the cell maintains a concentration of ATP much higher than that of ADP and phosphate, which makes ATP hydrolysis so much more favorable.

Nucleotides

Nucleotides are the building blocks of nucleic acids (RNA and DNA). Each nucleotide contains a **ribose** (or **deoxyribose**) **sugar** group; a **purine** or **pyrimidine base** joined to carbon number one of the ribose ring; and one, two, or three **phosphate units** joined to carbon five of the ribose ring. The nucleotide **a**denosine **tri**phosphate (ATP) plays a central role in cellular metabolism in addition to being an RNA precursor. Significantly more information about the function of the nucleic acids RNA and DNA will be provided in *MCAT Biology Review.*

ATP is the universal short-term energy storage molecule. It is a ribonucleotide (ribose is the sugar, as opposed to deoxyribose). Energy extracted from the oxidation of foodstuffs is immediately stored in the phospho-anhydride bonds of ATP. This energy is used to power cellular processes, and as we have already seen, it may also be used to synthesize glucose or fats, which are longer-term energy storage molecules. This applies to *all* living organisms, from bacteria to humans. Even some viruses carry ATP with them outside the host cell, though viruses cannot make their own ATP.

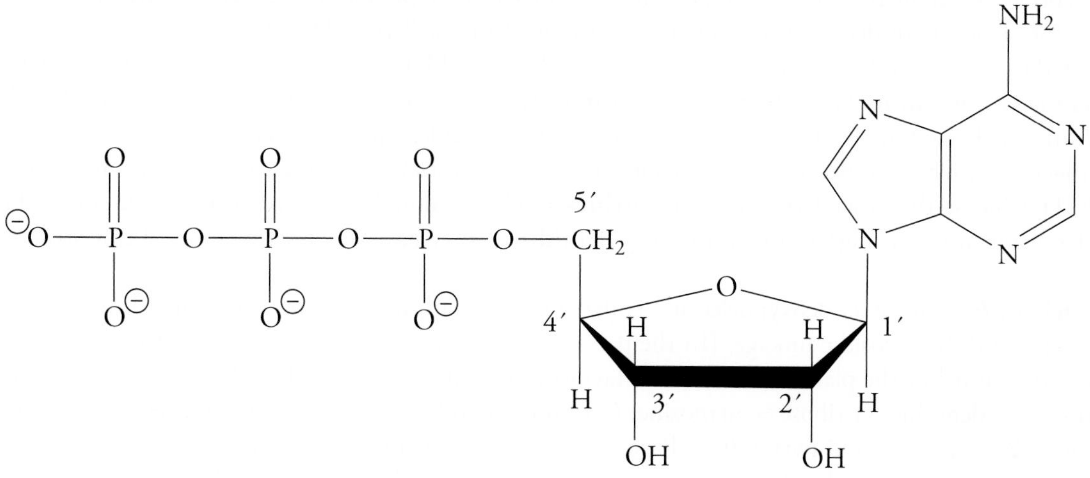

Figure 3   Adenosine Triphosphate (ATP)

The other nucleotides can also be used as energy, but they are used for this purpose far less often. GTP is used for energy in protein synthesis, and UTP is used to activate glucose-1-P in glycogenesis.

10.2 DNA STRUCTURE

General Overview

Understanding the structure of DNA provided in the Biology section (Part 3) provides great insight into its function, so let's start at the smallest level and work our way up. DNA is short for d̲e̲oxyribo̲nucleic a̲cid. DNA and RNA (r̲ibo̲nucleic a̲cid) are called **nucleic acids** because they are found in the nucleus and possess many acidic phosphate groups.

The building block of DNA is the d̲e̲oxyribo̲nucleoside 5' tr̲i̲p̲hosphate (dNTP, where N represents one of the four basic nucleosides). Deoxyadenosine 5' triphosphate (dATP) is shown in Figure 4. Deoxyribo-nucleotides are built from three components. The first is a simple monosaccharide, deoxyribose. [How does the structure of deoxyribose compare with that of ribose?[2]] In a dNTP, carbons on the ribose are referred to as 1', 2', and so on. The next component of the dNTP is an aromatic, nitrogenous base, namely **adenine** (A), **guanine** (G), **cytosine** (C), or **thymine** (T); see Figure 5. (Don't mix up the DNA base thymine with vitamin B_1, thiamine.) These aromatic molecules are bases because they contain several nitrogens that have free electron pairs capable of accepting protons. G and A are derived from a precursor called purine, so they are referred to as the **purines** and have a double-ring structure (a six-membered ring and a five-membered ring). C and T are the **pyrimidines**; they have single six-membered ring structure.[3]

A **nucleo*side*** is ribose (a deoxynucleoside is deoxyribose) with a purine or pyrimidine linked to the 1' carbon in a β-N-glycosidic linkage. [In the β-N-glycosidic linkage of a nucleoside, is the aromatic base above or is it below the plane of ribose in a Haworth projection?[4]] The nucleosides are named as follows: A-ribose = adenosine, G-ribose = guanosine, C-ribose = cytidine, T-ribose = thymidine, and U-ribose = uridine. Both purines and pyrimidines have abundant hydrogen bonding potential. [Will adenine and thymine H-bond with each other in dilute aqueous solution (0.1 *M*, for example)?[5]]

The final component of the deoxyribonucleotide building block of DNA is a phosphate group. **Nucleo*tides*** are phosphate esters of nucleosides, with one, two, or three phosphate groups joined to the ribose ring by the 5' hydroxy group. When nucleotides contain three phosphate residues, they may also be referred to as **deoxynucleoside triphosphates**; they are abbreviated **dNTP**, where d is for *deoxy* and N is for *nucleoside*. In individual nucleotides, N is replaced by A, G, C, T, or U. Because they contain acidic phosphates, the nucleotides may also be referred to by a name ending in "ylate." For example, TTP is thymidylate. The ubiquitous energy molecule, ATP, is a nucleotide which may be called adenylate (it's not deoxy).

---

[2] The 2' OH is missing in deoxyribose.

[3] A mnemonic for this is: Pyramids (pyrimidines) have sharp edges, so they CUT. The U stands for *uracil*, which is a pyrimidine found in RNA instead of T. Another mnemonic is CUT the Py.

[4] A beta linkage indicates that the anomeric carbon has a configuration with the attached group (a nitrogen of the aromatic ring of a purine or pyrimidine base) drawn *above* the plane of the ribose ring. Remember, it's better to β up!

[5] No. In dilute solution they will be H-bonded to water. However, H-bonds are the key determinant of the double-stranded structure of DNA; in DNA, the bases do not interact with water because DNA coiling places them inside the tube-like structure of the double helix, where they interact with each other.

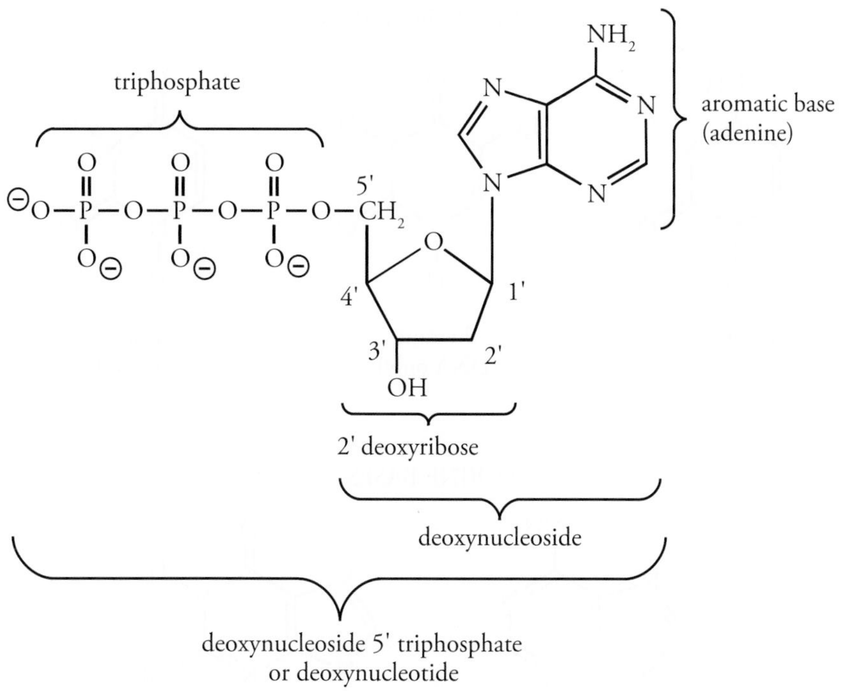

Figure 4 Deoxyadenosine Triphosphate (dATP)

The sugar-phosphate portion of the nucleotide is referred to as the **backbone** of the nucleic acid because it is invariant. The base is the variable portion of the building block. Thus, there are four different dNTPs, and they differ only in the aromatic base. [What is the backbone in protein, and what is the variable portion of the amino acid?[6] If an enzyme binds to a specific sequence of nucleotides in DNA, will the binding specificity be derived from interactions of portions of the polypeptide enzyme with the ribose and phosphate groups or with the purine and pyrimidine bases?[7]]

---

[6] Peptide bonds with a carbon between them are the backbone, and the R-group attached to the α carbon is the variable portion.

[7] Since the backbone is the same regardless of the nucleotide sequence, the specificity in binding must be derived from interactions with bases.

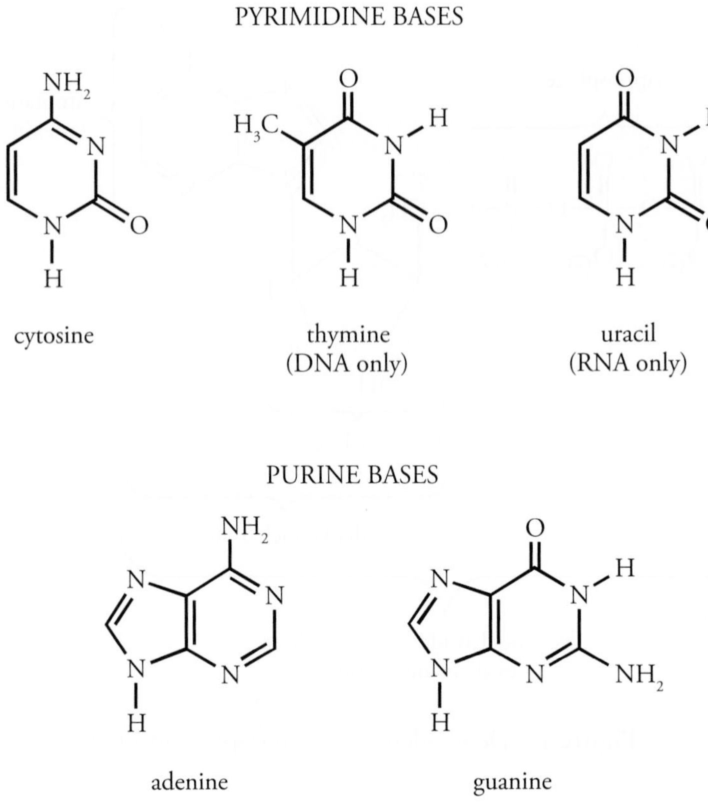

PYRIMIDINE BASES

cytosine thymine (DNA only) uracil (RNA only)

PURINE BASES

adenine guanine

Figure 5 Aromatic Bases of DNA and RNA

Polynucleotides

Nucleotides in nucleic acids are covalently linked by **phosphodiester bonds** between the 3' hydroxy group of the sugar in one nucleotide and the 5' phosphate group of the sugar in the next nucleotide (Figure 6). [What allows the polymerization of nucleotide triphosphates to be thermodynamically favorable?[8]] A polymer of several nucleotides linked together is termed an *oligo*nucleotide, and a polymer of many nucleotides is a *poly*-nucleotide. Since the only unique part of the nucleotide is the base, the sequence of a polynucleotide can be abbreviated by simply listing the bases attached to each nucleotide in the chain. The end of the chain with a free 5' phosphate group is written first in a polynucleotide, with other nucleotides in the chain indicated in the 5' to 3' direction. [Which of the nucleotides in the oligonucleotide ACGT has a free 3' hydroxy group?[9]]

---

[8] During polymerization of nucleoside triphosphates, pyrophosphate is hydrolyzed and released, making the reaction favorable and driving the polymerization forward.

[9] The T is written last and is therefore the 3' nucleotide, or the nucleotide with the free 3' hydroxy group.

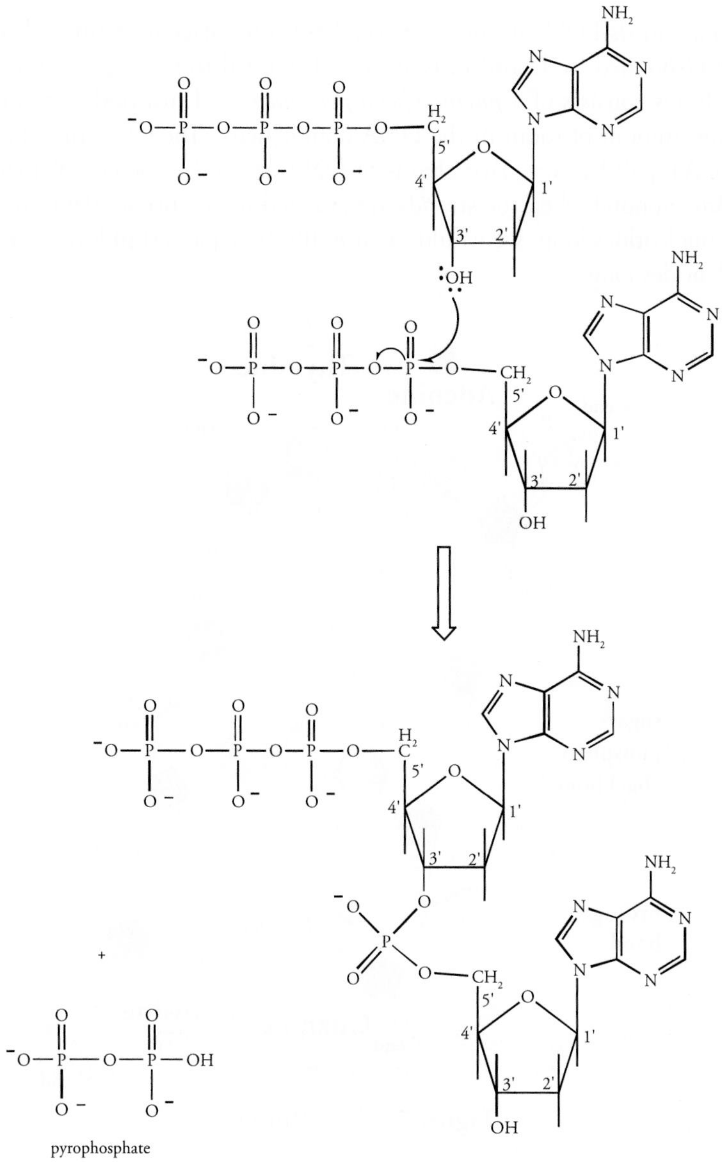

Figure 6   The Polymerization of Nucleotides

The Watson-Crick Model of DNA Structure

James Watson and Francis Crick (with the help of Maurice Wilkins and Rosalind Franklin) developed a model of the structure of DNA in the cell. According to the **Watson-Crick model**, cellular DNA is a right-handed double helix held together by hydrogen bonds and hydrophobic forces between bases. It is important to understand each facet of this model.

In the cell, DNA does not exist in the form of a single long polynucleotide. Instead, the DNA found in the nucleus is double-stranded (**ds**). In ds-DNA, two very long polynucleotide chains are hydrogen-bonded together in an **antiparallel orientation**. Antiparallel means the 5' end of one chain is paired with the 3' end of the other. [What common protein structure often depends on H-bonds between antiparallel chains?[10]] The H-bonds in ds-DNA are between the bases on adjacent chains. This H-bonding is very specific: A is always H-bonded to T, and G is always H-bonded to C (Figure 7). Note that this means an H-bonded pair always consists of a *purine plus a pyrimidine*.[11] Thus, both types of base pairs (AT or GC) take up the same amount of room in the DNA double helix. The GC pair is held together by three hydrogen bonds, the AT pair by two. Two chains of DNA are said to be complementary if the bases in each strand can hydrogen bond when the strands are oriented in an antiparallel fashion. If we are talking about ds-DNA 100 nucleotides long, we would say it is 100 base pairs (bp) long. A kbp (kilobase pair) is ds-DNA 1,000 nucleotides long.

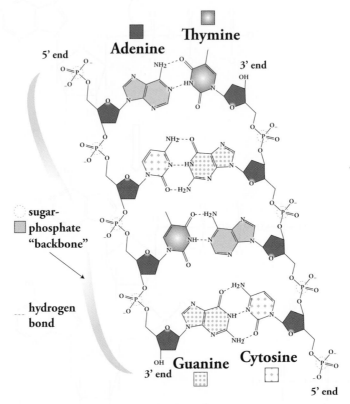

Figure 7 Base Pairing

The binding of two complementary strands of DNA into a double-stranded structure is termed **annealing**, or **hybridization**. The separation of strands is termed **melting**, or **denaturation**. The temperature at which a solution of DNA molecules is 50 percent melted is termed the T_m. [Would the T_m of ATTATCAT and its complementary strand be higher than, lower than, or equal to the melting temperature of AGTCGCAT and its complementary strand?[12] If you attached methyl groups to all the acidic phosphate oxygens along the length of a DNA double helix, would the chain have a higher or lower T_m than normal DNA?[13]]

---

[10] Antiparallel H-bonding is reminiscent of the β-pleated sheet, which is a common secondary structure (it can be quaternary, when two separate chains come together to form a sheet).

[11] This fact has a fringe benefit: we can calculate the number of purines if we know the number of pyrimidines. We can actually calculate several variables. Chargaff's Rule states that [A] = [T] and [G] = [C]; and [A] + [G] = [T] + [C].

[12] The T_m of the first oligonucleotide pair would be lower because it contains more AT pairs. A and T only form two hydrogen bonds, while G and C form three. Thus, it takes less kinetic energy to disrupt A-T rich ds-DNA than G-C rich ds-DNA.

[13] The charged phosphates electrostatically repel each other in normal DNA. Methyl esters will not be charged. The lack of electrostatic repulsion between the methyl ester backbones will increase the T_m, meaning that more kinetic energy will be required to melt the oligonucleotides.

- Which of the following is/are true about ds-DNA?[14]
    I. If the amount of G in a double helix is known, the amount of C can be calculated.
    II. If the fraction of purine nucleotides and the total molecular weight of a double helix are known, the amount of cytosine can be calculated.
    III. The two chains in a piece of ds-DNA containing mostly purines will be bonded together more tightly than the two chains in a piece of ds-DNA containing mostly pyrimidines.
    IV. The oligonucleotide ATGTAT is complementary to the oligonucleotide ATACAT.

There is another important detail about DNA structure: not only is it double stranded, it is also *coiled*. In ds-DNA, the two hydrogen-bonded antiparallel DNA strands form a **right-handed double helix** (meaning it corkscrews in a clockwise motion) with the bases on the interior and the ribose/phosphate backbone on the exterior. The double helix is stabilized by van der Waals interactions between the bases, which are stacked upon each other. Hydrophobic interactions between the bases are also very important in stabilizing the double helix. [But wait a minute. "Hydro*phobic* interactions between *bases*?" Isn't that a contradiction in terms? How can a *base* be hydro*phobic*?[15]] The bases lie in a plane, perpendicular to the length of the DNA molecule, stacked 3.4 angstroms (Å) apart from each other. The helix pattern repeats itself (i.e., completes a full turn) once every *34 angstroms*, which is every *10 base pairs*. While the length of a DNA double helix may vary enormously, from a few Å in an oligonucleotide to macroscopic lengths in a chromosome, the width is always 20 Å. [If a human chromosome has 9×10^7 base pairs, how long would the chromosome be if it were stretched out completely?[16]]

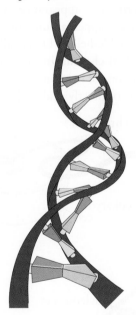

Figure 8 A Small Section of a DNA Double Helix

---

[14] **Item I: True.** For every G, there is a C; and for every A there is a T. Item II: False. The ratio of purines to pyrimidines is always the same (50:50) since each purine is paired with a pyrimidine. In order to calculate the amount of any one base, you have to know the ratio of AT to GC pairs. Item III: False. Again, the ratio of purines to pyrimidines is always the same—50:50. However, two chains containing mostly GC pairs will bond more tightly than two chains containing mostly AT pairs, since GC pairs are held together by 3 H-bonds, while AT pairs have only 2. **Item IV: True.** Remember, the strands are antiparallel: A and T pair, G and C pair, and the 5' end is always written first.

[15] Once a purine is H-bonded to a pyrimidine, most of the polar nature of the individual bases disappears because the charge dipoles are occupied in H-bonds.

[16] Since one angstrom is 10^{-10} meter, the length is $(3.4 \times 10^{-10}$ meters/base pair$)(9 \times 10^7$ base pairs$) = 30 \times 10^{-3}$ meters = 30 millimeters.

Chromosome Structure and Packing

The sum total of an organism's genetic information is called its **genome**. Eukaryotic genomes are composed of several large pieces of linear ds-*DNA*; each piece of ds-DNA is called a **chromosome**. Humans have 46 chromosomes, 23 of which are inherited from each parent. Prokaryotic (bacterial) genomes are composed of a **single circular chromosome**. Viral genomes may be linear or circular DNA or RNA. The human genome consists of over 10^9 base pairs, while bacterial genomes contain only 10^6 base pairs. But there is no direct correlation between genome size and evolutionary sophistication, since the organisms with the largest known genomes are amphibians. Much of the size difference in higher eukaryotic genomes is the result of repetitive DNA that has no known function.

If the DNA remained as a simple double helix floating free in the cell, it would be very bulky and fragile. Prokaryotes have a distinctive mechanism for making their single circular chromosome more compact and sturdy. An enzyme called **DNA gyrase** uses the energy of ATP to twist the gigantic circular molecule. Gyrase functions by breaking the DNA and twisting the two sides of the circle around each other. The resulting structure is a twisted circle that is composed of ds-DNA. As discussed above, the two strands are already coiled, forming a helix. The twists created by DNA gyrase are called **supercoils**, since they are coils of a structure that is already coiled.

Since eukaryotes have even more DNA in their genome than prokaryotes, the eukaryotic genome requires denser packaging to fit within the cell (Figure 9). To accomplish this, eukaryotic DNA is wrapped around globular proteins called **histones**. After being wrapped around histones, but before being completely packed away, DNA has the microscopic appearance of beads on a string. The beads are called **nucleosomes**; they are composed of DNA wrapped around an octamer of histones (a group of eight). The string between the beads is a length of double-helical DNA called linker DNA and is bound by a single linker histone. Fully packed DNA is called **chromatin**; it is composed of closely stacked nucleosomes. [Based on your knowledge of the interactions of macromolecules and the chemical composition of DNA, do you suppose that histones mostly basic or mostly acidic?[17]]

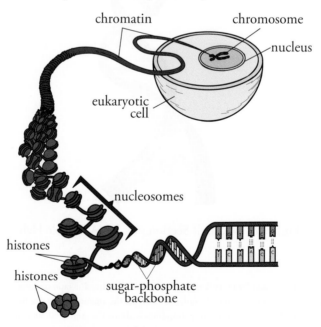

Figure 9 DNA Packaging

---

[17] They're mostly basic, since they must be attracted to the acidic exterior of the DNA double helix. This basicity is supplied by the amino acids arginine and lysine, which are unusually abundant in histones.

The following flow summarizes the structure of DNA in the nucleus: **Deoxyribose** → *add base* → **nucleoside** → *add three phosphates* → **nucleotide** → *polymerize with loss of two phosphates* → **oligonucleotide** → *continue polymerization* → **single-stranded polynucleotide** → *two complete chains H-bond in antiparallel orientation* → **ds DNA chain** → *coiling occurs* → **ds helix** → *wrap around histones* → **nucleosomes** → *complete packaging* → **chromatin**.

To look for patterns and morphology, chromosomes can be stained with chemicals. Usually, condensed metaphase chromosomes are used, as they are compact and easier to see. When chromosomes are treated, distinct light and dark regions become visible. The darker regions are denser, and are called **heterochromatin**. Heterochromatin is rich in repeats (see below). The lighter regions are less dense and are called **euchromatin**. Density gives a sense of DNA coiling or compactness, and these patterns are constant and heritable. It's now known that the lighter regions have higher transcription rates and therefore higher gene activity. The looser packing makes DNA accessible to enzymes and proteins.

Giemsa stain can also be used, and it produces what are called "G-banding patterns." Here too, darker staining regions are more dense than lighter staining regions. Chromosome bands are constant and specific to each chromosome, which means they can be used for diagnostic purposes (where cytologists look at chromosome structure). Banding patterns have also been linked to DNA replication, as it's been shown that lighter staining regions start replication earlier than darker staining regions. Again, this is likely due to accessibility of the DNA. Giemsa stains are most often used to produce karyotypes, as shown in Figure 10.

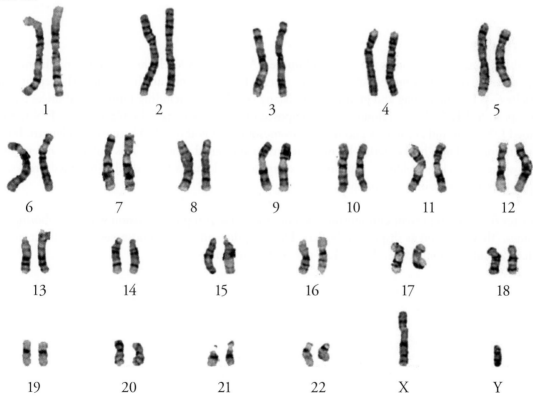

Figure 10   Giemsa Stain (a karyotype)

Centromeres

A centromere is the region of the chromosome to which spindle fibers attach during cell division. The fibers attach via **kinetochores**, multiprotein complexes that act as anchor attachment sites for spindle fibers. Other protein complexes also bind the centromere after DNA replication to keep sister chromatids attached to each other. Centromeres are made of heterochromatin and repetitive DNA sequences. Chromosomes have p (short) and q (long) arms, and the centromere position defines the ratio between the two (Figure 11).

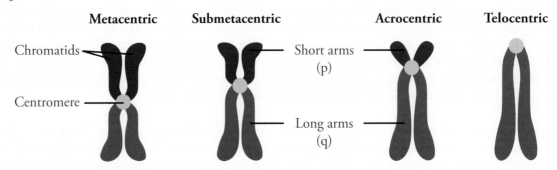

Figure 11 Centromere Positions

Telomeres

The ends of linear chromosomes are called **telomeres**. At the DNA level, these regions are distinguished by the presence of distinct nucleotide sequences repeated 50 to several hundred times. The repeated unit is usually 6–8 base pairs long and guanine-rich. Many vertebrates (including humans and mice) have the same repeat: 5'-TTAGGG-3'. Telomeres are composed of both single- and double-stranded DNA. Single-stranded DNA is found at the very end of the chromosome and is about 300 base pairs in length. It loops around to form a knot, held together by many telomere-associated proteins. This stabilizes the end of the chromosome; specialized telomere cap proteins distinguish telomeres from double-stranded breaks, and this prevents activation of repair pathways.

Telomeres function to prevent chromosome deterioration and also prevent fusion with neighboring chromosomes. They function as disposable buffers, blocking the ends of chromosomes. Since most prokaryotes have circular genomes, their DNA does not contain telomeres.

10.3 CHARACTERISTICS OF RNA

RNA is chemically distinct from DNA in three important ways:

1) RNA is **single-stranded**, except in some viruses.
2) RNA contains **uracil** instead of thymine.
3) The pentose ring in RNA is **ribose** rather than 2' deoxyribose.

As a result of this last difference, the RNA polymer is less stable, because the 2' hydroxyl can nucleophilically attack the backbone phosphate group of an RNA chain, causing hydrolysis when the remainder of the chain acts as leaving group. This cannot occur in DNA because there is no 2' hydroxyl. [Why is the stability of RNA relatively unimportant?[18]] This chemical property has a big impact in molecular biology labs, where DNA samples are stable at a range of temperatures for a relatively long period of time, but high quality RNA is difficult to extract and is only stable for a short time.

There are several different types of RNA, each with a unique role.

Coding RNA

Messenger RNA (mRNA), is the only type of coding RNA. This molecule carries genetic information to the ribosome, where it can be translated into protein (more information about translation can be found in the Biology section of this book).

Messenger RNA is constantly produced and degraded, according to the cell's need for the protein encoded by each piece of mRNA. In fact, this is the principal means by which cells regulate the amount of each particular protein they synthesize. Note that in eukaryotes, the first RNA transcribed from DNA is an immature or precursor to mRNA called **heterogeneous nuclear RNA** (hnRNA). Processing events (such as addition of a cap and tail and splicing) are required for hnRNA to become mature mRNA. Since prokaryotes do not process their primary transcripts, hnRNA is only found in eukaryotes.

Non-Coding RNA

Non-coding RNA (ncRNA) is a functional RNA that is not translated into a protein. The human genome codes for thousands of ncRNAs, and there are several types. The two major types to know for the MCAT are transfer RNA (tRNA) and ribosomal RNA (rRNA).

---

[18] Because a cell's DNA is necessary for the cell's entire life. RNA is a transient molecule that is transcribed, translated, and destroyed. As a matter of fact, the reason RNA contains uracil also has to do with the reduced need for fidelity in transcription as compared to replication. Without getting into the details, thymine is easier for DNA repair systems to work with, while uracil is much less energy-costly to make. So RNA has uracil, DNA has thymine.

Transfer RNA (tRNA) is responsible for translating the genetic code. Transfer RNA carries amino acids from the cytoplasm to the ribosome to be added to a growing protein. The structure of tRNA and how it does its job is discussed in in the Biology section of this book. [What is the minimum number of tRNAs in a given cell? What would be the maximum possible?[19]]

Ribosomal RNA (rRNA) is the major component of the ribosome. Humans have only four different types of rRNA molecules (18S, 5.8S, 28S, and 5S), though almost all of the RNA made in a given cell is rRNA. All rRNAs serve as components of the ribosome, along with many polypeptide chains. One rRNA provides the catalytic function of the ribosome, which is a little odd. In most other cases, enzymes are made from polypeptides. Catalytic RNAs are also called **ribozymes** (or ribonucleic acid enzymes), since they are capable of performing specific biochemical reactions, similar to protein enzymes.

Some other interesting non-coding RNAs include the following:

- **Small nuclear RNA** (snRNA) molecules (150 nucleotides) associate with proteins to form snRNP (small nuclear ribonucleic particles) complexes in the spliceosome.
- **MicroRNA** (miRNA) and **small interfering RNA** (siRNA) function in RNA interference (RNAi), a form of post-transcriptional regulation of gene expression. Both can bind specific mRNA molecules to either increase or decrease translation.

---

[19] Each tRNA must recognize a codon on mRNA and respond by delivering the appropriate amino acid to the ribosome. There are 20 different amino acids, so there at least 20 different tRNAs. However, there are 61 possible codons, so there could be as many as 61 different tRNAs. The actual number is between 20 and 61, because the third nucleotide of the codon is often not needed for specificity of the amino acid.

Part 3

MCAT Biology

Chapter 11
Molecular Biology

11.1 GENOME STRUCTURE AND GENOMIC VARIATIONS

The human genome contains 24 different chromosomes (22 autosomes, plus two different sex chromosomes), 3.2 billion base pairs, and codes for about 21,000 genes. It has numerous regions with high transcription rates, separated by long stretches of intergenic space. **Intergenic regions** are composed of noncoding DNA; they may direct the assembly of specific chromatin structure, and can contribute to the regulation of nearby genes, but many have no known function. Tandem repeats and transposons (see next page) are major components of intergenic regions.

Genomic regions with high transcription rates are rich in genes. A gene is a DNA sequence that encodes a gene product. It includes both regulatory regions (such as promoters and transcription stop sites), and a region that codes for either a protein or a non-coding RNA (see Section 10.3).

Genomic Variations

- **Single Nucleotide Polymorphisms:** single nucleotide changes once in every 1,000 base pairs in the human genome; SNPs, pronounced "snips," are essentially mutations.
- **Copy Number Variation:** structural variations in the genome that lead to different copies of DNA sections. Large regions of the genome (10^3 to 10^6 base pairs) can be duplicated (increasing copy number) or deleted (decreasing copy number).
- **Repeated Sequences—Tandem Repeats:** short sequences of nucleotides are repeated one right after the other, from as little as three to over 100 times. The human genome has over a thousand regions of tandem repeats.
- **Repeated Sequences:—Transposons:** mobile genetic elements that can jump around the genome. Transposons can cause mutations and chromosome changes (such as inversions, deletions, and rearrangements), and these will be discussed in Section 11.4.

11.2 THE ROLE OF DNA

DNA encodes and transmits the genetic information passed down from parents to offspring. Before 1944 it was generally believed that protein, rather than DNA, carried genetic information, since proteins have an "alphabet" of 20 letters (the amino acids), while DNA's "alphabet" has only 4 letters (the four nucleotides). But in that year, Oswald Avery showed that DNA was the active agent in bacterial transformation. In short, this means he proved that pure DNA from one type of *E. coli* bacteria could transform *E. coli* of another type, causing it to acquire the genetic nature of the first type. Later Hershey and Chase proved that DNA was the active chemical in the infection of *E. coli* bacteria by bacteriophage T2.

The Genetic Code

DNA contains sequences of nucleotides known as **genes** that serve as **templates** for the production of another nucleic acid known as RNA. The process of reading DNA and writing the information as RNA is termed **transcription**. This can generate either a final gene product (as in the case of all non-coding RNAs, discussed below), or a messenger molecule. The messenger RNA (mRNA) is then read, and the information is used to construct protein. The synthesis of proteins using RNA as a template is termed **translation**, and is accomplished by the **ribosome**, which is a massive enzyme composed of many proteins and pieces of RNA (known as ribosomal RNA or rRNA).[1]

The overall process looks like this: DNA → RNA → protein. This unidirectional flow equation represents the **Central Dogma** (fundamental law) of molecular biology. This is the mechanism whereby inherited *information* is used to create actual *objects*, namely enzymes and structural proteins.

This language used by DNA and mRNA to specify the building blocks of proteins is known as the **Genetic Code**. The alphabet of the genetic code contains only four letters (A, T, G, C). How can four letters specify the ingredients of the multitude of proteins in every cell? [What is the smallest "word" size that would allow this four-letter alphabet to encode twenty different amino acids?[2]] A number of experiments confirmed that the genetic code is written in three-letter words, each of which codes for a particular amino acid. A nucleic acid word (3 nucleotide letters) is referred to as a **codon**.

The genetic code is represented in Figure 1. The first nucleotide in a codon is given at the left, the second on top, and the third on the right. At the intersection of these three nucleotides is the amino acid called for by that codon.

1st Position (5' End)	2nd Position				3rd Position (3' End)
	U	**C**	**A**	**G**	
U	Phe	Ser	Tyr	Cys	U
	Phe	Ser	Tyr	Cys	C
	Leu	Ser	**Stop**	**Stop**	A
	Leu	Ser	**Stop**	Trp	G
C	Leu	Pro	His	Arg	U
	Leu	Pro	His	Arg	C
	Leu	Pro	Gln	Arg	A
	Leu	Pro	Gln	Arg	G
A	Ile	Thr	Asn	Ser	U
	Ile	Thr	Asn	Ser	C
	Ile	Thr	Lys	Arg	A
	Met	Thr	Lys	Arg	G
G	Val	Ala	Asp	Gly	U
	Val	Ala	Asp	Gly	C
	Val	Ala	Glu	Gly	A
	Val	Ala	Glu	Gly	G

Figure 1   The Genetic Code

[1]   To *transcribe* a letter is to listen to spoken words and write them down as printed text. The message doesn't change, and the language, English, doesn't change. To *translate* a letter is to change it from one language to another. Cellular transcription is the process whereby a code is read from a nucleic acid (DNA) and written in the language of another nucleic acid (RNA), so the language is the same. In cellular translation, nucleic acids are read and polypeptides are written, so here the language does change.

[2]   With four nucleotides, if a "word" (codon) is two nucleotides long, there are $4^2 = 16$ possible codons; too few to specify 20 unique amino acids. However, there are $4^3 = 64$ possible 3-letter "words," and 64 is more than enough different codons to specify 20 unique amino acids. Thus, three nucleotides is the minimum codon size.

- The genetic code was studied by experimenters using a cell-free protein synthesis system. All of the materials necessary for protein synthesis (ribosomes, amino acids, tRNA, GTP, ATP) were purified and placed in a beaker. Then synthetic RNA was added, and protein was translated from this template. For example, when synthetic RNA containing only cytosine (CCCCC…) was added, polypeptides containing only proline (polyproline) resulted. What kind of synthetic RNA would give rise to a mixture of polyproline, polyhistidine, and polythreonine?[3]

There are 64 codons. Sixty-one of them specify amino acids; the remaining three are called **stop codons**. Their function is to notify the ribosome that the protein is complete and cause it to stop reading the mRNA. Stop codons are also called **nonsense codons**, since they don't code for any amino acid. Note that most of the twenty amino acids can be coded for by more than one codon. Often, all four of the codons with the same first two nucleotides (for example, CU_) encode the same amino acid. [If the last nucleotide in the codon CUU is changed in a gene that codes for a protein, will the protein be affected?[4]] Two or more codons coding for the same amino acid are known as **synonyms**. Because it has such synonyms, the genetic code is said to be **degenerate**. However, it is very important to realize that though an amino acid may be specified by several codons, *each codon specifies only a single amino acid*. This means that each piece of DNA can be interpreted only one way: the code has no **ambiguity**.

11.3 DNA REPLICATION

The DNA genome is the control center of the cell. When mitosis produces two identical daughter cells from one parental cell, each daughter must have the same genome as the parent. Hence, cell division requires **DNA replication**. This is an enzymatic process that occurs during **S** (synthesis) **phase** in interphase of the cell cycle.

There is only one logical way to make a new piece of DNA that is identical to the old one: copy it. The old DNA is called **parental** DNA, and the new is called **daughter** DNA.

Experiments done by Meselson and Stahl in 1958 aimed to determine if DNA replication is semiconservative, conservative, or dispersive (Figure 2). In *conservative* replication, the parental ds-DNA would remain as-is while an entirely new double-stranded genome was created. The *dispersive* theory said that both copies of the genomes were composed of scattered pieces of new and old DNA. Meselson and Stahl showed that replication is semiconservative; after replication, one strand of the new double helix is parental (old) and one strand is newly synthesized daughter DNA.

---

[3] The RNA would have to be CCACCACCACCACCACCACCAC.... This would yield polyproline if read as CCA, CCA, CCA. But if it were read as CAC, CAC, CAC, it would give rise to polyhistidine. If it were read ACC, ACC, ACC, it would encode polythreonine.

[4] No, since CUN codes for leucine, regardless of what N is. Notice that switching the 3rd nucleotide in the majority of codons will have no effect.

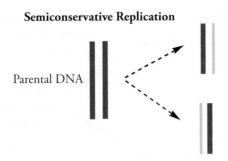

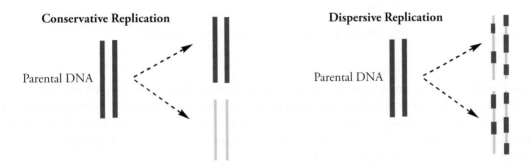

Figure 2   Meselson-Stahl Experiments

Let's begin a list of things to memorize here:

1) **DNA replication is semiconservative.**
   Individual strands of the double-stranded parent are pulled apart, then a new daughter strand is synthesized using the parental DNA as a template to copy from.[5] [What is the relationship between a parent or template strand and its daughter strand?[6]]

When it is not being replicated, DNA is tightly coiled. The replication process cannot begin unless the double helix is uncoiled and separated into two single strands. The enzyme that unwinds the double helix and separates the strands is called helicase. [Would you expect helicase to use the energy of ATP hydrolysis to do its job?[7]] The place where the helicase begins to unwind is not random. It is a specific location (sequence of nucleotides) on the chromosome called the **origin of replication** (abbreviated ORI).

When helicase unwinds the helix at the origin of replication, the helix gets wound more tightly upstream and downstream from this point.[8] The chromosome would get tangled and eventually break, except that enzymes called **topoisomerases** cut one or both of the strands and unwrap the helix, releasing the excess tension created by the helicases. Another potential problem is that single-stranded DNA is much less stable than ds-DNA. **Single-strand binding proteins (SSBPs)** protect DNA that has been unpackaged in preparation for replication and help keep the strands separated. The separated strands are referred to as an **open complex**. Replication may now begin.

---

[5]   A template is something that is copied. The metal plates used in printing presses are an example.

[6]   DNA strands are complementary to one another, so the daughter strand is complementary to its template.

[7]   Yes. Separating the strands requires the breaking of many H-bonds.

[8]   Imagine two long ropes wound around each other. What happens if you pull them apart in the middle?

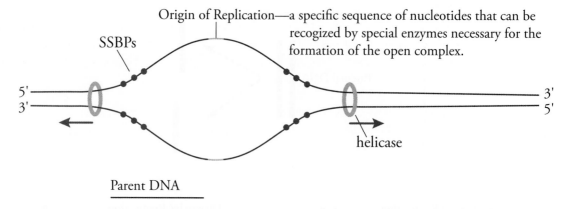

Origin of Replication—a specific sequence of nucleotides that can be recogized by special enzymes necessary for the formation of the open complex.

SSBPs

5'
3'

3'
5'

helicase

Parent DNA

Figure 3   Initiation—The Open Complex

An RNA primer must be synthesized for each template strand. This is accomplished by a set of proteins called the primosome, of which the central component is an RNA polymerase called **primase**. Primer synthesis is important because the next enzyme, DNA polymerase, cannot start a new DNA chain from scratch. It can only add nucleotides to an existing nucleotide chain. The RNA primer is usually 8–12 nucleotides long, and it is later replaced by DNA.

Daughter DNA is created as a growing polymer. **DNA polymerase** (DNA pol) catalyzes the elongation of the daughter strand using the parental template, and it elongates the primer by adding dNTPs to its 3' end. [The template strand is read in what direction?[9]] DNA pol is part of a large complex of proteins called the replisome. Other accessory proteins in this complex help DNA polymerase and allow it to polymerize DNA quickly. The prokaryotic replisome contains 13 components, and the eukaryotic replisome contains 27 proteins; additional complexity in the eukaryotic system is required because replication machinery must also unwind DNA from histone proteins.

Rapid elongation of the daughter strands follows. Since the two template strands are antiparallel, the two primers will elongate toward opposite ends of the chromosome. After a while it looks like this:

Origin of Replication

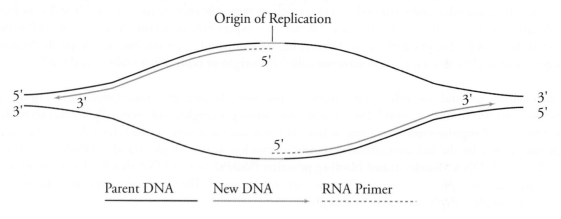

5'

5'
3'

3'

3'

3'
5'

5'

Parent DNA   New DNA   RNA Primer

Figure 4   Elongation

---

⁹   If the daughter is made 5' to 3', and the two strands have to end up antiparallel, the template must be read 3' to 5'.

DNA polymerase checks each new nucleotide to make sure it forms a correct base-pair before it is incorporated in the growing polymer. The thermodynamic driving force for the polymerization reaction is the removal and hydrolysis of pyrophosphate ($P_2O_7^{4-}$) from each dNTP added to the chain. Here are some more replication rules to memorize:

2) **Polymerization occurs in the 5' to 3' direction, without exception.** This means the existing chain is always lengthened by the addition of a nucleotide to the 3' end of the chain. There is never 3' to 5' polymerase activity.

3) **DNA pol requires a *template*.** It cannot make a DNA chain from scratch but must copy an old chain. This makes sense because it would be pretty useless if DNA pol just made a strand of DNA randomly, without copying a template.

4) **DNA pol requires a *primer*.** It cannot start a new nucleotide chain.

- Can DNA polymerase make the following partially double-stranded structure completely double stranded in the presence of excess nucleotides, using the top strand as a primer?[10]

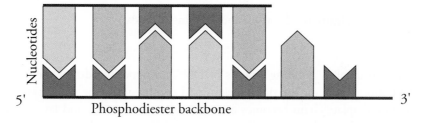

Replication proceeds along in both directions away from the origin of replication. Both template strands are read 3' to 5' while daughter strands are elongated 5' to 3'. The areas where the parental double helix continues to unwind are called the **replication forks.** Let's split the picture on the previous page (Figure 4) and look at an enlargement of the right side:

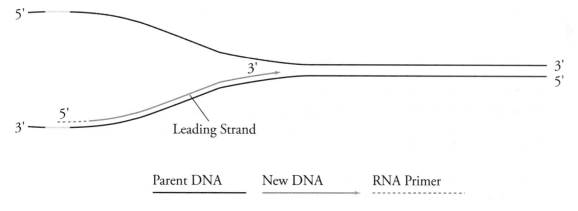

Figure 5   Leading Strand

---

[10] No. The DNA strands are antiparallel, meaning that the upper strand would have to be extended in a 3' to 5' direction, which is impossible. Note that the phrase "in the presence of excess nucleotides" is extraneous. It just means there are plenty of building blocks around. Typical MCAT smokescreen.

The problem is that chain elongation can only proceed in one direction, 5' to 3', but in order to replicate the right half of the top chain and the left half of the bottom one continuously, we would have to go in the opposite direction. Here's the solution:

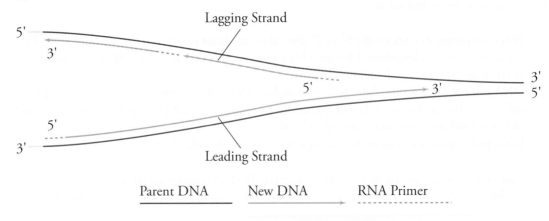

Figure 6   Leading and Lagging Strands

The solution to this problem involves building strands of DNA on opposite sides of the ORI using different methods. As the bottom chain on the right is elongated continuously, the replication fork widens. After a good bit of the top template chain becomes exposed, primase comes in and lays down a primer, which DNA pol can elongate. Then, when the replication fork widens again and more of the top template becomes exposed, these events are repeated. The bottom daughter on the right side, and the top daughter on the left side are called the **leading strands** because they elongate continuously right into the widening replication fork. The top daughter on the right, and the bottom daughter on the left are called the **lagging strands** because they must wait until the replication fork widens before beginning to polymerize. The small chunks of DNA comprising the lagging strand are called **Okazaki fragments**, after their discoverer. [As the replication forks grow, what role does helicase play?[11]] Let's continue our memory-list:

5) **Replication forks grow away from the origin in both directions.** Each replication fork contains a **leading strand** and a **lagging strand**.
6) Replication of the leading strand is **continuous** and leads into the replication fork, while replication of the lagging strand is **discontinuous**, resulting in Okazaki fragments.
7) Eventually **all RNA primers are replaced by DNA**, and the **fragments are joined by an enzyme called DNA ligase**.

DNA Polymerase

DNA polymerase can rapidly build DNA and is able to add tens of thousands of nucleotides before falling off the template. It is therefore said to be *processive*.

Eukaryotes have several different DNA polymerase enzymes, and their mechanisms of action are complex. You do not need to worry about this complexity.

---

[11] Helicase must continue to unwind the double helix and separate the strands for replication to continue beyond the fork.

Prokaryotes on the other hand have five types of DNA polymerases, called DNA polymerase I, II, III, IV, and V. You should definitely know the functions of DNA pol III and DNA pol I:

1) **DNA pol III** is responsible for the super-fast, super-accurate elongation of the leading strand. It has 5' to 3' polymerase activity as well as 3' to 5' exonuclease[12] activity. This is when the enzyme moves backwards to chop off the nucleotide it just added, if it was incorrect; the ability to correct mistakes in this way is known as **proofreading function**. It has no known function in repair and so is considered a replicative enzyme.

2) **DNA pol I** starts adding nucleotides at the RNA primer; this is 5' to 3' polymerase activity. Because it can only add 15–20 nucleotides per second, DNA pol III usually takes over about 400 base pairs downstream from the ORI. DNA pol I is also capable of 3' to 5' exonuclease activity (proofreading). DNA pol I removes the RNA primer via 5' to 3' exonuclease activity, while simultaneously leaving behind new DNA in __[13] activity. Finally, DNA pol I is important for excision repair (see below).

The functions of DNA pol II, IV, and V are less important to know for the MCAT:

3) DNA pol II has 5' to 3' polymerase activity, and 3' to 5' exonuclease proofreading function. It participates in DNA repair pathways and is used as a backup for DNA pol III.

4) DNA pol IV and DNA pol V have similar characteristics. They are error prone in 5' to 3' polymerase activity, but they function to stall other polymerase enzymes at replication forks when DNA repair pathways have been activated. This is an important part of the prokaryotic checkpoint pathway. This enzyme has additional repair functions as well.

If a bacterium possesses a mutation in the gene for DNA polymerase III, resulting in an enzyme without the 3' to 5' exonuclease activity, will mutations occur more often than in bacteria with a normal DNA polymerase gene?[14]

Prokaryotic vs. Eukaryotic Replication

Prokaryotes have only one chromosome, and this one chromosome has only one origin. Because the chromosome is circular, as replication proceeds the partially duplicated genome begins to look like the Greek letter θ (theta). Hence, the replication of prokaryotes is said to proceed by the **theta mechanism** and is referred to as **theta replication** (see Figure 7).

---

[12] **Exonuclease** means "cutting a nucleic acid chain at the end." An **endonuclease** will cut a polynucleotide acid chain in the middle of the chain, usually at a particular sequence. Two important types of endonucleases are: **repair enzymes** that remove chemically damaged DNA from the chain, and **restriction enzymes**, which are endonucleases found in bacteria. Their role is to destroy the DNA of infecting viruses, thus restricting the host range of the virus.

[13] 5' to 3' polymerase; remember, all polymerization is 5' to 3'.

[14] Yes. The 3' to 5' exonuclease activity is the polymerase's way of editing its work. Without this editing function, many more point mutations would occur due to the incorporation of wrong nucleotides. The normal polymerase is remarkably adept at sensing correct base pairing and removing bases that don't belong.

11.3

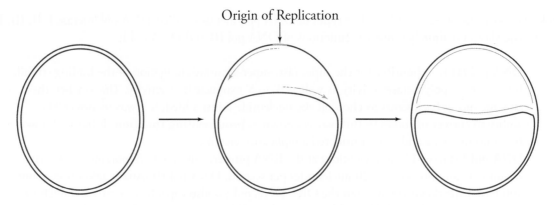

Origin of Replication

Figure 7   Theta (θ) Replication

In eukaryotic replication, each chromosome has several origins. This is necessary because eukaryotic chromosomes are so huge that replicating them from a single origin would be too slow. As the many replication forks continue to widen, they create an appearance of bubbles along the DNA strand, so they are referred to as "replication bubbles." Eventually the replication forks meet, and the many daughter strands are ligated together.

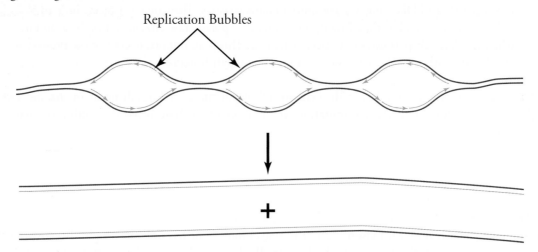

Replication Bubbles

+

Figure 8   Eukaryotic Replication

Replicating Telomeres

DNA polymerase can only build DNA in one direction (5' to 3'), and it requires both a template and a primer. These requirements lead to a roadblock at chromosome ends. Eventually there will be no place on the lagging strand to lay down a primer, and primers close to the end of DNA cannot be replaced with DNA because there is nothing on the other side (DNA polymerase usually uses a previous length of upstream DNA to replace the primer, but this isn't available at the end of a chromosome). This means that DNA replication machinery is unable to replicate sequences at the very ends of chromosomes, and after each round of the cell cycle and DNA replication, the ends of chromosomes shorten. **Telomeres** are disposable repeats at the end of chromosomes. They are consumed and shortened during cell division, becoming between 50 and 200 base pairs shorter.

When telomeres become *too* short, they reach a critical length where the chromosome can no longer replicate. As a consequence, cells can activate DNA repair pathways, enter a senescent state (where they are alive but not dividing), or activate apoptosis (pre-programmed cell death). The *Hayflick limit* is the number of times a normal human cell type can divide until telomere length stops cell division. Many age-related diseases are linked to telomere shortening.

Telomerase is an enzyme that adds repetitive nucleotide sequences to the ends of chromosomes and therefore lengthens telomeres. Telomerase is a ribonucleoprotein complex, containing an RNA primer and reverse transcriptase enzyme. Reverse transcriptases read RNA templates and generate DNA. In humans, the RNA template is 3'-CCCAATCCC-5', and this allows for chromosome extension, one DNA repeat (5'-TTAGGG-3') at a time (Figure 9). The telomerase complex continuously polymerizes, then translocates, allowing extension of six-nucleotide telomere repeats.

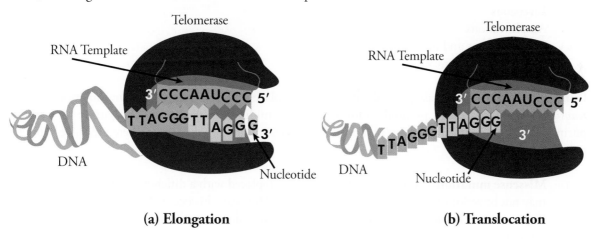

(a) **Elongation**   (b) **Translocation**

Figure 9   Telomerase and Telomere Lengthening

In most organisms, telomerase is only expressed in the germ line, embryonic stem cells, and some white blood cells. However, cancer cells can also express telomerase, which can help the cells immortalize. Telomere extension allows the cells to bypass senescence and apoptosis, and can therefore contribute to their transformation to a precancerous state.

11.4   GENETIC MUTATION

Genetic mutation refers to any alteration of the DNA sequence of an organism's genome. These can be inherited or acquired throughout life. Mutations that can be passed onto offspring are called germline mutations, since they occur in the germ cells (which give rise to gametes). Somatic mutations occur in somatic (non-gametic) cells and are not passed onto offspring. In other words, somatic mutations can have a major effect on an individual, but they will not be passed on to future individuals in that population. Our cells have evolved elaborate repair pathways to help deal with mutations.

Causes of Mutation

There are many causes of mutation. Most are induced by an environmental factor or chemical, however, they can also occur spontaneously. Causes include physical mutagens (such as ionizing or UV radiation), chemical mutagens (such as compounds that look like bases but are not, for example, ethidium bromide), and biological mutagens (such as viruses or faulty DNA pol enzymes).

11.4

Types of Mutations

Based on structure, there are seven kinds of mutations:

1) Point mutations
2) Insertions
3) Deletions
4) Inversions
5) Amplifications
6) Translocations and rearrangements
7) Loss of heterozygosity

Point mutations are single base pair substitutions (A in place of G, for example). Point mutations can be *transitions* (substitution of a pyrimidine for another pyrimidine or substitution of a purine for another purine) or *transversions* (substitution of a purine for a pyrimidine or vice versa). There are three types of point mutations:

1) **Missense mutation**: causes one amino acid to be replaced with a different amino acid. This may not be serious if the amino acids are similar. [How can this occur?[15]]
2) **Nonsense mutation**: a stop codon replaces a regular codon and prematurely shortens the protein.
3) **Silent mutation**: a codon is changed into a new codon for the same amino acid, so there is no change in the protein's amino acid sequence.

Insertion refers to the addition of one or more extra nucleotides into the DNA sequence, and deletion is the removal of nucleotides from the sequence. Both of these mutations can cause a shift in the reading frame. For example, AAACCCACC is read as AAA, CCC, ACC. It would code for Lys-Pro-Thr. Inserting an extra G into the first codon could produce this: AGAACCCACC. This would be read AGA, ACC, CAC, C. It now codes for Arg-Thr-His (plus there's an extra C). Not only has the first codon and amino acid changed, the whole gene will be read differently and all amino acids in the protein from that point on will change. Mutations that cause a change in the reading frame are called **frameshift mutations**. Generally speaking, frameshift mutations are very serious. Note that a frameshift can lead to premature termination of translation (yielding an incomplete polypeptide) if it results in the presence of an abnormal stop codon. [Are all insertions and deletions frameshift mutations?[16]]

---

[15] For example, substituting a small hydrophobe such as valine for another small hydrophobe like leucine will probably cause little disruption of protein structure. Another way of defining conservative mutations is that they cause changes in primary structure but do not affect secondary, tertiary, or quaternary structure.

[16] No. If you insert or delete one whole codon or several whole codons, you add or remove amino acids to the polypeptide without changing the reading frame.

In addition to mutations at individual nucleotides, larger-scale mutations are also common. Insertions and deletions can involve thousands of bases. An **inversion** is when a segment of a chromosome is reversed end to end. The chromosome undergoes breakage and rearrangement within itself (Figure 10).

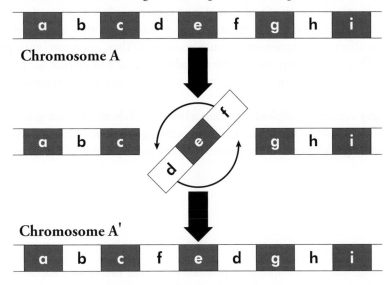

Figure 10 Chromosome Inversion

Chromosome amplification is when a segment of a chromosome is duplicated. This is similar to copy number variations mentioned above. **Translocations** result when recombination occurs between non-homologous chromosomes (Figure 11). This can create a gene fusion, where a new gene product is made from parts of two genes that were not previously connected. This is a common occurrence in many types of cancer. Translocations can be balanced (where no genetic information is lost), or unbalanced (where genetic information is lost or gained).

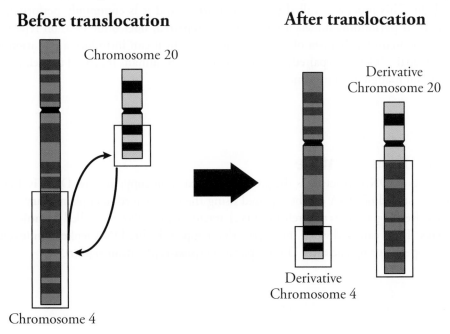

Figure 11 Chromosome Amplification

11.5

Transposons were introduced in Section 11.1. All transposons contain a gene that codes for a protein called transposase. This enzyme has "cut and paste" activity that catalyzes mobilization of the transposon (excision from the donor site) and integration into a new genetic location (the acceptor site). Sometimes the transposon sequence is complete excised and moved, and sometimes it is duplicated and moved, while still maintained at the original location. When transposons are mobilized, they can insert in any part of the genome, and this can affect gene expression or cause mutations. They can jump into a promoter and turn gene expression off. They could jump into a protein-coding region and disrupt (or mutate) the sequence. They can also jump into regulatory parts of the genome and ramp up gene expression at a nearby site.

Loss of heterozygosity occurs in a diploid organism when one allele of a certain gene is lost, either due to deletion or a recombination event. This makes the locus hemizygous: there is only one gene copy in a diploid organism. If the remaining allele is mutant or defective, all normal expression of this gene product is lost.

11.5 DNA REPAIR

Extensive DNA damage can induce apoptosis in eukaryotes, but before this happens, cells try to repair the DNA damage. This is important so that defective DNA isn't passed on to daughter cells. There are several types of DNA repair.

Direct Reversal

Many types of DNA damage are irreversible and require repair pathways to fix the damage. However, a few can be directly reversed. For example, some enzymes can repair UV-induced pyrimidine photodimers using visible light. This process is called photoreactivation, and it is commonly performed by bacteria and many plants. If pyrimidine dimers are not directly repaired, nucleotide excision repair can be used instead. This is the main mechanism of repair in humans, but it can introduce a mutation when trying to complete the repair. If left unrepaired, pyrimidine dimers in humans may lead to melanoma, a type of very dangerous and malignant skin tumor.

Homology-Dependent Repair

One of the benefits of DNA structure is the presence of a back-up copy; because DNA is double stranded, mutations on one strand of DNA can be repaired using the undamaged, complementary information on the other strand. Repair pathways that rely on this characteristic of DNA are called **homology-dependent repair pathways**. These can be divided into repair that happens before DNA replication (**excision repair**), or repair that happens during and after DNA replication (**post-replication repair**).

Excision Repair

Excision repair involves removing defective bases or nucleotides and replacing them. If these bases are not repaired, they can induce mutations during DNA replication, since replication machinery cannot pair them properly.

Post-Replication Repair

The **mismatch repair pathway** (MMR) targets mismatched base pairs that were not repaired by DNA polymerase proofreading during replication. To do this, mispaired bases must be identified and fixed, but the crucial question is: which base is the correct one and which is the mistake? For example, if DNA contains an AC base pair, is the adenine correct and C should be removed and replaced with T? Or is the cytosine correct and A should be removed and replaced with G?

Some bacteria use genome methylation to help differentiate between the older DNA template strand and the newly synthesized daughter strand. Methylation takes a while to complete, which means that shortly after DNA synthesis, the parental template strand will be labeled with methylated bases and the new daughter strand will not. Bacterial machinery can read these methyl tags and know which base is the correct one (the one on the older strand) and which needs to be replaced (the newer one).

Other prokaryotes and most eukaryotes use a different system, where the newly synthesized strand is recognized by the free 3'-terminus on the leading strand, or by the presence of gaps between Okazaki fragments on the lagging strand.

Double-Strand Break Repair

DNA double-strand breaks (DSBs) can be caused by reactive oxygen species, ionizing radiation, UV light, or chemical agents. Cells have two pathways to help in DSB repair: homologous recombination and nonhomologous end-joining. The goal of both is to reattach and fuse chromosomes that have come apart because of DSB. If done incorrectly, this can lead to deletions (where genetic information is lost) or translocations (where chromosome segments move to other chromosomes).

Homologous Recombination

After DNA replication, the genome contains identical sister chromatids. Homologous recombination is a process where one sister chromatid can help repair a DSB in the other. First, the DSB is identified and trimmed at 5' ends to generate single-stranded DNA (Figure 12). This is done by nucleases (which break phosphodiester bonds) and helicase (to unwind the DNA). Many proteins bind these ends and start a search of the genome to find a sister chromatid region that is complementary to the single-stranded DNA. Once found, the complementary sequences are used as a template to repair and connect the broken chromatid. This requires a "joint molecule," where damaged and undamaged sister chromatids cross over. DNA polymerase and ligase build a corrected DNA strand.

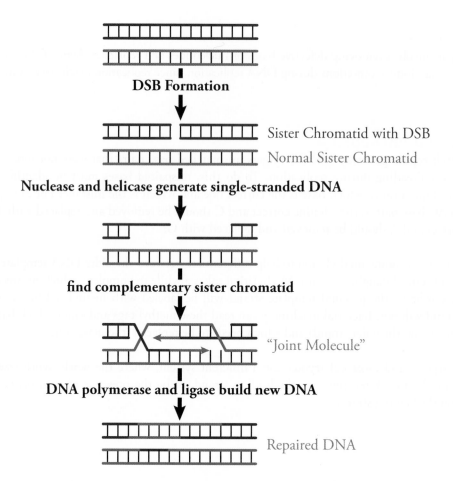

Sister Chromatid with DSB

Normal Sister Chromatid

"Joint Molecule"

Repaired DNA

Figure 12   Homologous Recombination to Repair Double-Strand Breaks

Nonhomologous End Joining

Cells that aren't actively growing or cycling through the cell cycle don't have the option of using sister chromatids to repair DSBs in an error-free way. Since DNA replication isn't happening, there is no chromosome backup to use. In this case, even a poorly repaired chromosome is better than one with a DSB, since chromosome breaks can lead to rearrangements.

Nonhomologous end joining is used to accomplish repair in this case. This process is common in eukaryotes but relatively uncommon in prokaryotes. First, broken ends are stabilized and processed, then DNA ligase connects the fragments. Nothing about this process requires specificity; the goal is just to reconnect broken chromosomes. Often, this can result in base pairs being lost or chromosomes being connected in an abnormal way.

11.6   GENE EXPRESSION: TRANSCRIPTION

Gene expression refers to the process whereby the information contained in genes begins to have effects in the cell. The Central Dogma tells us that genetic information must be written in the form of RNA (i.e., it must be **transcribed**); and then it must be expressed as protein (i.e., it must be **translated**). Hence, the logical place to begin our discussion of gene expression is with the nature of RNA and transcription.

Characteristics of RNA

As discussed previously, RNA is chemically distinct from DNA in three important ways:

1) RNA is **single-stranded**, except in some viruses.
2) RNA contains **uracil** instead of thymine.
3) The pentose ring in RNA is **ribose** rather than 2' deoxyribose.

As a result of this last difference, the RNA polymer is less stable, because the 2' hydroxyl can nucleophilically attack the backbone phosphate group of an RNA chain, causing hydrolysis when the remainder of the chain acts as leaving group. This cannot occur in DNA, since there is no 2' hydroxyl. Anticancer drugs often seek to block growth of rapidly dividing cells by inhibiting production of thymine. [Why is this an attractive target for cancer therapy?[17]] This chemical property has a big impact in molecular biology labs, where DNA samples are stable at a range of temperatures for a relatively long period of time, but high quality RNA is difficult to extract and is only stable for a short time.

There are several different types of RNA, each with a unique role.

Coding RNA

You are already familiar with **messenger RNA** (mRNA), the only type of coding RNA. This molecule carries genetic information to the ribosome, where it can be translated into protein; each unique polypeptide is created according to the sequence of codons on a particular piece of mRNA, which was transcribed from a particular gene. To allow for this, each mRNA has several regions. The 5' region is not translated into protein (it is called the 5' untranslated region, or **5'UTR**), but it is important in initiation and regulation. Following the 5'UTR is the region that codes for a protein. This starts at a start codon and ends at a stop codon, and it is called the **open reading frame** (ORF). The 3' end of the mRNA (after the stop codon) isn't translated into protein, but it often contains regulatory regions that influence post-transcriptional gene expression (see Section 11.7).

Eukaryotic mRNA is usually **monocistronic** and obeys the "one gene, one protein" principle. This means that each piece of mRNA encodes only one polypeptide (and so contains one ORF). Hence, there are as many different mRNAs as there are proteins. Because each mRNA can be read many times, each transcript can be used to make many copies of its polypeptide.

---

[17] All cells require RNA production, even if they are not growing, in order to continually replenish degraded RNA. RNA contains the bases cytosine, guanine, uracil, and adenine, but only DNA contains thymine. Thus, if thymine production is blocked, only DNA *replication* will be inhibited and only rapidly dividing cells such as cancer cells will be affected. Unfortunately, some normal cells in the body normally divide a lot (such as lining cells of the gut and hair follicles), explaining the side effects of chemotherapy.

11.6

In contrast, prokaryotic mRNA often codes for more than one polypeptide and is termed **polycistronic**. Different open reading frames on the same polycistronic mRNA are generally related in function. Translation termination and initiation sequences are found between the ORFs. The termination information helps finish the previous peptide chain, and initiation information helps start translation of the next open reading frame on the transcript.

Messenger RNA is constantly produced and degraded, according to the cell's need for the protein encoded by each piece of mRNA. In fact, this is the principal means whereby cells regulate the amount of each particular protein they synthesize. This is an important point that will be emphasized later. Note that in eukaryotes, the first RNA transcribed from DNA is an immature or precursor to mRNA called **heterogeneous nuclear RNA** (hnRNA). Processing events (such as addition of a cap and tail, and splicing) are required for hnRNA to become mature mRNA. Since prokaryotes do not process their primary transcripts, hnRNA is only found in eukaryotes.

Non-Coding RNA

Non-coding RNA (ncRNA) is a functional RNA that is not translated into a protein. The human genome codes for thousands of ncRNAs, and there are several types. The two major types to know for the MCAT are transfer RNA (tRNA) and ribosomal RNA (rRNA).

Transfer RNA (tRNA) is responsible for translating the genetic code. Transfer RNA carries amino acids from the cytoplasm to the ribosome to be added to a growing protein.

Ribosomal RNA (rRNA) Humans have four different types of rRNA molecules (18S, 5.8S, 28S and 5S). All rRNAs serve as components of the ribosome, along with many polypeptide chains. One rRNA provides the catalytic function of the ribosome, which is a little odd. In most other cases, enzymes are made from polypeptides. Catalytic RNAs are also called **ribozymes**.

Replication vs. Transcription

Transcription is the synthesis of RNA (usually mRNA, tRNA, or rRNA) using DNA as the template. The word *transcription* indicates that in the process of reading and writing information, the language does not change. Information is transferred from one polynucleotide to another. This should lead you to expect transcription to be fairly similar to replication. And it is.

Both replication and transcription involve **template-driven polymerization**. [Because of this, the RNA transcript produced in transcription is __[18] to the DNA template, just as the daughter strand produced in replication was.] The *driving force* for both processes is the removal and subsequent hydrolysis of pyrophosphate from each nucleotide added to the chain, with the existing chain acting as nucleophile. [Transcription, like replication, can occur only in the __[19] direction. Do the polymerase enzymes in both replication and transcription require a primer?[20]] Another important difference between transcription and DNA replication is that RNA polymerase lacks exonuclease activity; in other words, it cannot correct its errors. Thus, transcription is a lower fidelity process than replication.

---

[18] complementary

[19] 5' to 3'

[20] No, RNA pol does not require a primer. Remember, the primer in replication is a piece of RNA, made by an RNA polymerase.

Another similarity is that transcription, like replication, begins at a specific spot on the chromosome. The name of the site where transcription starts (the **start site**) is different from the name of the place where replication begins, __.[21] The sequence of nucleotides on a chromosome that activates RNA polymerase to begin the process of transcription is called the **promoter**, and the point where RNA polymerization actually *starts* is called the start site. In fact, from this point forward, just about every event in transcription is given a different name from the events in replication.

Reference Points in Transcription

Before we discuss the mechanics of transcription, we need to clarify a few reference points (see Figure 13). We noted previously that the chromosome is referred to as the *template*, not *parent*. Only one of the strands of the DNA template encodes a particular mRNA molecule. The strand that is actually transcribed is called the **template**, **non-coding**, **transcribed**, or **antisense strand**; it is complementary to the transcript. The other DNA strand is called the **coding** or **sense strand**; it has the same sequence as the transcript (except it has T in place of U). It is customary to say that transcription starts at a point and proceeds **downstream**, which means toward the 3' end of the coding strand and transcript. **Upstream** means toward the 5' end of the coding strand, beyond the 5' end of the transcript. Upstream nucleotide sequences are referred to using negative numbers, and downstream sequences are referred to using positive numbers. The first nucleotide on the template strand that is actually transcribed is called the start site. The corresponding nucleotide on the coding strand is given the number +1. As we'll see below, regulatory sequences on the chromosome are referred to by where they occur on the coding strand.

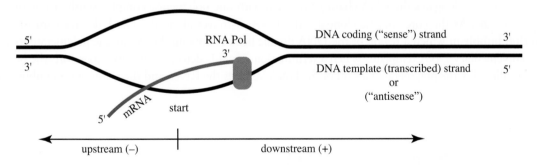

Figure 13 Reference Points in Transcription

---

[21] the origin

Prokaryotic Transcription

It is important to understand all the vocabulary and general principles presented above. In this section and the next, we will present some more detailed information.

In bacteria (prokaryotes), all types of RNA are made by the same RNA polymerase. Prokaryotic RNA polymerase is a large enzyme complex consisting of five subunits. This is the **core enzyme** responsible for rapid elongation of the transcript. However, the core enzyme alone cannot initiate transcription. An additional subunit termed the **sigma factor** (σ) is required to form what is sometimes referred to as the **holoenzyme** (*holo* = complete), which is responsible for initiation.

Transcription occurs in three stages: **initiation**, **elongation**, and **termination**. Initiation occurs when RNA polymerase holoenzyme binds to a promoter. The typical bacterial promoter contains two primary sequences: the **Pribnow box** at −10 and the **−35 sequence**. Holoenzyme scans along the chromosome like a train on a railroad track until it recognizes a promoter and then stops, forming a **closed complex**. The RNA polymerase must unwind a portion of the DNA double helix before it can begin to synthesize RNA. The RNA polymerase bound at the promoter with a region of single-stranded DNA is termed the **open complex**. Once the open complex has formed, transcription can begin.

The sigma factor plays two roles in helping the polymerase find promoters. The first is to greatly increase the ability of RNA polymerase to recognize promoters. The second is to decrease the nonspecific affinity of holoenzyme for DNA. Once the open complex and several phosphodiester bonds have been formed, the sigma factor is no longer necessary and leaves the RNA polymerase complex.

The core enzyme elongates the RNA chain *processively*, with one polymerase complex synthesizing an entire RNA molecule. As the core enzyme elongates the RNA, it moves along the DNA downstream in a **transcription bubble** in which a region of the DNA double helix is unwound to allow the polymerase to access the complementary DNA template. When a termination signal is detected, in some cases with the help of a protein called rho, the polymerase falls off of the DNA, releases the RNA, and the transcription bubble closes.

Comparing Prokaryotic and Eukaryotic Transcription

Eukaryotic and prokaryotic transcription are similar, but you need to be aware of four major differences.

Location

Eukaryotic means "true-kernelled." Prokaryotic means "before-the-kernel." The **karyon** (kernel) is, of course, the nucleus. The fact that prokaryotes have no nucleus means transcription occurs free in the cytoplasm, in the same compartment where translation occurs, and transcription and translation can occur *simultaneously*. Eukaryotes must transcribe their mRNA in the nucleus, then modify it (see below), then transport it across the nuclear membrane to the cytoplasm where it can be translated. Transcription and translation in eukaryotes *do not* occur simultaneously.

Another important difference between prokaryotic and eukaryotic gene expression is that the primary transcript in prokaryotes is mRNA. In other words, the product of transcription by prokaryotic RNA polymerase is ready to be translated. In fact, translation of prokaryotic mRNA begins before transcription is completed!

In contrast, the eukaryotic primary transcript (hnRNA made by RNA pol II, see below for info on eukaryotic RNA polymerases) is modified extensively before translation (Figure 23 on page 222). The most important example is **splicing**. Eukaryotic DNA has non-coding sequences intervening between the segments that actually code for proteins. Sometimes these intervening sequences contain enhancers or other regulatory sequences, and they can be quite long. _Int_ervening sequences in the RNA are called **introns**. Protein-coding regions of the RNA are termed **ex**ons because they actually get _ex_pressed. Before the RNA can be translated, introns must be removed and exons joined together; this is accomplished via splicing.

Splicing is mediated by the **spliceosome**, a complex that contains over 100 proteins and 5 small nuclear RNA (snRNA) molecules. About half the proteins stably bind snRNAs, and these form three small nuclear ribonucleic particles (snRNPs). Each snRNP is therefore made of proteins and snRNAs. The spliceosome assembles around each intron that needs to be removed. This happens in a series of steps, where different snRNP components are recruited and released as the reaction proceeds. The complex undergoes many conformational changes to attain catalytic activity.

Two splicing reactions are catalyzed by the spliceosome. The first reaction causes the intron to form a looped structure, then the second reaction joins the two exons (Figure 14) and releases the loop.

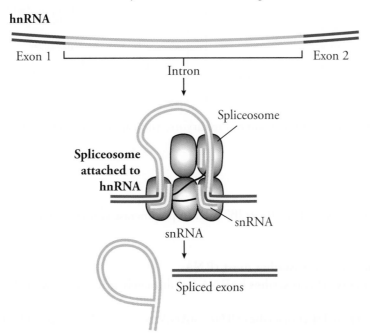

Figure 14   Mechanism of Splicing

For a given gene, there are often different options or patterns of splicing, a phenomenon called **alternative splicing**. There are many different common patterns. One gene could have different promoters in the 5' region, there can be alternative 5' exons or 3' exons, and some exons can be included or skipped. Finally, there could be mutually exclusive exons, where sometimes one is included and sometimes the other is kept. These patterns lead to different mRNAs being made from one DNA gene sequence; the mRNAs can be different in length and sequence. Shuffling exons in this way is one way to increase the complexity of gene expression.

Eukaryotic hnRNA must be modified in two other ways before translation can occur. A tag is added to each end of the molecule: a **5' cap** and a **3' poly-A tail**. The 5' cap is a methylated guanine nucleotide stuck on the 5' end [which is the end made __ (first or last?)[22]]. The poly-A tail is a string of several hundred adenine nucleotides. The cap is essential for translation, while both the cap and the poly-A tail are important in preventing digestion of the mRNA by exonucleases that are free in the cell.

- Why would active exonucleases be floating free in the cell?[23]

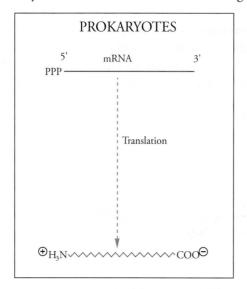 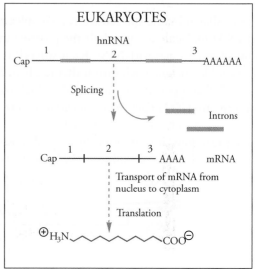

Figure 15 Comparison of Prokaryotic and Eukaryotic Gene Expression

RNA Polymerase

In prokaryotes, all RNA is made by the $\alpha 2\beta\beta'\sigma$ RNA polymerase complex. In eukaryotes, there are many different RNA polymerases.

- **RNA polymerase I transcribes most rRNA.**
- **RNA polymerase II transcribes hnRNA** (so ultimately mRNA), most snRNA, and some miRNA.
- **RNA polymerase III transcribes tRNA**, siRNA, some miRNA, and a subset of rRNA.

Please note: In our discussion of replication you learned about many *prokaryotic DNA* polymerases. In contrast, here you learned about many eukaryotic RNA polymerases. Don't get mixed up!

---

[22] It is made first, since transcription proceeds from 5' to 3'.

[23] Two conceivable reasons: 1) mRNA has a very short lifespan; it is degraded rapidly, and more must be made if the protein is still needed. Note that this is consistent with the idea that regulation of gene expression occurs primarily at the transcriptional level since this is more efficient. 2) Viruses may inject RNA into the cell. If it does not have the correct cap and tail modifications, exonucleases will destroy it.

11.7 GENE EXPRESSION: TRANSLATION

Translation is the synthesis of polypeptides according to the amino acid sequence dictated by the sequence of codons in mRNA. During translation, an mRNA molecule attaches to a ribosome at a specific codon, and the appropriate amino acid is delivered by a tRNA molecule. Then the second amino acid is delivered by another tRNA. Then the ribosome binds the two amino acids together, creating a dipeptide. This process is repeated until the polypeptide is complete, at which point the ribosome drops the mRNA and the new polypeptide departs.

Transfer RNA (tRNA)

Each tRNA is composed of a single transcript produced by RNA polymerase III. The tertiary structure of every tRNA molecule is similar. tRNAs have a stem-and-loop structure stabilized by hydrogen bonds between bases on neighboring segments of the RNA chain (Figures 16 and 17). Several modified nucleotides are found in tRNA (for example, dihydrouridine). One end of the structure is responsible for recognizing the mRNA codon to be translated. This is the **anticodon**, a sequence of three ribonucleotides that is complementary to the mRNA codon the tRNA translates. A key step in translation is *specific base pairing between the tRNA anticodon and the mRNA codon*. It is this specificity that dictates which amino acid of the twenty will be added to a growing polypeptide chain by the ribosome. The other end of the tRNA molecule has the **amino acid acceptor site**, which is where the amino acid is attached to the tRNA. [If you analyzed a thousand tRNA molecules, which region would you expect to vary the most?[24]]. Each tRNA can be named according to the amino acid it's specific for. For example, a tRNA for valine would be written $tRNA_{Val}$. When the amino acid is attached, the tRNA is written this way: $Val\text{-}tRNA_{Val}$.

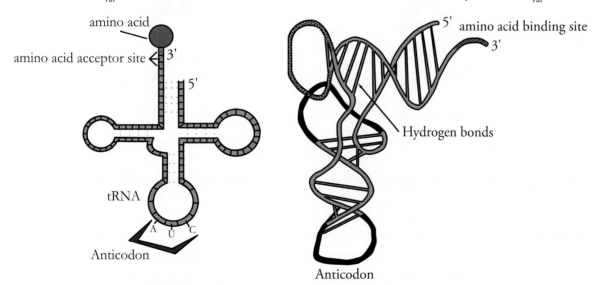

Figure 16   Cloverleaf (Two-Dimensional) Structure of tRNA

Figure 17   Three-Dimensional Structure of tRNA

---

[24] The anticodon is different for each of the different tRNA molecules. Part of the rest of the molecule varies from one tRNA to the next, but about 60 percent is constant. The amino acid binding site is always the same: CCA (at the 3' end of the tRNA molecule).

tRNA molecules often contain nitrogenous bases in many positions that have been covalently modified. Base methylation is particularly common. Some specific examples are inosine (derived from adenine), pseudouridine (derived from uracil), or lysidine (derived from cytosine). Inosine in particular plays an important role in wobble base pairing.

The Wobble Hypothesis

Using the standard genetic code, you would guess that organisms have 61 distinct tRNA molecules to recognize the 61 amino acid-coding codons possible in mRNA. In actual fact, most organisms have fewer than 45 different types of tRNAs, meaning some anticodons must pair with more than one codon. Francis Crick's **Wobble Hypothesis** explains this, and it states that the first two codon-anticodon pairs obey normal base pairing rules, but the third position is more flexible (Figure 18). This allows for non-traditional pairing and explains why a smaller number of tRNAs are possible.

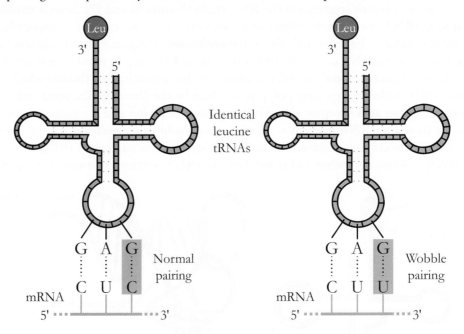

Figure 18   Wobble Base Pairing Between a tRNA Anticodon and an mRNA Codon

A modified inosine base (I) at the 5' end of the anticodon is particularly wobbly, as it can bond to three different codon bases (A, U or C). Some common wobble pairing combinations are:

5' Base in Anticodon (tRNA)	3' Base in Codon (mRNA)
G	C (Watson-Crick base) or U (wobble base)
C	G
A	U
U	A (Watson-Crick base) or G (wobble base)
I	A, U, or C (all wobble bases)

In other words, the most common wobble base pairs are guanine-uracil, inosine-uracil, inosine-adenine, and inosine-cytosine (G-U, I-U, I-A, and I-C). Both the wobble base pair and the normal Watson-Crick base pair have similar thermodynamic stabilities.

Amino Acid Activation

Peptide bond formation during protein synthesis is a process that requires a lot of energy because the peptide bond has unfavorable thermodynamics ($\Delta G > 0$) and slow kinetics (high activation energy). Reaction coupling is used to power the process: two high-energy phosphate bonds are hydrolyzed to provide the energy to attach an amino acid to its tRNA molecule. This process is called **tRNA loading** or **amino acid activation**, and it is useful because breaking the aminoacyl-tRNA bond will drive peptide bond formation forward. Amino acid activation occurs in several steps:

11.7

1) An amino acid is attached to AMP to form *aminoacyl* AMP. In this reaction, the nucleophile is the acidic oxygen of the amino acid, and the leaving group is PP_i.
2) The pyrophosphate leaving group is hydrolyzed to 2 orthophosphates. This reaction is highly favorable ($\Delta G \ll 0$).
3) tRNA loading, an unfavorable reaction, is driven forward by the destruction of the high-energy aminoacyl—AMP bond created in Step 1.

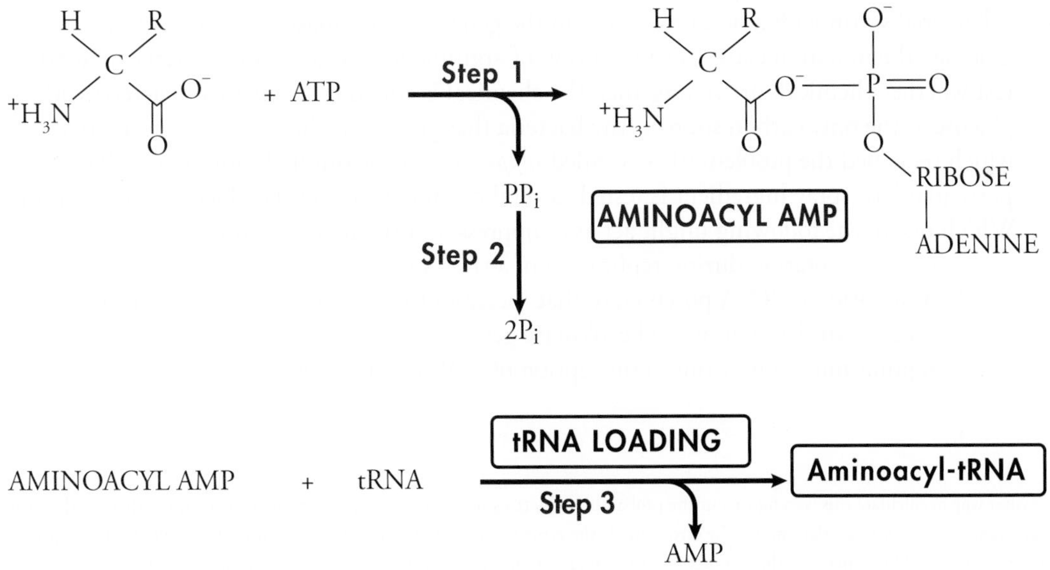

Figure 19   Amino Acid Activation as an Example of Reaction Coupling
Note: water as a reactant has been left out of all reactions in this figure.

Overall, amino acid activation requires 2 ATP equivalents because it uses two high-energy bonds. An ATP equivalent is a single high-energy phosphate bond. You can get 2 ATP equivalents by hydrolyzing 2 ATP to 2 ADP + 2 P_i or by hydrolyzing 1 ATP to AMP + 2 P_i.

Eventually, the bond between the amino acid and the tRNA molecule will be broken. This hydrolysis will power peptide bond formation: the nitrogen of another amino acid will nucleophilically attack the carbonyl carbon of this amino acid, and tRNA will be the leaving group.

Aminoacyl-tRNA Synthetases

We have stated that incorporation of the appropriate amino acid in a growing polypeptide depends on the delivery of the correct amino acid by a specific tRNA. But we also noted that the amino acid acceptor sites of all tRNA molecules are the same. How is the attachment of the appropriate amino acid to each tRNA molecule accomplished? **Aminoacyl-tRNA synthetase enzymes** are specific to each amino acid, and there is at least one aminoacyl-tRNA synthetase for every amino acid. This family of enzymes recognizes both the tRNA and the amino acid, based on their three-dimensional structures. They are highly specific, which is important because joining the wrong amino acid to a tRNA would result in the wrong amino acid being incorporated into a polypeptide. Given that some amino acids differ only by a single methyl group, this specificity is quite amazing. Aminoacyl-tRNA synthetases also function with a very low error rate. [If there is a 1/1000 error rate in amino acid incorporation, what percentage of polypeptides that are 500 amino acid residues long will not contain any errors?[25]]

Overall then, **amino acid activation** serves two functions. One is specific and accurate amino acid delivery, and the other is thermodynamic activation of the amino acid.

- A bacterial strain with a point mutation in the gene for hexokinase is not able to metabolize glucose. The mutation causes a substitution of arginine for serine. These bacteria are used to test whether chemicals are mutagenic. The chemical is added to a culture of bacteria with glucose as the only carbon source. Any bacteria that grow must have undergone a mutation which remedied the problem (this is called *suppression* of the original mutation). When a particular hair spray ingredient is tested, several colonies grow on the glucose-only medium. Which one of the following might act as a suppressor of the first mutation?[26]
  - A) A point mutation during replication of a tRNA gene
  - B) A mutation in RNA polymerase that increases the rate of promoter recognition
  - C) A base pair deletion in the hexokinase gene
  - D) A point mutation during transcription of a tRNA molecule

---

[25] The easiest way to calculate this is to figure out the probability of getting *all* amino acids in the protein correct, in other words, we must use the *non*-error rate for our calculation, not the error rate. If the error rate is 1/1000, then the non-error rate is 999/1000. The probability of having no errors is $.999^n$, where n = the number of amino acid residues. In other words, a single amino acid has .999 probability, or 99.9% probability of being correct. Two amino acids correct in a row have a $.999 \times .999$ probability $(.999^2)$, or .998, or 99.8% probability of happening. Continuing in this manner, a 500-amino acid protein has a $.999^{500}$ probability of being entirely correct, or .606, approximately a 60% probability. Longer proteins have a higher chance of containing errors.

[26] A single base change in the anticodon of the tRNA for arginine could cause it to recognize the codon for serine. If that happened in the mutant bacteria, problems might ensue, but one good result would be that the correct amino acid would be incorporated at the mutated site in hexokinase (choice **A** is correct; note that point mutations in tRNA genes are actually a common means of suppression in bacteria). Increasing the rate at which RNA polymerase recognizes the promoter might increase the rate of transcription, but it would not fix a mutant enzyme (choice B is wrong), and a base pair deletion in the hexokinase gene would cause a frameshift mutation and a serious significant change in protein structure and function (choice C is wrong). A point mutation during transcription of a tRNA molecule might have a temporary effect on a single bacterium, but it would not be passed on to its progeny; remember that only DNA mutations have lasting effects and that errors made during transcription are generally insignificant (choice D is wrong).

The Ribosome

The ribosome is composed of many polypeptides and rRNA chains held together in a massive quaternary structure. Ribosomes float around in the cytoplasm, and each has a small subunit and a large subunit. The unit of measurement is the Svedberg, or S, unit. Svedbergs are a sedimentation rate, that is, how quickly something will sink in a gradient during centrifugation, and the units are not additive.

The prokaryotic ribosome sediments in a gradient at a rate of 70S, so it is referred to as the **70S ribosome** (Figure 20). It is composed of a 30S small subunit and a 50S large subunit. The small subunit is made of a 16S rRNA and 21 peptides. Two rRNA molecules (23S and 5S) and 31 peptides make up the large subunit.

Eukaryotes have an **80S ribosome**. It also has a small and large subunit. The large subunit has three rRNA molecules (5S, 5.8S, and 28S) and 46 peptides and sediments in a gradient at a rate of 60S. The small subunit has 33 peptides and one rRNA (18S) and sediments in a gradient at a rate of 40S.

11.7

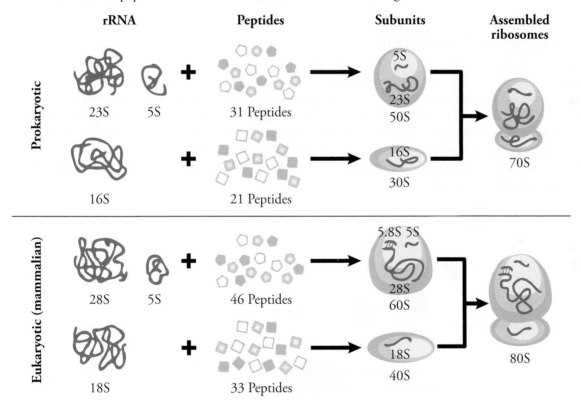

Figure 20   Ribosome Components

In both prokaryotes and eukaryotes, the complete ribosome (both subunits together) has three special binding sites. The **A site** (*a*minoacyl-tRNA site) is where each new tRNA delivers its amino acid. The **P site** (*p*eptidyl-tRNA site) is where the growing polypeptide chain, still attached to a tRNA, is located during translation. The **E site** (*e*xit-tRNA site) is where a now-empty tRNA sits prior to its release from the ribosome. [During translation, the next codon to be translated is exposed in the __[27].] tRNAs move through the sites from $\mathbf{A} \rightarrow \mathbf{P} \rightarrow \mathbf{E}$.

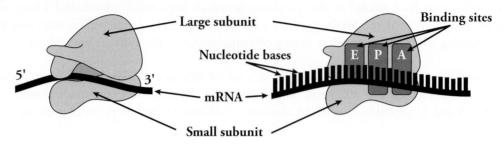

Figure 21   The Ribosome

Prokaryotic Translation

In prokaryotes, translation occurs in the same compartment and at the same time as transcription. In other words, *while the mRNA is being made* ribosomes attach and begin translating it. [That means that the first end of the mRNA to be translated is 5' or 3'?[28]] Note that it says ribosome**s** above. Several ribosomes attach to the mRNA and translate it simultaneously (see Figure 22; you may hear the term *polyribosome* used to describe this arrangement; polyribosomes are seen in both prokaryotes and eukaryotes). [You figured out the direction of translation on the mRNA from what you already know. Do you have any previous knowledge that would help you answer this: Does translation always begin at the 5' end of the mRNA, or somewhere up the chain?[29]]

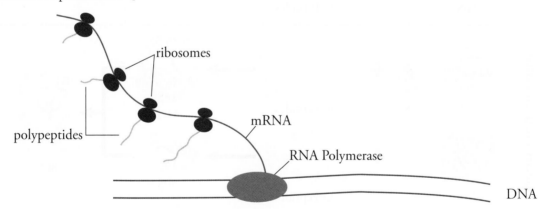

Figure 22   A Prokaryotic Polyribosome

Because prokaryotes often have polycistronic mRNAs, their ribosomes can also start translation in the middle of the chain. This means termination and initiation sequences are found between each ORF. Even for the first open reading frame on a transcript, translation doesn't begin right at the 5' end. An upstream

---

[27] A site, since this is where the next amino acid to be added must bind.

[28] 5' first, since the mRNA is made 5' end first. Transcription and translation go in the same direction on mRNA.

[29] It does not always occur at the very end. You can deduce this from the fact that mRNA is polycistronic. If there are more than one translation start site on the mRNA, they can't all be at the 5' end.

regulatory sequence is essential for initiation, just as in transcription. Here, instead of a promoter, we have a **ribosome binding site**, also known as the **Shine-Dalgarno sequence**, located at −10 (ten ribonucleotides upstream, or on the 5æ side of the start codon). The Shine-Dalgarno sequence is complementary to a pyrimidine rich region on the small subunit, and thus helps position the initiation machinery on the transcript.

Like transcription, translation has three distinct stages: initiation, elongation, and termination. Many antibiotics function by inhibiting a particular stage.[30]

Initiation starts with the small ribosomal subunit (30S) binding two initiation proteins called IF1 and IF3. This complex then binds the mRNA transcript. Next, the first aminoacyl-tRNA joins, along with a third initiation factor called IF2, which is also bound to one GTP. Finally, the 50S subunit completes the complex. This process is powered by the hydrolysis of one GTP molecule.[31] The first aminoacyl-tRNA is special; it is called the **initiator tRNA**, abbreviated **fMet-tRNA$_{fMet}$**. The "fMet" stands for *formylmethionine*, which is a modified methionine used as the first amino acid in all prokaryotic proteins.[32] The initiator tRNA sits in the P site of the 70S ribosome, hydrogen-bonded with the **start codon**. [What is the start codon? Does this codon initiate translation wherever it appears?[33]] Before elongation, all initiation factors dissociate from the complex.

Elongation, a three-step cycle, may now begin. In the first step, the second aminoacyl-tRNA enters the A site and hydrogen bonds with the second codon. This process requires the hydrolysis of one phosphate from GTP. In the second step, the **peptidyl transferase** activity of the large ribosomal subunit (the 23S rRNA) catalyzes the formation of a peptide bond between fMet and the second amino acid. The amino group of amino acid #2 acts as nucleophile, and tRNA$_{fMet}$ is the leaving group; it dissociates from the ribosome. A new dipeptide is now attached to tRNA #2. Now you can figure out the direction of translation from the point of view of the polypeptide; you won't have to memorize it.[34] The third step is **translocation**, in which tRNA #1 (now empty) moves into the E site, tRNA #2 (holding the growing peptide) moves into the P site, and the next codon to be translated moves into the A site, and this process costs one GTP. The new dipeptide is still attached to tRNA #2, and tRNA #2 is still H-bonded to codon #2. The presence of tRNA #1 in the E site (still H-bonded to codon #1) is thought to help maintain the reading frame of the mRNA (disruption of tRNA binding to the E site results in an increase in the number of frameshift mutations in the resulting protein). [Does the ribosome move relative to the mRNA during translocation?[35]] These three steps repeat over and over again, connecting amino acids in the order their codons appear along the mRNA strand (and thus appear in the A site).

Termination occurs when a stop codon appears in the A site. Instead of a tRNA, a **release factor** now enters the A site. This causes the peptidyl transferase to hydrolyze the bond between the last tRNA and the completed polypeptide. Finally, the ribosome separates into its subunits and releases both mRNA and polypeptide.

---

[30] For example, streptomycin and tetracycline bind to the 30S subunit of the prokaryotic ribosome. Chloramphenicol and erythromycin bind to the 50S subunit.

[31] This may seem odd, as ATP is normally the energy molecule. But a high energy phosphate is a high energy phosphate. Another example is the GTP produced in the Krebs cycle.

[32] In fact, cells of our immune system release cytotoxins when they sniff out fMet, because this chemical is a sure sign that bacteria are busily translating.

[33] Refer to the genetic code table. The codon for methionine is AUG; that's the start codon. It only initiates translation when it is preceded by a Shine-Dalgarno sequence (prokaryotes).

[34] The direction of synthesis is N → C, since the N of amino acid #2 binds to the C of #1. As the polypeptide elongates, its N terminus will come snaking out of the ribosome.

[35] It must, if the tRNA remains H-bonded to the mRNA while moving to another spot in the ribosome.

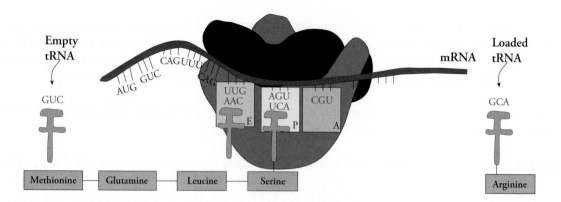

Figure 23   Translation Elongation

Let's focus for a moment on the energetics of translation. Why doesn't peptide bond formation require GTP hydrolysis, like the other steps in translation?[36] You should be able to answer questions like this: How many high energy phosphate bonds are required to make a 50 amino acid polypeptide chain, including the energy used to activate amino acids to aminoacyl-tRNAs?[37]

Eukaryotic Translation

There are several differences between eukaryotic and prokaryotic translation. Many of these have already been mentioned: the ribosome is larger (80S) and has different components than the prokaryotic ribosome, the mRNA must be processed before it can be translated (spliced, with cap and tail added), and the N-terminal amino acid is different (Met instead of fMet). Also remember that eukaryotic mRNA must not only be spliced, capped, and tailed, but it also requires transport from nucleus to cytoplasm, thus transcription and translation *cannot* proceed simultaneously.

Eukaryotes do not use the Shine-Dalgarno sequence to initiate translation. There are 5' UTR sequences in eukaryotes that function in starting translation; a common one is the *Kozak sequence*, which is a consensus sequence typically located a few nucleotides before the start codon.

---

[36] Because the bond between each amino acid and its tRNA is a high energy bond whose hydrolysis drives peptide bond formation. Remember that the aminoacyl-tRNA bond was formed using the energy of two phosphate bonds from ATP.

[37] There are two phosphate bonds hydrolyzed per amino acid to make the aminoacyl-tRNAs, or 100 for the 50 amino acid polypeptide. Two phosphate bonds are required for each elongation step, one for the entrance of each new aminoacyl-tRNA into the ribosomal A site and the other for translocation. Since there are 49 elongation steps for a 50-amino acid protein, 98 high energy bonds are hydrolyzed during elongation. Finally, one GTP is hydrolyzed during initiation to position the first tRNA and mRNA on the ribosome, and one GTP is hydrolyzed in termination. Thus, a total of 200 high-energy bonds are required for the translation of a 50-amino acid protein. In other words, it costs $4n$ high-energy bonds to make a peptide chain, where n is the number of amino acids in the chain.

Eukaryotic translation begins with formation of the initiation complex. First, a 43S pre-initiation complex forms, composed of the 40S small ribosomal submit, Met-tRNA$_{Met}$, and several proteins called eukaryotic initiation factors (or eIFs). Next, this assembled complex is recruited to the 5' capped end of the transcript, by an initiation complex of proteins (including other eIF proteins). Additional proteins are recruited (such as a polyA tail binding protein) and the initiation complex starts scanning the mRNA from the 5' end, looking for a start codon. Once the start codon has been found, the large ribosomal subunit (60S) is recruited and translation can begin.

Eukaryotes have two elongation factors. Additional elongation factors are required to facilitate peptide bond formation. [Are the nascent (newly formed) polypeptide chains emerging from a polyribosome in a eukaryote all the same?[38]] Eukaryotic translation termination involves two release factors to release the completed polypeptide.

- Which one of the following pairs of processes may occur simultaneously on the same RNA molecule in a eukaryotic cell?[39]
    A) Translation and transcription
    B) Transcription and splicing
    C) Splicing and translation
    D) Messenger RNA degradation and transcription

Cap-Independent Translation

It was long thought that all eukaryotic translation started at the 5' end of an mRNA. In other words, all eukaryotic transcripts were assumed to be monocistronic and coded for only one polypeptide chain. It is true that this mechanism is by far the major one in eukaryotic cells. Because of the important role of 5' mRNA cap recognition, it's called **cap-dependent translation**.

However, it's recently been discovered that eukaryotes are sometimes capable of starting translation in the middle of an mRNA molecule, a process called **cap-independent translation** (because the beginning of translation doesn't require the 5' cap of the mRNA). To do this, the transcript must have an internal ribosome entry site, or IRES. This is a specialized nucleotide sequence, and it was first discovered in viruses. Since then, IRESs have been found in a number of eukaryotic transcripts. Most code for proteins that help the cell deal with stress or help activate apoptosis. In other words, the IRESs found so far make sure the cell can make essential proteins when under sub-optimal growth conditions. Cells under stress generally inhibit translation (via inhibiting translation initiation), and cap-independent translation allows the cell to make proteins when doing so is crucial for survival or programmed cell death. Activation of translation using an IRES requires different proteins than normal initiation.

---

[38] In eukaryotes, the answer is: yes, always, because eukaryotic mRNA is monocistronic. In prokaryotes, however, different polypeptides may be translated from a single piece of mRNA, since prokaryotic mRNA is polycistronic.

[39] In order for processes in eukaryotes to occur simultaneously, they must occur in the same compartment. Transcription and splicing both occur in the nucleus and could therefore occur simultaneously (choice **B** is correct). Translation occurs in the cytoplasm while transcription and splicing occur in the nucleus, thus translation cannot occur at the same time as either of these processes (choices A and C are wrong). mRNA degradation and transcription cannot occur at the same time; if this were true no mRNA molecules would survive to be translated (choice D is wrong).

11.8 CONTROLLING GENE EXPRESSION

Adult humans have over 220 different types of cells, all with the same genome, but with different attributes such as morphology, lifespan, function, ability to secrete, response to signaling molecules, mobility, etc. These changes are due to differences in gene expression and protein function. In each cell type, some genes are expressed and others are silenced, further, genes that are expressed can have different levels of expression, where in one cell type the gene is expressed at a high level (to produce lots of ncRNA or protein), and in a different cell type the same gene is expressed at a low level. They can also have varying activity, stability, and half-life. These variations in gene expression can be altered using many different mechanisms:

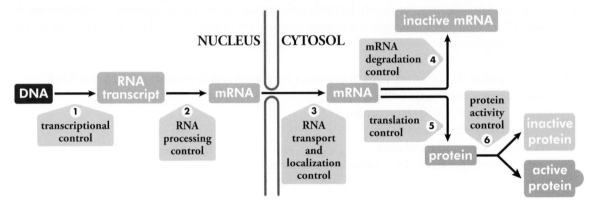

Figure 24 Mechanisms of Controlling Gene Expression in Eukaryotes

Transcription is the principle site of the regulation of gene expression in both eukaryotes and prokaryotes. This means that the amount of each protein made in every cell is affected by the amount of mRNA that gets transcribed. Gene expression can also be controlled epigenetically. Broadly speaking, **epigenetics** focuses on changes in gene expression that are not due to changes in DNA sequences, but are either heritable or have a long-term effect. The three most commonly studied areas in this field are DNA methylation, chromatin remodeling, and RNA interference.

Controlling Gene Expression at the DNA Level

DNA Methylation and Chromatin Remodeling

Both prokaryotic and eukaryotic DNA can be covalently modified by adding a methyl group. Bacteria methylate new DNA shortly after synthesis, and the brief delay is useful in mismatch repair pathways (see above). Methylation can also control gene expression in prokaryotes, either by promoting or inhibiting transcription.

Eukaryotic DNA methylation has been found in every vertebrate genome studied so far. Broadly speaking, it plays an important role in controlling gene expression (especially during embryonic development), and has also been implicated in several diseases. DNA methylation turns off eukaryotic gene expression two ways:

1) Methylation physically blocks the gene from transcriptional proteins.
2) Certain proteins bind methylated CpG groups and recruit chromatin remodeling proteins that change the winding of DNA around histones.

- Regulation of a gene is examined *in vitro* in the presence and absence of chromatin assembly, and in the presence and absence of a sequence-specific regulator of transcription. Transcription is quantitated after the experiment and the following results are obtained:

	Sequence-Specific Factor	DNA	Relative Amount of Transcription
1.	None	unpackaged	0.74
2.	None	packaged	0.07
3.	Present	unpackaged	1.0
4.	Present	packaged	0.59

Which one of the following conclusions can be drawn from this experiment?[40]

A) The degree of activation by the sequence-specific factor is greater in the presence of chromatin assembly than in its absence.
B) The sequence-specific factor acts to repress transcription.
C) The histones increase the rate of transcription.
D) The sequence-specific factor increases the rate of transition from a closed complex to an open complex.

Gene Dose

One way to increase gene expression is to increase the copy number of a gene by amplification. Increasing gene dose will allow a cell to make large quantities of the corresponding protein. Similarly, gene deletion causes a decrease in gene expression. Both are examples of copy number variation, discussed earlier in Section 11.1.

Imprinting

Genomic imprinting is when only one allele of a gene is expressed. Imprinting is a dynamic process and can change from generation to generation. In other words, a gene that is imprinted in an adult may be "unimprinted" and expressed in that adult's offspring. This observation led to the notion that imprinting is an epigenetic process. Silencing of a certain gene involves DNA methylation, histone modification, and binding of long ncRNAs (non-coding RNAs). These epigenetic marks are established in the germline and are maintained throughout life and mitotic divisions.

X Chromosome Inactivation

Female mammals have two X chromosomes, one of which is active (called Xa) and one of which is silenced, or inactive (and is called Xi). In humans, X-inactivation occurs early in development, at the blastocyst stage. Each cell in the inner cell mass randomly inactivates an X chromosome, and this decision is irreversible. This means every cell derived from each cell in the inner cell mass will have the same X chromosome inactivated,

---

[40] A quick glance at the data indicates that transcription is increased in the presence of the sequence-specific factor (compare lines 1 and 2 with lines 3 and 4; choice B is wrong) and that histones decrease the rate of transcription (packaged DNA has a lower rate of transcription than unpackaged; choice C is wrong). Looking closer, it appears that the sequence specific factor causes an approximate 8-fold increase in the transcription rate of packaged DNA (compare lines 2 and 4), but it doesn't even double the rate of transcription of unpackaged DNA (compare lines 1 and 3). It might be that this occurs because the factor increases the rate of transition to an open complex, but there is no data to support this (choice **A** is a better answer than choice D). Don't confuse "open complex" (which means separated DNA strands) with "unpackaged" (which means not wrapped around histones).

however, because each cell makes its own decision, an adult can have different X chromosomes inactivated in different tissues and cells. Because of X-inactivation, all humans have the same number of gene products for the X chromosome; males have only one X chromosome, and females have only one *active* X chromosome. Xi is very condensed and packaged in heterochromatin. It has high levels of DNA methylation.

Controlling Gene Expression at the RNA Level: Regulation of Transcription in Prokaryotes

Regulation of transcription is the primary method of regulation of gene expression in prokaryotes. One simple mechanism of transcriptional regulation in bacteria is that some promoters are simply stronger than others. The problem with this mechanism of regulation is that it is "pre-set" and cannot respond to changing conditions within the cell. Bacteria also possess far more complex regulatory mechanisms, which activate or suppress transcription depending on current needs for specific gene products. For example, bacteria only produce the enzyme β-galactosidase and other proteins required for lactose catabolism when lactose is present. [Assuming these protein products do not have a harmful effect on the cell, what advantage might there be in turning off the genes when the protein products are not required?[41]]

- Are the terms *polypeptide enzyme* and *gene product* synonymous? Or are there gene products that are not polypeptide enzymes? Are there polypeptides which are not enzymes?[42]

Enzymes involved in anabolism (biosynthesis) should be produced when the item they help make (their product) is scarce. Enzymes involved in catabolism (degradative metabolism) should be produced when the item they help breakdown (their substrate) is abundant, such as food. Thus there are two basic ways we can imagine how transcription is regulated. The transcription of enzymes involved in biosynthetic pathways should be inhibited by their product. The transcription of enzymes involved in catabolic pathways should be automatically inhibited whenever the substrate is not around and activated when it is. That is in fact exactly what happens. Anabolic enzymes whose transcription is inhibited in the presence of excess amounts of product are **repressible**. Catabolic enzymes whose transcription can be stimulated by the abundance of a substrate are called **inducible enzymes**.[43]

There are two common examples of this. The **lac operon** is inducible, since the enzymes it codes for are part of lactose catabolism, and the **trp operon** is repressible, since the enzymes it codes for mediate tryptophan biosynthesis or anabolism. An operon has two components, a coding sequence for enzymes, and upstream regulatory sequences or control sites. Operons may also include genes for regulatory proteins, such as repressors or activators, but don't have to. These genes can be located elsewhere in the genome and typically have their own promoters.

---

[41] It takes a great deal of ATP to synthesize RNA and protein, so it's more energy-efficient to transcribe and translate only the proteins that are needed.

[42] They are not synonymous. All polypeptides are gene products, but some gene products are not polypeptides and some polypeptides are not enzymes. Transfer RNA and rRNA are gene products, but not polypeptides. Microfilaments and other elements of the cytoskeleton, as well as collagen and many other polypeptides, are not enzymes.

[43] So note: The default for repressible systems is "ON"; for inducible systems the default is "OFF."

The Lac Operon

The lac operon contains several components:

1) *P* region: the promoter site on DNA to which RNA polymerase binds to initiate transcription of *Y*, *Z*, and *A* genes
2) *O* region: the operator site to which the Lac repressor binds
3) *Z* gene: codes for the enzyme β-galactosidase, which cleaves lactose into glucose and galactose
4) *Y* gene: codes for permease, a protein which transports lactose into the cell
5) *A* gene: codes for transacetylase, an enzyme which transfers an acetyl group from acetyl-CoA to β-galactosides (note that this function is not required for lactose metabolism)

Additionally, there are two genes, each with their own promoter, that code for proteins important in the regulation of the lac operon:

1) *crp* gene: located at a distant site, this gene codes for a catabolite activator protein (CAP) and helps couple the lac operon to glucose levels in the cell
2) *I* gene: located at a distant site, this gene codes for the Lac repressor protein

11.8

So overall, there are five protein coding genes and two regulatory sequences. Both *crp* and *I* have their own promoters. The protein products of these two genes control gene expression of *Z*, *Y*, and *A*.

Bacterial cells preferentially use glucose as an energy source. This means that in the presence of glucose, the lac operon will be off, or expressed at low amounts (see Figures 25 and 26). This is mediated by the CAP and repressor proteins. Glucose levels control a protein called adenylyl cyclase, which converts ATP to cAMP. In high glucose conditions, adenylyl cyclase is inactivated and cAMP levels are very low. In low glucose conditions, the opposite is true: adenylyl cyclase is activated and cAMP levels are high. CAP binds cAMP and this complex binds the promoter of the lac operon (Figure 27 on page 229). This helps activate RNA polymerase at the lac operon and contributes to the operon being turned on when glucose levels are low.

The *I* gene codes for a repressor protein, which binds the operator of the lac operon. This prevents RNA pol from binding the promoter and transcribing *Z*, *Y*, and *A* genes, thereby blocking transcription of the operon when lactose is absent (Figure 25). The repressor protein can also bind lactose, and this blocks its activity on the operator. This binding is allosteric, meaning it happens at a distant site from operator binding. It causes a conformational change in the tertiary structure of the repressor protein, such that it is no longer capable of binding to the operator. As a consequence, it falls off the DNA (Figures 26 and 27).

High transcription of *Z*, *Y*, and *A* genes occurs when glucose is absent and lactose is present (Figure 27). Low glucose results in an increased amount of cAMP, which binds to CAP and helps activate RNA polymerase activity at the lac operon. Lactose presence means the Lac repressor protein is unable to bind the lac operator and negatively regulate transcription; thus the polycistronic mRNA is transcribed at high levels. When the supply of lactose becomes very scarce, there isn't enough to bind to the repressors, and most of the repressor proteins return to their original structure. They now rebind to the operator, decreasing transcription of *Z*, *Y*, and *A* genes.

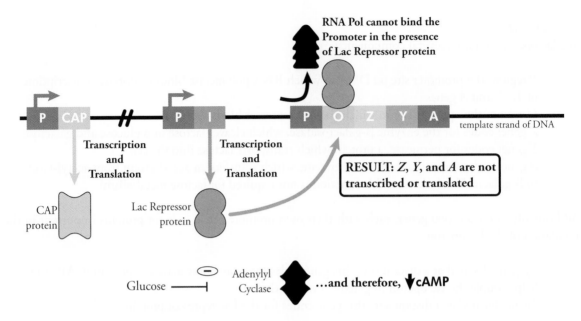

Figure 25   The Lac Operon in the Presence of Glucose and Absence of Lactose

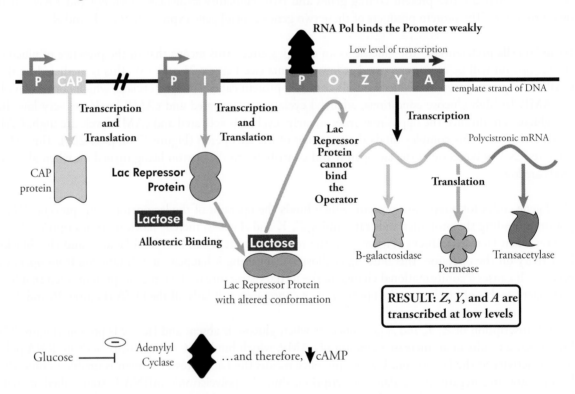

Figure 26   The Lac Operon in the Presence of both Glucose and Lactose

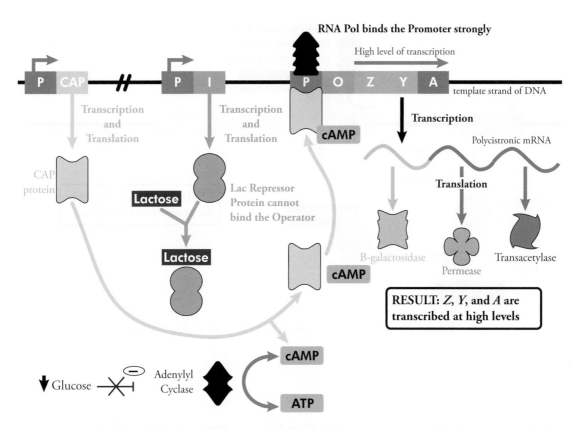

Figure 27 The Lac Operon in the Absence of Glucose and Presence of Lactose

- If the operator is mutated so that the lac repressor can no longer bind, what effect will this have on transcription?[44]

  A) Transcription of Gene Z will be activated, and Genes Y and A will not be affected.
  B) None of the genes will be transcribed, regardless of the presence or absence of lac repressor.
  C) Transcription will still be activated by lactose.
  D) All three genes will be expressed constitutively, regardless of the presence of lactose.

The Trp Operon

Bacteria use a five enzyme synthetic pathway to make the amino acid tryptophan from chorismic acid. In the presence of tryptophan, there is little point in making these enzymes, which are also co-localized in an operon.

The repressor protein is coded by the trpR gene (Figure 28). The repressor binds tryptophan when it is present, and the two together then bind the operator, to turn off transcription of the other five trp genes. In the absence of tryptophan, the bacterial cell must make its own. With no tryptophan present, the repressor protein cannot bind the operator. Without this block, RNA polymerase transcribes the five genes in the trp operon, and the five gene products allow the cell to make tryptophan. This is an example of anabolic repressible transcription.

---

[44] If the repressor cannot bind to the operator, nothing will prevent RNA polymerase from transcribing all the genes on the operon in an unregulated, constitutive (or continuous) fashion (choice **D** is true, and choice B is false). All genes on the operon are expressed or repressed together (choice A is false), and lactose will no longer have any effect (the expression of the genes is unregulated, so choice C is false).

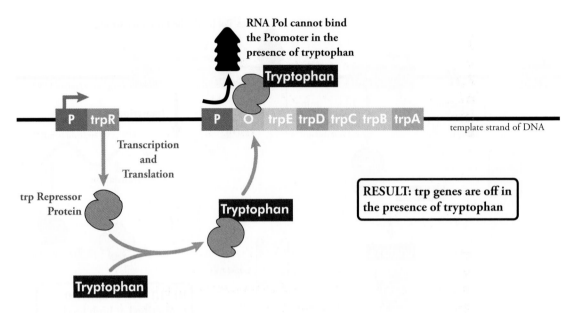

Figure 28 The Trp Operon in the Presence of Tryptophan

Control of Gene Expression at the RNA Level: Regulation of Transcription in Eukaryotes

Given the complexity of eukaryotes compared to prokaryotes, it is not surprising that the regulation of eukaryotic transcription is also more complex. Most of this regulation happens at initiation.

For protein-coding genes, there are upstream control elements (UCEs), usually about 200 bases upstream of the initiation site, a core promoter containing binding sites for the basal transcription complex and RNA polymerase II (about 50 bases upstream of the transcription start site), and a TATA box at –25. The TATA box is a highly conserved DNA recognition sequence for the TATA box binding protein (TBP). Binding of TBP to the TATA box initiates transcription complex assembly at the promoter.

Enhancer sequences in DNA are bound by **activator proteins**, and this is another kind of transcriptional regulation. The enhancer may be located many thousands of base pairs away from a promoter (either upstream or downstream) and still regulate transcription. This is likely done by DNA looping so enhancers and their activator proteins can get close to transcriptional machinery.

Eukaryotes also have **gene repressor proteins**, which inhibit transcription; this can also be done by modifying chromatin structure. *Transcription factors* have DNA-binding domains and are crucial in transcription regulation. They can bind promoters or other regulatory sequences. In fact, in many cases, transcription levels in eukaryotes are controlled by huge committees of proteins. This produces a combinatorial effect, where each protein contributes to regulation, and can itself be regulated. These complex networks help link transcription to cell signaling and status. The binding of transcriptional machinery to DNA is often regulated by extracellular signals. For example, steroid hormones bind to receptors in the cell, and this sends the receptor to the nucleus. The complex binds DNA to regulate transcription. [If a mutation in a eukaryotic fat cell reduces the level of several proteins related to fat metabolism, does this mean the proteins are encoded by the same mRNA?[45]]

Beyond regulating the initiation of transcription, eukaryotes employ several other methods of transcriptional regulation, including:

- **RNA Translocation**: mRNA transcripts must be exported from the nucleus to the cytoplasm and can also be transported to different areas of the cell. They are translationally silent while this is happening. This system is especially important in cells that have a high level of polarity, where one area or end of the cell is distinctly different from the other. For example, neurons have polarity, and some transcripts are transported to the dendrites, while others stay in the soma. This is a way of controlling gene expression: mRNA transcripts aren't translated into proteins until they are localized properly in the cell.
- **mRNA Surveillance**: Cells closely monitor mRNA molecules to ensure that only high-quality mRNA transcripts are read by the ribosome. Defective transcripts (such as those with premature stop codons, or those without stop codons at all) and stalled transcripts (where the ribosome is stalled in translation) are degraded.
- **RNA Interference**: RNA interference (RNAi) is a way to silence gene expression after a transcript has been made. It is mediated by miRNA and siRNA (Section 11.6). Generally speaking, the siRNAs bind complementary sequences on mRNAs, and this ds-RNA is then degraded. The amount of transcript in the cell decreases, and gene expression is thus negatively regulated.

11.8

Control of Gene Expression at the Protein Level: Translation Initiation

We've already discussed the complex process of assembling translational machinery. In both prokaryotes and eukaryotes, this is a highly regulated process that links protein synthesis with upstream signaling pathways. Otherwise there is little control at the level of translation.

Post-Translational Modification

Newly synthesized proteins released from the ribosome are rarely able to function. They need to be correctly folded, modified or processed, and transported to where they function in the cell. These modifications are called post-translational events, since they occur after protein synthesis.

Protein Folding

Folding a new protein into its correct three-dimensional shape is accomplished by a family of proteins called **chaperones**. These proteins are found across all types of organisms (from bacteria to plants to mammals), and they also function in assembly or folding of other macromolecular structures.

---

45 No, it does not. Eukaryotic mRNA is monocistronic. A more likely explanation is that a number of different genes located throughout the genome have related regulatory sequences that bind the same sequence-specific transcription factors. This is the means used by eukaryotes to achieve coordinated expression of genes. Related proteins are clumped together on the same piece of mRNA in prokaryotes only.

Covalent Modification

Many proteins are covalently modified. For example, the addition of a fatty acid can target a protein to a membrane (either the plasma membrane or an organelle membrane).

Smaller chemical groups can also be added. For example, proteins can be:

- acetylated
- formylated
- alkylated
- glycosylated
- phosphorylated
- sulphated

Processing

Many proteins require cleavage of some sort to become mature or functional. Protein precursors are often used when the mature protein may be dangerous to the organism. Because the precursor is already made, it allows large quantities of mature protein to be available on short notice. Enzyme precursors are called **zymogens** or **proenzymes**.

A well-known example of post-translational processing is insulin. Insulin is made from a prohormone (Figure 29); preproinsulin is the primary translational product of the gene. To form proinsulin, an N-terminus signal peptide is removed and disulphide bonds form, in the endoplasmic reticulum. Three cleavage events are necessary to process proinsulin; these cleavage events occur in a secretory vesicle.

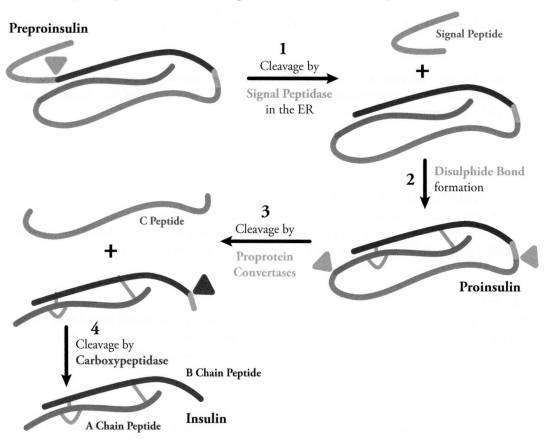

Figure 29 Insulin Processing: An Example of Post-Translational Modification

11.9 RETURN TO GENE STRUCTURE: A SUMMARY

Now that we have been through all the processes that a cell uses to turn a gene into a protein, and control this process, let's review the components (Figure 30). Transcription begins at a start site, but it needs a promoter upstream of this. It ends at a termination signal. The RNA transcript contains the open reading frame (which goes from start codon to stop codon), as well as both 5' and 3' regulatory regions.

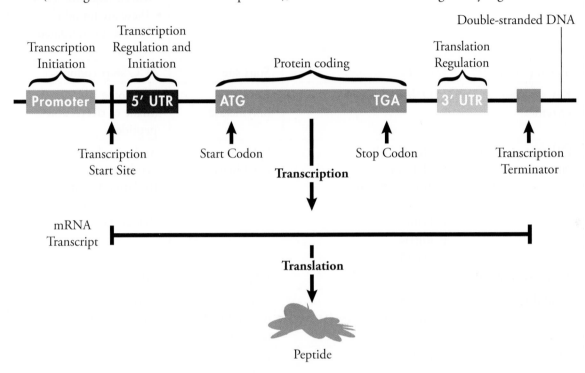

Figure 30   Gene Structure and Protein Expression

DNA replication, transcription, and translation have many similarities and some differences, and these are summarized in Table 1.

11.9

	DNA Replication	Transcription	Translation
Signal to get ready	ORI	Promoter	• Shine-Dalgarno (prok) • Kozak sequence (euk) • These are found in 5'UTR (untranslated region)
Signal to start	ORI	Start site	AUG start codon
Key synthesis enzyme	DNA polymerase	RNA polymerase	Ribosome (made of rRNA and peptides)
Other important enzymes	DnaA/ORC Helicase Topoisomerase SSBPs Primase Ligase Telomerase	Spliceosome machinery	Aminoacyl tRNA synthetases Initiation factors Elongation factors Release factors
Template molecule	DNA	DNA	mRNA
Read direction	3' to 5' on the DNA template	3' to 5' on the DNA template	5' to 3' on the RNA template
Molecule synthesized	DNA	RNA (mRNA in prok, hnRNA in euk)	Peptides
Build direction	5' to 3'	5' to 3'	N-terminus to C-terminus
Prokaryotic location	Cytoplasm	Cytoplasm	Cytoplasm
Eukaryotic location	Nucleus	Nucleus	Cytoplasm
Signal to stop	When the replication bubbles or newly synthesized strands meet and are ligated together	Transcription stop sequence or poly-A sequence	Stop codon (UAG, UGA, UAA)

Table 1   A Review of Molecular Biology Processes

Chapter 12
Microbiology

12.1 VIRUSES

Viruses infect all life forms on earth, including plants, animals, protists, and bacteria. A virus is an **obligate intracellular parasite**. As such, they are only able (*obligated*) to reproduce within (*intra*) cells. While within cells, viruses have some of the attributes of living organisms, such as the ability to reproduce; but outside cells, viruses are without activity. Viruses on their own are unable to perform any of the chemical reactions characteristic of life, such as synthesis of ATP and macromolecules.[1] *Viruses are not cells or even living organisms.* To reproduce, they commandeer the cellular machinery of the host they infect and use it to manufacture copies of themselves. In the final analysis, a virus is nothing more than a package of nucleic acid that says: "Pick me up and reproduce me." Remember this crucial definition: a virus is an obligate intracellular parasite that relies on host machinery whenever possible. In the following sections, we will look at some of the variations on this basic theme.

- Cyanide (an inhibitor of the electron transport chain) is added to a culture of virus-infected mammalian cells. The virus has none of the components of electron transport nor any other proteins that are inhibited by cyanide. Which one of the following best describes the effect of cyanide?[2]
  - A) The mammalian cells will die, and all viruses will be destroyed as well, regardless of their stage of development.
  - B) Mammalian cells are killed, and viral replication halted, but the culture remains infectious.
  - C) Mammalian cells stop growing, and viral replication is unaffected.
  - D) Mammalian cells continue to grow, but viral replication is halted.

Viral Structure and Function

The structure of viruses reflects their life cycle. In general, all viruses possess a nucleic acid genome packaged in a protein shell. The exterior protein packaging helps to convey the genome from one cell to infect other cells. Once in a cell, the viral genome directs the production of new copies of the genome and of the protein packaging needed to produce more virus. However, the nature of the genome, the protein packaging, and the viral life cycle vary tremendously between different viruses.

A viral genome may consist of either DNA *or* RNA that is either single- *or* double-stranded and is either linear *or* circular. Viruses utilize virtually every conceivable form of nucleic acid as their genome. However, a given type of virus can have only one type of nucleic acid as its genome, and a mature virus does not contain nucleic acid other than its genome. [If the ratio of adenine to thymine in a DNA virus is not one to one, what can be said about the genome of this virus?[3]]

---

[1] Note, however, that some viruses store some ATP in their capsids. They acquired this ATP from the previous host and typically use it to power penetration (see below).

[2] The mammalian cells are directly dependent on the ATP generated by the electron transport chain, so if cyanide inhibits the electron transport chain, the mammalian cells will die (choice D is wrong). The viruses are dependent on the mammalian cells for the ATP and enzymes needed for replication, so if the mammalian cells die, viral replication will stop (choice C is wrong). However, any viruses that had already completed the replication process when the cyanide was added will not be affected, and will remain infectious (choice **B** is correct, and choice A is wrong).

[3] Adenine base pairs with thymine in double-stranded DNA. Thus, for every A there should be one T for a one to one ratio of A to T. If the ratio differs from this, the genome must be single-stranded DNA, or RNA, which has no T.

A factor that influences all viral genomes, regardless of the form of the nucleic acid used as genome, is size as a limiting factor. Viruses are much smaller than the hosts they infect, both prokaryotic and eukaryotic. Figure 1 depicts the relative size of a **bacteriophage** (a virus that infects bacteria) and its host.

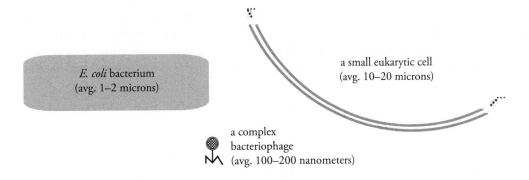

Figure 1   The Relative Size of a Virus

Not only are viruses small, but the exterior protein shell of a virus is typically a rigid structure of fixed size that cannot expand to accommodate a larger genome. To adapt to this size constraint, viral genomes have evolved to be extremely economical. One adaptation is for the viral genome to carry very few genes and for the virus to rely on host-encoded proteins for transcription, translation, and replication. [How do the ribosomes used to translate viral proteins compare to host ribosomes?[4]] Another adaptation found in viral genomes is the ability to encode more than one protein in a given length of genome. A virus can accomplish this feat by utilizing more than one reading frame within a piece of DNA so that genes may overlap with each other.

- A 1000 base pair region of viral genome is found to encode two polypeptides unrelated in amino acid sequence during infection of eukaryotic cells. If one of these polypeptides is 250 amino acids in length and the other is 300, what is the best explanation for this?[5]
    - A) A missense mutation
    - B) Viruses use a different genetic code than eukaryotes do
    - C) Overlapping multiple reading frames
    - D) The polypeptides are splicing variants

---

[4] Viruses use host ribosomes. Viral and host proteins are translated by the same ribosomes.

[5] The problem is that the virus must contain at least 750 bp (250 amino acids) and 900 bp (300 amino acids) of genetic information for unrelated polypeptides in 1000 bp of DNA. The only way to do this is overlapping multiple reading frames (choice C).

Surrounding the viral nucleic acid genome is a protein coat called the **capsid**. The capsid provides the external morphology that is used to classify viruses. It is made from a repeating pattern of only a few protein building blocks. *Helical* capsids are rod-shaped, while *polyhedral* capsids are multiple-sided geometric figures with regular surfaces. Complex viruses may contain a mixture of shapes. For example, the T4 bacteriophage has a helical sheath and a polyhedral head (Figure 2). This virus is commonly used in research; its host is the bacterium *E. coli*. The genome is located within the capsid **head**. Other parts of the capsid are used during infection of the host. The **tail fibers** attach to the surface of the host cell, as does the **base plate**. The **sheath** contracts using the energy of stored ATP, injecting the genome into the host. [Why might a bacteriophage inject its DNA, while animal viruses do not?[6]]

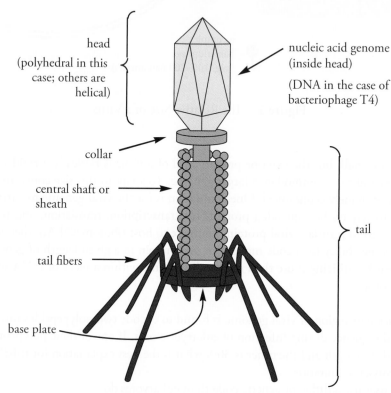

head
(polyhedral in this
case; others are
helical)

nucleic acid genome
(inside head)

(DNA in the case of
bacteriophage T4)

collar

central shaft or
sheath

tail

tail fibers

base plate

Figure 2   Bacteriophage T4

---

[6] Phage must puncture the bacterial cell wall, while animal viruses can be internalized whole into animal cells (since they do not have a cell wall).

The most important thing to understand is that the entire viral capsid is composed of protein, while the viral genome is composed of nucleic acid (DNA or RNA). Most viruses are not as structurally complex as the bacteriophage shown in Figure 2. See Figure 3 for more examples.

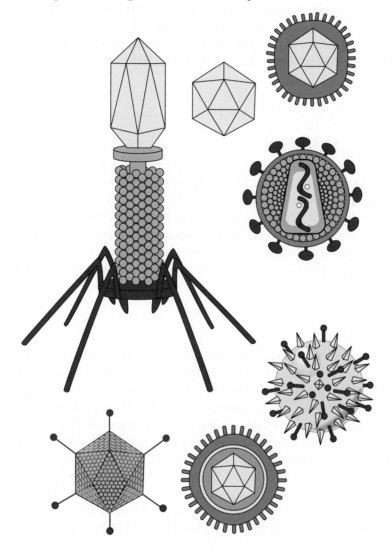

Figure 3   A Variety of Viruses

Many animal viruses also possess an **envelope** that surrounds the capsid. This is a membrane on the exterior of the virus derived from the membrane of the host cell. It contains phospholipids, proteins, and carbohydrates from the host membrane, in addition to proteins encoded by the viral genome. Enveloped viruses acquire this covering by **budding** through the host cell membrane. To infect a new host, some enveloped viruses fuse their envelope with the host's plasma membrane, which leaves the de-enveloped capsid inside the host cell. Viruses which do not have envelopes are called **naked viruses**. All phages and plant viruses are naked. [Can you imagine why this might be true?[7]]

---

[7]   Remember, viruses acquire envelopes by budding through host membranes. Phages and plant viruses infect hosts that possess cell walls. When viruses begin to exit the cell, the cell wall is destroyed, and host membranes rupture. Hence, there is no membrane through which the remaining viruses must bud; they simply escape in a lytic explosion.

Whether enveloped or naked, the surface of a virus determines what host cells it can infect. Viral infection is not a random process, but highly specific. A virus binds to a specific receptor on the cell surface as the first step in infection. After binding, the virus will be internalized, either by fusion with the plasma membrane or by receptor-mediated endocytosis. Only cells with a receptor that matches the virus will become infected, explaining why only specific species or specific cell types are susceptible to infection. The viral surface is also important for recognition by our immune system. [If antibodies to a viral capsid protein are ineffective in blocking infection, what might this indicate about the virus?[8]]

Bacteriophage Life Cycles

Since viruses lack the ability to produce energy and replicate on their own, they use the machinery of the cell they infect to carry out these processes. The viral genome contains genes that redirect the infected cell to produce viral products. The first step is binding to the exterior of a bacterial cell in a process termed **attachment** or **adsorption**. The next step is injection of the viral genome into the host cell in a process termed **penetration** or **eclipse**. It is called "eclipse" because the capsid remains on the outer surface of the bacterium while the genome disappears into the cell, removing infectious virus from the media. From this point forward a phage follows one of two different paths: it enters either the **lytic cycle** or the **lysogenic cycle**.

The Lytic Cycle of Phages

As soon as the phage genome has entered the host cell, host polymerases and/or ribosomes begin to rapidly transcribe and translate it. One of the first viral gene products made is sometimes an enzyme called **hydrolase**, a hydrolytic enzyme that degrades the entire host genome. (Hydrolase is an example of an **early gene**; one of a group of genes that are expressed immediately after infection and which includes any special enzymes required to express viral genes.) Then multiple copies of the phage genome are produced (using the dNTPs resulting from degradation of the host genome), as well as an abundance of capsid proteins. Next, each new capsid automatically assembles itself around a new genome. Finally, an enzyme called **lysozyme** is produced. An example of a **late gene**, lysozyme is also present in human tears and saliva. It destroys the bacterial cell wall. Because osmotic pressure is no longer counteracted by the protection of the cell wall, the host bacterium bursts ("lyses," hence the name *lytic*), releasing about 100 progeny viruses, which can begin another round of the cycle (see Figure 4). [If lysozyme were an early gene, would this be advantageous to the virus?[9]]

---

[8] It suggests that the virus is enveloped, so the antibody cannot reach its epitope on the capsid surface.

[9] No. The host cell would lyse before the phage had time to replicate and assemble.

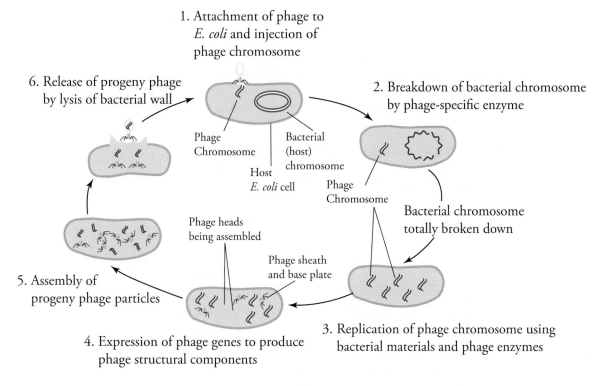

1. Attachment of phage to *E. coli* and injection of phage chromosome

6. Release of progeny phage by lysis of bacterial wall

2. Breakdown of bacterial chromosome by phage-specific enzyme

Phage Chromosome

Bacterial (host) chromosome

Host *E. coli* cell

Phage Chromosome

Bacterial chromosome totally broken down

Phage heads being assembled

Phage sheath and base plate

5. Assembly of progeny phage particles

4. Expression of phage genes to produce phage structural components

3. Replication of phage chromosome using bacterial materials and phage enzymes

Figure 4 The Lytic Cycle

- When phage are first added to a bacterial culture, the number of infective viruses initially decreases before it later increases. Why does this occur?[10]
- Bacteria cultured in the presence of ^{35}S-labeled cysteine and ^{32}P-labeled phosphates are infected with phage T4. When phage from this culture are used to infect a new nonradiolabeled bacterial culture, which of the isotopes will be found in the interior of the newly-infected bacteria?[11]

The Lysogenic Cycle of Phages

The lytic cycle is an efficient way for a virus to rapidly increase its numbers. It presents a problem though: all host cells are destroyed. This is an evolutionary disadvantage. Some viruses are cleverer: they enter the **lysogenic cycle**. Upon infection, the phage genome is incorporated into the bacterial genome and is now referred to as a **prophage**; the host is now called a **lysogen** (Figure 5). The prophage is silent; its genes are not expressed, and viral progeny are not produced. This dormancy is due to the fact that transcription of phage genes is blocked by a phage-encoded repressor protein that binds to specific DNA elements in phage promoters (operators). The cleverness of the lysogenic cycle lies in the fact that every time the host cell reproduces itself, the prophage is reproduced too. Eventually, the prophage becomes activated. It now removes itself from the host genome (in a process called **excision**) and enters the lytic cycle.

One potential consequence of the lysogenic cycle is that when the viral genome activates, excising itself from the host genome, it may take part of the host genome along with it. When the virus replicates, the

---

[10] The initial decrease is due to the simple fact that many phage have injected their genomes into hosts and are no longer infectious.

[11] The ^{35}S cysteine will be incorporated into viral coat proteins and the ^{32}P phosphate will be incorporated into the viral nucleic acid genome in newly released viral particles. (Proteins contain no P, and nucleic acids contain no S.) When these viruses infect bacteria, their nucleic acids are injected into the bacteria while the capsid proteins remain on the exterior, which means that only the ^{32}P will be found in the interior of the newly infected cells.

small piece of host genome will be replicated and packaged with the viral genome. In subsequent infections, the virus will integrate the "stolen" host DNA along with its own genome into the new host's genome. The presence of the new DNA will become evident if it codes for a trait that the newly-infected host did not previously possess, such as the ability to metabolize galactose. This process is called **transduction**. [Why would a bacterial gene, carried with a virus and integrated with viral genes into a new bacterial genome, not be repressed along with the viral genes during lysogeny?[12]]

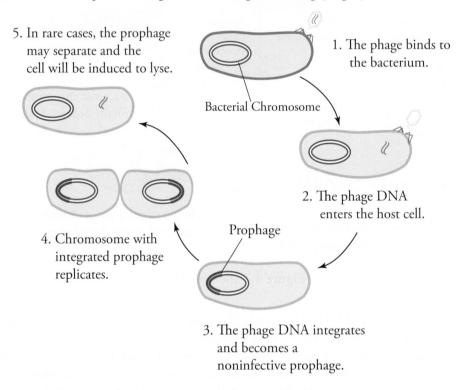

5. In rare cases, the prophage may separate and the cell will be induced to lyse.

1. The phage binds to the bacterium.

Bacterial Chromosome

2. The phage DNA enters the host cell.

Prophage

4. Chromosome with integrated prophage replicates.

3. The phage DNA integrates and becomes a noninfective prophage.

Figure 5   The Lysogenic Cycle

Replication of Animal Viruses

There are a number of differences between phages and viruses which infect animal cells. (Animal viruses don't have a special name like "phage.") The general outline of the viral life cycle, however, remains the same. The virus must specifically bind to a proper host cell, release its genetic material into the host, take over host machinery, replicate its genome, synthesize capsid components, assemble itself, and finally escape to infect a new cell.

Animal cells have proteins on the surface of their plasma membranes that serve as specific receptors for viruses. These receptors play a role in normal cellular function; they do not exist simply for the benefit of the virus. Part of the tissue-specificity of animal viruses is due to the distribution of receptors necessary for adsorption. For example, the binding of the HIV virus protein gp120 to a T cell membrane protein termed CD4 is one of the first steps in HIV infection.

---

[12] Prophage latency results from a viral repressor protein binding to viral DNA in a sequence-specific manner. The specific DNA sequence to which the repressor binds is present in the viral genes but not in the bacterial genes, so the bacterial gene can be expressed while the viral genes are repressed.

- Would treatment of an HIV-infected person with a soluble form of CD4 protein affect the infectivity of the virus?[13]
- Mutation of the cell-surface receptor that viruses attach to would be a means for an organism to become resistant to viral infection. Why is this mechanism not common?[14]
- Treatment of an enveloped animal virus with a mild detergent solubilizes several proteins from the virus, although the genome does not become accessible. Which one of the following is consistent with this scenario?[15]
    - A) Some of the proteins that are released by detergent may be encoded by the genome of the infected cell.
    - B) The infectivity of the virus is not affected by detergent treatment.
    - C) The proteins released by detergent are capsid proteins.
    - D) All the proteins released by the detergent are encoded by the viral genome.

The next step in the infection of an animal cell is penetration into the cell, just as in bacterial infection by a phage. Many animal viruses enter cells by **endocytosis** (a process whereby the host cell engulfs the virus and internalizes it). [Why don't phages enter their hosts by endocytosis?[16]] Once inside the host, the viral genome is *uncoated*, meaning it is released from the capsid. Alternatively, some viruses fuse with the plasma membrane to release virus into the cytoplasm. From this point, an animal virus may enter either a lytic cycle, a lytic-like cycle called the productive cycle, or a lysogenic cycle.

The lytic cycle in animal viruses is the same as in phages. The **productive cycle** is similar to the lytic cycle but does not destroy the host cell. It is possible because enveloped viruses exit the host cell by *budding through the host's cell membrane*, becoming coated with this membrane in the process. Budding does not necessarily destroy a cell since the lipid bilayer membrane can reseal as the virus leaves. Finally, in the animal virus lysogenic cycle the dormant form of the viral genome is called a **provirus** (analogous to a prophage). For example, Herpes simplex I is the virus that causes oral herpes. After infection, it may remain dormant as a provirus for an indefinite period of time. Then one day, usually when the host encounters stress (lack of sleep, upcoming professional school entrance exams), the virus reactivates.

Viral Genomes

The nature of the genome is perhaps the most important of the factors that determine viral uniqueness, and it has important consequences for how infection by each virus proceeds. In the following discussion, we will look at a few viral genomes with an eye to *what proteins the virus must encode or actually carry in its capsid based on its genome type*. Our purpose is not to provide new information, but rather to demonstrate what conclusions can be drawn from what you already know (typical MCAT passage material).

---

[13] Yes, it would. The soluble CD4 protein would bind to the virus's CD4 receptor (gp120) and block attachment of the virus to the T cells.

[14] Two reasons: 1) The receptor has a specific role in the normal physiology of the host, which a mutation might compromise. 2) Viruses generally evolve so rapidly that they can keep up with any changes in the host, but this is not an absolute rule. Cells of our immune system keep us alive by keeping up with most microorganisms' tricks.

[15] The detergent solubilized the viral envelope (choice C is wrong). As stated in the text, some envelop proteins are encoded by the virus and some are derived from the host's membranes during budding (choice **A** is correct, and choice D is wrong). Removal of envelope proteins will impair viral adsorption and reduce infectivity (choice B is wrong).

[16] Bacteria do not perform endocytosis, in part because they have a rigid cell wall which does not permit them to.

[+] RNA Viruses

—must *encode* RNA-dependent RNA pol (and do not have to carry it).

A (+) RNA virus, with a single-stranded RNA genome, is the simplest imaginable type of viral genome. As soon as the (+) RNA genome is in the host cell, host ribosomes begin to translate it, creating viral proteins. The viral genome acts directly as mRNA. The technical way to describe this scenario is to say the genome is **infective**, meaning injecting an isolated genome into the host cell will result in virus production. In order for the virus to replicate itself, one of the proteins it encodes must be an **RNA-dependent RNA polymerase**, the role of which is __?[17] (+) RNA viruses cause the common cold, polio, and rubella. [Will an infectious virus be produced if the genome of an enveloped (+) strand RNA virus is added to an extract prepared from the cytoplasm of eukaryotic cells that retains translational activity but lacks DNA replication or transcription of host genes?[18] If a viral genome is (+) strand RNA, what is used as a template by the RNA-dependent RNA polymerase?[19]]

[−] RNA Viruses

—must *carry* RNA-dependent RNA pol (and, of course, encode it too).

The genome of a (−) RNA virus is *complementary* to the piece of RNA that encodes viral proteins. In other words, the genome of a (−) RNA virus is the template for viral mRNA production. If host ribosomes translate (−) RNA, useless polypeptides will be made. Hence, the virus must not only encode an RNA-dependent RNA polymerase, it must actually carry one with it in the capsid. When the virus enters the host cell, this enzyme will create a (+) strand from the (−) genome. Then the viral life cycle can proceed. (−) RNA viruses cause rabies, measles, mumps, and influenza. [Do (−) strand RNA viruses use host enzymes to catalyze RNA production in transcription or in replication of the genome?[20]]

Retroviruses

—must *encode* reverse transcriptase.

HIV, the virus that causes AIDS, and HTLV (Human T cell Leukemia Virus) are examples of retroviruses. These are (+) RNA viruses which undergo lysogeny. In other words, they integrate into the host genome as proviruses. In order to integrate into our double-stranded DNA genome, a viral genome must also be composed of double-stranded DNA. Since these viral genomes enter the cell in an RNA form, they must undergo **reverse transcription** to make DNA from an RNA template. This snubbing of the central dogma is accomplished by an **RNA-dependent DNA polymerase** ("*reverse transcriptase*") encoded by the viral genome. Retroviruses are theoretically not required to carry this enzyme, only to encode it. [Why?[21]]

---

[17] to copy the RNA genome for viral replication; the host never makes RNA from RNA.

[18] No. The (+) strand RNA virus will be able to produce viral genome and proteins, but progeny will not be able to acquire the envelope they need to be infectious.

[19] To make (+) strand copies of the genome, the virus needs the complementary strand as a template: the (−) strand RNA. Thus, the RNA-dependent RNA polymerase produces a (−) strand intermediate before generating new (+) strand genomes.

[20] Neither. Viral RNA-dependent RNA polymerase first makes (+) strand as mRNA and then uses the (+) strand as the template to replicate new (−) strand genomes.

[21] Because the viral RNA genome can be translated by host ribosomes; thus, reverse transcriptase may be made after the viral genome enters the host. It just so happens that HIV does carry its reverse transcriptase within its capsid. You should understand why this is not a theoretical necessity.

Double-stranded DNA Viruses
—often *encode* enzymes required for dNTP synthesis and DNA replication.

These viruses often have large genomes that include genes for enzymes involved in deoxyribonucleotide synthesis (which we do whenever we make DNA) and DNA replication. [Given the limited information that viruses may contain in their genomes, why carry around genes for an enzyme possessed by the host?[22] Why don't RNA viruses do this?[23] Some DNA viruses induce infected host cells to enter mitosis and may even override cellular inhibition of cell division so strongly that the cell becomes cancerous; what is the advantage to the virus of inducing host-cell division?[24]]

12.2   SUBVIRAL PARTICLES
Some infectious agents are even smaller and simpler than viruses and are termed **subviral particles**. These include prions and viroids.

Prions
As infectious agents, prions do not strictly follow the Central Dogma because they are self-replicating proteins [Why does this violate the Central Dogma?[25]]. The prion itself is a misfolded version of a protein that already exists (see Figure 6).

---

[22] The host cell will only make dNTPs in preparation for replication. If the virus wants to reproduce without waiting for the host to do so, it must encode its own enzymes for the synthesis of DNA building blocks.

[23] Transcription is always occurring in all cells, so NTPs (not dNTPs) are always present.

[24] To replicate, the DNA virus must either provide all of the necessary components (such as dNTPs) itself, infect a cell that is already dividing, or induce the cell it infects to enter mitosis and produce the ingredients for DNA synthesis.

[25] The Central Dogma states that information flows in its nucleotide form from DNA to RNA (transcription), and then in its amino acid form from RNA to protein (translation). Prions take both transcription and translation out of the process and have proteins being shaped based on other proteins, hence the term "self-replicating."

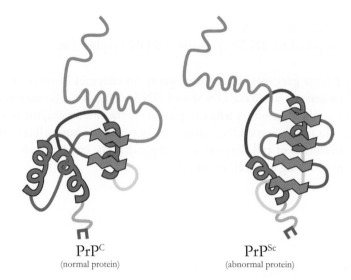

PrP^C
(normal protein)

PrP^Sc
(abnormal protein)

Figure 6 Comparison of the PrP^C structure to the PrP^Sc structure

When the normally folded protein (designated PrP^C) comes into contact with the prion (designated PrP^Sc), the prion acts as a template; the shape of the normal protein is altered and it too becomes infectious. Prions are responsible for a class of diseases in mammals referred to as the **transmissible spongiform encephalopathies** (TSEs). These diseases cause degeneration in the nervous system, especially the brain where characteristic holes develop, and are always fatal. The misfolded proteins are found in the nervous tissues and are very resistant to degradation by chemicals or heat, making them hard to destroy. Prion diseases are transmitted when tissue containing the abnormal proteins is ingested.

Prion diseases can also be genetically linked, through mutations in the gene that codes for the prion protein. For example, fatal familial insomnia (FFI) is an autosomal dominant condition inherited on chromosome 20, and Creutzfeldt Jakob disease (CJD) is also inherited. It is also possible for these diseases to arise spontaneously (through mutation) in someone with no prior family history. In general, however, prion diseases are very rare, striking only 1–2 people per million.

Whether transmitted, inherited, or spontaneously arising, prion diseases are characterized by their very long incubation periods, which can be several months to years in animals and several years to decades in humans. The misfolded proteins cause the destruction of neurons, particularly in the central nervous system, leading to loss of coordination, dementia, and death. Diagnosis is difficult, in part because of the long incubation periods and in part because the symptoms can be indicative of other conditions.

Viroids

Viroids consist of a short piece of circular, single-stranded RNA (200–400 bases long) with extensive self-complementarity (i.e., it can base-pair with itself to create some regions that are double-stranded; see Figure 7). Generally they do not code for proteins and they lack capsids. Some viroids are catalytic ribozymes, while others, when replicated, produce siRNAs that can silence normal gene expression. Replication of some viroids shares similarity to the replication of RNA viruses.

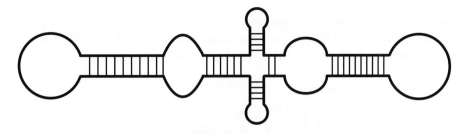

Figure 7   Structure of a viroid showing double-stranded regions

Most of the diseases caused by viroids are found in plants. The only human disease linked to viroids is Hepatitis D. The Hepatitis D viroid can only enter hepatocytes (liver cells) if it is contained in a capsid with a binding protein; since viroids do not have capsids, successful Hepatitis D infection required coinfection with Hepatitis B, from which it derives its capsid.

12.3   PROKARYOTES (DOMAIN BACTERIA)

Cell Theory

Advances in microbiology have been made possible by advancing technologies in magnification. Once humans were able to utilize basic, if crude, microscopy, the cell as the monomer of tissues and organs could be studied. In 1655, this led the English scientist, Robert Hooke, to define the Cell Theory based on his studies of cork. Its tenets are as follows:

1) All living organisms are composed of one or more cells and their products.
2) Cells are the monomer for any organism.
3) New cells arise from pre-existing, living cells.

All living organisms (which does not include viruses) can be classified as either **prokaryotes** or **eukaryotes**. The classification of organisms into these groups is based on examination of their internal cellular structure. Representatives from both groups are able to carry out the basic biochemical processes of photosynthesis, the Krebs cycle, and oxidative phosphorylation to produce ATP. The primary feature of prokaryotes that distinguishes them from eukaryotes is that they do not contain **membrane-bound organelles** (nucleus, mitochondria, lysosomes, etc.). *Prokaryote* means "before the nucleus," and the lack of a nucleus indicates that prokaryotes are evolutionarily the oldest domains. Unlike viruses, however, prokaryotes possess all of the machinery required for life. They are true cells, true living organisms. The prokaryotes include **bacteria**, **archea** (extremophiles), and **blue-green algae** (cyanobacteria).

The classification of living organisms, **taxonomy**, is an important part of biology because it is used to determine the evolutionary relationship of organisms to one another. The largest taxonomic division is the **domain**. There are three recognized domains: Bacteria, Archea, and Eukarya. Domains Bacteria and Archea include prokaryotic organisms, and Domain Eukarya includes eukaryotic organisms. Each domain can be further subdivided into **kingdoms**. Currently there are three well-recognized eukaryotic kingdoms (Animalia, Plantae, and Fungi), and great debate over the number of kingdoms that should be present in the other prokaryotic domains and in the single-celled eukaryotes (protists).

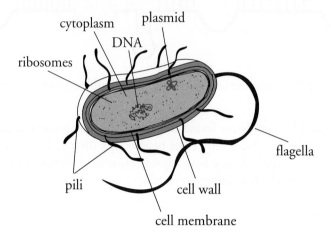

Figure 8 A Prokaryote

Bacterial Structure and Classification

Contents of the Cytoplasm

Unlike a eukaryotic cell, there are *no membrane-bound organelles* in prokaryotic cells (note that ribosomes, which are *not* membrane-bound, *are* found in bacteria). The prokaryotic genome is a single double-stranded circular DNA chromosome. It is not located in a nucleus and is not associated with histone proteins, as the eukaryotic genome is. In bacteria, transcription and translation occur in the same place, at the same time. Ribosomes begin to translate mRNA before it is completely transcribed. Many ribosomes translating a single piece of mRNA form a structure known as a **polyribosome**.[26]

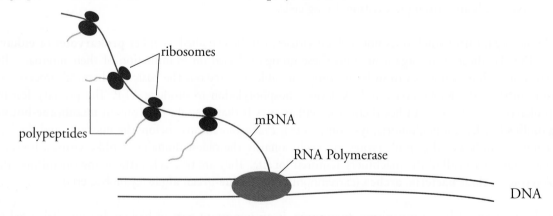

Figure 9 A Prokaryotic Polyribosome

---

[26] The 5' end of the mRNA polymer is free, since elongation of mRNA proceeds 5' to 3'. Proteins are made N to C, so the free end of the polypeptides is the N terminus.

Remember that the bacterial ribosome is structurally different from the eukaryotic ribosome, though both function the same way. The differences allow us to prescribe various antibiotics which interfere with bacterial translation without disrupting our own.

One last genetic element that can be found in prokaryotic cells is the **plasmid**. This is a circular piece of double-stranded DNA which is much smaller than the genome. Plasmids are referred to as **extrachromosomal genetic elements**. They often encode gene products which may confer an advantage upon a bacterium carrying the plasmid, for example, antibiotic-resistance genes. Many plasmids are capable of autonomous replication, which means that a single plasmid molecule within a bacterial cell may cause itself to be replicated into many copies. Plasmids are important not only because they may encode advantageous gene products, but also because they orchestrate bacterial exchange of genetic information, or **conjugation**, which is discussed below.

Bacterial Shape

Bacteria are often classified according to their shape. The three shapes and their proper names are organized in the following table:

Shape	Proper name (plural)	Proper name (singular)
round	cocci	coccus
rod-shaped	bacilli	bacillus
spiral-shaped	spirochetes or spirilla	spirochete, spirillum

Table 1 Bacterial Classification by Shape

The Cell Membrane and the Cell Wall

The bacterial cytoplasm is bounded by a lipid bilayer which is similar to our own plasma membrane. Outside the lipid bilayer is a rigid cell wall. It provides support for the cell, preventing lysis due to osmotic pressure. The bacterial cell wall is composed of **peptidoglycan**. It contains cross-linked chains made of sugars and amino acids, including D-alanine, which is not found in animal cells (our amino acids have the L configuration). The bacterial cell wall is the target of many antibiotics, such as penicillin. The enzyme *lysozyme*, which is found in tears and saliva and made by lytic viruses, destroys the peptidoglycan in the bacterial cell wall, resulting in an osmotically fragile structure called a **protoplast**. [Would a protoplast moved from salt water to fresh water shrivel or burst?[27]]

Gram Staining of the Cell Wall

This method of classification is derived from the extent to which bacteria turn color in a procedure termed **Gram staining**. The two groupings are **Gram-positive**, which stain strongly (a dark purple color) and **Gram-negative** bacteria, which stain weakly (a light pink color).

Gram-positive bacteria have a thick peptidoglycan layer outside of the cell membrane and no other layer beyond this. Gram-negative bacteria have a thinner layer of peptidoglycan in the cell wall but have an additional outer layer containing lipopolysaccharide. The intermediate space in Gram-negative bacteria between the cell membrane and the outer layer is termed the **periplasmic space**, in which are sometimes found

---

[27] It would burst, since water would flow into the cell by osmosis.

enzymes that degrade antibiotics (see Figure 10). The increased protection of Gram-negative bacteria from the environment is reflected in their weak staining, as well as in their increased resistance to antibiotics.

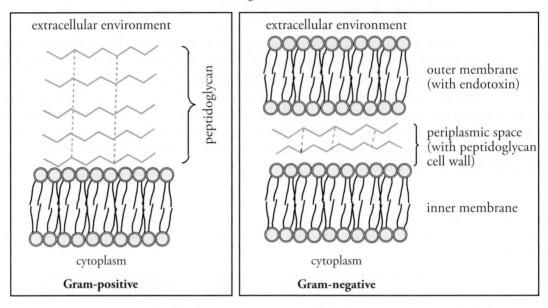

Figure 10   Gram-positive vs. Gram-negative Bacteria

The Capsule

Another attribute which only some bacteria have is the **capsule** or **glycocalyx**. This is a sticky layer of polysaccharide "goo" surrounding the bacterial cell and often surrounding an entire colony of bacteria. It makes bacteria more difficult for immune system cells to eradicate. It also enables bacteria to adhere to smooth surfaces such as rocks in a stream or the lining of the human respiratory tract.

Flagella

Another item only some bacteria have are long, whip-like filaments known as **flagella**, which are involved in bacterial motility. A bacterium which possesses one or more flagella is said to be **motile**, because flagella are the only means of bacterial locomotion. Bacteria may be **monotrichous** (meaning they have a flagellum located at only one end), **amphitrichous** (meaning they have a flagellum located at both ends), or **peritrichous** (meaning that they have multiple flagella). The following is which?[28]

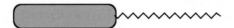

The structure of the flagellum is fairly complicated, with components encoded by over 35 genes, but it can be broken down into a few major components: the **filament**, the **hook**, and the **basal structure** (Figure 11). The basal structure contains a number of rings that anchor the flagellum to the inner and outer membrane (for a Gram-negative bacterium) and serve to rotate the **rod** and the rest of the attached flagellum in either a clockwise or counterclockwise manner. The most important thing to remember about the prokaryotic flagellum is that its structure is different from the eukaryotic one.

---

[28] Monotrichous

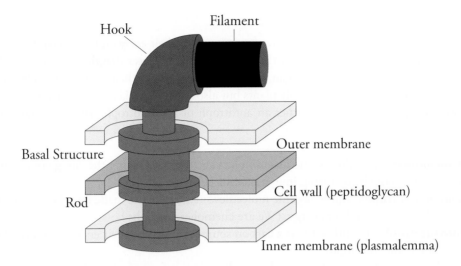

Figure 11 The Prokaryotic Flagellum

Pili

Pili are long projections on the bacterial surface involved in attaching to different surfaces. The **sex pilus** is a special pilus attaching F⁺ (male) and F⁻ (female) bacteria which facilitates the formation of **conjugation bridges** (discussed below). **Fimbriae** are smaller structures that are not involved in locomotion or conjugation but are involved in adhering to surfaces. [What other bacterial structure is involved in adhering to surfaces? Is it possible that the fimbriae play a role in infection by pathogenic organisms?[29]]

Bacterial Growth Requirements and Classification

Temperature

Another characteristic used to categorize bacteria is their ability to tolerate environmental variables, such as temperature. Though bacteria as a group can grow at a wide range of temperatures, each species has an optimal growth temperature. If the temperature is too high or too low, bacteria fail to grow and may be killed, hence the use of boiling to kill bacteria and refrigeration to slow bacterial growth and prevent food spoilage. Most bacteria favor mild temperatures similar to the ones that humans and other organisms favor (30°C); they are called **mesophiles** (moderate temperature lovers). **Thermophiles** (heat lovers) can survive at temperatures up to 100°C in boiling hot springs or near geothermal vents in the ocean floor. Bacteria that thrive at very low temperatures (near 0°C) are termed **psychrophiles** (cold lovers).

---

[29] The capsule, or glycocalyx is also involved in adherence. And yes, fimbriae do play a role in infection, by facilitating adhesion to cells so that the bacteria can colonize a tissue.

Nutrition

Bacteria can be classified according to their *carbon source* and their *energy source*. "**Troph**" is a Latin root meaning "eat." **Autotrophs** utilize CO_2 as their carbon source. **Heterotrophs** rely on organic nutrients (glucose, for example) created by other organisms. **Chemotrophs** get their energy from chemicals. **Phototrophs** get their energy from light; not only plants but also some bacteria do this. Each bacterium is either a chemotroph or a phototroph and is either an autotroph or a heterotroph. There are thus four types of bacteria:

1) **Chemoautotrophs** build organic macromolecules from CO_2 using the energy of chemicals. They obtain energy by oxidizing inorganic molecules like H_2S.

2) **Chemoheterotrophs** require organic molecules such as glucose made by other organisms as their carbon source and for energy. (We are chemoheterotrophs.)

3) **Photoautotrophs** use only CO_2 as a carbon source and obtain their energy from the Sun. (Plants are photoautotrophs.)

4) **Photoheterotrophs** are odd in that the get their energy from the Sun, like plants, but require an organic molecule made by another organism as their carbon source.

- A bacterium that causes an infection in the bloodstream of humans is most likely to be classified as which one of the following?[30]
  A) Chemoautotroph
  B) Photoautotroph
  C) Chemoheterotroph
  D) Photoheterotroph

- Which one of the following categories best describes an organism which uses sunlight to drive ATP production but cannot incorporate carbon dioxide into sugars?[31]
  A) Chemoautotroph
  B) Photoautotroph
  C) Chemoheterotroph
  D) Photoheterotroph

Growth Media

The environment in which bacteria grow is the **medium** (plural: **media**). In the lab, the most common solid medium is agar, a firm transparent gel made from seaweed. Bacteria live in the agar but do not metabolize it. The agar is usually kept in a clear plastic plate called a **Petri dish**, and the process of putting bacteria on such a plate is called **plating**. When one bacterium is plated onto a dish, if it grows, it will eventually give rise to many progeny in an isolated spot called a **colony**. **Minimal medium** contains nothing but glucose (in addition to the agar). More key terms: A **wild-type** bacterium (or a wild-type strain) is one which possesses all the characteristics normal to that particular species. The dense growth of bacteria seen in laboratory Petri dishes is known as a bacterial **lawn**. A **plaque** is a clear area in the lawn. Plaques result from death of bacteria and are caused by lytic viruses or toxins.

---

[30] Since there's no sunlight in the bloodstream, choice B and choice D are out. If it's a parasite, it most likely uses some of our chemicals, so it must be a heterotroph, which eliminates choice A. The answer is choice **C**.

[31] The ability to use sunlight indicates that the organism is a phototroph, and the inability to use carbon dioxide as a carbon source indicates that it is a heterotroph—it must use organic molecules as a carbon source. The answer is choice **D**.

Bacteria can reproduce very rapidly, provided that the conditions of their environment are favorable and nutrients are abundant. The **doubling time** is the amount of time required for a population of bacteria to double its number. It ranges from a minimum of 20 minutes for *E. coli* to a day or more for slow growers, such as the bacteria responsible for tuberculosis and leprosy. The doubling time of a bacterial species will vary, depending upon the availability of nutrients and other environmental factors.

One other important term in bacterial nutrition is **auxotroph** (don't confuse this term with *auto*troph). This is a bacterium which cannot survive on minimal medium because it can't synthesize a molecule it needs to live. Hence, it requires an *aux*iliary *troph*ic substance to live. For instance, a bacterium which is auxotrophic for arginine won't form a colony when plated onto minimal medium, but if the medium is supplemented with arginine, a colony will form. This arginine auxotrophy is denoted arg⁻. Auxotrophy results from a mutation in a gene coding for an enzyme in a synthetic pathway.

Bacteria can be differentiated not only by what substances they require, but also by what substances they are capable of metabolizing for energy. For instance, a strain of bacteria may be capable of surviving on minimal medium that has the disaccharide lactose as the only carbon source (no glucose). This would be denoted lac⁺. Mutation in a gene for the enzyme lactase would impair the bacterium's ability to survive on lactose-only medium. A bacterial strain incapable of growing with lactose as its only carbon source would be denoted lac⁻. Genetic exchange between bacteria by means of conjugation, transduction, or transformation (discussed on page 256) can remedy these disabilities.

Oxygen Utilization and Tolerance

Oxygen metabolism is *aerobic* metabolism. Bacteria which require oxygen are called **obligate aerobes**. Bacteria which do not require oxygen are called **anaerobes**. There are three subcategories: **facultative anaerobes** will use oxygen when it's around, but don't need it. **Tolerant anaerobes** can grow in the presence or absence of oxygen but do not use it in their metabolism. **Obligate anaerobes** are poisoned by oxygen. This is because they lack certain enzymes necessary for the detoxification of free radicals which form spontaneously whenever oxygen is around. Obligate anaerobes commonly infect wounds.

- If a bacterium cannot use oxygen as an electron acceptor, is it an obligate anaerobe, a tolerant anaerobe, a facultative anaerobe, or is it not possible to distinguish based on the information given?[32]

- A sample of bacteria is evenly mixed into a cool liquid agar nutrient mix in the absence of oxygen and then poured into a glass-walled tube that is open to the atmosphere on top. When the agar mix cools, it solidifies, and bacterial growth is observed as shown below. How would you classify the bacteria in terms of oxygen utilization and tolerance? (*Note:* Agar is practically impermeable to oxygen.)[33]

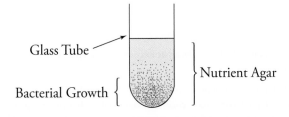

Glass Tube

Bacterial Growth

Nutrient Agar

---

[32] The bacterium cannot be a facultative anaerobe, since the question states it cannot use O_2. It could be either an obligate or a tolerant anaerobe depending on its ability to neutralize harmful oxygen free radicals.

[33] Since the bacteria grew only at the bottom of the tube, farthest away from any oxygen, this indicates that they could only grow in the absence of oxygen. Thus, they are obligate anaerobes.

12.3

Fermentation vs. Respiration

To briefly review, respiration is glucose catabolism with use of an inorganic electron acceptor such as oxygen. In contrast, fermentation is glucose catabolism which does not use an electron acceptor such as O_2; instead, a reduced by-product of glucose catabolism such as lactate or ethanol is given off as waste. [Why is fermentation necessary whenever an external electron acceptor is not used?[34]]

Anaerobic Respiration

This is not a contradiction in terms! It refers to glucose metabolism with electron transport and oxidative phosphorylation relying on an external electron acceptor *other than* O_2. For example, instead of reducing O_2 to H_2O, some anaerobic bacteria reduce SO_4^{2-} to H_2S, or CO_2 to CH_4. Nitrate (NO_3^-) is another possible electron acceptor.

- In an experiment, facultative anaerobic bacteria that are growing on glucose in air are shifted to anaerobic conditions. If they continue to grow at the same rate while producing lactic acid, then the rate of glucose consumption will:[35]
    A) increase 16 fold.
    B) decrease 16 fold.
    C) decrease 2 fold.
    D) not change.

Bacterial Life Cycle

Bacteria reproduce asexually. In asexual reproduction, there is no meiosis, no meiotic generation of haploid gametes, and no fusion of gametes to form a new individual organism. Instead, each bacterium grows in size until it has synthesized enough cellular components for two cells rather than one, replicates its genome, then divides in two. This process in bacteria is also known as **binary fission** (fission means "to split"). [In prokaryotes, does reproduction increase genetic diversity?[36] How is asexual reproduction in a eukaryote different from asexual reproduction in a prokaryote?[37]] Although bacteria do not reproduce sexually, they do possess a mechanism, termed **conjugation**, for exchanging genetic information (more on this later).

---

[34] Because NAD$^+$ must be regenerated from NADH for glycolysis to continue. In fermentation, the electrons are passed from NADH to a molecule other than O_2, such as pyruvic acid.

[35] Aerobic respiration produces 32 ATP per glucose in prokaryotes compared to only 2 ATP per glucose in fermentation. If the rate of growth is to remain the same, the rate of ATP production must remain the same to drive biosynthetic pathways forward. Since fermentation produces 1/16 the amount of ATP per glucose, the rate of glucose consumption must increase sixteen fold to maintain the rate of growth at the same level. The answer is choice **A**. (In reality the growth rate would probably decrease.)

[36] No. Each daughter cell is identical to the parent cell (assuming no mutation took place).

[37] In eukaryotes, asexual reproduction occurs through mitosis. Prokaryotes do not go through mitosis.

Growth of bacterial populations is described in stages (see Figure 12). Under ideal conditions, bacterial population growth is exponential, meaning that the number of bacterial cells increases exponentially with time. This also means the log of the population size grows linearly with time, hence the name **log phase.** [If 10 bacteria in log phase are placed in ideal growth conditions and the doubling time is 20 minutes, how many bacteria will there be after three hours?[38]]

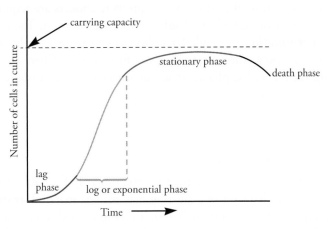

Figure 12   Bacterial Reproduction

Prior to achieving exponential growth, bacteria that were not previously growing undergo a **lag phase**, during which cell division does not occur even if the growth conditions are ideal.

- If growth conditions are ideal, why wouldn't cell division occur immediately?[39]
- Will bacteria that are transferred from a culture that is in log phase to a fresh new culture show a lag phase?[40]

As metabolites in the growth medium are depleted, and metabolic waste products accumulate, the bacterial population passes from log phase to **stationary phase**, in which cells cease to divide for lack of nutrients. The maximum population at the stationary phase is referred to as the **carrying capacity** for that environment. In the last stages of the stationary phase, cell death may occur as a result of the medium's inability to support growth. [If bacteria are grown in a medium with glucose as the main source of energy, when will the glycolytic pathway be more active: during the lag phase or during the stationary phase?[41]]

---

[38] Since three hours is equal to 180 minutes, the bacteria will divide nine times. Therefore, one bacterium will produce 2^9 = 512 bacteria after nine divisions. Since there are 10 bacteria initially, the total after four hours will be 10×2^9 = 5,120.

[39] Cells that are not growing are not actively producing components that are needed for cell division, such as dNTPs. The lag period is a time when biosynthetic pathways are very actively producing new cellular components so that cells can then begin to divide.

[40] No, since they will have all the gear necessary for population growth at the ready.

[41] The bacteria will use glucose during the lag phase to produce ATP and cellular machinery. During this period, glucose is abundant, and the cell is actively performing biosynthesis, so glycolysis is very active. During the stationary phase, however, the glucose will be depleted, and the rate of metabolism will have slowed dramatically, so the rate of glycolysis will decrease as well.

12.3

Endospore Formation

Some types of Gram-positive bacteria, such as the bacteria responsible for botulism, form **endospores** under unfavorable growth conditions. Endospores have tough, thick external shells comprised of peptidoglycan. Within the endospore are found the genome, ribosomes, and RNA which are required for the spore to become metabolically active when conditions become favorable. Endospores are able to survive temperatures above 100°C, which is why autoclaves or pressure cookers are required to completely sterilize liquids and substances that cannot be heated sufficiently in a dry oven. The metabolic reactivation of an endospore is termed **germination**. A single bacterium is able to form only one spore per cell. Thus, bacteria cannot increase their population through spore formation. [When are bacteria most likely to form endospores: during lag phase, log phase, or stationary phase? Is endospore formation a means for bacteria to reproduce?[42]]

Genetic Exchange Between Bacteria

Bacteria reproduce asexually, but genetic exchange is evolutionarily favorable because it fosters genetic diversity. Bacteria have three mechanisms of acquiring new genetic material: **transduction**, **transformation**, and **conjugation**. Note that none of these has anything to do with reproduction! Transduction was discussed in Section 12.1 under "lysogenic cycle"; it is the transfer of genomic DNA from one bacterium to another by a lysogenic phage. Transformation refers to a peculiar phenomenon: if pure DNA is added to a bacterial culture, the bacteria internalize the DNA in certain conditions and gain any genetic information in the DNA. Conjugation appears most likely to be related to normal bacterial function, however.

Conjugation

In conjugation, bacteria make physical contact and form a bridge between the cells. One cell copies DNA, and this copy is transferred through the bridge to the other cell. A key to bacterial conjugation is an extrachromosomal element known as the **F (fertility) factor**. Bacteria that have the F factor are **male**, or **F⁺**, and will transfer the F factor to female cells. Bacteria that do not contain the F factor are **female**, **F⁻**, and will receive the F factor from male cells to become male. [If all cells in a population are F⁺, will conjugation occur?[43]]

The F factor is a single circular DNA molecule. Although much smaller than the bacterial chromosome, the F factor contains several genes, many of which are involved in conjugation itself. After the male cell produces sex pili and the pili contact a female cell, a **conjugation bridge** forms. The F factor is replicated and transferred from the F⁺ to the F⁻ cell. DNA transfer between F⁺ and F⁻ cells is unidirectional; it occurs in one direction only (see Figure 13).

Although the F factor is an extrachromosomal element, it does sometimes become integrated into the bacterial chromosomes through recombination. A cell with the F factor integrated into its genome is called an **Hfr (high frequency of recombination) cell**. [Will an Hfr cell undergo conjugation with an F⁻ cell?[44]] When an Hfr cell performs conjugation, replication of the F factor DNA occurs as in F⁺ cells with the extra chromosomal F factor. Since the F factor DNA is integrated in the bacterial genome in Hfr cells, replication of F factor DNA continues into bacterial genes, and these too can be transferred into the F⁻ cell (see Figure 13).

---

[42] Stationary. Forming an endospore is like hibernating, not reproducing. Bacteria do it in order to sleep through the bad times.

[43] No. Conjugation occurs only between F⁺ (male) and F⁻ (female).

[44] Yes. All of the genes of the F factor are still present and expressed normally in the Hfr cell.

- If bacteria contain only one copy of the bacterial genome, how can recombination occur?[45]
- If the F factor in an Hfr strain integrates near a gene required for lactose metabolism, is it likely that other genes involved in lactose metabolism will be transferred during conjugation at the same time?[46]

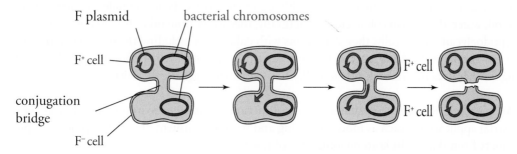

a) Conjugation and transfer of an F plasmid from an F+ donor to an F− recipient

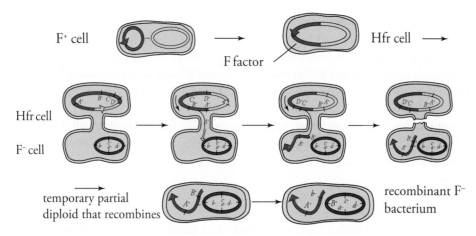

b) Conjugation and transfer of part of the bacterial chromosome from an Hfr donor to an F− recipient, resulting in recombination

Figure 13   Conjugation

Conjugation Mapping

Hfr bacteria provide a mechanism of mapping the bacterial genome. By allowing Hfr cells to conjugate in the lab and stopping the conjugation process after different time intervals, researchers can figure out the order of the genes on the bacterial chromosome by analyzing recipient cells to see what genes were transferred.

---

[45] When an Hfr cell conjugates with an F− cell and transfers a portion of the bacterial chromosomes, the F− cell will have two copies of some genes, and recombination can occur between the two copies.

[46] Yes. Genes for proteins of related functions are often adjacent to each other in prokaryotes (in operons) and so will transfer to an F− cell together.

Domain Archaea

Though all bacteria are prokaryotes, not all prokaryotes are equal. Certain prokaryotes belong to the domain *Archaea*, to be distinguished from the more "typical" bacteria (or eubacteria) which we have just discussed. The Archaea are the organisms that live in the world's most extreme environments, including hot springs, thermal vents, and hypersaline environments (although they can also be found in less extreme environments, such as soil, water, the human colon, etc.). Structurally, they differ from other bacteria because their cell wall lacks peptidoglycan. Genetically, they share traits with eukaryotes including the presence of introns and the use of many similar mRNA sequences. However, since they are single celled, they do reproduce via fission or budding. [What does this mean for their ability to increase their genetic diversity?[47]]

Since Archaea have to produce enzymes that can function in extreme environments, they are of great use in industrial applications, such as food processing and sewage treatment. The development of applications for products from these cells is an ongoing area of research.

Parasitic Bacteria

Parasitic bacteria can either be *obligate*, meaning that they must be inside a host cell to replicate, or *facultative*, meaning that they can live and replicate inside or outside of a host cell. In either case, the designation as a **parasite** means that damage is being done to the host cell. However, in order to ensure a continued supply of energy and cellular materials needed to survive and reproduce, parasitic bacteria need to modulate the course of that damage. [How is this model similar to viruses?[48]]

T cells (lymphocytes involved in immunity) are responsible for monitoring cellular contents; people who are T cell deficient have a hard time fighting off these types of bacterial infections, just as they would also struggle with viral infections.

Symbiotic Bacteria

Symbiotic bacteria coexist with a host, where both the bacterial cell and the host cell derive a benefit. An example of this would be the *Rhizobia* genus, which is responsible for the fixing of nitrogen in the nodules that exist on the roots of legumes. Without these bacteria the legume plants would not be able to grow, as they would be unable to derive the necessary nitrogen from the soil on their own. Due to their close relationship with their host cells, these bacteria often have smaller genomes with a more limited number of cellular products that are made, since the host cells can provide some of what the bacteria need. This can often mean that the symbiotic bacteria do not survive long outside of the host environment.

---

[47] Archaea would need to use separate strategies to increase their genetic diversity, just like eubacteria. The ability to become more genetically diverse would not be built into reproduction as it is in humans, in part because meiosis is not occurring.

[48] Viruses are obligate intracellular parasites. They do not have the option to replicate outside of a host cell, but must also balance the damage that is done to the host cell against what is needed for more virus to be made.

Chapter 13
Eukaryotic Cells

13.1   INTRODUCTION

It would be impossible to understand medicine without sound knowledge of the eukaryotic cell. You should be able to explain the function of each item labeled in Figure 1 below. Our discussion will be based on the animal cell. Fungi, plants, and protists are not covered on the MCAT.

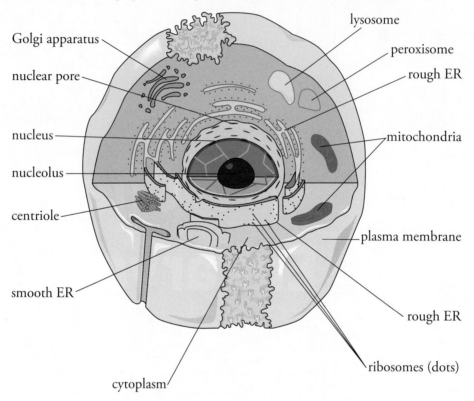

Figure 1   The Eukaryotic Cell

13.2 THE ORGANELLES

An **organelle** is a small structure within a cell that carries out specific cellular functions. Most organelles are bounded by their own lipid bilayer membrane. The membrane helps to seal off the contents of the organelle from the rest of the cytoplasm and control what enters and exits. A summary of the major animal cell organelles is given in the table below.

Organelle	Function (number of membranes surrounding)
nucleus	contain & protect DNA, transcription, partial assembly of ribosomes (2)
mitochondria	produce ATP via the Krebs cycle and oxidative phosphorylation (2)
ribosomes	synthesize proteins (0)
RER	location of synthesis/modification of secretory, membrane-bound & organelle proteins (1)
SER	detoxification & glycogen breakdown in liver; steroid synthesis in gonads (1)
Golgi apparatus	modification & sorting of protein, some synthesis (1)
lysosomes	contain acid hydrolases which digest various substances (1)
peroxisomes	metabolize lipids & toxins using H_2O_2 (1)

Table 1   Animal Cell Organelles

The Nucleus

One of the primary features of eukaryotic cells distinguishing them from prokaryotic cells is the **nucleus**. The nucleus contains the genome surrounded by the **nuclear envelope** that separates the contents of the nucleus into a distinct compartment, isolated from other organelles and from the cytoplasm. In eukaryotes, replication, transcription, and splicing occur in the nucleus, while translation occurs in the cytoplasm.

- If an enzyme that degrades mRNA is injected into the cytoplasm of a cell and all translation ceases, is the cell prokaryotic or eukaryotic?[1]
- When an enzyme that degrades DNA (DNase) is incubated with intact DNA isolated from an organism, the DNA is degraded. But when DNase is injected into the cytoplasm of cells from the same organism, no effect on the genome is observed. Which one of the following is the best explanation for this?[2]
    - A) The cell is a prokaryote; therefore, the genome is inaccessible to cytoplasmic enzymes.
    - B) The cell is a prokaryote; therefore, the circular genome is resistant to DNase.
    - C) The cell is a eukaryote; therefore, the genome is inaccessible to cytoplasmic enzymes.
    - D) The cell is a eukaryote; therefore, the linear genome is resistant to DNase.

---

[1] It could be either. mRNA and translation are found in the cytoplasm of both prokaryotes and eukaryotes, so the cell could be either.

[2] The isolated genome and the genome in the cell respond differently, so the key is not the circular or linear nature of the genome (choices B and D are wrong). The key is that in prokaryotes the injected cytoplasmic DNase will have access to the genome to degrade since they are in the same compartment, while in eukaryotes the DNase will not have access to the genome unless it enters the nucleus (choice **C** is the best choice).

The Genome

Eukaryotic genomes are organized into linear molecules of double-stranded DNA; the large size of the typical eukaryotic genome appears to make it necessary to split the genome into pieces, each a separate linear DNA molecule, termed a **chromosome**. Yeast have 4 different chromosomes, while there are 23 different human chromosomes. Since humans and most adult animals are diploid, they have two copies of each chromosome. Chromosomes have a **centromere** near the middle to ensure that newly replicated chromosomes are sorted properly during cell division, one copy to each daughter cell. Each eukaryotic chromosome also has special structures at both ends termed **telomeres**. Telomeres have large numbers of repeats of a specific DNA sequence and, with the help of a special DNA polymerase termed *telomerase*, maintain the ends of the linear chromosomes during DNA replication.

Within each chromosome is also a portion of the many thousands of genes in the genome as a whole. Genes can be mapped genetically and physically to the chromosome they reside on and to a specific location on that chromosome, a **locus**. The expression of eukaryotic genes is regulated by specific promoter and enhancer elements of that gene, but can also be affected by the position of the gene on the chromosome. Some regions of a chromosome are folded into densely packed chromatin, termed **heterochromatin**, within which genes tend to be inaccessible and turned off. Other regions known as **euchromatin** are more loosely packed (although still packaged into chromatin) and allow genes to be activated (see Chapter 10).

Finally, the nucleus is not a loose membrane bag with DNA floating inside. If nuclei are treated with DNase and with detergent, an insoluble mesh of protein, known as the **nuclear matrix** or **nuclear scaffold**, is left behind. The DNA in chromosomes is attached to the matrix at specific sites, and these (in some cases) appear to be involved in regulating gene expression or in limiting the effects of promoters and enhancers to discrete chromosomal regions known as domains. The role of the nuclear matrix is an area of ongoing research.

The Nucleolus

The **nucleolus** ("little nucleus") is a region within the nucleus which functions as a ribosome factory. There is no membrane separating the nucleolus from the rest of the nucleus. It consists of loops of DNA, RNA polymerases, rRNA, and the protein components of the ribosome. [Would you expect the nucleolus to be larger in cells that are actively synthesizing protein, or in quiescent cells?[3]]

The nucleolus is the site of transcription of rRNA by RNA pol I. Transcription of mRNA and tRNA is performed by other polymerases in other areas of the nucleus. The ribosome is partially assembled while still in the nucleolus. The protein components of the ribosome are not produced in the nucleolus; they are transported into the nucleus from the cytoplasm (remember that *all* translation takes place in the cytoplasm). After partial assembly, the ribosome is exported from the nucleus, remaining inactive until assembly is completed in the cytoplasm. This may serve to prevent translation of hnRNA.

---

[3] The nucleolus is largest in cells that are producing large amounts of protein. The increased size reflects increased synthesis of ribosomes.

The Nuclear Envelope

Surrounding the nucleus and separating it from the cytoplasm is the **nuclear envelope**, composed of two lipid bilayer membranes. The inner nuclear membrane is the surface of the envelope facing the nuclear interior, and the outer nuclear membrane faces the cytoplasm. The membrane of the endoplasmic reticulum is at points continuous with the outer nuclear membrane, making the interior of the ER (the **lumen** of the ER) contiguous with the space between the two nuclear membranes.

The nuclear envelope is punctuated with large **nuclear pores** that allow the passage of material into and out of the nucleus (see Figures 2 and 3). Molecules that are smaller than 60 kilodaltons, including small proteins, can freely diffuse from the cytoplasm into the nucleus through the nuclear pores. Larger proteins cannot pass freely through nuclear pores and are excluded from the nuclear interior unless they contain a sequence of basic amino acids called a **nuclear localization sequence**. Proteins with a nuclear localization sequence are translated on cytoplasmic ribosomes and then imported into the nucleus by specific transport mechanisms. It also appears likely that RNA is transported out of the nucleus by a specific transport system rather than freely diffusing into the cytoplasm. [If a 15 kD protein has a nuclear localization sequence that is then deleted from its gene, will the mutated protein still be found in the nucleus?[4]]

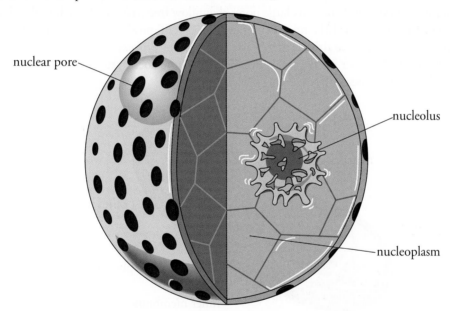

Figure 2   The Nucleus, Showing Pores

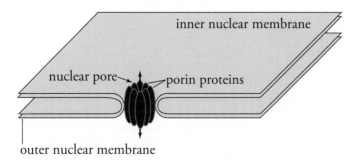

Figure 3   A Nuclear Pore Close-Up

---

[4] Yes. The protein is small enough that it can still pass through the nuclear pores by diffusion even without a nuclear localization sequence.

- Which one of the following proteins would NOT be found within the nucleus?[5]
    - A) A protein component of the large ribosomal subunit
    - B) A factor required for splicing
    - C) A histone
    - D) An aminoacyl tRNA synthetase

Mitochondria

Mitochondria are the site of oxidative phosphorylation (discussed in more detail in Chapter 8). The interior of mitochondria, the **matrix**, is bounded by the inner and outer mitochondrial membranes (see Figure 4). The matrix contains pyruvate dehydrogenase and the enzymes of the Krebs cycle. The inner membrane is the location of the electron transport chain and ATP synthase and is the site of the proton gradient used to drive ATP synthesis by ATP synthase. The inner membrane is impermeable to the free diffusion of polar substances, like protons, and is folded into the matrix in projections called **cristae**. The outer membrane is smooth and contains large pores that allow free passage of small molecules. The space between the membranes is called the intermembrane space. ATP produced within mitochondria is transported out into the cytoplasm to drive a great variety of cellular processes. [Why is the inner membrane folded into cristae?[6] If the inner membrane is impermeable, how does pyruvate get into the matrix where pyruvate dehydrogenase is located?[7]]

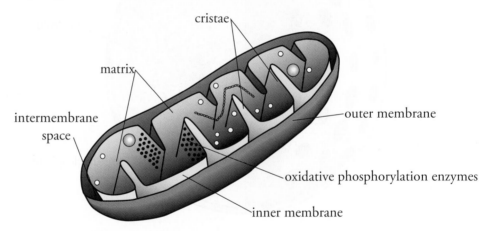

Figure 4   The Mitochondrion

---

[5] Aminoacyl tRNA synthetases are enzymes that function in the cytoplasm to attach amino acids to their respective tRNAs. They are never needed in the nucleus and would not be found there (choice **D** is correct). The protein components of ribosomes are synthesized in the cytoplasm and then imported into the nucleus to be assembled in the nucleolus (choice A would be found in the nucleus and can be eliminated). Splicing occurs in the nucleus, so anything involved in splicing would be found there (choice B can be eliminated). Histones are used for DNA packaging and would be found in the nucleus (choice C can be eliminated).

[6] The folding of the membrane increases its surface area and allows for increased electron transport and ATP synthesis per mitochondrion. (Folding is used elsewhere to increase surface area, such as in the kidney tubules and the lining of the small intestine.)

[7] Pyruvate is transported through the inner mitochondrial membrane by a specific protein in the membrane.

Mitochondria possess their own genome which is far smaller than the cellular genome and consists of a single circular DNA molecule. It encodes rRNA, tRNA, and several proteins, including some components of the electron transport chain and parts of the ATP synthase complex although most mitochondrial proteins are encoded by nuclear genes. Even more curious, mitochondria use a different system of transcription and translation than nuclear genes do. This includes a unique genetic code and unique RNA polymerases, DNA replication machinery, ribosomes, and aminoacyl-tRNA synthetases. In order to explain the fact that mitochondria possess a second system of inheritance, investigators have postulated that mitochondria originated as independent unicellular organisms living within larger cells. This is known as the **endosymbiotic theory** of mitochondrial evolution (*endo* = within; *symbiotic* = living together). In fact, if you compare a mitochondrion to a Gram-negative bacterium, you'll note that they look pretty similar. Pay attention to where the enzymes of electron transport are located and the genome shape.[8] Because many unique mitochondrial polypeptides are encoded by the cellular genome and not the mitochondrial genome, it has been suggested that the genes coding for these proteins may have been transferred to the nuclear genome over time.

Mitochondria exhibit **maternal inheritance**. This means that mitochondria are inherited only from the mother, since the cytoplasm of the egg becomes the cytoplasm of the zygote. (The sperm contributes only genomic [nuclear] DNA.)

Endoplasmic Reticulum (ER)

The **endoplasmic reticulum** (**ER**) is a large system of folded membrane accounting for over half of the membrane of some cells. There are two types of ER (see Figure 5): **rough ER** and **smooth ER**, each with distinct functions. The rough ER is called rough due to the large number of ribosomes bound to its surface; it is the site of protein synthesis for proteins targeted to enter the secretory pathway. The smooth ER is not actively involved in protein processing but can contain enzymes involved in steroid hormone biosynthesis (gonads) or in the degradation of environmental toxins (liver). The membrane of the endoplasmic reticulum is joined with the outer nuclear membrane in places, meaning that the space within the nuclear membranes is continuous with the interior of the ER (the ER **lumen**). The rough ER plays a key role directing protein traffic to different parts of the cell.

---

[8] Remember that bacterial electron transport depends on a proton gradient across the cell membrane. In a Gram-negative bacterium, this membrane would correspond to the mitochondrial inner membrane.

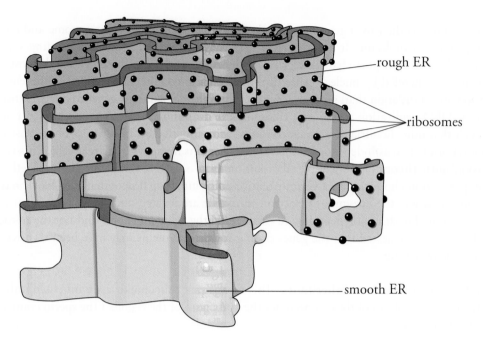

Figure 5 The ER

The Rough ER and the Secretory Pathway

There are two sites of protein synthesis in the eukaryotic cell: either on ribosomes free in the cytoplasm or on ribosomes bound to the surface of the rough ER. Proteins translated on free cytoplasmic ribosomes are headed toward peroxisomes, mitochondria, the nucleus, or will remain in the cytoplasm. Proteins synthesized on the rough ER will end up either 1) secreted into the extracellular environment, 2) as integral plasma membrane proteins, or 3) in the membrane or interior of the ER, Golgi apparatus, or lysosomes. Membrane-bound vesicles pass between these cellular compartments. Since the membranes of these organelles communicate through the traffic of vesicles, the interior of the ER, the Golgi apparatus, lysosomes, and the extracellular environment are in a sense contiguous. Proteins synthesized on the rough ER are transported in vesicles that bud from the ER to the Golgi apparatus, then to the plasma membrane or lysosome. A secreted protein that enters the ER lumen is separated by a membrane from the cytoplasm until the protein leaves the cell.

Whether a protein is translated on the rough ER is determined by the sequence of the protein itself. All proteins start translation in the cytoplasm; however, some proteins (secreted proteins and lysosomal proteins) have an amino acid sequence at their N-terminus called a **signal sequence.** The signal sequence of a nascent polypeptide is recognized by the **signal recognition particle** (**SRP**), which binds to the ribosome. The rough ER has SRP receptors that dock the ribosome-SRP complex on the cytoplasmic surface (along with the nascent polypeptide and mRNA). Translation then pushes the polypeptide, signal peptide first, into the ER lumen. After translation is complete, the signal peptide is removed from the polypeptide by a signal peptidase in the ER lumen. For secreted proteins, once the signal sequence is removed, the protein is transported in the interior of vesicles through the Golgi apparatus to the plasma membrane, where it is released by exocytosis into the extracellular environment.

- The mRNA for a secreted protein encodes a longer protein than is actually observed in the cellular exterior. Why?[9]
    - A) The protein was cleaved by a cytoplasmic protease.
    - B) The mRNA was not spliced properly.
    - C) The gene encoding the protein contained a nonsense mutation.
    - D) The signal sequence of the protein was removed in the rough ER.

Integral membrane proteins are processed slightly differently. Integral membrane proteins have sections of hydrophobic amino acid residues called **transmembrane domains** that pass through lipid bilayer membranes. The transmembrane domains are essentially signal sequences that are found in the interior of the protein (that is, not at the N-terminus). They are *not* removed after translation. A single polypeptide can have several transmembrane domains passing back and forth through a membrane. During translation, the transmembrane domains are threaded through the ER membrane. The protein is then transported in vesicles to the Golgi apparatus and plasma membrane in the same manner as a secreted protein (see Figure 6). [For a protein in the plasma membrane, does the portion of the protein projecting out of the ER membrane end up facing the cytoplasm or the cellular exterior?[10]]

Additional functions of the rough ER include the initial post-translational modification of proteins. Although glycosylation (the addition of saccharides to proteins) is usually associated with the Golgi apparatus, some glycosylation occurs in the lumen of the ER. Disulfide bond formation also occurs in the ER lumen.

Two last notes about protein traffic throughout the cell: First, the default target for proteins that go through the secretory path is the plasma membrane. **Targeting signals** are needed if a protein going through that path needs to end up elsewhere (e.g., the Golgi, the ER, the lysosome). Second, proteins that are made in the cytoplasm but need to be sent to an organelle that is not part of the secretory path (e.g., the nucleus, mitochondria, or peroxisomes) require sequences called **localization signals**. The table on the next page summarizes protein traffic.

---

[9] The only way a protein can be smaller than would be expected from its mRNA would be if some post-translational modification were to occur (choice **D** is correct). Choices B and C are pre-translational modifications and would not account for a size difference between mRNA and protein, and since secreted proteins are synthesized on the rough ER, they are inaccessible to cytoplasmic proteases (so choice A is wrong).

[10] The cytoplasm.

13.2

Protein Final Destination	Signal Sequence?	Localization Signal?	Transmembrane Domains?	Targeting Signal?	Example
Secreted	Yes	No	No	No	Antibodies, Neurotransmitters, Peptide hormones
Plasma Membrane	Yes	No	Yes	No	Receptors, channels
Lysosome	Yes	No	No	Yes	Acid hydrolases
Rough ER	Yes	No	No	Yes	Enzymes required for protein modification
Smooth ER	Yes	No	No	Yes	Enzymes required for lipid synthesis
Golgi Apparatus	Yes	No	No	Yes	Enzymes required for protein modification
Cytoplasm	No	No	No	No	Glycolysis enzymes
Nucleus	No	Yes	No	No	Histones, DNA/RNA polymerase
Mitochondria	No	Yes	No	No	PDC/Krebs cycle enzymes
Peroxisome	No	Yes	No	No	Catalase

Table 2   Summary of Cellular Protein Traffic

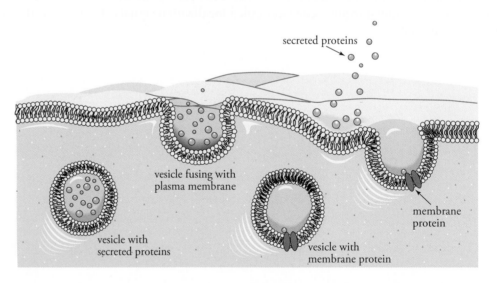

Figure 6   The Secretory Pathway—Secreted Proteins and Integral Membrane Proteins

The Golgi Apparatus

The Golgi apparatus is a group of membranous sacs stacked together like collapsed basketballs (see Figure 7). It has the following functions:

1) Modification of proteins made in the RER; especially important is the modification of oligo-saccharide chains
2) Sorting and sending proteins to their correct destinations
3) The Golgi also synthesizes certain macromolecules, such as polysaccharides to be secreted.

The vesicle traffic to and from the Golgi apparatus is mostly unidirectional; the membrane-bound or secreted proteins that are to be sorted and modified enter at one defined region and exit at another. (Traffic is said to be *mostly* unidirectional because on occasion, proteins that are supposed to reside in the ER accidentally escape, and they must be returned to the ER from the Golgi. This is called "retrograde traffic.") Each region of the Golgi has different enzymes and a different microscopic appearance. The portion of the Golgi nearest the rough ER is called the *cis* stack, and the part farthest from the rough ER is the *trans* stack. The *medial* stack is in the middle.[11] Vesicles from the ER fuse with the *cis* stack. The proteins in these vesicles are then modified and transferred to the *medial* stack, where they are further modified before passing to the *trans* stack. Proteins leave the Golgi at the *trans* face in transport vesicles. [If vesicle fusion with the *cis* Golgi was inhibited, could plasma membrane proteins still reach the cell surface?[12]] The route taken by a protein is determined by signals within the protein that determine which vesicle a protein is sorted into in the *trans* Golgi.

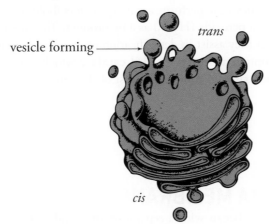

vesicle forming

trans

cis

Figure 7 The Golgi Apparatus

---

[11] Note that *cis* means "near," as in a *cis* double bond. *Trans* means "far." *Medial* means "in the middle." Also note that the order is alphabetical: *cis-medial-trans*.

[12] No. Secretory proteins must proceed via a specific path: from the ER to the *cis* Golgi to the medial and *trans* Golgi and from there to the cell surface.

Lysosomes

Lyse means cut. The **lysosome** is a membrane-bound organelle that is responsible for the degradation of biological macromolecules by hydrolysis. Lysosome proteins are made in the RER, modified in the Golgi, and released in their final form from the *trans* face of the Golgi. Organelles such as mitochondria that have been damaged or are no longer functional may be degraded in lysosomes in a process termed **autophagy** (self-eating). Lysosomes also degrade large particulate matter engulfed by the cell by **phagocytosis** (cell eating). For example, **macrophages** of the immune system engulf bacteria and viruses. The particle or microorganism ends up in a **phagocytic vesicle**, which will fuse with a lysosome. After hydrolysis, the lysosome will release molecular building blocks into the cytoplasm for reuse.

The enzymes responsible for degradation in lysosomes are called **acid hydrolases**. This name reflects the fact that these enzymes only hydrolyze substrates when they are in an acidic environment. This is a safety mechanism. The pH of the lysosome is around 5, so the acid hydrolases are active. But the pH of the cytoplasm is 7.4. If a lysosome ruptures, its enzymes will not damage the cell because the acidic fluid will be diluted, and the acid hydrolases will be inactivated. However, if many lysosomes rupture at once, the cell may be destroyed.

Peroxisomes

Peroxisomes are small organelles that perform a variety of metabolic tasks. The peroxisome contains enzymes that produce hydrogen peroxide (H_2O_2) as a by-product. They are essential for lipid breakdown in many cell types. In the liver they assist in detoxification of drugs and chemicals. H_2O_2 is a dangerous chemical, but peroxisomes contain an enzyme called **catalase** which converts it to $H_2O + O_2$. Separating these activities into the peroxisomes protects the rest of the cell from damage by peroxides or oxygen radicals.

13.3   THE PLASMA MEMBRANE

The evolution of life most likely began with a separation of "inside" from "outside." Once this had occurred, processes in the cell could increase their orderliness despite the entropic chaos of the surroundings. An alternate hypothesis is that life began with self-replicating RNA floating free in the ocean. As it grew more complex, this early genome would require protection. In any case, the separation of the cytoplasm from the extracellular environment was a major milestone in evolution. Bacteria, plants, and fungi accomplish this by forming a cell membrane and a cell wall (made of peptidoglycan, cellulose, and chitin, respectively). Eukaryotic animal cells have no cell wall and thus rely on the cell membrane as the only boundary between inside and outside. And they must devise another means of structural support: just as chordates have a bony endoskeleton instead of the primitive exoskeleton arthropods have, animal cells rely on an internal cytoskeleton instead of an external cell wall. Further problems arise in multicellular eukaryotes. Not only must each cell maintain its structural integrity, but it must also interact with its neighbors in an organized fashion. In the following discussion, we will study how each of these goals is accomplished.

Membrane Structure

All of the membranes of the cell are composed of **lipid bilayer** membranes. The three most common lipids in eukaryotic membranes are **phospholipids**, **glycolipids**, and **cholesterol**, of which phospholipids are the most abundant. An example of a phospholipid is *phosphatidyl choline* (see Figure 8) with two long hydrophobic fatty acids esterified to glycerol, along with a charged phosphoryl choline group. Thus, phospholipids have portions that are distinctly hydrophilic and hydrophobic. Glycolipids, with fatty acids groups and carbohydrate side chains, also have hydrophilic and hydrophobic regions. When fatty acids or phospholipids are mixed with water, they spontaneously arrange themselves with the hydrophobic tails facing the interior to avoid contact with water and the hydrophilic regions facing outward toward water (see Figure 9). Fatty acids form small micelles, but, due to steric hindrance, phospholipids arrange themselves spontaneously into **lipid bilayer membranes**. Since the lipid bilayer is the lowest energy state for these molecules, the bilayer membrane can reseal and repair itself if a small portion of membrane is removed.

The interior of the lipid bilayer membrane is very hydrophobic, with water largely excluded. Hydrophilic molecules such as ions, carbohydrates, and amino acids are not soluble in this environment, making the membrane a barrier to the passage of these molecules. Nonpolar molecules such as CO_2, O_2, and steroid hormones can cross the membrane easily. Water can also pass through the membrane but does so through specialized protein channels.

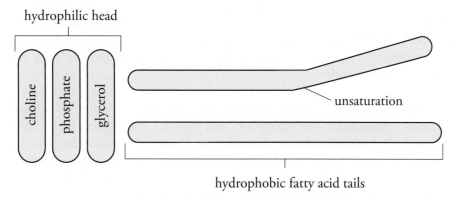

Figure 8 Phosphatidyl Choline, a Phospholipid

- Which one of the following statements best describes the physical characteristics of phospholipids?[13]
    A) Negatively charged at pH 7 and therefore entirely hydrophilic
    B) Hydrophobic
    C) Partially hydrophilic and partially hydrophobic
    D) Positively charged at pH 7 and therefore entirely hydrophilic

---

[13] Choice **C.** Phospholipids have hydrophobic components (fatty acid acyl chains) and hydrophilic components (phosphate and choline, for example, in phosphatidyl choline).

13.3

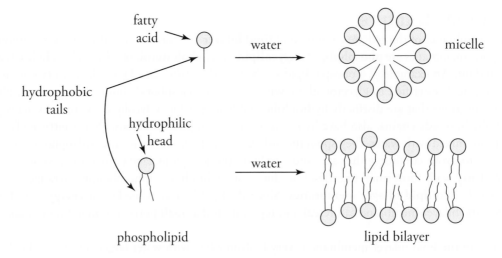

Figure 9 Lipid Behavior in an Aqueous Solvent

In addition to lipids, proteins are a major component of membranes. In some cases, such as the mitochondrial inner membrane, there is a higher protein than lipid concentration. Some proteins act to mediate interactions of the cell with other cells. Other proteins, called **cell-surface receptors**, bind extracellular signaling molecules such as hormones and relay these signals into the cell so that it can respond accordingly. **Channel proteins** selectively allow ions or molecules to cross the membrane. Each of these types of membrane protein is discussed below.

In general, membrane proteins are classified as peripheral or integral (see Figure 10). **Integral membrane proteins** are actually embedded in the membrane, held there by hydrophobic interactions. Membrane-crossing regions are called **transmembrane domains** (see Figure 11). Integral membrane proteins may have a complex pattern of transmembrane domains and portions not within the membrane. **Peripheral membrane proteins** are not embedded in the membrane at all, but rather are stuck to integral membrane proteins, held there by hydrogen bonding and electrostatic interactions.

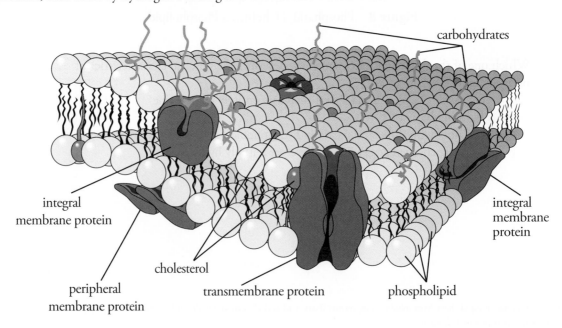

Figure 10 Membrane Proteins

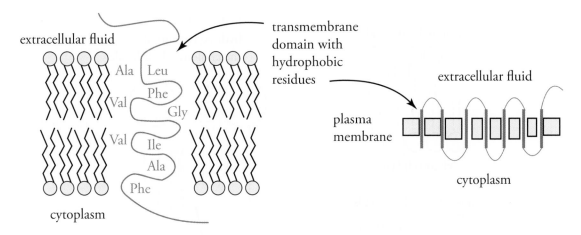

Figure 11   Transmembrane Domains

The current understanding of membrane dynamics is termed the **fluid mosaic model**, because the membrane is seen as a mosaic of lipids and proteins which are free to move back and forth fluidly. According to this model, lipids and proteins are free to diffuse laterally, in two-dimensions, but are **not free to flip-flop**. Phospholipid head groups and hydrophilic protein domains are restricted from entering the hydrophobic membrane interior just as hydrophilic molecules in the extracellular space are. Hence, the membrane is said to have **polarity**. This just means that the inside face and the outside face remain different. We have already discussed one such difference: All glycosylations are found on the extracellular face. So the "fluid" in "fluid mosaic" means that things are free to move back and forth, but in two dimensions only. One exception is that some proteins are anchored to the cytoskeleton and thus cannot move in any direction.

- Phospholipids can be covalently attached to a fluorescent tag and then integrated into a lipid bilayer. If one cell has a red fluorescent tagged lipid in its plasma membrane and another cell has a green fluorescent tagged lipid in its membrane, what will happen if the two cells are fused together?[14]

The fluidity of a membrane is affected by the composition of lipids in the membrane (see Figure 12). The hydrophobic van der Waals interactions between the fatty acid side chains are a major determinant of membrane fluidity. Saturated fatty acids, lacking any double bonds, have a very straight structure and pack tightly in the membrane, with strong van der Waals forces between side chains. Unsaturated fatty acids, with one or more double bonds, have a kinked structure and pack in the membrane interior more loosely. Cholesterol also plays a key role in maintaining optimal membrane fluidity by fitting into the membrane interior. [If the percentage of unsaturated fatty acids in a membrane is decreased, will membrane fluidity increase or decrease at body temperature?[15]]

---

[14] After a short period of time, the red and green tagged lipids will diffuse laterally and mix. An even distribution of the tags will be seen across the surface of the new hybrid cell.

[15] Unsaturated fatty acids, with a kinked structure, have fewer van der Waals interactions, and therefore allow a more fluid membrane structure. Decreasing the unsaturated fatty acids will decrease membrane fluidity.

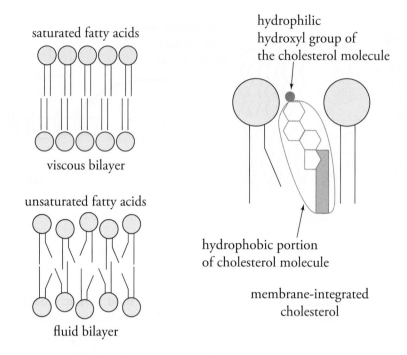

Figure 12 Factors Affecting Membrane Fluidity

13.4 TRANSMEMBRANE TRANSPORT

The cell requires membranes to act as barriers to diffusion but also requires the transport of many different substances across membranes. Integral membrane proteins transport material through membranes that cannot diffuse on their own across membranes. Transport across a membrane can be either **passive** (does not require cellular energy) or **active** (requires cellular energy). Before we discuss movements across membranes, let's review basic rules about concentration, ionizability, colligative properties, and diffusion and osmosis.

Concentration Measurements

Molarity (*M*) expresses the concentration of a solution in terms of moles of solute per volume (in liters) of solution:

$$\text{Molarity } (M) = \frac{\text{\# moles of solute}}{\text{\# liters of solution}}$$

Concentration is denoted by enclosing the solute in brackets. For instance, "$[Na^+] = 1.0\ M$" indicates a solution whose concentration is equivalent to 1 mole of sodium ions per liter of solution.

Molality (*m*) expresses concentration in terms of moles of solute per *mass* (in kilograms) of solvent:

$$\text{Molality } (m) = \frac{\text{\# moles of solute}}{\text{\# kg of solvent}}$$

Molality is particularly useful when measuring properties that involve temperature because, unlike molarity, molality does not change with temperature. And, since a liter of water has a mass of one kilogram, the molar and molal concentrations of dilute aqueous solutions are nearly the same. This is particularly true in biological systems, where the volume (essentially a cell) is very small and the solvent is always water.

Mole fraction simply expresses the fraction of moles of a given substance (which we'll denote here by S) relative to the total moles in a solution:

$$\text{mole fraction of S} = X_S = \frac{\text{\# moles of substance S}}{\text{total \# moles in solution}}$$

Mole fraction is a useful way to express concentration when more than one solute is present.

Electrolytes

When ionic substances dissolve, they **dissociate** into ions. Free ions in a solution are called **electrolytes** because the solution can conduct electricity. Some salts dissociate completely into individual ions, while others only partially dissociate (that is, a certain percentage of the ions will remain paired, sticking close to each other rather than being independent and fully surrounded by solvent). Solutes that dissociate completely (like ionic substances) are called **strong electrolytes**, and those that remain ion-paired to some extent are called **weak electrolytes**. (Covalent compounds that don't dissociate into ions are **nonelectrolytes**.) Solutions of strong electrolytes are better conductors of electricity than those of weak electrolytes.

Different ionic compounds will dissociate into different numbers of particles. Some won't dissociate at all, and others will break up into several ions. The **van't Hoff** (or **ionizability**) **factor** (*i*) tells us how many ions one unit of a substance will produce in a solution. For example,

- $C_6H_{12}O_6$ is non-ionic, so it does not dissociate. Therefore, $i = 1$.
  (Note: The van't Hoff factor for almost all biomolecules—hormones, proteins, steroids, etc.—is 1.)
- NaCl dissociates into Na^+ and Cl^-. Therefore, $i = 2$.
- HNO_3 dissociates into H^+ and NO_3^-. Therefore, $i = 2$.
- $CaCl_2$ dissociates into Ca^{2+} and $2\ Cl^-$. Therefore, $i = 3$.

Colligative Properties

Colligative properties depend on the *number* of solute particles in the solution rather than the *type* of particle. For example, when any solute is dissolved into a solvent, the boiling point, freezing point, and vapor pressure of the solution will be different from those of the pure solvent. For colligative properties, *the identity of the particle is not important.* That is, for a 1 *M* solution of *any* solute, the change in a colligative property will be the same no matter what the size, type, or charge of the solute particles. Remember to consider the van't Hoff factor when accounting for particles: one mole of sucrose ($i = 1$) will have the same number of particles *in solution* as 0.5 mol of NaCl ($i = 2$), and therefore will have the same effect on a colligative property. Thus, we can consider the effective concentration to be the product iM (or im); this is the concentration of particles present.

The four colligative properties we'll study for the MCAT are vapor-pressure depression, boiling-point elevation, freezing-point depression, and osmotic pressure.

Vapor-Pressure Depression

Think about being at the ocean or a lake in the summer. The air is always more humid (moist) than in the middle of a parking lot. Why? Because some of the water molecules gain enough energy to get into the gas phase, so we see a dynamic equilibrium setup between the molecules in the liquid phase and the molecules in the gas (vapor) phase.

Vapor pressure is the pressure exerted by the gaseous phase of a liquid that evaporated from the exposed surface of the liquid. The weaker a substance's intermolecular forces, the higher its vapor pressure and the more easily it evaporates. For example, if we compare diethyl ether, $H_5C_2OC_2H_5$, and water, we notice that while water undergoes hydrogen bonding, diethyl ether does not, so despite its greater molecular mass, diethyl ether will vaporize more easily and have a higher vapor pressure than water. Easily vaporized liquids—liquids with *high* vapor pressure—like diethyl ether are said to be **volatile.**

Now let's think about what happens to vapor pressure when the liquid contains a dissolved solute. The solute molecules are attached to solvent molecules and act as "anchors." As a result, more energy is required to enter the gas phase since the solvent molecules need to break away from their interactions with the solute before they can enter the gas phase. In fact, the boiling point of a liquid is defined as the temperature at which the vapor pressure of the solution is equal to the atmospheric pressure over the solution. Thus, at sea level, where the atmospheric pressure is 760 torr, the solution must have a vapor pressure of 760 torr in order to boil. Adding more solute to the same solution will decrease its vapor pressure. Boiling will still take place when vapor pressure is 760 torr, but more heat will have to be supplied to reach this vapor pressure, and thus the solution will boil at a higher temperature. For example, salted water (say, for cooking spaghetti) boils at a higher temperature than unsalted water.

Boiling-Point Elevation

When a liquid boils, the molecules in the liquid acquire enough energy to overcome the intermolecular forces and break free into the gas phase. The liquid molecules escape as a vapor at the surface between the liquid and air. But what happens when a non-volatile solute is added to the liquid? As described before, the solute particles are attached to solvent molecules and act as "anchors." As a result, more energy is required since you not only have to convert the solvent into the gas phase, but you first have to break the interaction with the solute. What happens to the boiling point? In order for the molecules to escape, they need more energy than they did without the solute. This translates into an elevation of the boiling point. The increase in boiling point is directly related to the number of particles in solution and the type of solvent. For a given solvent (again, in biological systems this is always water), the more solute particles, the greater the boiling-point elevation. Also, you have to consider that some compounds dissociate when they dissolve, so the equation for boiling-point elevation includes the van't Hoff factor, i:

Boiling-Point Elevation

$$\Delta T_b = k_b i m$$

In this equation, k_b is the solvent's boiling-point elevation constant, i is the solute's van't Hoff factor, and m is the molal concentration of the solution. For water, $k_b \approx 0.5°C/m$.

Freezing-Point Depression

What happens when we add a solute to a liquid, then try to freeze the solution? Solids are held together by attractive intermolecular forces. During freezing, the molecules in a liquid will assemble into an orderly, tightly packed array. However, the presence of solute particles will interfere with efficient arrangement of the solvent molecules into a solid lattice. As a result, a liquid will be less able to achieve a solid state when a solute is present, and the freezing point of the solution will decrease. (Or, equivalently, the melting point of a solid containing a solute is decreased.) The good news is that the formula for freezing-point depression has exactly the same form as the formula for boiling-point elevation, except that the temperature is going down instead of up (that is, the equation for freezing-point *depression* has a *minus* sign, whereas the equation for boiling-point *elevation* has a *plus* sign).

Freezing-Point Depression

$$\Delta T_f = -k_f i m$$

In this equation, k_f is the solvent's freezing-point depression constant, i is the solute's van't Hoff factor, and m is the molal concentration of the solution. For water, $k_f \approx 1.9°C/m$.

- Addition of concentrated sulfuric acid to pure water will result in:[16]
  - A) vapor-pressure depression.
  - B) boiling-point elevation.
  - C) freezing-point depression.
  - D) all of the above.

---

[16] The addition of a solute to a liquid always results in the effects of all the colligative properties simultaneously. Therefore, choice **D** is the answer.

Review of Diffusion and Osmosis

Diffusion is the tendency for liquids and gases to fully occupy the available volume (Figure 13). Particles in the liquid or gas phase are in constant motion, depending on temperature. If all particles are concentrated in one portion of a container, we have an orderly situation, which is unfavorable according to the Second Law of Thermodynamics (law of entropy). The constant thermal motion of particles in the cell leads to their spreading out to occupy all available space, which maximizes entropy. A solute will always diffuse *down its concentration gradient*, which means *from high to low concentration*. Diffusion continues until the solute is evenly distributed throughout the available volume. At this point, movement of solute back and forth continues, but no net movement occurs.

Osmosis is a special type of diffusion in which solvent diffuses rather than solute (Figure 13). For example, if a chamber containing water and a chamber containing a solution of sucrose are connected directly, sucrose will diffuse throughout the entire volume until a uniform concentration is reached. However, if the two chambers are separated by a **semipermeable membrane** that allows water but not sucrose to cross, then diffusion of sucrose between the chambers cannot occur. In this case, osmosis draws water into the sucrose chamber to reduce the sucrose concentration as well as the volume in the water chamber. Ignoring gravity, water will flow into the sucrose chamber until the concentration is the same across the membrane. The plasma membrane of the cell is a semipermeable membrane that allows water—but not most polar solutes—to cross by osmosis. [If a cell is placed in a hypertonic solution (solute concentration higher than in the cell), what will happen to the cell?[17]]

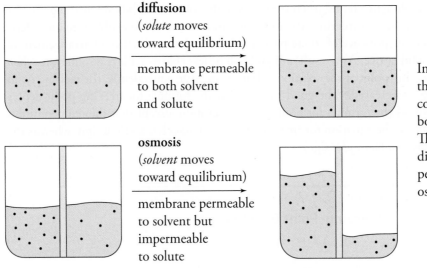

diffusion
(*solute* moves toward equilibrium)

membrane permeable to both solvent and solute

osmosis
(*solvent* moves toward equilibrium)

membrane permeable to solvent but impermeable to solute

In both diffusion and osmosis, the final result is that solute concentrations are the same on both sides of the membrane. The only difference is that in diffusion the membrane is permeable to solute and in osmosis it is not.

Figure 13   Diffusion and Osmosis

The term **tonicity** is used to describe osmotic gradients. If the environment is **isotonic** to the cell, the solute concentration is the same inside and outside. A **hypertonic** solution has more total dissolved solutes than the cell, a **hypotonic** solution has less. You may also hear the terms **isoosmotic**, **hyperosmotic**, and **hypoosmotic**.

---

[17] Water will flow out of the cell through the plasma membrane until the cell volume decreases to the point that the cell crenates (shrivels).

Osmotic Pressure

Osmosis describes the net movement of water across a semipermeable membrane from a region of low solute concentration to a region of higher solute concentration in an effort to dilute the higher concentration solution. The semipermeable membrane prohibits the transfer of solutes, but it allows water to transverse through it. In the following figure, the net movement of water will be to the right:

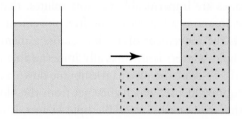

Osmotic pressure (Π) can be defined as the pressure it would take to *stop* osmosis from occurring. If a pressure gauge were added to the same system, osmotic pressure could be measured.

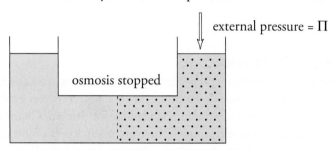

external pressure = Π

osmosis stopped

The osmotic pressure of a solution is given by the **van't Hoff equation**:

$$\Pi = MiRT$$

where Π is osmotic pressure in atm, M is the molarity of the solution, i is the van't Hoff factor, R is the universal gas constant (0.0821 L-atm/K-mol), and T is the temperature in kelvins.

Again, changes in osmotic pressure are affected only by the number of particles in solution (taking into account the van't Hoff factor), not by the identity of those particles.

Now let's continue the discussion on movements across the cell membrane.

Passive Transport

Passive transport is a biochemical term that means diffusion. It refers to *any thermodynamically favorable movement of solute across a membrane.* Another way to phrase this is to say that passive transport is any movement of solute *down a gradient*. No energy is required since the concentration gradient drives movement of the solute. There are two types of passive transport: simple diffusion and facilitated diffusion.

Simple Diffusion

Simple diffusion is diffusion of a solute through a membrane without help from a protein. For example, because they are hydrophobic, steroid hormones are free to move back and forth across the membrane by simple diffusion as pushed by concentration gradients.

However, lipid bilayer membranes are impermeable to most solutes; that is one of the main functions of membranes. The plasma membrane is a barrier to the free movement of all large and/or hydrophilic solutes. **Facilitated diffusion** is the movement of a solute across a membrane, down a gradient, when the membrane itself (the pure lipid bilayer) is intrinsically impermeable to that solute. Specific integral membrane proteins allow material to cross the plasma membrane down a gradient in facilitated diffusion. For example, red blood cells require glucose, which they get from the bloodstream. However, glucose is a bulky hydrophilic molecule that cannot cross the RBC lipid bilayer. Instead, it must be shuttled across by a particular protein in the RBC plasma membrane. There are two well-characterized types of proteins which serve this sort of function: **channel proteins** and **carrier proteins**. Channels and carriers give the membrane its essential feature of **selective permeability**; permeability to *some* things despite impermeability to *most* things.

Facilitated Diffusion: Channels

Channel proteins in the plasma membrane allow material that cannot pass through the membrane by simple diffusion to flow through the plasma membrane down a concentration gradient. Channels do this by forming a narrow opening in the membrane surrounded by the protein. Channels are very selective in what passes through the opening in the membrane. There are many kinds of ion channels, each of which allows the passage of only one type of ion through the channel down a gradient (see Figure 14). All cells have potassium ion channels, for example, that allow only potassium (and not sodium) to flow through the plasma membrane down a gradient. Ion channels are said to be **gated** if the channel is open in response to specific environmental stimuli. A channel that opens in response to a change in the electrical potential across the membrane is called a **voltage-gated** ion channel. One that opens in response to binding of a specific molecule like a neurotransmitter is called a **ligand-gated** ion channel. The regulation of membrane potential by gated ion channels plays a key role in the nervous system. [Can ion channels move ions against an electrochemical gradient?[18]]

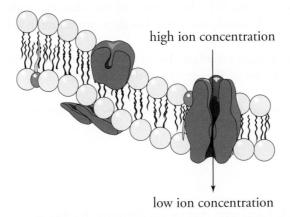

high ion concentration

low ion concentration

Figure 14   An Ion Channel

---

[18] No. Ion channels are only involved in facilitated diffusion, the movement of molecules down an electrochemical gradient with the help of a protein.

13.4

Facilitated Diffusion: Carriers

Carrier proteins also can transport molecules through membranes by facilitated diffusion, but they do so by a mechanism different from that of ion channels. Carrier proteins do not form a tunnel through membranes like ion channels do. Instead, carriers appear to bind the molecule to be transported at one side of the membrane and then undergo a conformational change to move the molecule to the other side of the membrane. Some carriers, called **uniports**, transport only one molecule across the membrane at a time (see Figure 15). Other carriers termed **symports** carry two substances across a membrane in the same direction. **Antiports**, on the other hand, carry two substances in opposite directions.

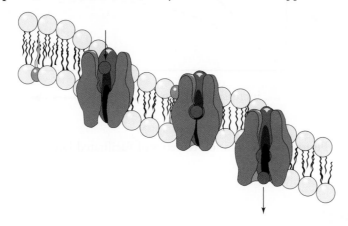

Figure 15   A Uniport

Pores and Porins

A **pore** is a tube through the membrane which is so large that it is *not selective* for any particular molecule. Rather, all molecules below a certain size may pass. (Also, a molecule which is just barely small enough to cross may not cross if it has the wrong charge on its surface.) Pores are formed by polypeptides known as **porins**. You are already familiar with several examples of pores. We have studied pores in the double nuclear membrane, the outer mitochondrial membrane, and the Gram-negative bacterial outer membrane. The eukaryotic plasma membrane does not have pores, because pores destroy the barrier function of the membrane, allowing solutes in the cytoplasm to freely diffuse out of the cell.

Kinetic Concerns

Simple diffusion can be distinguished from all forms of facilitated diffusion by the kinetics of the process. The rate of simple diffusion is limited only by the surface area of the membrane and the size of the driving force (gradient). Facilitated diffusion, however, depends on a finite number of integral membrane proteins. Hence, it exhibits saturation kinetics. Increasing the driving force for facilitated diffusion increases the rate of diffusion (the **flux**), but only to a point. Then all the transport proteins become saturated, and no further increase in flux is possible (Figure 16).

13.4

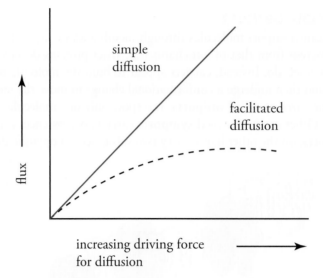

Figure 16 Saturation Kinetics of Facilitated Diffusion

Active Transport

Active transport is the movement of molecules through the plasma membrane against a gradient. Active transport requires energy input, since it is working against a gradient, and always involves a protein. The gradient being pumped against is not necessarily just a concentration gradient; for charged molecules, like ions, it can also involve electric potentials that form a combined electrochemical gradient. The form of energy input used to drive movement of molecules against an electrochemical gradient varies. In **primary active transport**, the transport of a molecule is coupled to ATP hydrolysis. In **secondary active transport**, the transport process is not coupled *directly* to ATP hydrolysis. Instead, ATP is first used to create a gradient, then the potential energy in that gradient is used to drive the transport of some other molecule across the membrane. Since ATP is not used in the actual transport of the "other" molecule, the ATP use is described as *indirect*. For example, the transport of glucose into some cells is driven *against the glucose* concentration gradient by the cotransport of sodium ions *down the sodium* electrochemical gradient, previously established by an ATPase pump. A common mechanism driving secondary active transport of many different molecules involves coupling transport to the flow of sodium ions down a gradient.

- If a protein moves sodium ions across the plasma membrane down an electrochemical gradient, what form of transport is this?[19]
  - A) Simple diffusion
  - B) Facilitated diffusion
  - C) Primary active transport
  - D) Secondary active transport

---

[19] Facilitated diffusion is the movement of molecules down a gradient with the help of a protein (choice **B** is correct). Membrane proteins are not required for simple diffusion (choice A is wrong), and active transport involves moving things *against* their gradients (choices C and D are wrong). Note also that in secondary active transport, the ion movement down its gradient must be coupled to the movement of some other molecule against *its* gradient.

The Na⁺/K⁺ ATPase and the Resting Membrane Potential

The Na⁺/K⁺ ATPase is a transmembrane protein in the plasma membrane of all cells in the body. The activity provided by this protein is to pump 3 Na⁺ out of the cell, 2 K⁺ into the cell, and to hydrolyze one ATP in the process (Figure 17). The sodium that is pumped out of the cell stays outside, since the plasma membrane is impermeable to sodium ions. Some of the potassium ions which are pumped into the cell are able to leak back out, however, through **potassium leak channels**. Potassium flows down its concentration gradient out of the cell through leak channels. The movement of ions out of the cell helps the cell to maintain osmotic balance with its surroundings. As potassium leaves the cell through the leak channels, the movement of positive charge out of the cell creates an electric potential across the plasma membrane with a net negative charge on the interior of the cell. This potential created by the Na⁺/K⁺ ATPase is known as the **resting membrane potential**. The concentration gradient of high sodium outside of the cell established by the Na⁺/K⁺ ATPase is the driving force behind **secondary active transport** of many different molecules, including sugars and amino acids. To summarize, the activity of the Na⁺/K⁺ ATPase is important in three ways:

1) to maintain osmotic balance between the cellular interior and exterior
2) to establish the resting membrane potential
3) to provide the sodium concentration gradient used to drive secondary active transport

- If an inhibitor of Na⁺/K⁺ ATPase is added to cells, which of the following may occur?[20]
  A) The cell will shrink and lose water.
  B) The interior of the cell will become less negatively charged.
  C) Secondary active transport processes will compensate for the loss of primary active transport.
  D) The cell will begin to proliferate.

---

[20] The Na⁺/K⁺ ATPase is required to establish the resting membrane potential in which the cellular interior has a negative charge. It pumps out one net positive ion. If this net positive ion stays inside the cell, the resting potential becomes less negative (choice **B** is correct). Since the interior of the cell is now more charged, the cell will have a tendency to take on water by osmosis, and it will swell (choice A is wrong). Secondary active transport depends on the gradient established by primary active transport (the Na⁺/K⁺ pump). If the pump is shut down, the gradient won't be established, and secondary active transport will also stop (choice C is wrong). The Na⁺/K⁺ ATPase has nothing to do with cellular proliferation (choice D is wrong).

13.4

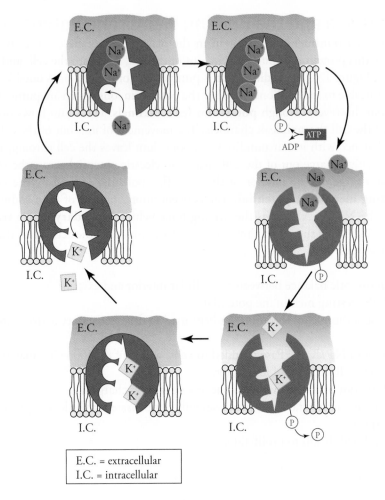

E.C. = extracellular
I.C. = intracellular

Figure 17 The Na⁺/K⁺ ATPase

How do we know exactly how the resting membrane potential is generated? For instance, how can we state with confidence that the electrogenicity of the Na⁺/K⁺ pump is far less important than the passive efflux of potassium in the generation of the RMP?

The answers were determined using experiments. An artificial cell with no pumps and no channels in its membrane would have identical concentrations and charges inside and outside. An artificial cell with potassium leak channels but no active transporters would also obviously have no gradients across its membrane.

What about an artificial cell with Na⁺/K⁺ ATPase pumps and normal cellular concentrations of ATP and ADP + P_i but no potassium leak channels? Here is where experimentation was necessary. In this situation, the resting membrane potential is determined only by the electrogenicity of the Na⁺/K⁺ pump. The RMP in such a system turns out to be about –10 mV.

When K⁺ leak channels are added to the membrane (in addition to the Na⁺/K⁺ ATPase pumps and normal cellular concentrations of ATP and ADP + P_i), the RMP is measured at the normal cellular level, around –70 mV.

The following table gives the concentrations of Na^+, K^+, and Cl^- inside and outside the cell. Know trends; don't memorize numbers.

Ion	Intracellular Conc. (mM)	Extracellular Conc. (mM)
Na^+	10	142
K^+	140	4
Cl^-	4	110
Ca^{2+}	0.0001	2.4

Table 3   Concentrations of Ions Inside/Outside Cell

Endocytosis and Exocytosis

Another mechanism used to transport material through the plasma membrane is within membrane-bound vesicles that fuse with the membrane (see Figure 18). **Exocytosis** is a process to transport material outside of the cell in which a vesicle in the cytoplasm fuses with the plasma membrane, and the contents of the vesicle are expelled into the extracellular space. The materials released are products secreted by the cell, such as hormones and digestive enzymes.

Endocytosis is the opposite of exocytosis: generally, materials are taken into the cell by an invagination of a piece of the cell membrane to form a vesicle. Again, the cytoplasm is not allowed to mix with the extracellular environment. The new vesicle which is formed is called an **endosome**. There are three types of endocytosis:

1) Phagocytosis
2) Pinocytosis
3) Receptor-mediated endocytosis

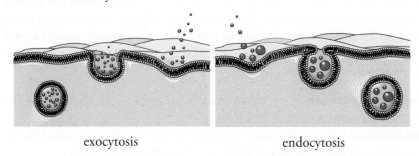

exocytosis   endocytosis

Figure 18   Endo- and Exocytosis

Phagocytosis means "cell eating." It refers to the nonspecific uptake of large particulate matter into a phagocytic vesicle, which later merges with a lysosome. Thus, the phagocytosed material will be broken down. The prime example of phagocytic human cells are macrophages ("big eaters") of the immune system, which engulf and destroy viruses and bacteria. (*Note:* This is *not* an invagination.)

Pinocytosis (cell drinking) is the nonspecific uptake of small molecules and extracellular fluid via invagination. Primitive eukaryotic cells obtain nutrition in this manner, but virtually all eukaryotic cells participate in pinocytosis.

Receptor-mediated endocytosis, on the other hand, is very specific. The site of endocytosis is marked by pits coated with the molecule **clathrin** (inside the cell) and with **receptors** that bind to a specific molecule (outside the cell). An important example is the uptake of cholesterol from the blood. Cholesterol is transported in the blood in large particles called lipoproteins. Cells obtain some of the cholesterol they require by receptor-mediated endocytosis of these lipoproteins. If they are not removed from the blood, cholesterol accumulates in the bloodstream, sticking to the inner walls of arteries. This results in **atherosclerosis** (a buildup of plaque on the walls of the arteries). [Does clathrin recognize and bind to lipoproteins?[21]] When the receptor-lipoprotein complex internalizes, it is taken into a vesicle that is termed an endosome. Lipoproteins are taken from the endosome to a lysosome where the cholesterol is released from the lipoprotein and the lipoprotein is degraded. The lipoprotein receptor is returned to the cell surface where it may again bind a lipoprotein. [How is receptor-mediated endocytosis similar to and different from active transport?[22]]

13.5   OTHER STRUCTURAL ELEMENTS OF THE CELL

Cell-Surface Receptors

Receptors form an important class of integral membrane proteins that transmit signals from the extracellular space into the cytoplasm. Each receptor binds a particular molecule in a highly specific lock-and-key interaction. The molecule that serves as the key for a given receptor is termed the **ligand**. The ligand is generally a hormone or a neurotransmitter. The binding of a ligand to its receptor on the extracellular surface of the plasma membrane triggers a response within the cell, a process termed **signal transduction**. There are three main types of signal-transducing cell-surface receptors: ligand-gated ion channels, catalytic receptors, and G-protein-linked receptors.

- **Ligand-gated ion channels** in the plasma membrane open an ion channel upon binding a particular neurotransmitter.
- **Catalytic receptors** have an enzymatic active site on the cytoplasmic side of the membrane. Enzyme activity is initiated by ligand binding at the extracellular surface.
- A **G-protein-linked receptor** does not directly transduce its signal, but transmits it into the cell with the aid of a **second messenger**. This is a chemical signal that relays instructions from the cell surface to enzymes in the cytoplasm. The most important second messenger is **cyclic AMP** (**cAMP**). Second messengers such as cAMP allow a much greater signal than the receptor alone can produce (see Figure 19).

---

[21] No. Clathrin is a fibrous protein inside the cell that associates with the cytoplasmic portions of the cell-surface receptors that bind lipoproteins.

[22] Both import a particular substance. One difference is that in endocytosis the substance ends up sealed in an endosome, whereas in active transport the substance is just dumped into the cytoplasm.

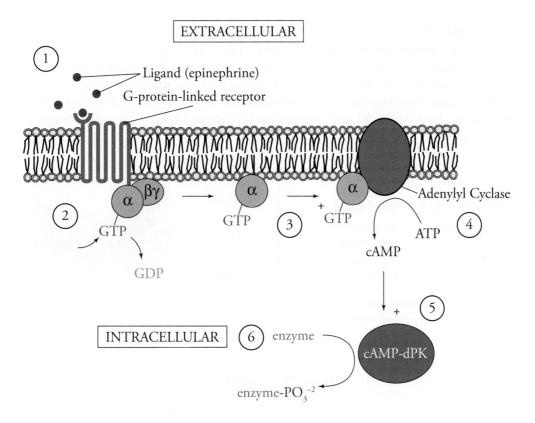

Figure 19   G-Protein Mediated Signal Transduction Stimulated by Epinephrine

1) Epinephrine arrives at the cell surface and binds to a specific G-protein-linked receptor.
2) The cytoplasmic portion of the receptor activates G-proteins, causing GDP to dissociate and GTP to bind in its place.
3) The activated G-proteins diffuse through the membrane and activate adenylyl cyclase.
4) Adenylyl cyclase makes cAMP from ATP.
5) cAMP activates cAMP-dependent protein kinases (cAMP-dPK) in the cytoplasm.
6) cAMP-dPK phosphorylates certain enzymes, with the end result being mobilization of energy. For example, enzymes necessary for glycogen breakdown will be activated, while enzymes necessary for glycogen synthesis will be inactivated, by cAMP-dPK phosphorylation.

There are different types of G-protein-linked receptors. The one depicted above is a **s**timulatory one. Its G-protein would be denoted **G**$_s$. Inhibitory G-protein-linked receptors activate **i**nhibitory G-proteins (**G**$_i$) which serve to *inactivate* adenylyl cyclase instead of activating it. In this way, different hormones can modulate each other's effects.

There are also G-protein-linked receptors which have nothing to do with cAMP. Instead, their G-proteins activate an enzyme called phospholipase C, initiating a different second messenger cascade, which results in an increase in cytoplasmic Ca^{2+} levels. The common theme shared by all G-protein-based signal transduction systems is their reliance on a G-protein, which is a signaling molecule that binds GTP. You should understand these key notions: cAMP as a second messenger, signal transduction, and signal amplification. The remaining details are not important for the MCAT; read for concepts, not memory.

The Cytoskeleton

The animal cell **cytoskeleton** provides the structural support supplied by the cell wall in bacteria, plants, and fungi. It also allows movement of the cell and its appendages (cilia and flagella) and transport of substances within the cell. Animal cells have an internal cytoskeleton composed of three types of proteins: **microtubules**, **intermediate filaments**, and **microfilaments** (see Figure 20). Microtubules are the thickest, microfilaments the thinnest. All three are composed of noncovalently polymerized proteins; in other words, they are a massive example of quaternary protein structure.

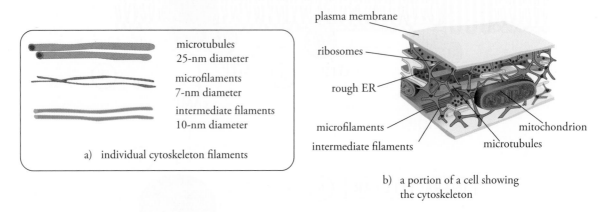

Figure 20   Cytoskeleton

Microtubules

The **microtubule** is a hollow rod composed of two globular proteins: α-**tubulin** and β-**tubulin**, polymerized noncovalently. Once formed, the microtubule can elongate by adding αβ-tubulin dimers to one end. The other end cannot elongate, because it is anchored to the **microtubule organizing center** (**MTOC**), located near the nucleus. Microtubules are dynamic and can get longer or shorter by adding or removing tubulin monomers from the end.

Within the MTOC is a pair of **centrioles** (see Figure 21). Each centriole is composed of a ring of nine microtubule triplets. When cell division occurs, the centrioles duplicate themselves, and then one pair moves to each end of the cell. During mitosis, microtubules radiating out from the centrioles attach to the replicated chromosomes and pull them apart. The microtubules that radiate out from the centrioles during mitosis are called the **aster**, because they are star-shaped. The microtubules connecting the chromosomes to the aster are **polar fibers**. The whole assembly is called the **mitotic spindle**. The centromere of each chromosome contains a **kinetochore** which is attached to the spindle by tiny microtubules called **kinetochore fibers**.

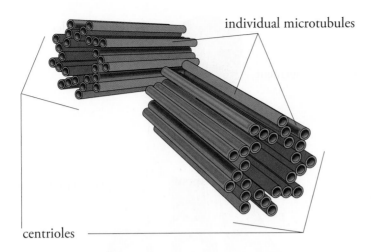

individual microtubules

centrioles

Figure 21   A Pair of Centrioles

In mitosis, the MTOC is essential, but the centrioles are not. There are two major pieces of evidence for this: 1) Plant cells lack centrioles but still undergo mitosis; 2) Experimenters have succeeded in removing the centrioles from animal cells, and the cells were still able to undergo mitosis.

Microtubules also mediate transport of substances within the cell. In nerve cells, materials are transported from the cell body to the axon terminus on a microtubule railroad. The transport process is driven by proteins that hydrolyze ATP and act as molecular motors along the microtubule.

Eukaryotic Cilia and Flagella

Cilia are small "hairs" on the cell surface which move fluids past the cell surface. For example, cilia on lining cells of the human respiratory tract continually sweep mucus toward the mouth in a mechanism termed the **mucociliary escalator**. A **flagellum** is a large "tail" which moves the cell by wiggling. The only human cell which has a flagellum is the __.[23] Cilia are small and flagella are long, but they have the same structure, with a "**9 + 2**" arrangement of microtubules (see Figure 22). Nine pairs of microtubules form a ring around two lone microtubules in the center. Each microtubule is bound to its neighbor by a contractile protein called **dynein** which causes movement of the filaments past one another. The cilium or flagellum is anchored to the plasma membrane by a **basal body**, which has the same structure as a centriole (a ring of nine triplets of microtubules). Remember that the prokaryotic flagellum is different in structure, and its motion is driven by a different mechanism.

---

[23] sperm

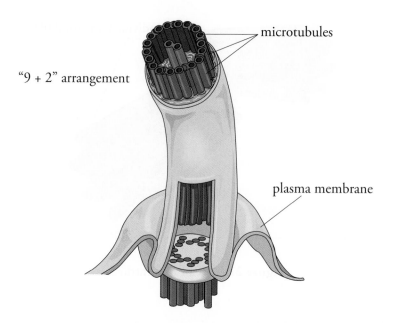

"9 + 2" arrangement

microtubules

plasma membrane

Figure 22 The Base of a Cilium or Flagellum

Microfilaments

Microfilaments are rods formed in the cytoplasm from polymerization of the globular protein **actin**. Actin monomers form a chain, and then two chains wrap around each other to form an actin filament. Microfilaments are dynamic and are responsible for gross movements of the entire cell, such as pinching the dividing parent cell into two daughters during cell division, and **amoeboid movement**. Amoeboid movement involves changes in the cytoplasmic structure which cause cytoplasm and the rest of the cell to flow in one direction.

Intermediate Filaments

Intermediate filaments are named for their thickness, which is between that of microtubules and microfilaments. Unlike microtubules and microfilaments, intermediate filaments are heterogeneous, composed of a wide range of polypeptides. Another difference is that intermediate filaments are more permanent, whereas microfilaments and microtubules are often disassembled and reassembled as needed by the cell. Intermediate filaments appear to be involved in providing strong cell structure, such as in resisting mechanical stress.

Cell Adhesion and Cell Junctions

In some tissues, cells are tightly bound to each other. For example, the intestinal wall is lined with a type of tissue called **epithelium**. The layer of epithelial cells in the gut forms a tight seal, preventing items from moving freely between the intestinal lumen and the body; this is accomplished by **tight junctions**. Epithelial cells in the skin are held together tightly but do not form a complete seal; this is accomplished by **desmosomes**. Some specialized cell types, such as heart muscle cells, are connected by holes called **gap junctions** that allow ions to flow back and forth between them.

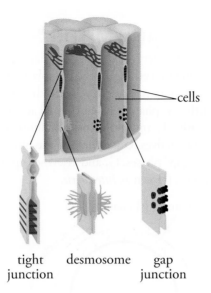

tight   desmosome   gap
junction   junction

cells

Figure 23   Cell Junctions

Tight junctions are also termed *occluding junctions* because they do not just join cells at one point, but form a seal between the membranes of adjacent cells that blocks the flow of molecules across the entire cell layer. They are not spots where cells are stuck together, but rather bands running all the way around the cells. Intestinal epithelial cells are involved in the active transport of glucose and other molecules from one side of epithelium to the other. A tight seal between these cells is required to prevent the two compartments from mixing. Tight junctions also block the flow of molecules within the plane of the plasma membrane. For example, the surface of the plasma membrane facing the intestinal lumen, termed the **apical** surface, has different membrane proteins than the plasma membrane on the other side of the cell facing the tissues beneath, called the **basolateral** surface.

Desmosomes do not form a seal, but merely hold cells together; they are also known as *spot desmosomes* because they are concise points, not bands all the way around the cell. The desmosome is composed of fibers that span the plasma membranes of two cells. Inside each cell, the desmosome is anchored to the plasma membrane by a plaque formed by the protein **keratin**.

Gap junctions form pore-like connections between adjacent cells, allowing the two cells' cytoplasms to mix. The connection is large enough to permit the exchange of solutes such as ions, amino acids, and carbohydrates, but not polypeptides and organelles. Gap junctions in smooth muscle and cardiac muscle allow the membrane depolarization of an action potential to pass directly from one cell to another.

13.6 THE CELL CYCLE AND MITOSIS

Our cells must reproduce themselves in order to replace lost or damaged cells so that tissues can grow. Cells reproduce themselves by first doubling everything in the cytoplasm and the genome and then splitting in half. Some cells continually go through a cycle of growth and division, which is traditionally discussed in four phases (see Figure 24). **S** (**synthesis**) phase is when the cell actively replicates its genome, as described in Chapter 11. **M phase** includes **mitosis** and **cytokinesis**. Mitosis is the partitioning of cellular components (genes, organelles, etc.) into two halves. Cytokinesis is the physical process of cell division. Between M phase and S phase, there are two "gap" phases, G_1 and G_2. The gap phases plus S phase together form the part of the cell cycle between divisions, known as *interphase*.

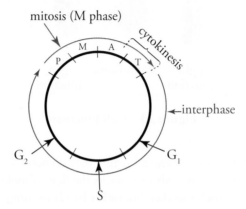

Figure 24 The Cell Cycle

The cell spends most of its time in interphase, busily metabolizing and synthesizing materials. Some cells are permanently stuck in interphase (G_0). In fact, the more specialized a cell becomes, the less likely it is to remain capable of reproducing itself.

During interphase, the genome is spread out in a form that is not visible with a light microscope without special stains, and DNA is accessible to the enzymes of replication. By the end of S phase, the nucleus contains two complete copies of the genome. The cell now has twice the normal amount of DNA.

Mitosis is divided into four phases: **prophase**, **metaphase**, **anaphase**, and **telophase**. The first sign of prophase is that the genome becomes visible upon condensing into densely-packed chromosomes, instead of diffuse chromatin. Observing a human cell under the light microscope at the beginning of prophase, one can see 46 differently-shaped chromosomes. Upon closer observation, one notes that each chromosome actually consists of two identical particles joined at a centromere. These two particles are the two copies of a chromosome, known as **sister chromatids**. When mitosis is complete, each new daughter cell will have 46 chromosomes, each consisting of a single chromatid, separated from its sister. Spending a little more time staring at the nucleus, you might notice that the jumble of 46 chromatid pairs actually consists of 23 **homologous pairs** of identical-appearing sister chromatid pairs (23 pairs of pairs). Homologous chromosomes are different copies of the same chromosome, one from your mother and the other from your father. To repeat:

Sister chromatids are identical copies of a chromosome, attached to each other at the centromere. Homologous chromosomes are equivalent but nonidentical and do not come anywhere near each other during mitosis.

Other important events occur during prophase. The nucleolus disappears, the spindle and kinetochore fibers appear, and the centriole pairs begin to move to opposite ends of the cell. So now the cell has two MTOCs, called **asters** (stars) because of the star-like appearance of microtubules radiating out. Also at the end of prophase, the nuclear envelope converts itself into many tiny vesicles.

Metaphase is simple: all the chromosomes line up at the center of the cell, forming the **metaphase plate**. The chromosomes line up in the center of the cell because the kinetochore of each sister chromatid is attached to spindle fibers that attach to MTOC at opposite ends of the cell. So each member of a pair of chromatids is pulled toward the opposite pole of the cell.

During anaphase, the spindle fibers shorten, and the centromeres of each sister chromatid pair are pulled apart. The cell elongates, and cytokinesis begins with the formation of a **cleavage furrow**, which is accomplished by a ring of actin filaments that encircle the cell and contract.

In telophase (*telos* is Greek for "end"), a nuclear membrane forms around the bunch of chromosomes at each end of the cell, the chromosomes decondense, and a nucleolus becomes visible within each new daughter nucleus. Each daughter nucleus has $2n$ chromosomes. Cytokinesis is complete, and the cell is split in two (see Figure 25).

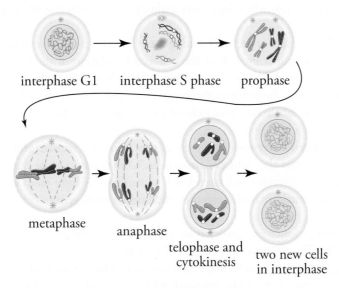

interphase G1   interphase S phase   prophase

metaphase   anaphase   telophase and cytokinesis   two new cells in interphase

Figure 25   The Phases of Mitosis

13.7 CANCER, ONCOGENES, AND TUMOR SUPPRESSORS

Inappropriate cell division (that is, cells that have lost control of the cell cycle) can have disastrous consequences. A mutation in a protein that is normally involved in regulating progression through the cell cycle can result in unregulated cell division and cancer. Cancer means "crab," as in the zodiac sign. The name derives from the observation that malignant tumors grow into the surrounding tissue, embedding themselves like clawed crabs.

- In normal eukaryotic cells, mitosis will not begin until the entire genome is replicated. If this inhibition is removed so that mitosis begins during S-phase, which one of the following would occur?[24]
    - A) The cells would grow more quickly.
    - B) The genome would become fragmented and incomplete.
    - C) The cells would display unregulated, cancerous growth.
    - D) The genome would be temporarily incomplete in each daughter cell, but DNA repair will fill in the missing gaps.

Cancers can present as malignant solid tumors or in a more diffuse cellular state, such as leukemia, a cancer occurring in the bone marrow where improper leukocytes are formed and circulated.

Mutated genes that induce cancer are termed **oncogenes** ("onco-" is a prefix denoting cancer). Normally, these genes are required for proper growth of the cell and regulation of the cell cycle. Oncogenes, then, are genes that can convert normal cells into cancerous cells. Sometimes these are abnormal versions of standard cellular growth genes. Sometimes the genes enter the cell because of a viral infection. In fact, the first identified oncogene, labeled *src*, was isolated from a retrovirus found in chickens.

Protooncogenes are the normal versions of the genes that allow for regular growth patterns, but can be converted into oncogenes under the right circumstances. Conversion may be due to mutation or because of exposure to a mutagen. Ultraviolet radiation (such as sunlight or light from tanning booths) and various chemicals (such as benzene) are both examples of common mutagens.

Tumor suppressor genes produce proteins that are the inherent defense system to prevent the conversion of cells into cancer cells. The two primary means of cancer prevention are to (a) detect damage to the genome and halt cell growth and division until the damage can be repaired, or (b) to trigger programmed cell death if the damage is too severe to be repaired. **p53** is an example of a product of a common tumor suppressor gene. Though normally at low levels in cells, its production is scaled up when genetic damage or oncogene activity is detected, and if sufficient repair is not possible, p53 will cause the cell to die in a process referred to as **apoptosis**.

---

[24] If the genome is not completely replicated and condensed prior to mitosis, it will be torn during cell division. Each daughter cell will receive only pieces of the genome rather than the complete genome and will not be able to survive (choice **B** is correct, and choices A and C are wrong). DNA repair systems can only repair sequence errors or minor structural problems; this problem would be too large to fix (choice D is wrong).

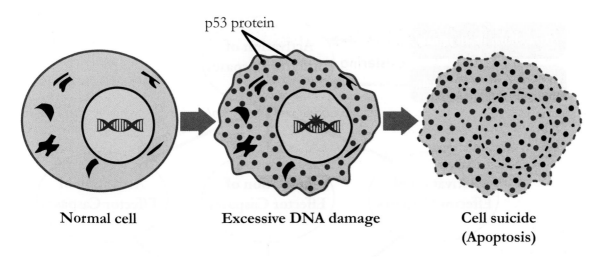

p53 protein

Normal cell   **Excessive DNA damage**   **Cell suicide (Apoptosis)**

Figure 26   Representation of p53 triggering apoptosis

Apoptosis

Apoptosis, or programmed cell death, allows a cell to shrink and die while simultaneously minimizing damage to neighboring cells and limiting the exposure of other cells to its cytosolic contents. The death of a cell is triggered by a stressor which may be external (such as nitric oxide, a toxin, or cytokines) or internal (such as when the level of the p53 tumor suppressor protein reaches a critical level).

The process of apoptosis begins with the shrinking of the cell and the disassembly of the cytoskeleton. While the cellular infrastructure is taken apart, the nuclear envelope breaks down and the genome is broken into pieces. A different profile of cell surface proteins emerges, thus signaling various phagocytic cells, including macrophages, to finish deconstructing and clearing away the dead cell.

A family of proteases, referred to as **caspases**, is responsible for carrying out the events of apoptosis. They have a cysteine in their active site and they cleave their target proteins at aspartic acid sites, hence their name (*c-asp*-ases). Caspases, like all potentially damaging enzymes, are produced in their inactive form as *procaspases*. Twelve different caspases have been identified in humans, and they are generally grouped into two categories, initiators and effectors. **Initiator caspases** respond to extra- or intracellular death signals by clustering together; this clustering allows them to activate each other. The activation of the initiators leads to the activation of the effector caspases in a cascade of activation. **Effector caspases** then cleave a variety of cellular proteins to trigger apoptosis.

14.1 INTRODUCTION TO GENETICS

Genetics is the science that describes the inheritance of traits from one generation to another. At the origin of genetics, patterns of inheritance were observed to follow certain predictable patterns, as described by Mendel's laws. The reasons for these patterns of inheritance were to remain a mystery until the nature of DNA as the genetic material was known. Today we can use our knowledge of DNA and the cell to understand Mendel's laws at the molecular level.

Genes and Alleles

One of the basic tenets of genetics is that children inherit traits from both parents. Humans have a life cycle in which life begins with a diploid cell, the zygote. Diploid organisms (or cells) have two copies of the genome in each cell, while haploid cells have one copy of the genome. In sexual reproduction, the diploid zygote is produced by fusion of two haploid gametes: a haploid ovum from the mother and a haploid spermatozoon from the father. The zygote then goes through many mitotic divisions to develop into an adult, with half of the genetic material in each cell from each parent. The adult, male or female, produces haploid gametes by meiotic cell division to repeat the life cycle once again.

The development of a zygote into an adult and the maintenance of adult cells and tissues requires many thousands of different gene products. All of these gene products are encoded in the genome and inherited from mother and father. The **gene**, a length of DNA coding for a particular gene product, is the fundamental unit of inheritance. [Are gene products always proteins?[1]] The genes are distributed among the chromosomes that compose the genome, and every gene can be pinpointed to a specific location called the **locus** (plural: **loci**) on a specific chromosome. [Can each physical trait of an organism be mapped to a single given locus?[2]]

The human genome is split into 24 different chromosomes: 22 of these are autosomes (non-sex chromosomes) and 2 are sex chromosomes (or allosomes, X and Y). Each human has 23 pairs of chromosomes (22 autosomes and a pair of sex chromosomes), for a total of 46 chromosomes. One chromosome of each pair is from the mother and one is from the father. The two nonidentical copies of a chromosome are called **homologous chromosomes**. Although these two copies look the same when examined at the crudest level under a microscope, and although they contain the same genes, the copies of the genes in the two homologous chromosomes may differ in their DNA sequence. Different versions of a gene, called **alleles**, may carry out the gene's function differently. Since a person carries two copies of every gene, one on each homologous chromosome, a person could potentially carry two different alleles. Individuals carrying different alleles of a gene will often have traits that allow the inheritance of alleles to be followed. [Is it possible for there to be more than two different alleles of a specific gene?[3]]

---

[1] No. tRNA and rRNA genes, as well as other small nuclear RNA genes, do not encode polypeptides.

[2] No. Every gene is located at a specific locus, but physical traits, particularly complex traits, like weight or height, can be controlled by many different genes and therefore do not map to a single locus, but to many.

[3] Yes, there can be many versions (alleles) of a particular gene. Under normal circumstances, however, one individual cannot have more than two of those different alleles, since they have only two copies of a gene (one on each homologous chromosome). An exception is when an individual is polyploid for a certain chromosome (i.e., they have more than two homologous chromosomes, for example in Down syndrome and Klinefelter syndrome).

- Which one of the following is true if an individual has two different alleles at a given locus?[4]
  A) The individual has two phenotypes, e.g., one brown eye and one blue.
  B) There are two alleles in one place on one particular chromosome.
  C) Two siblings have different appearances.
  D) There is a different allele on each of the two members of a homologous pair.

Genotype vs. Phenotype

The **genotype** is the DNA sequence of the alleles a person carries. A person carrying two different alleles at a given locus is called a **heterozygote**, while an individual carrying two identical alleles is called a **homozygote**. The expression of alleles often is different in heterozygotes and homozygotes.

The **phenotype** is the physical expression of the genotype. For example, the phenotype of a gene involved in hair color may be brown or blond. Since there are many different kinds of alleles, there are different ways these alleles can be expressed in the phenotype. If an allele is the one expressed in the phenotype, regardless of what the second allele carried is, the expressed allele is referred to as **dominant**. An allele that is not expressed in the heterozygous state is referred to as **recessive**. For example, consider a heterozygous organism in which one allele encodes the functional version of an enzyme, while the second allele encodes an inactive version of that enzyme. Upon observation, it is noted that the organism's enzymes are all functional; then the functional-enzyme allele is *dominant* and the inactive-enzyme allele is *recessive*. Since recessive alleles are not expressed in heterozygotes, it is not always possible to tell the genotype of an individual based solely on the phenotype. [Can a haploid organism like an adult fungus have recessive alleles?[5]]

There are certain conventions used in denoting genotypes in genetics that are useful to know. The alleles of a gene are usually denoted by letters. For example, for a gene called "curly," a dominant allele may be denoted by the capital letter *C* and a recessive allele may be denoted by the lower case letter *c*. A heterozygote is referred to as *Cc*, while homozygotes would be either *CC* or *cc*. More complex situations require more complex conventions, but most questions probably only involve two alleles at a locus. [If the dominant allele for curly (*C*) results in curly hair and the recessive allele (*c*) causes straight hair, what are the phenotypes of *CC*, *Cc*, and *cc* individuals?[6]]

---

[4] An individual with two different alleles at a given locus has one allele on one chromosome and the other allele on its homologous partner (so choice **D** is correct, and choice B is not possible). While choice A may be possible, it is an exceedingly complex phenomenon and not discernible from the information given. The question discusses a single individual, not a pair of siblings (eliminating choice C).

[5] No. If there is only one copy of a gene, then that is the copy which determines the phenotype.

[6] *CC* and *Cc* individuals have curly hair, and *cc* individuals have straight hair. Only homozygous recessive individuals express recessive traits. In the heterozygote, the presence of the recessive allele is masked by the dominant allele, so there are only two different phenotypes, although there are three different genotypes. This type of interaction between alleles is called **classical dominance**.

14.2 MEIOSIS

Mitotic cell division produces two daughter cells that are identical to the parent. However, the production of haploid cells such as gametes from a diploid cell requires a type of cell division that reduces the number of copies of each chromosome from two to one; this method of cell division is called **meiosis**. In males, meiosis occurs in the testes with haploid spermatozoa as the end result; in females, meiosis in the ovaries produces ova. (*Note*: This is not always the case, and while meiosis begins in the ovaries, it is completed only after fertilization; see Chapter 19 for a further discussion on oogenesis.) Specialized cells termed **spermatogonia** in males and **oogonia** in females undergo meiosis. Spermatogenesis and oogenesis share the same basic features of meiosis but differ in many of the specific features of gamete production. Meiosis itself will be discussed in this chapter, while the specifics of spermatogenesis and oogenesis will be discussed in Chapter 19.

Mitosis and meiosis are similar in many respects. Mitosis and meiosis are both preceded by one round of replication of the genome (S phase), leaving a diploid cell with replicated chromosomes (effectively 4 copies of the genome) (Figure 1). The different phases in cell division are referred to by the same names (prophase, metaphase, anaphase, and telophase) in both meiosis and mitosis and are mechanistically very similar. The primary difference between meiosis and mitosis is that replication of the genome is followed by one round of cell division in mitosis and two rounds of cell division in meiosis, **meiosis I** and **meiosis II** (Figure 2). Another important difference is that in meiosis, recombination occurs between homologous chromosomes.

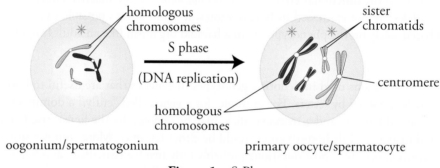

Figure 1   S-Phase

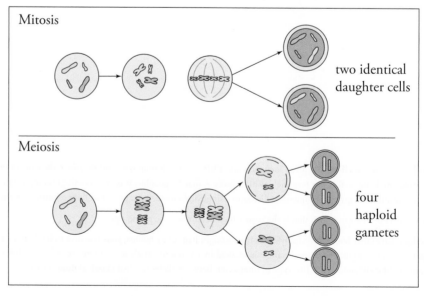

Figure 2   Mitosis vs. Meiosis

The first step in meiosis is **prophase I** (Figure 3). To depict meiosis, we will use a hypothetical model organism with a diploid genome with two different (nonhomologous) chromosomes (Figures 3–6).

- How many chromosomes are present in a cell from this organism during prophase I of meiosis?[7]

As in mitotic prophase, chromosomes condense in meiotic prophase I, and then the nuclear envelope breaks down. Unlike mitosis, however, homologous chromosomes pair with each other during meiotic prophase I in **synapsis**. Homologous chromosomes align themselves very precisely with each other in synapsis, with the two copies of each gene on two different chromosomes brought closely together. The paired homologous chromosomes are called a **bivalent** or **tetrad**.

When the DNA is aligned properly, it can then be cut precisely at the same location on homologous chromosomes. Genes are then swapped between the pair, and the chromosomes are realigned (Figure 3). This process is known as **crossing over** or **recombination** (Figure 4). Due to the extreme complexity of crossing over, meiotic prophase takes the most time in meiosis, days sometimes. Recombination during meiosis is an important source of genetic variation during sexual reproduction.

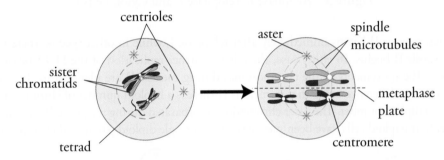

Figure 3   Prophase I and Metaphase I

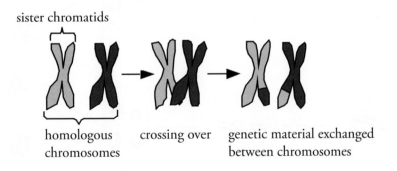

Figure 4   Crossing Over (Recombination)

After prophase I is **metaphase I**. In meiotic metaphase I, alignment along the metaphase plate occurs, as in mitosis. The difference is that in meiotic metaphase I, the *tetrads* are aligned at the center of the

---

[7]   The cells of the organism are diploid, with two versions of each of the two chromosomes, or four chromosomes total. After DNA synthesis, during prophase I, the cell still has four chromosomes; however, the chromosomes are replicated (now made of two pieces of DNA each) and held together at the centromere. Thus, each of the four chromosomes consists of two replicated sister chromatids (and the cell has a total of eight sister chromatids).

cell (the metaphase plate), whereas in mitosis, *sister chromatids* are aligned on the metaphase plate. In **anaphase I**, homologous chromosomes separate, and sister chromatids remain together (Figure 5). The cell then divides into two cells during **telophase I** (Figure 5). *It is important to note that at this point the cells are considered to be haploid.* Each cell has a single set of chromosomes. The chromosomes, however, are still replicated (still exist as a pair of sister chromatids). The whole point to the second set of meiotic divisions is to separate the sister chromatids so that each cell has a single set of unreplicated chromosomes.

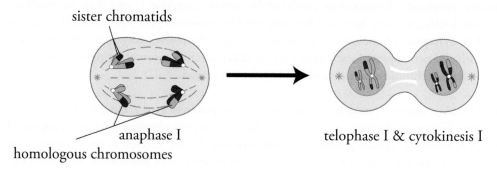

Figure 5   Anaphase I, Telophase I, and Cytokinesis I

In some species, meiosis II begins immediately after telophase I, while in other species, there is a period of time before meiosis II begins. In either case, there is no further replication of the DNA before the second set of divisions. The movements of the chromosomes during meiosis II are identical to the movements in mitosis, with the sole difference being that in meiosis II there is a haploid number of chromosomes, while in mitosis there is a diploid number. The sister chromatids are separated during anaphase II, and after telophase II is complete, four haploid cells have been produced from a single diploid parent cell (Figure 6).

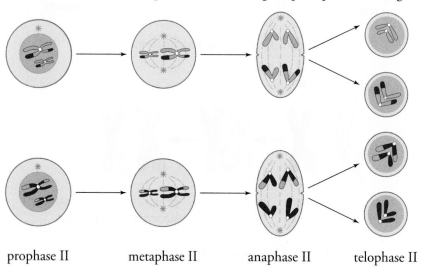

Figure 6   Meiosis II

- Which of the following occur in both meiosis and mitosis?[8]
  - I. Separation of sister chromatids on microtubules
  - II. Pairing of homologous chromosomes
  - III. Alignment of individual chromosomes at the metaphase plate

  - A) I only
  - B) II only
  - C) I and III
  - D) II and III

- If cells are blocked in meiotic metaphase II and prevented from moving on in meiosis, which one of the following will be prevented?[9]
  - A) Crossing over
  - B) Separation of homologous chromosomes
  - C) Separation of sister chromatids
  - D) Breakdown of the nuclear envelope

Nondisjunction

Sometimes during meiosis I homologous chromosomes fail to separate, and sometimes during meiosis II sister chromatids fail to separate. Such a failure of chromosomes to separate correctly during meiosis is called **nondisjunction**. [If two homologous chromosomes of chromosome #12 fail to separate during meiosis I, how many copies of chromosome #12 will the resulting gametes have?[10]] Gametes resulting from nondisjunction will have two copies or no copies of a given chromosome. Such a gamete can fuse with a normal gamete to create a zygote with either three copies of a chromosome (**trisomy**) or one copy of a chromosome (**monosomy**).

The genetic defect caused when an entire chromosome is either added or removed is usually so great that a zygote with either trisomy or monosomy cannot develop into a normal individual. There are examples in which nondisjunction is not lethal in humans, although it results in significant developmental abnormalities. Trisomy of chromosome #21 results in Down syndrome, with intellectual disability and abnormal growth. Nondisjunction of the sex chromosomes is also generally not lethal during development. Individuals who have only one X chromosome and no Y, for example, have Turner syndrome, with external female appearance but underdeveloped ovaries and sterility. Individuals with nondisjunction of the sex chromosomes will develop to have male appearance if they have at least one Y, no matter how many X chromosomes are present, and will have female genitalia if only X chromosomes are present. Most will be sterile, however, and many will suffer intellectual disability. [In an individual with Down syndrome, are

---

[8] **Item I is true**: The spindle separates sister chromatids during both (choices B and D can be eliminated). Note that neither of the remaining answer choices includes Item II, so Item II must be false, and we can ignore it. **Item III is true:** Alignment of individual chromosomes along the metaphase plate occurs during metaphase of mitosis and during metaphase II of meiosis. Note that Item II is in fact false: pairing of homologous chromosomes only occurs during prophase I of meiosis.

[9] Crossing over occurs during prophase I, separation of homologous chromosomes occurs during anaphase I, and nuclear envelope breakdown occurs during prophase I and sometimes prophase II (choices A, B, and D are false). Only separation of sister chromatids occurs after metaphase II, in anaphase II. Answer: choice **C**.

[10] If the homologous chromosomes do not separate in meiosis I, then one daughter cell from this division will have four copies of this chromosome and the other cell will have none. In meiosis II, sister chromatids will separate, leaving two gametes with two copies of the chromosome and two gametes with no copies of the chromosome.

the defects in development caused by an absence of genetic information?[11] If not, why does trisomy of this chromosome or other chromosomes have such dramatic effects?[12]]

14.3 MENDELIAN GENETICS

Gregor Mendel described the statistical behavior of the inheritance of traits in pea plants long before the nature of DNA and chromosomes was known. Unlike Mendel, however, we are now familiar with the molecular basis of genetics in meiosis and genes, and the laws of genetics that Mendel formulated can now be presented with insight based on this knowledge. Although Mendelian genetics generally only involves the simplest patterns of inheritance, it forms the foundation for understanding more complicated situations.

Mendel observed that traits were governed by pairs of hereditary material (alleles). The first of Mendel's laws, the **Law of Segregation**, states that the two alleles of an individual are separated and passed on to the next generation singly. [At what stage during meiosis are different alleles of a gene separated?[13]] Mendel's second law, the **Law of Independent Assortment**, states that the alleles of one gene will separate into gametes independently of alleles for another gene. We will illustrate these principles using the garden pea plant, but the principles apply equally well to humans.

A trait that can be studied in the pea plant is the color of the pea. We can call G the allele for green color, while g is the allele for yellow pea color. Mating between plants, a **cross**, is used as a tool in genetics to discern genotypes by looking at the phenotypes of progeny from a cross. A **pure-breeding strain** of yellow or green peas consistently yields progeny of the same color when mated within the strain. For example, if mating yellow plants with yellow plants always produces yellow progeny, yellow is a pure-breeding strain. [Can anything be deduced about the genotype of the pure-breeding strain of yellow peas?[14] If a pure-breeding yellow and pure-breeding green strain are crossed, and all of the progeny are green, what does this indicate about the expression of the yellow and green alleles?[15]] Let's assume that G is the dominant allele of the color gene, and g is the recessive allele. [Is it possible to deduce the genotype of a pea plant at the color gene if it is green?[16]] If a green plant is encountered, a **testcross** can be performed to deduce the genotype of the plant. A testcross is when one individual is crossed to another individual that has a homozygous (or pure-breeding) recessive genotype. The presence of all recessive alleles in one parent allows alleles from the other parent to be displayed phenotypically. The progeny of a testcross are called the F_1 **generation**. [If a green plant is testcrossed with a pure-breeding yellow strain, and some of the F_1 generation are yellow while others are green, what is the genotype of the original green plant?[17]] The results of a testcross are dependent on statistics and follow Mendel's laws.

---

[11] There is no information missing in a person with trisomy. All of the chromosomes are present, and there is no reason to believe that any of the genes on these chromosomes are deleted or mutated to render them inactive.

[12] The problem with trisomy appears not to be that genetic information is missing, but that there is *too much* present. A mechanism involved might be gene dosage. Genes are regulated to produce the right amount of each gene product. In trisomy, many genes are present in one more copy than usual, resulting in greater quantities of the gene products encoded on this chromosome. The extra quantities of so many gene products, even if they are normal in sequence, can have dramatic consequences.

[13] During meiosis I, at the time when homologous chromosome separate.

[14] If a strain always produces the same trait when mated with itself, it is likely to be homozygous for the trait. The pure-breeding yellow pea is homozygous for the yellow allele g of the color gene.

[15] The two strains were both pure-breeding and could only produce gametes containing one type of allele. All of the progeny would be the Gg genotype. If all progeny are green, then the green allele is dominant and the yellow allele is recessive.

[16] No. A green plant could either be heterozygous Gg or homozygous GG.

[17] The original pea is heterozygous Gg.

The principle of segregation can be illustrated with the color gene described above for the pea. If a pea is heterozygous *Gg*, its gametes will contain either the *G* allele or the *g* allele, but never both. The probability that a gamete in the heterozygote will contain one allele or the other is 50%, completely random. To illustrate the law of independent assortment, we need to introduce a second gene, one that controls the shape of the pea. *W* is the dominant allele, resulting in wrinkled peas, while *w* is the recessive allele, resulting in smooth peas in homozygous *ww* plants. According to the Law of Independent Assortment, the genes for the color of peas and the shape of peas are passed from one generation to another independently. The nature of the shape gene in a given gamete does not depend on and is not influenced by the color gene, if independent assortment is true. [If an individual is heterozygous at the color gene, *Gg*, and heterozygous at the shape gene, *Ww*, what are the chances that a gamete containing the *G* allele will also contain the *W* allele?[18]]

The Punnett Square

It is possible to predict the results of a cross between two individuals using the Laws of Segregation and Independent Assortment. Determining the result can be complex, however, so a visual tool called the **Punnett square** is often employed to make the process simpler. Let's use a simple square first, with only one trait involved (Figure 7); we will then tackle a more complicated problem with two different traits (Figure 8).

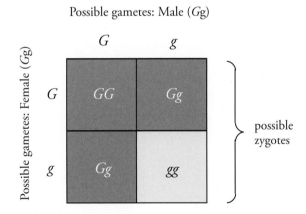

Figure 7   A Punnett Square Involving One Gene

In Figure 7, a Punnett square depicts a cross between two pea plants that are heterozygous for the color gene, with *G* the dominant green allele and *g* the recessive yellow allele. To draw a Punnett square, the following steps are involved:

Step 1: Determine the gametes that are possible from each parent in the cross.
Step 2: Draw a square with the possible gametes from each parent on two sides.
Step 3: Fill in the square with the zygote genotypes that would result from each possible combination of gamete.
Step 4: Determine the phenotype of each genotype.
Step 5: Find the probability of each genotype and each phenotype.

---

[18] According to independent assortment, the segregation of one gene does not depend on segregation of another. The chances of a gamete containing the *W* allele are 50%, regardless of the identity of the color allele.

- In the situation shown in Figure 7, which one of the following will be true?[19]
  - A) 25% of the offspring will be green, and 75% will be yellow.
  - B) 50% of the offspring will be green, and 50% will be yellow.
  - C) 75% of the offspring will be green, and 25% will be yellow.
  - D) 100% of the offspring will be green.

A more complicated Punnett square is needed to look at two traits during a cross. In Figure 8, a cross is performed between Plant 1, heterozygous at the color gene (*Gg*), and Plant 2, also heterozygous at the color gene. Plant 1 is also homozygous for the dominant allele of the shape gene (wrinkled peas), while Plant 2 is homozygous for the recessive allele (smooth). [What are the phenotypes of the plants being crossed?[20]] The same steps are followed to construct the Punnett square in Figure 8 as the one in Figure 7. First, determine the possible gametes for each pea plant being crossed. (In this case, there are really two possible gamete types from each parent, so the box could be simplified to have only two gametes on a side). Then, determine the possible combinations of gametes that could join to form zygotes and the phenotypes and frequencies of the F_1 generation. [What percentage of the F_1 generation will have smooth peas?[21] What percentage of peas will be green and wrinkled?[22] Yellow and wrinkled?[23] The cross depicted in Figure 8 was performed and produced 77 green wrinkled plants and 20 yellow wrinkled plants; why do these results not agree exactly with the ratios predicted in the Punnett square?[24]] Independent assortment and the principle of segregation are assumptions built into this Punnett square.

---

[19] If *G* (green allele) is dominant, then both *GG* homozygotes and *Gg* heterozygotes will be green, while only *gg* homozygotes will be yellow. 25% of the offspring in Figure 8 will be *GG* homozygotes, and 50% will be *Gg* heterozygotes, so a total of 75% of the offspring will be green (choice **C**).

[20] Plant 1 has green wrinkled peas, while Plant 2 has green smooth peas.

[21] All peas receive one *w* allele and one *W* allele, so all are wrinkled *Ww* heterozygotes (i.e., 0% are smooth).

[22] All F_1 peas are wrinkled and 75% are green, so 75% are green and wrinkled.

[23] All F_1 peas are wrinkled and 25% are yellow, so 25% are yellow and wrinkled.

[24] The results obtained in reality rarely agree exactly with the predicted result. If the results differ slightly from the prediction, the most likely explanation is statistical variability. The more progeny from the cross, the closer the result should be to the prediction.

14.3

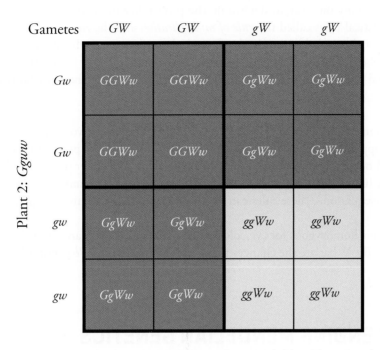

Plant 1: *GgWW*

Figure 8 A Punnett Square Depicting a Cross with Two Traits Involved

- In the cross depicted in Figure 8, how does the shape gene affect inheritance of the alleles for the color gene?[25]
    - A) The percentage of green peas is increased by the shape gene.
    - B) The shape gene has no effect on the inheritance of the alleles for the color gene.
    - C) The percentage of green peas is decreased by the shape gene.
    - D) The shape gene prevents segregation of the alleles for the color gene.

- If a green wrinkled plant from the F_1 generation in Figure 8 is crossed with a pure-breeding yellow smooth pea plant, what phenotypes are possible?[26]
- If any yellow smooth progeny are observed in this testcross, what does this indicate about the genotype of the F_1 plant?[27]

---

[25] Independent assortment and the principle of segregation are inherent in the Punnett square. There is no reason to believe that these are not followed, making choice **B** the best response. Choices A, C, and D all assume that either independent assortment or segregation did not occur.

[26] There are two different genotypes possible for the green wrinkled phenotype in the F_1 generation: *GGWw* or *GgWw*. The best way to determine all possible phenotypes in the cross is to draw a Punnett square for both of these potential genotypes:

If the F_1 plant is *GGWw*:

	GW	GW	Gw	Gw
gw	GgWw	GgWw	Ggww	Ggww

If the F_1 plant is *GgWw*:

	GW	Gw	gW	gw
gw	GgWw	Ggww	ggWw	ggww

Two genotypes are produced in equal ratios:
50% *GgWw* = green wrinkled phenotype
50% *Ggww* = green smooth

Four genotypes are produced:
25% *GgWw* = green wrinkled phenotype
25% *Ggww* = green smooth
25% *ggWw* = yellow wrinkled
25% *ggww* = yellow smooth

[27] If yellow smooth progeny are observed, the F_1 plant must be *GgWw*.

The Rules of Probability

Punnett squares are only one way to determine the probability of an outcome in a cross. Another way involves using statistical rules called the *rule of multiplication* and the *rule of addition*. The **rule of multiplication** states that the probability of both of two independent events happening can be found by multiplying the odds of either event alone. For example, if the probability of being struck by lightning is 1 in a million (10^{-6}) and the probability of winning the lottery is 10^{-7}, then the probability of both happening is the product: $10^{-6} \times 10^{-7} = 10^{-13}$.

The **rule of addition** can be used to calculate the chances of *either* of two events happening. The chance of either A or B happening is equal to the probability of A added to the probability of B, minus the probability of A and B occurring together. For example, the chance of either getting hit by lightning *or* winning the lottery is $10^{-6} + 10^{-7} = 1.1 \times 10^{-6}$. (*Note*: The product of 10^{-6} and 10^{-7} is so small that it can be neglected from the equation.) These rules can be a shortcut to using a Punnett square in some problems.

- A man that is homozygous for eye color, *bb*, is married to a woman who is heterozygous at the same gene: *Bb*. What are the chances that a child will have the *Bb* genotype and be a boy?[28]

14.4   EXTENDING MENDELIAN GENETICS

Mendel first started his work using mice, but abandoned rodents (either because of the mess involved, or because of the questionable ethics of a monk studying breeding schemes). In picking pea plants instead, he made a fortuitous decision. The traits he chose to study are (for the most part) controlled by a single gene with two alleles each. These two alleles have one completely dominant to the other, and therefore a simple relationship between genotype and phenotype. Although Mendel's peas all displayed very simple patterns of inheritance, the inheritance of traits is often more complicated.

Incomplete Dominance

Some alleles of genes display neither dominant nor recessive patterns of expression. If the phenotype of a heterozygote is a blended mix of both alleles, this is called **incomplete dominance**, and the alleles for that trait are given different, upper-case letters. For example, if a gene for flower color has two incompletely dominant alleles, *R* could be used to indicate the allele for red color and *W* to indicate the allele for white color. [If a gene for flower color has two alleles, *R* (red) and *r* (white), and *R* is dominant while *r* is recessive, what is the phenotype of *Rr* heterozygotes?[29] If *R* and *W* display incomplete dominance, what is the phenotype of *RW* heterozygotes?[30] How many phenotypes are possible if *R* and *W* display incomplete dominance?[31]]

---

[28] Without drawing a Punnett square, it is possible to see that all children must receive at least one *b* allele (from the father), and 50% of the children will receive the *B* allele from the mother; thus, 50% of the children will be *Bb*. The odds of a boy are 50%. Therefore, the odds a child is both a boy and has the *Bb* genotype are, by the rule of multiplication, 0.5 × 0.5 = 0.25, or 25%.

[29] *Rr* heterozygotes will have the phenotype of the dominant allele: red.

[30] In this case, *RW* heterozygotes will be neither red nor white, but a blend of the two: pink.

[31] Three phenotypes and three genotypes: *RR* (red), *RW* (pink), and *WW* (white).

Codominance

Codominance is a slightly different situation, in which two alleles are both expressed but are not blended. For example, the alleles of the gene for ABO blood group antigens that are found on the surface of red blood cells display codominance. Each of the alleles is expressed on red blood cells, regardless of the second allele in the cell. There are three alleles for the ABO blood group antigens: I^A, I^B, and i. The alleles I^A and I^B are codominant and will be expressed regardless of the second allele, while i is recessive to both I^A and I^B. The alleles I^A and I^B cause type A or type B antigens to be expressed, while i does not cause antigen expression.

- What is the phenotype of an individual heterozygous for the I^A and I^B alleles?[32]
- What is the phenotype of an individual heterozygous for I^B and i?[33]
- If a woman heterozygous for type A blood marries a man who is heterozygous for type B blood, what are the possible genotypes (and blood types) of their children?[34]

The other main antigen used in blood typing is the Rh (rhesus) factor. The expression of this antigen follows a classically dominant pattern; $Rh^D Rh^D$ and $Rh^D Rh^d$ (also seen as RR and Rr) genotypes lead to the expression of this protein on the surface of the red cell (Rh positive), and the $Rh^d Rh^d$ (or rr) genotype leads to the absence of the protein (Rh negative).

Although Mendel's peas all displayed very simple patterns of inheritance, there are often many complications in the inheritance of traits. For example:

Pleiotropism: A gene is said to have pleiotropic effects if its expression alters many different, seemingly unrelated aspects of the organism's total phenotype. For example, a mutation in a gene may cause altered development of heart, bone, and inner ears.

Polygenism: Complex traits that are influenced by many different genes are called polygenic. These traits tend to display a range of phenotypes in a continuous distribution. For example, height is polygenic and is influenced by genes for growth factors, receptors, hormones, bone deposition, muscle development, energy utilization, and so on.

Penetrance: Penetrance describes the likelihood that a person with a given genotype will express the expected phenotype. While many traits are completely penetrant (all individuals with a given allele or mutation display the phenotype), there is a spectrum of options: alleles or mutations can also have high, incomplete, or low penetrance.

Epistasis: This refers to a situation where expression of alleles for one gene is dependent on a different gene. For example, a gene for curly hair cannot be expressed if a different gene causes baldness.

- 100 people are homozygous for an allele that is implicated in cancer, but only 20 develop cancer. What are potential explanations for why only some people express a gene out of a broader population with the same genotype?[35]

---

[32] The red blood cells will express both type A and type B antigens, so the blood type will be AB.

[33] The red blood cells will express type B antigen only, and the blood type will be B.

[34] Because they are both heterozygous, the woman's genotype is $I^A i$ and the man's genotype is $I^B i$. Thus, their children could be $I^A I^B$ (type AB), $I^A i$ (type A), $I^B i$ (type B), or ii (type O).

[35] The trait of cancer development is probably polygenic, so it does not display simple patterns of inheritance. Cancer development is also influenced by the environment, such as exposure to carcinogens, further complicating the penetrance of the genotype.

- In one strain of mouse, homozygotes for an allele of a gene develop heart defects, while in another strain of mouse, homozygotes with the same allele develop normally. Heterozygotes develop normally in both strains. What is the most likely explanation for the difference between the two strains?[36]
    - A) The allele is recessive.
    - B) The development of the heart defect is influenced by more than one locus.
    - C) The allele has pleiotropic effects on development.
    - D) The allele is codominant.

The Sex Chromosomes

Early in the twentieth century it was observed that women have twenty-three pairs of chromosomes that are homologous, while men have only twenty-two pairs of chromosomes that match in appearance. The two chromosomes in men that did not match each other were termed the **X** and the **Y chromosomes** because of their appearance during mitosis (Figure 9). Males have an X and a Y, while females have two X chromosomes. The presence of a Y chromosome in humans (genotype XY) is a key factor in the determination of the sex of an embryo, and subsequent development into a male. The absence of a Y (genotype XX) results in a female as the default developmental pathway. During meiosis, females generate gametes that contain an X chromosome; males generate gametes with either an X or a Y chromosome, meaning that it is the *male* gamete that determines the gender of an embryo (Figure 10).

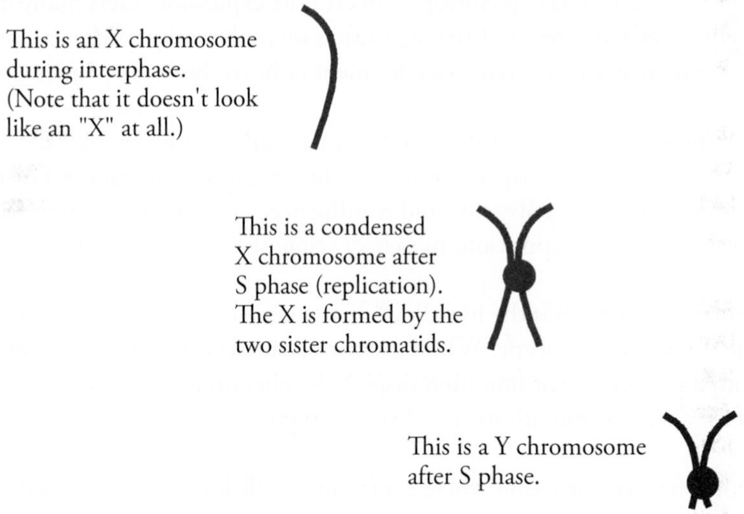

This is an X chromosome during interphase. (Note that it doesn't look like an "X" at all.)

This is a condensed X chromosome after S phase (replication). The X is formed by the two sister chromatids.

This is a Y chromosome after S phase.

Figure 9   The Sex Chromosomes

---

[36] The key variable must not lie within the allele itself, since this remains the same (so choices A and D are wrong). The genetic background of the two different strains of mice must affect whether or not the heart defect phenotype is expressed. Further, only one defect is observed (so it can't be pleitropic; choice C is wrong). Therefore, the heart defect phenotype must be influenced by some other locus that is different in the two strains of mice, making choice **B** the best answer.

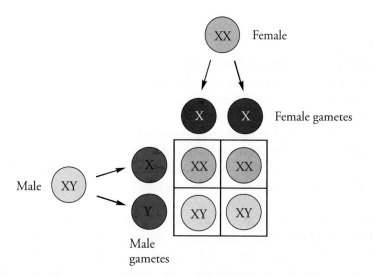

Figure 10   Determination of the Zygote's Sexual Genotype

The sex chromosomes also play a key role in the inheritance of other traits that are not directly involved in sexual development. Much of what has been discussed about inheritance was dependent on the assumption that there are two copies of every chromosome and therefore two copies of every gene in each cell. This is true for genes found on every pair of chromosomes except for one pair: the sex chromosomes. Genes that lie on the X chromosome will be present in two copies in females but only in one copy in males. [What pattern of expression will a recessive allele on the X chromosome display in males?[37]] Traits that are determined by genes on the X or Y chromosome are called **sex-linked traits** because of their unique patterns of expression and inheritance. The inheritance of traits coded by genes on sex chromosomes will be covered in Section 14.6.

---

[37] In males, recessive alleles on the X chromosome are always expressed, since no other allele is present that can mask the recessive allele.

14.5 LINKAGE

The traits that Mendel studied and based the law of independent assortment on were located on separate chromosomes. Genes that are located on the *same* chromosome may not display independent assortment, however. The failure of genes to display independent assortment is called **linkage**.

- If eye color is controlled by a gene on chromosome #11 and the hair color locus is located on chromosome #14, do these genes assort independently?[38]
- If the portion of chromosome #14 containing the hair color gene is translocated onto chromosome #11, will these genes still assort independently?[39]

If genes are located very close to each other on the same chromosome, then they will probably *not* be inherited independently of each other. Let's illustrate this with a pea gene for height and two alleles of the height gene, tall (*T*) and short (*t*), with the *T* allele dominant and the *t* allele recessive. If the height gene and the color gene are very near each other on the same chromosome, then the alleles of these genes on a specific chromosome will probably assort together into gametes during meiosis (Figure 11). This limits the possible combinations of the alleles in the gametes.

*TtG*g Individual: Independent Assortment

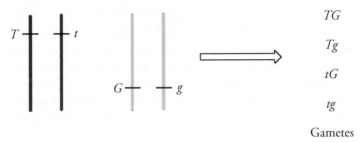

*TtG*g Individual: Linkage

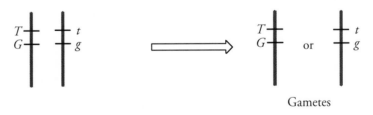

OR

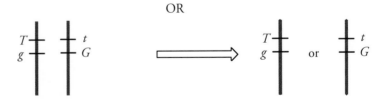

Figure 11   Linkage of Alleles during Meiosis

---

[38] Yes, they will. Assortment of nonhomologous chromosomes into gametes is random during meiosis.

[39] A translocation occurs when a piece of one chromosome is moved onto another chromosome. The two genes are then found on the same chromosome and may not assort independently.

- If the color gene and the height gene display linkage, is it possible to predict the possible gametes of a *TTgg* individual?[40] of a *TtGg* individual?[41]

To know how alleles that display linkage assort during meiosis, it may be necessary to know which alleles were on a chromosome together. As seen in Figure 11, there are two possible ways the height and color genes could be linked. The dominant alleles of two different genes can be linked together on the same chromosome (*TG*), the recessive alleles of two different genes can be linked (*tg*), or one dominant and one recessive allele can be linked (*Tg* and *tG*).

With genes that are found on the same chromosome, the design of a Punnett square is slightly different. The possible gametes are limited since they cannot assort independently. Consider a cross between a homozygous *ttgg* pea plant and a double-heterozygous plant with both dominant alleles on one chromosome and both recessive alleles located together on another chromosome. They can only make a limited number of different gametes, not the four possible combinations of alleles that would be found if the genes were on different chromosomes. A Punnett square will help to illustrate linkage in this example (Figure 12).

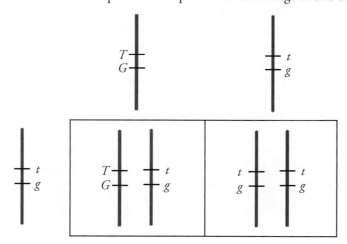

Figure 12   Assortment of Linked Genes

- What are the phenotypes of the F_1 progeny in the cross in Figure 12?[42]
- If a tall green pea from the F_1 progeny is crossed with a pure-breeding short yellow plant, what phenotypes will be observed and in what ratios?[43]
- If height and color genes were not linked, what ratios of phenotypes would be observed in a cross between a *TtGg* and a *ttgg* individual?[44]

---

[40] Yes. A *TTgg* individual can only make *Tg* gametes, regardless of whether the genes are on the same chromosome or not.

[41] No. To predict how these traits will assort, it is necessary to know which alleles are present together on the same chromosome.

[42] There are only two phenotypes: 50% tall green and 50% short yellow.

[43] The pure-breeding short yellow plant can only have *tg* gametes. The tall green plant can make only two types of alleles, the same gametes shown for its parent. The results of the backcross will be the same as for the original cross in Figure 12, with 50% tall green and 50% short yellow plants.

[44] The *ttgg* individual can make only *tg* gametes. The *TtGg* individual can make four different types of gametes if the genes are not linked: *TG*, *Tg*, *tG*, and *tg*. The genotypes and phenotypes of the cross will be 25% *TtGg* (tall green), 25% *Ttgg* (tall yellow), 25% *ttGg* (short green), and 25% *ttgg* (short yellow).

14.5

- Assume all of the characteristics already introduced for the height, color, and shape pea genes that have been used as examples. The height and color genes are located near each other on the same chromosome and display complete linkage, but the shape gene is located on a different chromosome. If an individual with a *TtGgWw* genotype and the *T* and *g* alleles on the same chromosome is crossed with a *ttGgWw* individual, what result will be observed?[45]

  A) All tall peas will be wrinkled.
  B) All wrinkled peas will be tall.
  C) All yellow peas will be tall.
  D) All tall peas will be yellow.

Linkage and Recombination

Linkage is the exception to the law of independent assortment. When genes are located on the same chromosome, they will display linkage and will not assort independently. Meiotic recombination provides the exception to linkage. During the formation of gametes, meiotic recombination between homologous chromosomes can separate alleles that were located on the same chromosome. In the example in Figure 13, three genes are located on the same chromosome. Prior to recombination, *ABC* were found on one chromosome and *abc* were found on the homologous chromosome. [What combinations of alleles will be found in gametes in the absence of recombination?[46]] Recombination produces new combinations of alleles not found in the parent and also allows genes located on the same chromosome to assort independently.

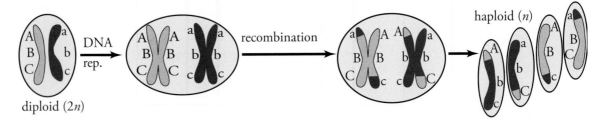

Figure 13   Recombination—Another Look

The example of the height and color genes in pea plants will help to illustrate linkage and the effects of recombination on patterns of inheritance. As before, the height and color genes are located on the same chromosome. There are two alleles of the height gene, dominant *T* (tall) and recessive *t* (short) and two alleles of the color gene, dominant *G* (green) and recessive *g* (yellow). The following cross is performed: a pure-breeding tall green plant is crossed with a pure-breeding short yellow plant. [What phenotypes are predicted in this cross if linkage is complete?[47]] A pea plant from this cross is then self-pollinated (crossed

---

[45] The gene for shape (wrinkled vs. smooth) is on a different chromosome than the other two genes, so there is no correlation between the wrinkled trait and the other traits (eliminating choices A and B). To be yellow, a pea must be homozygous *gg*. One of the *g* alleles must come from the chromosome with *T* and *g* together, making all yellow plants tall (choice **C** is correct). Some of the *Tg* gametes will join with *tG* gametes from the *ttGg* individual, meaning that some plants are tall and green (choice D is wrong). Drawing a Punnett Square can help to solve this problem.

[46] *ABC* or *abc* genotypes

[47] Only one phenotype. The F_1 generation will all receive a *TG* chromosome from the pure-breeding tall green parent and a *tg* chromosome from the pure-breeding short yellow parent.

with itself) to produce an F_2 generation. [If linkage is complete, what genotypes and phenotypes will be observed in the F_2 generation?[48] If the genes assort completely randomly, what genotypes and phenotypes will be observed in the F_2 generation?[49]] The F_2 generation in this cross was observed to have the following plants: 30 tall green plants, 9 short yellow plants, 2 tall yellow plants, and 1 short green plant. [Which of these phenotypes are recombinant phenotypes?[50]] Often in a cross involving genes on the same chromosome, the result will be intermediate between independent assortment and complete linkage. The reason for this is that recombination occurs between the genes during meiosis of *some* of the gametes but not *all* of the gametes. [If it is known that two genes are located on the same chromosome but during a cross they assort completely randomly, how can this be?[51]]

The frequency of recombination between two genes on a chromosome is proportional to the physical distance between the genes along the linear length of the DNA molecule. [Does recombination occur between genes more frequently if they are near each other or far apart?[52]] The farther apart two genes are on a chromosome, the more likely recombination will occur between the genes during meiosis. If the genes are located far enough apart, recombination will occur so frequently between the genes that they will no longer display linkage and will assort as independently as if they were on separate chromosomes. The **frequency of recombination** is given as the *number of recombinant phenotypes* resulting from a cross *divided by the total number of progeny.*

$$\text{RF} = \text{recombination frequency} = \frac{\text{number of recombinants}}{\text{total number of offspring}}$$

Since the frequency of recombination is proportional to the physical distance of genes from each other, it can be used as a tool to map genes in relation to each other on chromosomes.

---

[48] 75% tall green and 25% short yellow. Try a Punnett square to verify this result, remembering to assort alleles together into gametes.

[49] 9:3:3:1 of tall green, tall yellow, short green, and short yellow, respectively. This is a classical Mendelian ratio observed when heterozygotes at two alleles are crossed.

[50] The tall yellow and short green phenotypes would not be observed if linkage was complete (as in #56). The only way to produce these phenotypes is if a small number of gametes received chromosomes in which the *TG* and *tg* alleles were separated from each other by recombination, so these are the recombinant phenotypes.

[51] If the genes are on the same chromosome, but are far apart from one another, then recombination occurs frequently. The genes will assort randomly during meiosis and will not display any linkage even though they are on the same chromosome.

[52] The farther two genes are away from each other, the greater the odds that recombination will occur between them.

Example 14-1: The height and color gene in pea plants are on the same chromosome as a third gene for big or small flowers. The alleles of flower size are a dominant *B* (big) and a recessive *b* (small). The color gene (*G*, green or *g*, yellow) is studied in relation to the flower size gene. In the first cross, pure-breeding homozygous *BBGG* plants are crossed with *bbgg* plants. [What is the phenotype of the F_1 progeny?[53]] An F_1 progeny is then crossed with a *bbgg* plant and the following phenotypes observed: 44 big flower green plants, 40 small flower yellow plants, 8 big flower yellow plants, and 8 small flower green plants.

- Which of these are recombinant phenotypes?[54]
- What is the frequency of recombination between the genes?[55]
- What is the maximal frequency of recombination?[56]
- In another cross, the frequency of recombination between the flower size and height genes is examined and found to be 10 recombinant plants out of 100 progeny. Is the height gene or the color gene closer to the flower size gene?[57]
- Assume that hair color in humans is determined by a gene for which there are two alleles: *B* or brown, which is dominant, and *b* or blond, which is recessive. The hair color gene is located on the same chromosome as another gene that determines the strength of bones, and the two genes are very close together. The alleles of the bone strength gene are *S*, the dominant sturdy bone allele, and *s*, the recessive fragile bone allele. Jose and Tonya have dark hair and sturdy bones. One of their children has brown hair and fragile bones. One grandparent of Jose and one grandparent of Tonya had fragile bones and blond hair, while the remaining grandparents were homozygous for brown hair and sturdy bones. Which of the following is/are true?[58]

  I.   The child of Jose and Tonya represents a recombinant phenotype.
  II. All of the children of Jose and Tonya must have fragile bones.
  III. Jose and Tonya may have other children with blond hair and fragile bones.

  A) I only
  B) II only
  C) I and III only
  D) II and III only

---

[53] The F_1 progeny are all *BbGg* genotype and therefore are big flower green plants.

[54] Big flower yellow plants and small flower green plants can only be produced through recombination between the flower size and color genes.

[55] The frequency of recombination is 16 recombinant phenotypes out of 100 progeny = 16%.

[56] The maximal frequency of recombination would be when there was no linkage and the genes assorted independently. In this case there would be 25% big flower yellow plants and 25% small flower green plants, or 50% maximal frequency of recombination.

[57] There is less recombination between the height and flower size genes (10% frequency) than between the color and flower size genes (16%), so the height gene is closer to the flower size gene than the color gene is.

[58] **Item I is true:** The simplest explanation is that the grandparent on each side passed on the fragile allele and the blond allele, but recombination occurred, so that the fragile and blond alleles assorted independently. Item II is false: Jose and Tonya both have the dominant sturdy bone gene in at least one copy, so some children are likely to have sturdy bones. **Item III is true:** Both Jose and Tonya may have one chromosome with the blond allele and the fragile bone allele linked. If so, a nonrecombinant phenotype would be blond/fragile. The answer is choice **C**.

Example 14-2: In fruit flies, curly wings (*C*) are dominant to flat wings (*c*) and extra bristles (*E*) are dominant to normal bristles (*e*). A pure-breeding fly with curly wings and extra bristles is mated to a pure-breeding fly with flat wings and normal bristles. Two of the F1 flies are then mated to produce an F2 generation. The following phenotypes are observed in the F2 generation:

Phenotype	Number
Curly wings, extra bristles	173
Flat wings, normal bristles	22
Curly wings, normal bristles	59
Flat wings, extra bristles	64

All of the following are true EXCEPT:
  A) this is the expected distribution for a dihybrid cross.
  B) the genes for wing shape and bristle style are linked.
  C) if an F2 fly with flat wings and normal bristles were mated to an F1 fly, approximately 25% of the progeny flies would have flat wings and normal bristles.
  D) all the F2 flies with flat wings and normal bristles are pure-breeding.

Solution: "Pure-breeding" means "homozygous," so the original flies must have the genotypes *CCEE* and *ccee*, and all of the F1 flies have the genotype *CcEe*. The cross between two F1 flies is therefore a dihybrid cross: *CcEe* x *CcEe*, and if the genes are not linked, the expected phenotype ratio from that cross is 9:3:3:1. In other words, in the F2 generation there should be nine flies with both dominant traits (curly wings and extra bristles), three flies that are dominant for the first trait and recessive for the second (curly wings and normal bristles), three flies that are recessive for the first trait and dominant for the second (flat wings and extra bristles), and one fly that has both recessive traits (flat wings and normal bristles).

	CE	*Ce*	*cE*	*ce*
CE	*CCEE*	*CCEe*	*CcEE*	*CcEe*
Ce	*CCEe*	*CCee*	*CcEe*	*Ccee*
Ce	*CcEE*	*CcEe*	*ccEE*	*ccEe*
ce	*CcEe*	*Ccee*	*ccEe*	*CCee*

This is in fact the ratio that we see in the F2 generation (choice A is true and can be eliminated), which means that the genes are not linked (choice **B** is false and is the correct answer choice). If the genes were linked, we would see fewer of the recombinant flies (curly wings/normal bristles and flat wings/extra bristles) than we do, and more of the original phenotypes (curly wings/extra bristles and flat wings/normal bristles). If an F2 with flat wings and normal bristles (*ccee*) were mated to an F1 fly (*CcEe*) we would see an equal distribution of all four phenotypes:

	CE	*Ce*	*cE*	*ce*
ce	*CcEe*	*Ccee*	*ccEe*	*ccee*

so 25% of the resulting progeny would have flat wings and normal bristles (choice C is true and can be eliminated). Any fly with flat wings and normal bristles must be pure-breeding, since they must be homozygous recessive for both traits (*ccee*, choice D is true and can be eliminated).

14.6 INHERITANCE PATTERNS

There are six inheritance patterns that you should be familiar with: autosomal recessive, autosomal dominant, mitochondrial, Y-linked, X-linked recessive, and X-linked dominant. In this section, each will be described and then a summary table is presented.

Autosomal traits are caused by genetic variation on the autosomes (the 22 pairs of non-sex chromosomes in humans). These traits can be **autosomal dominant** (in which case a single copy of the allele will confer the trait or disease phenotype) or **autosomal recessive** (in which case two copies of the allele are required for the affected phenotype). Both tend to affect males and females equally; in other words, there is no sex bias for these traits.

There is a small, haploid DNA genome inside the mitochondria and humans inherit this genome from their mothers. This is because the sperm contributes only nuclear chromosomes to the zygote; the ovum contributes nuclear chromosomes and the rest of the cellular material including the organelles. There are some traits that are inherited via the mitochondrial genome, although these **mitochondrial traits** are rare. Luckily, they are fairly easy to spot because affected females have all affected offspring (sons and daughters). Affected individuals must have an affected mother, and affected males cannot have any affected offspring. An individual cannot inherit mitochondrial traits from their father.

Traits that are determined by genes located on the X or Y chromosome are called **sex-linked traits** and display unusual patterns of inheritance. Traits encoded by genes on the Y chromosome (Y-linked traits) would only be passed from male parents to male children. [Would it be possible for a father to pass a Y-linked trait to female children?[59] Can males be carriers of recessive Y-linked traits without expressing them?[60]] Y-linked traits are quite rare, because the Y chromosome is small and contains a relatively small number of genes. Many of the genes on the Y-chromosome function in sex determination.

X-linked traits are observed quite frequently and can be X-linked recessive or X-linked dominant. There are several well-studied examples of X-linked recessive traits that are common in the human population; hemophilia is an example. Women are often carriers of X-linked recessive alleles but will only express recessive X-linked traits when they are homozygous. Men have only one copy of genes on the X chromosome and as a result, they *always* express recessive X-linked alleles. [From which parent do males receive X-linked traits?[61]] These traits tend to affect males more than females.

Red-green colorblindness, an X-linked trait, is caused by a defect in a visual pigment gene on the X chromosome. The allele that is responsible for colorblindness is a pigment gene that does not produce functional protein. The colorblindness allele, like many recessive traits carried in the population, is not expressed in heterozygotes. Colorblindness is unusual in women but fairly common in men. Females have two copies of the gene, so will not express the trait if they are heterozygotes, while males have only one X chromosome and so will always express the allele whenever they receive it. [A man is colorblind, and his wife is homozygous normal for genes encoding visual pigment proteins. What will be the phenotypes and genotypes of sons and of daughters of this couple?[62]]

---

[59] No. Females never have a Y chromosome and so can never carry or express a Y-linked trait.

[60] No. Y-linked traits are carried in only one copy, since there is only one Y chromosome per cell. If a male carries a recessive Y-linked trait, he will express it.

[61] Since males receive their X chromosome from their mother (and their Y chromosome from their father), they receive X-linked traits from their mother.

[62] Sons will have a normal phenotype and carry one copy of the normal gene. Daughters will carry one normal gene and one recessive color-blindness allele and will have the normal phenotype.

X-linked dominant traits are harder to identify. A female will display an X-linked dominant phenotype if she has one or two copies of the allele on her X chromosomes. A male will express the phenotype if he inherited the affected allele from his mother. While these traits still tend to affect males more than females, this trend is less obvious than for X-linked recessive traits.

Table 1 summarizes the six inheritance patterns you should be familiar with, and it lists some strategies you can use to distinguish between them.

Inheritance Pattern	Identification Techniques	Unaffected Genotypes	Affected Genotypes
Autosomal recessive	• Can skip generations (affected individuals can have unaffected parents) • Number of affected males is usually equal to the number of affected females	AA Aa	aa
Autosomal dominant	• Does not skip generations (affected individuals must have an affected parent) • Number of affected males is usually equal to number of affected females • An affected parent passes the trait to either all or half of offspring	aa	AA Aa
Mitochondrial	• Maternal inheritance • Affected female has all affected children • Affected male cannot pass the trait onto his children • Unaffected female cannot have affected children	a	A
Y-linked	• Affects male only; females never have the trait • Affected father has all affected sons • Unaffected father cannot have an affected son	XY^a	XY^A
X-linked recessive	• Can skip generations (affected individuals can have unaffected parents) • Tend to affect males more than females • Unaffected females can have affected sons • Affected female has all affected sons, but can have both affected and unaffected daughters	$X^A X^A$ $X^A X^a$ $X^A Y$	$X^a X^a$ $X^a Y$
X-linked dominant	• Hardest to identify • Does not skip generations (affected individuals must have an affected parent) • Usually affects males more than females • Affected fathers have all affected daughters • Affected mothers can have unaffected sons (and unaffected daughters), and pass the trait equally to sons and daughters	$X^a X^a$ $X^a Y$	$X^A X^A$ $X^A X^a$ $X^A Y$

Table 1   Summary of Inheritance Patterns

- Two mouse genes located on the X chromosome are being studied. The alleles of the genes are:
  Fuzzy hair: F, dominant (normal hair) and f, recessive (fuzzy hair)
  Extra toes: E, dominant (extra toes), and e, recessive (normal toes)
  A female with normal hair and extra toes is crossed with a male with normal hair and extra toes. The progeny have the following phenotypes:

Phenotype	Male	Female
Normal hair, extra toes	46	100
Normal hair, normal toes	4	0
Fuzzy hair, extra toes	5	0
Fuzzy hair, normal toes	45	0

14.7

Which one of the following is true concerning this experiment?[63]
  A) Males have a higher rate of recombination than females do.
  B) In the absence of recombination, all males would have normal hair and extra toes.
  C) The rate of recombination on the X chromosome is the same in males and females.
  D) Both males and females have recombinant genotypes, but only males have recombinant phenotypes.

---

[63] The genotype of the male parent must be X^{FE} Y. The predominance of the normal hair-extra toes and fuzzy hair-normal toes phenotypes in the F_1 generation indicates that the female parent must have one X chromosome with both dominant alleles together, and one X chromosome with both recessive alleles together, in other words, her genotype must be $X^{FE} X^{fe}$. The fuzzy hair-extra toes and normal hair-normal toes phenotypes are much less common and must be the result of recombination in the female parent, producing X^{Fe} and X^{fE} chromosomes. Note that recombination between the X and Y chromosomes in males is not possible due to the fact that the X and Y carry different genes (choices A and C are wrong). If recombination had not occurred in the female parent, all F_1 males would have received either X^{FE} or X^{fe}, giving both normal hair-extra toes and fuzzy hair-normal toes phenotypes (choice B is wrong). Choice **D** is the correct answer: the F_1 females must also have recombinant genotypes on the X chromosomes they received from their mother, but every F_1 female also received both dominant alleles on the X chromosome they received from their father. Thus, only the dominant phenotypes are seen in the F_1 females.

14.7 POPULATION GENETICS

Population genetics describes the inheritance of traits in populations over time. The word *population* has a specific meaning in this setting: *a population consists of members of a species that mate and reproduce with each other.* [If a group of sea turtles lives most of the year dispersed over a large area of ocean without contact with each other but congregate once a year to reproduce, is this group a population?[64]] To a population geneticist, each individual is merely a temporary carrier of the alleles in a population.

In population genetics, the units of genetic inheritance are alleles of genes, just as in Mendelian genetics. However, in population genetics, alleles are examined across the entire population rather than in individuals. The sum total of all genetic information in a population is called the **gene pool**. The frequency of an allele in a population is a key variable used to describe the gene pool. [If there are 5000 hippos in a population, out of which there are 100 homozygotes of an autosomal allele h and 400 heterozygotes, what is the frequency of the h allele in the population?[65] If 20% of the population is heterozygous for an allele Q and 10% is homozygous, what will be the frequency of the allele in the population?[66]]

Hardy-Weinberg in Population Genetics

Population genetics does not simply describe the gene pool of a population but attempts to predict the gene pool of a population in the future. The **Hardy-Weinberg Law** states that the *frequencies of alleles in the gene pool of a population will not change over time*, provided that a number of assumptions are true:

1) There is no mutation.
2) There is no migration.
3) There is no natural selection.
4) There is random mating.
5) The population is sufficiently large to prevent random drift in allele frequencies.

What Hardy-Weinberg means at the molecular level is that segregation of alleles, independent assortment, and recombination during meiosis can alter the combinations of alleles in gametes but cannot increase or decrease the frequency of an allele in the gametes of one individual or the gametes of the population as a whole.

- If 100 homozygous green pea plants and 100 homozygous yellow pea plants are crossed, 1000 green pea plants are produced. Does this mean that the yellow alleles disappeared from the population?[67]

---

[64] Yes. A population does not need to live with each other, only to reproduce sexually with each other.

[65] The allele frequency is the number of copies of a specific allele divided by the total number of copies of the gene in the population. If there are 5000 hippos, and each has 2 copies of the gene, there are 10,000 copies of the gene in the population. There are 100 homozygotes of the h allele, each with 2 copies of it, and 400 heterozygotes with one h allele, for a total of 600 h alleles in the population. Thus, the frequency of the h allele is 600/10000 = 0.06.

[66] In this case, the number of individuals in the population is not provided, but it is not needed. The total number of alleles is 100%. The frequency of the allele is 0.5 × (20% heterozygotes) + 10% homozygotes = 20%.

[67] The yellow alleles are still there (but in the heterozygous state), so they do not appear in the phenotype.

- What is the frequency of the yellow allele in the gene pool of the progeny?[68]
- If the green peas from the F_1 generation are allowed to mate randomly within the population, and there is no mutation, migration, natural selection, or random drift, what will be the frequency of the yellow allele in the population after four generations?[69]

The Hardy-Weinberg law has also been translated into mathematical terms. Assuming that there are two alleles of a gene in a population, the letter p is used to represent the frequency of the dominant allele, and the letter q is used to represent the frequency of the recessive allele. Since there are only two alleles, the following fundamental equation must be true:

$$p + q = 1$$

Based on allele frequency, it is possible to calculate the proportion of genotypes in a population. Take a situation where the frequency of a dominant allele, G, equals p and the frequency of a recessive allele, g, equals q. If the equation above is squared on both sides, it becomes:

$$(p + q)^2 = 1$$

$$p^2 + 2pq + q^2 = 1$$

where

$$p^2 = \text{the frequency of the } GG \text{ genotype}$$

$$2pq = \text{the frequency of the } Gg \text{ genotype}$$

$$q^2 = \text{the frequency of the } gg \text{ genotype}$$

- If the frequency of the G allele is 0.25 in a population of 1000 mice, determine the number of individuals who are Gg heterozygotes if there is random mating but no migration, mutation, random drift, or natural selection.[70]
- If allele frequencies in a population are constant, and genotype frequencies can be calculated from allele frequencies, how will genotype frequencies vary over time?[71]

After one generation, a population will reach **Hardy-Weinberg equilibrium**, in which allele frequencies no longer change. Since allele frequencies do not change, and genotype frequencies can be calculated from allele frequencies, it follows that genotype frequencies also do not change over time.

---

[68] The frequency of the yellow allele will be 50%, just as it was in the parents. None of the alleles in a population were destroyed, so the frequency is the same as in the parental generation.

[69] According to Hardy-Weinberg, there will be no change in the frequency of the allele. The frequency of the yellow allele will still be 50% after four generations.

[70] If the frequency of the G allele (p) is 0.25, then the frequency of the g allele (q) must be 0.75, since $p + q = 1$. The frequency of the heterozygotes in the population will be $2pq = 2(0.25)(0.75) = 0.375$. Therefore, the number of individuals in this population who are heterozygotes will be $0.375 \times 1000 = 375$.

[71] Genotype frequencies as well as allele frequencies will remain constant according to Hardy-Weinberg.

Hardy-Weinberg in the Real World

Hardy-Weinberg requires a number of assumptions in order to be true. The assumptions, as presented earlier, are that in a population there is random mating and no mutation, migration, natural selection, or random drift. Thus, Hardy-Weinberg describes a highly idealized set of conditions required to prevent alleles from being added or removed from a population. In reality, it is not possible for a population to meet all of the conditions required by Hardy-Weinberg.

1) **Mutation**: Mutation is inevitable in a population. Even if there are no chemical mutagens or radiation, inherent errors by DNA polymerase would over time cause mutations and introduce new alleles in a population.
2) **Migration**: If migration occurs, animals leaving or entering the population will carry alleles with them and disturb the Hardy-Weinberg equilibrium.
3) **Natural Selection**: For there to be no natural selection, there would have to be unlimited resources, no predation, no disease, and so on. This is not a set of conditions encountered in the real world.
4) **Non-random Mating**: If individuals pick their mates preferentially based on one or more traits, alleles that cause those traits will be passed on preferentially from one generation to another.
5) **Random Drift**: If a population becomes very small, it cannot contain as great a variety of alleles. In a very small population, random events can alter allele frequencies significantly and have a large influence on future generations.

14.8

14.8   EVOLUTION BY NATURAL SELECTION

At one time, life on Earth was generally viewed as static and unchanging, but we now know that this is not the case. Over the geologic span of Earth's history, many species have arisen, changed over millions of years, given rise to new species, and died out. These changes in life on Earth are called **evolution**. Although he did not arrive at his theory alone, Charles Darwin played an important role in shaping modern thought by proposing natural selection as the mechanism that drives evolution. **Natural selection** is an interaction between organisms and their environment that causes differential reproduction of different phenotypes and thereby alters the gene pool of a population. In essence the theory of evolution by natural selection is this:

1) In a population, there are heritable differences between individuals.
2) Heritable traits (alleles of genes) produce traits (phenotypes) that affect the ability of an organism to survive and have offspring.
3) Some individuals have phenotypes that allow them to survive longer, be healthier, and have more offspring than others.
4) Individuals with phenotypes that allow them to have more offspring will pass on their alleles more frequently than those with phenotypes that have fewer offspring.
5) Over time, those alleles that lead to more offspring are passed on more frequently and become more abundant, while other alleles become less abundant in the gene pool.
6) Changes in allele frequency are the basis of evolution in species and populations.

To put it simply, evolution occurs when natural selection acts on genetic variation to drive changes in the genetic composition of a population. A key term in evolution is **fitness**. In evolutionary terms, fitness is not how well an animal is physically adapted to a niche in the environment, or how well it can feed itself, but how successful it is in passing on its alleles to future generations. The way to have greater fitness is by having more offspring that pass on their alleles to future generations of the population. Some species achieve greater fitness through sheer numbers of progeny produced, who are then left to fend for themselves. Other species have fewer progeny, but protect and nurture the young to maturity.

- If an allele of a gene causes cancer in elderly polar bears after their reproductive years have passed, how will it affect the fitness of bears carrying the allele?[72]
- If a recessive allele causes sterility in homozygotes, how will it affect the fitness of heterozygotes?[73]
- A group of mice are infected with recombinant virus in bone marrow cells that allows the mice to live longer. The mice are then released into a wild population. Will natural selection act to increase the life span of the population?[74]
- Which of the following will have greater fitness: a fish that has two offspring and protects and nurtures its young to maturity, or a fish that has 10 offspring and abandons them, resulting in the death of 8 young fish before maturity?[75]

14.8

Sources of Genetic Diversity

Natural selection acts on the genetic diversity in a population to alter allele frequencies, causing evolution. Genetic diversity in a population is a requirement for natural selection to occur. [If a population of sea otters contains only one allele of a gene that protects against cold, can natural selection drive evolution of this trait?[76] Can natural selection cause new alleles to appear in the population?[77]] Natural selection does not introduce genetic diversity, however; it can act only on existing diversity to alter allele frequencies.

There are two sources of genetic variation in a population: *new alleles* and *new combinations of existing alleles*. New alleles are the result of mutations in the genome. New combinations of alleles are generated during sexual reproduction as a result of independent assortment, recombination, and segregation during meiosis. By increasing and maintaining genetic variation in a population, sexual reproduction allows for greater capacity for adaptation of a population to changing environmental conditions.

- If a mutation occurs in a muscle cell of an individual who then has many progeny, does this mutation increase genetic variation in the population?[78]
- If a population of flowers loses the ability to reproduce sexually and reproduces only asexually, how will this affect natural selection in the population?[79]

---

[72] The allele will not affect fitness. The bears will only be affected at a time when they can no longer have offspring, so it will not affect the ability of bears to transmit their alleles to future generations.

[73] If the allele is truly recessive, it will not affect fitness at all. Natural selection can act only on phenotypes, not genotypes.

[74] No. Natural selection only acts on heritable traits. Infected bone marrow cells will not be passed on in the germ line to the next generation, so the long life span of these mice is not a heritable trait.

[75] The fish will technically have the same fitness, since both will contribute to the gene pool of future generations equally.

[76] If there is only one allele, then there is no variability that natural selection can act on, and no way that allele frequencies can change to cause evolution.

[77] No. Natural selection can only alter the frequency of existing alleles, not create new alleles.

[78] No. Mutation must occur in the germ line to introduce a new allele into a population. A mutation in a somatic cell cannot be passed on to the next generation.

[79] If the flowers can only reproduce asexually, then they have lost the ability of meiosis to generate new combinations of alleles and new genetic variation for natural selection to act on.

Modes of Natural Selection

Natural selection can occur in many different manners and have different effects in a population. The following are a few examples:

1) **Directional Selection:** Polygenic traits often follow a bell-shaped curve of expression, with most individuals clustered around the average and some members of a population trailing off in either direction away from the average. If natural selection removes those at one extreme, the population average over time will move in the other direction. Example: Giraffes get taller as all short giraffes die for lack of food.

2) **Divergent Selection:** Rather than removing the extreme members in the distribution of a trait in a population, natural selection removes the members near the average, leaving those at either end. Over time, divergent selection will split the population in two and perhaps lead to a new species. Example: Small deer are selected for because they can hide, and large deer are selected because they can fight, but mid-sized deer are too big to hide and too small to fight.

3) **Stabilizing Selection:** Both extremes of a trait are selected against, driving the population closer to the average. Example: Birds that are too large or too small are eliminated from a population because they cannot mate.

4) **Artificial Selection:** Humans intervene in the mating of many animals and plants, using artificial selection to achieve desired traits through controlled mating. Example: The pets and crop plants we have are the result of many generations of artificial selection.

5) **Sexual Selection:** Animals often do not choose mates randomly, but have evolved elaborate rituals and physical displays that play a key role in attracting and choosing a mate. Example: Some birds have bright plumage to attract a mate, even at the cost of increased predation.

6) **Kin Selection:** Natural selection does not always act on individuals. Animals that live socially often share alleles with other individuals and will sacrifice themselves for the sake of the alleles they share with another individual. Example: A female lion sacrifices herself to save her sister's children.

14.9 THE SPECIES CONCEPT AND SPECIATION

A **species** is a group of organisms which are capable of reproducing with each other sexually. (Other criteria, such as morphology, are used to classify species that only reproduce asexually.) [What's the difference between a population and a species?[80]] Two individuals are not members of the same biological species if they cannot mate and produce fit offspring. [When a horse mates with a donkey a mule is born. Mules are healthy animals with long life spans, but they are sterile. Are horses and donkeys members of the same species?[81]] **Reproductive isolation** keeps existing species separate. There are two types of reproductive isolation: **prezygotic** and **postzygotic**.

Prezygotic barriers prevent the formation of a hybrid zygote. Such barriers may be:

• Ecological: individuals who could otherwise mate live in different habitats, and thus cannot access each other
• Temporal: individuals mate at different times of the day, season, or year
• Behavioral: some species require special rituals or courtship behaviors before mating can occur

---

[80] Members of a species *can* mate and produce fit offspring. Members of a population *do*. Remember it this way: a population is a subset of a species.

[81] No, since their offspring are unfit (unable to reproduce).

- Mechanical: reproductive structures or genital organs of two individuals are not compatible (even if they court and attempt copulation)
- Gametic: sperm from one species cannot fertilize the egg of a different species due incompatibilities in the sperm-egg recognition system, discussed in Chapter 19

Postzygotic barriers to hybridization prevent the development, survival, or reproduction of hybrid individuals (those that arise from a mating between two different species), and thus prevent gene flow if fertilization between two different species does occur. There are three types of postzygotic barriers:

- Hybrid inviability: hybrid offspring do not develop or mature normally, and normally die in the embryonic stage
- Hybrid sterility: a hybrid individual is born and develops normally, but does not produce normal gametes, and thus is incapable of breeding (e.g., a mule, offspring of a mating between a horse and a donkey, is sterile)
- Hybrid breakdown: when two hybrids mate successfully to produce a hybrid offspring, but this second generation hybrid is somehow biologically defective

Cladogenesis (the creation of a new species that branches off from the existing species) has left traces which taxonomists use to classify organisms. **Homologous structures** are physical features shared by two different species as a result of a common ancestor. For example, bird wings have five bony supports which resemble distorted human fingers, and dog paws also resemble distorted human hands. The explanation is that dogs, birds, and people all have a common ancestor which had five-toed feet. **Analogous structures** serve the same function in two different species, but *not* due to common ancestry. The flagellum of the human sperm and bacterial flagella are an example; they have entirely different structures from different organisms yet play the same role in motility.

14.10 TAXONOMY

Taxonomy is the science of biological classification, originated by Carolus Linnaeus in the eighteenth century. He devised the **binomial classification** system we use today, in which each organism is given two names: genus and species. The binomial name of an organism is written in italics (or is underlined) with the genus capitalized and the species not, as in *Homo sapiens* (man the wise). There are eight principal taxonomic categories: **domain**, **kingdom**, **phylum**, **class**, **order**, **family**, **genus**, and **species**.[82] You should know how humans are classified and the defining characteristics of each category. Table 2 on the next page provides a general summary.

---

[82] A mnemonic goes: "Dumb King Philip Came Over From Greece Sunday" (or "Dumb King Phil Came Over For Great Spaghetti.").

Domain	Bacteria	Archaea	Eukarya			
Kingdom	Eubacteria	Archaea	Protista	Fungi	Plantae	Animalia
Cell wall	peptidoglycan	polysaccharides and proteins, but no peptidoglycan	optional and varied	chitin	cellulose	none
Organelles	none	none	Typical eukaryotic organelles such as: nucleus, RER, SER, Golgi, peroxisome, lysosomes, chloroplasts, vacuoles, mitochondria, etc.			
Chromosomes	1 circular ds DNA	1 circular ds DNA	several linear ds DNA chromosomes			
Life cycle	asexual repro. (binary fission)	asexual repro. (binary fission)	varied (sexual and asexual)	varied (sexual and asexual)	mostly sexual reproduction	mostly sexual reproduction
Ploidy and Cellularity	Unicellular	Unicellular	Mostly unicellular	Mostly multicellular and mostly haploid	Multicellular, alternates between haploid and diploid	Multicellular and diploid
Cellular motility	flagella	flagella	amoeboid or flagellar	non-motile	some flagellated sperm	amoeboid or flagellar
Cilia/flagella	unique structure	unique structure	characteristic 9 + 2 arrangement of microtubules			
Nutrition	varied, absorptive	varied, absorptive	varied	chemo-hetero., absorptive	most photoauto. w/ chlorophyll	chemo-hetero., ingestive
Glycolysis/ ATP	All living organisms perform glycolysis & use ATP. All kingdoms contain at least some members which perform oxidative phosphorylation.					
Examples	bacteria & blue-green algae	Archaea (extremophiles)	*Plasmodium* plankton, algae, kelp, seaweed	yeasts, molds, mushrooms, truffles	trees, flowers, mosses, ferns	sponges, worms, mollusks, insects, reptiles, birds, mammals

Table 2   Taxonomic Characteristics

14.10

Domain Bacteria and Domain Archaea were both previously classified into Kingdom Monera. Because of huge diversity in these organisms, they have since been separated into two domains, and for these organisms, the kingdom and domain are the same.

14.11   THE ORIGIN OF LIFE

Based on radioisotope dating, the earth is thought to be 4.5 billion years old. All life evolved from prokaryotes. The oldest fossils are 3.5 billion-year-old outlines of primitive prokaryotic cell walls found in stromatolites (layered mats formed by colonies of prokaryotes).

The atmosphere of the young Earth was different from today's atmosphere. The predominant gases then were probably H_2O, CO, CO_2, and N_2. The most important thing to note here is the absence of O_2. It is thought that the early atmosphere was a **reducing environment**, where electron donors were prevalent. Oxygen is an electron acceptor, and as such, tends to break organic bonds. In this early world, simple organic molecules, or monomers ("single units") could form spontaneously. The energy for this synthesis was provided by lightning, radioactive decay, volcanic activity, or the Sun's radiation. Laboratory recreations of the early environment result in the spontaneous formation of amino acids, carbohydrates, lipids, and ribonucleotides, as well as other organic compounds.

Spontaneous polymerization of these monomers can also be observed in the lab (including spontaneous polymerization of ribonucleotides). No enzymes were present when this was occurring for the first time in nature, but it is thought that metal ions on the surface of rocks and especially clay acted as catalysts. This is known as **abiotic synthesis**. Polypeptides made in this way are called **proteinoids**.

Proteinoids in water spontaneously form droplets called **microspheres**. When lipids are added to the solution, **liposomes** form, with lipids forming a layer on the surface of proteins. A more complex particle known as a **coacervate** includes polypeptides, nucleic acids, and polysaccharides. Coacervates made with pre-existing enzymes are capable of catalyzing reactions. Microspheres, liposomes, and coacervates are collectively referred to as **protobionts**.

Protobionts resemble cells in that they contain a protected inner environment and perform chemical reactions. They can also reproduce to a certain extent: when they grow too large, they split in half. What is lacking, however, is an organized mechanism of heredity. This was first provided by RNA. As noted above, RNA chains form spontaneously in the appropriate solution. Even more interesting is the observation that single-stranded RNA chains can be self-replicating. A daughter chain lines up on the parent by base pairing and then spontaneously polymerizes with a surprisingly low error rate. A nonspecific catalyst such as a metal ion can further increase the efficiency of RNA self-replication.

Somehow a mechanism evolved for polypeptides to be copied from early RNA genes. You already know about the inherent tendency for phospholipids to form lipid bilayers. Given all this information, it's not too hard to imagine true cells evolving from a primordial soup at the dawn of time. The last step in the evolution of the earliest cells would have been the switch from RNA to DNA as the genetic material. DNA is more stable due to its 2′-deoxy structure and also due to the fact that it spontaneously forms a compact double-stranded helix.

Chapter 15
The Nervous and
Endocrine Systems

15.1 NEURONAL STRUCTURE AND FUNCTION

Neurons are specialized cells that transmit and process information from one part of the body to another. This information takes the form of electrochemical impulses known as **action potentials**. The action potential is a localized area of depolarization of the plasma membrane that travels in a wave-like manner along an axon. When an action potential reaches the end of an axon at a synapse, the signal is transformed into a chemical signal with the release of neurotransmitter into the synaptic cleft, a process called **synaptic transmission** (Section 15.2). The information of many synapses feeding into a neuron is integrated to determine whether that neuron will in turn fire an action potential. In this way, the action of many individual neurons is integrated to work together in the nervous system as a whole.

Structure of the Neuron

The basic functional and structural unit of the nervous system is the **neuron** (Figure 1). The structure of these cells is highly specialized to transmit and process **action potentials**, the electrochemical signals of the nervous system (Figure 3). Neurons have a central cell body, the **soma**, which contains the nucleus and is where most of the biosynthetic activity of the cell takes place. Slender projections, termed **axons** and **dendrites**, extend from the cell body. Neurons have only one axon (as long as a meter in some cases), but most possess many dendrites. Neurons with one dendrite are termed **bipolar**; those with many dendrites are **multipolar**. Neurons generally carry action potentials in one direction, with dendrites receiving signals and axons carrying action potentials away from the cell body. Axons can branch multiple times and terminate in **synaptic knobs** that form connections with target cells. When action potentials travel down an axon and reach the synaptic knob, chemical messengers are released and travel across a very small gap called the **synaptic cleft** to the target cell. The nature of the action potential and the transmission of signals across the synaptic cleft are key aspects of nervous system function. [In Figure 1, in what direction does an action potential travel in the axon shown?[1] What's the difference between a neuron and a nerve?[2]]

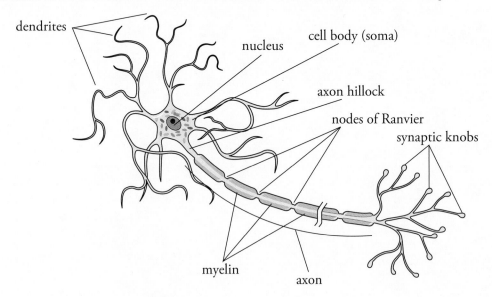

Figure 1   A Multipolar Neuron

---

[1]   Action potentials travel from the cell body down the axon, or from left to right in Figure 1.

[2]   A neuron is a single cell. A nerve is a large bundle of many different axons from different neurons.

The Action Potential

The Resting Membrane Potential

The **resting membrane potential** is an electric potential across the plasma membrane of approximately –70 millivolts (mV), with the interior of the cell negatively charged with respect to the exterior of the cell. Two primary membrane proteins are required to establish the resting membrane potential: the Na⁺/K⁺ ATPase and the potassium leak channels. The **Na⁺/K⁺ ATPase** pumps three sodium ions out of the cell and two potassium ions into the cell with the hydrolysis of one ATP molecule. [What form of transport is carried out by the Na⁺/K⁺ ATPase?[3]] The result is a sodium gradient with high sodium outside of the cell and a potassium gradient with high potassium inside the cell. **Leak channels** are channels that are open all the time and that simply allow ions to "leak" across the membrane according to their gradient. Potassium leak channels allow potassium, but no other ions, to flow down their gradient out of the cell. The combined loss of many positive ions through Na⁺/K⁺ ATPases and the potassium leak channels leaves the interior of the cell with a net negative charge, approximately 70 mV more negative than the exterior of the cell; this difference is the resting membrane potential. Note that there are very few sodium leak channels in the membrane (the ratio of K⁺ leak channels to Na⁺ leak channels is about 100:1), so the cell membrane is virtually impermeable to sodium.

- If the potassium leak channels are blocked, what will happen to the membrane potential?[4]
- What would happen to the membrane potential if sodium ions were allowed to flow down their concentration gradient?[5]

The resting membrane potential establishes a negative charge along the interior of axons (along with the rest of the neuronal interior). Thus, the cells can be described as **polarized**; negative on the inside and positive on the outside. An action potential is a disturbance in this membrane potential, a wave of **depolarization** of the plasma membrane that travels along an axon. Depolarization is a change in the membrane potential from the resting membrane potential of approximately –70 mV to a less negative, or even positive, potential. After depolarization, **repolarization** returns the membrane potential to normal. The change in membrane potential during passage of an action potential is caused by movement of ions into and out of the neuron through ion channels. The action potential is therefore not strictly an electrical impulse, like electrons moving in a copper telephone wire, but an electro*chemical* impulse.

Depolarization

Key proteins in the propagation of action potentials are the **voltage-gated sodium channels** located in the plasma membrane of the axon. In response to a change in the membrane potential, these ion channels open to allow sodium ions to flow down their gradient into the cell and depolarize that section of membrane. [What is the effect of opening the voltage-gated sodium channels on the membrane potential?[6]] These channels are opened by depolarization of the membrane from the resting potential of –70 mV to a **threshold potential** of approximately –50 mV. Once this threshold is reached, the channels are opened

---

[3] The Na⁺/K⁺ ATPase uses ATP to drive transport against a gradient; this is primary active transport.

[4] The flow of potassium out of the cell makes the interior of the cell more negatively charged. Blocking the potassium leak channels would reduce the magnitude of the resting membrane potential, making the interior of the cell less negative.

[5] Sodium ions would flow into the cell and reduce the potential across the plasma membrane, making the interior of the cell less negative and even relatively positive if enough ions flow into the cell.

[6] Sodium (positively charged) flows into the cell, down its concentration gradient, making the interior of the cell less negatively charged, or even positively charged.

fully, but they are closed below the threshold and do not allow the passage of any ions through the channel. When the channels open, sodium flows into the cell, down its concentration gradient, depolarizing that section of the membrane to about +35 mV before inactivating. Some of the sodium ions flow down the interior of the axon, slightly depolarizing the neighboring section of membrane. When the depolarization in the next section of membrane reaches threshold, those voltage-gated sodium channels open as well, passing the depolarization down the axon (Figure 2). [Once an action potential is initiated in an axon, can it be stopped?[7]]

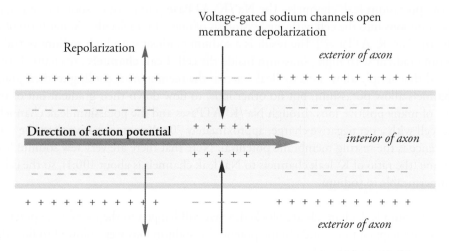

Figure 2   The Action Potential is a Wave of Membrane Depolarization

- Which one of the following can cause the interior of the neuron to have a momentary positive charge?[8]
    A) Opening of potassium leak channels
    B) Activity of the Na+/K+ ATPase
    C) Opening of voltage-gated sodium channels
    D) Opening of voltage-gated potassium channels

Repolarization

With the opening of voltage-gated sodium channels, sodium flows into the cell and depolarizes the membrane to positive values. As the wave of depolarization passes through a region of membrane, however, the membrane does not remain depolarized (Figure 2).

---

[7] No, it cannot. Action potentials are continually renewed at each point in the axon as they travel. Assuming there are enough voltage-gated channels, once an action potential starts, it will propagate without a change in amplitude (size) until it reaches a synapse.

[8] Choices A, B, and D all make the interior of the cell more negative. Choice **C** is the answer. Voltage-gated sodium channels can make the interior of the cell momentarily positive during passage of an action potential.

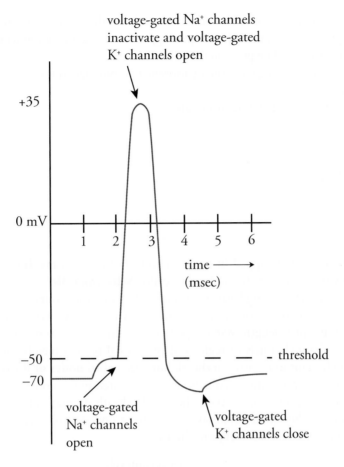

Figure 3 The Action Potential at a Single Location

After depolarization, the membrane is **repolarized**, re-establishing the original resting membrane potential. A number of factors combine to produce this effect:

1) Voltage-gated sodium channels **inactivate** very quickly after they open, shutting off the flow of sodium into the cell. The channels remain inactivated until the membrane potential nears resting values again.

2) Voltage-gated potassium channels open more slowly than the voltage-gated sodium channels and stay open longer. Voltage-gated potassium channels open in response to membrane depolarization. As potassium leaves the cell down its concentration gradient, the membrane potential returns to negative values, actually overshooting the resting potential by about 20 mV (to about −90 mV). At this point the voltage-gated potassium channels close.

3) Potassium leak channels and the Na^+/K^+ ATPase continue to function (as they always do) to bring the membrane back to resting potential. These factors alone would repolarize the membrane potential even without the voltage-gated potassium channels, but it would take a lot longer.

- If a neuron were stimulated to fire an action potential in the presence of a toxin that prevents voltage-gated potassium channels from opening, which of the following will occur?[9]
    - I. Depolarization will be prevented.
    - II. It will take much longer for the membrane to repolarize to the normal resting membrane potential.
    - III. The Na⁺/K⁺ ATPase will be inactivated.

    A) I only
    B) II only
    C) I and II only
    D) II and III only

Saltatory Conduction

The axons of many neurons are wrapped in an insulating sheath called **myelin** (Figure 4). The myelin sheath is not created by the neuron itself, but by cells called **Schwann cells**[10], a type of glial cell, that exist in conjunction with neurons, wrapping layers of specialized membrane around the axons. No ions can enter or exit a neuron where the axonal membrane is covered with myelin. [Would an axon be able to conduct action potentials if its entire length were wrapped in myelin?[11]] There is no membrane depolarization and no voltage-gated sodium channels in regions of the axonal plasma membrane that are wrapped in myelin. There are periodic gaps in the myelin sheath however, called **nodes of Ranvier** (Figures 1, 4, and 5). Voltage-gated sodium and potassium channels are concentrated in the nodes of Ranvier in myelinated axons. Rather than impeding action potentials, the myelin sheath dramatically speeds the movement of action potentials by forcing the action potential to jump from node to node. This rapid jumping conduction in myelinated axons is termed **saltatory conduction**.

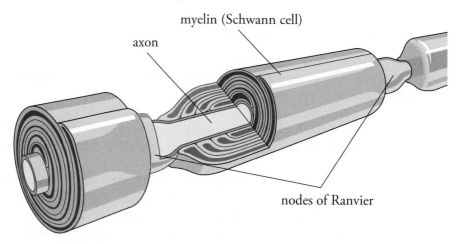

Figure 4   A Schwann Cell Wrapping an Axon with Myelin

---

[9] Item I is false: Depolarization is caused by the opening of voltage-gated Na⁺ channels; since these channels are not affected, depolarization should occur normally. **Item II is true:** The opening of voltage-gated K⁺ channels allows K⁺ ions to flow out of the cell, quickly repolarizing it. If these channels could not open, repolarization would take much longer, as it would rely on the inactivation of voltage-gated Na⁺ channels and the work of the Na⁺/K⁺ ATPase. Item III is false: The Na⁺/K⁺ ATPase will work harder than ever. The answer is choice **B**.

[10] Schwann cells are found in the peripheral nervous system (PNS). In the central nervous system (CNS), myelination of axons is accomplished via similar cells called oligodendrocytes.

[11] No. The action potential requires the movement of ions across the plasma membrane to create a wave of depolarization.

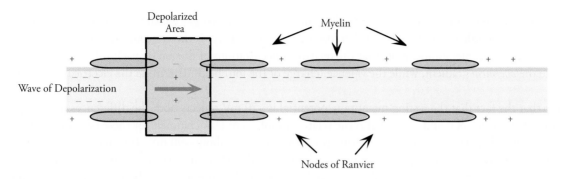

Figure 5 Propagation of the AP in a Myelinated Axon (cross section)

Glial Cells

As mentioned before, the myelin sheath is formed by a type of glial cell called a Schwann cell. However, Schwann cells are not the only type of glial cell. **Glial cells** are specialized, non-neuronal cells that typically provide structural and metabolic support to neurons (Table 1). Glia maintain a resting membrane potential but do not generate action potentials.

Cell Type	Location	Primary Functions
Schwann cells	PNS	Form myelin—increase speed of conduction of APs along axon
Oligodendrocytes	CNS	Form myelin—increase speed of conduction of APs along axon
Astrocytes	CNS	Guide neuronal development Regulate synaptic communication via regulation of neurotransmitter levels
Microglia	CNS	Remove dead cells and debris
Ependymal cells	CNS	Produce and circulate cerebrospinal fluid

Table 1 Types of Glial Cells and Their Functions

Equilibrium Potentials

During the action potential, the movement of Na⁺ and K⁺ ions across the membrane through the voltage-gated channels is *passive*; driven by gradients. The **equilibrium potential** is the membrane potential at which this driving force (the gradient) does not exist; in other words, there would be no net movement of ions across the membrane.

The equilibrium potential for any ion is based on the electrochemical gradient for that ion across the membrane, and it can be predicted by the **Nernst equation**:

$$E_{ion} = \frac{RT}{zF} \ln \frac{[X]_{outside}}{[X]_{inside}}$$

where E_{ion} is the equilibrium potential for the ion, R is the universal gas constant, T is the temperature (in Kelvin), z is the valence of the ion, F is Faraday's constant, and [X] is the concentration of the ion on each side of the plasma membrane. Note that the relative concentrations of the ion on each side of the membrane create the *chemical* gradient, while the valence (charge of the ion) helps determine the electrical gradient.

Note that the fact that the resting membrane potential is –70 mV reflects both the differences in the equilibrium potentials for Na⁺ and K⁺, and also the relative numbers of leak channels for these two ions. If the cell were completely permeable to K⁺, the resting potential would be about –90 mV. The fact that the resting potential is *very close* to the K⁺ equilibrium potential indicates that there are a large number of K⁺ leak channels in the membrane; the cell at rest is almost completely permeable to potassium. However, the resting potential is slightly more positive than –90 mV, indicating that there are a few Na⁺ leak channels allowing Na⁺ in. Not very many Na⁺ leak channels, though, or the resting potential would be much more positive; closer to the Na⁺ equilibrium potential. (This is in fact what we see when the cell *does* become completely permeable to Na⁺ at the beginning of the action potential; the membrane potential shoots upward to +35 mV.)

The Refractory Period

Action potentials can pass through a neuron extremely rapidly, thousands each second, but there is an upper limit to how soon a neuron can conduct an action potential after another has passed. The passage of one action potential makes the neuron nonresponsive to membrane depolarization and unable to transmit another action potential, or **refractory**, for a short period of time. There are two phases of the refractory period, caused by two different factors. During the **absolute refractory period**, a neuron will not fire another action potential no matter how strong a membrane depolarization is induced. During this time, the voltage-gated sodium channels have been *inactivated* (not the same as *closed*) after depolarization. They will not be able to be opened again until the membrane potential reaches the resting potential and the Na⁺ channels have returned to their "closed" state. During the **relative refractory period**, a neuron can be induced to transmit an action potential, but the depolarization required is greater than normal because the membrane is **hyperpolarized**. When repolarization occurs, there is a brief period in which the membrane potential is more negative than the resting potential (Figure 3) caused by voltage-gated potassium channels that have not closed yet. Because it is further from threshold, a greater stimulus is required to open the voltage-gated sodium channels to start an action potential.

15.2   SYNAPTIC TRANSMISSION

A **synapse** is a junction between the axon terminus of a neuron and the dendrites, soma, or axon of a second neuron. It can also be a junction between the axon terminus of a neuron and an organ. There are two types of synapses: electrical and chemical. **Electrical synapses** occur when the cytoplasms of two cells are joined by gap junctions. If two cells are joined by an electrical synapse, an action potential will spread directly from one cell to the other. Electrical synapses are not common in the nervous system, although they are quite important in propagating action potentials in smooth muscle and cardiac muscle. In the nervous system, **chemical synapses** are found at the ends of axons where they meet their target cell; here, an action potential is converted into a chemical signal. The following steps are involved in the transmission of a signal across a chemical synapse in the nervous system (Figure 6), as well as at the junctions of neurons with other cell types, such as skeletal muscle cells:

1) An action potential reaches the end of an axon, the synaptic knob.
2) Depolarization of the presynaptic membrane opens voltage-gated calcium channels.
3) Calcium influx into the presynaptic cell causes exocytosis of neurotransmitter stored in secretory vesicles.
4) Neurotransmitter molecules diffuse across the narrow synaptic cleft (small space between cells).
5) Neurotransmitter binds to receptor proteins in the postsynaptic membrane. These receptors are ligand-gated ion channels.
6) The opening of these ion channels in the postsynaptic cell alters the membrane polarization.
7) If the membrane depolarization of the postsynaptic cell reaches the threshold of voltage-gated sodium channels, an action potential is initiated.
8) Neurotransmitter in the synaptic cleft is degraded and/or removed to terminate the signal.

Presynaptic Neuron
1. Voltage-gated calcium channels open
2. Influx of calcium
3. Exocytosis of secretory vesicle
4. Release of neurotransmitter into synaptic cleft

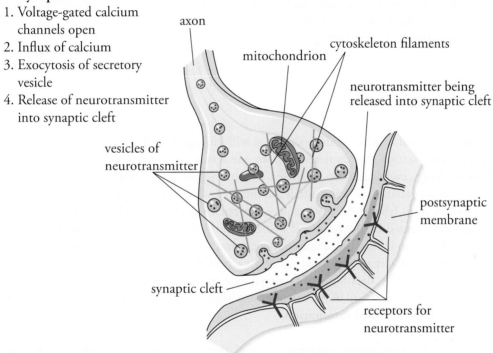

Postsynaptic Neuron
1. Neurotransmitter binds to ligand-gated ion channel.
2. Ions enter postsynaptic cell.
3. Membrane polarization is increased or decreased.

Figure 6   A Typical Synapse

There are several different neurotransmitters and neurotransmitter receptors. Some of the other neurotransmitters are **gamma-aminobutyric acid (GABA)**, **serotonin**, **dopamine**, and **norepinephrine**. If a neurotransmitter, such as acetylcholine, opens a channel that depolarizes the postsynaptic membrane, the neurotransmitter is termed **excitatory**. Other neurotransmitters, however, have the opposite effect, making the postsynaptic membrane potential more negative than the resting potential, or hyperpolarized.

Neurotransmitters that induce hyperpolarization of the postsynaptic membrane are termed **inhibitory**. (Note, however, that ultimately it is not the *neurotransmitter* that determines the effect on the postsynaptic cell, it is the *receptor* for that neurotransmitter and its associated ion channel. The same neurotransmitter can be excitatory in some cases and inhibitory in others.) Each presynaptic neuron can release only one type of neurotransmitter, although a postsynaptic neuron may respond to many different neurotransmitters.

- If a neurotransmitter causes the entry of chloride into the postsynaptic cell, is the neurotransmitter excitatory or inhibitory?[12]

- If an inhibitor of acetylcholinesterase is added to a neuromuscular junction, then the postsynaptic membrane will:[13]
    A) be depolarized by action potentials more frequently.
    B) be depolarized longer with each action potential.
    C) be resistant to depolarization.
    D) spontaneously depolarize.

Summation

Once an action potential is initiated in a neuron, it will propagate to the end of the axon at a speed and magnitude of depolarization that do not vary from one action potential to another. The action potential is an "**all-or-nothing**" event. The key regulated step in the nervous system is whether or not a neuron will fire an action potential. Action potentials are initiated when the postsynaptic membrane reaches the threshold depolarization (about -50 mV) required to open voltage-gated sodium channels. The postsynaptic depolarization caused by the release of neurotransmitter by one action potential at one synapse is not generally sufficient to induce this degree of depolarization. A postsynaptic neuron has many different neurons with synapses leading to it, however, and each of these synapses can release neurotransmitter many times per second. The "decision" by a postsynaptic neuron whether to fire an action potential is determined by adding the effect of all of the synapses impinging on a neuron, both excitatory and inhibitory. This addition of stimuli is termed **summation**.

Excitatory neurotransmitters cause postsynaptic depolarization, or **excitatory postsynaptic potentials** (**EPSPs**), while inhibitory neurotransmitters cause **inhibitory postsynaptic potentials** (**IPSPs**). One form of summation is **temporal summation**, in which a presynaptic neuron fires action potentials so rapidly that the EPSPs or IPSPs pile up on top of each other. If they are EPSPs, the additive effect might be enough to reach the threshold depolarization required to start a postsynaptic action potential. If they are IPSPs, the postsynaptic cell will hyperpolarize, moving further and further away from threshold, effectively becoming inhibited. The other form of summation is **spatial summation**, in which the EPSPs and IPSPs from all of the synapses on the postsynaptic membrane are summed at a given moment in time. If the total of all EPSPs and IPSPs causes the postsynaptic membrane to reach the threshold voltage, an action potential will be fired.

---

[12] Chloride ions are negatively charged. The entry of chloride ions into the cell will make the postsynaptic potential more negative, or hyperpolarized, so the neurotransmitter is inhibitory.

[13] Choice **B** is the correct answer. If acetylcholinesterase is inhibited, acetylcholine will remain in the synaptic cleft longer, and acetylcholine-gated sodium channels will remain open longer with each action potential that reaches the synapse. If the sodium channels are open longer, the depolarization of the postsynaptic membrane will last longer.

- In which one of the following ways can a presynaptic neuron increase the intensity of signal it transmits?[14]
  - A) Increase the size of presynaptic action potentials
  - B) Increase the frequency of action potentials
  - C) Change the type of neurotransmitter it releases
  - D) Change the speed of action potential propagation

15.3 FUNCTIONAL ORGANIZATION OF THE HUMAN NERVOUS SYSTEM

The nervous system must receive information, decide what to do with it, and cause muscles or glands to act upon that decision. Receiving information is the **sensory** function of the nervous system (carried out by the peripheral nervous system, or **PNS**), processing the information is the **integrative** function (carried out by the central nervous system, or **CNS**), and acting on it is the **motor** function (also carried out by the PNS).[15] **Motor neurons** carry information from the nervous system toward organs that can act upon that information, known as **effectors**. [What are the two categories of effector organs?[16]] Notice that "motor" neurons do not lead only "to muscle." Motor neurons, which carry information away from the central nervous system and innervate effectors, are called **efferent** neurons (remember, efferents go to effectors). **Sensory neurons**, which carry information toward the central nervous system, are called **afferent** neurons.

Reflexes

The simplest example of nervous system activity is the **reflex**. This is a direct motor response to sensory input which occurs without conscious thought. In fact, it usually occurs without any involvement of the brain at all. In the simplest example, a sensory neuron transmits an action potential to a synapse with a motor neuron in the spinal cord, which causes an action to occur. For example, in the **muscle stretch reflex**, a sensory neuron detects stretching of a muscle (Figure 7). The sensory neuron has a long dendrite and a long axon, which transmits an impulse to a motor neuron cell body in the spinal cord. The motor neuron's long axon synapses with the muscle that was stretched and causes it to contract. That is why the quadriceps (thigh) muscle contracts when the patellar tendon is stretched by tapping with a reflex hammer. A reflex such as this one, involving only two neurons and one synapse, is known as a **monosynaptic reflex arc.**

Something else also happens when a physician taps the patellar tendon. Not only does the quadriceps

---

[14] A neuron cannot change the size of action potentials it transmits, but it can increase the *number* of action potentials it transmits in a given amount of time (the *frequency* of action potentials). The increased frequency of action potentials will add up through temporal summation in the postsynaptic cell to produce an increased response (choice **B** is correct). Action potentials are all-or-nothing once they are started. The magnitude of membrane depolarization during propagation of the action potential does not change (choice A is wrong). A neuron can release only one type of neurotransmitter and does not change this (choice C is wrong), and the speed of propagation cannot be varied from one action potential to the next (choice D is wrong).

[15] More detailed information about the anatomy and functions of the CNS and PNS will be presented later in this chapter.

[16] Muscles and glands

contract, but the hamstring also *relaxes*. If it did not, the leg would not be able to extend (straighten). The sensory neuron (that detects stretch) synapses with not only a motor neuron for the quadriceps, but also with an **inhibitory interneuron**. This is a short neuron which forms an inhibitory synapse with a motor neuron innervating the hamstring muscle. When the sensory neuron is stimulated by stretch, it stimulates both the quadriceps motor neuron and the inhibitory interneuron to the hamstring motor neuron. As a result, the quadriceps contracts and the hamstring relaxes. An interneuron is the simplest example of the integrative role of the nervous system. Concurrent relaxation of the hamstring and contraction of the quadriceps is an example of **reciprocal inhibition**.

- If a reflex occurs without the involvement of the brain, how are we aware of the action?[17]

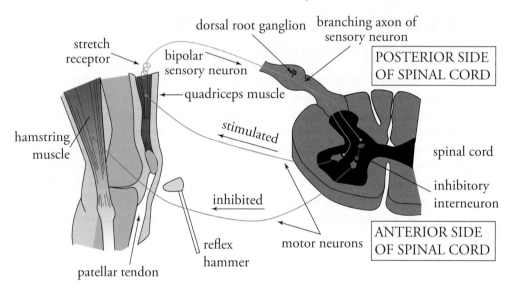

Figure 7 The Muscle Stretch Reflex

Large-Scale Functional Organization

The peripheral nervous system can be subdivided into several functional divisions (Figure 8). The portion of this system concerned with conscious sensation and deliberate, voluntary movement of **skeletal muscle** is the **somatic** division. The portion concerned with digestion, metabolism, circulation, perspiration, and other involuntary processes is the **autonomic** division. The somatic and autonomic divisions both include afferent and efferent functions, although the sources of sensory input and the target of efferent nerves are different. The efferent portion of the autonomic division is further split into two subdivisions: **sympathetic** and **parasympathetic**. When the sympathetic system is activated, the body is prepared for "fight or flight." When the parasympathetic system is activated, the body is prepared to "rest and digest." Table 2 summarizes the main effects of the autonomic system. Notice that many sympathetic effects result from release of epinephrine into the bloodstream by the adrenal medulla. The parasympathetic system prepares you to rest and digest food.

---

[17] Two ways: First, the sensory neuron also branches to form a synapse with a neuron leading to the brain. Second, other sensory information is received after the action is taken.

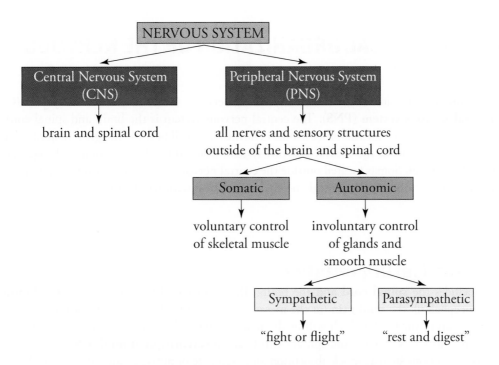

Figure 8 Overall Organization of the Nervous System

Organ or System	Parasympathetic: rest and digest	Sympathetic: fight or flight
digestive system: glands	stimulation	inhibition
motility	stimulation (stimulates digestion)	inhibition (inhibits digestion)
sphincters	relaxation	contraction
urinary system: bladder	contraction (stimulates urination)	relaxation (inhibits urination)
urethral sphincter	relaxation (stimulates urination)	contraction (inhibits urination)
bronchial smooth muscle	constriction (closes airways)	relaxation (opens airways)
cardiovascular system		
heart rate and contractility	decreased	increased
blood flow to skeletal muscle	—	increased
skin	—	sweating and general vasoconstriction
eye: pupil	constriction	dilation
muscles controlling lens	accommodation for near vision	accommodation for far vision
adrenal medulla	—	release of epinephrine
genitals	erection / lubrication	ejaculation / orgasm

Table 2 Effects of the Autonomic Nervous System

15.4 ANATOMICAL ORGANIZATION OF THE NERVOUS SYSTEM

The main anatomical division of the nervous system is between the **central nervous system** (**CNS**) and the **peripheral nervous system** (**PNS**). The central nervous system is the brain and spinal cord. The peripheral nervous system includes all other axons, dendrites, and cell bodies. The great majority of neuronal cell bodies are found within the central nervous system. Sometimes they are bunched together to form structures called **nuclei.** Somas located outside the central nervous system are found in bunches known as **ganglia**. The anatomy of both the central and the peripheral system will be presented.

CNS Anatomical Organization

The CNS includes the **spinal cord** and the brain. The brain has three subdivisions: the **hindbrain** (or the rhombencephalon), the **midbrain** (or the mesencephalon), and the **forebrain** (or the prosencephalon). These four regions of the CNS (which will be discussed individually below) perform increasingly complex functions. The entire CNS (brain and spinal cord) floats in **cerebrospinal fluid** (**CSF**), a clear liquid that serves various functions such as shock absorption and exchange of nutrients and waste with the CNS.

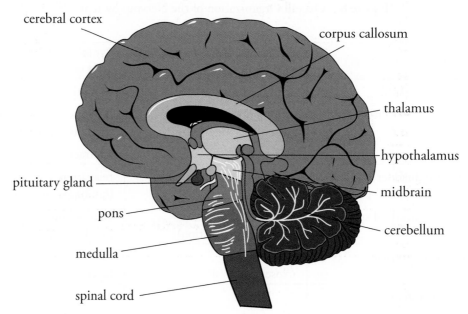

Figure 9   Organization of the CNS (cross-section of the brain)

1) The spinal cord is connected to the brain and is protected by the CSF and the vertebral column. It is a pathway for information to and from the brain. Most sensory data is relayed to the brain for integration, but the spinal cord is also a site for information integration and processing. The spinal cord is responsible for simple spinal reflexes (like the muscle stretch reflex) and is also involved in primitive processes such as walking, urination, and sex organ function.

2) The hindbrain includes the medulla, the pons, and the cerebellum.
- The **medulla** (or medulla oblongata) is located below the pons and is the area of the brain that connects to the spinal cord. It functions in relaying information between other areas of the brain, and it regulates vital autonomic functions such as blood pressure and digestive functions (including vomiting). Also, the respiratory rhythmicity centers are found here.
- The **pons** is located below the midbrain and above the medulla oblongata. It is the connection point between the brain stem and the cerebellum (see below). The pons controls some autonomic functions and coordinates movement; it plays a role in balance and antigravity posture.
- The **cerebellum** (or "little brain") is located behind the pons and below the cerebral hemispheres. It is an integrating center where complex movements are coordinated. An instruction for movement from the forebrain must be sent to the cerebellum, where the billions of decisions necessary for smooth execution of the movement are made. Damage to the cerebellum results in poor hand-eye coordination and balance. Both the cerebellum and the pons receive information from the vestibular apparatus in the inner ear, which monitors acceleration and position relative to gravity.

3) The midbrain is a relay for visual and auditory information and contains much of the reticular activating system (RAS), which is responsible for arousal or wakefulness.

Another term you should be familiar with is **brainstem**. Together, the medulla, pons, and midbrain constitute the brainstem, which contains important processing centers and relays information to or from the cerebellum and cerebrum.

4) The forebrain includes the **diencephalon** and the **telencephalon**.
  a) The diencephalon includes the thalamus and hypothalamus:
- The thalamus is located near the middle of the brain below the cerebral hemispheres and above the midbrain. It contains relay and processing centers for sensory information.
- The hypothalamus interacts directly with many parts of the brain. It contains centers for controlling emotions and autonomic functions, and it has a major role in hormone production and release. It is the primary link between the nervous and the endocrine systems, and by controlling the pituitary gland is the fundamental control center for the endocrine system (discussed later in this chapter).
  b) All parts of the CNS up to and including the diencephalon form a single symmetrical stalk, but the telencephalon consists of two separate cerebral hemispheres. Generally speaking, the areas of the left and right hemispheres have the same functions. However, the left hemisphere primarily controls the motor functions of the right side of the body, and the right hemisphere controls those of the left side. Also, in most people, the left side of the brain is said to be dominant. It is generally responsible for speech. The right hemisphere is more concerned with visual-spatial reasoning and music.
- The **cerebral hemispheres** are connected by a thick bundle of axons called the **corpus callosum**. A person with a cut corpus callosum has two independent cerebral cortices and to a certain extent two independent minds!
- The **cerebrum** is the largest region of the human brain and consists of the large, paired cerebral hemispheres. The hemispheres of the cerebrum consist of the **cerebral cortex** (an outer layer of gray matter) plus an inner core of white matter connecting the cortex to the diencephalon. The gray matter is composed of trillions of somas; the white matter is composed of myelinated axons. (Most axons in the CNS and PNS are myelinated.) The cerebral hemispheres are responsible for conscious thought processes and

intellectual functions. They also play a role in processing somatic sensory and motor information. The cerebral cortex is divided into four pairs of lobes, each of which is devoted to specific functions:

i) the **frontal lobes** initiate all voluntary movement and are involved in complex reasoning skills and problem solving.

ii) the **parietal lobes** are involved in general sensations (such as touch, temperature, pressure, vibration, etc.) and in gustation (taste).

iii) the **temporal lobes** process auditory and olfactory sensation and are involved in short-term memory, language comprehension, and emotion.

iv) the **occipital lobes** process visual sensation.

Figure 10 shows some of the more important cortical areas.

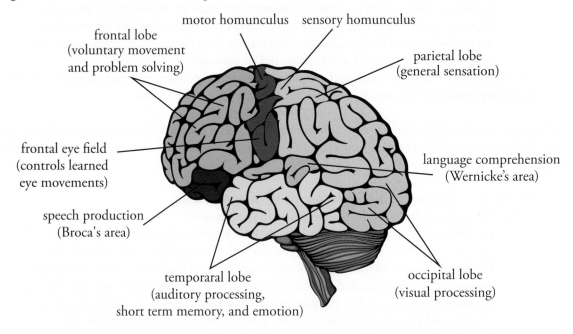

Figure 10   Principal Areas of the Cerebral Cortex

Two last regions of the brain deserve mention:

- The **basal nuclei** (also called the "cerebral nuclei" and previously known as the basal ganglia) are composed of gray matter and are located deep within the cerebral hemispheres. They include several functional subdivisions, but broadly function in voluntary motor control and procedural learning related to habits. The basal nuclei and cerebellum work together to process and coordinate movement initiated by the primary motor cortex; the basal nuclei are inhibitory (preventing excess movement), while the cerebellum is excitatory.

- The **limbic system** is located between the cerebrum and the diencephalon. It includes several substructures (such as the amygdala, the cingulate gyrus, and the hippocampus) and works closely with parts of the cerebrum, diencephalon, and midbrain. The limbic system is important in emotion and memory.

The information above describes the general functions of each region of the brain. Table 3 summarizes the brain functions and provides a little more specific detail for each region.

Structure	General Function	Specific Functions
Spinal cord	Simple reflexes	• controls simple stretch and tendon reflexes • controls primitive processes such as walking, urination, and sex organ function
Medulla	Involuntary functions	• controls autonomic processes such as blood pressure, blood flow, heart rate, respiratory rate, swallowing, vomiting • controls reflex reactions such as coughing or sneezing • relays sensory information to the cerebellum and the thalamus
Pons	Relay station and balance	• controls antigravity posture and balance • connects spinal cord and medulla with upper regions of brain • relays information to the cerebellum and thalamus
Cerebellum	Movement coordination	• integrating center • coordination of complex movement, balance and posture, muscle tone, spatial equilibrium
Midbrain	Eye movement	• integration of visual and auditory information • visual and auditory reflexes • wakefulness and consciousness • coordinates information on posture and muscle tone
Thalamus	Integrating center and relay station	• relay center for somatic (conscious) sensation • relays information between spinal cord and cerebral cortex
Hypo-thalamus	Homeostasis and behavior	• controls homeostatic functions (such as temperature regulation, fluid balance, appetite) through both neural and hormonal regulation • controls primitive emotions such as anger, rage, and sex drive • controls the pituitary gland
Basal nuclei	Movement	• regulate body movement and muscle tone • coordination of learned movement patterns • general pattern of rhythmic movements (such as controlling the cycle of arm and leg movements when walking) • subconscious adjustments of conscious movements
Limbic system	Emotion, memory, and learning	• controls emotional states • links conscious and unconscious portions of the brain • helps with memory storage and retrieval

15.4

Structure	General Function	Specific Functions
Cerebral cortex	Perception, skeletal muscle movement, memory, attention, thought, language, and consciousness	• divided into four lobes (frontal, parietal, temporal, and occipital) with specialized subfunctions • perception and processing of the special senses (vision, hearing, smell, taste, touch) • conscious thought processes and planning, awareness, and sensation • intellectual function (intelligence, learning, reading, communication) • abstract thought and reasoning • memory storage and retrieval • initiation and coordination of voluntary movement • complex motor patterns • language (speech production and understanding) • personality
Corpus callosum	Connection	• connects the left and right cerebral hemispheres

Table 3 Summary of Brain Functions

The motor and sensory regions of the cortex are organized such that a particular small area of cortex controls a particular body part. A larger area is devoted to a body part which requires more motor control or more sensation (Figure 11). For example, more cortex is devoted to the lips than to the entire leg. The body parts represented on the cortex can be sketched. The drawing looks like a distorted person, known as a **homunculus** (little man).

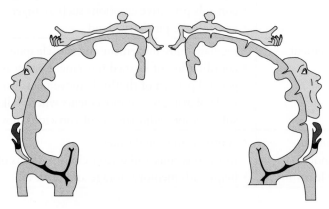

Figure 11 The Sensory Homunculus

Neurotransmitters

Neurotransmitters can generally be divided into excitatory transmitters, which increase the likelihood of the postsynaptic neuron firing, and inhibitory neurotransmitters, which decrease the likelihood of firing. Although, be careful! The actual function of each neurotransmitter varies widely based on the part of the nervous system or part of the brain where it is active, and how it interacts with other neurotransmitters.

Neurotransmitter	Primary Functions
Dopamine	• Reward, mood, pleasure, smooth motor movements, focus and attention • Shortages can lead to depression, lethargy, and difficulty coordinating motion
Serotonin	• Mood, digestion, sleep, memory, sexual desire • Shortages can lead to aggression, compulsive behavior, overeating, and depression
Melatonin	• Circadian rhythm, sleepiness, sleep initiation (melatonin is technically a "neurotransmitter-like substance") • Shortages can lead to insomnia
Gamma Aminobutyric Acid (GABA)	• Primary inhibitory neurotransmitter in the brain • Shortages can lead to stress and anxiety, depression, ADHD, Panic Disorders, and a host of other disorders
Acetylcholine	• Excitation at neuromuscular junction, parasympathetic nervous system activity • Shortages can lead to dysfunction of the GI tract and paralysis
Epinephrine (adrenaline) and norepinephrine (noradrenaline)	• Two similar molecules both involved in fight or flight response, sympathetic nervous system activation (both are hormones and neurotransmitters) • Shortages can lead to fatigue, lack of focus, apathy
Glutamate	• Primary excitatory neurotransmitter in the brain, learning, memory, long-term potentiation • Shortages can lead to fatigue, low concentration and energy

Table 4   Summary of Neurotransmitters

PNS Anatomical Organization

All neurons entering and exiting the CNS are carried by 12 pairs of **cranial nerves** and 31 pairs of **spinal nerves**. Cranial nerves convey sensory and motor information to and from the brainstem. Spinal nerves convey sensory and motor information to and from the spinal cord. The different functional divisions of the nervous system have different anatomical organizations (Figure 12).

The **vagus nerve** is an important example of a cranial nerve, and one that you should be familiar with for the MCAT. The effects of this nerve upon the heart and GI tract are to decrease the heart rate and increase GI activity; as such it is part of the *parasympathetic division* of the autonomic nervous system. It is a bundle of axons that end in ganglia on the surface of the heart, stomach, and other visceral organs. The many axons constituting the vagus nerve are preganglionic and come from cell bodies located in the CNS. On the surface of the heart and stomach they synapse with postganglionic neurons. The detailed terminology in this paragraph will make more sense to you as you read through the next couple of sections.

Somatic PNS Anatomy

The somatic system has a simple organization:

- *All* somatic motor neurons innervate skeletal muscle cells, use ACh as their neurotransmitter, and have their cell bodies in the brain stem or the ventral (front) portion of the spinal cord.

- *All* somatic sensory neurons have a long dendrite extending from a sensory receptor toward the soma, which is located just outside the CNS in a **dorsal root ganglion**. The dorsal root ganglion is a bunch of somatic (and autonomic) sensory neuron cell bodies located just dorsal to (to the back of) the spinal cord. There is a pair of dorsal root ganglia for every segment of the spinal cord, and thus the dorsal root ganglia form a chain along the dorsal (back) aspect of the vertebral column. The dorsal root ganglia are protected within the vertebral column but are outside the **meninges** (protective sheath of the brain and cord) and thus outside the CNS. An axon extends from the somatic sensory neuron's soma into the spinal cord. In all somatic sensory neurons, the first synapse is in the CNS; depending on the type of sensory information conveyed, the axon either synapses in the cord, or stretches all the way up to the brain stem before its first synapse!

Autonomic PNS Anatomy

Anatomical organization of autonomic efferents is a bit more complex.[18] The efferents of the sympathetic and parasympathetic systems consist of two neurons: a preganglionic and a postganglionic neuron. The **preganglionic neuron** has its cell body in the brainstem or spinal cord. It sends an axon to an autonomic ganglion, located outside the spinal column. In the ganglion, this axon synapses with a **postganglionic neuron**. The postganglionic neuron sends an axon to an effector (smooth muscle or gland). *All* autonomic preganglionic neurons release acetylcholine as their neurotransmitter. *All* parasympathetic postganglionic neurons also release acetylcholine. Nearly all sympathetic postganglionic neurons release norepinephrine (NE, also known as noradrenaline) as their neurotransmitter.

---

[18] The anatomy of autonomic sensory neurons (afferents) is poorly defined and will not be on the MCAT.

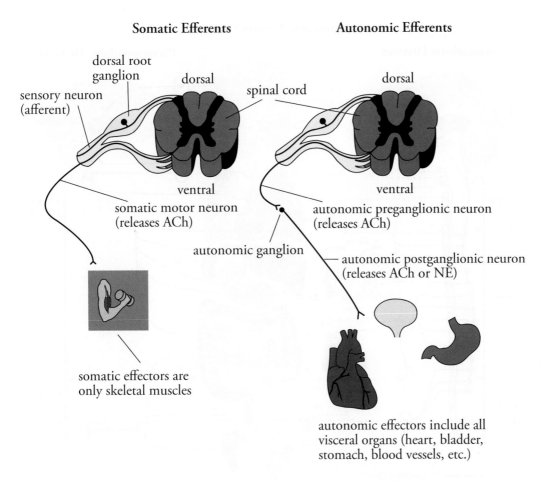

Somatic Efferents

Autonomic Efferents

Figure 12   Anatomical Organization of PNS Efferents

All sympathetic preganglionic efferent neurons have their cell bodies in the thoracic (chest) or lumbar (lower back) regions of the spinal cord. Hence, the sympathetic system is also referred to as the *thoracolumbar system*. The parasympathetic system is known as the *craniosacral system*, because all of its preganglionic neurons have cell bodies in the brainstem (which is in the head or cranium) or in the lowest portion of the spinal cord, the sacral portion. In the sympathetic system, the preganglionic axon is relatively short, and there are only a few ganglia; these sympathetic ganglia are quite large. The sympathetic postganglionic cell sends a long axon to the effector. In contrast, the parasympathetic preganglionic neuron sends a long axon to a small ganglion which is close to the effector. For example, parasympathetic ganglia controlling the intestines are located on the outer wall of the gut. The parasympathetic postganglionic neuron has a very short axon, since the cell body is close to the target. These differences are visualized in Figure 13 and summarized in Table 5.

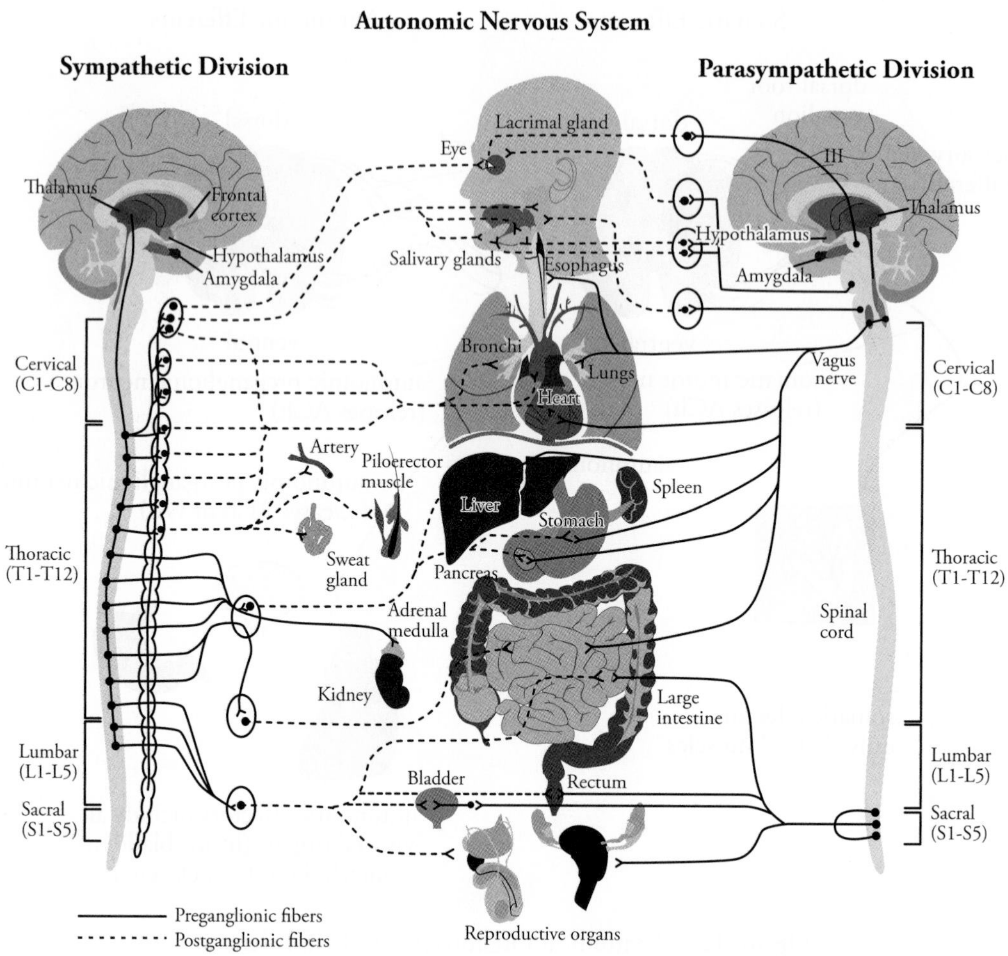

Autonomic Nervous System

Figure 13 Pre- and Post-Ganglionic Fibers of the Autonomic Nervous System

The autonomic afferent (sensory) neurons are similar to the somatic afferent neurons with one exception: they can synapse in the PNS (at the autonomic ganglia) with autonomic efferent neurons in what is known as a "short reflex." (Recall that the first synapse of somatic afferent neurons is in the CNS.)

	Sympathetic	Parasympathetic
General function	fight or flight, mobilize energy	rest and digest, store energy
Location of preganglionic soma	thoracolumbar = thoracic and lumbar spinal cord	craniosacral = brainstem ("cranial") and sacral spinal cord
Preganglionic axon neurotransmitter = acetylcholine (ACh)	short	long
Ganglia	close to cord, far from target	far from cord, close to target
Postganglionic axon (usual neurotransmitter)	long (norepinephrine [NE])	short (acetylcholine [ACh])

Table 5 Sympathetic vs. Parasympathetic

The Adrenal Medulla

The **adrenal gland** is named for its location: "Ad-" connotes "above," and "renal" refers to the kidney. There are two adrenal glands, one above each kidney. The adrenal has an inner portion known as the **medulla** and an outer portion known as the **cortex**. The cortex is an important endocrine gland, secreting **glucocorticoids** (the main one is cortisol), **mineralocorticoids** (the main one is aldosterone), and some sex hormones.

The adrenal medulla, however, is part of the sympathetic nervous system. It is embryologically derived from sympathetic postganglionic neurons and is directly innervated by sympathetic preganglionic neurons. Upon activation of the sympathetic system, the adrenal gland is stimulated to release **epinephrine**, also known as **adrenaline**. Epinephrine is a slightly modified version of *nor*epinephrine, the neurotransmitter released by sympathetic postganglionic neurons. Epinephrine is a hormone because it is released into the bloodstream by a ductless gland. But in many ways it behaves like a neurotransmitter. It elicits its effects very rapidly, and the effects are quite short-lived. Ongoing release of epinephrine from the adrenal medulla during fight-or-flight situations prolongs and enhances the effects of the sympathetic neurons. In general, epinephrine's effects are those listed in Table 5 for the sympathetic system. Stimulation of the heart is an especially important effect.

15.5   SENSATION AND PERCEPTION

Sensation is the process by which we receive information from the world around us. Sensory receptors detect data, both internally (from within the body) and externally (from the environment), and send this information to the central nervous system for processing. Sensation is the act of receiving information, while perception is the act of organizing, assimilating, and interpreting the sensory input into useful and meaningful information.

Types of Sensory Receptors

Sensory receptors are designed to detect one type of stimulus from either the interior of the body or the external environment. Each sensory receptor receives only one kind of information and transmits that information to sensory neurons, which can in turn convey it to the central nervous system. Sensory receptors that detect stimuli from the outside world are **exteroceptors** and receptors that respond to internal stimuli are **interoceptors**. A more important distinction between sensory receptors is based on the type of stimulus they detect. The types of sensory receptors are listed below.

1) **Mechanoreceptors** respond to mechanical disturbances. For example, **Pacinian corpuscles** are pressure sensors located deep in the skin. Another important mechanoreceptor is the **auditory hair cell**. This is a specialized cell found in the cochlea of the inner ear. It detects vibrations caused by sound waves.

2) **Chemoreceptors** respond to particular chemicals. For example, **olfactory receptors** detect airborne chemicals and allow us to smell things. Taste buds are **gustatory receptors**. Autonomic chemoreceptors in the walls of the carotid and aortic arteries respond to changes in arterial pH, PCO_2, and PO_2 levels.

3) **Nociceptors** are pain receptors. They are stimulated by tissue injury. Nociceptors are the simplest type of sensory receptor, generally consisting of a free nerve ending that detects chemical signs of tissue damage.

4) **Thermoreceptors** are stimulated by changes in temperature. There are autonomic and somatic examples.

5) **Electromagnetic receptors** are stimulated by electromagnetic waves. In humans, the only examples are the rod and cone cells of the retina of the eye (also termed **photoreceptors**).

15.5

Encoding of Sensory Stimuli

All sensory receptors need to encode relevant information regarding the nature of the stimulus being detected. There are four properties that need to be communicated to the CNS:

1) Stimulus **modality** is the type of stimulus. As mentioned above, the CNS determines the stimulus modality based on which type of receptor is firing.

2) Stimulus **location** is communicated by the receptive field of the sensory receptor sending the signal. Localization of a stimulus can be improved by overlapping receptive fields of neighboring receptors. This works like a Venn diagram, and it allows the brain to localize a stimulus activating neighboring receptors to the area in which their receptive fields overlap. Discrimination between two separate stimuli can be improved by lateral inhibition of neighboring receptors.

3) Stimulus **intensity** is coded by the frequency of action potentials. The *dynamic range*, or range of intensities that can be detected by sensory receptors, can be expanded by range fractionation—including multiple groups of receptors with limited ranges to detect a wider range overall. One example of this phenomenon is human cone cells responding to different but overlapping ranges of wavelengths to detect the full visual spectrum of light.

4) Stimulus **duration** may or may not be coded explicitly. *Tonic receptors* fire action potentials as long as the stimulus continues. However, these receptors are subject to adaptation, and the frequency of action potentials decreases as the stimulus continues at the same level (see below). *Phasic receptors* only fire action potentials when the stimulus begins, and they do not explicitly communicate the duration of the stimulus. These receptors are important for communicating changes in stimuli, and essentially adapt immediately if a stimulus continues at the same level.

The ability to adapt to a stimulus is an important property of sensory receptors. This allows the brain to tune out unimportant information from the environment. **Adaptation** is a decrease in firing frequency when the intensity of a stimulus remains constant. For example, if you walk into a kitchen where someone is baking bread, the bread odor molecules stimulate your olfactory receptors to a great degree and you smell the bread baking. But if you remain in the kitchen for a few minutes, you stop smelling the bread; the continuous input to the olfactory receptors causes them to stop firing even though the odor molecules are still present.

Proprioceptors

This is a broad category including many different types of receptors. **Proprioception** refers to awareness of self (awareness of body part position). An important example of a proprioceptor is the **muscle spindle**, a mechanoreceptor. This is a sensory organ specialized to detect muscle stretch. You are already familiar with it because it is the receptor that senses muscle stretch in the deep tendon reflex. Other proprioceptors include **Golgi tendon organs**, which monitor tension in the tendons, and **joint capsule receptors**, which detect pressure, tension, and movement in the joints. By monitoring the activity of the musculoskeletal system, the proprioceptive component of the somatic sensory system allows us to know the positions of our body parts. This is most important during activity, when precise feedback is essential for coordinated motion. [What portion of the CNS would you expect to require input from proprioceptors?[19]]

Gustation and Olfaction

Taste and smell are senses that rely on chemoreceptors in the mouth and nasal passages. **Gustation** is taste, and **olfaction** is smell. Much of what is assumed to be taste is actually smell. (Try eating with a bad head cold.) In fact, taste receptors (known as **taste buds**) can only distinguish five flavors: sweet (glucose), salty (Na^+), bitter (basic), sour (acidic), and umami (amino acids and nucleotides). Each taste bud responds most strongly to one of these five stimuli. The taste bud is composed of a bunch of specialized epithelial cells, shaped roughly like an onion. In its center is a **taste pore**, with **taste hairs** that detect food chemicals. Information about taste is transmitted by cranial nerves to an area of the brain's temporal lobe not far from where the brain receives olfactory information.

Olfaction is accomplished by olfactory receptors in the roof of the **nasopharynx** (nasal cavity). The receptors detect airborne chemicals that dissolve in the mucus covering the nasal membrane. Humans can distinguish thousands of different smells. Olfactory nerves project directly to the **olfactory bulbs** of the brain. The olfactory bulbs are located in the temporal lobe of the brain near the limbic system, an area important for memory and emotion (which may explain why certain smells can bring back vivid memories and feelings).

Hearing and the Vestibular System

Structure of the Ear

The **auricle** or **pinna** and the external **auditory canal** comprise the **outer ear**. The **middle ear** is divided from the outer ear by the **tympanic membrane** or eardrum. The middle ear consists of the **ossicles**, three small bones called the **malleus** (hammer), the **incus** (anvil), and the **stapes** (stirrup). The stapes attaches to the **oval window**, a membrane that divides the middle and **inner ear**. Structures of the inner ear include the **cochlea**, the **semicircular canals**, the **utricle**, and the **saccule**. The semicircular canals together with the utricle and saccule are important to the sense of balance. The **round window** is a membrane-covered hole in the cochlea near the oval window. It releases excess pressure. The **Eustachian tube** (also known as the **auditory tube**) is a passageway from the back of the throat to the middle ear. It functions to equalize the pressure on both sides of the eardrum and is the cause of the "ear popping" one experiences at high altitudes or underwater.

---

[19] The cerebellum, which is responsible for motor coordination.

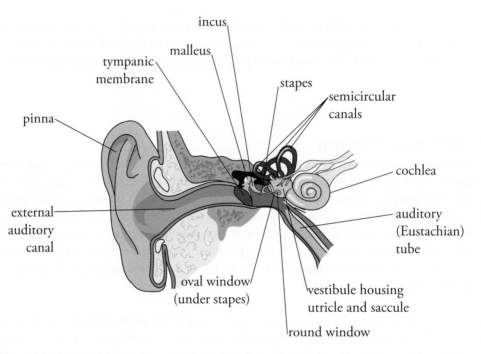

Figure 14 The Ear

Mechanism of Hearing

Sound waves enter the external ear to pass into the auditory canal, causing the eardrum to vibrate. The malleus attached to the eardrum receives the vibrations, which are passed on to the incus and then to the stapes. The bones of the middle ear are arranged in such a way that they amplify sound vibrations passing through the middle ear. The stapes is the innermost of the three middle-ear bones, contacting the oval window. Vibration of the oval window creates pressure waves in the **perilymph** and **endolymph**, the fluids in the cochlea. Note that sound vibrations are first conveyed through air, next through bone, and then through liquid before being sensed. The pressure waves in the endolymph cause vibration of the **basilar membrane**, a thin membrane extending throughout the coiled length of the cochlea. The basilar membrane is covered with the auditory receptor cells known as **hair cells**. These cells have **cilia** (hairs) projecting from their apical (top) surfaces (opposite the basilar membrane). The hairs contact the **tectorial membrane** (tectorial means "roof"), and when the basilar membrane moves, the hairs are dragged across the tectorial membrane and they bend. This displacement opens ion channels in the hair cells, which results in neurotransmitter release. Dendrites from bipolar auditory afferent neurons are stimulated by this neurotransmitter, and thus sound vibrations are converted to nerve impulses. The basilar membrane, hair cells, and tectorial membrane together are known as the **organ of Corti**. The outer ear and middle ear convey sound waves to the cochlea, and the organ of Corti in the cochlea is the primary site at which auditory stimuli are detected.

Summary: From Sound to Hearing

sound waves → auricle → external auditory canal → tympanic membrane → malleus → incus → stapes → oval window → perilymph → endolymph → basilar membrane → auditory hair cells → tectorial membrane → neurotransmitters stimulate bipolar auditory neurons → brain → perception

---

Pitch (frequency) of sound is distinguished by which *regions* of the basilar membrane vibrate, stimulating different auditory neurons. The basilar membrane is narrow, thick, and sturdy near the oval window and gradually becomes wider, thin, and floppy near the apex of the cochlea. Low frequency (long wavelength) sounds stimulate hair cells at the apex of the cochlear duct, farthest away from the oval window, while high-pitched sounds stimulate hair cells at the base of the cochlea, near the oval window. **Loudness** of sound is distinguished by the *amplitude* of vibration. Larger vibrations cause more frequent action potentials in auditory neurons.

Locating the source of sound is also an important adaptive function. Having two ears allows for stereophonic (or three-dimensional) hearing. The auditory system can determine the source of a sound based on the difference detected between the two ears. For example, if a horn blasts to your right, your right ear will receive the sound waves slightly sooner and slightly more intensely than your left ear. Sound stimuli are processed in the **auditory cortex**, located in the temporal lobe of the brain.

In humans, audition is highly adaptive. While we are able to hear a wide range of sounds, those sounds with frequencies within the range corresponding to the human voice are heard best, and we are able to differentiate variations among human voices. For example, when answering the phone, you will recognize your mom's voice within a fraction of a second.

- If a sensory neuron leading from the ear to the brain fires an action potential more rapidly, how will the brain perceive this change?[20]
- If the bones of the middle ear are unable to move, would this impair the detection of sound by conductance through bone?[21]

Equilibrium and Balance

The vestibular complex is made up of the three **semicircular canals**, the **utricle**, the **saccule**, and the **ampullae**. All are essentially tubes filled with endolymph, and like the cochlea, they contain hair cells that detect motion. However, their function is to detect not sound, but rather rotational acceleration of the head. They are innervated by afferent neurons which send balance information to the pons, cerebellum, and other areas. The vestibular complex monitors both static equilibrium and linear acceleration, which contribute to your sense of balance.

Vision: Structure and Function

The eye is the structure designed to detect visual stimuli. The structures of the eye first form an image on the retina, which detects light and converts the stimuli into action potentials to send to the brain. Light enters the eye by passing through the **cornea**, the clear portion at the front of the eye. Light is bent or **refracted** as it passes through the cornea (which is highly curved and thus acts as a lens), since the refractive index of the cornea is higher than that of air. The cornea is continuous at its borders with the white of the eye, the **sclera**. Beneath the sclera is a layer called the **choroid**. It contains darkly-pigmented cells;

---

[20] More rapid firing of a cochlear neuron indicates an increase in volume of sound. If the pitch changed, a different set of neurons would fire action potentials.

[21] The bones of the middle ear serve to conduct vibration from the outer ear to the liquid within the cochlea but are not involved directly in detecting sound. Bone conductance can still stimulate the cochlea and result in hearing if the middle ear is nonfunctional.

this pigmentation absorbs excess light within the eye. Beneath the choroid is the **retina**, the surface upon which light is focused.

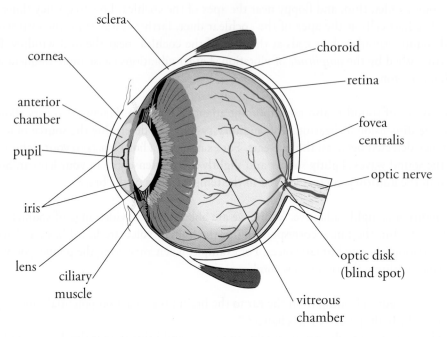

Figure 15   The Eye

Just inside the cornea is the **anterior chamber** (front chamber), which contains a fluid termed **aqueous humor**. At the back of the anterior chamber is a membrane called the **iris** with an opening called the **pupil**. The iris is the colored part of the eye, and muscles in the iris regulate the diameter of the pupil. Just behind the iris is the **posterior chamber**, also containing aqueous humor. In the back part of the posterior chamber is the **lens**. Its role is to fine-tune the angle of incoming light so that the beams are perfectly focused upon the retina. The curvature of the lens (and thus its refractive power) is varied by the **ciliary muscle**.

Light passes through the **vitreous chamber** en route from the lens to the retina. This chamber contains a thick, jelly-like fluid called **vitreous humor**. The retina is located at the back of the eye. It contains electro-magnetic receptor cells (photoreceptors) known as **rods** and **cones** which are responsible for detecting light. The rods and cones synapse with nerve cells called **bipolar cells**. In accordance with the name "bipolar," these cells have only one axon and one dendrite. The bipolar cells in turn synapse with **ganglion cells**, whose axons comprise the **optic nerve**, which travels from each eye toward the occipital lobe of the brain where complex analysis of a visual image occurs. In Figure 16, you may notice that light has to pass through two layers of neurons before it can reach the rods and cones. The neurons are fine enough to not significantly obstruct incoming rays.

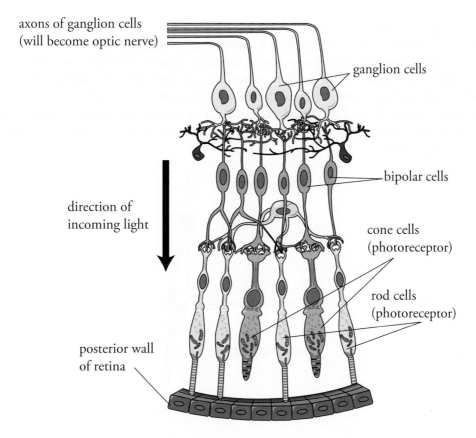

Figure 16   Organization of the Retina

The point on the retina where many axons from ganglion cells converge to form the optic nerve is the **optic disk**. It is also known as the **blind spot** (Figure 17) because it contains no photoreceptors. Another special region of the retina is the **macula**. In the center of the macula is the **fovea centralis** (focal point), which contains only cones and is responsible for extreme visual acuity. When you stare directly at something, you focus its image on the fovea.

A   ●   ●   B

Cover your left eye and focus your right eye on dot A while holding the page about 5 inches away from your face. Move the page forward and back. You will find that at a certain distance, dot B becomes invisible. You are placing dot A on the fovea by focusing on it, and at the correct distance, dot B becomes focused on the blind spot.

Figure 17   Demonstrating the Blind Spot

The Photoreceptors: Rods and Cones

Rods and cones, named because of their shapes, contain special pigment proteins that change their tertiary structure upon absorbing light. Each protein, called an **opsin**, is bound to one molecule of **retinal**, which is derived from vitamin A. In the dark, when the rods and cones are resting, retinal has several *trans* double bonds and one *cis* double bond. In this conformation, retinal and its associated opsin keep a sodium channel open. The cell remains depolarized. Upon absorbing a photon of light, retinal is converted to the **all-trans form**. This triggers a series of reactions that ultimately closes the sodium channel, and the cell hyperpolarizes.

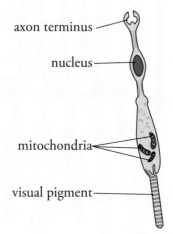

Figure 18 Rod Cell Structure

Rods and cones synapse on bipolar cells. Because of their depolarization in the dark, both types of photoreceptors release the neurotransmitter **glutamate** onto the bipolar cells, inhibiting them from firing. Upon the absorption of a photon of light and subsequent hyperpolarization, photoreceptors release less glutamate, or stop releasing it altogether.

The effect on the bipolar cells varies. Some bipolar cells are "on center" and are inhibited by glutamate. This means that when the photoreceptor is in the dark and releasing glutamate, the on-center bipolar cell releases very little or no neurotransmitter. However when the photoreceptor is in the light (light is ON the center) and stops releasing glutamate, the inhibition of the on-center bipolar cell stops, and the bipolar cell increases its release of neurotransmitter. "Off center" bipolar cells work in the opposite manner; they are stimulated by the glutamate released when the photoreceptor is in the dark, and inhibited when glutamate stops being released in the light. All of the axons of the ganglion cells together make up the optic nerve to the brain.

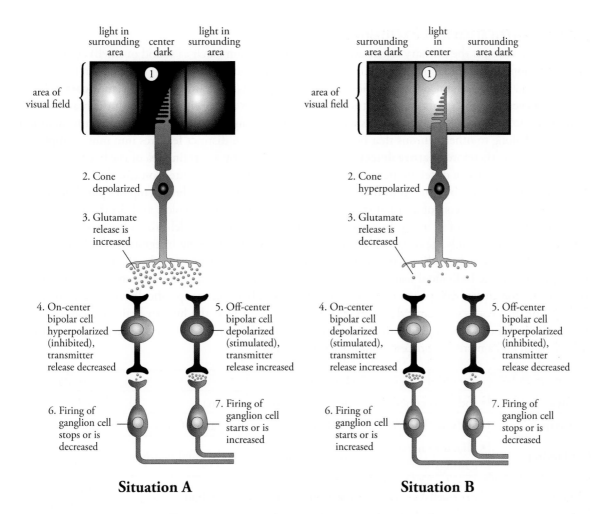

15.5

Figure 19 On-Center Off-Center Bipolar Cells

Night vision is accomplished by the rods, which are more sensitive to dim light and motion and are more concentrated in the periphery of the retina. Cones require abundant light and are responsible for color vision and high-acuity vision, and hence are more concentrated in the fovea.[22] Color vision depends on the presence of three different types of cones. One is specialized to absorb blue light, one absorbs green, and one absorbs red. [What physical difference allows this functional difference?[23]] The brain perceives hues by integrating the relative input of these three basic stimuli.

---

[22] Remember: *Cones—Color—a*C*uity.*

[23] Each type of cone makes a particular pigment protein that is specialized to change conformation when light of the appropriate frequency strikes it.

Vision: Information Processing

For humans, vision is the primary sense; even if other information (such as sound or smell) counters visual information, we are more likely to "believe our eyes." The processing of visual information is extremely complex, and highly reliant on expectations and past experience. Neurons in the **visual cortex** fire in response to very specific information; feature-detecting neurons are specific neurons in the brain that fire in response to particular visual features, such as lines, edges, angles, and movement. This information is then passed along to other neurons that begin to assimilate these distinct features into more complex objects, and so on. Therefore, **feature detection theory** explains why a certain area of the brain is activated when looking at a face, a different area is activated when looking at the letters on this page, etc. In order to process vast amounts of visual information quickly and effectively, our brain employs **parallel processing**, whereby many aspects of a visual stimulus (such as form, motion, color, and depth) are processed simultaneously instead of in a step-by-step or serial fashion. [Note: parallel processing is also employed for other stimuli as well.] The occipital lobe constructs a holistic image by integrating all of the separate elements of an object, in addition to accessing stored information. For example, the brain is simultaneously processing the individual features of an image, while also accessing stored information, to rapidly come to the conclusion that you are not only viewing a face, but you are specifically viewing your mom's face. All of this requires a tremendous amount of resources; in fact, the human brain dedicates approximately 30% of the cortex to processing visual information, while only 8% is devoted to processing touch information, and a mere 3% processes auditory information!

Modality	Receptor	Receptor type	Organ	Stimulus
Vision	• rods and cones	• electromagnetic	• retina	• light
Hearing	• auditory hair cells	• mechanoreceptor	• organ of Corti	• vibration
Olfaction	• olfactory nerve endings	• chemoreceptor	• individual neurons	• airborne chemicals
Taste	• taste cells	• chemoreceptor	• taste bud	• food chemicals
Touch (a few examples)	• Pacinian corpuscles • free nerve endings • temperature receptors	• mechanoreceptor • nociceptor • thermoreceptor	• skin	• pressure • pain • temperature
Interoception (two examples)	• aortic arch baroreceptors • pH receptors	• baroreceptor • chemoreceptor	• aortic arch • aortic arch / medulla oblongata	• blood pressure • pH

Table 6 Summary of Sensory Modalities

General Sensory Processing

Absolute Thresholds

We are very sensitive to certain types of stimuli. The minimum stimulus intensity required to activate a sensory receptor 50% of the time (and thus detect the sensation) is called the **absolute threshold**. In other words, for each special sense, the 50% recognition point defines the absolute threshold. (Note that this threshold can vary between individuals and different organisms—the absolute smell threshold for a human and a dog differs greatly.) Absolute thresholds also vary with age. For example, as we age, we gradually lose our ability to detect higher-pitched sounds. [What is the anatomical reason for this?[24]]

Difference Thresholds

Absolute thresholds are important for detecting the presence or absence of stimuli, but the ability to determine the change or difference in stimuli is also vital. The **difference threshold** (also called the *just noticeable difference*, or JND) is the minimum noticeable difference between any two sensory stimuli, 50% of the time. The magnitude of the initial stimulus influences the difference threshold; for example, if you lift a one pound weight and a two pound weight, the difference will be obvious, but if you lift a 100 pound weight and 101 pound weight, you probably won't be able to tell the difference. Indeed, **Weber's Law** dictates that two stimuli must differ by a constant *proportion* in order for their difference to be perceptible. Interestingly, the exact proportion varies by stimulus; but for humans, two objects must differ in weight by 2% [in the weight example above, what is the minimum weight needed to detect a difference between it and the 100 pound weight?[25]], two lights must differ in intensity by 8%, and two tones must differ in frequency by 0.3%.

15.6 THE ENDOCRINE SYSTEM

The nervous system and endocrine system represent the two major control systems of the body. The nervous system is fast-acting with relatively short-term effects, whereas the endocrine system takes longer to communicate signals but has generally longer lasting effects. These two control systems are interconnected, as neurons can signal the release of hormones from endocrine glands. [What is an example of this involving the adrenal medulla?[26]] A primary connection between the nervous and endocrine systems is the *hypothalamic-pituitary axis*, which is described in more detail below.

Hormone Types: Transport and Mechanisms of Action

While the nervous system regulates cellular function from instant to instant, the endocrine system regulates physiology (especially metabolism) over a period of hours to days. The nervous system communicates via the extremely rapid action potential. The signal of the endocrine system is the **hormone**, defined as a molecule which is *secreted into the bloodstream* by an endocrine gland, and which has its effects upon *distant* target cells possessing the appropriate receptor. An **endocrine gland** is a *ductless* gland whose secretory products are picked up by capillaries supplying blood to the region. (In contrast, **exocrine glands** secrete their products into the external environment by way of ducts, which empty into the gastrointestinal lumen or the external world.) A **hormone receptor** is a polypeptide that possesses a ligand-specific binding site. Binding of ligand (hormone) to the site causes the receptor to modify target cell activity.

---

[24] Loud sounds can mechanically harm the hair cells, causing them to die. When this occurs, the hair cell can no longer send sound signals to the brain. In people, once a hair cell dies, it will never regrow. The hair cells that detect higher frequency sounds are the smallest and the most easily damaged; therefore, as people age and more hair cells are damaged and lost, hearing loss occurs. Since the smallest hair cells are the ones most likely lost, loss of sensitivity to high-pitched sounds is common in older people.

[25] 102 pounds, which is 2% heavier than 100 pounds.

[26] The sympathetic nervous system directly innervates the adrenal medulla to stimulate the release of epinephrine.

Tissue-specificity of hormone action is determined by whether the cells of a tissue have the appropriate receptor.

Hormones can be grouped into one of two classes. *Hydrophilic* hormones, such as **peptides** and **amino-acid derivatives**, must bind to receptors on the cell surface, while *hydrophobic* hormones, such as the **steroid hormones**, bind to receptors in the cellular interior.

Peptide Hormones

Peptide hormones are synthesized into the rough ER and modified in the Golgi. Then they are stored in vesicles until needed, when they are released by exocytosis. In the bloodstream they dissolve in the plasma, since they are hydrophilic. Their hydrophilicity also means they cannot cross biological membranes and thus are required to communicate with the interior of the target cell by way of a second messenger cascade, discussed in Chapter 12. To briefly review, the peptide hormone is a first messenger which must bind to a cell-surface receptor. The receptor is a polypeptide with a domain on the inner surface of the plasma membrane that contains the ability to catalytically activate a second messenger. The end result of second messenger activation is that the function of proteins in the cytoplasm is changed. A key feature of second messenger cascades is signal amplification, which allows a few activated receptors to change the activity of many enzymes in the cytoplasm.

Because peptide hormones modify the activity of existing enzymes in the cytoplasm, their effects are exerted rapidly, minutes to hours from the time of secretion. Also, the duration of their effects is brief.

There are two subgroups within the peptide hormone category: polypeptides and amino acid derivatives. An example of a polypeptide hormone is insulin, which has a complex tertiary structure involving disulfide bridges. Amino acid derivatives, as their name implies, are derived from single amino acids and contain no peptide bonds. For example, tyrosine is the parent amino acid for the catecholamines (which include epinephrine) and the thyroid hormones.

Steroid Hormones

Steroids are hydrophobic molecules synthesized from cholesterol in the smooth endoplasmic reticulum. Due to their hydrophobicity, steroids can freely diffuse through biological membranes. Thus, they are not stored but rather diffuse into the bloodstream as soon as they are made. If a steroid hormone is not needed, it will not be made. Steroids' hydrophobicity also means they cannot be dissolved in the plasma. Instead, they journey through the bloodstream stuck to proteins in the plasma, such as albumin. [What holds the steroid bound to a plasma protein?[27]] The small, hydrophobic steroid hormone exerts its effects upon target cells by *diffusing through the plasma membrane to bind with a receptor in the cytoplasm.* Once it has bound its ligand, the steroid hormone-receptor complex is transported into the nucleus, where it acts as a sequence-specific regulator of transcription. Because steroid hormones must modify transcription to change the *amount* and/or *type* of proteins in the cell, their effects are exerted slowly, over a period of days, and persist for days to weeks.

Steroids regulating sexuality, reproduction, and development are secreted by the testes, ovaries, and placenta. Steroids regulating water balance and other processes are secreted by the adrenal cortex. All other endocrine glands secrete peptide hormones. (Note that although thyroid hormone is derived from an amino acid, its mechanism of action more closely resembles that of the steroid hormones.)

---

[27] No bond—just hydrophobic interactions

	Peptides	Steroids
Structure	hydrophilic, large (polypeptides) or small (amino acid derivatives)	hydrophobic, small
Site of synthesis	rough ER	smooth ER
Regulation of release	stored in vesicles until a signal for secretion is received	synthesized only when needed and then used immediately, not stored
Transport in bloodstream	free	stuck to protein carrier
Specificity	only target cells have appropriate surface receptors (exception: thyroxine = cytoplasmic)	only target cells have appropriate cytoplasmic receptors
Mechanism of effect	bind to receptors that generate second messengers which result in modification of *enzyme activity*	bind to receptors that alter *gene expression* by regulating DNA transcription
Timing of effect	rapid, short-lived	slow, long-lasting

Table 7   Peptide vs. Steroid Hormones

15.6

Organization and Regulation of the Human Endocrine System

The endocrine system has many different roles. Hormones are essential for gamete synthesis, ovulation, pregnancy, growth, sexual development, and overall level of metabolic activity. Despite this diversity of function, endocrine activity is harmoniously orchestrated. Maintenance of order in such a complex system might seem impossible to accomplish in a preplanned manner. Regulation of the endocrine system is not preplanned or rigidly structured, but is instead generally automatic. Hormone levels rise and fall as dictated by physiological needs. The endocrine system is ordered yet dynamic. This flexible, automatic orderliness is attributable to feedback regulation. The amount of a hormone secreted is controlled not by a preformulated plan but rather by changes in the variable the hormone is responsible for controlling.

An example of feedback regulation is the interaction between the hormone calcitonin and serum $[Ca^{2+}]$. The function of calcitonin is to prevent serum $[Ca^{2+}]$ from peaking above normal levels, and the amount of calcitonin secreted is directly proportional to increases in serum $[Ca^{2+}]$ above normal. When serum $[Ca^{2+}]$ becomes elevated, calcitonin is secreted. Then when serum $[Ca^{2+}]$ levels fall, calcitonin secretion stops. The falling serum $[Ca^{2+}]$ level (*that which is regulated*) feeds back to the cells which secrete calcitonin (*regulators*). The serum $[Ca^{2+}]$ level is a **physiological endpoint** that must be maintained at constant levels. This demonstrates the role of the endocrine system in maintaining **homeostasis**, or physiological consistency.

An advantage of the endocrine system and its feedback regulation is that very complex arrays of variables can be controlled automatically. It's as if the variables controlled themselves. However, some integration (a central control mechanism) is necessary. Superimposed upon the hormonal regulation of physiological endpoints is another layer of regulation: hormones that regulate hormones. Such meta-regulators are known as **tropic hormones**.

For example, adrenocorticotropic hormone (ACTH) is secreted by the anterior pituitary. The role of ACTH is to stimulate increased activity of the portion of the adrenal gland called the **cortex**, which is responsible for secreting cortisol (among other steroid hormones). ACTH is a tropic hormone because it does not directly affect physiological endpoints, but merely regulates another regulator (cortisol). Feedback regulation applies to tropic hormones as well as to direct regulators of physiological endpoints; the level of ACTH is influenced by the level of cortisol. When cortisol is needed, ACTH is secreted, and when the serum [cortisol] increases sufficiently, ACTH secretion slows.

You may have noticed that in both of our examples the effect of feedback was *inhibitory*: the result of hormone secretion inhibits further secretion. Inhibitory feedback is called **negative feedback** or **feedback inhibition**. Most feedback in the endocrine system (and if you remember, most biochemical feedback) is negative.

15.6

There is yet another layer of control. Many of the functions of the endocrine system depend on instructions from the brain. The portion of the brain which controls much of the endocrine system is the **hypothalamus**, located at the center of the brain. The hypothalamus controls the endocrine system by releasing tropic hormones that regulate other tropic hormones, called **releasing and inhibiting factors** or **releasing and inhibiting hormones**.

For example (Figure 20), the hypothalamus secretes corticotropin releasing hormone (CRH, also known as CRF, where "F" stands for factor). The role of CRH is to cause increased secretion of ACTH. Just as ACTH secretion is regulated by feedback inhibition from cortisol, CRH secretion, too, is inhibited by cortisol. You begin to see that regulatory pathways in the endocrine system can get pretty complex.

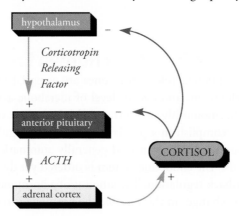

Figure 20 Feedback Regulation of Cortisol Secretion

The hypothalamus exerts its control of the pituitary by secreting its hormones into the bloodstream, just like any other endocrine gland; what's unique is that a special miniature circulatory system is provided for efficient transport of hypothalamic releasing and inhibiting factors to the anterior pituitary. This blood supply is known as the **hypothalamic-pituitary portal system**. You will also hear the term *hypothalamic-hypophysial portal system*. **Hypophysis** is another name for the pituitary gland.

A Note on Portal Systems: As a general rule, blood leaving the heart moves through only one capillary bed before returning to the heart, since the pressure drops substantially in capillaries. A portal system, however, consists of two capillary beds in sequence, allowing for direct communication between nearby structures. The two portal systems you need to understand are: the hypothalamic-pituitary portal system and the hepatic portal system (from the gastrointestinal tract to the liver (Chapter 16).

One more bit of background information is necessary before we can delve into specific hormones. The pituitary gland has two halves: front (*anterior*) and back (*posterior*); see Figure 21. The **anterior pituitary** is also called the **adenohypophysis** and the **posterior pituitary** is also known as the **neurohypophysis**. It is important to understand the difference. The anterior pituitary is a normal endocrine gland, and it is controlled by hypothalamic releasing and inhibiting factors (essentially tropic hormones). The posterior pituitary is composed of axons which descend from the hypothalamus. These hypothalamic neurons that send axons down to the posterior pituitary are an example of **neuroendocrine cells**, neurons which secrete hormones into the bloodstream. The hormones of the posterior pituitary are ADH (antidiuretic hormone or vasopressin), which causes the kidney to retain water during times of thirst, and oxytocin, which causes milk let-down for nursing as well as uterine contractions during labor.

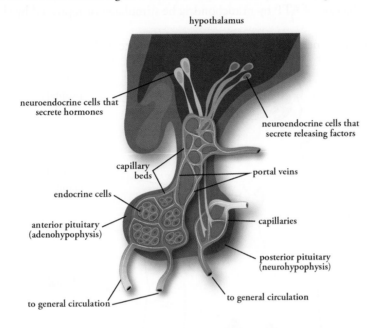

Figure 21   The Hypothalamic-Pituitary Control Axis

Major Glands and Their Hormones

The major hormones and glands of the endocrine system are listed in Table 8. Many of these hormones will be discussed in detail in later chapters. Insulin and glucagon will be discussed in the chapter on digestion and energy metabolism (Chapter 17). Testosterone, estrogen, progesterone, FSH, and LH will be presented in the chapter on reproductive biology (Chapter 19). The function of epinephrine has already been presented as part of the sympathetic nervous system response. In general, the hormones are involved in development of the body and in maintenance of constant conditions, homeostasis, in the adult. [Is epinephrine secreted by a duct into the bloodstream?[28]]

Thyroid hormone and **cortisol** have broad effects on metabolism and energy usage. Thyroid hormone is produced from the amino acid tyrosine in the thyroid gland and comes in two forms, with three or four iodine atoms per molecule. The production of thyroid hormone is increased by thyroid stimulating hormone (TSH) from the anterior pituitary, which is regulated by the hypothalamus and the central nervous system in turn. The mechanism of action of thyroid hormone is to bind to a receptor in the cytoplasm of cells that then regulates transcription in the nucleus. The effect of this regulation is to increase the overall metabolic rate and body temperature, and, in children, to stimulate growth. Exposure to cold can increase the production

---

[28] No. Endocrine glands are ductless and do not release hormones via ducts. Hormones are released directly into the bloodstream.

of thyroid hormone. Cortisol is secreted by the adrenal cortex in response to ACTH from the pituitary. In general, the effects of cortisol tend to help the body deal with stress. Cortisol helps to mobilize glycogen and fat stores to provide energy during stress and also increases the consumption of proteins for energy. These effects are essential, since removal of the adrenal cortex can result in the death of animals exposed to even a small stress. Long-term high levels of cortisol tend to have negative effects, however, including suppression of the immune system.

- Would an inhibitor of protein synthesis block the action of thyroid hormone?[29]
- Would the production of ATP by mitochondria be stimulated or repressed by thyroid hormone?[30]
- Would thyroid hormone affect isolated mitochondria directly?[31]

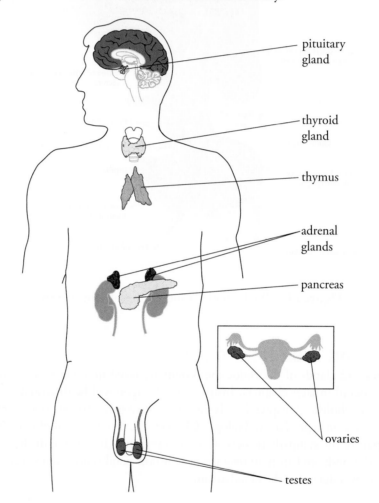

Figure 22 The Major Endocrine Glands

---

[29] Yes. Thyroid hormone binds to a receptor that regulates transcription. The mRNA stimulated by thyroid hormone receptor in the nucleus must be processed and translated before the effects of thyroid hormone can become evident.

[30] Thyroid hormone stimulates the basal metabolic rate throughout the body. More ATP will be consumed, so the mitochondria are stimulated to make more ATP.

[31] No. Thyroid hormone affects mitochondria *indirectly*, through the regulation of nuclear genes.

Gland	Hormone (class)	Target/effect
Hypothalamus	releasing and inhibiting factors (peptides)	anterior pituitary/modify activity
Anterior pituitary	growth hormone (GH) (peptide)	↑ bone & muscle growth, ↑ cell turnover rate
	prolactin (peptide)	mammary gland/milk production
tropic	thyroid stimulating hormone (TSH) (peptide)	thyroid/↑ synthesis & release of TH
	adrenocorticotropic hormone (ACTH) (peptide)	↑ growth & secretory activity of adrenal cortex
gonadotropic	luteinizing hormone (LH) (peptide)	ovary/ovulation, testes/testosterone synth.
	follicle stimulating hormone (FSH) (peptide)	ovary/follicle development, testes/spermatogenesis
Posterior pituitary	antidiuretic hormone (ADH, vasopressin) (peptide)	kidney/water retention
	oxytocin (peptide)	breast/milk letdown, uterus/contraction
Thyroid	thyroid hormone (TH, thyroxine) (modified amino acid)	child: necessary for physical & mental development; adult: ↑ metabolic rate & temp.
thyroid C cells	calcitonin (peptide)	bone, kidney; lowers serum $[Ca^{2+}]$
Parathyroids	parathyroid hormone (PTH) (peptide)	bone, kidney, small intestine/raises serum $[Ca^{2+}]$
Thymus	thymosin (children only) (peptide)	T cell development during childhood
Adrenal medulla	epinephrine (modified amino acid)	sympathetic stress response (rapid)
Adrenal cortex	cortisol ("glucocorticoid") (steroid)	longer-term stress response; ↑ blood [glucose]; ↑ protein catabolism; ↓ inflammation & immunity; many other
	aldosterone ("mineralocorticoid") (steroid)	kidney/↑ Na^+ reabsorption to b.p.
	sex steroids	not normally important, but an adrenal tumor can overproduce these, causing masculinization or feminization
Endocrine pancreas (islets of Langerhans)	insulin (β cells secrete) (peptide) —absent or ineffective in diabetes mellitus	↓ blood [glucose]/↑ glycogen & fat storage
	glucagon (α cells secrete) (peptide)	↑ blood [glucose]/↓ glycogen & fat storage
	somatostatin (SS—δ cells secrete) (peptide)	inhibits many digestive processes
Testes	testosterone (steroid)	male characteristics, spermatogenesis
Ovaries/placenta	estrogen (steroid)	female characteristics, endometrial growth
	progesterone (steroid)	endometrial secretion, pregnancy
Heart	atrial natriuretic factor (ANF) (peptide)	kidney/↑ urination to ↓ blood pressure
Kidney	erythropoietin (peptide)	bone marrow/↑ RBC synthesis

Table 8 Summary of the Hormones of the Endocrine System

15.6

Chapter 16
The Circulatory, Respiratory, Lymphatic, and Immune Systems

16.1 OVERVIEW OF THE CIRCULATORY SYSTEM

The cells of a multicellular organism have the same basic requirements as unicellular organisms. Living so close to billions of other cells has many advantages, but there are drawbacks too. Each cell must compete with its neighbors for nutrients and oxygen and must also cope with the waste products that are inevitable in so dense a civilization. Other requirements of community living are efficient communication and homeostasis. The circulatory system addresses these problems by accomplishing the following goals:

1) Distribute nutrients from the digestive tract, liver, and adipose (fat) tissue.
2) Transport oxygen from the lungs to the entire body and carbon dioxide from the tissues to the lungs.
3) Transport metabolic waste products from tissues to the excretory system (i.e., the kidneys).
4) Transport hormones from endocrine glands to targets and provide feedback.
5) Maintain homeostasis of body temperature.
6) *Hemostasis* (blood clotting). This does not address a need of a multicellular organism *per se*, but rather is necessitated by the presence of the circulatory system itself.

The flow of blood through a tissue is known as **perfusion**. Inadequate blood flow, known as **ischemia**, results in tissue damage due to shortages of O_2 and nutrients and buildup of metabolic wastes. When adequate circulation is present but the supply of oxygen is reduced, a tissue is said to suffer from **hypoxia**.

Components of the Circulatory System

The functions of the circulatory system involve transport of blood throughout the body and exchange of material between the blood and tissues. The **heart** is a muscular pump that forces blood through a branching series of vessels to the lungs and the rest of the body. Vessels that carry blood away from the heart at high pressure are **arteries**, and vessels that carry blood back toward the heart at low pressure are **veins**. As arteries pass farther from the heart, the pressure of blood decreases, and they branch into increasingly smaller arteries called **arterioles**. The arterioles then pass into the **capillaries**, very small vessels, often just wide enough for a single blood cell to pass. Arterioles have smooth muscle in their walls that can act as a control valve to restrict or increase the flow of blood into the capillaries of tissues. The capillaries have thin walls made of a single layer of cells, and they are designed to allow the exchange of material between the blood and tissues. After passing through capillaries, blood collects in small veins called **venules**, then into the veins leading back to the heart. Except for the largest vessels near the heart, veins lack a muscular wall. From the heart, the blood can be pumped out once again through the arteries to the capillaries in the tissues.

- If the arterioles constrict in a tissue, will material diffuse through the wall of the arterioles into the tissue?[1]

The inner lining of all blood vessels is formed by a thin layer of **endothelial cells**; the walls of capillaries are formed from a single layer of such cells. These cells have important roles in a number of vascular functions such as:

- vasodilation and vasoconstriction
- inflammation

---

[1] No. All exchange of material between the blood and tissues must occur in capillaries. The walls of arterioles are too thick and muscular for exchange to occur.

- angiogenesis (the formation of new blood vessels)
- thrombosis (blood clotting)

Endothelial cell dysfunction can lead to a number of pathogenic conditions, such as hypercholesterolemia, hypertension, inappropriate clot formation, and coronary artery disease and atherosclerosis; in fact, endothelial cell dysfunction is key to the development of atherosclerosis, and it predates any clinical vascular signs by several years.

To achieve both efficient oxygenation of blood in the lungs and transport of oxygenated blood to the tissues, the heart has evolved in humans to have two sides separated by a thick wall to pump blood in two separate circuits. The right side of the heart pumps blood to the lungs, and the left side of the heart pumps blood to the rest of the body. The flow of blood from the heart to the lungs and back to the heart is the **pulmonary circulation**, and the flow of blood from the heart to the rest of the body and back again is the **systemic circulation** (Figure 1).

By having two separate circulations, most blood passes through only one set of capillaries before returning to the heart. There are exceptions to this, however: **portal systems**. In the hepatic portal system, blood passes first through capillaries in the intestine, then collects in veins to travel to the liver, where the vessels branch and the blood passes again through capillaries. Another example is the hypothalamic-hypophysial portal system, in which blood passes through capillaries in the hypothalamus to the portal veins, then to capillaries in the pituitary. The portal systems evolved as direct transport systems, to transport nutrients directly from the intestine to the liver or hormones from the hypothalamus to the pituitary, without passing through the whole body.

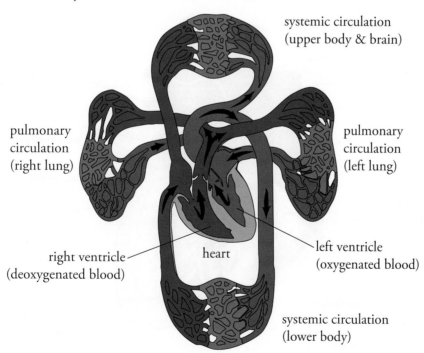

systemic circulation
(upper body & brain)

pulmonary
circulation
(right lung)

pulmonary
circulation
(left lung)

right ventricle
(deoxygenated blood)

heart

left ventricle
(oxygenated blood)

systemic circulation
(lower body)

Figure 1 Pulmonary and Systemic Circuits

16.2   THE HEART

The heart has two kinds of chambers involved in pumping blood, the **atria** and the **ventricles** (Figure 2). The atria are reservoirs or "waiting rooms" where blood can collect from the veins before getting pumped into the ventricles. The muscular ventricles pump blood out of the heart at high pressures into the arteries. The systemic circulation and the pulmonary circulation are separated within the heart, so the right and left sides of the heart each have one atrium and one ventricle. The right atrium receives deoxygenated blood from the systemic circulation (from the large veins: the **inferior vena cava** and the **superior vena cava**) and pumps it into the right ventricle. From the right ventricle, blood passes through the pulmonary artery to the lungs. Oxygenated blood from the lungs returns through the pulmonary veins to the left atrium and is pumped into the left ventricle before being pumped out of the heart in a single large artery, the **aorta**, to the systemic circulation.

- Do all of the arteries of the body carry oxygenated blood?[2]

- Based on the above, you can conclude that blood flows:[3]
  - A) from the lungs into the right atrium, since the right side of the heart deals with deoxygenated blood.
  - B) from the right ventricle to the right atrium, since the atrium is a low-pressure chamber.
  - C) from the right atrium to the left ventricle, since the right side of the heart deals with deoxygenated blood and the left side must pump blood to the body.
  - D) from the lungs into the left atrium and from there to the left ventricle, since the left side of the heart deals with oxygenated blood.

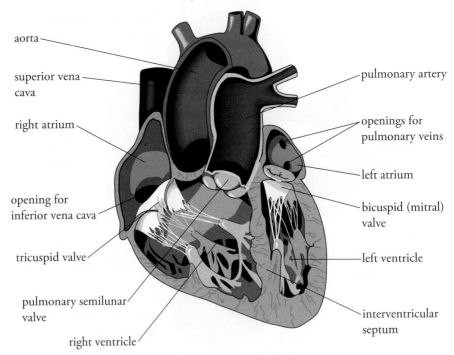

Figure 2   The Heart

---

[2] No. The pulmonary artery carries deoxygenated blood from the heart to the lungs.

[3] Oxygenated blood flows from the lungs to the left atrium (choice A is wrong), then to the left ventricle (choice **D** is right, and choice C is wrong). The atrium is a low pressure chamber, however, blood flow from the ventricles to the atria is prevented by the atrioventricular valves (choice B is wrong).

Valves

Valves are necessary to ensure one-way flow through the circulatory system. Valves in the heart are especially important, since the pressure differentials there are so extreme. In particular, ventricular pressure is very high and atrial pressure is lower. Hence, an **atrioventricular valve** (**AV valve**) between each ventricle and its atrium is necessary to prevent backflow.

The AV valve between the left atrium and the left ventricle is the **bicuspid** (or **mitral**) **valve**. [The mitral valve must withstand enormous pressures. What would happen if it ruptured?[4]] The AV valve between the right atrium and the right ventricle is the **tricuspid valve**. [What valve prevents blood flow between the left ventricle and the right ventricle?[5]]

Another set of valves is needed between the large arteries and the ventricles; these are the **pulmonary** and **aortic semilunar valves**. [Since the ventricles are ultra-high pressure chambers, why is it necessary to put valves between them and the arteries?[6]] Together these two valves are known simply as the *semilunar valves*.

There are also valves throughout the venous system. This is necessary because in passing through capillaries, blood loses its pressure. Hence, there is not much of a driving force pushing it toward the heart. Contraction of skeletal muscle becomes important, because normal body movements push and squeeze the veins, pressurizing venous blood and pushing it along. Venous valves prevent backflow; as long as the valves hold up, the blood moves toward the heart.

The Cardiac Cycle

The heart contracts, then relaxes, in a cycle which ends only in death. The left and right sides of the heart proceed through the same cycle at the same time. The cardiac cycle is divided into two periods, **diastole** and **systole** (pronounced dy-AS-toe-lee and SIS-toe-lee). During diastole, the ventricles are relaxed, and blood is able to flow into them from the atria. In fact, the atria contract during diastole, to propel blood into the ventricles more rapidly. [How strong is atrial compared to ventricular contraction?[7]] At the end of diastole, the ventricles contract, initiating systole. The ensuing buildup of pressure causes the AV valves to slam shut. Over the next few milliseconds, the pressure in the ventricles increases rapidly, until the semilunar valves fly open and blood rushes into the aorta and pulmonary artery. Systole is the period of time during which the ventricles are contracting, beginning at the "lub" sound and ending at the "dup." At the end of systole, the ventricles are nearly empty[8] and stop contracting. As a result, the pressure inside falls rapidly, and blood begins to flow backward, from the pulmonary artery into the right ventricle, and from the aorta into the left ventricle. But very little backflow actually occurs, because the semilunar valves slam shut when the pressure in the ventricles becomes lower than the pressure in the great arteries. At this point, the heart has completed a full cardiac cycle and is back in diastole.

---

[4] The left ventricle would pump blood in both directions; out the aorta and back into the left atrium. The result will be elevated pulmonary blood pressure and pulmonary edema.

[5] None! The two ventricles are separated by a thick muscular wall. Remember: the left and right halves are separate.

[6] The ventricles are only pressurized while contracting. When they are not contracting, they must have a very low pressure so that blood can flow into them from the atria. Without the semilunar valves (that close while the ventricles are relaxed), blood could backflow and re-enter the ventricles from the arteries, rather than proceeding through the systemic and pulmonic circuits.

[7] Much weaker. The atria really only contract to ensure that most of the blood they contain passes into the ventricles. In contrast, the ventricles must propel blood through arteries, capillary beds, and veins. Hence, the muscular walls of the atria are much thinner than those of the ventricles.

[8] Actually, only about 2/3 of the blood is normally ejected from the ventricle; this is the **ejection fraction**.

- Which one of the following is true during diastole?[9]
  - A) The bicuspid valve is closed.
  - B) Blood does not flow through the aortic valve.
  - C) Both semilunar valves are open.
  - D) Pressure in the atria is low, and thus the atria fill with blood from the vena cava and pulmonary arteries.

Heart Sounds, Heart Rate, and Cardiac Output

The "lub-dup" of the heartbeat is produced by valves slamming shut. The "lub" results from the closure of the AV valves at the beginning of systole, and the "dup" is the sound of the semilunar valves closing at the end of systole. [Based on this, which is longer: systole or diastole?[10]]

The **heart rate** (HR) or **pulse** is the number of times the "lub-dup" cardiac cycle is repeated per minute. The normal pulse rate is about one beat per second, ranging from 45 beats per minute (b.p.m.) in athletes to 80 or more beats per minute in the elderly and in children. The explanation for this variation is that a stronger heart pumps more blood each time it contracts, and thus may beat fewer times per minute and still provide adequate circulation. Athletes have strong hearts, while children and the elderly have weaker hearts. The amount of blood pumped with each systole is known as the **stroke volume** (SV). The total amount of blood pumped per minute is termed the **cardiac output** (CO), defined by the equation

$$\text{cardiac output (L/min)} = \text{stroke volume (L/beat)} \times \text{heart rate (beats/min)}$$
$$CO = SV \times HR$$

- An overweight child weighing 110 pounds, a female athlete weighing 110 pounds, and an elderly man weighing 110 pounds all require a cardiac output of about 5 L/min. But the child and the old man have a stroke volume of 1/16 L, while the athlete's stroke volume is 1/9 L. How can the child and the old man supply enough blood to their bodies?[11]

The Frank-Starling Mechanism and Venous Return

There are several ways to increase cardiac output. One is increasing heart rate, as we saw above. Also, a stronger heart has a larger stroke volume and is capable of a greater cardiac output. Another mechanism of increased stroke volume is termed the **Frank-Starling mechanism**. If the heart muscle is stretched, it will contract more forcefully. How can the heart muscle be stretched? By filling it with more blood, of course. The return of blood to the heart by the vena cava is termed **venous return**. If venous return is increased, the heart fills more. As a result, its muscle fibers are stretched, and they respond by contracting more

---

[9] During diastole the ventricles are relaxing and filling. The bicuspid valve separates the left atrium from the left ventricle, and it must be open to allow blood to flow into the left ventricle (choice A is wrong). The pressure in the ventricles during diastole is lower than arterial pressure, so blood tries to backflow into the ventricles but closes the semilunar valves (aortic and pulmonary; choice **B** is correct, and choice C is wrong). While it is true that the atrial pressure is low during diastole and blood flows in from the vena cava, the pulmonary arteries carry blood away from the heart and toward the lungs (choice D is wrong).

[10] Diastole is longer, since it occupies the space between *lub-dup* and *lub-dup*. Systole is shorter, since it occupies the space between *lub* and *dup*.

[11] The athlete's heart can provide the necessary cardiac output by pumping at a leisurely rate of 45 beats per minute. But the hearts of the child and old man will have to work hard to pump enough blood; their pulses will be 80 beats per minute.

forcefully. The result is that a larger volume of blood enters the heart *and* the heart contracts better. The stroke volume can be increased significantly in this manner. The control of cardiac output in this manner is largely automatic: the more blood the heart receives from the tissues, the more it pumps out to the tissues.

Cardiac Muscle

The force of contraction in the ventricles and atria is generated by the cardiac muscle cells that form the muscular walls of the chambers of the heart. All muscle cells, including those of cardiac muscle, share with neurons the ability to propagate an action potential across their surface. The action potential in all muscle cells, as in neurons, is a wave of depolarization of the plasma membrane.

A difference between neurons and cardiac muscle cells is that cardiac muscle is a **functional syncytium**. A syncytium is a tissue in which the cytoplasm of different cells can communicate via gap junctions. In cardiac muscle, the gap junctions are found in the **intercalated disks**, the connections between cardiac muscle cells. The depolarization of a cardiac muscle cell can be communicated directly through the cytoplasm to neighboring cardiac muscle cells through these gap junctions. (Recall that this is an example of an electrical synapse; there are no chemical synapses between cardiac muscle cells.) As a result, once an action potential starts, it spreads in a wave of depolarization throughout the cardiac muscle tissue in the atria or the ventricles. The atria and the ventricles are separate syncytia. The action potential in the heart is transmitted from the atrial syncytium to the ventricles by the **cardiac conduction system**. Transmission of the action potential is delayed slightly as it passes through the part of the conduction system known as the AV node (Figure 5).

Voltage-gated sodium channels, also called **fast sodium channels**, play an important role in cardiac muscle, as in neurons, but, in addition, another type of voltage-gated channel, the **slow calcium channel**, is involved in the cardiac muscle action potential. Like all voltage-gated channels, these channels open in response to a change in membrane potential to a specific voltage (the threshold voltage) and, when open, allow the passage of calcium down its gradient. These channels also stay open longer than the fast sodium channels do, causing the membrane depolarization to last longer in cardiac muscle than in neurons, producing a plateau phase (Figure 4).

The nature of the action potential in cardiac muscle affects the function of this tissue. Cardiac cells, like all cells with an excitable membrane, have a period during and just after the action potential during which they are refractory to new action potentials. Another result of the long depolarization in cardiac muscle is that the contraction of muscle lasts a long time, strengthening the force with which blood is expelled. To maximize the entry of calcium in the cell, cardiac muscle has involutions of the membrane called **T tubules**. The action potentials travel down along T tubules, allow the entry of calcium from the extracellular environment, and also induce the sarcoplasmic reticulum to release calcium. The combination of intracellular and extracellular calcium causes the contraction of actin-myosin fibers. [Will the absolute refractory period, during which a cell will not fire an action potential, be longer in cardiac or neuronal cells?[12] Will the strength of contraction by cardiac muscle be affected by the extracellular concentration of calcium ions?[13]]

---

[12] The absolute refractory period is the period during the action potential in which a new action potential cannot be induced. If the membrane is still depolarized as part of an action potential, it will be refractory to new action potentials. Cardiac muscle action potentials last much longer than neuronal (or skeletal muscle) action potentials, and will therefore have a longer absolute refractory period.

[13] Yes. A significant portion of the calcium that stimulates contraction comes from the extracellular pool, entering the cell as part of the action potential.

Rhythmic Excitation of the Heart

Once an action potential is initiated, it will spread throughout the cardiac muscle of the heart. Interestingly, the heart is *not* stimulated to contract by neuronal or hormonal influences, although these can change the rate and strength of contraction (the **contractility** of the heart). Isolated cardiac muscle cells will in some circumstances continue contracting on their own, free of any external influences. So, what initiates the action potential in heart tissue? The initiation of each action potential that starts each cardiac cycle occurs automatically from within the heart itself, in a special region of the right atrium called the **sinoatrial (SA) node**. Under normal circumstances, the cells of the SA node act as the **pacemaker of the heart**. The SA node exhibits automaticity and its action potential is commonly divided into 3 separate phases; Phase 0, Phase 3, and Phase 4. (*Note*: Other cardiac myocytes (muscle cells) additionally have Phases 1 and 2, but the SA node does *not*; see Figure 3.)

The SA node is unique in that it has an *unstable resting potential* (not really resting, huh?). This is **Phase 4** (automatic slow depolarization) and is caused by special **sodium leak channels** that are responsible for its rhythmic, automatic excitation. This inward sodium leak brings the cell potential to the threshold for voltage-gated calcium channels; when they open they cause **Phase 0**, the upstroke of the pacemaker potential. It is caused mainly by an inward flow of Ca^{2+}. (*Note*: Skeletal muscle cells and other myocytes depolarize because of a Na^+ influx, not Ca^{2+} like the SA node.) This Ca^{2+} drives the membrane potential of the SA nodal cells toward the positive Ca^{2+} equilibrium potential. Note also that the Ca^{2+} channels operate more slowly than the Na^+ channels, leading to a more gradual upsweep in the action potential.

Phase 3 is repolarization. It is caused by closure of the Ca^{2+} channels and opening of the K^+ channels, leading to an outward flow of K^+ from the cell. This loss of positively charged K^+ ions drives the membrane potential back down toward the negative K^+ equilibrium potential.

The SA node cells transmit their action potential through intercalated discs to the rest of the conduction cells in the heart (as well as to the atrial myocytes), repolarize, then start the process over again, repeated once per heartbeat for the life of the individual (Figure 3).

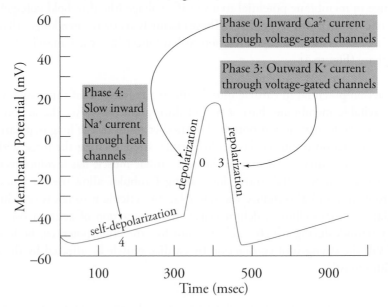

Figure 3   The Pacemaker Potential of the SA Node

Note that while several regions of the heart can spontaneously depolarize (for example, the AV node, Purkinje fibers), the SA node has the most Na⁺ leak channels of all of the conduction system. Thus, it reaches threshold before any other region of the heart does, and, sets the rate of heart contraction (that's why it's called the "**pacemaker**" of the heart). When the SA nodal cells are injured or the pathway of atrial depolarization is blocked, these other regions of the heart will take over the pacemaking responsibility, but pace the heart at a slower rate.

The cardiac muscle cells of the heart have an action potential that differs from the SA node and the other conduction system cells. These muscle cells have a resting membrane potential of about –90 mV (very close to the K⁺ equilibrium potential). The action potentials here have a long duration, up to 300 milliseconds normally. The phases of the action potential in these cells are Phases 0–4 (see Figure 4).

Phase 0 (depolarization) is again the upstroke of the action potential and is caused by the transient increase in Na⁺ conductance (just like in neurons). Action potentials propagating through the intercalated discs stimulate myocytes to reach threshold for voltage-gated Na⁺ channels. Once threshold is reached, the Na⁺ channels open and Na⁺ rushes into the cell.

In **Phase 1** (initial repolarization), the Na⁺ channels inactivate and K⁺ channels open. This leads to an efflux of K⁺ and a slight drop in cell potential. Furthermore, the increased potential due to the initial Na⁺ influx causes the opening of voltage-gated Ca²⁺ channels; this leads to **Phase 2**, the **plateau** phase. During the plateau, the influx of Ca²⁺ ions balance the K⁺ efflux from phase one, leading to a transient equilibrium in cell potential.

Phase 3 (repolarization) occurs when the Ca²⁺ channels close and the K⁺ channels continue to allow K⁺ to leave the cell (again, this is just like in neurons). **Phase 4** (the resting membrane potential) is the period during which inward and outward current are equal. Remember, this is dictated by action of the Na⁺/K⁺ ATPase and slow K⁺ leak channels.

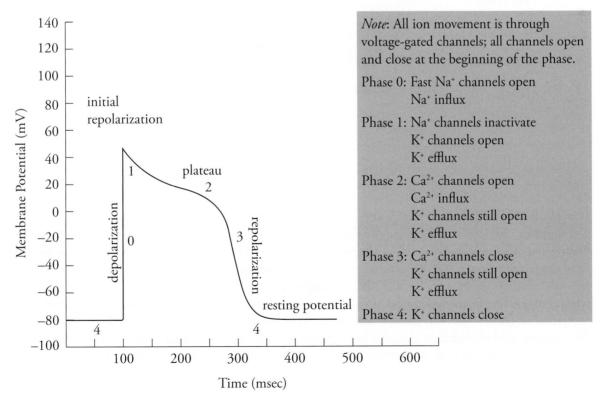

Note: All ion movement is through voltage-gated channels; all channels open and close at the beginning of the phase.

Phase 0: Fast Na⁺ channels open
    Na⁺ influx

Phase 1: Na⁺ channels inactivate
    K⁺ channels open
    K⁺ efflux

Phase 2: Ca²⁺ channels open
    Ca²⁺ influx
    K⁺ channels still open
    K⁺ efflux

Phase 3: Ca²⁺ channels close
    K⁺ channels still open
    K⁺ efflux

Phase 4: K⁺ channels close

Figure 4 Phases of the Membrane Potential in a Cardiac Muscle Cell

Thus, each heartbeat begins as an action potential in the **sinoatrial (SA) node** then spreads throughout the atria, causing them to contract and fill the ventricles with blood. The action potential also spreads down the special conduction pathway that transmits action potentials very rapidly without contracting. The pathway connects the SA node to the **atrioventricular (AV) node**. Since this pathway connects the two nodes, it is referred to as the **internodal tract**. Note that while the impulse travels to the AV node almost instantaneously, it spreads through the atria more slowly, because contracting heart muscle cells pass the impulse more slowly than specialized conduction fibers. At the AV node, the impulse is delayed slightly, then passes from the node to the ventricles via the conduction pathway again. This part of the conduction pathway is known as the **AV bundle (bundle of His)**. The AV bundle divides into the **right** and **left bundle branches**, then into the **Purkinje fibers**, which allow the impulse to spread rapidly and evenly over both ventricles. Note that the Purkinje fibers spread over the inferior portion of the ventricles (paradoxically called the "apex" of the heart). The result is that this region of the ventricles contracts first, and blood is pushed toward the superior region of the heart (paradoxically called the "base"), where the valves and arteries are (Figure 5).

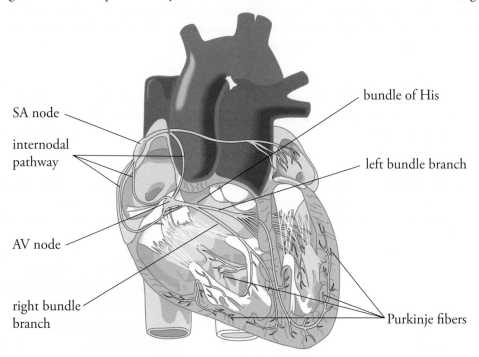

Figure 5   The Cardiac Conduction System

Regulation of the Heart by the Autonomic Nervous System

The autonomic nervous system does not initiate action potentials in the heart, but it does regulate the rate of contraction. The intrinsic firing rate of the SA node is about 120 beats per minute. The reason the normal heart rate is only about 60–80 beats/minute is that the parasympathetic nervous system continually inhibits depolarization of the SA node. In particular, the **vagus nerve** (a cranial nerve) contains preganglionic axons which synapse in ganglia near the SA node. The postganglionic neurons innervate the SA node, releasing acetylcholine (ACh). The ACh inhibits depolarization by binding to receptors on the cells of the SA node. The constant level of inhibition provided by the vagus nerve is known as **vagal tone**. In summary, the role of the *parasympathetic* system in controlling the heart is to modulate the rate by *inhibiting rapid automaticity*.

The sympathetic system can also influence the heart. At rest, however, most nervous input is from the vagus. The sympathetic system kicks in when increased cardiac output is needed during a "fight or flight" response. The sympathetic system affects the heart in two ways. First, sympathetic postganglionic neurons directly innervate the heart, releasing norepinephrine. Second, epinephrine secreted by the adrenal medulla binds to receptors on cardiac muscle cells. The effect of sympathetic activation is stimulatory. The heart rate increases, and so does the force of contraction.

16.3   HEMODYNAMICS

Resistance

Hemodynamics is the study of blood flow. The driving force for blood flow is a difference in pressure from arteries to veins. The force opposing flow is friction, which results when blood squeezes through many tiny branching vessels. The technical term for this opposing force is **resistance**. Ohm's Law summarizes the relationship between these variables: $\Delta P = Q \times R$. Here, ΔP is the pressure gradient (in mm Hg) from the arterial system to the venous system, Q stands for blood flow (or cardiac output) in L/min, and R denotes resistance. The usefulness of this simple equation is twofold: first, it shows us that blood pressure is directly proportional to both cardiac output and peripheral resistance. If either of these change, blood pressure changes similarly. [How would an increase in stroke volume change blood pressure?[14]] Second, it shows us that if we want to change blood flow, we can only change it by changing either the pressure or the resistance; those are the only independent variables in the equation.

We know that pressure can be varied by increasing the *force* (thus changing the stroke volume) or *rate* (beats per minute) of cardiac contraction. What about resistance? The principal determinant of resistance is the degree of constriction of arteriolar smooth muscle, also known as **precapillary sphincters**. If arteriolar smooth muscles contract, it becomes more difficult for blood to flow from arteries into capillaries; that is, the resistance goes up. The resistance of the entire systemic circuit is easily calculated using the above equation in the form $R = \Delta P/Q$. We can measure ΔP and Q, then solve for R. This quantity is known as the **peripheral resistance**.

The sympathetic nervous system controls the peripheral resistance. A certain amount of pressure in the arterial system is always desirable; otherwise not all tissues would be perfused. This basal level of pressure is provided by a constant level of norepinephrine released by millions of sympathetic postganglionic axons innervating precapillary sphincters. This constant nervous input is known as **adrenergic tone**. (Adrenergic means sympathetic; the word comes from adrenaline, which is another name for epinephrine.) [Why might tense, stressed out people tend to have high blood pressure?[15]]

The sympathetic system can increase the overall peripheral resistance, thus increasing blood pressure. It can also specifically divert blood away from one tissue so that another is preferentially perfused. In particular, sympathetic activation causes precapillary sphincters in the gut to contract, while arterioles supplying skeletal muscle are allowed to relax. The result is that blood flow is diverted from the gut to skeletal muscle, which facilitates the fight or flight response.

---

[14] Recall that CO = SV × HR, therefore an increase in stroke volume would increase cardiac output. Since blood pressure and cardiac output are directly proportional, an increase in cardiac output would increase blood pressure as well.

[15] Tension and stress are similar to fear. Both involve activation of the sympathetic nervous system.

Blood Pressure

When physicians measure blood pressure, what they are actually measuring is **systemic arterial pressure**. This is the force per unit area exerted by blood upon the walls of arteries. You may recall that a typical blood pressure reading looks like this: 120/80, pronounced "120 over 80." What do the two numbers mean? 120 mm Hg is the **systolic pressure**, and 80 mm Hg is the **diastolic pressure**. In other words, 120 mm Hg is the highest pressure that ever occurs in the circulatory system of this particular patient during the time the blood pressure is being measured. This level is attained as the ventricles contract (that is, during systole). 80 mm Hg is as low as the pressure gets between heartbeats (that is, during diastole) during the measurement.

It is important to emphasize the last sentence: this is the lowest *arterial* pressure occurring at any time during the cardiac cycle. You must realize that throughout the cardiac cycle, the pressure in the vena cava is about *zero* mm Hg. The highest pressures in the circulatory system are achieved in the left ventricle, aorta, and other large arteries. But every large artery branches, giving rise to many arterioles, and every arteriole gives rise to many capillaries. The result of all this branching is that the pressure generated by the heart is dissipated (Figure 6). By the time blood reaches the vena cava, it depends on valves to prevent backflow because the driving pressure is negligible.

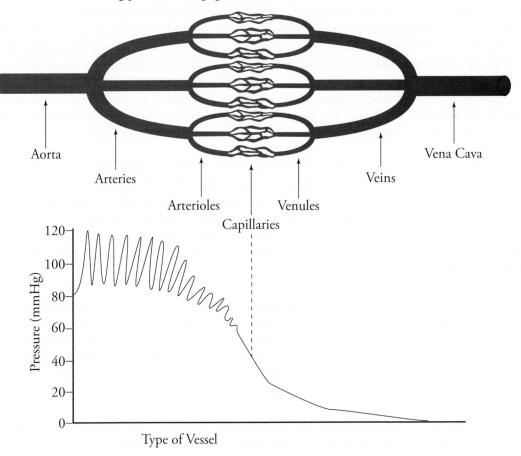

Figure 6 Pressures Throughout the Circulatory System

Why is the diastolic arterial pressure as high as it is? In other words, between heartbeats, why does the arterial pressure remain elevated? Without the heart contracting, wouldn't you expect the pressure to fall rapidly? This is the reason arteries are highly elastic and muscular. When the heart contracts, the arteries distend like balloons. During diastole, the arteries exert pressure on the blood, just as an inflated balloon exerts pressure on the air it contains. This maintains diastolic pressure, which is important because it provides a continued driving force for blood.

Local Autoregulation

The nervous system does not control blood flow to every single region of the body. The amount of feedback information this would require would be huge. Instead, tissues in need of extra blood flow are able to requisition it themselves. This phenomenon is known as **local autoregulation**. The mechanism is simple: certain metabolic wastes have a direct effect on arteriolar smooth muscle, causing it to relax. Hence, when a tissue is underperfused, wastes build up, and vasodilation occurs automatically. Autoregulation is the principal determinant of coronary blood flow (blood supply to the heart); it generally overrides nervous input.

16.4 COMPONENTS OF BLOOD

Blood has a liquid portion called **plasma**, and a portion which is composed of cells. The cellular elements of blood are known as **formed elements**. Plasma accounts for 55 percent of the volume of blood, and consists of the following items dissolved in water: electrolytes, buffers, sugars, blood proteins, lipoproteins, CO_2, O_2, and metabolic waste products. **Electrolytes** refer to Na^+, K^+, Cl^-, Ca^{2+}, and Mg^{2+} ions. **Buffers** in the blood maintain a constant pH of 7.4; the principal blood buffer is bicarbonate (HCO_3^-).

The principal sugar in the blood is glucose. A constant concentration must be maintained so that all the cells of the body receive adequate nutrition. The blood proteins, most of which are made by the liver, include albumin, immunoglobulins (antibodies), fibrinogen, and lipoproteins. **Albumin** is essential for maintenance of **oncotic pressure** (osmotic pressure in the capillaries due only to plasma proteins). The **immunoglobulins** are a key part of the immune system (Section 16.12). **Fibrinogen** is essential for blood clotting (hemostasis). **Lipoproteins** are large particles consisting of fats, cholesterol, and carrier proteins. Their role is to transport lipids in the bloodstream. CO_2 and O_2 are involved in respiration, of course. However, CO_2 is also important for its role in buffering the blood. The principal *metabolic waste product* is **urea**, a breakdown product of amino acids. Urea is basically a carrier of excess nitrogen. There are other important waste products too, such as **bilirubin**, a breakdown product of heme (the oxygen-binding moiety of hemoglobin, discussed below).

By centrifuging whole blood, one can separate the plasma from the formed elements, as shown on the following page. The volume of blood occupied by the red blood cells (**erythrocytes**) is known as the **hematocrit** (Figure 7). The normal hematocrit in adult males is 40–45 percent; in females it is lower, approximately 35–40 percent. White blood cells (**leukocytes**) and platelets account for a small volume (about 1 percent). All the formed elements of the blood develop from special cells in the bone marrow, known as **bone marrow stem cells**.

If whole blood is allowed to clot, one is left with a solid clot plus a clear fluid known as **serum**. Hence, serum is similar to plasma except that it lacks all the proteins involved in clotting.

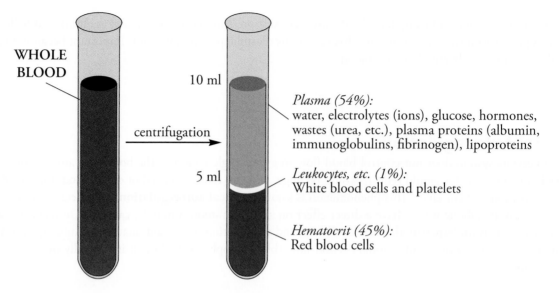

Figure 7 The Hematocrit and the Components of Blood

Erythrocytes (Red Blood Cells—RBCs)

The hormone **erythropoietin** (made in the kidney) stimulates RBC production in the bone marrow. Aged RBCs are eaten by phagocytes in the spleen and liver.

The erythrocyte is a cell, but it has no nucleus or other organelles such as mitochondria. However, it does require the energy of ATP for processes such as ion pumping and basic maintenance of cell structure during its 120-day lifetime in the bloodstream. Lacking mitochondria, the RBC relies on glycolysis for ATP synthesis. The purpose of the RBC is to transport O_2 to the tissues from the lungs and CO_2 from the tissues to the lungs. Hence, it requires a large surface area for gas exchange. A high surface-to-volume ratio is achieved by the RBC's flat, biconcave shape (like a deflated basketball or a throat lozenge, see Figure 8). The RBC is able to carry oxygen because it contains millions of molecules of **hemoglobin** (more on hemoglobin later).

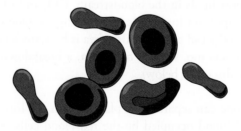

Figure 8 Red Blood Cells (Erythrocytes)

Blood Typing

Blood typing is the classification of a person's blood based on the presence or absence of certain surface antigens on their red blood cells. The two most important blood group antigens are the **ABO blood group** and the **Rh blood group**. The ABO blood group consists of glycoproteins that are coded for by three different alleles: I^A, I^B, and i. These alleles and their genotypes and phenotypes were discussed in more detail in Chapter 14 (Genetics and Evolution).

The other main antigen used in blood typing is the Rh (rhesus) factor. The expression of this antigen follows a classically dominant pattern: RR and Rr genotypes lead to the expression of the protein on the surface of the red blood cell (Rh positive), and the rr genotype leads to the absence of the protein (Rh negative). The combinations of the ABO alleles and the Rh alleles (and the respective antigens they code for) determine the overall blood type of an individual. Table 1 summarizes these blood types.

	$I^A I^A$ or $I^A i$	$I^B I^B$ or $I^B i$	$I^A I^B$	ii
RR or Rr	type A+	type B+	type AB+	type O+
rr	type A−	type B−	type AB−	type O−

Table 1 Blood Group Genotypes and Phenotypes

Determining blood type is critical when performing blood transfusions. Antibodies to the A and B antigens are produced early in infancy and can cause clumping and destruction of red blood cells bearing the incorrect antigen (called a **transfusion reaction**). For example, a person with A+ blood produces anti-B antibodies; if transfused with type B blood, these antibodies will clump and destroy the donated type B cells, possibly leading to the death of the recipient. Note that this early production of antibodies without prior exposure to the antigen is unusual; typically the immune system must be exposed to a foreign protein before it produces antibodies against it.

Antibodies to the Rh antigen do not develop unless a person with Rh− blood is exposed to Rh+ blood, an event called "sensitization"; note that this is the typical response of the immune system to a foreign protein (antigen). Subsequent exposure to Rh+ blood can then result in a transfusion reaction. This is particularly dangerous in the case of an Rh− mother carrying an Rh+ baby. Typically, if it is the first baby, there are no complications (unless the mother had been previously sensitized); the mother's blood and the baby's blood do not mix during pregnancy. However, on delivery, some Rh+ cells from the child can mix with the mother's Rh− blood and lead to her sensitization. Future Rh+ babies are then at risk, since the anti-Rh antibodies can cross the placental barrier to clump and/or destroy the Rh+ baby's red blood cells. This is known as **hemolytic disease of the newborn** or *erythroblastosis fetalis*, and can be fatal. Injection of the mother at the time of birth with anti-Rh antibodies can clump and lead to the destruction of any stray Rh+ cells from the baby; this can prevent sensitization of the mother and protect any future unborn Rh+ children.

Two special blood types are AB+ and O−. Type AB+ individuals do not make antibodies to any of the blood group antigens, since their red blood cells possess all three of the antigens. Thus, type AB+ individuals are known as "**universal recipients**" because they can receive any of the other blood types without complication. Type O− individuals do not possess any of the surface antigens that could trigger a reaction in an individual with a different blood type. Thus, O− individuals are known as "universal donors" because they can donate blood to any of the other blood types, typically without complication. (Note that type O− individuals do make anti-A and anti-B antibodies, and these can sometimes cause issues in recipients. It is always best to match blood types between donors and recipients when possible.)

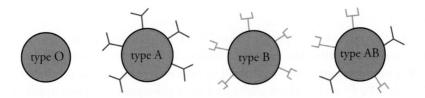

Figure 9 RBC Surface Antigens

Leukocytes

The white blood cell's role is to fight infection and dispose of debris. All white blood cells are large complex cells with all the normal eukaryotic cell structures (nucleus, mitochondria, etc.). Some white blood cells (**macrophages** and **neutrophils**) move by amoeboid motility (crawling). This is important because they are able to squeeze out of capillary intercellular junctions (spaces between capillary endothelial cells) and can therefore roam free in the tissues, hunting for foreign particles and pathogens. Some white blood cells exhibit **chemotaxis**, which means movement directed by chemical stimuli. The chemical stimuli can be toxins and waste products released by pathogens, or can be chemical signals released from other white blood cells. There are six types of white blood cells (Table 2).

Cell	Role
monocytes:	
macrophage	phagocytose debris and microorganisms; amoeboid motility; chemotaxis
lymphocytes:	
B cell	mature into *plasma cell* and produce antibodies
T cell	kill virus-infected cells, tumor cells, and reject tissue grafts; also control immune response
granulocytes:	
neutrophil	phagocytose bacteria resulting in pus; amoeboid motility; chemotaxis
eosinophil	destroy parasites; allergic reactions
basophil	store and release histamine; allergic reactions

Table 2 Roles of the Six Types of Leukocytes

Platelets and Hemostasis

Like red blood cells, platelets have no nuclei and a limited lifespan. They are derived from the fragmentation of large bone marrow cells called **megakaryocytes**, which are derived from the same stem cells that give rise to red blood cells and white blood cells. The function of platelets is to aggregate at the site of damage to a blood vessel wall, forming a **platelet plug**. This immediately helps stop bleeding. **Hemostasis** is a term for the body's mechanism of preventing bleeding.

The other component of the hemostatic response is **fibrin**. This is a threadlike protein which forms a mesh that holds the platelet plug together. When the fibrin mesh dries, it becomes a scab, which seals and protects the wound. The plasma protein **fibrinogen** is converted into fibrin by a protein called **thrombin** when bleeding occurs. A blood clot, or **thrombus**, is a scab circulating in the bloodstream. Calcium as well as many accessory proteins are necessary for the activation of thrombin and fibrinogen. Several of the proteins depend on vitamin K for their function. Defects in these proteins result in **hemophilia** ("loving to bleed"), an X-linked recessive group of diseases involving excessive bleeding.

16.5   TRANSPORT OF GASES

Oxygen

Oxygen is too hydrophobic to dissolve in the plasma in significant quantities. Hence, RBCs are used to bind and carry O_2. RBCs are able to carry oxygen because they contain millions of molecules of **hemoglobin** (Hb). This is a complex protein composed of four polypeptide subunits. Each subunit contains one molecule of **heme**, which is a large multi-ring structure that has a single iron atom bound at its center. The role of heme with its iron atom is to bind O_2. Since each hemoglobin has four subunits and each subunit has one heme, each molecule of hemoglobin can carry four molecules of oxygen. Hemoglobin has some important properties which make it an excellent oxygen carrier.

The four subunits of hemoglobin do not bind oxygen independently of each other. When none of the subunits have oxygen bound, all four subunits assume a **tense** conformation that has a relatively low affinity for oxygen. (A *conformation* is a specific three-dimensional structure of a protein.) When one of the subunits binds oxygen, its conformation changes from a tense to a **relaxed** state that has a higher affinity for oxygen. The change in the three-dimensional structure of the subunit with oxygen bound is then communicated to the other subunits through contacts between the polypeptides to alter their conformation and increase their affinity for oxygen as well. Thus, hemoglobin is said to bind oxygen **cooperatively**.

- Myoglobin is a molecule with a structure very similar to hemoglobin, but with a single subunit that has one binding site. Does myoglobin display cooperativity in oxygen binding?[16]
- If binding of oxygen is cooperative, is it saturable?[17]
- Does hemoglobin have higher affinity for oxygen in the tissues or in the lungs?[18]

This has monumental significance for the ability of the blood to transport oxygen efficiently. The level of O_2 in active tissues is very low, because they use it in oxidative phosphorylation. Hence, in the tissues, hemoglobin has low affinity for oxygen and tends to release any oxygen which it carries. The level of O_2 in the lungs is of course very high. Hence, when a red blood cell is passing through a capillary in the lungs, the hemoglobin it contains will have higher affinity due to cooperative binding and will tend to

---

[16] Cooperativity requires more than one binding site in a protein so that one binding site can alter the affinity of another. Myoglobin cannot be cooperative in oxygen binding since it has only one binding site.

[17] There are a limited number of binding sites, even if they are cooperative, so binding will be saturated at a high concentration (partial pressure) of oxygen. There is a limit to the oxygen carrying capacity of the blood.

[18] At higher partial pressure of oxygen, more of the hemoglobin protein will have at least one of the subunits occupied with oxygen. Since binding is cooperative, the more oxygen that is bound, the higher the affinity for oxygen. The partial pressure of oxygen is higher in the lungs than in the tissues, so hemoglobin will have higher affinity for oxygen in the lungs.

bind oxygen very strongly. The result is that a lot of oxygen is picked up by RBCs in the lungs, and most of it is released as they pass through active tissues that need oxygen. This is an amazing example of how structural biochemistry determines physiology (or vice versa).

There is even more complexity to the hemoglobin story. It turns out that certain factors stabilize the tense configuration (which has a low O_2 affinity). These factors are:

1) decreased pH,
2) increased P_{CO_2} (level of CO_2 in the blood), and
3) increased temperature.

The fact that these factors stabilize tense hemoglobin and thus reduce its oxygen affinity is known as the **Bohr effect**. This system is truly incredible when you realize that these three factors perfectly characterize the environment within active tissues.

The affinity of hemoglobin for oxygen can be quantified by measurement of the fraction of O_2-binding sites which have bound O_2. If hemoglobin is in the relaxed configuration, then as more oxygen becomes available, much more of it will be bound up. But if it is in the tense configuration, the tendency to bind oxygen is reduced, and less will be bound. This can be described mathematically using the notion of **percent saturation (% sat.)**:

$$\% \text{ sat.} = (\# \text{ of } O_2 \text{ molecules bound}) \div (\# \text{ of } O_2 \text{ binding sites}) \times 100\%$$

- At a given P_{O_2}, which has a higher % sat.: tense or relaxed hemoglobin?[19]

This information can be depicted graphically, using an **O_2-Hemoglobin Dissociation Curve**, which plots % sat. vs. P_{O_2} (Figure 10). The sigmoidal shape of the curve resembles the behavior of cooperative enzymes.

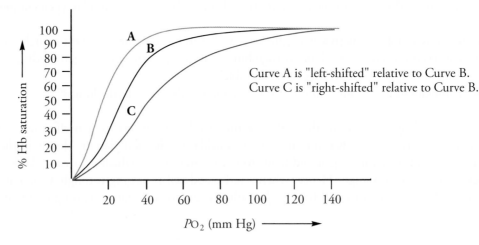

Curve A is "left-shifted" relative to Curve B.
Curve C is "right-shifted" relative to Curve B.

Figure 10 O_2-Hemoglobin Dissociation Curves

---

[19] Relaxed, since it has a higher affinity. This just means that at any O_2 level, relaxed hemoglobin will bind more O_2 than tense hemoglobin will.

Answer all of the following questions about Figure 10 before looking at the footnote.[20]

- Curve _____ represents Hb with the highest affinity of all.
- Curve C could be the result of _____.
- Curve A would most likely be seen in what region of the body?
- Why do all the curves level off?

Carbon Dioxide

Carbon dioxide is transported in the blood in three ways:

1) 73% of CO_2 transport is accomplished by the conversion of CO_2 to **carbonic acid**, which can dissociate into **bicarbonate** and a **proton** according to this reaction: $CO_2 + H_2O \rightleftharpoons H_2CO_3 \rightleftharpoons HCO_3^- + H^+$. These compounds are extremely water-soluble and are thus easily carried in the blood. The conversion of CO_2 into carbonic acid is catalyzed by an RBC enzyme called **carbonic anhydrase**. Remember that this reaction is also important as the principal plasma pH buffer.

2) Some CO_2 (~20%) is transported by simply being stuck onto hemoglobin. It does *not* bind to the oxygen-binding sites, but rather to other sites on the protein. Binding of CO_2 to hemoglobin is important in the Bohr effect because it stabilizes tense Hb.

3) CO_2 is somewhat more water-soluble than O_2, so a fair amount (~7%) can be dissolved in the blood and carried from the tissues to the lungs. Virtually no oxygen can be dissolved in the blood.

Exchange of Substances Across the Capillary Wall

The capillaries are the site of exchange between the blood and tissues. To facilitate exchange, capillaries have walls of only a single layer of flattened endothelial cells, and there are spaces (**intercellular clefts**) between the endothelial cells which make up the capillary wall. Three types of substances must be able to pass through the clefts: nutrients, wastes, and white blood cells. We will discuss each of these in turn. [Is it necessary for O_2 and CO_2 to pass through the clefts?[21]]

There are three main types of nutrients: amino acids, glucose, and lipids. Amino acids and glucose are absorbed from the digestive tract and carried by a special vein called the **hepatic portal vein** to the liver. It is called a *portal vein* because it connects two capillary beds: the one in the intestinal wall and the one inside the liver. The liver stores amino acids and glucose, and it releases them into the bloodstream as needed. From the bloodstream they can pass through capillary clefts into the tissues. The journey of lipids through the bloodstream is different. Fats are absorbed from the intestine and packaged into

---

[20] Curve A is farthest to the left and thus represents the highest affinity. Curve C could be the result of the Bohr effect. At a given O_2 level, the hemoglobin studied in Curve C has less of a tendency to bind oxygen (a lower affinity). Curve A would most likely be seen in the lungs, where there is plenty of oxygen and relaxed hemoglobin predominates. All the curves level off because 100% is the maximum degree of saturation; all the hemoglobin molecules become completely saturated.

[21] No, they can pass straight through any cell by simple diffusion.

16.5

chylomicrons, which are a type of lipoprotein. The chylomicrons enter tiny lymphatic vessels in the intestinal wall called **lacteals**. The lacteals empty into larger lymphatics, which eventually drain into a large vein near the neck. Hence, dietary fats bypass the hepatic vein. The result is that after eating a fatty meal, a person's blood will appear milky. (The term for this is **lipemia**, which means "lipids flowing in the blood.") The chylomicrons are taken up by the liver and converted into another type of lipoprotein, which is released into the bloodstream. This lipoprotein carries fats to **adipocytes** (fat cells) for storage. When fats are to be used for energy, adipocyte triglycerides are hydrolyzed, and free fatty acids are released into the bloodstream. They pass easily through capillary pores and thus can be picked up by cells of various tissues.

Many wastes are produced during cellular metabolism. They diffuse through the capillary walls into the bloodstream. The liver removes many wastes and converts them into forms which can be excreted in the feces. Such compounds are passed into the gut as **bile**. Other wastes are excreted directly by the kidneys.

White blood cells must be able to pass out of capillaries in order to patrol the tissues for invading microorganisms. Two of the six types of white blood cell can squeeze through the clefts: the _____ and the _____. These are large cells which depend on _____ in order to fit through the clefts, which are too small to allow RBCs to pass.[22]

It is also important to realize that water has a great tendency to flow out of capillaries, through the clefts. There are two reasons: 1) the hydrostatic pressure (fluid pressure) created by the heart simply tends to squeeze water out of the capillaries, and 2) the high osmolarity of the tissues tends to draw water out of the bloodstream. The circulatory system deals with this problem by giving the plasma a high osmolarity. [Would dissolving NaCl in the plasma accomplish this?[23]] Plasma osmolarity is provided by high concentrations of large plasma proteins, mainly albumin. Albumin is too large and rigid to pass through the clefts, so it remains in the capillaries and keeps water there too. The osmotic pressure provided by plasma proteins is given a special name: **oncotic pressure**. However, some water does leak out, resulting in an interesting cycle.

1) At the beginning of the capillary, the hydrostatic pressure is high. The result is that water squeezes out into the tissues.
2) As water continues to leave the capillary, the relative concentration of plasma proteins increases.
3) At the end of the capillary the hydrostatic pressure is quite low, but since the blood is now very concentrated, the oncotic pressure is very high. As a result, water flows back into the capillary from the tissues.

Thus, some water is lost into the tissues, but due to the oncotic pressure of the plasma proteins, the net loss is normally low.

•   Albumin is made in the liver. Alcoholics with diseased livers make insufficient amounts of albumin, and thus have insufficient plasma oncotic pressure. What would be the effect on the body?[24]

---

[22] Macrophages and neutrophils can squeeze through the clefts, even though they are larger than RBCs, because they are capable of *amoeboid motility*, as noted in Table 2. RBCs are not capable of independent motility.

[23] No, because salts can freely pass out of the capillaries.

[24] The result is systemic edema (swelling, or fluid collection), including the limbs, abdomen, and lungs.

16.6 FUNCTIONS OF THE RESPIRATORY SYSTEM

Single-cell eukaryotes that require oxygen to perform oxidative phosphorylation can acquire it by simple diffusion of oxygen from the surrounding medium. Even simple multicellular organisms such as coelenterates (jellyfish and hydra) can still receive sufficient oxygen by diffusion between cells and the environment. Larger organisms, such as the vertebrates, evolved a respiratory system to exchange O_2 and CO_2 between the atmosphere and the blood and a circulatory system to transport those gases between the respiratory system and the rest of the tissues of the body. Note that at the cellular level, all organisms exchange respiratory gases via simple diffusion across the plasma membrane. However, the respiratory system ensures the efficient delivery of O_2 and removal of CO_2 for all cells in a complex, multicellular animal.

The simple movement of air into and out of the lungs is properly called **ventilation**, whereas the actual exchange of gases (between either the lungs and the blood or the blood and the other tissues of the body) is called **respiration**. The parts of the respiratory system that participate *only* in ventilation are referred to as the **conduction zone**, and the parts that participate in actual gas exchange are referred to as the **respiratory zone**. Additional tasks performed by the respiratory system include the following:

1) *pH regulation*. In the blood, CO_2 is converted to carbonic acid by the RBC enzyme carbonic anhydrase. When CO_2 is exhaled by the lungs, the amount of carbonic acid in the blood is decreased, as a result, the pH of the blood increases (becomes more alkaline). ***Hyperventilation*** (too much breathing) causes alkalinization of the blood, known as **respiratory alkalosis**. ***Hypoventilation*** (too little breathing) causes acidification of the blood, or **respiratory acidosis**. [Which organ regulates pH over a period of hours to days?[25]]

2) *Thermoregulation*. Breathing can result in significant heat loss. Heat loss from the respiratory system occurs through **evaporative water loss**, which functions under the same principles as sweating.

3) *Protection from disease and particulate matter*. The lungs provide a large moist surface where chemicals and pathogens can do harm. The **mucociliary escalator** and alveolar macrophages, discussed later, protect us from harmful inhaled particles.

---

[25] The kidney

16.7   ANATOMY OF THE RESPIRATORY SYSTEM

The Conduction Zone

As mentioned previously, the part of the respiratory system designed only to allow gases to enter and exit the system is called the conduction zone (Figure 11). Inhaled air follows this pathway: **nose → nasal cavity → pharynx → larynx → trachea → bronchi → terminal bronchioles → respiratory bronchioles → alveolar ducts → alveoli** (the respiratory bronchioles, alveolar ducts, and alveoli are parts of the respiratory zone and will be discussed later). The nose is important for warming, humidifying, and filtering inhaled air; nasal hairs and sticky mucus act as filters. The nasal cavity is an open space within the nose. The pharynx is the throat (a common pathway for air and food) at the bottom of which is the larynx. The larynx has three functions: 1) it is made entirely of cartilage and thus keeps the airway open, 2) it contains the **epiglottis**, which seals the trachea during swallowing to prevent the entry of food, and 3) it contains the **vocal cords**, which are folds of tissue positioned to partially block the flow of air and vibrate, thereby producing sound. The **trachea** is a passageway which must remain open to permit air flow. Rings of cartilage prevent its collapse. The trachea branches into two **primary bronchi**, each of which supplies one lung. Each bronchus branches repeatedly to supply the entire lung. Collapse of bronchi is prevented by small plates of cartilage. Very small bronchi are called **bronchioles**. They are about 1 mm wide and contain no cartilage. Their walls are made of smooth muscle, which allows their diameters to be regulated to adjust airflow into the system. The smallest (and final) branches of the conduction zone are aptly called the **terminal bronchioles**.

The smooth muscle of the walls of the terminal bronchioles is too thick to allow adequate diffusion of gases; this is why no gas exchange occurs in this region. The conduction zone is strictly for ventilation.

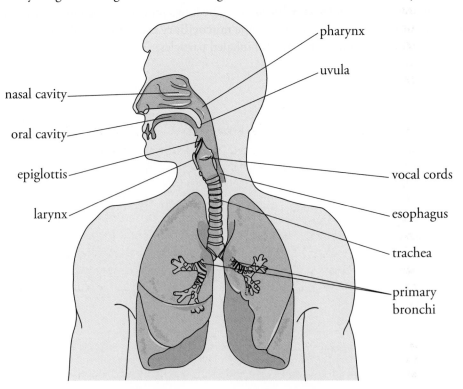

Figure 11   The Conduction Zone

The Respiratory Zone

The region of the system where gas exchange occurs is the respiratory zone (Figure 12). The actual structure across which gases diffuse is called the **alveolus** (plural: **alveoli**). Alveoli are tiny sacs with very thin walls (they're so thin that they're transparent!). The wall of the alveolus is only one cell thick, except where capillaries pass across its outer surface. The duct leading to the alveoli is called an **alveolar duct**, and its walls are entirely made of alveoli. The alveolar duct branches off a **respiratory bronchiole**. This is a tube made of smooth muscle, just like the terminal bronchioles, but with one important difference: the respiratory bronchiole has a few alveoli scattered in its walls. This allows it to perform gas exchange, so it is part of the respiratory zone.

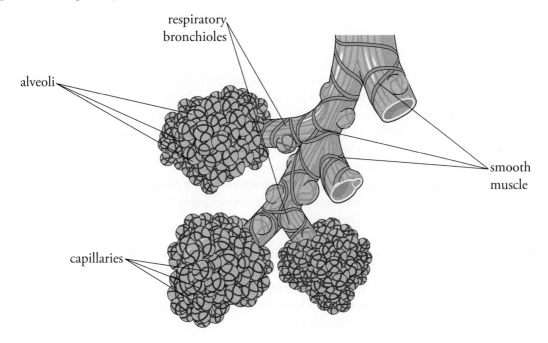

Figure 12   The Respiratory Zone

The Respiratory Epithelium: Protection from Disease and Particulate Matter

The entire respiratory tract is lined by epithelial cells. From the nose all the way down to the bronchioles, the epithelial cells are tall **columnar** (column-shaped) cells. They are too thick to assist in gas exchange; they merely provide a conduit for air. Some of these cells are specialized to secrete a layer of sticky mucus and are called **goblet cells** (just like in the gastrointestinal tract). The columnar epithelial cells of the upper respiratory tract have cilia on their apical surfaces which constantly sweep the layer of mucus toward the pharynx, where mucus containing pathogens and inhaled particles can be swallowed or coughed out. This system is known as the **mucociliary escalator**. [What would be the advantage of swallowing pathogens and particles?[26]]

---

[26] Gastric acidity destroys many pathogens. Also, particles which would likely harm the delicate alveoli are unlikely to harm the tough lining of the GI tract.

The alveoli, alveolar ducts, and the smallest bronchioles (respiratory bronchioles) are involved in gas exchange. Oxygen and CO_2 must be able to diffuse across the layer of epithelial cells in order to pass freely between the bloodstream and the air in the lungs. Tall columnar cells with cilia would be too large to permit rapid diffusion. Hence, gas-exchanging surfaces are lined with a single layer of thin, delicate squamous epithelial cells. (Squamous means flat.) A single layer of squamous epithelial cells is called *simple squamous epithelium*. It would also be unacceptable to have a layer of mucus covering the gas exchange surface, so another method of protection from disease and inhaled particles is necessary. Alveolar macrophages fill this role by patrolling the alveoli, engulfing foreign particles.

Surfactant

16.7

Imagine a bee hive made of tissue paper. If you put it in a steamy bathroom, what would happen? Would all the small air spaces remain filled with air? No, the hive would collapse into a wet ball, because the mutual attraction of water molecules would overcome the flimsy support structure provided by the fine paper fibers. The tendency of water molecules to clump together creates **surface tension**, which is the force that causes wet hydrophilic surfaces (e.g., the tissue paper) to stick together in the presence of air. Think of it this way: air is hydrophobic, so hydrophilic substances in the presence of air tend to clump together. Now imagine a bee hive made of thin wax paper. If you put it into a steamy room, does it collapse? No, because the wax on the surface of the paper prevents adjacent pieces of paper from being strongly attracted. In other words, the wax destroys the surface tension.

The alveoli are as fine and delicate as tissue paper, and they too tend to collapse due to surface tension (Figure 13). This problem is solved by a soapy substance called **surfactant** (*surf*ace *act*ive substance), which coats the alveoli. Just like the wax in our example above, surfactant reduces surface tension. Surfactant is a complex mixture of phospholipids, proteins, and ions secreted by cells in the alveolar wall. [Is it likely that these are the principal lining cells of the alveolar wall?[27]]

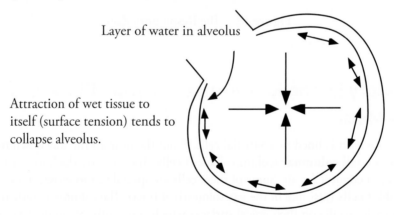

Layer of water in alveolus

Attraction of wet tissue to itself (surface tension) tends to collapse alveolus.

Figure 13   Surface Tension in an Alveolus

---

[27] No, the principal cells of the alveolar wall are thin, squamous cells designed to allow diffusion of gases. Cells which actively secrete substances (i.e., surfactant) are large, metabolically active cells with many mitochondria. The basic alveolar lining cells (simple squamous epithelium) are called Type 1 alveolar cells. The fat (cuboidal) epithelial cells that secrete surfactant are called Type 2 alveolar cells.

- There is not sufficient surfactant within a fetus' lungs until about the eighth month of gestation, so some premature infants lack the protective effects of surfactant when they are born. Which of the following statements best describes resulting effects upon respiration in "preemies" (babies born prematurely)?[28]
    - A) Surface tension would be abnormally low.
    - B) The alveoli would collapse.
    - C) Oxygen would be unable to diffuse through water.
    - D) Respiration is unnecessary, since the infant is dependent on the mother.

16.8 PULMONARY VENTILATION

Pulmonary ventilation is the circulation of air into and out of the lungs to continually replace the gases in the alveoli with those in the atmosphere. The drawing of air into the lungs is termed **inspiration**, and the movement of air out of the lungs is termed **expiration**. Inspiration is an active process driven by the contraction of the diaphragm, which enlarges the chest cavity (and the lungs along with the chest cavity) when drawing air in. Passive expiration is driven by the elastic recoil of the lungs and does not require active muscle contraction. These processes will be described in more detail below.

The Pleural Space and Lung Elasticity

The lungs are large elastic bags that tend to collapse in upon themselves if removed from the chest cavity. The structures of the chest prevent this collapse, however, and they allow the lungs to remain inflated during inspiration and expiration. The lungs are not directly connected to the chest wall, however. Each lung is surrounded by two membranes, or **pleura**: the **parietal pleura**, which lines the inside of the chest cavity, and the **visceral pleura**, which lines the surface of the lungs (Figure 14). Between the two pleura is a very narrow space called the **pleural space**. The pressure in the pleural space (the **pleural pressure**) is negative, meaning that the two pleural membranes are drawn tightly together by a vacuum. This negative pressure keeps the outer surface of the lungs drawn up against the inside of the chest wall. Additionally, a thin layer of fluid between the two pleura helps hold them together through surface tension.

---

[28] In the absence of surfactant, surface tension would be high (choice A is wrong), and the alveoli would collapse on every exhalation like tissue-paper beehives (choice **B** is correct). It would take an enormous exertion to reopen the collapsed alveoli to get any air (oxygen) into them; the result is poor oxygen delivery to the alveoli and thus to the blood (for this reason, preemies are typically kept on ventilators until their surfactant levels are higher and they are stronger in general). Note that oxygen has some ability to diffuse through water, but choice C is wrong mostly due to irrelevance. It's not as though in the absence of surfactant the lungs suddenly fill with water. Respiration is always necessary once a baby is born; this question specifically refers to infants born prematurely (choice D is wrong).

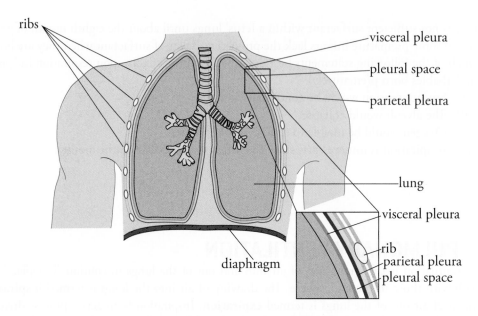

ribs

visceral pleura

pleural space

parietal pleura

lung

visceral pleura

rib

parietal pleura

pleural space

diaphragm

Figure 14 The Lungs and Pleura

- If the pleural space is punctured, opening it to the external atmosphere, which one of the following will occur?[29]
  - A) Fluid will leak out of the pleural space.
  - B) Air will leak out of the pleural space.
  - C) Air will leak into the pleural space.
  - D) Since the pressure within the pleural space is equal to atmospheric pressure during expiration, nothing will happen.

Inspiration is caused by muscular expansion of the chest wall, which draws the lungs outward (expands them) and causes air to enter the system. The lungs expand along with the chest due to the negative pressure in the pleural space. The expansion of the chest during inspiration is driven primarily by contraction of the **diaphragm**, a large skeletal muscle that is stretched below the ribs between the abdomen and the chest cavity. When resting, the diaphragm is shaped like a dome, bulging upward into the chest cavity. When it contracts, the diaphragm flattens and draws the chest cavity downward, forcing it and the lungs (which are stuck to the inside wall of the chest cavity) to expand. The external **intercostal muscles** between the ribs also contract during inspiration, pulling the ribs upward and further expanding the chest cavity. Inspiration is an *active* process, requiring contraction of muscles to occur.

Resting expiration, by contrast, is a *passive* process (no muscle contraction required). When the diaphragm and rib muscles relax, the elastic recoil of the lungs draws the chest cavity inward, reducing the volume of the lungs and pushing air out of the system into the atmosphere. During exertion (or at other times when a more forcible exhalation is required), contraction of abdominal muscles helps the expiration process by pressing upward on the diaphragm, further shrinking the size of the lungs and forcing more air out. This is called a **forced expiration** and is an active process.

---

[29] The pleural space is always at negative pressure, or the lung would collapse. If the pleural pressure is negative, and an opening to the atmosphere is made, then air will rush into the pleural space and the lungs will collapse. The correct answer is choice **C**. (Note that choice A will probably also occur, but the amount of fluid is so minimal as to be insignificant. Choice C is the better choice.)

The pressure of air in the alveoli and the pleural pressure vary during inspiration and expiration. During inspiration, the following steps occur:

1) The diaphragm contracts and flattens (moves downward).
2) The volume of the chest cavity expands.
3) The pleural pressure decreases, becoming more negative.
4) The lungs expand outward.
5) The pressure in the alveoli becomes negative.
6) Air enters the lungs and the alveoli.

The opposite steps occur during expiration. Typically inspiration and expiration are not consciously controlled although they are mediated by voluntary muscle (which means we *can* control the processes if we want to!).

- What would be the result of a hole in the lung that allowed inhaled air to flow into the pleural cavity?[30]

16.8

Pulmonary Ventilation: Volumes and Capacities

Spirometry is the measurement of the volume of air entering or exiting the lungs at the various stages of ventilation.[31] A **spirometer** is a device used for these measurements. Data can be plotted on a **spirometric graph** (Figure 15). The volumes and capacities defined below should be familiar to you but do *not* need to be memorized.

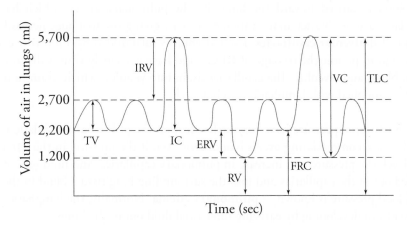

Figure 15 Lung Volumes and Capacities

The **tidal volume (TV)** is the amount of air that moves in and out of the lungs with normal light breathing and is equal to about 10 percent of the total volume of the lungs (0.5 liters out of 5–6 liters). The **expiratory reserve volume (ERV)** is the volume of air that can be expired after a passive resting expiration. The **inspiratory reserve volume (IRV)** is the volume of air that can be inspired after a relaxed inspiration.

---

[30] A hole in the lung would allow air to flow into the pleural cavity, just like a hole from the pleural space to the exterior. This would cause the lung to collapse, because negative pleural pressure is the only significant force opposing lung collapse. Inspiration would be impossible.

[31] *Spir-* is from re*spir*ation.

The **functional residual capacity** (**FRC**) is the volume of air left in the lungs after a resting expiration. The **inspiratory capacity** (**IC**) is the maximal volume of air which can be inhaled after a resting expiration. The **residual volume** (**RV**) is the amount of air that remains in the lungs after the strongest possible expiration. The **vital capacity** (**VC**) is the maximum amount of air that can be forced out of the lungs after first taking the deepest possible breath. The **total lung capacity** (**TLC**) is the vital capacity plus the residual volume (TLC = VC + RV).

- Is the total volume of the lungs exchanged with each breath?[32]

- In emphysema, lung elasticity is greatly reduced. Each of the following occurs EXCEPT:[33]
  A) Residual volume increases.
  B) Total lung capacity increases.
  C) Resting expiration becomes active instead of passive.
  D) Pleural pressure becomes more negative.

16.9 GAS EXCHANGE

The Pulmonary Circulation

Deoxygenated blood is carried toward the lungs by the pulmonary artery, which has left and right branches. These large arteries branch many times, eventually giving rise to a huge network of **pulmonary capillaries**, also called **alveolar capillaries**. Each alveolus is surrounded by a few tiny capillaries, which are just wide enough to permit the passage of RBCs, and have extremely thin walls to permit diffusion of gases between blood and alveolus. The capillaries drain into venules, which drain into the pulmonary veins. The lungs are supplied with lymphatic vessels as well.

Small increases in left atrial pressure have very little effect on the pulmonary circulation because pulmonary veins can dilate, accommodating excess blood. However, if the pressure in the left atrium increases above a certain level, the pressure will increase in pulmonary capillaries, and fluid (essentially blood plasma) will be forced out of the capillaries and into the surrounding lung tissue. Fluid in the lungs resulting from increased blood pressure is known as **pulmonary edema**. Normally, the lymphatic system prevents pulmonary edema from developing by carrying interstitial fluid out of the lungs.

---

[32] No, some air always remains in the lungs; the FRC during relaxed breathing or the RV during deep breathing.

[33] Typically, when the lungs are stretched on inspiration, elastic recoil draws them inward and leads to expiration. The loss of elasticity means that the lungs do not want to recoil as strongly (or at all) and remain in their stretched position (choice B would occur and can be eliminated). Thus, expiration is not as efficient and more air remains in the lungs after expiration than normal (choice A would occur and can be eliminated). In order to make expiration more efficient, contraction of internal intercostal and abdominal muscles must be used to compress the chest cavity and push air out (choice C would occur and can be eliminated). Even at rest, alveoli are typically stretched somewhat and elastic recoil tends to draw them inward; this helps creates the negative pleural pressure. However, if lung elasticity is reduced, there is less of a force drawing them inward, and the pleural pressure would be less negative, not more (choice **D** would not occur and is the correct answer choice).

- Which of the following may result from increased pulmonary capillary hydrostatic pressure?[34]

    I. Accumulation of interstitial fluid in the lungs
    II. Fluid accumulation in the alveoli
    III. Decreased oxygenation of the blood due to excess fluid slowing O_2 diffusion

    A) I and II only
    B) I and III only
    C) II and III only
    D) I, II, and III

The lungs are "designed" to expose a large amount of blood to a large amount of air. Hence, the primary property of the lung is its enormous surface area, close to that of a tennis court. The goal is to allow O_2 from the atmosphere to diffuse into pulmonary capillaries, where it is bound by hemoglobin in RBCs. Simultaneously, CO_2 diffuses from the blood to the alveolar gas.

Air is a complex mixture of many gases, with nitrogen and oxygen as its primary components and other gases such as water vapor and carbon dioxide forming small percentages of the total (Table 3). In cities, poisons such as carbon monoxide may attain significant concentrations (partial pressures).

Gas	% of atmosphere
N_2	80%
O_2	20%
H_2O	0.5%
CO_2	0.04%

Table 3 Approximate Atmospheric Gas Compositions

Each gas that is part of a mixture contributes to the total pressure of the mixture in proportion to its abundance. The contribution of each individual gas to the total pressure is termed the **partial pressure**. The partial pressure of Gas X is abbreviated P_X. For example, P_{O_2} designates the partial pressure of oxygen. [If the total atmospheric pressure is 760 torr, what is the partial pressure of oxygen (P_{O_2}) in the atmosphere?[35]] The total pressure is the sum of all partial pressures.

Henry's Law

Gases in the air equilibrate with gases in liquids. If you place a beaker of water in a room, after a time, the gases in the room will diffuse into the water. Hence, partial pressures are also used to describe the amount of gases carried in the bloodstream.

In order to diffuse into a cell, gas molecules from the air must dissolve into a liquid (e.g., extracellular fluid). According to **Henry's Law**, the amount of gas that will dissolve into liquid is dependent on the partial pressure of that gas as well as the solubility of that gas in the liquid. If we use oxygen as an example, Henry's Law states:

---

[34] If the hydrostatic pressure is high enough, all of these will result (choice D).

[35] Oxygen forms 20% of the atmosphere (Table 3). The partial pressure of oxygen in the atmosphere is 20% of 760 torr, or about 150 torr.

$$[O_2] = P_{O_2} \times S_{O_2}$$

where $[O_2]$ is the concentration of dissolved oxygen, P_{O_2} is the partial pressure of oxygen in the air above the fluid, and S_{O_2} is the solubility of oxygen in that liquid. Thus, an increase in pressure increases the amount of gas dissolved in a liquid.

Note that gases become less soluble in liquids as temperatures increase; this is why a soda goes flat faster on a hot day, and it is why a goldfish will gulp for air when the water is too warm. [Scuba divers breathe pressurized air. Why do they have to worry about nitrogen bubbles forming in the extracellular fluid if they ascend too quickly?[36]]

In the lungs, oxygen and carbon dioxide diffuse between the alveolar air and blood in the alveolar capillaries (Figure 16). The driving force for the exchange of gases in the lungs is the difference in partial pressures between the alveolar air and the blood. For diffusion to occur (from the air to the blood), gases must first pass across the alveolar epithelium, then through the interstitial liquid, and finally across the capillary endothelium. These three barriers to diffusion together form the **respiratory membrane** (the pathway is obviously reversed for diffusion from the blood to the air). [Do the lipid membranes of the alveolar and capillary cells act as barriers to the diffusion of oxygen and carbon dioxide?[37]]

16.9

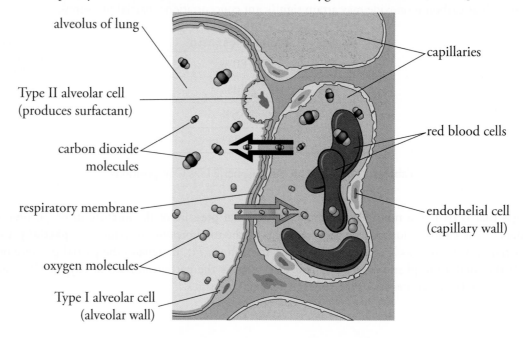

Figure 16   Diffusion of Gases Between an Alveolus and a Capillary

---

[36] Gases are more soluble in liquids at high pressures. At depth, gases dissolve into the blood and extracellular fluids more readily because of the high pressure of the surrounding water. If a diver ascends too quickly, the gases come out of solution before they can be transported to the respiratory system. This results in air bubbles that primarily contain nitrogen, the most abundant gas in the air we breathe. These bubbles tend to form most abundantly at the joints and cause decompression sickness, a painful condition commonly known as "the bends." To treat decompression sickness, afflicted divers are put into a hyperbaric (high pressure) chamber to redissolve the gases before slowly restoring the tissues to atmospheric pressure.

[37] No, lipid bilayers do not act as barriers to the diffusion of such small hydrophobic molecules.

As blood passes through the alveolar capillaries, the oxygen pressure gradient between the alveolar air and the blood drives the net diffusion of oxygen into the blood. The arterial P_{O_2} is denoted P_aO_2.

- Is the P_{O_2} at the arterial end of pulmonary capillaries greater than, less than, or equal to the P_{O_2} in the venous end?[38]

- Although the partial pressures of oxygen and nitrogen in the atmosphere are relatively constant, the partial pressure of water vapor can vary considerably. If water vapor in the atmosphere increases, which one of the following will occur?[39]
    - A) The total atmospheric pressure will increase.
    - B) The partial pressures of oxygen and nitrogen will decrease.
    - C) The partial pressure of oxygen will decrease, and the partial pressure of nitrogen will increase.
    - D) The partial pressure of oxygen will increase, and the partial pressure of nitrogen will decrease.

16.10 REGULATION OF VENTILATION RATE

Proper regulation of the rate and depth of breathing is essential. Although breathing can be voluntarily controlled for short periods of time, it is normally an involuntary process directed by the **respiratory control center** in the medulla of the brain stem. The stimuli that affect ventilation rate are both mechanical and chemical (Table 4).

The principal chemical stimuli that affect ventilation rate are increased P_{CO_2}, decreased pH, and decreased P_{O_2} (with CO_2 and pH being the primary regulators and O_2 secondary). These variables are monitored by special autonomic sensory receptors. **Peripheral chemoreceptors** are located in the aorta and the carotid arteries and monitor the P_{CO_2}, pH, and P_{O_2} of the blood, while **central chemoreceptors** are found in the medullary respiratory control center, and monitor P_{CO_2} and pH of the cerebrospinal fluid (CSF). Recall that pH and P_{CO_2} are connected through the carbonic acid buffer system of the blood (discussed briefly in Chapter 16).

$$CO_2 + H_2O \rightleftharpoons H_2CO_3 \rightleftharpoons H^+ + HCO_3^-$$

---

[38] Less than. Deoxygenated blood (P_{O_2} = 40 torr) enters the pulmonary system in the pulmonary artery. As the deoxygenated blood passes through the capillaries, it becomes increasingly oxygenated until it emerges at the venous end equilibrated with the alveolar oxygen pressure (P_{O_2} = 100 torr).

[39] Total atmospheric pressure is defined as the force exerted against a surface due to the weight of the air above that surface, thus it is determined primarily by gravitational forces and changes very little (choice A is wrong). Partial pressure, however, is defined as the portion of total pressure due to a particular gas. Thus, if the partial pressure of water increases (and since the total pressure remains the same), the relative partial pressures of oxygen and nitrogen would have to decrease (choice **B** is correct, and choices C and D are wrong).

Respiration eliminates CO_2 from the body. Thus, changes in ventilation rate can have rapid effects on pH due to the decrease or increase in P_{CO_2} and the resulting shift to maintain the above equilibrium. For example, a person hyperventilating during an anxiety attack can have an elevated pH. [Why do we give these folks a paper bag to breathe into?[40]] A person whose ventilation rate has been reduced due to extreme alcohol intoxication can become acidotic. Similarly, changes in pH can be compensated for by increasing or decreasing ventilation rate. For example, diabetics who are acidotic due to the metabolism of proteins and fats instead of glucose will have an increased ventilation rate to remove CO_2 and increase pH.

Mechanical stimuli that affect ventilation rate include physical stretching of the lungs and irritants. The mechanical stretching of lung tissue stimulates stretch receptors that inhibit further excitatory signals from the respiratory center to the muscles involved in inspiration. The walls of bronchi and larger bronchioles contain smooth muscle. Contraction of this smooth muscle is known as **bronchoconstriction**. Irritation of the inner lining of the lung stimulates irritant receptors, and reflexive contraction of bronchial smooth muscle prevents irritants from continuing to enter the passageways.

There are also **irritant receptors** in the lung that trigger coughing and/or bronchoconstriction when an irritating chemical (such as smoke) is detected.

Stimulus	Receptor	Effect
stretch of lung	stretch receptor in lung	inhibits inspiration
↑P_{CO_2}	peripheral chemoreceptors and medullary respiratory center	increased P_{CO_2} causes ↓pH via carbonic anhydrase; the ↓pH is what is actually sensed (see below)
↓pH	as above	increases respiratory rate
↓P_{O_2}	peripheral chemoreceptors	increases respiratory rate
chemical irritation	irritant receptor in lung	coughing and/or bronchoconstriction

Table 4 Factors that Regulate Ventilation Rate

16.10

---

[40] Breathing into a paper bag forces them to rebreathe their exhaled CO_2. This pushes the equilibrium of the equation to the right and brings pH back down to normal.

16.11   THE LYMPHATIC SYSTEM

The lymphatic system (Figure 17) is a one-way flow system which begins with tiny lymphatic capillaries in all the tissues of the body that merge to form larger lymphatic vessels. These merge to form large lymphatic ducts. Lymphatic vessels have valves, and the larger lymphatic ducts have smooth muscles in their walls. As a result, the lymphatic system acts like a suction pump to retrieve water, proteins, and white blood cells from the tissues. The fluid in lymphatic vessels is called **lymph**. The lymph is filtered by numerous **lymph nodes**. The lymph nodes are an important part of the immune system because they contain millions of white blood cells that can initiate an immune response against anything foreign that may have been picked up in the lymph. The large lymphatic ducts merge to form the **thoracic duct**, which is the largest lymphatic vessel, located in the chest. The thoracic duct empties into a large vein near the neck. Also, lymphatic vessels from the intestines dump dietary fats in the form of chylomicrons into the thoracic duct.

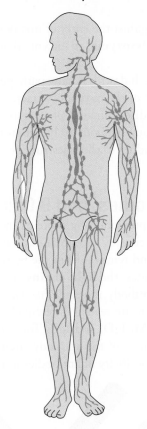

Figure 17   The Lymphatic System: Vessels and Lymph Nodes

16.11

16.12 THE IMMUNE SYSTEM

The interior of the body provides a warm, protective, nourishing environment where micro-organisms can flourish. We could not survive without a versatile and efficient immune system to destroy invaders without destroying the body itself. There are three types of immunity: innate, humoral, and cell-mediated.

Innate Immunity

Innate immunity refers to the general, non-specific protection the body provides against various invaders. The simplest example of innate immunity is the barrier to the outside world known as **skin**. The skin prevents many types of pathogens from infecting us. Here is a list of the principal components of innate immunity:

1) The skin is an excellent barrier against the entry of microorganisms.
2) Tears, saliva, and blood contain **lysozyme**, an enzyme that kills some bacteria by destroying their cell walls.
3) The extreme acidity of the stomach destroys many pathogens which are ingested with food or swallowed after being passed out of the respiratory tract.
4) Macrophages and neutrophils indiscriminately phagocytize microorganisms.[41]
5) The **complement system** is a group of about 20 blood proteins that can nonspecifically bind to the surface of foreign cells, leading to their destruction.

Humoral Immunity, Antibodies, and B Cells

Humoral immunity refers to specific protection by proteins in the plasma called **antibodies** (**Ab**) or **immunoglobulins** (**Ig**). Antibodies specifically recognize and bind to microorganisms (or other foreign particles), leading to their destruction and removal from the body. Each antibody molecule is composed of two copies of two different polypeptides, the **light chains** and the **heavy chains**, joined by disulfide bonds (Figure 18). In addition, each antibody molecule has two regions, the **constant region** and the **variable (antigen binding) region**. There are several different classes of immunoglobulins, differentiated by their constant regions: IgG, IgA, IgM, IgD, and IgE. The classes of immunoglobulins have slightly different functions (see Table 5); with most of the antibody circulating in plasma in the IgG class. The variable regions are responsible for the specificity of antibodies in recognizing foreign particles.

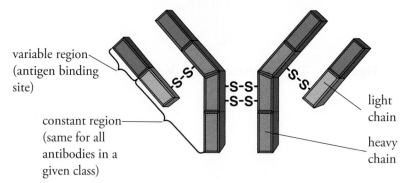

Figure 18 Antibody Structure

---

[41] Do not confuse this portion of innate immunity with cell-mediated immunity. You are correct to notice that cells are involved, but this activity is placed in the "innate" category because we are referring to non-specific phagocytosis. Humoral and cell-mediated immunity are highly specific. One other subtlety: when a macrophage eats an antigen which has been coated with specific antibodies, we are dealing with humoral immunity; this is different from the indiscriminate, nonspecific pathogen phagocytosis discussed above.

Constant Region Class	Location in Body	Function
IgM	blood and B cell surface	Involved in initial immune response; pentameric structure in blood, monomeric structure on B cell as antigen receptor
IgG	blood	Involved in ongoing immune response; the majority of antibody in the blood is IgG; can also cross the placental barrier
IgD	B cell surface	Serves with IgM as antigen receptor on B cells
IgA	secretions (saliva, mucus, tears, breast milk, etc.)	Secreted in breast milk; helps protect newborns, dimeric structure
IgE	blood	Involved in allergic reactions

Table 5   Classes of Antibodies

Each antibody forms a unique variable region that has a different binding specificity. The molecule that an antibody binds to is known as the **antigen** (**Ag**). Examples of antigens are viral capsid proteins, bacterial surface proteins, and toxins in the bloodstream (such as tetanus toxin). The specificity of antigen binding is determined by the fit of antigen in a small three-dimensional cleft formed by the variable region of the antibody molecule (Figure 18). Why might an antibody that binds tightly to a small region of a protein, five amino acids out of 200, have very low affinity for the same five amino acids of the protein when presented as an isolated peptide?[42] Antigens are often large molecules which have many different recognition sites for different antibodies. The small site that an antibody recognizes within a larger molecule is called an **epitope**. Very small molecules often do not elicit the production of antibodies on their own but will when bound to an antigenic large molecule like a protein. The protein in this case is called a **carrier**, and the small molecule that becomes antigenic is known as a **hapten**. When antibody binds to an antigen, the following can contribute to removal of the antigen from the body:

1) Binding of antibody may directly inactivate the antigen. For example, binding of antibody to a viral coat protein may prevent the virus from binding to cells.
2) Binding of antibody can induce phagocytosis of a particle by macrophages and neutrophils.
3) The presence of antibodies on the surface of a cell can activate the complement system to form holes in the cell membrane and lyse the cell.

Antibodies are produced by a type of lymphocyte called **B cells**. Antibodies produced by an individual B cell can recognize only one specific antigen, but B cells in general produce antibodies that recognize an immense array of antigens. Immature B cells are derived from precursor stem cells in the bone marrow. The genes that encode antibody proteins are assembled by recombination from many small segments during B cell development. Thus, there are many different B cell clones, each with a different variable region. The immature B cells express antibody molecules on their surface. When antigen binds to the antibody on the surface of a specific immature B cell, that cell is stimulated to proliferate and differentiate into two kinds of cells: **plasma cells** and **memory cells**. Plasma cells actively produce and secrete antibody protein into

16.12

---

[42] In the intact protein the five amino acids assume a specific three-dimensional conformation that is recognized well by the antibody. The five amino acids as a small peptide, however, will not fold the same way and probably would not be as well recognized by the antibody.

the plasma. Memory cells are produced from the same clone and have the same variable regions, but they do not secrete antibody; they are like pre-activated, dormant B cells. The memory cells remain dormant, sometimes for years, waiting for the same antigen to reappear. If it does, the memory cells *then* become activated, and start producing antibody very quickly; so quickly that no symptoms of illness appear. This method of selecting B cells with specific antigen binding is called **clonal selection**. [In general, every cell of the body is said to possess the same copy of the genome. Is this true in the immune system?[43]]

- Which one of the following best describes the mechanism by which production of specific antibody is achieved in response to antigen exposure?[44]
  - A) Immature B cell clones expressing several different antibody genes select for one gene and turn off expression of the others.
  - B) Antigen stimulates proliferation of a specific B cell clone expressing a single antibody protein that recognizes that antigen.
  - C) The variable regions of antibody proteins on an immature B cell clone form a pocket around the antigen, and the antibody genes are recombined to fit the bound antigen.
  - D) Antibody light and heavy chains are mixed on each B cell's surface in different combinations to produce different antigen recognition.

The first time a person encounters an antigen during an infection, it can take a week or more for B cells to proliferate and secrete significant levels of antibody. This is known as the **primary immune response** and is too slow to prevent symptoms of the infection from occurring. The immune response to the same antigen the second time a person is exposed, the **secondary immune response**, is much swifter and stronger, so much so that symptoms never develop, and the person is said to "be immune." This immunity can last for years and is due to the presence of the memory cells produced during the first infection. **Vaccination** is used to improve the response to infection by exposing the immune system to an antigen associated with a virus or bacterium, thus building up the secondary immune response if the live pathogen is encountered in the future. [Vaccination against some viruses is ineffective in preventing future infection, while it is highly effective against other viruses. Does the failure of vaccination to protect against some viruses indicate a failure in the ability to produce memory cells?[45]]

16.12

---

[43] No. Recombination during development of B cells and T cells makes these an exception to the generalization that every cell contains the whole genome.

[44] Choice **B** is correct. The two key features of clonal selection in B cells are 1) recombination during development to produce many clones, each with a single antigen recognition specificity, and 2) selection of a clone out of the many clones based on specific recognition of antigen by preexisting antibody genes.

[45] No. It is probably the result of mutation by the virus. Vaccination against one form of virus and production of memory cells will not protect against a virus if the viral antigen mutates so that it is no longer recognized by the immune system.

Cell-Mediated Immunity and the T Cell

There are two types of **T cells**: **T helpers** ("CD4 cells") and **T killers** (cytotoxic T cells, "CD8 cells"). The role of the T helper is to activate B cells, T killer cells, and other cells of the immune system. Hence, the T helper is the central controller of the whole immune response. It communicates with other cells by releasing special hormones called **lymphokines** and **interleukins**.[46] The T helper cell is the host of HIV, the virus that causes AIDS.

The role of the T killer cell is to *destroy abnormal host cells*, namely:
1) Virus-infected host cells
2) Cancer cells
3) Foreign cells such as the cells of a skin graft given by an incompatible donor

The "T" in "T cell" stands for **thymus**. T cells are named after this gland because this is where they develop during childhood. Trillions of different T cells are produced in the bone marrow during childhood. Each of these is specific for a particular antigen, just as with B cells. [If a T cell is specific for an antigen, does that mean it releases antibodies that bind to the antigen?[47]] The protein on the T cell surface that can bind antigen is the **T cell receptor**.

The function of T cells is exceedingly complex. As a brief introduction, the way a T cell recognizes a bad cell is by "examining" (binding to) proteins on its surface. One important group of cell-surface proteins is known as the **major histocompatibility complex** (**MHC**). Our cells are all programmed to have MHC proteins on their surfaces so that the immune system can keep an eye on what is going on inside every cell. There are two kinds of MHCs, known as MHC class I and MHC class II, or simply **MHC I** and **MHC II**. MHC I proteins are found on the surface of every nucleated cell in the body. Their role is to randomly pick up peptides from the inside of the cell and display them on the cell surface. This allows T cells to monitor cellular contents. For example, if a cell is infected with a virus, one of its class I MHC complexes will display a piece of a virus-specific protein. When a T killer cell detects the viral protein (by binding to it) displayed on the cell's MHC I, it becomes activated and will proliferate.

16.12

The role of MHC II is more complex. Only certain special cells have MHC II. These cells are known as **antigen-presenting cells** (**APCs**). The antigen-presenting cells include macrophages and B cells. Their role is to phagocytize particles or cells, chop them up, and display fragments using the MHC II display system, which T helpers then recognize (bind to). After a T helper is activated by antigen displayed in MHC II, it will activate B cells (and stimulate proliferation of T killer cells) that are specific for that antigen. The activated B cells mature into plasma cells and secrete antibodies specific for the antigen. The complexity of this process helps explain why the primary immune response takes a week or more.

- Can a T helper cell become activated after encountering a foreign particle floating in the blood? If so, how? If not, why not, and what else is required?[48]

Note that full activation of T cells only occurs when the T cell binds to both antigen (displayed on MHC I or II) and the MHC molecule itself.

---

[46] *Lympho-* is short for lymphocytes, and *-kine* means move or activate. *Inter-* means between, and *-leukin* is for leukocytes or white blood cells.

[47] No, only B cells make antibodies. If a T helper is specific for an antigen, it will activate B cells or T killers to destroy it.

[48] No, T helpers are only activated by antigen presented on MHC II. For a foreign particle to activate a helper T cell, the particle must first be displayed by an antigen-presenting cell (macrophage or B cell). The antigen-presenting cell must phagocytize the particle, hydrolyze it into fragments in a lysosome, and allow it to bind to an MHC II which will be displayed on the cell surface.

Other Tissues Involved in the Immune Response

The **bone marrow** is the site of synthesis of all the cells of the blood from a common progenitor. The cell which gives rise to all the various blood cells is called the bone marrow stem cell. **Lymph nodes** were discussed earlier in this chapter. The **spleen** filters the blood and is a site of immune cell interactions, just like lymph nodes. The spleen also destroys aged RBCs. The **thymus** is the site of T cell maturation. The thymus shrinks in size in adults since the maturation of the immune system and T cells is most active in children. The **tonsils** are masses of lymphatic tissue in the back of the throat that help "catch" pathogens which enter the body through respiration or ingestion. The **appendix** is very similar to the tonsils, both in structure and function, and is found near the beginning of the large intestine. Neither the appendix nor the tonsils are required for survival and are often removed if they become infected.

16.13   AUTOIMMUNITY

Ideally, the immune system will only recognize and destroy foreign antigen; it should ignore (not become activated against) all normal proteins and cell structures; this is called **tolerance**. However, the production of these trillions of different B cells and T cells with different receptors is random, and as a result, many of them will be specific for normal molecules found in the human body, or *self* antigens. Thus, B cells and T cells must go through a selection process in order to eliminate any self-reactive cells.

For B cells, this generally occurs in the bone marrow, but it can also occur in lymph nodes. An immature B cell whose surface receptor binds to normal cell surface proteins (for example, MHCs or other proteins on a macrophage or other bone marrow cell) is induced to die through apoptosis. Those whose surface receptors bind to normal soluble proteins (for example, hemoglobin or lipoproteins) do not go through apoptosis, but become unresponsive or **anergic**. Only those B cells whose surface receptors bind to no normal proteins during maturation are released into the circulation. For T cells, the process is similar, but it occurs in the thymus or in the lymph nodes; immature T cells whose antigen receptors bind normal proteins become anergic. The result of this is that billions of B and T cells survive, but billions of others do not. The ones that survive go on to proliferate if stimulated by antigen in the proper context, each producing a group of identical B or T cells, all specific for a particular antigen. Such a group is known as a **B cell or T cell clone**. Clonal selection in response to antigen recognition is similar in B and T cells.

It is very important to get rid of all cells specific for self-antigen, because such cells can cause an **autoimmune reaction**, in which the immune system attacks normal body cells or proteins. Obviously, this would cause problems as normal body structures become inflamed or destroyed. Some autoimmune diseases include type I diabetes mellitus, rheumatoid arthritis, Graves' disease, myasthenia gravis, and celiac disease. Autoimmune diseases are often treated with immunosuppressant drugs or with steroids to reduce the inflammatory response.

16.13

Chapter 17
The Excretory and Digestive Systems

17.1   THE EXCRETORY SYSTEM OVERVIEW

Excretion is the disposal of waste products. "The excretory system" generally refers to the kidneys, even though the liver, large intestine, and skin are involved in excretion too. Let's begin by summarizing the excretory roles of these organs, to see where the kidneys fit into the picture.

Liver

The **liver** is responsible for excreting many wastes by chemically modifying them and releasing them into bile (discussed later in this chapter). In particular, the liver deals with hydrophobic or large waste products, which cannot be filtered out by the kidney. (The kidney can only eliminate small hydrophils dissolved in plasma.) For example, in the liver, old heme units are broken down into bilirubin which is then tagged with a molecule called glucuronate; the resulting bilirubin glucuronate is excreted with bile.

The liver is also very important in excretion because it synthesizes **urea** (Figure 1) and releases it into the bloodstream. Urea is a carrier of excess nitrogen resulting from protein breakdown. Excess nitrogen must be converted to urea because free ammonia is toxic. Urea derives its name from the fact that it is excreted in urine.

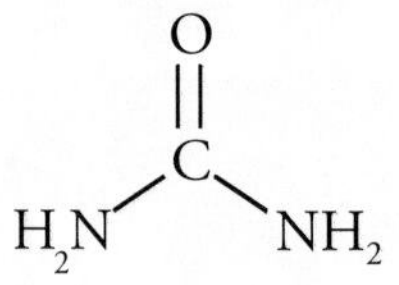

$$\underset{H_2N}{}\overset{\overset{\displaystyle O}{\|}}{\underset{}{C}}\underset{NH_2}{}$$

Figure 1   Urea

Colon

The **large intestine** reabsorbs water and ions (sodium, calcium, etc.) from feces. In this sense, it doesn't really excrete anything, but merely processes wastes already destined for excretion. However, the colon is also capable of excreting excess ions (e.g., sodium, chloride, calcium) into the feces, using active transport.

Skin

The skin produces sweat, which contains water, ions, and urea. In other words, sweat is similar to urine. In this sense, the skin is an excretory organ. However, sweating is not primarily controlled by the amount of waste that needs to be excreted, but rather by temperature and level of sympathetic nervous system activity. Therefore, the excretory role of the skin is secondary.

Kidneys

The final responsibility for excretion of hydrophilic wastes lies with the kidneys. Substances which must be excreted in the urine include urea, sodium, bicarbonate, and water. "But wait," you say, "sodium, bicarbonate and water aren't waste products!" Actually, they sometimes are wastes, when they are present at abnormally high concentrations. You begin to see that the kidney is not like the colon, a passive container for wastes waiting to be excreted. It is a sensitive regulator that must keep concentrations at *optimum levels*, as opposed to simply dumping things.

This is the homeostatic role of the kidneys. **Homeostasis** refers to the constancy of physiological variables. For example, the normal serum Na^+ concentration is 142 mEq/L. Variations in this level greater than 15 percent are fatal due to dysfunction of neurons, cardiac muscle cells, and other cell types. There are other components to homeostasis which the kidney does not control (e.g., temperature maintenance).

Excretory and Homeostatic Roles of the Kidney

1) Excretion of hydrophilic wastes
2) Maintenance of constant solute concentration and constant pH
3) Maintenance of constant fluid volume (important for blood pressure and cardiac output)

As a simplification, we can say that these goals are accomplished via three processes:

- The first process is **filtration**. This entails the passage of pressurized blood over a filter (like a coffee filter). Cells and proteins remain in the blood (like coffee grinds), while water and small molecules are squeezed out into the **renal tubule** (like java). During filtration, water, waste products, and also useful small molecules such as glucose are filtered into the renal tubule. The fluid in the tubule is called **filtrate**, and it will eventually be made into urine.
- The second process is **selective reabsorption**. Here we take back useful items (glucose, water, amino acids), while leaving wastes and some water in the tubule.
- The third process is **secretion**. This involves the addition of substances to the filtrate. Secretion can increase the rate at which substances are eliminated from the blood; because not only are the substance filtered out, more of them are added to the filtrate *after* filtration.

The last step in urine formation is **concentration and dilution**. This involves the selective reabsorption of water, and it is where we decide whether to make concentrated urine or dilute urine. After this step, whatever remains in the renal tubule gets excreted as urine.

17.2 ANATOMY AND FUNCTION OF THE URINARY SYSTEM

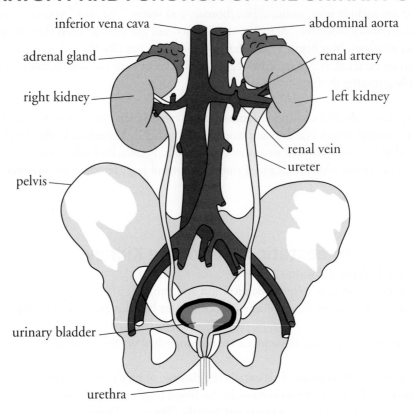

Figure 2 Gross Anatomy of the Urinary System

Each kidney is a filtration system that removes unwanted materials from the blood and passes them to the bladder for storage and eventual elimination. Blood enters the kidney from a large **renal artery**, which is a direct branch of the lower portion of the aorta (the abdominal aorta). Purified blood is returned to the circulatory system by the large **renal vein**, which empties into the inferior vena cava. Urine leaves each kidney in a **ureter**, which empties into the **urinary bladder**. The bladder is a muscular organ which stretches as it fills with urine. When it becomes full, signals of urgency are sent to the brain. There are two sphincters controlling release of urine from the bladder: an **internal sphincter** made of smooth (involuntary) muscle and an **external sphincter** made of skeletal (voluntary) muscle. The internal sphincter relaxes reflexively (and the bladder contracts) when the bladder wall is stretched. If a person decides the time is appropriate, they can relax the external sphincter, allowing urine to flow from the bladder into the urethra and out of the body.

A frontal section (separating front from back) through the kidney demonstrates its internal anatomy (Figure 3). The outer region is known as the **cortex**, and the inner region is the **medulla**. The **medullary pyramids** are pyramid-shaped striations within the medulla. This appearance is due to the presence of many **collecting ducts**. Urine empties from the collecting ducts and leaves the medulla at the tip of a pyramid, known as a **papilla** (plural: **papillae**). Each papilla empties into a space called a **calyx** (plural: **calyces**). The calyces converge to form the **renal pelvis**, which is a large space where urine collects. The renal pelvis empties into the ureter.

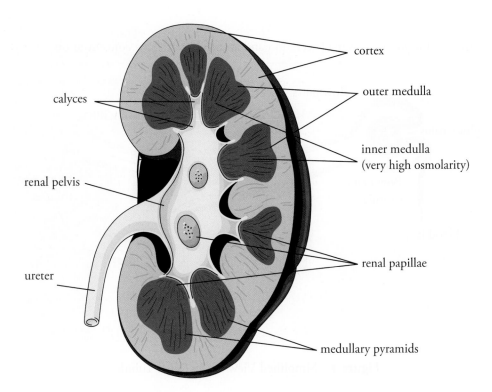

Figure 3 Internal Anatomy of the Kidney

Simplified Microscopic Anatomy and Function

The functional unit of the kidney is the **nephron**. It consists of two components:

1) A rounded region surrounding the capillaries where filtration takes place, known as the **capsule**, and

2) a coiled tube known as the **renal tubule** (Figure 4). The tubule receives filtrate from the capillaries in the capsule at one end and empties into a **collecting duct** at the other end. The collecting duct dumps urine into the renal pelvis.

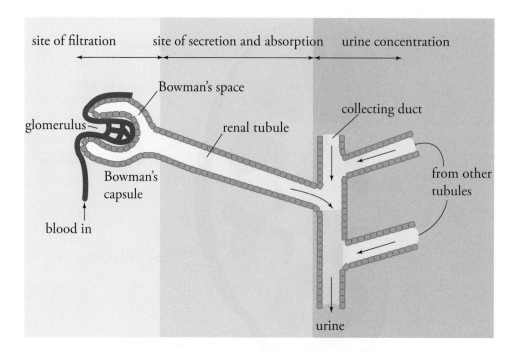

Figure 4 Simplified View of the Renal Tubule

Many blood vessels surround the nephron. They carry arterial blood toward the capillaries of the capsule for filtration, then surround the tubule to carry filtered blood and reabsorbed substances away from the tubule (Figure 5).

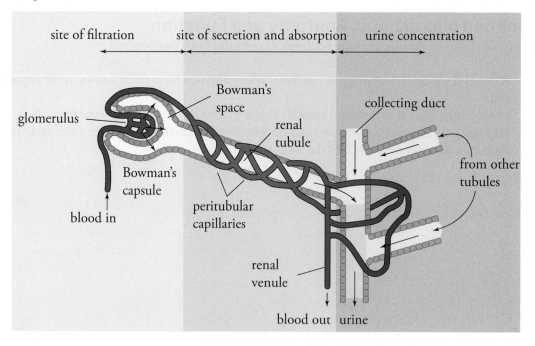

Figure 5 Simplified View of the Renal Tubule Plus Blood Vessels

The pictures above depict most of the structures responsible for the three processes involved in urine formation. Let's go through the steps again, but this time in more detail.

Filtration

Blood from the renal artery flows into an **afferent arteriole**, which branches into a ball of capillaries known as the **glomerulus**. From there the blood flows into an **efferent arteriole**. Constriction of the efferent arteriole results in high pressure in the glomerulus, which causes fluid (essentially blood plasma) to leak out of the glomerular capillaries. The fluid passes through a filter known as the **glomerular basement membrane** and enters **Bowman's capsule**. As you can see from the figures, the lumen of Bowman's capsule is continuous with the lumen of the rest of the tubule. Substances which are too large to pass through the glomerular basement membrane are not filtered; they remain in the blood in the glomerular capillaries and drain into the efferent arteriole.[1] Examples are blood cells and plasma proteins.

- Which of the following are NOT present in the filtrate in Bowman's capsule in concentrations similar to those seen in blood?[2]
  - I.   Albumin (a plasma protein)
  - II. Glucose
  - III. Sodium

  - A) I only
  - B) I and II only
  - C) II and III only
  - D) I, II, and III

Selective Reabsorption

The filtrate in the tubule consists of water and small hydrophilic molecules such as sugars, amino acids, and urea. Some of these substances must be returned to the bloodstream. They are extracted from the tubule, often via active transport, and picked up by **peritubular capillaries**, which drain into venules that lead to the renal vein. For example, glucose is actively transported out of the filtrate and returned to the bloodstream by a cotransporter identical to the one involved in glucose absorption in the small intestine. A lot (most) of the reabsorption occurs in the part of the tubule nearest to Bowman's capsule, called the **proximal convoluted tubule** (**PCT**). All solute movement in the PCT is accompanied by water movement. As a result, a lot of water reabsorption occurs in this region also; roughly 70% of the volume of the filtrate is reabsorbed here. The amount (final volume) of urine we make is determined by much smaller fluxes taking place in the distal nephron. This makes sense if you think about it: about 5% of our circulating blood is continuously being filtered out of the glomerulus, and most of this must be taken back. Note that reabsorption in the PCT is selective in that it chooses what to reabsorb, but it is not overly regulated, since it reabsorbs "as much as possible," not a certain amount.

Selective reabsorption takes place further along the nephron as well, in the **distal convoluted tubule** (**DCT**). Reabsorption in this location is more regulated than in the PCT, usually via hormones (see below, under "Concentration and Dilution").

---

[1]   The glomerular basement membrane is actually a layer lining *each capillary* of the glomerulus.

[2]   **Item I: True.** Plasma proteins are too large to pass through the filter. Item II: False. Glucose passes through into the filtrate and must be reclaimed during selective reabsorption. Item III: False. Sodium also passes into the filtrate. It will be reclaimed or left in the filtrate to be urinated out, depending on physiological needs. The correct answer is choice **A**.

Secretion

Secretion is the movement of substances into the filtrate (usually via active transport) thus increasing the rate at which they are removed from the plasma. Not everything that needs to be removed from the blood gets filtered out at the glomerulus; secretion is a "back-up" method that ensures what needs to be eliminated, gets eliminated. As with reabsorption, secretion occurs all along the tubule; however, unlike reabsorption, most secretion takes place in the DCT and the collecting duct. Note also that this is the primary way that many drugs and toxins are deposited in the urine.

Concentration and Dilution

Before filtrate is discarded into the ureter as urine, adjustments are made so that the urine volume and osmolarity are appropriate. This occurs in the last part of the tubule, known as the **distal nephron** (meaning the most distant part of the tubule), which includes the **DCT** and the **collecting duct**. It is controlled by two hormones: **ADH** and **aldosterone**.

1) *ADH:* When you are dehydrated, the *volume of fluid* in the bloodstream is low and the *solute concentration* in the blood is high. Hence, you need to make small amounts of highly concentrated urine. Under these conditions (low blood volume and high blood osmolarity), **antidiuretic hormone (ADH** or **vasopressin)** is released by the posterior pituitary. This prevents **diuresis** (water loss in the urine) by increasing water reabsorption in the distal nephron. This is accomplished by making the distal nephron (primarily the collecting duct) permeable to water. (Without ADH, this region is impermeable to water. Note that this is the first time we have encountered a layer in the body which is impermeable to water.) As a result, water flows out of the filtrate into the tissue of the kidney, where it is picked up by the peritubular capillaries, and thus returned to the blood. [Why would water tend to flow out of the tubule into the tissue of the kidney?[3]] A drop in blood pressure can also trigger ADH release (renal regulation of blood pressure will be discussed below).

    After drinking a lot of water, the plasma volume is too high, and a large volume of dilute urine is necessary. In this case, no ADH is secreted. The result is that the collecting duct is not permeable to water. This means that any water in the filtrate remains in the tubule and is lost in the urine, or *diuresed*.

2) *Aldosterone:* When the blood *pressure* is low, **aldosterone** is released by the adrenal cortex. It causes increased reabsorption of Na⁺ by the distal nephron. The result is increased plasma osmolarity, which leads to increased thirst and water retention, which raises the blood pressure. (The fact that increased serum [Na⁺] increases blood pressure is the reason people with high blood pressure have to avoid salty foods.) When the blood pressure is high, aldosterone is not released. As a result, sodium is lost in the urine. Plasma osmolarity (and eventually blood pressure) falls. Other triggers for the release of aldosterone are low blood osmolarity, low blood volume, and **angiotensin II** (discussed later in this chapter).

ADH and aldosterone work together to increase blood pressure. First, aldosterone causes sodium reabsorption, which results in increased plasma osmolarity. This causes ADH to be secreted, which results in increased water reabsorption and thus increased plasma volume.

---

[3] The renal medulla has a very high osmolarity, which causes water to exit the tubule by osmosis. This will shortly be discussed in more detail.

Actual Microscopic Anatomy and Function

Up to this point we have presented a conceptual outline of kidney function, and we have referred to a simplified nephron, depicted as a straight tube. But the nephron is more complex than that (Figure 6). Bowman's capsule empties into the first part of the tubule, known as the proximal convoluted tubule (PCT). Again, proximal means "near" (near the glomerulus), and convoluted just means twisting and turning. Both Bowman's capsule and the PCT are located in the **renal cortex**, the outer layer of the kidney. The PCT empties into the next region of the nephron, known as the **loop of Henle**. This is a long loop that dips down into the **renal medulla**, the inner part of the kidney. The part that heads into the medulla is called the **descending limb of the loop of Henle**, and the part that heads back out toward the cortex is the **ascending limb**. The descending limb is thin walled, but part of the ascending limb is thin and the other part is thick. These are referred to simply as the *thin ascending limb* and the *thick ascending limb* of the loop of Henle. As we continue down the tubule, the loop of Henle becomes the distal convoluted tubule (DCT). The DCT dumps into a **collecting duct**. Many collecting ducts merge to form larger tributaries which empty into renal calyces. Figure 6 shows the actual anatomy and function of the nephron. You should familiarize yourself with the information in the picture, but this level of detail is too advanced to warrant extensive discussion. The conceptual material presented above is more typical of MCAT questions.

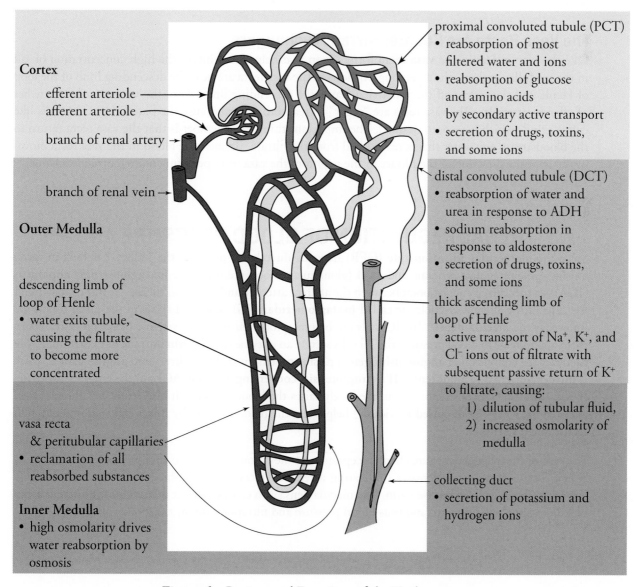

Figure 6 Regions and Functions of the Nephron

The Loop of Henle Is a Countercurrent Multiplier

Although we do not intend to go into too much detail on renal physiology, one concept is important to mention: the notion of a **countercurrent multiplier**. The significance of the loop of Henle is that the ascending and descending limbs go in opposite directions and have different permeabilities. The descending limb is permeable to water, but not to ions. Hence, water exits the descending limb, flowing into the high-osmolarity medullary interstitium.[4] Thus, the filtrate becomes concentrated. The thin ascending limb is *not* permeable to water, but it passively loses ions from the high-osmolarity filtrate into the renal medullary interstitium. Additionally, the thick ascending limb actively transports salt out of the filtrate into the medullary interstitium, and the medullary interstitium becomes *very* salty. This is important because the medulla will suck water out of the collecting duct by osmosis whenever the collecting duct is permeable to water (for example, in the presence of ADH).

Don't spend too much time pondering over this now (you will in medical school). Just remember that *the loop of Henle is a countercurrent multiplier that makes the medulla very salty, and this facilitates water reabsorption from the collecting duct. This is how the kidney is capable of making urine with a much higher osmolarity than plasma.*

The Vasa Recta Are Countercurrent Exchangers

Like the loop of Henle, the **vasa recta** form a loop that helps to maintain the high concentration of salt in the medulla. In short, the ascending portions of the vasa recta are near the descending limb of the loop of Henle and thus carry off the water that leaves the descending limb. Also, the vasa recta are branches of efferent arterioles. The vasa recta are "eager" to reabsorb water because the blood they contain is like coffee grinds which have been drained. The important thing to remember is that the vasa recta return to the bloodstream any water that is reabsorbed from the filtrate. Because the blood in the vasa recta moves in the opposite direction of the filtrate in the nephron, the vasa recta perform countercurrent exchange.

17.3   RENAL REGULATION OF BLOOD PRESSURE AND PH

Since the **glomerular filtration rate** (**GFR**) depends directly on pressure, the kidney has built-in mechanisms to help regulate systemic and local (glomerular) blood pressure. The **juxtaglomerular apparatus** (**JGA**) is a specialized contact point between the afferent arteriole and the distal tubule. At this contact point, the cells in the afferent arteriole are called **juxtaglomerular** (**JG**) **cells**, and those in the distal tubule are known as the **macula densa**. The JG cells are baroreceptors that monitor systemic blood pressure. When there is a decrease in blood pressure, the JG cells secrete an enzyme called **renin** into the bloodstream. Renin catalyzes the conversion of **angiotensinogen** (a plasma protein made by the liver) into **angiotensin I,** which is further converted to **angiotensin II** by **angiotensin-converting enzyme** (**ACE**) in the lungs. Angiotensin II is a powerful vasoconstrictor that immediately raises the blood pressure. It also stimulates the release of aldosterone, which (as discussed previously) helps raise the blood pressure by increasing sodium (and, indirectly, water) retention.

The cells of the macula densa are chemoreceptors, and they monitor filtrate osmolarity in the distal tubule. When filtrate osmolarity decreases (indicating a reduced filtration rate), the cells of the macula densa stimulate the JG cells to release renin. The macula densa also causes a direct dilation of the afferent arteriole, increasing blood flow to (and thus blood pressure and filtration rate in) the glomerulus.

---

[4]   *Interstitium* is a generic word for "tissue." It literally means "an in-between region"; in this case it means tissue in-between renal tubules.

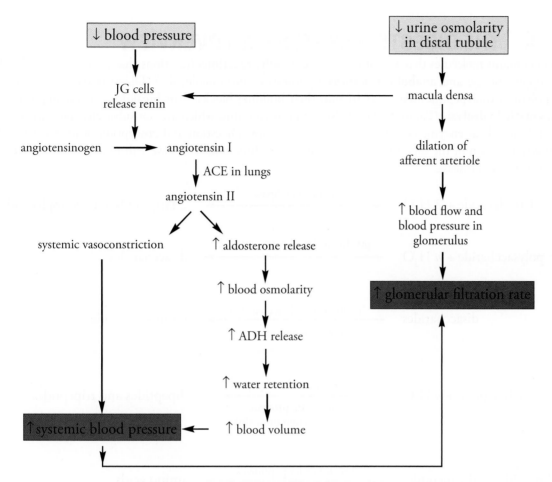

Figure 7   Regulation of Blood Pressure and GFR by the Kidney

Renal Regulation of pH

The kidney is essential for maintenance of constant blood pH. It accomplishes this by a very simple and direct mechanism: when the plasma pH is too high, HCO_3^- is excreted in the urine; when the plasma pH is too low, H^+ is excreted. We will not go into the details. Just be aware that the enzyme **carbonic anhydrase** is involved. It is found in epithelial cells throughout the nephron, except the flat (squamous) cells of the thin parts of the loop of Henle. Carbonic anhydrase catalyzes the conversion of CO_2 into carbonic acid (H_2CO_3), which dissociates into bicarbonate plus a proton. Once this reaction has taken place, the kidney can reabsorb or secrete bicarbonate or protons as needed. Generally speaking, protons are secreted and bicarbonate is reabsorbed; the amounts are adjusted to adjust pH. However, note that renal pH adjustments are slow, requiring several days to return plasma pH to normal after a disturbance.

17.4 THE DIGESTIVE SYSTEM—AN OVERVIEW

Food contains molecules that are substrates in **catabolic reactions** (reactions that break down molecules to supply energy) and **anabolic reactions** (synthesis of macromolecules). Digestion is the breakdown of polymers (polypeptides, fats, starch) into their building blocks. This breakdown is accomplished by **enzymatic hydrolysis** (Figure 8). Food also contains vitamins, which are not substrates, but rather serve a catalytic role as enzyme cofactors or prosthetic groups. Digestion and absorption of foodstuffs is the primary function of the digestive system. A secondary function, which we will touch on only briefly, is protection from disease.

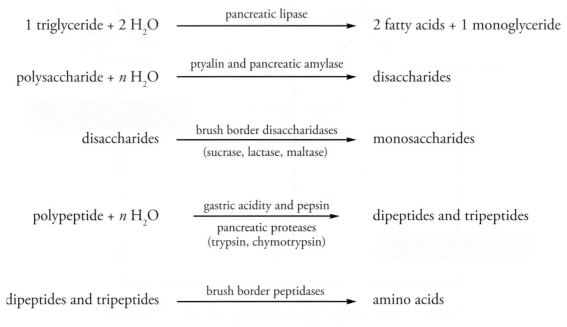

Figure 8 Enzymatic Hydrolysis of Biological Macromolecules

Digestion is accomplished along the **gastrointestinal (GI) tract**, also known as the **digestive tract**, the **alimentary canal**, or simply the **gut**. The GI tract is a long, muscular tube extending from the mouth to the anus. The inside of the gut is the **GI lumen**. The lumen is continuous with the space outside the body. (Food could go from the plate into the lumen and from there into the toilet bowl without ever contacting the bloodstream, the muscles, the bones, etc.) The GI lumen is a compartment where the usable components of foodstuffs are extracted, while wastes are left to be excreted as feces. The entire GI tract is composed of specific tissue layers which surround the lumen (Figure 9).

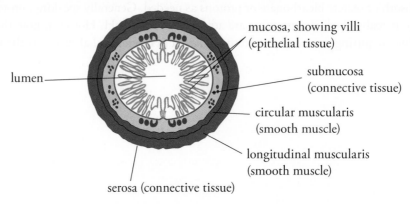

Figure 9 Layers of the GI Tract

GI Epithelium

Because it is exposed to substances from the outside world, the innermost lining of the lumen is composed of the same type of cells that line the outer surface of the body and the inner surface of the respiratory tract: epithelial cells. By definition, epithelial cells are attached to a **basement membrane**. The surface of the epithelial cell which faces into the lumen is the **apical surface** (apex means top; apical is the adjective). In the small intestine, the apical surfaces of these cells have outward folds of their plasma membrane called **microvilli** to increase their surface area. The apical surface is separated from the remainder of the cell surface by **tight junctions**, which are bands running all the way around the sides of epithelial cells, creating a barrier that separates body fluids from the extracellular environment. The sides and bottom of an epithelial cell form the surface opposite the lumen, known as the **basolateral** surface (Figure 10). As discussed below, specialized epithelial cells are responsible for most of the secretory activity of the GI tract.

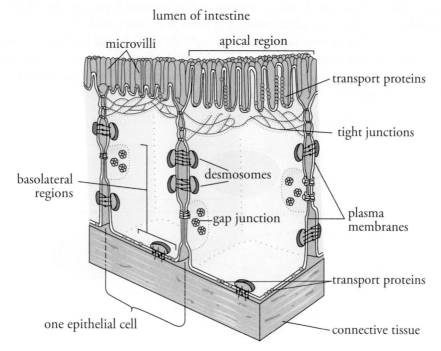

Figure 10   Epithelial Cells

GI Smooth Muscle

GI muscle is known as **smooth muscle** because of its smooth microscopic appearance. This contrasts with **striated muscle**, which appears striped under magnification. Skeletal (voluntary) muscle and cardiac (heart) muscle are striated. (The differences between smooth, skeletal, and cardiac muscle cells will be covered in Chapter 18.) Note in Figure 9 that there are two layers of smooth muscle lining the gut. The **longitudinal layer** runs along the gut lengthwise, while the **circular layer** encircles it.

GI motility refers to the rhythmic contraction of GI smooth muscle. It is determined by a complex interplay between five factors:

1)   Like cardiac muscle, GI smooth muscle exhibits *automaticity*. In other words, it contracts periodically without external stimulation, due to spontaneous depolarization.

2) Like cardiac muscle, GI smooth muscle is a **functional syncytium**, meaning that when one cell has an action potential and contracts, the impulse spreads to neighboring cells.

3) The GI tract contains its own massive nervous system, known as the **enteric nervous system**. The enteric nervous system plays a major role in controlling GI motility.

4) GI motility may be increased or decreased by hormonal input.

5) The parasympathetic nervous system stimulates motility and causes sphincters to relax (allowing the passage of food through the gut), while sympathetic stimulation does the opposite.

GI motility serves two purposes: mixing of food and movement of food down the gut. Mixing is accomplished by disordered contractions of GI smooth muscle, which result in churning motions. Movement of food down the GI tract is accomplished by an orderly form of contraction known as **peristalsis** (Figure 11). During peristalsis, contraction of circular smooth muscle at point A prevents food located at point B from moving backward. Then longitudinal muscles at point B contract, with the result being shortening of the gut so that it is pulled up over the food like a sock. As a result, the food moves toward point C. Then circular smooth muscles at point B contract to prevent the food from moving backward, and longitudinal muscles at point C contract, with the result being movement of food past point C, and so on. A ball of food moving through the GI tract is called a **bolus**.

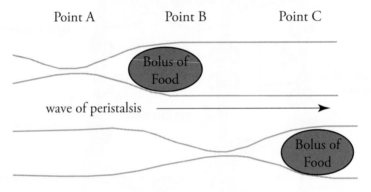

Figure 11 Peristalsis

Enteric Nervous System

The enteric nervous system is the branch of the **autonomic nervous system** that helps to control digestion via innervation of the gastrointestinal tract, pancreas, and gall bladder. Specifically, it helps to regulate local blood flow, gut movements, and the exchange of fluid from the gut to and from its lumen. This branch can operate independently of the other two branches of the autonomic nervous system, but both of those branches can modulate the activity of the enteric nervous system.

The enteric nervous system is made up of two networks of neurons: the **myenteric plexus** and the **submucosal plexus**. The myenteric plexus is found between the circular and longitudinal muscle layers and helps primarily to regulate gut motility. The submucosal plexus is found in the submucosa and helps to regulate enzyme secretion, gut blood flow, and ion/water balance in the lumen. In areas where these functions are minimal (for example, the esophagus or anus), the submucosal plexus is sparse.

17.4

GI Secretions

Generally speaking, GI secretion (release of enzymes, acid, bile, etc.) is stimulated by food in the gut and by the parasympathetic nervous system, and it is inhibited by sympathetic stimulation. There are two types of secretion: **endocrine** and **exocrine**. [What's the difference?[5]] Exocrine glands are composed of specialized epithelial cells, organized into sacs called **acini** (singular: **acinus**). Acinar cells secrete products which pass into ducts. It is important to keep the contrast between endocrine and exocrine in mind. Figure 12 shows the microscopic structure of an exocrine gland.

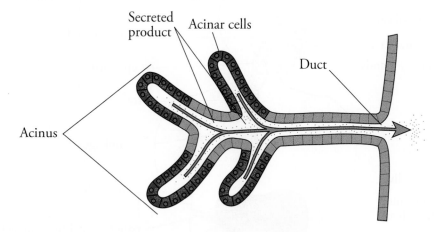

Figure 12 Exocrine Gland Structure

Most exocrine secretion in the GI tract is performed by exocrine glands within special digestive organs. These glands release enzymes into ducts (see Figure 12) that ultimately empty into the GI lumen. The digestive organs primarily involved in exocrine secretion include the liver, gallbladder, and pancreas. However, some exocrine secretion is performed by specialized individual epithelial cells in the wall of the gut itself. These cells are miniature exocrine glands, releasing secretions directly into the gut lumen. Important examples are the cells of the **gastric glands** in the stomach and specialized mucus-secreting cells called **goblet cells**. The gastric glands secrete acid and pepsinogen (a protease zymogen discussed below). Goblet cells are found along the entire GI tract. Mucus is a slimy liquid which protects and lubricates the gut; any body surface covered with mucus is known as a **mucus membrane**. One last secretion must be mentioned: water. Whenever a meal is to be digested, it must be dissolved in water. Hence, each day, gallons of water are secreted into the GI lumen. Most of it is reabsorbed in the small intestine, and the colon is responsible for reclaiming whatever water is left.

Endocrine secretion is also accomplished by both specialized organs (the pancreas) and by cells in the wall of the gut. Remember that endocrine secretions (hormones) do not empty into ducts but instead are picked up by nearby capillaries. In other words, you should realize that when the same organ has both endocrine and exocrine activities, these functions are accomplished by separate cells, which are usually grouped in such a way as to be microscopically distinguishable. For example, the two principal cell types in the pancreas are: 1) exocrine cells, referred to simply as **pancreatic acinar cells**, which are organized into acini that drain into ducts, and 2) endocrine cells clumped together in groups known as **islets of Langerhans**, which are supplied with capillaries.

---

[5] *Exocrine* glands secrete their products (digestive enzymes, etc.) into *ducts* that drain into the GI lumen. *Endocrine* glands are ductless glands; their secretions (hormones) are picked up by capillaries and thus enter the bloodstream.

17.5 THE GASTROINTESTINAL TRACT

Although the GI tract is a continuous tube, each portion is seen as a separate organ: mouth, pharynx, esophagus, etc. Here we will summarize the major structures and functions of each GI organ. The liver, gallbladder, and pancreas, known as **accessory organs**, are covered in Section 17.6.

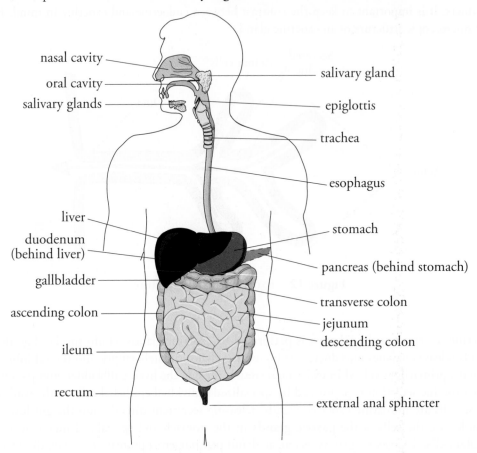

Figure 13 Organs of the Digestive System

Mouth

The mouth has three roles in the digestion of foodstuffs:

1) Fragmentation
2) Lubrication
3) Some enzymatic digestion

Fragmentation is accomplished by **mastication (chewing)**. The **incisors** (front teeth) are for cutting, the **cuspids** (canine teeth) are for tearing, and the **molars** are for grinding.

Lubrication and some digestion are accomplished by **saliva**, a viscous fluid secreted by salivary glands. Saliva contains **salivary amylase (ptyalin)**, which hydrolyzes starch, breaking it into fragments. The smallest fragment yielded by salivary amylase is the disaccharide; digestion to monosaccharides occurs only at the intestinal brush border (discussed below). Saliva also contains a small amount of **lingual lipase** for fat digestion. No digestion of proteins occurs in the mouth. Lastly, saliva also contains **lysozyme**, which attacks bacterial cell walls. Hence, the mouth also participates in innate immunity.

The muscles of the mouth and the muscular tongue are important for compacting chewed food into a smooth lump which can be swallowed, a **bolus**.

Pharynx and Esophagus

The **pharynx** is what we commonly call the throat. The pharynx contains the openings to two tubes: the **trachea** and the **esophagus**. The trachea is a cartilage-lined tube at the front of the neck which conveys air to and from the lungs. The esophagus is a muscular tube behind the trachea which conveys food and drink from the pharynx to the stomach. During swallowing, solids and liquids are excluded from the trachea by a flat cartilaginous flap, the **epiglottis**. A bolus of food passes through the pharynx, over the epiglottis, and into the esophagus, where it is conveyed to the stomach by peristalsis. Two muscular rings regulate movement of food through the esophagus. The **upper esophageal sphincter** is near the top of the esophagus, and the **lower esophageal sphincter** (also known as the **cardiac sphincter** since it is found near the heart) is at the end of the esophagus, at the entrance to the stomach. [Does the lower esophageal sphincter regulate movement of substances into or out of the esophagus?[6]]

Stomach

The stomach is a large hollow muscular organ which serves three purposes: partial digestion of food, regulated release of food into the small intestine, and destruction of microorganisms. The following list highlights some of the attributes and secretions that allow the stomach to accomplish these goals. **Gastric** is an adjective meaning "related to the stomach."

Acidity

Gastric pH is about 2, due to the secretion of HCl by parietal cells, located in the gastric mucosa. Effects of low gastric pH include: 1) destruction of microorganisms, 2) acid-catalyzed hydrolysis of many dietary proteins, and 3) conversion of pepsinogen to pepsin.

Pepsin

This is an enzyme secreted by **chief cells** in the stomach wall. It catalyzes proteolysis (protein breakdown). Pepsin is secreted as **pepsinogen**, which is an inactive precursor that must be converted to the active form (pepsin). As noted above, this conversion is catalyzed by gastric acidity. The secretion of an inactive precursor is a common theme in the GI tract; the inactive form is known as a **zymogen**. Most zymogens are activated by proteolysis (cleavage of the protein at a specific site that activates it).

---

[6] It is there to prevent reflux from the stomach into the esophagus. There is no reason to regulate movement of substances out of the esophagus into the stomach, since nothing is stored in the esophagus; it's just a conduit.

Motility

The stomach constantly churns food. Like chewing, this breaks up food particles so that they are exposed to gastric acidity and enzymes. Food mixed with gastric secretions is known as **chyme**.

Sphincters

The lower esophageal sphincter prevents reflux of chyme into the esophagus. The **pyloric sphincter** prevents the passage of food from the stomach into the duodenum. Opening of the pyloric sphincter (stomach emptying) is inhibited when the small intestine already has a large load of chyme. More specifically, stretching or excess acidity in the duodenum inhibits further stomach emptying, by causing the pyloric sphincter to contract. This effect is mediated both by nerves connecting the duodenum and stomach, and by hormones. The main hormone responsible is **cholecystokinin**, secreted by epithelial cells in the wall of the duodenum. [Is this hormone secreted into the lumen of the duodenum or into the lumen of the stomach?[7]]

Gastrin

This is a hormone secreted by cells in the stomach wall known as **G cells**. It stimulates acid and pepsin secretion and gastric motility. Gastrin secretion is stimulated by food in the stomach and by parasympathetic stimulation. The small molecule **histamine** (which is secreted in response both to stomach stretching and to gastrin) binds to parietal cells to stimulate acid release. The ulcer-healing drugs cimetidine (Tagamet) and ranitidine (Zantac) function by blocking the binding of histamine to its receptor (the "H_2 receptor") on parietal cells. This results in less gastric acidity, which allows ulcers to heal.

Small Intestine

Food leaving the stomach enters the small intestine, a tube which is about an inch wide and 10-feet long. (After death, it measures about 25 feet due to relaxation of longitudinal muscles.) The small intestine is divided into three segments: the **duodenum**, **jejunum**, and **ileum**. Digestion begins in the mouth (ptyalin), continues in the stomach, and is completed in the duodenum and jejunum. Absorption begins in the duodenum and continues throughout the small intestine. The anatomy and function of the small intestine are described below. In Section 17.7 we will detail the specific mechanisms of digestion and absorption of carbohydrates, proteins, and fats.

Surface Area

The key feature that allows the small intestine to accomplish absorption is its large surface area; this results from 1) length, 2) villi, and 3) microvilli. **Villi** (singular: **villus**) are macroscopic (multicellular) projections in the wall of the small intestine. **Microvilli** are microscopic foldings of the cell membranes of individual intestinal epithelial cells. The lumenal surface of the small intestine is known as the **brush border** due to the brush-like appearance of microvilli.

---

[7]   Neither! It's a hormone; by definition, it is secreted into the bloodstream.

The Intestinal Villus

The villus is a finger-like projection of the wall of the gut into the lumen. It has three very important structures:

1) The villus contains capillaries, which absorb dietary monosaccharides and amino acids. The capillaries merge to form veins, which merge to form the large **hepatic portal vein**, which transports blood containing amino acid and carbohydrate nutrients from the gut to the liver.

2) The villus also contains small lymphatic vessels called **lacteals**, which absorb dietary fats. The lacteals merge to form large lymphatic vessels, which transport dietary fats to the thoracic duct, which empties into the bloodstream.

3) **Peyer's patches** are part of the immune system. They are collections of lymphocytes dotting the villi that monitor GI contents and thus confer immunity to gut pathogens and toxins.

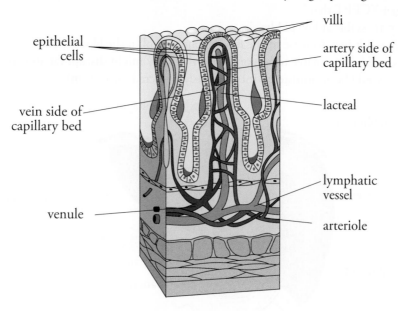

Figure 14   An Intestinal Villus

Bile and Pancreatic Secretions in the Duodenum

A key anatomical feature of the duodenum is that two ducts empty into it (Figure 15). One is the **pancreatic duct**, which delivers the exocrine secretions of the pancreas (digestive enzymes and bicarbonate). The other is the **common bile duct**, which delivers **bile**. This is a green fluid containing **bile acids**, which are made from cholesterol in the liver and are normally absorbed and recycled. Bile is stored in the **gallbladder** until it is needed. Bile has two functions: it is a vehicle for the disposal (excretion) of waste products by the liver, and it is essential for the digestion of fats, as discussed below. The bile duct and the pancreatic duct empty into the duodenum via the same orifice, known as the **sphincter of Oddi** (Figure 15).

- Bile acids secreted into the duodenum are normally reabsorbed in the ileum. Bile acid sequestrants are drugs which bind bile acids in the small intestine, causing them to remain in the GI lumen and eventually be excreted as feces. Each of the following is most likely true about such drugs EXCEPT that:[8]
    - A) they are stable at low pH levels.
    - B) they result in a decrease in the level of cholesterol in the bloodstream.
    - C) it would be reasonable to be concerned that they might disrupt fat absorption.
    - D) they would be administered intravenously (injected into a vein).

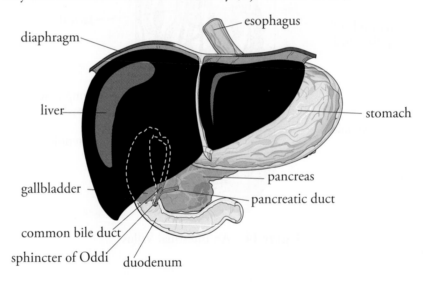

Figure 15 Anatomy around the Duodenum

Duodenal Enzymes

Some duodenal epithelial cells secrete enzymes. Duodenal **enterokinase** (also known as **enteropeptidase**) activates the pancreatic zymogen **trypsinogen** to trypsin (Section 17.6). Other duodenal enzymes are peculiar in that they are not truly secreted, but rather do their work inside or on the surface of the brush border epithelial cell. These duodenal enzymes are called **brush border enzymes**. Their role is to hydrolyze the smallest carbohydrates and proteins (like disaccharides and dipeptides) into monosaccharides and amino acids (Section 17.7).

---

[8] Since the drugs must pass through the stomach, they should be stable at low pH levels (choice A is true and can be eliminated). The text states that bile acids are made from cholesterol and normally recycled. It is reasonable to assume that blocking this recycling would require the conversion of more cholesterol into bile acids, which would lower the serum cholesterol level. This is in fact what bile acid sequestrants are used for (choice B is true and can be eliminated). It would be reasonable to be concerned about fat absorption, based on the fact that bile acids are necessary for this absorption, as stated in the text (choice C is true and can be eliminated). However, the drugs would have to be *swallowed* to end up within the GI lumen, not injected (choice **D** is false and is the correct answer choice).

Duodenal Hormones

Other duodenal epithelial cells secrete hormones. The three main duodenal hormones are **cholecystokinin (CCK)**, **secretin**, and **enterogastrone**. CCK is secreted in response to fats in the duodenum. It causes the pancreas to secrete digestive enzymes, stimulates gallbladder contraction (bile release), and decreases gastric motility. Note that all these processes cooperate to deal with fats in the duodenum, by digesting them and preventing further stomach emptying. Secretin is released in response to acid in the duodenum. It causes the pancreas to release large amounts of a high-pH aqueous buffer, namely HCO_3^- in water. This neutralizes HCl released by the stomach. Duodenal pH must be kept neutral or even slightly basic for pancreatic digestive enzymes to function. Enterogastrone decreases stomach emptying.

Jejunum and Ileum

Substances not absorbed in the duodenum must be absorbed in these lower segments of the small intestine. The lower small intestine performs special absorptive processes. For example, absorption of vitamin B_{12} occurs only in the ileum (and only when vitamin B_{12} is complexed with **intrinsic factor**, a glycoprotein secreted by the parietal cells of the stomach). A valve called the **ileocecal valve** separates the ileum from the cecum, which is the first part of the large intestine.

Colon (Large Intestine)

Like the rest of the intestine, the colon is a muscular tube. It is 3- or 4-feet long and several inches wide. Its role is to absorb water and minerals, and to form and store feces until the time of defecation. Abnormalities of colon function result in poor fluid absorption and diarrhea, which can cause dehydration and death. The first part of the colon is the **cecum**. Entrance of chyme into the cecum is controlled by the ileocecal valve. The **appendix** is a finger-like appendage of the cecum. It is composed primarily of lymphatic tissue and was mentioned in the preceding chapter. The last portion of the colon is called the **rectum**. Exit of feces (**defecation**) from the rectum occurs through the **anus**. Defecation is controlled by the **anal sphincter**, which has an internal portion and an external portion. The internal anal sphincter consists of smooth muscle, which is under autonomic control. The external anal sphincter consists of skeletal muscle and is under voluntary control. (Note that this is the same arrangement as seen in the urinary sphincters.) Most of the wastes from a meal are defecated about a day after it is eaten. However, the wastes from a meal are first present in stool after just a few hours and some residue of a meal is typically still present in the colon after several days.

The colon contains billions of bacteria of various species. Many are facultative or obligate anaerobes. Undigested materials are metabolized by colonic bacteria. This often results in gas, which is given off as a waste product of bacterial metabolism. **Colonic bacteria** are important for two reasons: 1) the presence of large numbers of normal bacteria helps keep dangerous bacteria from proliferating, due to competition for space and nutrients, and 2) colonic bacteria supply us with **vitamin K,** which is essential for blood clotting.

17.6 THE GI ACCESSORY ORGANS

The GI accessory organs are those that play a role in digestion, but are not actually part of the alimentary canal. They include the **pancreas**, **liver**, **gallbladder**, and the large **salivary glands** found outside the mouth. We have already discussed saliva, so the salivary glands will not be discussed further here. The pancreas and liver are essential for GI function. The gallbladder is not essential, but can become infected, obstructed, or cancerous, and is thus medically important.

Exocrine Pancreas

Pancreatic enzymes released into the duodenum are essential for digestion. **Pancreatic amylase** hydrolyzes polysaccharides to disaccharides. **Pancreatic lipase** hydrolyzes triglycerides at the surface of a micelle (see below, under "Liver and Gallbladder"). **Nucleases** hydrolyze dietary DNA and RNA. Several different **pancreatic proteases** are responsible for hydrolyzing polypeptides to di- and tripeptides. Pancreatic proteases are secreted in their inactive **zymogen** forms and must be activated by removal of a portion of the polypeptide chain. **Trypsinogen** is a zymogen which is converted to the active form, **trypsin**, by **enterokinase**, an intestinal enzyme. Other pancreatic enzymes are then activated by trypsin. These include **chymotrypsinogen** (active form: **chymotrypsin**), **procarboxypeptidase** (active form: **carboxypeptidase**), and **procollagenase** (active form: **collagenase**).

Control of the Exocrine Pancreas

Two hormones discussed previously help to control pancreatic secretion. **Cholecystokinin** (CCK) secreted into the bloodstream by the duodenum causes the pancreas to secrete enzymes. **Secretin**, also released by the duodenum, causes the pancreas to secrete water and bicarbonate (high pH). Parasympathetic nervous system activation increases pancreatic secretion; sympathetic activation reduces it.

Endocrine Pancreas

The endocrine pancreas consists of small regions within the pancreas known as **islets of Langerhans**. There are three types of cells in the islets, and each secretes a particular hormone into the bloodstream.

1) α cells secrete **glucagon** in response to low blood sugar. Glucagon functions to mobilize stored fuels by stimulating the liver to hydrolyze glycogen and release glucose into the bloodstream, and by stimulating adipocytes (fat cells) to release fats into the bloodstream.
2) β cells secrete **insulin** in response to elevated blood sugar (e.g., after a meal). Its effects are opposite those of glucagon: insulin stimulates the removal of glucose from the blood for storage as glycogen and fat.
3) δ cells secrete **somatostatin**. It inhibits many digestive processes.

Focus on Blood Glucose

1) **Lowering blood glucose:** Insulin is essential for life because it causes sugar to be removed from the bloodstream and stored. Diabetics lack insulin or have dysfunctional insulin receptors. Their blood sugar levels are extraordinarily high. The excess glucose directly destroys many physiological systems at the cellular level, including neurons, blood vessels, and the kidneys.

2) **Raising blood glucose:** Three hormones can raise the blood glucose level: glucagon (a polypeptide hormone from the pancreas), epinephrine (an amino acid derivative from the adrenal medulla), and cortisol (a steroid or glucocorticoid from the adrenal cortex). Note that of these three hormones, one is a steroid, one is a polypeptide, and one is an amino acid derivative. Also note that there is only one hormone that can lower blood glucose, while three different hormones can raise blood glucose. It makes sense to have many ways to raise blood glucose, and for it to be less easy to lower blood glucose, since low blood glucose levels are immediately fatal, while elevated blood glucose is harmless in the short term. (Over several years, however, it is harmful.)

- Which one of the following statements is true?[9]
    A) Insulin stimulates the release of glucose into the blood and also stimulates peristalsis in the small intestine.
    B) Gastrin stimulates stomach emptying and inhibits secretion of gastric acid.
    C) Cholecystokinin stimulates peristalsis in the intestine and inhibits stomach emptying.
    D) Glucagon stimulates the storage of glucose and stimulates small intestinal peristalsis.

17.6

Liver and Gallbladder

The exocrine secretory activity of the liver is simple: it secretes bile. The liver actually produces about 1 liter of bile a day. The principal ingredients of bile include bile acids (known as **bile salts** in the deprotonated—anionic—form), cholesterol, and bilirubin (from RBC breakdown). Bile emulsifies large fat particles in the duodenum, creating smaller clusters of fat particles called **micelles**. The smaller particles have a greater collective surface area than the large particles, and thus are more easily digested by hydrophilic lipases (from the pancreas). Also, bile helps fatty particles to diffuse across the intestinal mucosal membrane.

Bile made in the liver can go to one of two places: it is either directly secreted into the duodenum or is stored for later use in the **gallbladder**. Bile stored in the gallbladder is concentrated, and it is released when a fatty meal is eaten. A **gallstone** is a large crystal formed from bile made with ingredients in incorrect proportions.

The gallbladder itself has no secretory activity. Bile release from this organ is dictated by both the endocrine system and the nervous system. Both CCK (released by the duodenal cells) and the parasympathetic nervous system stimulate contraction of the gallbladder wall.

The liver plays a more complicated role in the *processing* of absorbed nutrients than it does in digestion (breakdown). In order to understand this process, it helps to consider the **hepatic portal system**. The liver receives blood from two places. First, it receives oxygenated blood from the hepatic arteries. Second, it receives venous blood draining the stomach and intestines through the **hepatic portal vein**. (Hepatic means "relating to the liver.") As this blood percolates through the liver, nutrients are extracted by hepatocytes (liver

---

9 Insulin stimulates the *removal* of glucose from the blood (choice A is false), gastrin *causes* acid secretion (choice B is false), and glucagon functions to *raise* blood glucose (choice D is false). Choice **C** is a true statement.

cells). The hepatocytes monitor the blood and make changes to the body's physiology based on what is and is not present (much as the hypothalamus does in the hypothalamic-pituitary portal system). For example, if blood glucose is low, the liver will initiate a cascade that leads to glycogen breakdown as well as new glucose production (gluconeogenesis). The free glucose can be released to raise blood glucose levels.

Both the liver and the skeletal muscles are capable of storing glucose as glycogen and subsequently breaking glycogen down when glucose is needed. However, only the liver is able to release free glucose to the bloodstream. The product of glycogen breakdown is glucose-6-phosphate; in order to move into the bloodstream, this product must be dephosphorylated, and only the liver contains the enzyme needed to accomplish this (glucose-6-phosphatase).

The waste products from protein catabolism (breakdown) are also regulated through the liver. When proteins are broken down into amino acids, and amino acids are broken down even further (e.g., to enter the Krebs cycle to generate ATP during starvation), nitrogenous by-products are released in the form of NH_3 (ammonia). Ammonia in high levels is toxic to the body, so it is transported to the liver where it is converted into urea. Urea is then absorbed into the bloodstream and excreted by the kidney in urine.

Lipid metabolism is assisted by the liver as well. Lipids exit the intestine and enter the lymphatic system in molecules called **chylomicrons**. Chylomicrons are degraded by lipases into triglycerides, glycerol, and cholesterol rich **chylomicron remnants**. These remnants are taken up by hepatocytes and combined with proteins to make lipoproteins (HDL, LDL, VLDL, etc.). These lipoproteins then re-enter the blood and are the source of cholesterol and triglycerides for the other tissues of the body.

Many important plasma proteins (such as albumin, globulins, fibrinogens, and other clotting factors necessary to stop bleeding) are made in the liver and secreted into the plasma. People with liver disease often have problems with sealing wounds due to a lack of clotting factors. They also have a tendency to swell up; the lack of albumin allows fluid to leave the bloodstream and enter the tissues.

Finally, the liver is the major center for drug and toxin detoxification in the body. The smooth ER in hepatocytes contains enzyme pathways that break down drugs and toxins into forms that are less toxic and more readily excreted by the renal and gastrointestinal systems. Interestingly, sometimes these same enzyme pathways in hepatocytes are used to convert some drugs into their active forms. Therefore, people with liver disease must have drug levels in their blood monitored closely when they are on medications that are affected by the detoxification system of the liver.

Hormonal Control of Appetite

The desire to eat between meals is subject to hormonal control. When the stomach is empty, gastric cells produce the hormone **ghrelin** to stimulate appetite. When the colon is full, the jejunum (lower intestine) produces **peptide YY** to reduce appetite. The hormone **leptin**, produced by white adipose tissue (fat), is an appetite suppressant that acts as an "adipostat"—maintaining stable lipid content in adipose tissue. Leptin is secreted in response to increased triglyceride levels, and it works to suppress appetite until appropriate levels are restored. All three of these hormones can affect multiple target tissues, but their effects on appetite are primarily mediated by the arcuate nucleus of the hypothalamus.

17.7   A DAY IN THE LIFE OF FOOD

In order to draw the above information together, let's trace the path of each of the three main types of dietary nutrients: carbohydrates, proteins, and fats.

Carbohydrates

You purchase a sourdough baguette and tear off a hunk. Chewing increases the bread's surface area, allowing it to soak up more saliva. Ptyalin hydrolyzes starch into fragments, while the tongue and cheeks form a bolus. As you swallow, the upper esophageal sphincter relaxes. Peristalsis carries the bolus to the stomach; the lower esophageal sphincter relaxes to let it pass. In the stomach, strong acid destroys most of the microorganisms which were present in the bread, while further hydrolyzing some polysaccharides. The stomach thoroughly churns the bread, forming acidic chyme, which is gradually released into the duodenum. In the duodenum, pancreatic amylase chops the polysaccharides into disaccharides, which diffuse to the intestinal brush border. Here the disaccharides are hydrolyzed to monosaccharides. Digestion is complete. Up to this point, none of the sugar composing the bread has entered your body; it remains on the lumenal side of GI epithelial tight junctions.

Since they are bulky and hydrophilic, monosaccharides must be taken up into the intestinal epithelial cell by active transport. An apical symport transports one sugar into the cell while allowing sodium to flow in, down its large concentration gradient (Figure 16). The large sodium concentration gradient is created by constant activity of Na^+/K^+ ATPases on the basolateral surface of the cell, pumping Na^+ out. As secondary active transport continues to pack the epithelial cell with monosaccharides, their concentration gets quite high. Hence, there is now a concentration gradient driving them out of the cell into nearby capillaries. This movement occurs by facilitated diffusion (uniports) at the basolateral surface of the cell. In the bloodstream, sugars dissolve into the plasma as it flows into the hepatic portal vein toward the liver.

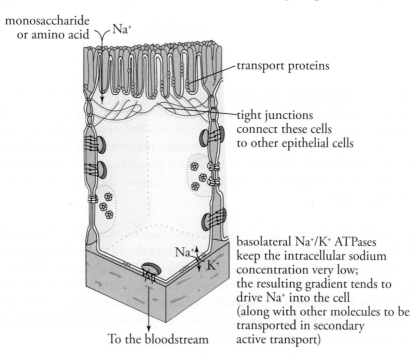

monosaccharide or amino acid — Na^+

transport proteins

tight junctions connect these cells to other epithelial cells

Na^+ K^+

basolateral Na^+/K^+ ATPases keep the intracellular sodium concentration very low; the resulting gradient tends to drive Na^+ into the cell (along with other molecules to be transported in secondary active transport)

To the bloodstream

Figure 16   Absorption of Hydrophilic Food Monomers

The liver takes up some of the sugars and begins to store them or use their energy. Nonetheless, the blood sugar level increases rather suddenly. When the pancreas is exposed to elevated blood glucose levels, the β cells of the islets of Langerhans secrete insulin. The insulin causes many different cells (liver, muscle, nerve, and fat cells) to take up, utilize, and store glucose. Soon the blood sugar level returns to normal, and you're ready for dessert.

Proteins

The next day, you're ready for a nice can of albacore in spring water.

In your mouth, the tuna is ground and mixed with saliva. No digestion of protein occurs in the mouth. A bolus is formed, and you swallow. Churning of the stomach mixes the tuna with acid, mucus, and enzymes. The low pH kills microorganisms and causes many peptide bonds to hydrolyze. Activated pepsin attacks polypeptides, breaking them into fragments. Chyme is gradually released into the duodenum.

Chyme in the duodenum causes duodenal epithelial cells to secrete CCK and secretin. As a result, the gallbladder releases concentrated bile and the pancreas secretes a basic (high pH) solution of bicarbonate plus digestive zymogens. In the gut, trypsinogen is activated to trypsin by enterokinase. Trypsin then activates other zymogens. The activated proteases go to work on polypeptides from the tuna until all that's left are dipeptides and tripeptides. These are hydrolyzed by brush border peptidases.

Amino acid absorption is similar to monosaccharide absorption: a secondary active transporter (symport) specific to each amino acid couples the uptake of an amino acid to the entrance of sodium into the cell, and a uniporter facilitates movement out of the intestinal epithelial cell into the interstitium. Just as with carbohydrates, the amino acid ends up in the liver, where it is catabolized for energy or used in synthesis (anabolism).

Fats

"Enough of sourdough and tuna fish!" you declare, as you enter an ice cream shop. The almost-pure triglycerides melt in your mouth and are swallowed. The stomach's churning mixes the triglycerides with acid and mucus to some extent, but because they are extremely hydrophobic, they end up just floating in a layer above the aqueous contents of the stomach. Eventually they are emptied into the duodenum where they stimulate CCK release into the bloodstream. Then the pancreas sends enzymes into the gut, via the sphincter of Oddi. But there is a problem: pancreatic lipase cannot digest the fats if they are organized into huge hydrophobic droplets.

Fortunately, CCK in the bloodstream also stimulates gallbladder contraction. This sends bile down the bile duct into the duodenum. Bile acids emulsify the lipids from the ice cream, forming tiny micelles. Then pancreatic lipase can go to work. It hydrolyzes triglycerides to monoglycerides plus free fatty acids, as shown in Figure 17. These move into intestinal epithelial cells by simple diffusion, which they are able to do thanks to their greasy hydrophobicity and small size. Once inside, they are converted back to triglycerides, which are packaged into **chylomicrons**. These are large particles composed of fats and proteins that are designed to transport fats in the bloodstream (Figure 17).

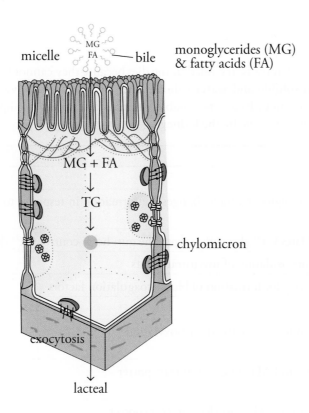

micelle — monoglycerides (MG) & fatty acids (FA)

bile

MG + FA

TG

chylomicron

exocytosis

lacteal

Figure 17   Fat Absorption

The chylomicrons do not enter intestinal blood capillaries. Instead, they enter tiny lymphatic capillaries known as **lacteals**. These merge to form larger lymphatic vessels, which eventually empty into the thoracic duct. This empties into a large vein near the heart. A few minutes after your sundae, huge amounts of fat are released from the thoracic duct directly into the bloodstream. Your plasma attains a milky yellow color which is easily noticeable when a blood sample is taken. The term for milky plasma is **lipemia**, meaning "fat in the blood."

The chylomicrons circulate throughout the body and are gradually whittled away by removal of fat. In particular, adipose and liver tissues contain the enzyme **lipoprotein lipase**, which hydrolyzes chylomicron triglycerides into monoglycerides and free fatty acids. These diffuse into adipocytes and liver cells, are remade into triglycerides, and then stored.

17.8 VITAMINS

Vitamins are nutrients which must be included in the diet because they cannot be synthesized in the body. They are divided into **fat-soluble** and **water-soluble** categories. Fat-soluble vitamins require bile acids for solubilization and absorption. Excess fat-soluble vitamins are stored in adipose tissue. Excess water-soluble vitamins are excreted in urine by the kidneys.

Vitamin	Function
fat-soluble	
A (retinol)	A visual pigment which changes conformation in response to light
D	Stimulates Ca^{2+} absorption from the gut; helps control Ca^{2+} deposition in bones
E	Prevents oxidation of unsaturated fats
K	Necessary for formation of blood coagulation factors
water-soluble	
B_1 (thiamine)	Needed for enzymatic decarboxylations
B_2 (riboflavin)	Made into FAD, an electron transporter
B_3 (niacin)	Made into NAD^+, an electron transporter
B_6 (pyridoxine)	A coenzyme involved in protein and amino acid metabolism
B_{12} (cobalamin)	A coenzyme involved in the reduction of nucleotides to deoxynucleotides
C (ascorbic acid)	Necessary for collagen formation; deficiency results in scurvy
Biotin	Prosthetic group essential for transport of CO_2 groups
Folate	Enzyme cofactor used in the transport of methylene groups; synthesis of purines and thymine; required for normal fetal nervous system development

Table 1 Vitamins

Chapter 18
The Musculoskeletal System and Skin

18.1 OVERVIEW OF MUSCLE TISSUE

There are three types of muscle which differ in cellular physiology, anatomy, and function. The type we are all familiar with is **skeletal muscle** (Section 15.3), which is also known as *voluntary* muscle, because its role is to contract in response to conscious intent. The next muscle type is called **cardiac muscle** because it is found only in the wall of the heart. Skeletal and cardiac muscle are said to be **striated** because of their microscopic appearance. The third type of muscle is **smooth muscle**, which is found in the walls of all hollow organs such as the GI tract, the urinary system, the uterus, etc. It is responsible for GI motility, constriction of blood vessels, uterine contractions, and so on. We have no conscious control over cardiac or smooth muscle because they are innervated only by the autonomic nervous system. The three types of muscle share some characteristics and differ in others. In Sections 18.3 and 18.4 we characterize cardiac and smooth muscle by comparison with skeletal muscle.

18.2 SKELETAL MUSCLE

Movement of Joints

Skeletal muscle provides voluntary movement of the body in response to stimulation by somatic motor neurons, but skeletal muscle alone cannot move the body. Skeletal muscle requires the framework of the bones of the skeleton for movement to occur. Skeletal muscles are attached at each end to two different bones. Muscles are often attached to bones by **tendons**, strong connective tissue formed primarily of collagen. By contracting, skeletal muscle can draw the points of attachment on the two bones closer together.

Structure of Skeletal Muscle

Each skeletal muscle is composed not only of muscle tissue, but also of connective tissue that holds the contractile tissue together in bundles called **fascicles** to allow flexibility within the muscle (Figure 1). Looking within each bundle, it is possible to see many fine **muscle fibers** (also called **myofibers**). Each muscle fiber is a single skeletal muscle cell. Skeletal muscle cells are **multinucleate syncytia** formed by the fusion of individual cells during development. They are innervated by a single nerve ending, and they stretch the entire length of the muscle. The myofiber has a cell membrane, called the **sarcolemma**, that is made of the plasma membrane and an additional layer of polysaccharide and collagen. This additional layer helps the cell to fuse with tendon fibers. Within each skeletal muscle cell (myofiber) are many smaller units called **myofibrils**. The myofibril in the muscle cell is like a specialized organelle; it is responsible for the striated appearance of skeletal muscle and generates the contractile force of skeletal muscle.

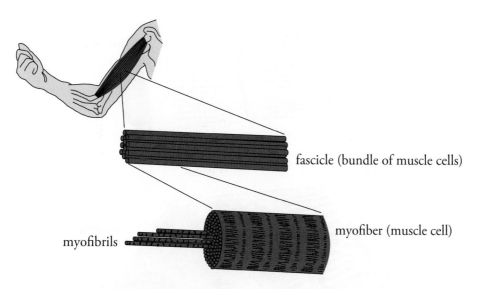

fascicle (bundle of muscle cells)

myofiber (muscle cell)

myofibrils

Figure 1 Levels of Skeletal Muscle Organization

The proteins in the myofibril that generate contraction are polymerized **actin** and **myosin**. Actin polymerizes to form **thin filaments** visible under the microscope, and myosin forms **thick filaments** (Figure 2). The striated appearance of skeletal muscle is due to the overlapping arrangement of bands of thick and thin filaments in **sarcomeres**. A myofibril is composed of many sarcomeres aligned end-to-end. Each sarcomere is bound by two **Z lines**. Thin filaments (actin) attach to each Z line and overlap with thick filaments (myosin) in the middle of each sarcomere; the thick filaments are not attached to the Z lines. The regions of the sarcomere composed only of thin filaments are referred to as the **I bands**. The full length of the thick filament represents the **A band** within each sarcomere; this includes both the overlapping regions of thick and thin filaments (where contraction is generated), as well as the region composed of only thick filaments (this is seen in resting sarcomeres only and is referred to as the **H zone**). See Figure 2.

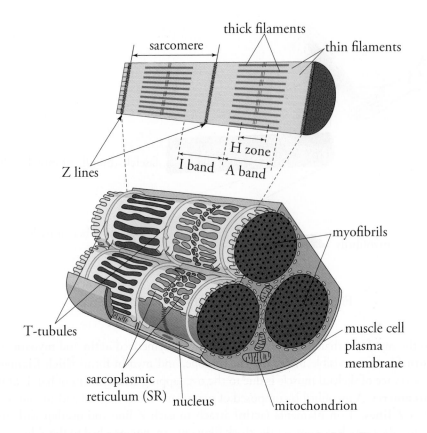

Figure 2 The Sarcomere and a Cross-Section of a Myofiber

The Sliding Filament Model of Muscle Contraction

Within each sarcomere, actin and myosin filaments overlap with each other (Figure 3). Contraction occurs when the thin and thick filaments slide across each other, drawing the Z lines of each sarcomere closer together and shortening the length of the muscle cell. [During muscle contraction, do the thin and thick filaments shorten?[1]] Filament sliding is powered by ATP hydrolysis. Myosin is an enzyme which uses the energy of ATP to create movement. (You will hear the term "myosin ATPase.") Each myosin monomer contains a **head** and a **tail**. The head attaches to a specific site on an actin molecule (the **myosin binding site**). When it is attached, myosin and actin are said to be connected by a **cross bridge**. Contraction occurs when the angle between the head and tail decreases. Filament sliding occurs in four steps. It is important to remember which step requires a new ATP molecule.

Steps of the contractile cycle:
1) Binding of the myosin head to a myosin binding site on actin, also known as **cross bridge formation**. At this stage, myosin has ADP and P_i bound.
2) The **power stroke**, in which the myosin head moves to a low-energy conformation and pulls the actin chain towards the center of the sarcomere. ADP is released.
3) Binding of a new ATP molecule is necessary for *release* of actin by the myosin head (key!).

---

[1]   No. The thin and thick filaments slide across each other to shorten the sarcomere without themselves changing in length.

4) ATP hydrolysis occurs immediately and the myosin head is *cocked* (set in a high-energy conformation, like the hammer of a gun). Another cycle begins when the myosin head binds to a new binding site on the thin filament.

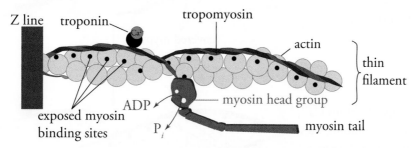

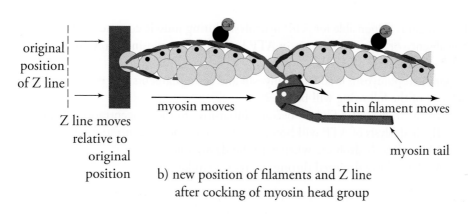

a) original position of filaments and myofibrils
prior to cocking of myosin head group

b) new position of filaments and Z line
after cocking of myosin head group

Figure 3   Filament Sliding

Excitation-Contraction Coupling in Skeletal Muscle

The above four steps in the contractile cycle occur spontaneously. In other words, if you put actin and myosin into a beaker and add ATP and Mg^{2+} (necessary for all reactions involving ATP), ATP will be hydrolyzed and the filaments will slide past one another. But in the myofiber, contraction occurs only when the cytoplasmic $[Ca^{2+}]$ increases. This is because in addition to polymerized actin, the thin filament contains the **troponin-tropomyosin complex** (Figure 4) that prevents contraction when Ca^{2+} is not present. **Tropomyosin** is a long fibrous protein that winds around the actin polymer, blocking all the myosin-binding sites. **Troponin** is a globular protein bound to the tropomyosin that can bind Ca^{2+}. When troponin binds Ca^{2+}, troponin undergoes a conformational change that moves tropomyosin out of the way, so that myosin heads can attach to actin and filament sliding can occur.

18.2

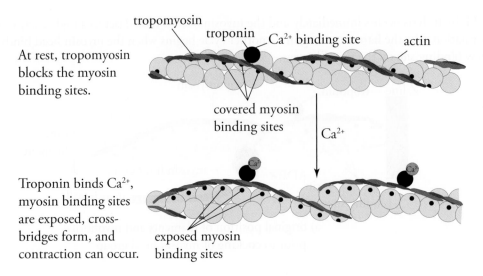

At rest, tropomyosin blocks the myosin binding sites.

Troponin binds Ca^{2+}, myosin binding sites are exposed, cross-bridges form, and contraction can occur.

Figure 4   The Troponin/Tropomyosin Complex

- What protein is responsible for ATP hydrolysis during muscle contraction?[2]
- In the absence of actin, which step in ATP hydrolysis by myosin is prevented, the hydrolysis of ATP or the release of ADP?[3]
- If troponin-tropomyosin is added to myosin and actin filaments in a test tube along with ATP, which one of the following will be true?[4]
  - A) The hydrolysis of ATP will become insensitive to the concentration of calcium.
  - B) The hydrolysis of ATP will become sensitive to the concentration of calcium.
  - C) ATP will be hydrolyzed when actin binds myosin.
  - D) ATP will be hydrolyzed during the power stroke.

The Neuromuscular Junction and Impulse Transmission

The **neuromuscular junction** (**NMJ**) is the synapse between an axon terminus (synaptic knob) and a myofiber. The NMJ is not a single point, but rather a long trough or invagination (infolding) of the cell membrane; the axon terminus is elongated to fill the long synaptic cleft. The purpose of this arrangement is to allow the neuron to depolarize a large region of the postsynaptic membrane at once. The postsynaptic membrane (the myofiber cell membrane) is known as the **motor end plate**. ACh is the neurotransmitter at the NMJ.

Impulse transmission at the NMJ is typical of chemical synaptic transmission: An action potential arrives at the axon terminus, triggering the opening of _____ channels; the resulting increase in _____

---

[2]   Myosin is the protein with the ATPase activity.

[3]   In the absence of actin, myosin can still hydrolyze ATP, but it cannot release ADP after hydrolysis.

[4]   Choice **B** is correct. Without troponin-tropomyosin, ATP hydrolysis will begin as soon as ATP, actin, and myosin are mixed. In the presence of troponin-tropomyosin, myosin cannot bind actin, but if calcium is added, the troponin-tropomyosin complex allows binding and ATP hydrolysis can occur once again.

triggers the _____ of acetylcholine.[5] The postsynaptic membrane contains ACh receptors, which are ligand-gated Na⁺ channels. The ACh must reach its receptor by diffusing across the synaptic cleft. Binding of ACh to its receptor results in a postsynaptic sodium influx, which depolarizes the postsynaptic membrane. This depolarization is known as an **end plate potential** (**EPP**). The smallest measurable EPP, caused by exocytosis of a single ACh vesicle, is known as a **miniature EPP** (**MEPP**).

ACh will continue to stimulate postsynaptic receptors until it is destroyed. This is accomplished by the enzyme **acetylcholinesterase**, which hydrolyzes ACh to choline plus an acetyl unit.

As in neurons, summation is required to initiate an AP in the postsynaptic cell. In other words, a single MEPP is insufficient to cause the myofiber to contract. When a sufficient EPP occurs, threshold is reached, and _____ channels open in the postsynaptic membrane.[6] This initiates an AP in the myofiber. The AP is propagated as in neurons, by a continuing wave of voltage-gated sodium channel opening. The shape of this AP on a graph is similar to the shape of the neuronal AP.

This AP must depolarize the entire myofiber if contraction is to occur. But there is a problem: action potentials occur only at the cell surface, because they are by nature a depolarization of the cell membrane. The myofiber is so thick that an AP on its surface will not depolarize its interior. The solution is to have deep invaginations of the cell membrane, which allow the AP to travel into the thick cell. These deep infoldings are called **transverse tubules** (**T-tubules**, see Figure 2).

Another specialized membrane in the myofiber is the **sarcoplasmic reticulum** (**SR**). This is a huge, specialized smooth endoplasmic reticulum, which enfolds each myofibril in the cell (Figure 2). The SR is specialized to sequester and release Ca^{2+}. Active transporters in the SR rapidly remove calcium from the *sarcoplasm* (myofiber cytoplasm). Then, when an AP travels down the T-tubular network, it depolarizes the cell, and with it, the SR. The SR contains voltage-gated Ca^{2+} channels, which allow Ca^{2+} to rush out of the SR into the sarcoplasm upon depolarization. The increase in sarcoplasmic $[Ca^{2+}]$ causes troponin-tropomyosin to change conformation, allowing myosin to bind actin. Actin and myosin fibers slide across each other, and the muscle fiber contracts. When the cell repolarizes, calcium is actively sequestered by the SR, and contraction is ended.

Mechanics of Contraction

The smallest measurable muscle contraction is known as a muscle **twitch**. The nervous system can increase the force of contraction in two ways.

1) **Motor unit recruitment**. A motor unit is a group of myofibers innervated by the branches of a single motor neuron's axon. A muscle twitch results from the activation of one motor neuron, and a larger twitch can be obtained by activating ("recruiting") more motor neurons (and thus more myofibers).

---

[5] An action potential arrives at the axon terminus, triggering the opening of **voltage-gated Ca^{2+}** channels; the resulting increase in **intracellular Ca^{2+}** triggers the **release of vesicles** of acetylcholine.

[6] voltage-gated sodium channels

2) **Frequency summation**. Each contraction ends when the SR returns the [Ca²⁺] to low resting levels. If a second contraction occurs rapidly enough, however, there is insufficient time for the Ca²⁺ to be sequestered by the SR, and the second contraction builds on the first. The force of contraction increases. A rapidly repeating series of stimulations results in the strongest possible contraction, known as tetanus. This is a normal occurrence which the nervous system uses to obtain strong contractions.[7]

- The central nervous system can increase the strength of skeletal muscle contraction by:[8]
  - A) increasing the size of action potentials in somatic motor neurons that innervate the muscle.
  - B) increasing the number of neurons that innervate each skeletal muscle cell.
  - C) increasing the number of motor neurons leading to a muscle that are firing action potentials.
  - D) decreasing firing by inhibitory neurons that innervate the skeletal muscle.

Energy Storage in the Myofiber

ATP provides the energy for contraction, and supplies must be regenerated by glucose catabolism. However, glycolysis and the TCA cycle are not fast enough to keep pace with the rapid ATP utilization during extended contraction. There is a need for an *intermediate-term* energy storage molecule. **Creatine phosphate** is that molecule. During contraction, its hydrolysis drives the regeneration of ATP from ADP + P$_i$.

Muscle is highly aerobic tissue, with abundant mitochondria. **Myoglobin** is a globular protein and is similar to one of the four subunits of hemoglobin. The role of myoglobin is to provide an oxygen reserve by taking O$_2$ from hemoglobin and then releasing it as needed.

Nonetheless, during prolonged contraction, the supply of oxygen runs low, and metabolism becomes anaerobic. Lactic acid is produced and moves into the bloodstream, causing a drop in pH. The liver picks up this lactate and converts it into pyruvate, which can be used in various pathways.

Cramps may result from exhaustion of energy supplies (temporary lack of ATP) in muscle cells. **Rigor mortis** is rigidity of skeletal muscles which occurs soon after death. It results from complete ATP exhaustion; without ATP, myosin heads cannot release actin, and the muscle can neither contract nor relax.

---

[7] Do not confuse this with the disease tetanus, caused by *tetanospasmin*, a bacterial toxin. The disease is an exaggerated, uncontrolled example of the normal process.

[8] Each muscle cell is innervated by a single neuron (choice B is wrong), and the more neurons that fire, the more muscle cells that will contract; the more muscle cells that contract, the greater the total force of contraction (choice **C** is correct). Action potentials are all-or-none events; the depolarization is the same size in a given neuron (choice A is wrong), and there are no inhibitory neurons that innervate the neuromuscular junction. Only acetylcholine, which is excitatory to muscle cells, is released at these synapses (choice D is wrong). (All motor neurons release a constant, small, baseline amount of ACh onto the muscle cell; this provides a baseline level of contraction that we commonly call "muscle tone." To inhibit a muscle, the amount of baseline ACh is reduced.)

Muscle Fiber Types

Skeletal muscle fibers generally fall into one of two categories, slow twitch fibers and fast twitch fibers. "Slow" and "fast" refer to their contractile speeds; slow twitch fibers take around three times as long as fast twitch fibers to reach their maximum tension after stimulation.

Type I Slow Twitch Fibers

These fibers are also known as **red slow twitch** or **red oxidative** fibers because of their high myoglobin content. They also have a much better blood supply than fast twitch fibers due to an extensive surrounding capillary network. The combination of good oxygen delivery from the blood stream and the ability to store oxygen on their myoglobin allows these fibers to maintain contraction for extended periods of time without fatigue. These are the fibers that allow marathoners and long distance cyclists to run or bike for hours at a time.

Type II Fast Twitch Fibers

These fibers actually fall into two subcategories according to their ability to resist fatigue. Both fiber types contract quickly, but Type IIA fast twitch fibers have more mitochondria than Type IIB fast twitch and are thus more fatigue resistant.

- *Type IIA:* also known as fast twitch oxidative fibers, these are somewhat resistant to fatigue. They cannot maintain activity for as long as slow twitch fibers can (only around 30 minutes or so), but far exceed the duration of use of the Type IIB fibers.
- *Type IIB:* also known as white fast twitch fibers due to their lack of mitochondria, these fibers contract very quickly with great force. However, they fatigue just as quickly, maxing out at around one minute of use. These are the fibers that provide the explosive force needed for jump shots and pole vaults.

Table 1 below compares the three fiber types.

Fiber type	Slow Twitch	Type IIA	Type IIB
Other names	Red slow twitch, red oxidative	Intermediate, fast twitch oxidative	White fast twitch
Speed of contraction	Slow	Intermediate	Very fast
Force generated	Low	Medium	High
Mitochondria	Many	Some	Very few
Capillaries	Very dense	Medium	Very few
Fatigue resistance	High Hours of use	Medium 30 minutes of use	Low 1 minute of use

Table 1 Comparison of Muscle Fiber Types

18.3   CARDIAC MUSCLE COMPARED TO SKELETAL MUSCLE

Cardiac muscle is similar to skeletal muscle in the following ways:

1) Thick and thin filaments are organized into sarcomeres. Hence, both cardiac and skeletal muscle are microscopically striated (striped).
2) T-tubules are present and serve the same function (transmission of APs into the interior of the large, thick cell).
3) Troponin-tropomyosin regulates contraction in the same way.

Cardiac muscle is *different* from skeletal muscle in some important ways:

1) Cardiac muscle cells are not structurally syncytial (they each have only one nucleus), while skeletal muscle cells are syncytial. But all the muscle cells of the heart are interconnected by gap junctions known as **intercalated disks**, which allow action potentials to propagate throughout the entire heart without allowing nuclei and cytoplasmic contents to be shared; only small items like ions can pass. Heart muscle is thus called a ***functional* syncytium** because it acts like a syncytium (but isn't really).
2) Cardiac muscle cells are each connected to several neighbors by intercalated disks.
3) Some of the calcium required for cardiac muscle-cell contraction comes from the extracellular environment, through the voltage-gated calcium channels. In skeletal muscle, all the calcium for contraction comes from the sarcoplasmic reticulum, an intracellular structure.
4) Cardiac muscle contraction does *not* depend on stimulation by motor neurons. In fact, the most important nerve releasing ACh at chemical synapses with the heart is inhibitory! This is the vagus nerve, a parasympathetic nerve. It synapses with the sinoatrial node, where it releases ACh to inhibit spontaneous depolarization (discussed below), with the result being a slower heart rate. Contrast this with skeletal muscle innervation, in which neurons release ACh to stimulate contraction. [If neurons don't trigger cardiac contraction, what does?[9]]
5) The AP in cardiac muscle depends not only on voltage-gated sodium channels (**fast sodium channels**, as in skeletal muscle), but also on voltage-gated calcium channels. These are called **slow channels** because they respond more slowly to threshold depolarization, opening later than the fast channels and taking longer to close. The voltage-gated calcium channels cause the cardiac AP to have the distinctive plateau shown in Figure 5.

---

[9]   Cardiac contraction is triggered by the sinoatrial node, which sets the pacing for the heart. This is discussed in Chapter 16.

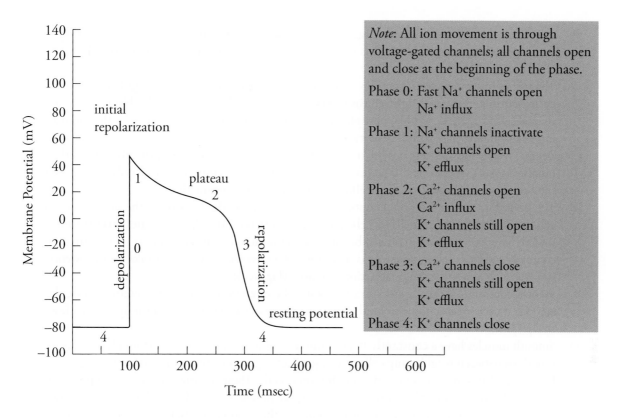

Figure 5 The Cardiac Muscle Cell Action Potential

The significance of the plateau phase is twofold: 1) a longer duration of contraction facilitates ventricular emptying (better ejection fraction), and 2) a longer refractory period helps prevent disorganized transmission of impulses throughout the heart and makes summation and tetanus impossible. This is advantageous because the heart must relax after each contraction. So remember, skeletal muscle cells and neurons have the same steeply-spiking AP, while cardiac muscle cells have a spike and a plateau. Figure 5 shows the phases of the cardiac action potential.

18.4 SMOOTH MUSCLE COMPARED TO SKELETAL MUSCLE

Smooth muscle is like skeletal muscle in that contraction is accomplished by sliding of actin and myosin filaments; the four-step contractile cycle is the same. Another similarity is that contraction is triggered by an increase in cytoplasmic [Ca^{2+}]. Like skeletal muscle cells, smooth muscle cells do not branch. However, smooth muscle is different from skeletal muscle in many ways:

1) Smooth muscle cells are much narrower and shorter than skeletal muscle cells.
2) T-tubules are *not* present. The smooth muscle cell is so small that they are unnecessary; a depolarization on the surface can depolarize the entire cell.
3) Each smooth muscle cell has only one nucleus and is connected to its neighbors by gap junctions (like cardiac muscle cells) which allow impulses to spread from cell to cell. Hence, both smooth and cardiac muscle are functional syncytia.

4) Thick and thin filaments are not organized into sarcomeres in smooth muscle. Instead they are dispersed in the cytoplasm. This is why the cell appears smooth instead of striated (no regular A band, H zone, etc.).

5) The troponin–tropomyosin complex is not present. Instead, contraction is regulated by **calmodulin** and **myosin light-chain kinase** (**MLCK**). In brief, calmodulin binds Ca^{2+} and then activates MLCK. MLCK phosphorylates a portion of the myosin molecule, thus activating its enzymatic/mechanical activity.

6) While skeletal muscles rely heavily on Ca^{2+} from sarcoplasmic reticulum, the SR in smooth muscles is poorly developed. It stores some Ca^{2+} that can be released upon depolarization, but the cell also relies heavily on extracellular stores of Ca^{2+} for contraction.

7) The smooth muscle cell action potential varies depending on the location of the smooth muscle cell. Most smooth muscle cells can elicit action potentials (also called **spike potentials**) similar to skeletal muscle action potentials, but since smooth muscle cells have almost no sodium fast channels and their action potential is determined by slow channels only, it takes ten to twenty times as long as a skeletal muscle action potential (Figure 6).

8) Some smooth muscle that must sustain prolonged contractions (such as the uterus or vascular smooth muscle) has action potentials similar to those of cardiac muscle, although with a less-sharp spike.

9) Smooth muscles have a constantly fluctuating resting potential. Ions pass through the gap junctions between neighboring cells, causing the changes in resting potential to propagate like waves through the connected smooth muscle cells. These fluctuations in resting potential are called "slow waves." Slow waves are NOT spike potentials and do NOT elicit muscle contractions, but they are necessary to help *coordinate* the action potentials. In response to local stimuli (e.g., stretching of smooth muscle in the gut wall due to a food bolus), neurotransmitter from parasympathetic neurons is released. The neurotransmitter binds to receptors on smooth muscle cells and primes them for an action potential by pushing their electrical potential closer to threshold. Slow waves then pass through these "primed" smooth muscle cells, they reach threshold, and undergo an action (spike) potential (Figure 6). The amplitude of these slow waves is increased by ACh and decreased by NE (e.g., stimulating the gut during a parasympathetic response, and slowing it down during a sympathetic one).

10) Like skeletal muscle, smooth muscles are innervated by motor neurons, but in the case of smooth muscle, they are *autonomic* motor neurons instead of somatic motor neurons. Individual neurons do activate smooth muscle cells (as in skeletal muscle), but, as mentioned previously, the action potential then spreads from cell to cell. (Recall that in skeletal muscle, each action potential is limited to one large myofiber, while the heart is one large functional syncytium in which each action potential spreads to every cell. Hence, regarding innervation and the spread of impulses, smooth muscle shares features of both skeletal and cardiac muscle.)

18.4

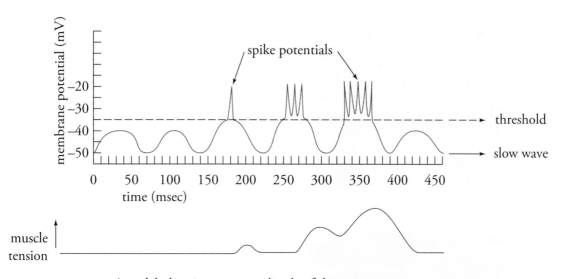

Acetylcholine increases amplitude of slow wave.
Norepinephrine decreases amplitude of slow wave.

Figure 6 The Smooth Muscle Cell Spike Potential and Slow Waves

Feature	Skeletal Muscle	Cardiac Muscle	Smooth Muscle
Appearance	Striated	Striated	No striations
Upstroke of action potential	Inward Na$^+$ current	Inward Ca^{2+} (SA node) Inward Na$^+$ (atria, ventricles, Purkinje)	Inward Na$^+$
Plateau	No	Yes (except for SA node)	No
Duration of AP	2–3 msec	150 msec (SA node) 300 msec (other cells)	20 msec
Calcium from	AP opens voltage-gated Ca^{2+} channels in SR, Ca^{2+} released from SR	AP opens voltage-gated Ca^{2+} channels, inward Ca^{2+} current during plateau Ca^{2+}-induced-Ca^{2+} release from SR	AP opens Ca^{2+} channels in cell membrane, inward Ca^{2+} current
Molecular basis for contraction	Ca^{2+} troponin binding	Ca^{2+} troponin binding	Ca^{2+} calmodulin binding, myosin light-chain kinase activation
Functional syncytium	No	Yes	Yes
Contraction dependent on extracellular Ca^{2+}	No	Partially	Yes

Table 2 Comparison of Skeletal, Cardiac, and Smooth Muscle

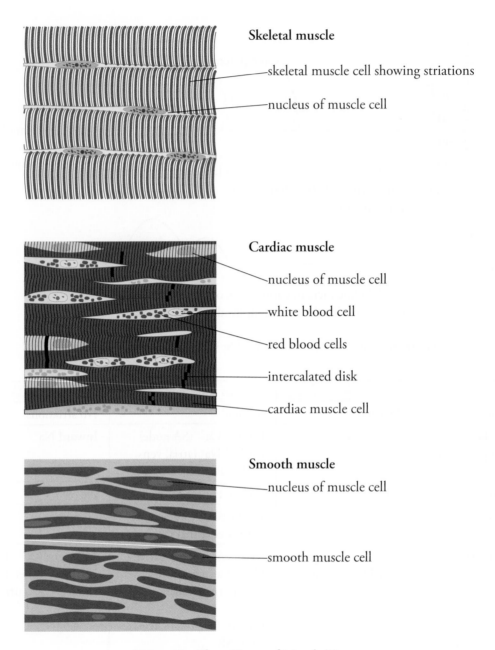

Figure 7   Three Types of Muscle Tissue

18.5 OVERVIEW OF THE SKELETAL SYSTEM

As vertebrates, we have an **endoskeleton** made of bone. This contrasts with the chitinous exoskeleton of arthropods. The vertebrate skeletal system serves five roles:

1) support the body,
2) provide the framework for movement,
3) protect vital organs (brain, heart, etc.),
4) store calcium, and
5) synthesize the formed elements of the blood (red blood cells, white blood cells, platelets). This occurs in the marrow of flat bones and is called **hematopoiesis**.

The vertebrate endoskeleton is divided into **axial** and **appendicular** components. The axial skeleton consists of the skull, the vertebral column, and the rib cage. All other bones are part of the appendicular skeleton (see Figure 8).

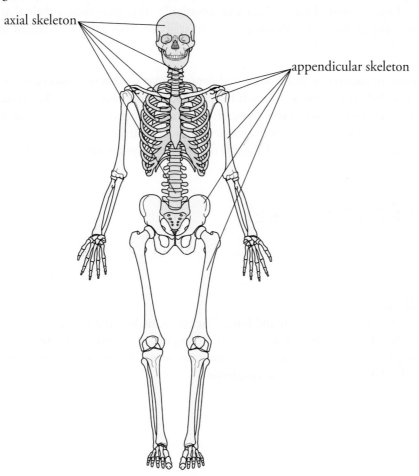

Figure 8 Axial and Appendicular Skeletons

18.6 CONNECTIVE TISSUE

Bone is an example of **connective tissue**. Connective tissue consists of cells and the materials they secrete. All connective tissue cells are derived from a single progenitor, the **fibroblast**. This name derives from its ability to secrete fibrous material such as **collagen**, a strong fibrous protein. Another important fibrous extracellular protein is **elastin**, which gives tissue the ability to stretch and regain its shape. Fibroblast-derived cells include **adipocytes** (fat cells), **chondrocytes** (cartilage cells), and **osteocytes** (bone cells).

Connective tissue differs from the other tissue types in the body (epithelial, muscle, and nervous tissue) because it is primarily extracellular material with a few cells scattered in it (the other three tissue types are the opposite; mostly cellular, with little extracellular material). The extracellular material is known as the **matrix** and consists of the fibers described above and **ground substance**, a thick, viscous material. The main ingredients of the ground substance are proteoglycans; these are large macropolymers consisting of a protein core with many attached carbohydrate chains. The carbohydrate chains are called glycosaminoglycans (GAGs) and like all carbohydrates, they are very hydrophilic. Hence, in the body, they are always surrounded by a large amount of water ("water of solvation"). This gives tissues their characteristic thickness and firmness. For example, dehydration results in saggy skin because of decreased hydration of the ground substance in the extracellular matrix.

There are two types of connective tissue: loose and dense. **Loose connective tissues** are basically packing tissues, and they include areolar tissue (the soft material located between most cells throughout the body) and adipose tissue (fat). **Dense connective tissue** refers to tissues that contain large amounts of fibers (especially collagen), such as tendons, ligaments, cartilage, and bone. Cartilage and bone are sometime classified as supportive connective tissues, because of the role they play in physical support of body structures.

18.7 BONE STRUCTURE

Macroscopic

There are two primary bone shapes: **flat** and **long**. Flat bones, such as the scapula, the ribs, and the bones of the skull, are the location of hematopoiesis and are important for protection of organs. The bones of the limbs are long bones, important for support and movement. The main shaft of a long bone is called the **diaphysis**. The flared end is called the **epiphysis**.

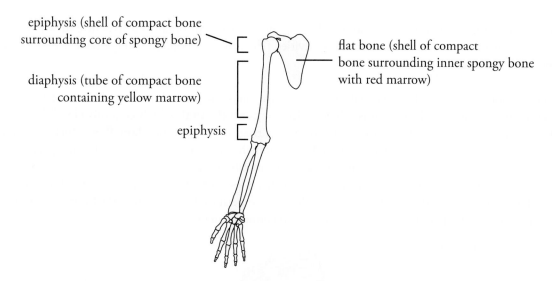

epiphysis (shell of compact bone surrounding core of spongy bone)

flat bone (shell of compact bone surrounding inner spongy bone with red marrow)

diaphysis (tube of compact bone containing yellow marrow)

epiphysis

Figure 9 Gross Anatomy of Bone

The general structure of bone may be either **compact** or **spongy**. As the names imply, compact bone is hard and dense, while spongy bone is porous. Spongy bone is always surrounded by a layer of compact bone. The diaphysis of long bones is a tube composed only of compact bone.

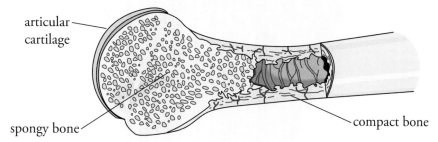

articular cartilage

spongy bone

compact bone

Figure 10 Compact and Spongy Bone

Bone marrow is non-bony material found in the shafts of long bones and in the pores of spongy bones. **Red marrow**, found in spongy bone within flat bones, is the site of hematopoiesis. Its activity increases in response to erythropoietin, a hormone made by the kidney. **Yellow marrow**, found in the shafts of long bones, is filled with fat and is inactive.

Microscopic

Bone is composed of two principal ingredients: collagen and **hydroxyapatite**, which is a solid material consisting of calcium phosphate crystals. During bone synthesis, collagen is laid down in a highly ordered structure. Then hydroxyapatite crystals form around the collagen framework, giving bone its characteristic strength and inflexibility.

Spongy bone under the microscope looks like a sponge. It has a disorganized structure in which many spikes of bone surround marrow-containing cavities. The spikes of bone in spongy bone are called **spicules** or **trabeculae**.

Compact bone has a specific organization (Figure 11). The basic unit of compact bone structure is the **osteon**. In the center of the osteon is a hole called the **central canal**, which contains blood, lymph vessels, and nerves. Surrounding the canal are concentric rings of bone termed **lamellae** (which just means "sheets" or "layers"). Tiny channels, or **canaliculi**, branch out from the central canal to spaces called **lacunae** ("lakes"). In each lacuna is an **osteocyte**, or mature bone cell. Osteocytes have long processes which extend down the canaliculi to contact other osteocytes through gap junctions. This allows the cells to exchange nutrients and waste through an otherwise impermeable membrane. **Perforating canals** are channels that run perpendicular to central canals to connect osteons.

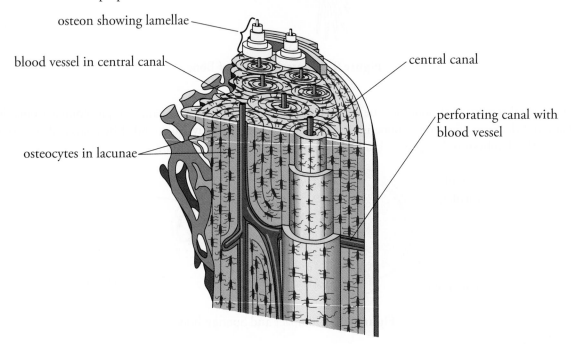

osteon showing lamellae

blood vessel in central canal

central canal

perforating canal with blood vessel

osteocytes in lacunae

Figure 11   Microscopic Structure of Compact Bone

18.8   TISSUES FOUND AT JOINTS

Cartilage

Cartilage is a strong but very flexible extracellular tissue secreted by cells called **chondrocytes**. There are three types of cartilage: hyaline, elastic, and fibrous. **Hyaline cartilage** is strong and somewhat flexible. The larynx and trachea are reinforced by hyaline cartilage, and joints are lined by hyaline cartilage known as **articular cartilage**, as shown in Figure 11. **Elastic cartilage** is found in structures (such as the outer ear and the epiglottis) that require support and more flexibility than hyaline cartilage can provide; it contains elastin. **Fibrous cartilage** is very rigid and is found in places where very strong support is needed, such as the pubic symphysis (the anterior connection of the pelvis) and the intervertebral disks of the spinal column. Cartilage is not innervated and does not contain blood vessels (it is **avascular**). It receives nutrition and immune protection from the surrounding fluid. [Why do cartilage injuries take a long time to heal?[10]]

Ligaments, Tendons, and Joints

Ligaments and tendons are strong tissues composed of dense connective tissue. **Ligaments** connect bones to other bones, and **tendons** connect bones to muscles. The point where one bone meets another is called a **joint**. Immovable joints, called **synarthroses**, are basically points where two bones are fused together. For example, the skull is formed from many fused bones. Slightly movable joints, called **amphiarthroses**, provide both movability and a great deal of support (*amphi-* means "both"). The vertebral joints are an example. Freely movable joints (i.e., most of the joints in the body) are called **diarthroses**. There are several types, for example, ball and socket (hip, shoulder), and hinge (elbow). All movable joints are supported by ligaments.

Movable joints are lubricated by **synovial fluid**, which is kept within the joint by the **synovial capsule**. The surfaces of the two bones that contact each other are perfectly smooth because they are lined by special **articular cartilage** (composed of hyaline cartilage). Like all cartilage, articular cartilage lacks blood vessels. Hence, it is easily damaged by overuse or infection. Inflammation of joints (**arthritis**) leads to destruction of the articular cartilage, which causes pain and stiffness.

---

[10]   Cells in cartilage are not directly supplied by blood and have a low rate of metabolism. Thus, they are slow to repair damage. Often the damaged cartilage is simply removed or repaired surgically.

19.1   THE MALE REPRODUCTIVE SYSTEM

Anatomy

The principal male reproductive structures that are visible on the outside of the body are the scrotum and the penis. The scrotum contains the male gonads, which are known as **testes** (testicles). The testes have two roles: 1) synthesis of sperm (**spermatogenesis**), and 2) secretion of male sex hormones (**androgens**, e.g., testosterone) into the bloodstream. More detail on these topics is given later. Here we will trace the path of a sperm from its origination to its final destination.

The sites of spermatogenesis within the testes are the **seminiferous tubules**. The walls of the seminiferous tubules are formed by cells called **sustentacular cells** (also known as *Sertoli cells*). Sustentacular cells protect and nurture the developing sperm, both physically and chemically; their role will be discussed in more detail below. The tissue between the seminiferous tubules is simply referred to as testicular interstitium.[1] Important cells found in the testicular interstitium are the **interstitial cells** (also known as Leydig cells). They are responsible for androgen (testosterone) synthesis.

The seminiferous tubules empty into the **epididymis**, a long coiled tube located on the posterior (back) of each testicle (Figure 1). The epididymis from each testicle empties into a **ductus deferens** (also call the *vas deferens*), which in turn leads to the **urethra** (the tube inside the penis). To get to the urethra, the ductus deferens leaves the scrotum and follows a peculiar path: it enters the **inguinal canal**, a tunnel that travels along the body wall toward the crest of the hip bone. (There are two inguinal canals, left and right.) From the inguinal canal, the ductus deferens enters the pelvic cavity. Near the back of the urinary bladder, it joins the duct of the seminal vesicle (discussed below) to form the **ejaculatory duct**. The ejaculatory ducts from both sides of the body then join the urethra.

A pair of glands known as **seminal vesicles** is located on the posterior surface of the bladder. They secrete about 60 percent of the total volume of the **semen** into the ejaculatory duct. Semen is a highly nourishing fluid for sperm and is produced by three separate glands: the seminal vesicles, the **prostate**, and the **bulbourethral glands**. These are collectively referred to as the **accessory glands** (see Table 1). The ejaculatory duct empties into the **urethra** as it passes through the prostate gland. One final set of glands, the bulbourethral glands, contributes to the semen near the beginning of the urethra.

Gland and secretions	Function of secretions	% of total ejaculate volume
Seminal vesicles—mostly fructose	Nourishment of sperm	60%
Prostate gland—fructose and a coagulant	Nourishment, allows semen to coagulate after ejaculation	35%
Bulbourethral glands—thick, alkaline mucus	Lubricate urethra, neutralize acids in male urethra and in female vagina	3%
Testes—sperm	Male gamete	2%

Table 1   The Accessory Glands

---

[1]   *Interstitium* is a term used to describe a thing or a region which is "between" other structures.

The urethra exits the body via the penis. Penile erection facilitates deposition of semen near the opening of the uterus during intercourse. Specialized **erectile tissue** in the penis allows erection. It is composed of modified veins and capillaries surrounded by a connective tissue sheath. Erection occurs when blood accumulates at high pressure in the erectile tissue. Three compartments contain erectile tissue: the **corpora cavernosa** (there are two of these) and the **corpus spongiosum** (only one).

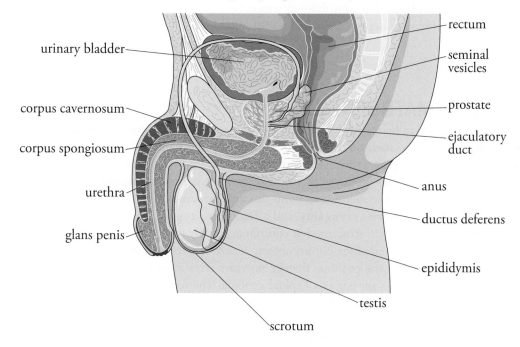

Figure 1   The Male Reproductive System

The Male Sexual Act

The three stages of the male sexual act are: arousal, orgasm, and resolution. These events are controlled by an integrating center in the spinal cord, which responds to physical stimulation and input from the brain. The cerebral cortex can activate this integrating center (as in sexual arousal during sleep) or inhibit it (anxiety interferes with sexual function).

Arousal is dependent upon parasympathetic nervous input and can be subdivided into two stages: erection and lubrication. **Erection** involves dilation of arteries supplying the erectile tissue. This causes swelling, which in turn obstructs venous outflow. This causes the erectile tissue to become pressurized with blood. **Lubrication** is also a function of the parasympathetic system. The bulbourethral glands secrete a viscous mucous which serves as a lubricant.

Stimulation by the sympathetic nervous system is required for **orgasm**, which can also be divided into two stages: emission and ejaculation. **Emission** refers to the propulsion of sperm (from the ductus deferens) and semen (from the accessory glands) into the urethra by contractions of the smooth muscle surrounding these organs. Emission is followed by **ejaculation**, in which the fluid (semen and sperm) is propelled out of the urethra by rhythmic contractions of muscles surrounding the base of the penis. Ejaculation is actually a reflex reaction caused by the presence of semen in the urethra. Emission and ejaculation together constitute the male orgasm.

Resolution, or a return to a normal, unstimulated state, is also controlled by the sympathetic nervous system. It is caused primarily by a constriction of the erectile arteries. This results in decreased blood flow to the erectile tissue and allows the veins to carry away the trapped blood, returning the penis to a flaccid state. This typically takes 2–3 minutes.

- Name the three glands that contribute to semen.[2]
- What is the difference between emission and ejaculation?[3]

19.2 SPERMATOGENESIS

What processes in a human being involve meiosis? Only one: **gametogenesis**. This is the process whereby **diploid germ cells** undergo **meiotic division** to produce **haploid gametes**. As discussed in Chapter 14, meiotic cell division fosters genetic diversity in the population (by independent assortment of genes and by recombination). The gametes produced by the male are known as **spermatozoa**, or *sperm*; females produce **ova**, or *eggs*. The role of the sperm is to swim through the female genital tract to reach the egg and fuse with it. This fusion is known as **syngamy**, and it results in a **zygote**. The gametes produced by males and females differ dramatically in structure but contribute equally to the genome of the zygote (except in the special case of the two different sex chromosomes, X and Y, given to male offspring). Although both gametes contribute equally to the genome, the egg provides *every other part of the zygote*, since the only part of the sperm which enters the egg is a haploid genome. The term for this is **maternal inheritance**. For instance, mitochondria are inherited maternally.

Sperm synthesis is called **spermatogenesis** (Figure 2). It begins at puberty and occurs in the testes throughout adult life. [Do females also make gametes throughout adult life?[4]] The seminiferous tubule is the site of spermatogenesis. The entire process of spermatogenesis occurs with the aid of the specialized sustentacular cells found in the wall of the seminiferous tubule. Immature sperm precursors are found in the outer wall of the tubule, and nearly-mature spermatozoa are deposited into the lumen; from there they are transported to the epididymis. The cells that give rise to spermatogonia (and to their female counterparts, oogonia) are known as **germ cells**; under the right conditions, they *germ*inate and give rise to a complete organism.

---

[2] Seminal vesicles, prostate, and bulbourethral glands

[3] Emission is the movement of sperm and semen components into the urethra; ejaculation is the movement of semen from the urethra out of the body.

[4] No. This is discussed in Section 19.6.

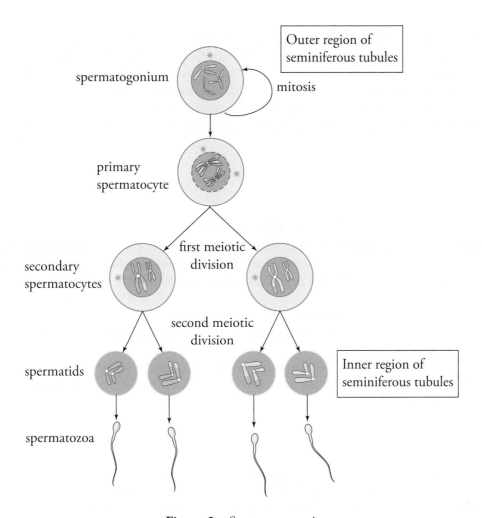

Figure 2   Spermatogenesis

- Do spermatogonia divide by mitosis or by meiosis?[5]
- How many mature sperm result from a single spermatogonium after it becomes committed to meiosis?[6]
- Which of the following statements is/are true?[7]
    - I.   During gametogenesis, sister chromatids remain paired with each other until anaphase of the second meiotic cell division.
    - II.   A difference between mitosis and meiosis is that mitosis requires DNA replication prior to cell division but meiosis does not.
    - III.   Recombination between sister chromatids during gametogenesis increases the genetic diversity of offspring.

---

[5]   Mitosis. Spermatogonia undergo the meiotic S phase (replicate the genome), but the stages which undergo the actual meiotic *divisions* are called spermatocytes. *All* gamete precursors with "cyte" in their name undergo a meiotic division.

[6]   Four haploid cells result from the reductive division (meiosis) of one diploid spermatogonium. Compare this to oogenesis.

[7]   **Item I: True.** Meiosis I involves the pairing, recombination, and separation of homologous chromosomes. Meiosis II is like mitosis, where sister chromatids separate. Item II: False. Both require DNA replication in a preceding S phase. Item III: False. Sister chromatids don't recombine, homologous chromosomes do. (Even if sister chromatids did recombine, it would make no difference since they are identical.)

Spermatids develop into spermatozoa in the seminiferous tubules with the aid of sustentacular cells. The DNA condenses, the cytoplasm shrinks, and the cell shape changes so that there is a **head**, containing the haploid nucleus and the acrosome, and a flagellum which forms the **tail**. There is also a **neck** region at the base of the tail, which contains many mitochondria. The **acrosome** is a compartment on the head of the sperm that contains hydrolytic enzymes required for penetration of the ovum's protective layers. **Bindin** is a protein on the sperm's surface that attaches to receptors on the zona pellucida surrounding the ovum (discussed below).

Hormonal Control of Spermatogenesis

Testosterone plays the essential role of stimulating division of spermatogonia. **Luteinizing hormone** (**LH**) stimulates the interstitial cells to secrete testosterone. **Follicle stimulating hormone** (**FSH**) stimulates the sustentacular cells. The hormone **inhibin** is secreted by sustentacular cells; its role is to inhibit FSH release.

- Which of the following is/are true?[8]
  - I. Luteinizing hormone reaches its target tissue through the hypothalamic-hypophysial portal system.
  - II. The absence of luteinizing hormone does not affect spermatogenesis.
  - III. Increased testosterone levels in the blood decrease the production of follicle stimulating hormone.

19.3 DEVELOPMENT OF THE MALE REPRODUCTIVE SYSTEM

The gender of a developing embryo is determined by its sex chromosomes, either XX in females or XY in males. During the early weeks of development, however, male and female embryos are indistinguishable. Early embryos, whether male or female, have undifferentiated gonads, and possess both **Wolffian ducts** that can develop into male internal genitalia (epididymis, seminal vesicles, and ductus deferens) and **Müllerian ducts** that can develop into female internal genitalia (uterine tubes, uterus and vagina). In the absence of a Y chromosome, Müllerian duct development occurs by default, and female internal genitalia result. Female *external* genitalia (labia, clitoris) are also the default; note that the external genitalia are not derived from the Müllerian ducts. Genetic information on the Y chromosome of XY embryos leads to the development of testes, which cause male internal and external genitalia to develop by producing testosterone and **Müllerian inhibiting factor** (**MIF**).

MIF is produced by the testes and causes regression of the Müllerian ducts; this prevents the development of female internal genitalia. Testosterone secretion by cells which will later give rise to the testes begins around week 7 of gestation. By week 9, testes are formed, and their interstitial cells supply testosterone. The testosterone that is responsible for the development of male external genitalia enters the systemic circulation and must be converted to **dihydrotestosterone** in target tissues in order to exert its effect (Figure 3).

---

[8] Item I: False. LH is secreted by the anterior pituitary and reaches its targets via the systemic circulation. GnRH reaches its target via the portal system. Item II: False. LH is necessary because it stimulates the interstitial cells to secrete testosterone, which is necessary for germ cell stimulation. **Item III: True.** Testosterone, estrogen, progesterone, and inhibin are all hormones which exert feedback inhibition upon the anterior pituitary and hypothalamus.

- If an XY genotype embryo fails to secrete testosterone, will it have testes or ovaries?[9]

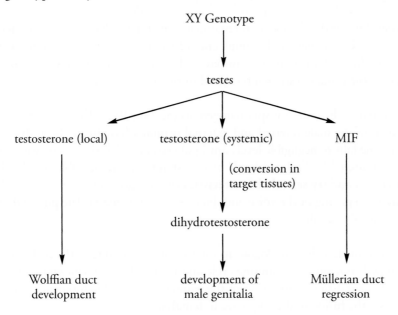

Figure 3 Control of Development of the Male Reproductive System

- Which one of the following would best characterize an embryo with an XY genotype that lacks the receptor for testosterone?[10]
  A) Testes, ductus deferens, and seminal vesicles are present; external genitalia are female.
  B) Ovaries, uterine tubes, and uterus are present; external genitalia are female.
  C) Testes are present; external genitalia are female; neither Müllerian nor Wolffian ducts develop.
  D) Testes and male external genitalia are present.

The development of the male and female reproductive systems is closely related. As described above, the three main fetal precursors of the reproductive organs are the Wolffian ducts, the Müllerian ducts, and the gonads. While the Wolffian ducts are the precursors of internal male genitalia, they essentially disappear in the female reproductive system. For the Müllerian ducts, this process is reversed; they essentially disappear in the male reproductive system and form the internal genitalia of the female system. Structures arising from these ducts tend to have the same function (for example, ductus deferens in males and the uterine tubes in females both carry gametes), but because they arise from different precursors, they are considered to be **analogous structures**.

---

[9] Testosterone is *produced by* the embryonic testes. Their development does not depend on testosterone. Hence, an XY embryo that didn't secrete testosterone would most likely have testes nonetheless.

[10] The XY genotype would lead to the development of testes (choice B is wrong), and the testes would produce MIF and testosterone. MIF would cause the degeneration of the Müllerian ducts, and no female internal genitalia would develop. However, the inability to respond to testosterone (because of the missing receptor) would prevent the development of the Wolffian ducts (choice A is wrong) as well as the male external genitalia (choice D is wrong). The external genitalia would default to female (choice **C** is correct).

19.4 ANDROGENS AND ESTROGENS

All hormones involved in the development and maintenance of male characteristics are termed **androgens**, while those involved in development and maintenance of female characteristics are termed **estrogens**. The primary androgen produced in the testes is testosterone. It is converted into dihydrotestosterone within the cells of target tissues. The primary estrogen produced in the ovaries is estradiol.

Testosterone is required in the testes for spermatogenesis (Section 19.2). The role of testosterone in the embryonic development of the male internal and external genitalia has already been discussed. After birth, the level of testosterone falls to negligible levels until puberty, at which time it increases and remains high for the remainder of adult life. Elevated levels of testosterone are responsible for the development and maintenance of male **secondary sexual characteristics** (maturation of the genitalia, male distribution of facial and body hair, deepening of the voice, and increased muscle mass). The pubertal growth spurt and fusion of the epiphyses also result.

The role of estrogen in the female is analogous to the role of testosterone in the male. Beginning at puberty, estrogen is required to regulate the uterine cycle and for the development and maintenance of female secondary sexual characteristics (maturation of the genitalia, breast development, wider hips, and pubic hair). Estrogen causes the fusion of the epiphyses in females.

- If testosterone levels are abnormally elevated during childhood, how will the height of the individual be affected?[11]
- How do androgens reach the cytoplasm to bind to cytoplasmic receptors?[12]

During puberty and adult life, sex steroid production is controlled by the hypothalamus and the anterior pituitary. **Gonadotropin releasing hormone (GnRH)** from the hypothalamus stimulates the pituitary to release the gonadotropins: follicle-stimulating hormone (FSH) and luteinizing hormone (LH). In men, LH acts on interstitial cells to stimulate testosterone production, and FSH stimulates the sustentacular cells. In women, FSH stimulates the granulosa cells to secrete estrogen, and LH simulates the formation of the corpus luteum and progesterone secretion. Feedback inhibition by the steroids inhibits the production of GnRH and LH and FSH. Inhibin, produced by sustentacular cells and the granulosa cells, provides further feedback regulation of FSH production (Figure 4).

---

[11] The child will undergo precocious puberty, involving an early growth spurt, so the child will be unusually tall. But then early fusion of the epiphyses will result in a shorter adult height than expected.

[12] These highly hydrophobic molecules can diffuse through the cell membrane and bind to cytoplasmic receptors.

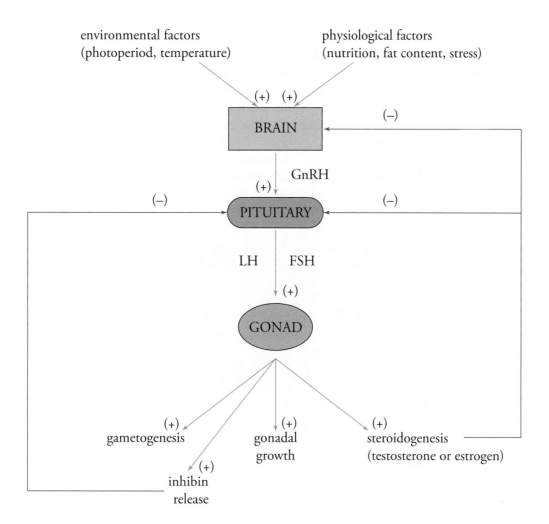

Figure 4 Regulation of Sex Steroid Production

19.5 THE FEMALE REPRODUCTIVE SYSTEM

Anatomy and Development

We mentioned in Section 19.3 that male and female genitalia are derived from a common undifferentiated precursor. Because of this, the structures of the female external genitalia are homologous to those of the male. In the female, the XX genotype leads to the formation of ovaries capable of secreting the female sex hormones (estrogens) instead of testes that secrete androgens. In the male, testosterone causes a pair of skin folds known as **labioscrotal swellings** to grow and fuse, forming the scrotum. In the female, without the influence of testosterone, the labioscrotal swellings form the **labia majora** of the vagina (labia = lips, majora = larger). The structure that gave rise to the penis in the male embryo becomes the **clitoris** in the female, located within the labia majora in the uppermost part of the vulva. Just beneath the clitoris is the **urethral opening**, where urine exits the body. Surrounding the urethral opening is another pair of skin folds called the **labia minora**.

The opening of the **vagina** is also found between the labia minora. The female internal genitalia (vagina, uterine tubes, uterus) are derived from the Müllerian ducts, so there are no homologous structures in the male. The vagina is a tube which would end in the pelvic cavity, except that another hollow organ, the **uterus**, opens into its upper portion. The part of the uterus which opens into the vagina is called the **cervix** ("neck," as in "cervical"). The innermost lining of the uterus (closest to the lumen) is the **endometrium**. It is responsible for nourishing a developing embryo, and in the absence of pregnancy is shed each month, producing menstrual bleeding. Surrounding the endometrium is the **myometrium**, which is a thick layer of smooth muscle comprising the wall of the uterus. The uterus ends in two **uterine tubes** (also called *fallopian tubes*), which extend into the pelvis on either side. Each uterine tube ends in a bunch of finger-like structures called **fimbriae**. The fimbriae brush up against the **ovary**, which is the female gonad. [At the time of ovulation, where does the oocyte come from and where does it go?[13]]

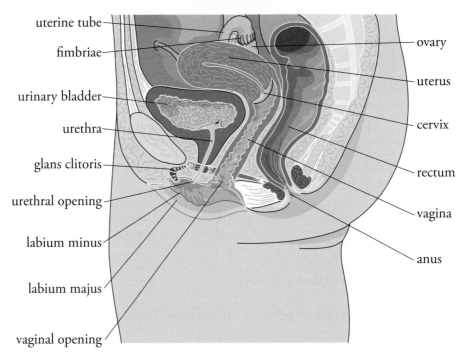

Figure 5   The Female Reproductive System

- What is the fate of the Wolffian ducts and their derivatives in the female?[14]
- Is estrogen production by the ovaries required for the development of the uterine tubes and uterus?[15]

---

[13] It emerges from the ovary (sometimes causing pain in the middle of the menstrual cycle) and must be swept into the uterine tube by a constant flow of fluid into the uterine tube caused by cilia.

[14] In the absence of testosterone, they atrophy.

[15] No, the Müllerian ducts develop into vagina, uterus, and uterine tubes by default as long as MIF is absent.

The Female Sexual Act

The stages are the same as in the male: **arousal**, **orgasm**, and **resolution**. The arousal stage, as in the male, is subdivided into erection and lubrication and is controlled by the parasympathetic nervous system. The clitoris and labia minora contain erectile tissue and become engorged with blood, just as in the male. Lubrication is provided by mucus secreted by **greater vestibular glands** and by the vaginal epithelium. Orgasm in the female is controlled by the sympathetic nervous system and involves muscle contractions, just as in the male, in addition to a widening of the cervix. (These events are thought to facilitate the movement of sperm into the uterus.) The female does not experience ejaculation. Resolution is also the same as in the male, controlled by the sympathetic system, but can take up to 20–30 minutes (compared to 2–3 minutes in the male).

19.6   OOGENESIS AND OVULATION

Oogenesis begins prenatally. In the ovary of a female fetus, germ cells divide mitotically to produce large numbers of **oogonia**. [How is this different from the male scenario?[16]] Oogonia not only undergo mitosis *in utero*, but they also enter the first phase of meiosis and are arrested in prophase I (as primary oocytes). The number of oogonia peaks at about 7 million at mid-gestation (20 weeks into the fetal life). At this time, mitosis ceases, conversion to primary oocytes begins, and there is a progressive loss of cells so that at birth there are only about 2 million primary oocytes. By puberty this number is further reduced to only about 400,000. Only about 400 oocytes are ever actually **ovulated** (released) in the average woman, and the remaining 99.9 percent will simply degenerate.

The primary oocytes formed in a female fetus can be frozen in prophase I of meiosis for decades, until they re-enter the meiotic cycle. Beginning at puberty and continuing on a monthly basis, hormonal changes in the woman's body stimulate completion of the first meiotic division and ovulation. This meiotic division yields a large secondary oocyte (containing all of the cytoplasm and organelles) and a small **polar body** (containing half the DNA, but no cytoplasm or organelles). The polar body (called the *first* polar body) remains in close proximity to the oocyte. The second meiotic division (i.e., completion of oogenesis) occurs *only if* the secondary oocyte is fertilized by a sperm; this division is also unequal, producing a large ovum and the second polar body. Note that if fertilization does occur, the nuclei from the sperm and egg do not fuse immediately. They must wait for the secondary oocyte to release the second polar body and finish maturing to an ootid and then an ovum. Finally, the two nuclei fuse, and a diploid (2*n*) zygote is formed.

- Is the secondary oocyte haploid?[17]
- When an oogonium undergoes meiosis, three cells result. How many of these are eggs, and why do only three cells result? (Meiosis results in four cells in the male.)[18]

Before we move on to a discussion of the menstrual cycle, you will need more background information on oogenesis. The primary oocyte is not an isolated cell. It is found in a clump of supporting cells called **granulosa cells**, and the entire structure (oocyte plus granulosa cells) is known as a **follicle**. The granulosa

---

[16] It only happens in *adult* males. Here, we're talking about events in the ovaries of a female while she's still in her mother's womb.

[17] Yes. After the first meiotic division, the cell is haploid; the homologous chromosomes have been separated. (They are, however, still replicated, hence the reason for meiosis II.)

[18] Only one egg results. The three cells which result are two polar bodies plus one ovum. There are only three because the first polar body does not divide. (In meiosis in the male, both cells derived from the first meiotic division go on to divide.)

cells assist in maturation. [What is the male counterpart of the granulosa cell?[19]] An immature primary oocyte is surrounded by a single layer of granulosa cells, forming a **primordial follicle**.

As the primordial follicle matures, the granulosa cells proliferate to form several layers around the oocyte, and the oocyte itself forms a protective layer of mucopolysaccharides termed the **zona pellucida**. There may be several follicles in the ovary; they are surrounded and separated by cells termed **thecal cells**. [What is the male counterpart of the thecal cells, and to which hormone do they respond?[20]] Of the several maturing follicles, only one progresses to the point of ovulation each month; all others degenerate. The mature follicle is known as a **Graafian follicle**. During ovulation, the Graafian follicle bursts, releasing the secondary oocyte with its zona pellucida and protective granulosa cells into the fallopian tube. At this point, the layer of granulosa cells surrounding the ovum is known as the **corona radiata**. The follicular cells remaining in the ovary after ovulation form a new structure called the **corpus luteum** (Figure 6).

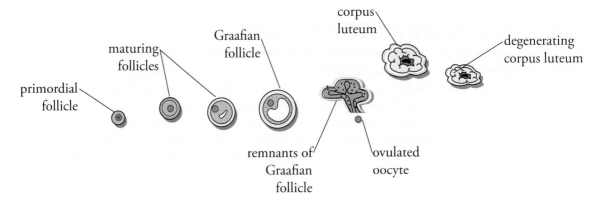

Figure 6   The Fate of a Follicle

Estrogen is made and secreted by the granulosa cells (with help from the thecal cells) during the first half of the menstrual cycle. Both estrogen and progesterone are secreted by the corpus luteum during the second half of the cycle. Estrogen is a steroid hormone that plays an important role in the development of female secondary sexual characteristics, in the menstrual cycle, and during pregnancy. Progesterone is also a steroid hormone involved in the hormonal regulation of the menstrual cycle and pregnancy, but with different effects than estrogen.

---

[19]   The cells that support and nurture developing spermatocytes are the sustentacular cells.

[20]   They are analogous to the testicular interstitial cells. Both interstitial and thecal cells are stimulated by LH.

19.7 THE MENSTRUAL CYCLE

The menstrual cycle is (on average) a 28-day cycle that includes events occurring in the ovary (discussed above and referred to as the **ovarian cycle**), as well as events occurring in the uterus (the shedding of the old endometrium and preparation of a new endometrium for potential pregnancy), referred to as the **uterine cycle**.

The Ovarian Cycle

The ovarian cycle can be subdivided into three phases:

1) During the **follicular phase**, a primary follicle matures and secretes estrogen. Maturation of the follicle is under the control of follicle stimulating hormone (FSH) from the anterior pituitary. The follicular phase lasts about 13 days.

2) In the **ovulatory phase**, a secondary oocyte is released from the ovary. This is triggered by a surge of luteinizing hormone (LH) from the anterior pituitary. The surge also causes the remnants of the follicle to become the corpus luteum. Ovulation typically occurs on day 14 of the cycle.

3) The **luteal phase** begins with full formation of the corpus luteum in the ovary. This structure secretes both estrogen and progesterone, and has a life span of about two weeks. The average length of the luteal phase is about 14 days.

The hormones secreted from the ovary during the ovarian cycle direct the uterine cycle.

The Uterine Cycle

The uterine cycle covers the same 28 days that were discussed above, but the focus is on the preparation of the endometrium for potential implantation of a fertilized egg. The uterine cycle can also be subdivided into three phases:

1) The first phase is **menstruation**, triggered by the degeneration of the corpus luteum and subsequent drop in estrogen and progesterone levels. The sharp decrease in these hormones causes the previous cycle's endometrial lining to slough out of the uterus, producing the bleeding associated with this time period. Menstruation typically lasts about 5 days.

2) During the **proliferative phase** of the menstrual cycle, estrogen produced by the follicle induces the proliferation of a new endometrium. This phase lasts about 9 days.

3) After ovulation the **secretory phase** occurs, in which estrogen and progesterone produced by the corpus luteum further increase development of the endometrium, including secretion of glycogen, lipids, and other material. If pregnancy does not occur, the death of the corpus luteum and decline in the secretion of estrogen and progesterone trigger menstruation once again. The secretory phase typically lasts about 14 days.

The menstrual cycle repeats every 28 days from puberty until menopause (at about age 50–60).

- At what stage of development is the endometrium when ovulation occurs?[21]
- Where is the secondary oocyte during the secretory phase?[22]

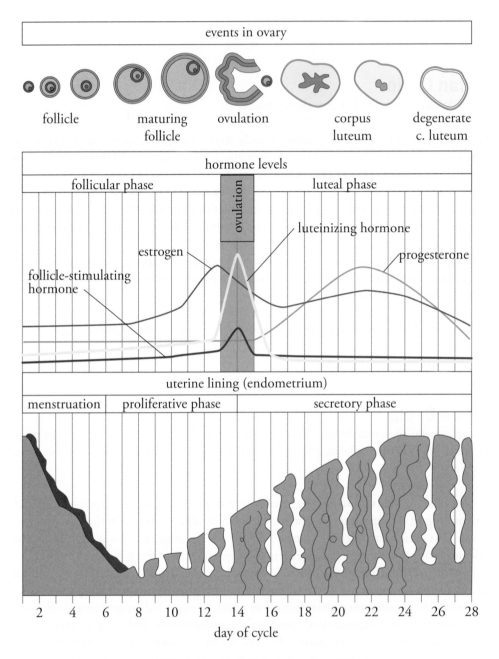

Figure 7   Summary of the Menstrual Cycle

---

[21] The endometrium is at the proliferative phase, under the influence of ovarian estrogen.

[22] The secondary oocyte is traveling down the uterine tube toward the uterus. If it fails to implant in the uterus, the secretory phase ends and menstruation begins.

19.8 HORMONAL CHANGES DURING PREGNANCY

There are still a couple of points we have not made completely clear: How can pregnancy occur if the uterine lining is lost each month, and why does the body discard the endometrium?

Recall that the physiological reason for endometrial shedding is a decrease in estrogen and progesterone levels, which occurs as the corpus luteum degenerates. Why does the corpus luteum degenerate? Due to a decrease in luteinizing hormone. Why does LH decrease? Due to feedback inhibition from the high levels of estrogen and progesterone secreted by the corpus luteum.

Let's begin with why LH levels decrease. During pregnancy, ovulation should be prevented. The way ovulation is prevented is for the constant high levels of estrogen and progesterone seen during pregnancy to inhibit secretion of LH by the pituitary; no LH surge, no ovulation. Constant high levels of estrogen inhibit LH release. The result is pregnancy without continued ovulation. The *secondary* result is the one we were trying to explain: when the corpus luteum secretes a lot of estrogen and progesterone during the menstrual cycle, LH levels drop, causing the corpus luteum to degenerate. The point is that the corpus luteum degenerates unless fertilization has occurred.

So how can pregnancy occur? If pregnancy is to occur, the endometrium must be maintained, because it is the site of gestation (i.e., where the embryo lives and is nourished). If fertilization takes place, a developing embryo becomes **implanted** in the endometrium within a few days, and a **placenta** begins to develop. The **chorion** is the portion of the placenta that is derived from the zygote. It secretes **human chorionic gonadotropin**, or **hCG**, which can take the place of LH in maintaining the corpus luteum. In the presence of hCG, the corpus luteum does not degenerate, the estrogen and progesterone levels stay elevated, and menstruation does not occur. This answers the question of *how* pregnancy can occur. hCG is the hormone tested for in pregnancy tests because its presence absolutely confirms the presence of an embryo.

- Which of the following occur(s) during the menstrual cycle immediately after ovulation?[23]
  - I. A drop in luteinizing hormone release from the anterior pituitary
  - II. Completion of the second meiotic cell division by the oocyte
  - III. Shedding of the endometrium

- As a woman ages, the number of follicles remaining in the ovaries decreases until ovulation ceases. At this point, termed **menopause**, the menstrual cycle no longer occurs. Which of the following occur(s) during menopause?[24]
  - I. FSH levels drop dramatically and stay low.
  - II. Estrogen levels are abnormally high.
  - III. LH levels are very high and stay high.

---

[23] **Item I: True.** The LH surge causes ovulation; once ovulation has occurred, LH levels fall significantly. Item II: False. Meiosis I is completed prior to ovulation. Meiosis II isn't completed until after fertilization. Item III: False. Ovulation occurs around day 14 of the cycle. Menstruation begins at day 1.

[24] In the absence of estrogen and progesterone secretion by follicles, there is no feedback inhibition of LH and FSH, so their levels are very high in postmenopausal women. Hence, only **item III is true.**

19.8

- Which of the following statements concerning the menstrual cycle is/are true?[25]
  - I. The proliferative phase of the endometrium coincides with the maturation of ovarian follicles.
  - II. The secretory phase of the endometrial cycle is dependent on the secretion of estrogen from cells surrounding secondary oocytes.
  - III. Luteinizing hormone levels are highest during the menstrual phase of the endometrial cycle.

19.9 FERTILIZATION AND CLEAVAGE

A secondary oocyte is ovulated and enters the uterine tube. It is surrounded by the **corona radiata** (a protective layer of granulosa cells) and the **zona pellucida** (located just outside the egg cell membrane). The oocyte will remain fertile for about a day. If intercourse occurs, sperm are deposited near the cervix and are activated, or **capacitated**. Sperm capacitation involves the dilution of inhibitory substances present in semen. The activated sperm will survive for two or three days. They swim through the uterus toward the secondary oocyte.

Fertilization is the fusion of a spermatozoon with the secondary oocyte (Figure 8). It normally occurs in the uterine tube. In order for fertilization to occur, a sperm must penetrate the corona radiata and bind to and penetrate the zona pellucida. It accomplishes this using the **acrosome reaction**. The **acrosome** is a large vesicle in the sperm head containing hydrolytic enzymes which are released by exocytosis. After the corona radiata has been penetrated, an **acrosomal process** containing actin elongates toward the zona pellucida. The acrosomal process has **bindin**, a species-specific protein which binds to receptors in the zona pellucida. Finally, the sperm and egg plasma membranes fuse, and the sperm nucleus enters the secondary oocyte. In about twenty minutes, the secondary oocyte completes meiosis II, giving rise to an ootid and the second polar body. The ootid matures rapidly, becoming an **ovum**. Then the sperm and egg nuclei fuse, and the new diploid cell is known as a **zygote**.

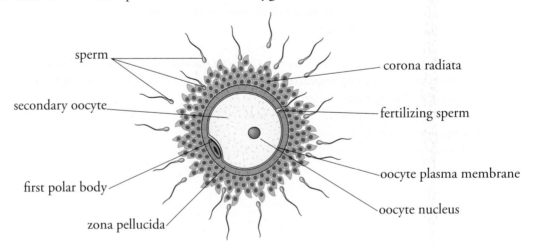

Figure 8 Fertilization

---

[25] **Item I: True.** This is explained in the text. Item II: False. It is secretion of estrogen and progesterone *by the corpus luteum* that drives the secretory phase. The corpus luteum is in the ovary, while the secondary oocyte is out in the uterine tube. Item III: False. The luteinizing hormone level peaks during the proliferative phase, since this is when ovulation occurs.

Penetration of an ovum by more than one sperm is known as **polyspermy**. It is normally prevented by the **fast block to polyspermy** and the **slow block to polyspermy**, which occur upon penetration of the egg by a spermatozoon. The fast block consists of a depolarization of the egg plasma membrane. This depolarization prevents other spermatozoa from fusing with the egg cell membrane. The slow block results from a Ca^{2+} influx caused by the initial depolarization. The slow block is also known as the **cortical reaction**. It has two components: swelling of the space between the zona pellucida and the plasma membrane and hardening of the zona pellucida. The Ca^{2+} influx has one other noteworthy effect. It causes increased metabolism and protein synthesis, referred to as **egg activation**.

Cleavage

The process of **embryogenesis** begins within hours of fertilization, but it proceeds slowly in humans. The first stage is **cleavage**, in which the zygote undergoes many cell divisions to produce a ball of cells known as the **morula**. The first cell division occurs about 36 hours after fertilization. [The morula is the same size as the zygote, which indicates that the dividing cells spend most of their time in what phases of the cell cycle?[26] During cleavage of the zygote, do homologous chromosomes physically interact with each other?[27]]

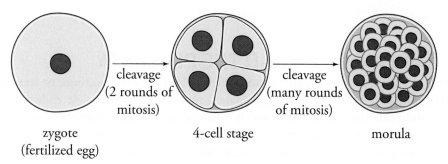

Figure 9 Cleavage

As cell divisions continue, the morula is transformed into a **blastocyst** (Figure 10). This process is known as **blastulation**. The blastocyst consists of a ring of cells called the **trophoblast** surrounding a cavity, and an **inner cell mass** adhering to the inside of the trophoblast at one end of the cavity. The **trophoblast** will give rise to the **chorion** (the zygote's contribution to the placenta). The inner cell mass will become the **embryo**.

- If two inner cell masses form in the blastula, what will the result be?[28]

---

[26] They must spend most of their time during the S (synthesis) and M (mitotic) phases, skipping the G_1 and G_2 (gap or growth) phases.

[27] No. Pairing of homologous chromosomes only takes place during meiosis, which only occurs during gametogenesis.

[28] The inner cell mass becomes the embryo. Two inner cell masses derived from a single zygote and enclosed by the same trophoblast will result in a pair of identical twins sharing the same placenta.

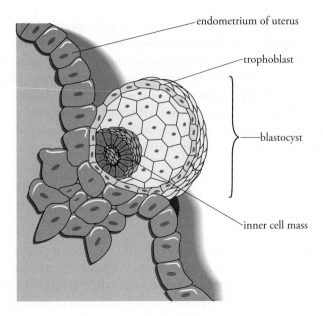

endometrium of uterus

trophoblast

blastocyst

inner cell mass

Figure 10 The Blastocyst at the Beginning of Implantation

19.10 IMPLANTATION AND THE PLACENTA

The developing blastocyst reaches the uterus and burrows into the endometrium, or **implants**, about a week after fertilization (Figure 10). The trophoblast secretes proteases that lyse endometrial cells. The blastocyst then sinks into the endometrium and is surrounded by it, absorbing nutrients through the trophoblast into the inner cell mass. The embryo receives a large part of its nutrition in this manner for the first few weeks of pregnancy. This is why the secretory phase of the endometrial cycle occurs: endometrial cells store glycogen, lipids, and other nutrients so that the early embryo may derive nourishment directly from the endometrium. Later, an organ develops which is specialized to facilitate exchange of nutrients, gases, and even antibodies between the maternal and embryonic bloodstreams: the **placenta**. Because it takes about three months for the placenta to develop, it is during the first trimester (three months) of pregnancy that hCG is essential for maintenance of the endometrium (Section 19.8).

• What happens if the corpus luteum is removed during the first trimester?[29]

During the last six months of pregnancy, the corpus luteum is no longer needed because the placenta itself secretes sufficient estrogen and progesterone for maintenance of the endometrium.

The development of the placenta involves the formation of **placental villi**. These are chorionic projections extending into the endometrium, into which fetal capillaries will grow. Surrounding the villi are sinuses (open spaces) filled with maternal blood. [Does oxygen-containing blood pass from the mother into the developing fetus?[30]]

---

[29] The woman menstruates, and the embryo is lost. Remember, the role of hCG is to substitute for LH in stimulating the corpus luteum. The role of the corpus luteum is to make estrogen and progesterone, which maintain the endometrium.

[30] No. The placenta is like a lung in that it facilitates exchange of substances between the two bloodstreams without allowing actual mixing.

The embryo is not the only important structure derived from the inner cell mass. There are three others: amnion, yolk sac, and allantois. The **amnion** surrounds a fluid-filled cavity which contains the developing embryo. Amniotic fluid is the "water" which "breaks" (is expelled) before birth. The **yolk sac** is the first site of red blood cell synthesis in the embryo. Finally, the **allantois** develops from the embryonic gut and forms the blood vessels of the umbilical cord, which transport blood between embryo and placenta.

- Each of the following has the same genome EXCEPT:[31]
  - A) Chorion
  - B) Amnion
  - C) Yolk sac
  - D) Endometrium

19.11 POST-IMPLANTATION DEVELOPMENT

We have examined embryogenesis from fertilization through blastulation. The next phase is **gastrulation**. Gastrulation is when the three **primary germ layers** (the **ectoderm**, the **mesoderm**, and the **endoderm**) become distinct.

In primitive organisms, the **blastula** (equivalent to blastocyst) is a hollow ball of cells, and gastrulation involves the **invagination** (involution) of these cells to form layers. Imagine pushing your fist into a big soft round balloon to create an inner layer (contacting your fist) and an outer layer (contacting the air). The inner layer is the endoderm, and the outer layer is the ectoderm. The mesoderm (middle layer) develops from the endoderm. The cavity (where your fist is) is primitive gut, or **archenteron**. The opening (where your wrist is) is the **blastopore**, and it will give rise to the anus. The whole structure is the **gastrula**. (Don't be confused: the *gastr*ula has a *blast*opore; the *blast*ula has no opening.)

In humans, things are a little different. The gastrula develops from a double layer of cells called the **embryonic disk**, instead of from a spherical blastula. But the end result is the same: three layers. You need to know what parts of the human body are derived from each layer.

Ectoderm	Mesoderm	Endoderm
• Entire nervous system • Pituitary gland (both lobes), adrenal medulla • Cornea and lens • Epidermis of skin and derivatives (hair, nails, sweat glands, sensory receptors) • Nasal, oral, anal epithelium	• All muscle, bone, and connective tissue • Entire cardiovascular and lymphatic system, including blood • Urogenital organs (kidneys, ureters, gonads, reproductive ducts) • Dermis of skin	• GI tract epithelium (except mouth and anus) • GI glands (liver, pancreas, etc.) • Respiratory epithelium • Epithelial lining of urogenital organs and ducts • Urinary bladder

Table 2 Fates of the Primary Germ Layers

[31] The chorion, amnion, and yolk sac are all derived from the inner cell mass of the blastula, and therefore must have the same genome (choices A, B, and C can be eliminated). However, the endometrium is derived from the mother (it is the inner lining of the uterus), and would have a different genome than the embryo (choice **D** is correct).

Pay attention to what *types* of thing are derived from each layer, and you'll see that it's relatively easy to memorize. One key thing to note is that **ectoderm** and *epithelium* are not synonymous. Epithelium outside the body (epidermis) is derived from ectoderm, but epithelium inside the body (gut lining) comes from endoderm.

- Which of the following statements is/are true?[32]
  - I. Oxygen must diffuse across the chorionic membrane to reach the fetus from the mother.
  - II. Transplantation of cells from the trophoblast of one embryo to the trophoblast of another embryo will result in an infant with a mixed genetic composition.
  - III. All of the cells of the blastocyst are functionally equivalent.

The next step after gastrulation is **neurulation**, the formation of the nervous system. It begins when a portion of the ectoderm differentiates into the **neural plate**. At the edges of the plate are the **neural crest cells**; these edges thicken and fold upward (the **neural folds**), leaving the bottom of the plate to form the neural tube. The neural tube ultimately develops into the central nervous system (brain and spinal cord). During that process, the neural crest cells separate from the neural tube and the overlying ectoderm (which ultimately becomes the epidermis), then migrate to different parts of the embryo to differentiate into a variety of cell types, including melanocytes, glial cells, the adrenal medulla, some peripheral neurons, and some facial connective tissue (Figure 11). The formation of the neural tube is induced by instructions from the underlying notochord, which is mesodermal in origin. It gives rise to the vertebral column.

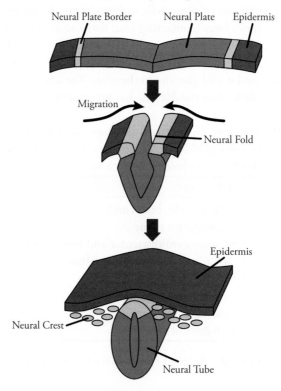

Figure 11 Neural Crest

---

[32] **Item I: True.** The chorion is part of the placenta. Item II: False. The trophoblast is derived from the outer cell mass and gives rise only to the chorion. The embryo is derived entirely from the inner cell mass. Item III: False. The trophoblast and the inner cell mass are both components of the blastocyst, and they have very different roles.

Neurulation is one component of **organogenesis**, the development of organ systems. By the eighth week of gestation, all major organ systems are present, and the **embryo** is now called a **fetus**. Even though the developmental process has attained staggering complexity, by the end of the first trimester the fetus is still only 5 cm long. [During which trimester is the developing human most sensitive to toxins such as drugs and radiation?[33]]

- A radioactive dye is detected only in the cells of placental villi. Weeks earlier, it must have been injected into the:[34]
    - A) inner cell mass.
    - B) trophoblast.
    - C) endometrium.
    - D) zygote.

Environment-Gene Interaction

During this early time period in development, the prenatal environment can play a significant role in gene expression. For example, a lack of folic acid in the mother's diet at this time can lead to significant defects in the formation of the neural tube and central nervous system. Certain illnesses in the mother can lead to issues in the fetus; influenza has been linked to schizophrenia and German measles to deafness, eye abnormalities, and heart defects. Hypoxia in utero, such as might be caused by maternal cigarette smoking (and the resultant vasoconstriction of uterine blood vessels) can lead to a reduction in grey matter development. Fetal alcohol syndrome due to excess maternal alcohol consumption can lead to stunted fetal growth, brain damage, and other behavioral and physical problems.

19.12 DIFFERENTIATION

The specialization of cell types during development is termed **differentiation** because as cells specialize they become different from their parent cells and from each other. By specializing, a cell becomes better able to perform a particular task, while becoming less adept at other tasks. For example, a sensory neuron is the best vehicle for the transmission of a nerve impulse over great distances, but it is quite incapable of obtaining nourishment on its own, or even of reproducing itself.

Primitive cells in the zygote and the morula have the potential to become any cell type in the blastocyst, including the trophoblast and the inner cell mass. They are therefore known as **totipotent** cells. Cells of the inner cell mass are more specialized and are called **pluripotent**. They can differentiate into any of the three primary germ layers (ectoderm, mesoderm, or endoderm) and therefore have the capability to become any of the 220 cells types that make up an adult human. However, they cannot contribute to the trophoblast of the blastocyst.

---

[33] During the first trimester, when the organs are being formed.

[34] The placenta is derived from the chorion, which is derived from the cells of the trophoblast, thus injecting a dye into the trophoblast would lead to its detection in the placental villi (choice **B** is correct). The inner cell mass ultimately becomes the embryo, thus dye injected into the inner cells mass would be detected in the embryo, not the placenta (choice A is wrong). The endometrium is derived from the mother and is only the site of implantation and placental development. It does not actually contribute to the placenta, thus dye injected into the endometrium would not be detected in the placenta (choice C is wrong). The zygote is the precursor to all embryonic and extraembryonic structures. Injecting a dye into the zygote would lead to its detection not only in the placenta, but also in the amnion, chorion, and embryo itself (choice D is wrong).

As development continues, cells continue to specialize. For example, after gastrulation, cells from the early embryonic germ layers are each considered **multipotent**. This means they can become many, but not all cell types. For example, cells of the mesoderm can differentiate into muscle and bone cells, but not into neurons or digestive epithelium.

In other words, totipotent cells differentiate into pluripotent cells, which specialize to become multipotent cells. Most cells in the adult have lost all potency and have become completely specialized mature cells, incapable of changing into other cell types. Adult stem cells are an exception to this.

Stem cells, because of their ability to become nearly any cell type in the body, are of great interest in research; they remain a potential source for regenerative medicine and tissue replacement after injury or disease. In humans, embryonic stem cells are the only pluripotent cells that have been found. These cells are isolated from the inner cell mass of the blastocyst.

Term	Definition	Examples
Totipotent	Can generate trophoblast and inner cell mass	zygote morula iPS cells
Pluripotent	Can differentiate into any of three primary germ layers Can generate all adult cell types (over 220)	inner cell mass of blastocyst (embryonic stem cells)
Multipotent	Can produce many (not all) cell types More differentiated than pluripotent Often tissue-specific	3 primary germ layers Adult Stem Cells
De-differentiation	Some cells can go backwards Example: Mature → Multipotent → Pluripotent → Totipotent	iPS cells cancer cells

Table 3

There is a certain point in the development of a cell at which the cell fate becomes fixed; at this point, the cell is said to be **determined**. Determination precedes differentiation. This means a cell is determined before it is visibly differentiated. Determination can be **induced** by a cell's environment, such as exposure to diffusible factors or neighboring cells, or it can be preprogrammed.

- During early embryonic development, cells near the developing notochord undergo an irreversible developmental choice to become skeletal muscle later in development, although they do not immediately change their appearance. This is an example of which of the following?[35]
  - A) Determination
  - B) Differentiation
  - C) Totipotency
  - D) Induction

---

[35] A cell whose fate is fixed is said to be determined, however if it has not yet undergone a change in appearance, it has not yet been differentiated (choice **A** is correct, and choice B is wrong). Since the cell is destined to become muscle, it is no longer totipotent (choice **C** is wrong). Although the cells are found near the notochord, there is no reason to assume the location is the reason for their determination. They could be cytoplasmically determined (choice D is wrong).

19.12

There is such a thing as **dedifferentiation**. This is the process whereby a specialized cell *un*specializes and may become totipotent. If a dedifferentiated cell proliferates in an uncontrolled manner, the result can be cancer. The most important lesson you can learn from the notion of dedifferentiation is that every cell has the same genome. The specialization of cell types is a function of things in the cytoplasm and maybe proteins and RNA in the nucleus, but no genetic changes normally take place during development and differentiation.

- Can you think of two exceptions to this rule, where a particular cell type normally has a unique genome?[36]

19.13   PREGNANCY

The early stages of development already discussed (gastrulation and neurulation) comprise the embryonic stage of development. These eight weeks comprise the majority of the first trimester; during this time all major organ systems appear. The stage of development from eight weeks until birth is known as the fetal stage. This stage covers the second and third trimesters of the pregnancy.

Second Trimester

During this time the organs and organ systems of the fetus continue to develop structurally and functionally. The fetus grows, typically reaching a weight of approximately 0.6 kg, and looks distinctly human.

Third Trimester

This is a stage of rapid fetal growth, including significant deposition of adipose tissue. Most of the organ systems become fully functional. A baby born 1–2 months early has a reasonably good chance of survival.

Maternal Experience

The demands placed on the mother's body increase significantly over the course of the pregnancy. Maternal respiratory rate increases to bring in additional oxygen and eliminate additional carbon dioxide. Blood volume in the mother increases by about 50% due to a drop in oxygen levels (because of the metabolic demands of the fetus) and a subsequent release of erythropoietin and renin. This is accompanied by an increase in glomerular filtration rate of a corresponding 50%. The demand for nutrients and vitamins increases by about 30%, the uterus undergoes a very significant increase in size, and the mammary glands increase in size. Additionally, secretory activity begins in the mammary glands, although this is not technically lactation.

---

[36] One exception is B cells and T cells of the immune system. They undergo gene (DNA!) rearrangements in the process of attaining antigen specificity. The other exception is gametes. They have unique genomes because of 1) reductive division with independent assortment, and 2) recombination.

19.14   BIRTH AND LACTATION

The technical term for birth is **parturition**. It is dependent on contraction of muscles in the uterine wall. The very high levels of progesterone secreted throughout pregnancy help to repress contractions in uterine muscle, but near the end of pregnancy, uterine excitability increases. This increased excitability is likely to be a result of several factors, including a change in the ratio of estrogen to progesterone, the presence of the hormone **oxytocin** secreted by the posterior pituitary, and mechanical stretching of the uterus and cervix.

Weak contractions of the uterus occur throughout pregnancy. As pregnancy reaches full term, however, rhythmic **labor contractions** begin. It is thought that the onset of labor contractions is the result of a positive feedback reflex: the increased pressure on the cervix crosses a threshold that causes the posterior pituitary to increase the secretion of oxytocin. Oxytocin causes the uterine contractions to increase in intensity, creating greater pressure on the cervix that stimulates still more oxytocin release and even stronger contractions.

The first stage of labor is dilation of the cervix. The second stage is the actual birth, involving movement of the baby through the cervix and birth canal, pushed by contraction of uterine (smooth) and abdominal (skeletal) muscle. The third stage is the expulsion of the placenta, after it separates from the wall of the uterus. Contractions of the uterus after birth help to minimize blood loss.

During pregnancy, milk production and secretion would be a waste of energy, but after parturition it is necessary. During puberty, estrogen stimulates the development of breasts in women. The increased levels of estrogen and progesterone secreted by the placenta during pregnancy cause the further development of glandular and adipose breast tissue. But while these hormones stimulate breast development, they inhibit the release of **prolactin** and thus the production of milk. After parturition, the levels of estrogen and progesterone fall and milk production begins. Every time suckling occurs, the pituitary gland is stimulated by the hypothalamus to release a large surge of prolactin, prolonging the ability of the breasts to secrete milk. If the mother stops breast-feeding the infant, prolactin levels fall and milk secretion ceases. The converse is also true: milk secretion can continue for years, as long as nursing continues. The breasts do not leak large amounts of milk when the infant is not nursing. This is because the posterior pituitary hormone **oxytocin** is necessary for **milk let-down** (release). Oxytocin is also released when suckling occurs.

19.14

Part 4

MCAT Psychology and Sociology

Chapter 20
Research Methods

In addition to psychology and sociology content at the first-year undergraduate level, the MCAT Psychology and Sociology section will also feature many questions that incorporate research methods and study design (about 20–25% of the section). These questions will require knowledge of the elementary aspects of social research, such as types of study design, especially the experimental method. Almost all Psychology/Sociology passages will contain a study, and the majority of these passages will contain at least one question in which you are asked to evaluate the study or make a prediction about the implications of the research. Fortunately, the amount of content associated with these questions is manageable, and is not heavy in statistics. What is required is knowledge of the common types of research conducted by social scientists, strengths and weaknesses of each method, and the types of conclusions that can reasonably be drawn from each.

20.1 EXPERIMENTAL DESIGN

Because the word "experiment" is often used interchangeably with research it is easy to forget that "experimental design" is a technical term for a *specific type* of research. For example, many different types of studies have shown that a Mediterranean diet (one rich in seafood, legumes, nuts, olive oil, fruits, and vegetables) is associated with cardiovascular health and longevity. However, to show that consuming a Mediterranean diet helps *cause*, or helps *lead to* cardiovascular health and longevity, an experimental design is needed.

To see why this is the case, imagine a study in which a team of social scientists creates a scale to measure the extent to which an individual follows the Mediterranean diet. When paired with a food frequency questionnaire, they assign a score for each individual from 1 (diet least resembles a traditional Mediterranean diet) to 12 (diet most resembles a traditional Mediterranean diet). Let's call it the Mediterranean Diet Index (MDI). They find that as individual MDI scores increase, so do measures of cardiovascular health. This, however, does not show that adherence to the Mediterranean Diet *leads to* improved health.

The team has found a positive correlation (discussed below) between the MDI and cardiovascular fitness, but correlation is not causation. Based on the findings, it is possible that people with a genetic predisposition towards cardiovascular health produce a profile of digestive enzymes that leads to a natural preference for a Mediterranean style diet. Or perhaps there is some third factor such as exercise or social support that leads to both greater cardiovascular health *and* preference for Mediterranean foods (see figure 1). To rule out these other possible explanations, the team must conduct a follow up study with an experimental design.

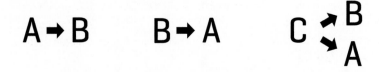

Figure 1 Possible causal relationships that could explain a correlation that is found between two variables, A and B.

There are several steps to good experimental design. To understand them, let's imagine the type of study the researchers might conduct, consider what an optimal design might look like for each step, and think about how flaws in the execution of each step might compromise the purpose of the experiment: to show a causal relationship between two variables, namely, to show that adherence to a Mediterranean diet leads to greater cardiovascular health.

1) <u>Select the population.</u> The first thing the researchers must agree on is the population of interest. Whom do they want to study? It may seem obvious that they would be interested in "all humans," however for various reasons this may not be the best group to select. For example, since many experiments in the social sciences are done by scholars at universities, let's suppose our team of researchers were all tenured at a University, Healthy Living U. Then the easiest way for the researchers to get a large sample at low cost would be to use students at Healthy Living U as participants in the experiment. Of course, our researchers would ideally like their findings to apply to everyone, but this would involve finding older (and younger) participants, incentivizing them to participate in the research, and following through to make sure they follow the experimental protocol correctly. Because this would be very taxing in terms of resources and logistics, the researchers decide that their population of interest will be healthy young adults in their early twenties.

Think about what this (very reasonable) decision about what population to study implies for later findings. If the researchers *do* find that Mediterranean diet adherence leads to cardiovascular health, can they say that this result is also true for individuals in their 50s or 60s? It very well might, but this conclusion now lies outside the scope of the Healthy Living U experiment. Follow-up studies would be needed to say for sure whether the effect also applies to older adults. The researchers have compromised the reach and scope of their experiment, but they now have the advantage of a large pool of willing participants that they can sample for their experiment.

2) <u>Operationalize the independent and dependent variables.</u> The **independent variable** is the variable manipulated by the research team. The **dependent variable** is the variable that is measured. In the correlational study described earlier, researchers found that high MDI scores were associated with better health. In this follow-up experimental study, the *causal* relationship that researchers want to test experimentally is whether eating a Mediterranean diet *leads to* greater cardiovascular health. The researchers must specify exactly what they mean by this. The independent variable in this experiment is adherence to a Mediterranean diet, and to qualify as an experiment design, this variable must be *directly manipulated* by the researchers. Researchers want to have maximum control over the experimental environment so that they can be sure that differences between the groups actually led to the effect, assuming one is measured. Good experimental design requires experiments that can be reproduced by other researchers, who may want to verify the results on their own or critique or adapt some aspect of the experiment. Precise definitions are key.

The researchers decide that they will work with the cafeteria on campus to serve a special diet to participants. They team up with a group of nutritionists to create a 6-month, 21-meal weekly diet plan that participants will be required to eat. Participants can also consume a preselected set of snacks and beverages in their dorm rooms, but these are provided and outside foods are not allowed. The diet the team constructs is such that it would score a perfect 12 on the MDI scale. Now, the independent variables are strictly operationalized, or specified.

The dependent variable in the experiment is cardiovascular health. This is the variable that the researchers will measure to see if their diet has an effect. To obtain rigorous results, the researchers must create an **operational definition**, a specification of precisely what they mean by each variable. The independent variable was operationalized as a very specific set of foods consumed over a 6-month period. The dependent variable must be equally well-defined, and must also meet the criteria of being **quantitative**, or numerical, as opposed to **qualitative**, or descriptive. Quantitative data will be necessary later to conduct statistical analyses that will test the research hypothesis. The researchers decide that the dependent variables they will measure are heart rate, blood pressure, peak oxygen uptake, aerobic recovery rate, blood glucose levels, and ejection fraction. Each of these will produce a numerical value that they will measure before and after the 6-month period. The difference in these values will test the effect of the dietary regiment on health.

These are strong operational definitions. Both the independent and dependent variable definitions are specific and replicable, and the dependent variable is sufficiently quantitative to allow for statistical analyses. However, notice that the researchers have introduced new limitations to the experiment. Look first at the independent variable. What if the Mediterranean diet really starts to be effective after many years? Perhaps our bodies have an adjustment period to any new dietary protocol and we only start to see benefits over timespans longer than 6 months. If that were the case, the present experiment would not pick up a result, and might wrongly conclude that the diet is ineffective. The operationalization of the dependent variable also introduced limitations. It is quantitative and rigorous; however, it only indirectly measures what we are really interested in: lowered risk of heart attack, increased longevity, and high life satisfaction. The variables the researchers selected can only *indirectly* suggest that the quality of life variables we really care about are improving. Again, good experimental design often involves making compromises to meet conditions or make conducting a study realistic.

It would be great if we could verify experimentally that eating a specific diet decreases the risk of heart attack and leads to increased longevity. However, let's reflect for a moment on how difficult that would be in practice. The Healthy Living U experiment we are developing is already shaping up to be *very* restrictive on participants, even though we have created a rather optimal scenario by defining variables so many participants who live in the research environment could be used. Imagine if we extended the dietary regiment for a lifetime, then measured average life expectancy and morbidity due to cardiovascular disease over the course of decades. This would be nearly impossible to accomplish in practice, but that is what we would need to do to conclusively show that the diet led to health benefits! To conduct experiments that are realistically feasible, the Healthy Living U researchers must compromise by narrowing the scope of their study and selecting measurable dependent variables like heart rate and blood pressure that *imply* cardiovascular health, rather than trying to measure cardiovascular morbidity and life expectancy directly.

The accumulation of knowledge is slow and laden with potential logical errors and fallacies, and correct conclusions can only be drawn with great rigor and attention to detail by many scientists over many, many years. When we think about the many challenges inherent to establishing causal relationships, it is incredible that we know as much as we do!

3) <u>Carefully select control and experimental groups.</u> The group of participants that receives treatment is the experimental group. To draw conclusions about the effect of the treatment, researchers need a **control** group, which acts as a point of reference and comparison.

Suppose the high-MDI 6-month diet leads to improvements for participants in each of the cardiovascular variables measured. This would seem to be a great success for the experiment, but it could not confirm the experimental hypothesis without a control group. For example, how would researchers know that being given *any* dietary regiment might not also have the same results? Imagine the discipline that would be inculcated in participants just because they were monitored by a team of scientists and given special attention and a special diet. This increased discipline and attention might motivate them to exercise more, sleep better, and be healthier in general, and eventually lead to improved health measures. The researchers need a point of comparison to rule this possibility out.

Assigning a control group is one of the most important aspects of experimental design. Without one, a study is not experimental and causal relationships cannot be drawn. Let's think about what type of control group would best answer the research question. Researchers want to show that eating a Mediterranean diet causes cardiovascular health. To show this, they need a control group that is as similar as possible to the experimental group, except for the variable of interest—the treatment.

The objective is to rule out **extraneous (or confounding) variables**, variables other than the treatment that could potentially explain an experimental result. What sorts of variables could affect the current experiment? Gender, age, and socioeconomic status might play a role. There might also be racial differences in responsiveness to the dietary regiment. Certainly exercise, BMI, and stress levels could play a role as well. If researchers agreed on this list of potential extraneous variables, they would carefully select groups that were homogenous in age, gender, race, status, serum cortisol levels, and BMI. To control for exercise, they might create a regulated regiment for both groups to follow. Still, they would not be done.

Remember that to optimize study design, the two groups must be *as similar as possible, or homogenous*. When evaluating research methodology in published articles, the care that researchers take to maintain homogeneity can seem extreme. However, many studies have shown that unexpected and seemingly unrelated variables can lead to an effect. One of the many phenomena that complicate social research and can lead to erroneous results is the **placebo effect**, the well-known fact that just *believing* that treatment is being administered can lead to a measurable result.

To help counter the placebo effect, studies must be **double blind**; neither the person administering treatment nor the participants truly know if they are assigned to the treatment or control groups. If we apply these considerations to the Healthy Living U experiment, then the control group needs their own special diet, with physiologists taking their readings, and special chefs to cook the meals in the cafeteria.

But before we start recruiting participants and conduct the study, we must take one more thing into account. The study is designed to test for the *Mediterranean* diet, specifically. To appropriately isolate this variable (also for ethical reasons, see below), researchers had better give a healthy alternative diet to the control group. A control group that is given pizza, burgers, and fries would not be a good point of reference, since any healthy diet would probably produce a relative benefit. The researchers might select a diet that scores a 6 on the MDI so it is relatively average in "Mediterranean-ness," but is known to also be composed of fresh, healthy foods. Then later, if a difference were measured, researchers could be relatively sure that this result was due to the Mediterranean diet specifically, and not just the effect of eating a healthy diet curated by a team of professional nutritionists.

Researchers can never account for *every* potential extraneous variable. Firstly, *any* variable could theoretically be a potential confound, so researchers must focus on the most likely candidates. Beyond that, it may not be possible to control for a variable even if researchers would like to. For example, there is one variable that the Healthy Living U team can't account for—education level. No matter what the team does, they cannot include individuals without high school diplomas in their study without severely complicating their procedure. The team must accept that education level might affect the results, but they cannot control for that at this moment. We can start to see why almost every paper in the social sciences, in the discussion section, contains a phrase to the effect of "further research is necessary."

4) <u>Randomly sample from the population.</u> Finally, researchers can start recruiting participants for the study. The sampling should be random: it should be equally likely for any member of the population to be a participant in the study. This is an ideal that is almost never accomplished in practice in the social sciences. For the Healthy Living U study, any healthy young adult in their early 20s should have an equal chance of participating in the study. However, since the study is done at a specific university, only students at that school can be used. One of the most common flaws in social research is the fact that most studies are done on undergraduate students, and results are then applied to the greater population. This is a dubious and highly precarious leap in logic.

Usually, participants in a study are incentivized in some way, which could range from monetary compensation to access to new treatments and medication. The team at Healthy Living U might use grades or gift cards as an incentive for students to participate. This introduces another potential problem to the study, **attrition**, participants dropping out of the study. If the reason that participants are dropping out is non-random, this might introduce an extraneous variable. For example, if the participants who end up dropping out do so because they tend to not follow through with things they sign up for, this personality characteristic may confound any conclusions that are drawn about their health and cardiovascular fitness.

5) <u>Randomly assign individuals to groups.</u> Once the individuals who will participate in the study have been incentivized and rounded up, it is time to assign them to the experimental and control groups. In a well-designed experiment, it should be equally likely that they are assigned to either group. In contrast to step 4, this one is relatively easy to pull off. Assignment is usually not perfectly random, but if scientists alternate assignments or use another randomization technique they will usually come close. In this study, there are many extraneous variables that the researchers decided to account for, so they might use a **randomized block technique**. In this technique, researchers evaluate where participants fall along the variables they wish to homogenize, then they randomly assign individuals from these groups so that the treatment and control group are similar along the variables of interest.

6) <u>Measure the results.</u> For this experiment, the dependent variable is a set of well-known physiological measurements with standardized collection procedures and error measures. More generally, if researchers are using a survey or relatively new instrument, they must check to make sure that their measurements are valid. The most important aspects of measurement for an experiment are that the dependent variable is quantitative, therefore measurable, and that instruments used are **reliable**, that they measure what they're supposed to and repeated measurements lead to similar results. This is often a point of consideration for psychological studies that might test dependent variables like mood, memory, and attitude that are hard to rigorously pin down. If surveys are used, for example, researchers should test the reliability of the instrument and be sure that they actually measure what they purport to.

7) <u>Test the Hypothesis.</u> Scientists and philosophers of science over the years have generally agreed that it is better to incorrectly conclude that there is no effect than to falsely suppose a result that does not actually exist. They have reached a consensus, much like the legal concept of "innocent until proven guilty," that it is better to reason from a point of skepticism. For this reason, scientists generally start with the **null hypothesis**: they assume that there is no causal relationship between the variables and any measured effect, if there is one, is due to chance. Then, they see if evidence from the experiment suggests that the null hypothesis is true or false. Taking this position places the "burden of proof" on the experimental hypothesis, the proposition that variations in the independent variable cause changes in the dependent variables.

To reject the null hypothesis, it is not satisfactory simply to observe a difference between two groups. After all, the observed difference may simply be due to chance. Even two identical groups or identical measures are subject to randomness, and can therefore produce different measures even if there is no fundamental difference. To see why, and to get an idea of how social scientists and statisticians conduct hypothesis testing, consider the following example.

Imagine you and a friend roll two dice (each a cube with six faces labeled from "1" to "6"). Even with two equivalent fair dice, it is not difficult to imagine that if you each roll once, you may obtain two different values. Suppose you roll a 3, and your friend rolls a 5. Should you conclude that your friend cheated, and is using an unfair die? Of course not. The difference in that individual roll could simply be due to chance. If the dice are fair, after many rolls, you will find that both your averages start to converge to the natural average, 3.5[1]. If, for example, you each roll 1,000 times, and your average score is 3.497 while your friend's average score is 3.501, you will conclude that the dice were fair and the slight difference measured is simply due to chance.

Likewise, if the Healthy Living U team of researchers find slight differences between the experimental and control groups in cardiovascular fitness, they will not rush to conclude that the difference was *significant*. In statistics and hypothesis testing, a **significant difference** is a measured difference between two groups that is large enough that it is probably not due to chance. The vagueness of this definition is intentional. It is up to the researchers to determine when the difference is big enough.

---

[1] The sum of the possible scores divided by the number of possibilities ([1 + 2 + 3 + 4 + 5 + 6]/6)

To see how this works in practice, let's return to the example of rolling die. Suppose that this time around, when you and your friend roll 1,000 times, your average is 3.506 and your friend's average is 3.813. Did your friend cheat? It is not immediately obvious whether it is reasonable for you to conclude that they did. Maybe they just got lucky. Although you can never be absolutely sure, using statistics it is possible to calculate the probability that your friend obtained this value using a fair die.

Now, suppose that you ran the necessary statistical tests and they show that the chance of the measured difference in die scores was 17%. What would you conclude? You might say, well, I don't want to wrongfully incriminate my friend, it is still reasonably probable that they got their score by chance. But what if the probability you found was 6%? 3%? 0.04%? At what point would you confront your friend and accuse them of cheating? It is not an easy decision to make, since whatever value you choose as the threshold point will inherently be arbitrary.

Scientists evaluating data from experiments have the same problem. They can never be certain that a difference measured in an experiment actually reflects a fundamental difference between the groups and is not just due to chance. They must arbitrarily pick a cutoff point at which it is reasonable to conclude "beyond reasonable doubt" that there was a difference. Conventionally, social scientists have decided that if the probability of an observed difference is found to be 5% (or 0.05) or less, this constitutes a significant difference. A **p-value** is a number from 0 to 1 that represents the probability that a difference observed in an experiment is due to chance. By convention, if (and only if) $p < 0.05$, scientists reject the null hypothesis. Other p-values such as 0.01 or 0.001 are also frequently used as the threshold for significance in some cases. To make sure that the experiment picks up an effect, it is necessary to have a large enough sample size, or number of participants. Usually 30 or more participants are necessary to meet the mathematical criteria needed to conduct statistical tests. A larger **sample size**, or number of participants, is usually preferred. This increases the **power** of the experiment, or the ability to pick up an effect if one is actually present.

Whatever researchers decide to do, they must select the significance threshold in advance, or they might be extremely tempted to "move the goalposts," or change the number so that their data reach significance. For the MCAT, make sure you know what p-values represent, and that a lower value suggests a stronger relationship.

Step:	Objective:	Common Flaws in Design:
1. Select the population	• Determine the population of interest • Consider what group will be pragmatic to sample	• Population is too restrictive, sampling all individuals of interest is not practical
2. Operationalize variables	• Determine the independent and dependent variables • Specify exactly what is meant by each • Make sure the dependent variable can be measured quantitatively within the parameters of the study	• Insufficient rigor in description • Execution of independent condition presents practical problems
3. Divide into groups	• Carefully select experimental and control groups • Homogenize the two groups • Isolate the treatment by controlling for potential extraneous variables	• Control group does not resemble treatment along important variables • Experiment is not double blind • Participants can guess the experiment, allowing a placebo effect to occur
4. Random sampling	• Make sure all members of the population are represented • Ideally each member has an equal chance of being selected, but this is often not possible	• Sampling is not truly random • Sample does not represent the population of interest
5. Random assignment	• Individuals who have been sampled are equally likely to be assigned to treatment or control • Consider matching along potential extraneous variables which have been pre-selected	• Groups are not properly matched • Assignment is not perfectly random
6. Measurement	• Make sure measurements are standardized • Make sure instruments are reliable	• Tools are not precise enough to pick up a result • Instruments used for measurement are not reliable
7. Test the hypothesis	• Use statistics to check for a significant difference • Assign a pre-established threshold at which the null hypothesis will be rejected	• Small sample size leads to insufficient power • Researchers do not set thresholds in advance and make after-the-fact conclusions that lead to logical fallacies

Figure 2   Summary of the Experiment by Researchers at Healthy Living U.

We started with a relatively simple research question about how a type of diet affects health. The steps we took show the difficulty in practice of executing true experimental design. Even after taking all these pains to optimize the experiment, we still had to accept several limitations in random sampling and reach of the study, to name just a few. Conducting social science experiments is often extremely time and resource intensive, and practical and ethical considerations often leave running an experimental design completely off the table when exploring a scientific question or hypothesis. Next, we'll summarize some of the primary challenges in experimental designs, then explore many of the other research designs that scientists can turn to if experimental design is too limiting or cumbersome. The payoff to conducting a well-designed experiment is huge: establishment of a causal relationship. However, it may not be the best way to approach a problem. First, let's summarize the problems that tend to come up in experimental methodology.

Example 20-1: 30 university students participate in a study on the effects of the use of a new memory technique on memory retention. In the first group, which consisted of participants who were paired with odd numbers in a number generator, each individual learned the memory technique watching a recorded video tutorial. Then, a separate staff member administered the memory test. This same staff member also administered the test to the second group, and did not know who was in each group. The second group was not taught a memory technique and began the study by sitting for the memory test. Statistical tests were conducted by comparing the number of items correctly recorded in the two groups, and results confirmed the experimental hypothesis. Which of the following elements of experimental design is missing?

    A) Random assignment
    B) Adequate control group
    C) Double-blind methodology
    D) Operationalized variables

Solution: The description of the study suggests that the control group is not optimal for the objective of the research being conducted. The control group receives no treatment during the first part of the study, which introduces confounds. It is possible that sitting participants down and doing any training program with them will help increase focus and concentration, and therefore memory. With the control group used, researchers cannot be sure that a difference between groups is actually due to use of the memory strategy (choice B is correct). The use of a number generator suggests that random assignment was used (choice A is wrong). The study design used a video recording and a staff member who did not know which group they were working with, meeting the criteria for double-blind methodology (choice C is wrong). The variables are operationalized since the tutorial characterizes the experimental group, and the score on the memory exam is the dependent variable (choice D is wrong).

Internal and External Validity and Ethical Considerations

As we took a step-by-step look at experimental design, we looked at some of the potential flaws that come up in experiments, and how they might compromise our ability to draw conclusions about the real world from our study. These flaws can be placed into two categories. In one case, the flaw or limitation might make it difficult to apply our conclusion to the real world. This is known as a flaw in **external validity**. For example, the fact that only students of Healthy Living U can participate in the study is a threat to external validity. We cannot be absolutely sure that a result that rejects the null hypothesis applies to *all* healthy young adults in their mid-twenties. The fact that no high school dropouts or PhD students were included could also threaten external validity, because we cannot be sure that the findings also apply to these educational brackets.

Another important threat to external validity in this experiment is the fact that there was a special diet, constructed by professional researchers, cooked by culinary professionals at a university, and monitored by a team of scientists. It is not realistic to expect an average person trying to eat an experimental diet to match the rigor of this group. For any of these reasons (and many others) an affirmative finding that a high-MDI diet leads to healthier outcomes might not apply to conditions outside the conditions of the study.

On the other hand, a limitation in the study might be such that the experiment is not "well done," and we cannot be sure about the conclusion because of some inherent flaw in the design. **Internal validity** is high if confounding variables have been considered and minimized, and the causal relationship between the independent and dependent variable can actually be established by the way the experiment was set up. What if researchers forgot to control for gender? What if the diet they selected did not actually represent a Mediterranean diet? What if they had participants in their control group eat unhealthy and processed foods? If any of these were true, they would confound the results and threaten internal validity. Below is a summary of the common threats to validity in social science experiments that appear frequently on the MCAT.

Impression Management	Participants adapt their responses based on social norms or perceived researcher expectations; self-fulfilling prophecy; methodology is not double-blind, Hawthorne Effect
Confounding Variables	Extraneous variables not accounted for in the study; another variable offers an alternative explanation for results; lack of a useful control
Lack of Reliability	Measurement tools do not measure what they purport to, lack consistency
Sampling Bias	Selection criteria is not random, Population used for sample does not meet conditions for statistical test (e.g., population is not normally distributed)
Attrition Effects	Participant fatigue; participants drop out of study

Figure 3 Threats to Internal Validity

Experiment doesn't reflect real world	Laboratory setups that don't translate to the real world, lack of generalizability
Selection Criteria	Too restrictive of inclusion/exclusion criteria for participants (i.e., sample is not representative)
Situational Effects	Situational effects: presence of laboratory conditions changes outcome (e.g., pre-test and post-test, presence of experimenter, claustrophobia in an MRI machine)
Lack of Statistical Power	Sample groups have high variability; sample size is too small

Figure 4 Threats to External Validity

Finally, all studies should consider the ethical implications of the procedures they implicate. This is true for experimental as well as non-experimental designs. We'll look more closely at other study types below, but ethical problems tend to arise more frequently in experimental designs because researchers are directly manipulating variables, not just observing what they see in nature. Suppose, for example, that the Healthy Living U team wanted to conduct a separate experiment to show that high-fat, high-sugar diets are more likely to cause heart disease. This would clearly be unethical. They would be intentionally administering a treatment that they believe is harmful to participants.

Some social science experiments of the early-20th century contained egregious ethical breaches and it was many years before researchers, institutions, and society gradually came to an agreement on the correct protocol for running experiments. Modern experiments must be cleared by an independent internal commission that considers ethics. They must also contain some type of **disclosure**, an outlining of the nature of the experiment to participants before they are subject to experimental procedures that clarifies incentives, expectations, and rights. Finally, experimental protocol should include **debriefing**, in which participants are told after the experiment exactly what was done and why the experiment was conducted. In some cases, particularly if the experiment may have triggered psychological vulnerability, participants may be offered access to treatment or counseling services.

Example 20-2: Based on the information presented, which of the following critiques of the Mediterranean Diet study is most appropriate?

    A) The study lacks generalizability, which threatens internal validity.
    B) The study contains potential confounds, which threatens external validity.
    C) The study lacks reliability, which threatens external validity.
    D) The study contains sampling bias, which threatens internal validity.

Solution: As discussed above, the study includes sampling bias, because participants all go to the same university, and may be different from the population of interest. Sampling bias is a threat to internal validity, since it introduces potential confounding variables (choice D is correct). Generalizability is a threat to external validity, not internal (choice A is wrong). Confounding variables are a threat to internal validity, not external (choice B is wrong). Reliability of measurement instruments is a threat to internal validity, not external (choice C is wrong).

20.2 NON-EXPERIMENTAL STUDIES

We have seen that experiments are difficult to conduct, sometimes prohibitively, and introduce many possible problems in validity and ethics. They are often worth the trouble. If they decide to use another type of study, researchers have many other types of design at their disposal. Each offers its own benefits and potential drawbacks. In general, non-experimental designs tend to offer the benefit of observing phenomena in a more naturalistic setting. This means that they may offer benefits in external validity. The tradeoff is reduced control of the variables of interest, which tends to reduce the internal validity.

Almost all Psychology/Sociology passages contain some type of study. This is what makes knowledge of research design such a high-yield skill set. About ¼ of passage-related questions will require knowledge of research methods, and most of these will be about experimental design. They will ask you to draw a conclusion, make a prediction, or identify a flaw. Questions that are not about experimental design tend to be more straightforward and require knowledge of the most common types of non-experimental research, how they are conducted, and the benefits and drawbacks of each. Below are the most frequently tested non-experimental research designs that appear on the MCAT.

1) Correlational Studies. Earlier we saw that a relationship between two variables such as diet and health did not necessarily imply causation. **Correlational studies** explore the relationship between two quantitative variables. The most commonly used type of correlation is the **Pearson Correlation**. A Pearson correlation assigns a number from –1 to +1 to a pair of variables. If the value is negative, we say that the two variables are negatively correlated. This means that if one increases, the other will decrease, and vice versa. On the other hand, a positive Pearson correlation represents a positive correlation, which means that as one variable increases, the other also increases, and if one variable decreases the other will also decrease. A value of zero indicates no correlation, or no relationship between the two variables. Significance testing can be combined with Pearson correlations to see if the computed correlation is likely to have occurred by chance, or not.

2) Ethnographic Studies. **Ethnographic studies** are a qualitative method in which researchers immerse themselves completely in the lives, culture, or way of life of the people they are studying. These studies tend to be lengthy and thorough and involve as little interference or intervention by the researchers as possible. The culture studied is often unique or remote in some way, or offers a special insight into the scientific question. A researcher interested in the effect of the Mediterranean diet on health might go to a remote Sicilian village and study the lives of the participants, scrutinizing their everyday lives and recording everything they possibly can over the span of several years.

3) Twin Studies. **Twin studies** are often run to test the relationship between nature and nurture. They are the best way to measure **heritability**, the extent to which differences in an observed trait is due to genetics versus the environment. For example, twin studies interested in the heritability of intelligence might look at correlations in IQ scores between monozygotic (identical) and fraternal (dizygotic) twins. It is reasonable to conclude that differences between these two correlations are due to genetics, since both twins share an environment. In contrast, an intelligence study might look at the difference in correlations between IQs of identical twins reared together versus reared apart. These differences would likely be due to the environment, since both sets of twins would share the same percentage of genes, namely 100.

4) Longitudinal Studies. Researchers may be interested in how individuals develop over time along some research method. The New York Longitudinal Study is a classic example of the **longitudinal method**, which involves periodically measuring a dependent variable over long time frames. The New York Longitudinal Study asked as simple research question: what effect does our disposition at birth have on the life we lead? To test this, researchers categorized newborns according to their disposition: were they agreeable or irritable, healthy or sickly, regular or irregular in biological functions? They then checked in on subjects over periodic intervals to see if temperament at birth predicted later outcomes. Longitudinal studies are costly, difficult to execute, and have high attrition rates. The potential benefit is they offer the ability to detail how an effect or factor develops over time.

5) Case Studies. **Case studies** involve in-depth exploration of one individual sample point, or case. Suppose that a researcher from Healthy Living U met a native Sicilian in her late 90s with extraordinary health and fitness. They might want to know everything possible about this person's diet and lifestyle to understand how she was able to obtain such a high level of fitness. They might look at dietary habits over time, exercise frequency, interaction with family, sleep patterns, and any other variable of interest that they can think of. They would then compile this data and offer a report for critique by the scientific community. This would offer an excellent way to thoroughly explore the potential causes that lead to a phenomena, but of course the limitation is that there is no isolation of variables and control over the conditions. It is also difficult to determine how the different variables involved in a phenomenon interact.

6) Phenomenological Studies. All of the studies we have discussed so far have involved researchers studying another individual or group of individuals. Another type of study could involve researchers studying themselves, or researchers recording individuals as they reported their own personal experience. **Phenomenological studies** are interested in describing phenomena, in using the introspective method to explore research questions. Hermann Ebbinghaus made many groundbreaking discoveries in learning and forgetting by taking detailed data and notes on his own performance. He would try to learn something new, and record detailed graphs on how he scored on memorization tasks, then later the rate at which he forgot. These investigations were phenomenological, they attempted to understand his own perceptions and understandings, rather than make a comparison between variables or draw a causal conclusion.

Example 20-3: A study investigates the relationship between heavy alcohol consumption and working memory. Which of the following results is most likely associated with the results of the study?

A) The experimental group has significantly more memory recall than controls.
B) The control group has significantly more memory recall than the experimental group.
C) A correlation of +0.42
D) A correlation of -0.06

Solution: It is important to note that an experimental design, in this case, would be unethical. It would involve randomly administering something harmful (heavy alcohol consumption) to participants. This eliminates choices A and B. An increase in alcohol consumption is associated with reduced memory, so the predicted correlation would be negative. This eliminates C, and choice D is correct.

Example 20-4: Which of the following results is needed to establish the internal validity of a study based on an assessment or inventory for depression that has not been previously used?

    I. A positive correlation among repeated administrations
    II. A negative correlation with other personality dimensions
    III. A positive correlation with other inventories of depression

    A) I only
    B) II only
    C) I and III only
    D) I, II, and III

Solution: A psychometric assessment tool should have test-retest consistency (independent administrations yield similar results) and consistency with other measures of depression is another important component of construct validity. Item I is true: this describes test-retest consistency (choice B is wrong). Item II is false: a negative correlation with other personality dimensions is not needed to demonstrate validity. This may be true for some dimensions which are known to be negatively correlated with depression, but not for dimensions which have no known correlation with depression or a positive correlation, like anxiety (choice A and choice D are wrong). Item III is true: this describes consistency with other assessments of depression (choice C is correct).

Chapter 21
Social Structure, Group Identity, and Self Identity

21.1   SOCIOLOGY: THEORETICAL APPROACHES

A **society** can be defined as a collection of individuals who share a culture (discussed more in depth later in this chapter) and live/interact with each other within a definable area. **Sociology** attempts to understand the behavior of societies. Sociology is the study of how individuals interact with, shape, and are subsequently shaped by, the society in which they live. Cultural influences are important in understanding individuals, and sociologists consider both the actions of individuals and patterns of behavior in groups. Four main sociological theories have been developed by sociologists to understand the behavior of societies.

Functionalism (also known as Structural Functionalism)

The oldest of the main theories of sociology, **functionalism**, conceptualizes society as a living organism with many different parts and organs, each of which has a distinct purpose. The approach focuses on the social functions of different structures by seeing what they contribute to society at large. For example, the contribution of our lungs to the body is to orchestrate the exchange of air. Similarly, we can think about the function of schools, churches, hospitals, and other social structures. Just like organs function interdependently to help the organism survive, social structures work together to sustain society. Similarly, just as an organism can thrive, evolve, and grow, or become disease-addled and die, so can society.

Émile Durkheim, considered one of the founders of sociology, was a pioneer of modern social research and established the field as separate and distinct from psychology and political philosophy. Durkheim was a major proponent of functionalism, and he believed that modern societies were more complex than primitive societies, where people all share a common language, values, and symbols. In modern society, he argued, people take on distinct roles, and rely upon each other to make the society function. Durkheim proposed that complex societies involved many different but interdependent parts working together to maintain stability, a type of **dynamic equilibrium** in which the structure of society is constantly changing, but also evolving in a way that maintains its health and stability. Healthy societies would be able to achieve and maintain this equilibrium, while unhealthy ones would not. Durkheim further believed that society should always be viewed holistically—as a collective of social facts rather than individuals. **Social facts** are the elements that serve some function in society, such as the laws, morals, values, religions, customs, rituals, and rules that make up a society.

When investigating social facts and their function in society, a distinction is made between manifest and latent functions. **Manifest functions** are the intended and obvious consequences of a social structure, while **latent functions** are unintended or less recognizable consequences, and they can be considered beneficial, neutral, or harmful. For example, the manifest function of a hospital may be to promote health in the populace, and a latent function may also be to reduce crime by creating more jobs in a community. It should be noted that not all of the effects of social structures are good. A **social dysfunction** is a process that has undesirable consequences, and it may actually reduce the stability of society. For example, the hospital may also increase an income gap between medical professionals in the community and others.

Conflict Theory

Unlike the functionalist perspective, which emphasizes the harmony of parts, **conflict theory** views society as a competition for limited resources. According to conflict theory, inequality in resources is inevitable in society, therefore, individuals will compete for social, political, and material resources like money, land, power, and leisure. Because of this inevitable inequality, certain groups and people will be able to amass more resources than others. Those with the most power and influence will maintain their positions of power by suppressing the advancement of others. This tension does not have to be violent, but it could occur as negotiations, debates, and disputes.

Karl Marx, who is closely identified with this theory, looked at the economic conflict between different social classes. Marx argued that societies progress through class struggle between those who own and control production, such as landowners and investors, and those who provide labor such as the working class and physical laborers. He believed that capitalism produced internal tensions which would ultimately lead to self-destruction of capitalist society, to be replaced by socialism. **Ludwig Gumplowicz** expanded upon Marx's ideas by proposing that society is shaped by war and conquest and that cultural and ethnic conflicts lead to certain groups becoming dominant over other groups. **Max Weber** agreed with Marx that inequalities in a capitalist system would lead to conflict, but he did not believe that the collapse of capitalism was inevitable; rather, he argued that there could be more than one source of conflict, such as conflict over inequalities in political power and social status. Weber also argued that there were several factors that moderated people's reaction to inequality, such as agreement with authority figures, high rates of social mobility, and low rates of class difference. Along with Émile Durkheim, Karl Marx and Max Weber are considered the fathers of sociology. More recently, conflict theory has been applied to inequalities between groups based on race and gender.

Symbolic Interactionism

While the first two perspectives look at society from a macro (big-picture) perspective, **symbolic interactionism** starts at the micro (close-up) level and sees society as the buildup of everyday interactions. This theory examines the relationship between individuals and society by focusing on communication, the exchange of information through language and symbols. Symbolic interactionism is particularly interested in the symbols that people use to contribute values and beliefs to others. For example, dress codes at the workplace can communicate a sense of whether the setting is casual or formal. A smile indicates that someone is pleased. All of these small social changes combined create our overall impression of society. Symbolic interactionism sees the individual as active in shaping her society, instead of merely being acted upon by society.

This theory analyzes society by addressing the subjective meanings that people impose upon objects, events, and behaviors. Subjective meaning is important because people behave based on what they *believe to be true*, whether or not it actually is true. However, there must also be some agreement as to what symbols mean for society to function, so there is also an objective component to the symbols that are used. People interpret one another's behaviors, and these collective interpretations form a social bond.

Symbolic Interactionism holds the principal of *meaning* to be the central aspect of human behavior: (1) humans ascribe *meaning* to things, and act toward those things based on their ascribed meaning; (2) *language* allows humans to generate meaning through social interaction with each other and society; and (3) humans modify meanings through an interpretive *thought* process.

A specific type of interactionist philosophy is called the **dramaturgical approach**. As the name suggests, this assumes that people are theatrical performers and that everyday life is a stage. Just as actors project a certain on-screen image, people in society choose what kind of image they want to communicate verbally and nonverbally to others. For example, a college student who lands a coveted internship downtown will project a different image while at her internship than she will in class, and an even different image still when hanging out with her friends at a bar, or visiting her family in her childhood home.

Social Constructionism

Social constructionism argues that people actively shape their reality through social interactions—therefore, reality is not inherent, but socially constructed. A major focus of social constructionism is to uncover the ways in which individuals and groups participate in the construction of their perceived social reality. A **social construct** is a concept or practice that is a construct of a group; essentially, everybody in society agrees to treat a certain aspect a certain way regardless of its inherent value. For example, money in itself is worthless—merely a piece of paper or metal—but because people have agreed that it is valuable, it has agreed-upon value. Originally, social constructionists claimed that everything could be seen as a social construct, since even objects such as a table or desk or scientific theories like gravity, plate tectonics, and calculus are learned and passed on through social interactions. However, most social constructionists today focus their attention on concepts that are not necessarily true in nature but have an agreed upon social meaning such as health, race, success, or citizenship. Another example of a frequently studied social construct is the institution of marriage. It is something that exists completely within the realm of human society and contains its own specific rules, morals, expectations, etc. Society creates certain ideas about how marriage is supposed to look, as well as how it is supposed to be fulfilled by individuals.

A major focus of social constructionists is the study of how individuals and groups participate in the construction of society and social reality. Social construction is a dynamic, ongoing process, which must be maintained, reaffirmed, and passed along to future generations. Take the example of marriage again. The social construct of marriage has a different set of beliefs and expectations than it did, say, 30 years ago. For example, societal views on divorce and same sex marriage are vastly different. This evolution of social constructs takes place through a process known as socialization. Rules and norms are not overarching, undeniable truths, but are socialized concepts. While many social constructs such as gender, sexual orientation, and income are often taken for granted, social constructionism focuses on the social process that drive the formation of these concepts that people may assume to be "real." Social constructionism researches both how social constructs evolve within a society (macro-level) and how social constructs are understood and adapted within individual and group interactions (micro-level).

In addition to the four main sociological theories, three other theories have also been influential in sociology and are widely studied as frameworks for understanding society.

Feminist Theory

Feminist theory is concerned with the social experiences of both men and women and the differences between these experiences (for example, manhood versus womanhood and masculine versus feminine). Feminist sociologists strive to understand both the social structures contributing to gender differences (macro-level) and the effects of gender differences on individual interactions (micro-level). Because gender is a social construct, rather than some innate difference between people, sociologists are interested in the processes that create gender inequalities. The feminist perspective uses this understanding to strive for a gender balance.

Rational Choice and Social Exchange Theories

Cost-benefit analysis is an important component of the decision-making process; individuals make rational economic decisions to minimize costs and maximize benefits (cost-effective decisions). Economic theories assume that behaviors are utilitarian. Both **rational choice** and **social exchange theories** have similar assumptions, such as the assumption that individuals have possible alternatives and the freedom of choice to make decisions about these alternatives. Furthermore, although these theories are rooted in economic ideas, the processes still operate within the common social structure and are considered social norms.

Rational choice theory is concerned with decision-making, and proposes that there is a simple instrumental reason for all choices—they provide the greatest reward at the lowest cost. In particular, rational choice is more concerned with measurable resources like time and money than subjective emotions, such as guilt. Because it is borrowed from economics, it is more concerned with extrinsic costs and rewards than intrinsic ones.

The related **social exchange theory** explores decisions within social interactions. The social exchange perspective explains that decisions regarding interactions are similar to rational choice theory; we assign punishments (costs) and rewards (benefits) to interactions and relationships, and prefer those with the greatest personal benefits. However, with social exchanges, while the exchanges are calculated and negotiated, the costs and rewards do not have to be economic in nature. Rational Rewards are those things with positive values; these benefits can be economic but are more often physical (a hug), psychological (support), or emotional (a smile). In contrast, punishments are those things with negative values; again, these costs can be economic but can also be physical (a shove), psychological (abandonment), or emotional (a frown).

Example 21-1: The glass escalator is a phenomenon that has been observed regarding men who work in fields in which they are statistically underrepresented relative to women. According to feminist theory, what do we expect would occur for men in these fields?

- A) Structural advantages within the career for advancement, and structural disadvantages in the form of stigmatization outside of the career
- B) Structural disadvantages within the career, and structural advantages in the form of cultural capital outside of the career
- C) Structural advantages within the career for advancement, and structural advantages in the form of cultural capital outside of the career
- D) Structural disadvantages within the career, and structural disadvantages in the form of stigmatization outside of the career

Solution: Feminist theory focuses on the unfair treatment of women with respect to men. Therefore, it would predict men would receive structural advantages within fields in which they are underrepresented. Research suggests that this is, in fact, the case (choices B and D are wrong). Another important component of feminist theory is the belief that strict gender roles and expectations have detrimental personal and societal consequences, and that these social norms are strictly enforced through stigmatization. Therefore, a feminist theorist would predict that men who work in fields that are perceived as feminine would face stigmatization outside of their careers (choice A is correct, and choice C is wrong).

21.2 SOCIAL INSTITUTIONS

Social institutions are a complex of roles, norms, and values organized into a relatively stable form that contributes to social order by governing the behavior of people. Social institutions provide predictability and organization for individuals within a society, and they mediate social behavior between people. Social institutions provide harmony, and they allow for specialization and differentiation of skills. Examples of social institutions in the United States include our educational systems, family, religions, government, and healthcare systems.

Family

Family is part of all human cultures. A family is a set of people related by blood, marriage, adoption, or some other agreed-upon relationship that signifies some responsibility to each other. Over history, families have tended to serve five functions.

1) Reproduction and the monitoring of sexual behavior
2) Protection
3) Socialization—passing down norms and values of society
4) Affection and companionship
5) Social status—social position is often based on family background and reputation

One way of conceptualizing family is to distinguish **nuclear family**, consisting of direct blood relations, like parents, children, and siblings from **extended family**, in which grandparents, aunts, uncles, and others are included. Across cultures and even within a culture, the members of the family that typically live together may vary.

There are many alternatives to the traditional nuclear family that consists of a husband and wife with their children. A few of the variations on this traditional model seen in the United States are described as follows:

1) **Cultural differences**: many cultures emphasize the importance of extended family, often living with grandparents, cousins, and other relatives. In some cases, "kin" who are non-blood related members of the community may be considered part of the family.
2) **Divorce**: the divorce rate has generally risen in the United States due to various factors. This has led to more nontraditional family structures, such as remarried and blended families, as well as single parent homes.
3) **Cohabitation**: there has been a large increase, especially among couples in their 20s and 30s in living together without getting married. These couples may be in a transitional phase heading toward marriage, or they may choose not to get married at all.
4) **Lesbian and gay relationships**: lesbian and gay couples might also engage in all of the same behaviors that a "traditionally" married couple might, including property ownership and raising children, and often turn to cohabitation in states that do not extend legal rights to lesbian and gay couples.

Education

Educational institutions have both manifest (stated) and latent (hidden) functions. Their manifest functions are to systematically pass down knowledge and to give status to those who have been educated. For example, patients trust doctors mainly because of the conferral of an awarded degree and subsequent licensure. This degree and licensure represents an agreed-upon amount of information, skills, and training acquired in order to practice medicine (something that was actually not always the case in the United States!). Latent functions are just as important; they include socialization, serving as agents of change, and maintaining social control.

As a social institution, schools transmit aspects of the dominant culture. Schooling also helps maintain the current social norms by training students on discipline expected in institutions like the workplace, training for particular vocations, and even redirecting students to fit norms.

While many forms of student socialization are intentional (manners, learning to talk only when called on, learning to work independently), there are other lessons learned in school known as the hidden curriculum. Students may be aware of the hidden curriculum because it can come into conflict with the manifest (stated) curriculum. For example, medical educators know that medical students experience a conflict between the stated values of their curriculum and the lived reality of hospital work they encounter during their third and fourth years. While students may have learned about the sanctity of patient care during their lectures, they often encounter hospital staff whose actions inadvertently teach them that patients are nuisances.

Another aspect of the hidden curriculum is the realization that school does not offer an equal opportunity to all. Certain benefits such as small class size, excellent teachers, and the availability of the latest technology and resources, often are based on socioeconomic status. Access to higher education, a key factor in getting a good job, is also highly dependent on family income. Level of education then continues to be influential in terms of power, respect, and social standing.

An example of these processes at work is the widening disparity between children from high-income neighborhoods and those from low-income neighborhoods, a type of educational segregation. In comparison with children from wealthier neighborhoods, children from poorer neighborhoods:

- tend to attend poorer schools
- are more likely to drop out of school before graduation and not attend college
- are more likely to seek vocational training or an Associate's degree
- are more likely to end up with lower-paying jobs

Each of these phenomena tend to perpetuate a cycle of poverty and are likely to contribute to increased inequality. Another aspect of the hidden curriculum is teacher expectancy. Research has shown that teachers tend to quickly form expectations of individual students, and once they have formed these expectations, they tend to act toward the student with their expectations in mind. If the student accepts the teacher's expectations as reasonable, the student will begin to perform in accordance with them, as well. This is known as teacher expectancy theory. Teacher expectancy often helps children exceed their own expectations of themselves—this is the ideal of education. However, teachers are not free of stereotypes, and their expectations can have the effect of underestimating students. When these students then perform to meet their teacher's low expectations of them, they reinforce the teacher's stereotypes and simultaneously miss out on the opportunities for upward mobility education can provide.

Religion

Organized religion is a social institution involving belief and practices. These practices are based on objects and ideas that are recognized as sacred, or extraordinary and worthy of reverence. The five major world religions are Christianity, Islam, Judaism, Hinduism, and Buddhism. The vast majority of people identify with one or more of these belief structures, although there are many other religions and many non-believers who do not identify with any religion.

From a functionalist standpoint, religion can create social cohesion (as well as dissent), and provide believers with meaning and purpose. Social cohesion is often experienced by members of religious groups due to the system of shared beliefs and values that it provides. Religious communities can be a source of emotional, spiritual, and material support in difficult times. However, religion can also be a source of social dissent, as a history of violence between religious factions indicates. Religion is a powerful social institution that can influence members of society in different ways depending on the context.

There are many individual differences among people who consider themselves members of a particular religion. **Religiosity** refers to the extent of influence of religion in a person's life. Some may be very devout, with the extreme form being **fundamentalists**, who adhere strictly to religious beliefs. Others may adhere more to the beliefs of the religion without the rituals or to the rituals without the beliefs.

Government and Economy

Our political and economic structures both influence and are influenced by social structure. Governments across the world derive their power from different places. The United States government is one based on **rational-legal authority**, legal rules and regulations are stipulated in a document like the Constitution. Many corporations, including healthcare organizations, work within this structure and are often organized in a similar way. Other governments around the world may derive power from **traditional authority**, power due to custom, tradition, or accepted practice. Still other leaders may be powerful due to **charismatic authority**, the power of their persuasion.

In addition to deriving power from rational-legal authority, our political and economic system is influenced greatly by capitalist ideals. **Capitalism** is an economic system in which resources and production are mainly privately owned, and goods/services are produced for a profit. It is thought that the advantages of capitalism are that it benefits the consumer by allowing for competition, emphasizes personal freedom, and increases efficiency through subdivision of labor, performance of tasks by individuals in specific roles, and economic scaling, mass production that lowers the price per unit, often through the use of industrial processes. Disadvantages include that overwhelming power amassed by corporations may lead to actions that are not in the best interest of the greater society.

Socialism is an economic system in which resources and production are collectively owned. Private property is limited and government intervenes to distribute resources. The primary criticism of socialist societies is that the economy is centrally controlled and run by the government. Among many reasons, historically this has been due to the fact that socializing property requires the seizure of private property, and has required authoritarian control to keep in the hands of government.

Most nations incorporate both capitalist and socialist ideas. **Welfare capitalism** is a system in which most of the economy is private with the exception of extensive social welfare programs to serve certain needs within society. **State capitalism** is a system in which companies are privately run, but work closely with the government in forming laws and regulations. Distinguishing among the different types of economy can be difficult, but often counties in Western Europe with privately owned companies and extensive social welfare programs are considered to operate under welfare capitalism while countries like Brazil and Russia, with massive state-run oil conglomerates are considered state capitalist economies.

Health and Medicine

Medicine is the social institution that governs health and illness, particularly with respect to diagnosis, treatment, and prevention of illness. Society plays a large role in defining health/illness and acceptable healthcare practices. The United States has experienced the spread of the medical model of disease, which emphasizes physical or medical factors as the cause of all illness. The process by which a condition comes to be reconceptualized as a disease with a medical diagnosis and a medical treatment is known as medicalization.

An alternate way of understanding illness is known as the social model of disease. The social model of disease emphasizes the effect one's social class, employment status, neighborhood, exposure to environmental toxins, diet, and other factors can have on a person's health. While someone working from the perspective of the medical model might look for the ultimate cause of a person's illness (for example, pneumonia resulting from exposure to the bacterium *streptococcus pneumoniae*), someone working from the social model would be attuned to a more proximate cause—something about the patient's life circumstances that put him/her at greater risk of exposure to the bacterium. Although the medical model remains the dominant form of clinical reasoning in medical care, there has been an emphasis on the biopsychosocial aspects of medical care (hence the presence of this material on the MCAT). This model aims to take into consideration the psychological, social, and cultural factors that influence health, including perception of illness, beliefs about health, community practices, etc., that may affect emotional states, medication compliance, and a multitude of other health-related outcomes.

In addition to defining health and illness, social pressures create the conditions for health and illness. Obesity is a larger problem in low-income areas in the United States, in large part due to the presence of food deserts. A **food desert** is an area where healthy, fresh food is difficult to find. A common definition of a food dessert is an area with no supermarkets within one mile where a large portion of the population does not have a car. In the United States, areas that fit these criteria are most commonly located the rural South and Appalachia, and disproportionately affect the poor. Food deserts are one of the factors that contribute to high obesity rates in parts of the United States. Other factors include social and cultural practices that encourage the consumption of low-quality, high-calorie food and do not encourage physical activity.

The **sick role** is a concept developed by American sociologist **Talcott Parsons**. According to this concept, when a person is ill, he/she is not able to be a contributing member of society. Being ill, from Parsons' point of view, is a type of deviance. For others to take up the extra work in this person's absence they must consider the person's illness to be legitimate—they must sanction this person's deviance by exempting him/her from normal social roles and by not blaming the person for his/her illness. In return, the person must fulfill the role obligations of an ill person: the person should seek medical care and the person should make a sincere attempt to get well.

When studying illness experience, sociologists are not just interested in the meanings people give to their illness, but also how the experience of being ill affects patients' daily lives—their ability to work, spend time with friends and family, and cultivate their selves. Illness experience is particularly important to consider in light of chronic disease. With a chronic disease, a patient can have no reasonable expectation of getting better; thus, she/he must adjust normal daily life to fit the constraints of the illness. This process can be isolating and destabilize one's sense of self, which is largely founded on the activities of normal life, hobbies and work, and one's relationships. Self-concept and daily activities reinforce each other, so illness experience encompasses both the individual's understanding of his/her condition as well as the material impact being ill has on the person's daily life.

21.3 CULTURE AND DEMOGRAPHICS

Culture

Culture refers to a shared way of life, including the beliefs and practices that a social group shares. Although cultures can vary a great deal, they are composed of some common elements. **Symbolic culture** consists of symbols that are recognized by people of the same culture. Symbols convey agreed-upon meaning, can communicate the values and norms of the culture, and include rituals, gestures, signs, and words that help people within a society communicate and understand each other. Symbols and rituals can differ between cultures, for example, some cultures celebrate the life of a deceased relative with a party while others mourn at a more somber funeral.

Material culture involves physical objects or artifacts. This includes clothing, hairstyles, food, and the design of homes. The importance placed on material objects can reflect the culture's values; for example, the American dream often includes a car, a symbol of mobility and independence. In contrast, **non-material culture** is specific to social thoughts and ideas, such as values. Note that symbolic culture can be either material or non-material.

Popular culture is a phrase used to describe features of culture that appeal to the masses, often those communicated through mass media such as radio and television. This is distinguished from **high culture**, which describes those features held in high esteem as exemplary.

While comparing different cultures is useful for noticing differences, some anthropologists assert that there are also some cultural **universals**—patterns or traits that are common to all people. Cultural universals tend to pertain to basic human survival and needs, such as securing food and shelter, and also pertain to events that every human experiences, including birth, death, and illness.

Two of the most crucial elements of culture are values and beliefs. People within a given culture tend to share common values and beliefs. **Values** can be defined as a culture's standard for evaluating what is good or bad, while **beliefs** are the convictions or principles that people hold, and do not necessarily have a value judgement attached. In order to promote societal values, laws, or rewards may be in place to encourage behavior in line with social values and discourage behavior counter to social values. **Norms** are the visible and invisible rules of social conduct within a society. Norms help define what types of behaviors are acceptable and in accordance with a society's values and beliefs.

Culture and Social Groups

Sociobiology is a study of how biology and evolution have affected human social behavior. Primarily, it applies Darwin's principle of natural selection to social behavior, suggesting there is a biological basis for many behaviors. That is, particular social behaviors persist over generations because they are adaptive for survival. For example, among mammals, sexual behavior often varies by sex because males tend to have a lower physiological costs associated with reproduction. In human societies, aggression may also manifest in different ways based on biological drives, with men committing more violent crimes than women.

Sociobiologists would look for a way to explain these differences by corroborating animal behavior with evolutionary adaptations and taking into account social factors.

Scientists also believe that the origins of culture lie in human evolution. Through time, humans in various societies evolved the ability to categorize and communicate human experience through the use of symbols (as discussed above). As these codified systems for communication were learned and taught to future generations, they began to develop independently of human evolution. While people living in different areas will likely develop their own unique cultures, culture can still be taught and learned. Therefore, anthropologists consider culture to be not just a product of human evolution, but a complement to it; it is a means of social adaptation to the natural world.

Social Construction and Transformation

Cultural diffusion is the transfer of elements of culture—social ideas and processes such as religious traditions—from one social group to another. This contributes to cultural similarities between different societies. Diffusion can also occur within a single culture, leading to some similarities in beliefs even in different levels of societies (such as among different classes). It can be direct or indirect, or sometimes even forced, as with cultural imperialism. The rate of diffusion has increased as a result of modern conveniences that offer opportunities for cross-cultural communication, like modern media and transportation. **Cultural transmission** is the process through which this information is spread across generations, or the mechanisms of learning. Learning is a social process that occurs through individual experiences in which we attach different meanings to different things; we then learn to remember and respond to these meanings.

Social constructionism suggests that our realities are produced and reproduced; elements of culture are not static. In some cases, **social change** occurs, in which societies experience a change in state. This can be subtle, like with the development of new linguistic phrases, or radical, like with **revolutions**, which involve fundamental changes and social restructuring. Transformative social changes, such as technological innovations, often challenge our understanding of the world because there is no social consensus about the new innovation; the creation of new social rules "lags" behind. This is described as **cultural lag**.

When individuals experience changes, such as social changes, that necessitate a period of adjustment, there is often **transition shock**. When this disorientation is the result of an individual being subjected to alternative cultures and foreign environments, such as through leisure travel or permanent relocation, it is called **culture shock**. Different cultures have different cuisines, fashions, languages, signs, etc., and individuals must grow accustomed to all of these changes. For example, the transition to medical school causes a definite reaction for most students; there is a feeling of "information overload" as the result of exposure to unfamiliar content and the disruption of people's previous schedules. **Reverse culture shock** involves the same experiences but upon an individual's return to their initial environment.

Sociocultural evolution is a set of theories describing the processes through which societies and cultures have progressed over time. Both individual behavior and social structures experience continuous transformation in response to their complex needs. Sociologists argue that these changes are the result of social factors, such as social interactions, rather than biological factors. Historical studies have revealed a lot of societies throughout time, but today, there exist just a couple hundred as the result of natural growths and declines. Two modern theories of sociocultural evolution, *modernization* and *sociobiology*, are discussed previously.

POPULATION STUDIES

Human **population** is the collection of people in a defined geographical area, and it also refers to the number of people in the area. Population studies are interested in demographic shifts. There is periodic population growth and population decline as a result of birth rates, death rates, and migration rates. The world as a whole is experiencing a period of population growth that is predicted to continue for many decades. Much of this growth is attributed to advances in agricultural production (the green revolution) and innovations in medicine that have contributed to changes in birth and death rates. In contrast, many industrialized countries are experiencing population due to declining birth rates.

There are concerns with population increases and decreases both. For example, in societies experiencing growth, there is concern of reaching **overpopulation**, at which point there are more people than can be sustained; in societies experiencing decline, there are concerns about maintaining economic success. The total possible population that can be supported with relevant resources and without significant negative effects in a given area is referred to as the **carrying capacity**. Populations tend to increase and decrease until **population equilibrium** is met at this maximum load.

Population projections are estimates of future populations made from mathematical extrapolations of previous data. Traditional projections are based on birth rates, death rates, and migration rates, and thus do not consider unpredicted effects on population, like the chance of catastrophes. The global population reached seven billion in 2011. Experts project an increase in this population until at least 2050 with upper estimates ranging from 9 to 11 billion despite decreases in worldwide fertility rates. The projections suggest that the greatest contributions will be made in less-developed regions.

Fertility and Mortality

Birth rates and death rates are often reported through statistical measures. The **crude birth rate** (CBR) is the annual number of births per 1,000 people in a population. Experts consider crude birth rates of 10–20 to be low and those of 40–50 to be high. The **crude death rate** (CDR) is the annual number of deaths per 1,000 persons in a population. Experts consider crude death rates below 10 to be low and those above 20 to be high. The **rate of population change** is the difference between the crude birth rate and crude death rate. There are also **age-specific birth rates** and **age-specific death rates**, which are the annual number of births or deaths per 1,000 persons in an age group.

The **general fertility rate** is the annual number of births per 1,000 women in a population. The more complicated measure of **total fertility rate** predicts the total number births per single woman in a population with the assumption that the woman experiences the current recorded age-specific fertility rates and reaches the end of her reproductive life. The **replacement fertility rate** is the fertility rate at which the population will remain balanced, and **sub-replacement fertility** indicates that the birth rate is less than the death rate, thus the population size will not be sustained. The **population-lag effect** refers to the fact that changes in total fertility rates are often not reflected in the birth rate for several generations. This is the result of **population momentum**, in which the children produced during periods of higher fertility rates reproduce; there are more women of reproductive age and thus more births overall, regardless of the number of births per women. Because crude birth rates do not consider age or sex differences, fertility rates offer a clearer idea of demographic trends. For example, fertility rates have increased in the older age groups as women pursue education and participate in the labor force at greater rates, thus beginning reproduction later in life.

Mortality refers to the death rate in a population, and this also includes both general and specific measures. This is distinguished from **morbidity**, which refers to the nature and extent of disease in a population; the **prevalence rate** measures the number of individuals experiencing a disease and the **incidence rate** measures the number of new cases of a disease. Reference to death rates in medicine often concern the **case fatality rate**, which measures deaths as the result of a set diagnosis or procedure, sometimes specific to the beginning or late stages. The current leading cause of death worldwide is ischemic heart disease, but there are also variations in causes of death by location; for example, age-related issues are a major cause of death in developed countries while malnutrition is a major cause of death in developing countries. There is an inverse correlation between a nation's crude death rate and its gross domestic product (GDP). The crude death rate is not sensitive to factors with a natural correlation to death, such as age structure. Thus, there are two additional common and reliable indicators of important qualities of life: the infant mortality rate and life expectancy. The **infant mortality rate** is the annual number of deaths per 1,000 infants under one year of age. **Life expectancy** is the number of years that an individual at a given age can expect to live at present mortality rates. Estimates of global life expectancies range from 36 to 79 years.

Developed regions tend to have lower birth rates and death rates. Factors contributing to decreasing crude birth rates include access to contraception, costs associated with raising a child, and other social changes. For example, teenage births are at a historical low in the United States and an increasing number of older couples are choosing to postpone reproduction, or to not reproduce at all. Factors contributing to decreasing crude death rates include improvements in agriculture, medicine, and sanitation.

Example 21-2: Data from most countries around the world show that women outlive men, on average, with the discrepancy varying considerably from country to country. Which of the following conclusions would a functionalist most likely reach to explain this result?

    A) Biologically, females have a genetic advantage over males due to the XX chromosomal structure, which duplicates sequences and reduces the risk of early death from genetic malfunctions.

    B) Men are conditioned under different sets of social norms within a patriarchal society, which encourage more risk-taking behaviors.

    C) Women play an important role as caregivers, so societies have evolved to encourage healthier habits in women.

    D) Evolution posits that females carry a higher biological cost to reproduction; therefore, males engage in high-risk behaviors to demonstrate relative evolutionary fitness to females who are more sexually selective.

Solution: When explaining social phenomena, functionalists place emphasis on the way different aspects within a society cohesively work together to form a whole. A functionalist would look for an explanation that focused on the social function of certain constructs. The role of women as caregivers could be one function that causes society to place an increased value on preserving healthier habits in older women (choice C is correct). Although the biological explanation is plausible, it does not fit specifically within a functionalist framework, because it does not emphasize social functions and social roles (choice A is wrong). Feminist theorists are more likely to emphasize the role of patriarchal society and strict gender roles (choice B is wrong). A focus on evolution and competition among males for a sexual partner is more likely to fit within the framework of Conflict Theory (choice D is wrong).

Migration

In addition to birth rates and death rates, population is also determined through rates of **migration**, the geographical movement of individuals, families, or other small or large groups of people. Migration implies the intention of permanent relocation ("settling down") and is thus distinct from non-permanent movement. For example, non-permanent travel for leisure, pilgrimage, or seasonal reasons and **nomadism**, which is a traditional method of continuous travel in search of natural resources as a method of sustenance ("hunting and gathering"), are not considered migration because there is no intention to settle. **External migration**, also referred to as cross-border or international migration, involves migration to another nation. Motivations for external migration are often economic or political in nature. **Internal migration** involves migration to another region of the same nation. Motivations for internal migration are often more economic in nature as individuals pursue better opportunities, such as education. Those who migrate to unsettled areas are **settlers** and those who migrate to settled areas as a result of displacement are **refugees**. More complicated is **colonization**, which involves migration to settled areas in which dominance is exerted over the indigenous state. **Immigration** involves entering a new area, and these people are called immigrants (and can be either legal or illegal residents); **emigration** involves leaving an old area, and these people are called emigrants. **Reverse migration**, or return migration, is the return of individuals to their former homes.

There are numerous historical theories describing the reasons for migration and its effects. **Push factors** are those things that are unattractive about an area and "push" people to leave. Push factors are often economic, political, or religious in form: active oppression of social groups; additional forms of prejudice and discrimination, such as housing discrimination; insufficient access to social resources, such as education, or social services to meet basic needs, such as shelter; widespread inequalities, such as health disparities; and so on. **Pull factors** are those things that are attractive about an area and "pull" people there. These are the opposite of push factors and often include positive opportunities for economic, political, or religious freedom and success. The interaction between push and pull factors contributes to the rates of migration. Migration also has an impact on the nation to which people move; for example, the cultural diffusion of new ideas.

Urban Growth, Decline, and Renewal

Internal migration includes the movement between rural and urban areas. The spatial distribution of individuals and social groups is an interest of **social geography**. **Urbanization** refers to the growth of urban areas (as people move from rural to urban areas) as the result of global change. Urbanization is tied to **industrialization**, the process through which societies transform from agrarian to industrial in nature. Cities tend to offer many employment opportunities, as well as being places where money and wealth are localized. Furthermore, people can access more social services in cities. This is related to **rural flight**, or rural exodus, which studies the migration from rural areas to urban areas from the other perspective. The widespread social changes associated with industrialization and urbanization during the eighteenth and nineteenth centuries are responsible for the start of the sociological tradition as a separate subject following the scientific method. The oldest theories were developed in an attempt to process these broad historical changes.

Suburbanization refers to population growth on the fringes of urban areas (as people move from urban areas to suburban areas). The **suburbs** are residential satellite communities located in the peripheral regions of major urban centers that are often connected to the cities in some fashion. Migration to these metropolitan regions is an example of **urban sprawl**, or the migration of people from urban areas to otherwise remote areas. The negative effects of urban sprawl include **urban blight**, which occurs when less functioning areas of large cities degrade as a result of urban decline. These forms of migration can thus lead to desolate properties, such as condemned houses, and the resulting dangerous conditions can contribute to an increase in crime levels in blighted areas. Those who remain in the blighted areas are often poor and have less access to social amenities and opportunities.

Gentrification refers to the renovation of urban areas (as people move from rural or suburban areas back to urban areas) in a process of urban renewal. Gentrification is often specific to the introduction of wealthier residents to the cities who then help to restore the existing infrastructure, which alters the region's demographics and economics. For example, the conversion of old industrial buildings to high end "loft-style" housing options brings new businesses to the area to serve the new middle class population. This causes much social change with both positive and negative effects; for example, it can increase the tax base, but it can also lead to the displacement of the original local people.

Theories of Population Change

There are multiple theories of population change. **Demographic transition** (DT) is the transition from overall higher to overall lower birth and death rates as a result of a country's development from a pre-industrial to industrial framework due to both economic and social changes; thus, both fertility and mortality rates decrease as in the transition from an agricultural to a manufacturing society. This has long-term effects, such as a stable population. The model includes specific stages of transition and, in general, developed countries are further along in this transition than developing countries, but most countries have started to experience changes in crude birth rate and crude death rate. However, the model is limited; for example, it does not consider additional social factors that affect birth rates, like religious influences.

Thomas Robert Malthus argued that population is the result of available resources for sustenance, such as productive farmland. Humans are inclined to reproduce and thus population growth is often exponential, especially during times of excess. However, **Malthusianism** states that the possible rate of population increase exceeds the possible rate of resource increase. This perspective resulted as a criticism of utopian views, explaining that the rules of nature make it impossible for population to increase unchecked without serious distress due to insufficient resources. A **Malthusian Catastrophe** occurs when the means of sustenance are not enough to support the population, resulting in population reduction through actual or predicted famine. **Neo-Malthusianism** is a movement based on these principles that advocates for population control in order to reduce the negative effects of population strain, such as environmental effects. Malthus found controlled populations to be more stable in terms of economics and standards of living in particular.

Demographic Structure

Researchers often use aggregate statistics to provide a demographic profile of a specific population (based on region or time). Demographics often focus on subsets of the population with the intent of describing the shared characteristics of members of these subsets.

Minorities are those demographic groups that are distinguished from the majority, who frequently occupy a disproportionate number of the positions of power and influence in a society. The **dominant groups** are those with the social power to assign these labels.

Demographic measures discussed below include age, gender, race and ethnicity, sexual orientation, and immigration status. However, there are many more examples of demographic interest, such as disabilities, languages, and socioeconomic characteristics (education, employment status, income, wealth, etc.).

Age

Years are the most common units of measurement for age, but months or even weeks are also used in certain situations, such as with infants. The most basic categories of age are described in the following ranges:

- **Juveniles (infants, children, preadolescents, and adolescents)**: 0–19 years
- **Early adults**: 20–39 years
- **Middle adults**: 40–59 years
- **Late adults**: 60+ years

However, additional descriptions are also used (for example, those aged 13–18 are called teenagers). **Age cohorts** are an example of statistical cohorts in which a group of subjects share the characteristic of age. These groups are used in longitudinal studies, also called **cohort studies**, which conduct research for extended periods of time to better understand the different perspectives of those in the cohort and those in the general population. Generational cohorts, or **generations**, are groups of people born in the same period. These distinct generations share specific experiences that become representative of the group (a popular example is Generation X). Demographic age profiles describe populations in terms of age groups. Populations with a proportionate distribution are the most stable. **Population aging** occurs when there is a disproportionate amount of older people in a population. This raises concerns such as health-care demands and provider shortages. **Ageism** is prejudice or discrimination against a person based on age, often against older people.

The concept of aging has both biological and social components. *Social aging* reflects the biological changes in a multidimensional process in which individuals experience complex emotional and social changes. Factors including active engagement, interpersonal relationships, personal control, and social support contribute to optimal aging and predict objective and subjective measures of well-being in adults. There are serious social implications of an aging population. Economic consequences of a rising median age include increased requirements for pension liabilities, retirement packages, and worker's compensation. In contrast, an increase in children leads to greater demands for social resources such as education.

The social significance of aging is considerable. For example, children and adults have different legal rights. Individuals receive different roles and statuses, as well as greater social opportunities, at certain milestones, such as the age of consent, drinking age, retirement age, smoking age, and voting age. These are sometimes called **rites of passage**; these rituals reflect important life transitions and also include more personal changes such as marriage. The courts also consider age in cases of criminal prosecution; the defense might argue that juveniles are not liable for their crimes due to a lack of social experiences and responsibilities.

Gender

Sex is a biological characteristic based on chromosomes, external genitalia, gonads, and hormones. Categories of sex are male (XY), female (XX), and intersex, which is applicable when a single sex cannot be identified. **Gender** is a social characteristic (a social construction) based on behavioral role expectations.

Gender is thought to be influenced by both nature and nurture. In terms of nature, biological measures can have behavioral effects (for example, hormones influence emotions). The natural sciences are interested in the consequences of biological differences between men and women on gender. In some cases, genetic abnormalities (such as the XXY chromosomal abnormality in Klinefelter's syndrome) might cause unexpected presentations when compared to the assumptions made from one's biological sex. In terms of nurture, our social surroundings have a profound effect on the development of our gender identities. The social sciences are interested in the consequences of social processes. **Gender roles** describe the social and behavioral expectations for men and women. These expectations are internalized and become connected to our self-identities (how we think about ourselves) and thus influence our behaviors. **Gender expression** is the external manifestation of these roles.

Transgender individuals have gender identities that are inconsistent with their biological sex divisions. Modern technologies allow the pursuit of anatomical and hormone adjustment through sex reassignment procedures. The term transsexual is sometimes used to describe individuals who have undergone such procedures.

Race and Ethnicity

Race and ethnicity are related concepts that are of much interest to sociologists because of their importance in human interactions; however, it is important to first understand the distinction between these two demographic characteristics. **Race** is a description of a distinct social group based on certain shared characteristics, such as physical or genetic similarities. According to the U.S. Census, the currently accepted race categories include Black/African American, White, Asian, American Indian/Alaska Native, Native Hawaiian/Other Pacific Islander, and "Other." **Ethnicity** is also a description of a distinct social group based on certain shared characteristics but these tend to be more social in nature, such as tradition, religion, language, food, or national history. The five largest ethnic groups are as follows: (1) Han Chinese, (2) Hindustani people, (3) Arabs, (4) Bengalis, and (5) Russians. This shows the distinction of ethnicities from nationalities. For example, Arab populations originate in the Arabian Peninsula, which includes several modern nations with the current five largest populations being in (1) Egypt, (2) Algeria, (3) Iraq, (4) Sudan, and (5) Morocco. In the reverse direction, in addition to Arab populations, Egypt also includes ethnic minorities, such as the Beja, Berber, Dom, and Nubian peoples.

Prejudices that hold that one race is inferior to another and actions that discriminate based on race are called **racism**. Sometimes racism is used to describe discrimination on an ethnic or cultural basis, independent of whether these differences are described as racial. The confusion largely stems from confusion about the definitions of the terms "race" and "ethnicity." Ethnocentrism is a related concept that describes biases that result when people look at issues from the perspective of a particular cultural background.

Sexual Orientation

Sexual orientation describes the direction of a person's romantic or sexual attraction or behavior. It is important to note that these categories are crude descriptions of attractions or behaviors, not of people themselves. There are three main sexual orientations.

- **Heterosexual**: the orientation toward the opposite gender or sex
- **Homosexual**: the orientation toward the same gender or sex
- **Bisexual**: the orientation toward both genders or sexes

Bisexual identities do not necessitate an equal attraction toward both genders and sexes; in some cases, there is a distinct, but not exclusive, sexual preference toward one gender or sex. Bisexual communities include those who are **pansexual** and attracted to people irrespective of gender or sex. Recent research suggests a fourth sexual orientation (asexual) but this is contended because others argue that it is actually the absence of a traditional sexual orientation. **Asexuality** involves the lack of sexual attraction. This is different from the decision to be abstinent or celibate for personal reasons, such as religious beliefs.

Heteronormative beliefs consider heterosexual to be the preferred sexual orientation, and they often enforce strict gender roles. The prejudice and discrimination against non-heterosexual individuals can be political, economic, religious, or social in nature. There are sometimes public sanctions, such as formal policies, reinforcing these beliefs. This has led to modern social movements for the recognition of legal rights, such as adoption rights, marriage rights, and health-care rights for same-sex couples.

There is much debate about the causes of sexual orientation, including both biological theories that consider factors like genetics and hormones and environmental theories that consider factors like parenting. There is some argument that non-heterosexual behavior is unnatural for certain reasons (for example, it does not permit reproduction). However, research suggests that sexual orientation is a human characteristic that is generally resistant to change, and it has been observed in naturalistic settings throughout the animal kingdom, from other primates to smaller mammals and fruit flies and worms.

Immigration Status

Immigration was introduced above as the migration of people to a new area. Immigration status is another common demographic measure. The United States has had four main periods of immigration, based on the social context, as well as the distinct demographics (ethnicities, nationalities, and races) of the migrants.

1) **The 17th and 18th centuries**: During this period, English colonists migrated to the United States (the colonial period). Indentured servants also migrated through this process, accounting for more than half of all immigrants from Europe during the period.
2) **The mid-19th century**: During this period, the most migrants came from northern Europe.
3) **The early 20th century**: During this period, the most migrants came from southern and Eastern Europe. For example, Jewish refugees moved to the United States in flight from the Nazi regime during World War II. The peak of European migration was 1907, after which the social context of the United States made conditions less suitable for immigration. The Great Depression, for example, led to a period of higher national emigration rates than immigration rates (this occurred in the early 1930s).
4) **The late 20th century (post-1965) to the present**: During this period, the majority of migrants have been from Asia and Latin America. In general, a plurality of immigrants are women in the 15 to 35 age range. It is common for people to migrate to areas with similar populations (such as areas populated with people of their ethnic background).

Immigration controls are formal policies that define and regulate who has the right to settle in an area. This is important because it restricts legal immigration, and it increases the need for economic and political resources to ensure an individual's success in migrating. Today, most legal immigration is granted on the basis of family reunification (this accounts for two-thirds of all cases), employment skills, and humanitarian reasons.

The shared experiences of immigrants are of concern to sociologists. These individuals are often mistreated, and in some cases their rights are violated in the immigration process. Immigrants are also a common target of prejudice and discrimination. Furthermore, immigrant status can have implications for social functioning due to the differences in the social conventions of developing and developed countries. For example, arranged marriages are more common in the East than in the West, which requires immigrants to reconcile these practices with the accepted traditions of their new homes.

DEMOGRAPHIC SHIFTS AND SOCIAL CHANGE

Globalization

Modern advancements in telecommunications and transportation have contributed to the rates of **globalization**, the process of increasing interdependence of societies and connections between people across the world. **Telecommunications**, in particular, use modern technologies to ease the challenges of communication across distances, and like most information and communication technologies, contribute to the integration of economical, political, and social processes worldwide. **Economic interdependence** can be thought of as the division of labor on a global scale; countries might have the demand for products without the internal means of production. The example of **outsourcing** involves the contracting of third parties for specific operations. This can be domestic or foreign, but the financial savings associated with foreign outsourcing have made it a focus of much opposition.

There are also cultural consequences of globalization as the sharing of cultures leads to more foreign choices, such as cuisines and media options. In some cases, this interchange can lead to the disintegration of local culture as new ideas are welcomed. Periods of **civil unrest**, or civil disorder, involve forms of collective behavior in which there is public expression of the group's concern, often in response to major social problems, like with political demonstrations and protests. **Terrorism** involves the use of violence with the intention to create fear in the target communities. There is no single form of terrorism: it can be committed for ideological, nationalistic, political, religious, or other reasons. The defining characteristic of terrorist acts is violence directed toward non-combatants.

21.4 STRATIFICATION

Stratification and Inequality

Social stratification refers to the way groups are organized into strata according to power, wealth, and income (among other things). People with the most resources comprise the top tiers of the stratification, while people with the least resources comprise the bottom tiers. The **caste system** describes a closed stratification where people are born into their social strata. On the other hand, the **class system** considers both social variables and individual initiative; the class system groups together people of similar wealth, income, education, etc., but the classes are open, meaning that people can strive to reach a higher class (or fall to a lower one). A **meritocracy** is another stratification system that uses merit (or personal effort) to establish social standing; this is an idealized system—no society solely stratifies based on effort.

Most sociologists define stratification in terms of socioeconomic status. **Socioeconomic status** (SES) can be defined in terms of power (the ability to get other people to do something), property (sum of possessions and income), and prestige (reputation in society).

Social mobility refers to the ability to move up or down within the social stratification system. **Upward mobility** refers to an increase in social class; **Downward mobility** refers to a decrease in social class. **Intergenerational mobility** occurs when there is an increase or decrease in social class between parents and children within a family, and **intragenerational mobility** describes the differences in social class between different members of the same generation.

Social reproduction refers to the structures and activities in place in a society that transmit and reinforce social inequality from one generation to the next. Cultural capital and social capital are two mechanisms by which social reproduction occurs. **Cultural capital** refers to the non-financial social assets that promote social mobility. Education is an excellent example of cultural capital. **Social capital** refers to the potential for social networks to facilitate upward social mobility. For example, if a young woman comes from an upper middle class family and wants to become a doctor, her mom might introduce her to a friend who is a doctor, who can give her some advice and set her up with a shadowing opportunity. Social capital is a powerful way to tap into vast networks of resources, but it can also serve to reinforce inequalities already present in society.

Residential segregation refers to the separation of groups into different neighborhoods; separation most often occurs due to racial differences, ethnic differences, and/or socioeconomic differences. Residential segregation is not based on laws, but rather enduring social patterns, which are attributed to suburbanization, discrimination, and personal preferences. **Environmental injustice** refers to the fact that people in poorer communities are more likely to be subjected to negative environmental impacts to their health and wellbeing, such as the building of a large, pollution-generating power plant near their neighborhoods. Environmental injustice and residential segregation are two factors that continue to perpetuate inequalities in society.

Global stratification compares the wealth, economic stability, and power of various countries. A comparison across the globe highlights the worldwide patterns of **global inequality**. **Relative poverty** is the inability to meet the average standard of living within a society, whereas **absolute poverty** is the inability to meet a bare minimum of basic necessities, including clean drinking water, food, safe housing, and reliable access to healthcare.

Example 21-3: Which of the following types of capital is related to socioeconomic status?

      I. Physical capital
    II. Cultural capital
  III. Social capital

    A) I only
    B) II only
    C) I and II only
    D) I, II, and III

Solution: Item I is true: income, savings, and physical property are all examples of physical capital (choice B is wrong). Item II is true: some non-financial attributes, such as education, are included in the assessment of socioeconomic status (choice A is wrong). Item III is true: social capital, related to who someone knows, is associated with socioeconomic status because social networks often provide a boost to power and prestige, two of the important components of socioeconomic status (choice D is correct, and choice C is wrong).

21.5 SELF-CONCEPT AND IDENTITY FORMATION

Self-concept or **self-identity** is broadly defined as the sum of an individual's knowledge and understanding of his- or herself. Differing from **self-consciousness**, which is awareness of one's self, self-concept includes physical, psychological, and social attributes, which can be influenced by the individual's attitudes, habits, beliefs, and ideas. For example, if you asked yourself the question "Who am I?" your responses would form the basis of your self-concept. Self-concept is how an individual defines him- or herself based on beliefs that person has about him- or herself, known as **self-schemas**. For example, an individual might hold the following self-concepts: female, African-American, student, smart, funny, future doctor.

Different Types of Identities

These qualities can be further divided into those that form personal identity and those that form social identity. **Personal identity** consists of one's own sense of personal attributes (in the example above, smart and funny constitute attributes of personal identity). **Social identity** consists of social definitions of who you are; these can include race, religion, gender, occupation, and such (in the example above, female, African-American, student, and future doctor constitute attributes of social identity). Thus, the "self" is a personal and social construction of beliefs. As a quick way to remember different aspects of one's identity, consider the ADRESSING framework: each letter stands for a different characteristic. These characteristics are age, disability status, religion, ethnicity/race, sexual orientation, socioeconomic status, indigenous background, national origin, and gender.

Old information that is consistent with one's self-concept is easy to remember, and new information coming in that is consistent with one's self-schemas is easily incorporated. This tendency to better remember information relevant to ourselves is known as the **self-reference effect**. Inconsistent information is more difficult. For example, if someone considers herself to be intelligent but receives an extremely low score on an exam, this would oppose her self-concept. Therefore, this person may choose to externalize the new information from her self-concept by attributing it to a lack of sleep or an unfair test.

The Role of Self-Esteem, Self-Efficacy, and Locus of Control in Self-Concept and Self-Identity

In addition to how the "self" is defined, there are three powerful influences on an individual's development of self-concept. These are self-efficacy, locus of control, and self-esteem.

1) **Self-efficacy** is a belief in one's own competence and effectiveness. It's how capable we believe we are of doing things. Self-efficacy can vary from task to task; an individual may have high self-efficacy for a math task and low self-efficacy for juggling.

2) **Locus of control** can be internal or external. Those with an **internal locus of control** believe they are able to influence outcomes through their own efforts and actions. Those with an **external locus of control** perceive outcomes as controlled by outside forces. In an extreme situation, in which people are exposed to situations in which they have no control, they may learn not to act because they believe it will not affect the outcome anyway. Even once this situation passes and they find themselves once again in arenas in which they can exert some control, this lack of action may persist. This phenomenon is known as **learned helplessness**. It has been shown that believing more in an internal locus of control can be empowering and lead to proactivity. An external locus of control and learned helplessness are characteristics of many depressed and oppressed people, and often result in passivity.

3) **Self-esteem** is one's overall self-evaluation of one's self-worth. Self-esteem is related to self-efficacy; self-efficacy can improve self-esteem if one has it for an activity that one values. However, if the activity is not one that is valued, it may not help self-esteem. Low self-esteem increases the risk of anxiety, depression, drug use, and suicide. However, inflated self-esteem is also present in gang members, terrorists, and bullies, and may be used to conceal inner insecurities.

Influence of Social Factors on Identity Formation

Influence of Individuals

Charles Cooley, an American sociologist, posited the idea of the **looking-glass self**, which is the idea that a person's sense of self develops from interpersonal interactions with others in society and the perceptions of others. According to this idea, people shape their self-concepts based on their understanding of how others perceive them. The looking-glass self begins at an early age and continues throughout. **George Herbert Mead**, another American sociologist, developed the idea of **social behaviorism**: The mind and self emerge through the process of communicating with others. The idea that the mind and self emerge through the social process of communication or use of symbols was the beginning of the **symbolic interactionism** school of sociology (mentioned earlier). Mead believed that there is a specific path to development of the self. During the preparatory stage, children merely imitate others, as they have no concept of how others see things. In the play stage, children take on the roles of others through playing (as when playing house and taking on the role of "mom"). During the game stage, children learn to consider multiple roles simultaneously, and they can understand the responsibilities of multiple roles. Finally, the child develops an understanding of the **generalized other**, the common behavioral expectations of general society. Mead also characterized the "me" and the "I." The "me" is how the individual believes the generalized other perceives it. The "me" could also be defined as the social self. The "I" is the response to the "me"; in other words, the "I" is the response of the individual to the attitudes of others. The "I" is the self as subject; the "me" is the self as object.

Influence of Culture and Socialization on Identity Formation

Socialization is the process through which people learn to be proficient and functional members of society; it is a lifelong, sociological process where people learn the attitudes, values, and beliefs that are reinforced by a particular culture. For older adults, this process often involves teaching the younger generation their way of life; for young children, it predominantly involves incorporating information from their surrounding culture as they form their personalities (the patterns for how they think and feel).

Norms

Every society has spoken or unspoken rules and expectations for the behavior of its members, called norms; social behaviors that follow these expectations and meet the ideal social standard, then, are described as **normative behavior**. They are reinforced in everyday social interactions by **sanctions**—rewards and punishments for behaviors that are in accord with or against norms. For example, in some nations, it is considered the norm to offer your food to others when eating in a public place. To offer food to a stranger on a bus in the United States, though, would likely result in a sanction such as a disapproving or uncomfortable look.

Norms can be classified in multiple ways, and one way is by formality. **Formal norms** are generally written down; laws are examples of formal norms. They are precisely defined, publicly presented, and often accompanied by strict penalties for those who violate them. **Informal norms** are generally understood but are less precise and often carry no specific punishments. One example is greeting an interviewer with a handshake (a norm in the United States). Not to do so does not carry a fine, but it may affect the interviewer's perception of the job candidate.

Another way of classifying norms is based on their importance. **Mores** ("more-ays") make up society's core values of right and wrong and so are often strictly enforced. For example, animal abuse and treason are actions that break mores in the United States and carry harsh penalties. **Folkways** are norms that are less important but shape everyday behavior (for example, styles of dress, ways of greeting).

In contrast, those behaviors that customs forbid are described as **taboo**. In the case of a taboo, the endorsement of the norm is so strong that its violation is considered forbidden and severely punishable through formal or non-formal methods. Taboo behaviors, in general, result in disgust toward the violator. There is often a moral or religious component to the taboo, and violation of the norm poses the threat of divine penalties.

Anomie

The normative effects of social values contribute to social cohesion and social norms are involved in maintaining order. In some cases, societies lack this cohesion and order. This is referred to as **anomie**, a concept that describes the social condition in which individuals are not provided with firm guidelines in relation to norms and values and there is minimal moral guidance or social ethic. For this reason, anomie is often thought of as a state of normlessness.

Cultural Assimilation

Assimilation and amalgamation are two possible outcomes of interactions between multiple cultures in the same space. **Assimilation** is the process in which an individual forsakes aspects of his or her own cultural tradition to adopt those of a different culture. Generally, this individual is a member of a minority group who is attempting to conform to the culture of the dominant group.

$$A + B + C \rightarrow A$$

In the diagram above, A is the dominant group that minority groups B and C work to imitate and become absorbed by. In order to assimilate, members of the minority group may make great personal sacrifices, such as changing their spoken languages, their religions, how they dress, and their personal values.

Amalgamation occurs when majority and minority groups combine to form a new group.

$$A + B + C \rightarrow D$$

In this case, a unique cultural group is formed that is distinct from any of the initial groups.

Multiculturalism

Multiculturalism or **pluralism** is a perspective that endorses equal standing for all cultural traditions. It promotes the idea of cultures coming together in a melting pot, rather than in a hierarchy. The United States, despite common description as a melting pot, includes elements of hierarchy. For example, English is the dominant language, and national holidays tend to reflect Eurocentrism.

$$A + B + C \rightarrow A + B + C$$

In true multiculturalism, each culture maintains its practices. It is especially apparent in cities such as New York where there exist pockets of separate cultures (Chinatown, Little Italy, Koreatown). As a practice, multiculturalism is under debate. Supporters say it increases diversity and helps empower minority groups. Opponents say it encourages segregation over unity by maintaining physical and social isolation and hinders cohesiveness of a society.

Subcultures

Bike enthusiasts, bartenders, and medical personnel are examples of groups that can be called subcultures. A **subculture** is a segment of society that shares a distinct pattern of traditions and values that differs from that of the larger society. As the name suggests, a subculture can be thought of as a culture existing within a larger, dominant culture. Members of a subculture do participate in many activities of the larger culture, but they also have unique behaviors and activities that are specific to their subculture.

21.6 POSITIVE AND NEGATIVE ELEMENTS OF SOCIAL INTERACTION

Attribution

Attribution theory is rooted in social psychology and attempts to explain how individuals view behavior, both our own behavior and the behavior of others. Given a set of circumstances, individuals attribute behavior to internal causes (**dispositional attribution**) or external causes (**situational attribution**). Imagine you are driving and someone cuts you off. You might think, "Wow, that driver is a real jerk." This would be a dispositional attribution, because the driver's behavior is attributed to an internal cause. On the other hand, you could alternatively think, "Wow, that driver must be in a hurry because of an emergency; maybe he just found out his mom is in the hospital." This would be a situational attribution.

What determines whether we attribute behavior to internal or external causes? There are three factors that influence this decision: consistency, distinctiveness, and consensus. To consider these, imagine a simple situation: you are walking past your friend, who looks angry and walks past you without saying hello.

1) **Consistency:** is anger consistent with how your friend typically acts? If it is, then you might explain it with internal causes (dispositional). If not, you might think there are external factors that explain it (situational).

2) **Distinctiveness:** is your friend angry toward everyone or just toward you? If your friend is angry toward everyone, the cause likely has to do with your friend (dispositional). If your friend is just angry toward you, it may be situational; maybe you did something.

3) **Consensus:** is your friend the only one angry or is everyone angry? If your friend is the only one angry, then it is more likely that the anger has something to do with your friend (dispositional). If everyone is angry, then it might be situational (the team lost the playoffs).

Note that the above attributions are guidelines reflecting how we might respond. Often, one domain independently is not enough to determine whether a behavior is situational or dispositional. For example, suppose your friend is always angry on Friday nights when you get together for drinks (consistency). This could be dispositional behavior, or it could be situational (for example, you meet your friend just after working a demanding shift with an abrasive supervisor). Clearly, attribution is not an exact science and is subject to many possible errors, and misattributions are common.

Attributional Biases

A common mistake in attribution is the **fundamental attribution error**, which is that we tend to underestimate the impact of a situation and overestimate the impact of a person's character or personality. Another way of saying this is that we tend to assume that people *are* how they act. Thus, we are more likely to think that the driver who cuts us off is a jerk in general, rather than assuming the driver acted that way because he has to rush to the hospital to be with his ailing mother. On the other hand, when we attribute our own actions to something, we tend to attribute external rather than internal causes. So if I cut someone off, it is because I had a good reason to. This tendency to blame our actions on the situation and blame the actions of others on their personalities is also called the **actor-observer bias**.

People tend to give themselves much more credit than they give others. We are wired to perceive ourselves favorably. The **self-serving bias** is the tendency to attribute successes to ourselves and our failures to others or the external environment. If we perform well academically, it is because we are smart and worked hard. If we perform poorly academically, it was because the test was unfair or the teacher graded too hard.

Similarly, we have a tendency to be optimistic and want to believe that the world is a good place. We want to believe that life can be predictable and that actions influence outcomes. The **optimism bias** is the belief that bad things happen to other people, but not to us. This goes hand-in-hand with the fact that we want to believe that life is fair, which also impacts how we think about others. The **just world phenomenon** is a tendency to believe that the world is fair and people get what they deserve. When bad things happen to others, it is the result of their actions or their failure to act, not because sometimes bad things happen to good people. Similarly, when good things happen to us, it is because we deserved it.

Another type of error that occurs when we make assumptions about others is the halo effect (or halo error). The **halo effect** is a tendency to believe that people have inherently good or bad natures, rather than looking at individual characteristics. Our overall impression of a person is influenced by how we feel or think about his or her character. For example, your overall impression of your neighbor might be "he is nice," therefore, you make other assumptions about him ("he must be a good dad"). The **physical attractiveness stereotype** is a specific type of halo effect; people tend to rate attractive individuals more favorably for personality traits and characteristics than they do those who are less attractive.

Self-Perceptions Shape our Perceptions of Others

Social perception involves the understanding of others in our social world; it is the initial information we process about other people in order to try to understand their mindsets and intentions. **Social cognition** is the ability of the brain to store and process information regarding social perception. Social perception is the process responsible for our judgments and impressions about other people, and it allows us to recognize how others impact us and predict how they might behave in given situations. We rely upon our social perception and cognition in order to interpret a range of socially relevant information, such as verbal and non-verbal communication, tone, facial expressions, and an understanding of the social relationships and social goals present in situations. Using social perception, we try to figure out what others are thinking. Sometimes our tendencies lead us to mistakes in social perception. A **false consensus** occurs when we assume that everyone else agrees with what we do (even though they may not). A **projection bias** happens when we assume others have the same beliefs we do. Since people have a tendency to look for similarities between themselves and others, they often assume congruence of beliefs even when this is unfounded.

Stereotypes, Prejudice, and Discrimination

Many people may not know the differences between the terms stereotype, prejudice, discrimination, and racism, but from a sociological perspective, it is important to know their meanings. **Stereotypes** are oversimplified ideas about groups of people, based on characteristics (race, gender, sexual orientation, religion, disability). Stereotypes can be positive ("X group is successful because they are hard workers") or negative ("Y group is poor because they are lazy").

Prejudice refers to the thoughts, attitudes, and feelings someone holds about a group that are not based on actual experience. As the name implies, prejudice is a prejudgment or biased thinking about a group and its members. The group that one is biased against can be one defined by race, age, gender, religion, or any other characteristic. While prejudice involves thinking a certain way, **discrimination** involves acting a certain way toward a group.

Institutional discrimination refers to unjust and discriminatory practices employed by large organizations that have been codified into operating procedures, processes, or institutional objectives. An example of institutional discrimination was the "don't ask, don't tell" policy of the U.S. military, which frowned upon openly gay men and women serving in the armed forces. In general, members of minority groups are much more likely to encounter institutional discrimination than members of majorities.

Emotion and Cognition in Prejudice

Emotion can play a role in feeding prejudices. At the core of prejudice is often fear or frustration. When someone is faced with something intimidating or unknown, especially if it is presumed to be blocking that person from some goal (frustration), hostility can be a natural reaction.

Attributional biases (described above), particularly the optimism bias and just-world belief, also suggest that we are more likely to believe that the world is fair and predictable, things happen for a reason, and people get what they deserve. Thus, the sick or disadvantaged often face prejudice because others believe that they have done something wrong that led them to be in their position. Thus, someone with HIV may face prejudice, including the assumption that he or she contracted the disease through irresponsible behavior, despite how the disease was actually transmitted.

Self-Fulfilling Prophecy and Stereotype Threat

These stereotypes can lead to behaviors that affirm the original stereotypes in what is known as a **self-fulfilling prophecy**. For example, if a college guy believes that the girls in a certain sorority are snobby and prudish, he may avoid engaging in conversations with the girls from that sorority at parties. Because he does not engage them in conversation, his opinion of them as snobby and prudish will probably be reinforced. People may also be affected by stereotypes they know others have of a group to which they belong. **Stereotype threat** refers to a self-fulfilling fear that one will be evaluated based on a negative stereotype.

Example 21-4: Students from lower economic status backgrounds demonstrate lower test scores than peers. Without knowing more detail on the cause of the discrepancies, which of the following is most consistent with the prediction of someone practicing a conflict theory approach?

    A) Prejudice
    B) Discrimination
    C) Teacher Expectancy
    D) Hidden Curriculum

Solution: Conflict theorists are most likely to focus on competition and oppression of disadvantaged groups, particularly groups that are low in socioeconomic status. Therefore, discrimination would be the most likely explanation (choice B is correct). Since discrimination is an action and prejudice is a belief, the conflict theorist would be more likely to believe that direct actions are the cause of the differences than beliefs, which may or may not be acted on (choice A is wrong). Teacher expectancy is often implicit, such that the teacher is not aware that they are acting on a belief, or that they are having an impact on the outcomes (choice C is wrong). The hidden curriculum relates to messages beyond the stated curriculum that are passed on in the classroom. While this could affect academic performance, it is not the most likely explanation a conflict theorist would give, because it does not suggest direct competition and structural oppression of disadvantaged groups (choice D is wrong).

Groups

A **group** is a collection of any number of people (as few as two) who regularly interact and identify with each other, sharing similar norms, values, and expectations. A team of neurologists may be considered a group, while the entire hospital staff may not be considered a group, if there is little interaction between departments. Within a social structure, groups are often the setting for social interaction and influence. Groups help clearly define social roles and statuses. People who exist in the same space but do not interact or share a common sense of identity make up an **aggregate**. For example, an MCAT study group that meets after class regularly at a coffee shop to prepare for the exam is a group. All of the people that frequent that coffee shop on a regular basis (but do not interact or share a common identity) are an aggregate. Similarly, people who share similar characteristics but are not otherwise tied together would be considered a **category**. All of the people studying for the MCAT this year make up a category of people.

Groups can be further divided into primary groups and secondary groups. **Primary groups** play a more important role in an individual's life; these groups are usually smaller and include those with whom the individual engages with in person, in long-term, emotional ways. A **secondary group** is larger and more impersonal, and members may interact for specific reasons for shorter periods of time. Primary groups serve **expressive functions** (meeting emotional needs) and secondary groups serve **instrumental functions** (meeting pragmatic needs). A family would be an example of a primary group (regardless of how family is defined), whereas the MCAT study group would be an example of a secondary group.

In-groups and out-groups are subcategories of primary and secondary groups. A group that an individual belongs to and believes to be an integral part of her identity is in an **in-group**. A group that an individual does not belong to is her **out-group**. Social identity theory asserts that when we categorize other people, we identify with some of them, who we consider our in-groups, and see differences with others, who we consider our out-groups. We tend to have favorable impressions of our in-groups because they bolster our social identities and self-esteem. People tend to have positive stereotypes about their own in-groups ("we are hard-working"). On the other hand, we may have more negative impressions of members of out-groups. Different can be seen as worse (for example, "I feel sorry for those who don't believe the same things I do"). People also tend to have more negative stereotypes about out-groups ("they are lazy"). In-groups and out-groups help to explain some negative human behaviors like exclusion and bullying.

A **reference group** is a standard measure that people compare themselves to. For example, peers who are also studying for the MCAT might be a reference group for you. This is a group you might compare yourself to. What are the people in this group studying? What classes are they taking? When are they taking the exam? To which medical schools are they applying? An individual can have multiple reference groups, and these different groups may convey different messages. For example, you might view your friends in class who are all taking the MCAT as one reference group, and your older sibling, who is in medical school, and his or her medical school friends as another reference group.

Furthermore, there are descriptions of group size. The number of people present within the group has consequences for group relations. The smallest social group, known as the dyad, contains two members. Dyadic interaction is often more intimate and intense than that in larger groups because there is no outside competition. However, the small size also requires active cooperation and participation from both members to be stable. In some cases of dyads, such as within marriages, there are laws that enforce the strength of the pair. Dyads can involve equal relationships, such as with monogamous romantic partners, or unequal relationships, such as with master-servant relationships. The next largest group, known as the triad, contains three members. In the dyad, there is a single relationship, but in the triad, there are three separate relationships, one between each pair of members.

Social Facilitation

Social psychology seeks to understand how people influence each other through their interactions. The most basic level of experience between members of society is "mere presence." **Mere presence** means that people are simply in each other's presence, either completing similar activities or apparently minding their own business. For example, the task of grocery shopping usually involves the mere presence of other shoppers, without direct engagement. What's fascinating is that it turns out the mere presence of others has a measurable effect on an individual's performance.

People tend to perform simple, well-learned tasks better when other people are present. For example, people can do simple math problems more quickly and run slightly faster when in the presence of others. However, on more complex tasks or tasks that are less practiced, individuals may perform worse in front of a group. Taken together, this finding has been called the **social facilitation effect**.

Deindividuation

When situations provide a high degree of arousal and a very low sense of responsibility, people may act in startling ways, surprising both to themselves at a later time and to others who know them closely. In these situations, people may lose their sense of restraint and their individual identity in exchange for identifying with a group or mob mentality, a situation called **deindividuation**. Its effects can be seen in examples ranging from atrocious acts during wartime to mosh pits at concerts.

Bystander Effect

The **Kitty Genovese** case involved the stabbing of a woman in New York City late at night. Although details of the case are more complicated, the incident was highlighted because of the perceived lack of effort of neighbors to help her while she cried for help. After her murder was discovered, detectives interviewed her neighbors and found that many of them had heard her cries for help, but no one had called the police. Time and again, the reason provided for a lack of action was that everyone assumed someone else had already called the police. Research spawned by this event revealed what is known as the **bystander effect**: the finding that a person is less likely to provide help when there are other bystanders. This occurs because the presence of bystanders creates a diffusion of responsibility—the responsibility to help does not clearly reside with one person in the group.

Social Loafing

Diffusion of responsibility can also occur when individuals are evaluated in groups, since there is a tendency to exert less effort than if evaluated individually, a phenomenon called **social loafing**.

Social facilitation and social loafing are both responses to the group situation and the task at hand. Which one tends to occur is based in part on evaluation. When being part of a group increases concerns over evaluation, social facilitation occurs. When being part of a group decreases concerns over evaluation, social loafing occurs. In order to fight against the threat of social loafing, companies in which people work in groups often use measures of group performance (for example, a store's total revenue) as well as of individual performance (for example, individual sales).

Group Polarization

We've seen how groups can influence one's performance, either by facilitating or hindering it based on circumstances. But how does group influence affect beliefs and opinions? It turns out that groups tend to intensify the preexisting views of their members—that is, the average view of a member of the group is accentuated. This tendency is called **group polarization**. It does NOT indicate that the group becomes more divided on an issue, but rather, suggests that the entire group tends toward more extreme versions of the average views they initially shared before discussion.

Groupthink

Pressure not to "rock the boat" in a group by providing a dissenting opinion can lead to what is known as groupthink. Although **groupthink** is a state of harmony within a group (because everyone is seemingly in a state of agreement), it can lead to some pretty terrible decisions. Groupthink manifests in a group when certain factors come together. Groups that are at risk tend to be overly friendly and cohesive, isolated from dissenting opinions, and have a directive leader whose decisions everyone tends to favor.

There are certain symptoms that are often clues to the presence of groupthink.

- The group is overly optimistic of its capabilities and has unquestioned belief in its stances—an overestimation of "might and right."
- The group becomes increasingly extreme by justifying its own decisions while demonizing those of opponents.
- Some members of the group prevent dissenting opinions from permeating the group by filtering out information and facts that go against the beliefs of the group (a process called **mindguarding**).
- There is pressure to conform, and so individuals censor their own opinions in favor of consensus, which creates an illusion of unanimity.

Stigma and Deviance

Complex social processes regulate social behaviors through positioning social norms as the correct method of action. However, there are cases where individuals do not conform to the expectations implicit in social structures. In contrast to normative behavior, non-normative behavior is viewed as incorrect because it challenges shared values and institutions, thus threatening social structure and cohesion. These behaviors are seen as abnormal and thus discouraged. Actions that violate the dominant social norms, whether formal or informal, are described as forms of deviance. In some cases, deviant behavior is seen as criminal, in which case it violates public policies; thus, studies of deviance are popular among criminologists. Society often devalues deviant members by assigning demeaning labels, called **stigma**.

Conformity and Obedience

There are two well-known experiments that sought to investigate the influence of conformity and obedience.

21.6

Solomon Asch wanted to test the effects of **group pressure** (or **peer pressure**) on individuals' behavior, so he designed a series of simple experiments where subjects would be asked to participate in a study on visual perception. In the experiment, subjects were asked to determine which of three lines was most similar to a comparison line (in the experiment, there was one line that was clearly identical to the comparison line and the other two were clearly longer). When subjects completed this task alone, they erred less than 1% of the time. When subjects were placed in a room with several other people that they thought were also participating in the study, but were actually **confederates** (meaning that they were part of the experiment), the results were quite different. On the first few tests, all of the confederates responded correctly. However, after a little while the confederates began all choosing one of the incorrect lines. What's interesting is that Asch found that more than one third of subjects conformed to the group by answering incorrectly. They chose to avoid the discomfort of being different, rather than trust their own judgment in answering. The phenomenon of adjusting behavior or thinking based on the behavior or thinking of others is called **conformity**.

Another commonly referenced experiment is **Stanley Milgram**'s study involving fake shocks. The participants in this study believed that they were in control of equipment that delivered shocks to a student who was attempting to pass a memory test. No shocks were actually used. A researcher was in the room and directed the participant to administer increasing levels of shock to this student, a confederate, by turning a dial whenever he or she answered incorrectly. The only contact the participant had with the student was to hear the student's voice from the other room. When shocks were given at particular levels, the participants would hear moans, shouts of pain, pounding on the walls, and after that, dead silence. Milgram found that participants in the study were surprisingly obedient to the researcher's demands that they continue to administer the shocks. Out of 40 subjects, few questioned the procedure before reaching 300 volts and 26 of the subjects continued all the way to the maximum 450 volts. The experiment speaks to the power of authority and the discomfort that being disobedient invokes.

There are three ways that behavior may be motivated by social influences.

1) *Compliance*: Compliant behavior is motivated by the desire to seek reward or to avoid punishment. There is likely to be a punishment for disobeying authority. Compliance is easily extinguished if rewards or punishments are removed.

2) *Identification*: Identification behavior is motivated by the desire to be like another person or group. A participant who conformed in Asch's experiment likely did not want to be disapproved of for choosing a different answer than the rest of the group. Identification endures as long as there is still a good relationship with the person or group being identified with and there are not convincing alternative viewpoints presented.

3) *Internalization*: Internalized behavior is motivated by values and beliefs that have been integrated into one's own value system. Someone who has internalized a value not to harm others may have objected to the shocks administered in Milgram's study. This is the most enduring motivation of the three.

There are several factors that influence conformity.

1) *Group Size:* A group doesn't have to be very large, but a group of 3–5 people will elicit more conformity than one with only 1–2 people.
2) *Unanimity:* There is a strong pressure not to dissent when everyone else agrees. However, if just one person disagrees, others are more likely to voice their real opinions.
3) *Cohesion:* An individual will more likely be swayed to agree with opinions that come from someone within a group with whom the individual identifies.
4) *Status:* Higher-status people have stronger influence on opinions.
5) *Accountability:* People tend to conform more when they must respond in front of others rather than in closed formats in which they cannot be held accountable for their opinions.
6) *No Prior Commitment:* Once people have made public commitments, they tend to stick to them. For example, once someone has taken a pledge to become a fraternity brother, he is more likely to follow the norms of that group.

21.7 SOCIAL INTERACTION AND SOCIAL BEHAVIOR

All social interactions take place within social structures, which are composed of five elements: statuses, social roles, groups (previously discussed), social networks, and organizations. These five elements are developed through the process of socialization, discussed earlier. Social interactions include things like expressing emotion, managing others' impressions of you, communicating, and other social behaviors.

Social Structures

Statuses and Roles

Status is a broad term in sociology that refers to all the socially defined positions within a society. These can include positions such as "president," "parent," "resident of Wisconsin," and "Republican." Needless to say, one person can hold multiple statuses at the same time. One's **master status** is the one that dominates the others and determines that individual's general position in society.

Statuses may be ascribed or achieved. **Ascribed statuses** are those that are assigned to a person by society regardless of the person's own efforts. For example, gender and race are ascribed statuses. **Achieved statuses** are considered to be due largely to the individual's efforts.

Roles

Social roles are expectations for people of a given social status. It is expected that doctors will possess strong medical knowledge and be intelligent. Role expectations can also come with ascribed statuses. There may be an expectation that a female is more likely to be a babysitter than a male. Roles help contribute to society's stability by making things more predictable.

However, roles can also be sources of tension in multiple ways. **Role conflict** happens when there is a conflict in society's expectations for *multiple statuses* held by the same person (for example, a male nurse or a gay priest). **Role strain** is when a *single status* results in conflicting expectations. For example, a homosexual man may feel pressure to avoid being "too gay" and also "not gay enough." **Role exit** is the process of disengaging from a role that has become closely tied to one's self-identity to take on another. Some examples include the transition from high school student to more independent college student living on campus with peers. Another would be transitioning from the workforce to retirement. These transitions are difficult because they involve the process of detaching from something significant, as well as embarking on something new and unknown.

21.7 Networks and Organizations

Networks

Think about the people you know. Now think about the people that those people know. As you keep extrapolating out to more distant connections, you can get a sense of your **social network**. A social network is a web of social relationships, including those in which a person is directly linked to others as well as those in which people are indirectly connected through others. Facebook is a popular online social network. Social networks are often based on groups that individuals belong to. Network ties may be weak, but they can be powerful resources in meeting people (for example, using a network like LinkedIn to find a job).

Organizations

Large, more impersonal groups that come together to pursue particular activities and meet goals efficiently are called **organizations**. They tend to be complex and hierarchically structured. Formal organizations can include businesses, governments, and religious groups. Organizations serve the purpose of increasing efficiency, predictability, control, and uniformity in society. They also allow knowledge to be passed down more easily, so that individual people become more replaceable. As an example, consider going to a McDonald's. Because this corporation is an organization, one may expect a particular experience and menu options regardless of who is actually working at that particular restaurant.

There are three types of organizations. **Utilitarian organizations** are those in which members get paid for their efforts, such as businesses. **Normative organizations** motivate membership based on morally relevant goals, for example, Mothers against Drunk Driving (MADD). **Coercive organizations** are those for which members do not have a choice in joining (for example, prisons). Like groups, organizations both are influenced by statuses and roles and help define statuses and roles.

Bureaucracy is a term used to describe an administrative body and the processes by which this body accomplishes work tasks. Bureaucracies rise from an advanced division of labor in which each worker does his or her small task. These tasks are presided over and coordinated by managers. A major theory of bureaucracy was developed by sociologist **Max Weber**, who considered bureaucracy to be a necessary aspect of modern society. Weber outlined the following characteristics of an ideal bureaucracy:

1) It covers a fixed area of activity.
2) It is hierarchically organized.

3) Workers have expert training in an area of specialty.
4) Organizational rank is impersonal, and advancement depends on technical qualification, rather than favoritism.
5) Workers follow set procedures to increase predictability and efficiency.

One major concept related to bureaucracy is rationalization.

Rationalization describes the process by which tasks are broken down into component parts to be efficiently accomplished by workers within the organization. Because the workers follow set procedures in completing tasks, it is easy to predict the outcome of the process. Manufacturers have taken advantage of these aspects of bureaucracy when designing production processes. Sociologist **George Ritzer** studied how rationalization could be applied to the design of McDonalds, restaurants to produce food quickly, and to produce uniform products across all franchises. He describes the rationalization of fast food production as McDonaldization. This process has four components that reflect the principles of bureaucracy: efficiency, calculability (assessing performance through quantity and/or speed of output), predictability, and control (automating work where possible in order to make results more predictable).

One paradoxical feature of organizations is that, although they may be founded to tackle challenges in new ways, as their organizational structure becomes more complex, it also becomes more conservative and less able to adapt. This pattern is known as the **Iron Law of Oligarchy**. Oligarchy means rule by an elite few, and it comes about through the very organization of the bureaucracy itself. Bureaucracies depend on increased centralization of tasks as one moves up the hierarchy. That is, there are many layers of managers in a bureaucracy, each one responsible for coordinating (centralizing) a set of tasks. The individuals who are responsible for coordinating the coordinators have the most power, and those individuals become an oligarchy at the top of the organizational structure. Furthermore, these oligarchs become specialized at their task (management), just as other members of the organization become specialists in their tasks. As discussed above, one downside to bureaucracy is that workers will fight to maintain control over their task and their established way of carrying it out. Thus, managers defend their position at the top of the organizational structure, thereby entrenching the oligarchy.

Social Interactions

Impression Management

In sociology and psychology, **impression management** or **self-presentation** is the conscious or unconscious process whereby people attempt to manage their own images by influencing the perceptions of others. This is achieved by controlling either the amount or type of information, or the social interaction. People construct images of themselves, and they want others to see them in certain lights. There are multiple impression management strategies that people employ. Assertive strategies for impression management include the use of active behaviors to shape our self-presentations, such as talking oneself up and showing off flashy status symbols to demonstrate a desired image. Defensive strategies for impression management include avoidance or self-handicapping. **Self-handicapping** is a strategy in which people create obstacles and excuses to avoid self-blame when they do poorly.

Front Stage Versus Back Stage Self

The **dramaturgical perspective** in sociology stems from symbolic interactionism and posits that we imagine ourselves as playing certain roles when interacting with others. This perspective uses the theater as a metaphor for the way we present ourselves; we base our presentations on cultural values, norms, and expectations, with the ultimate goal of presenting an acceptable self to others. Dramaturgical theory suggests that our identities are not necessarily stable, but dependent on our interactions with others; in this way, we constantly remake who we are, depending on the situations we are in. Social interaction can be broken into two types: front stage and back stage. In the **front stage**, we play a role and use impression management to craft the way we come across to other people. In the **back stage**, we can "let down our guard" and be ourselves. For example, the way you dress and behave at work (front stage) is different than your dress and behavior at home (back stage).

Verbal and Nonverbal Communication

Nonverbal communication involves all of the methods for communication that we use that do not include words. A majority of these cues are visual, but we employ other cues as well. Nonverbal communication includes gestures, touch, body language, eye contact, facial expressions, and a host of finer subtleties. The act of communicating verbally also employs a lot of nonverbal cues, such as pitch, volume, rate, intonation, and rhythm.

Social Behavior

Social behavior occurs between members of the same species within a given society. Specific social behaviors include attraction, aggression, attachment, and social support.

Attraction between members of the same species is a primary component of love, and it explains much about friendship, romantic relationships, and other close social relationships. Researchers in social psychology are particularly interested in studying human attraction because it helps to explain how much we like, dislike, or hate others. Research into human attraction has found that the following three characteristics foster attraction: proximity, physical attractiveness, and similarity.

Proximity (geographic nearness) is the most powerful predictor for friendship. Think of the people you consider your closest friends. How many of them shared a grade school classroom or a neighborhood with you growing up? How many people from your freshman dorm or living situation do you still consider to be close friends? People are more inclined to like, befriend, and even marry others from the same class, neighborhood, or office. People prefer repeated exposure to the same stimuli; this is known as the **mere exposure effect**. With certain exceptions, familiarity breeds fondness.

Appearance also has a powerful impact on attraction. Physical attractiveness is an important predictor of attraction; in fact, studies show that people rate physically attractive people higher on a number of characteristics and traits, indicating that physically attractive people are somehow more likeable. While many aspects of attractiveness vary across cultures, some appear to be culturally universal, such as youthful appearance in women (perhaps reflecting a biological constraint of fertility), and maturity, dominance, and affluence in men. Humans also tend to prefer average, symmetrical faces. Attractiveness is also influenced by personality traits; people believed to have positive personality traits are judged more attractive.

21.7

Similarity between people also impacts attraction. Friends and partners are likely to share common values, beliefs, interests, and attitudes. The more alike people are, the more their liking for each other endures over time.

Aggression

While attraction is an important unifying force in society, aggression is the opposite; a potentially destructive force to social relations. **Aggression** is broadly defined as behavior that is forceful, hostile, or attacking. In sociology, aggression is considered something that is intended to cause harm or promote social dominance within a group. While aggression is employed for a variety of reasons by humans today (competitive sports, war, getting ahead at work), in non-human animals it is generally employed as a means for protecting resources, such as food, territory, and mates.

Many psychological and social factors are thought to trigger aggression in humans. The **frustration-aggression principle** suggests that when someone is blocked form achieving a goal, this frustration can trigger anger, which can lead to aggression. Other frustrating stimuli, such as physical pain, unpleasant odors, and hot temperatures can also lead to aggression. Aggression is more likely to occur in situations in which prior experience has somehow promoted aggression.

Social Support

Social support is a major determinant of health and wellbeing for humans and other animals. Family relationships provide comfort, and close relationships are predictive of health outcomes. Happily married people live longer, healthier lives, regardless of age, sex, and race. People who have social support have been shown to engage in healthier behaviors; they are less likely to smoke, more likely to exercise, and report a better capacity to cope with adversity and stress. Interestingly, social support is not confined to human-human interactions. People with dogs or other pets also reap some of the benefits of social support.

Biological Explanations of Social Behavior in Animals

Many animals also exhibit a wide range of social behavior. Some species (such as ants, bees, and wasps) engage in highly organized and hierarchical social behaviors, with each individual playing a specific role within the group. Most mammals also engage in social behavior, and many interesting phenomena have been elucidated by studying how mammals interact with members of their own species.

Inclusive Fitness and Altruism

The **inclusive fitness** of an organism is its ability to pass on its genes, including its own offspring and the offspring of relatives. It proposes that an organism can improve its overall genetic success through altruistic social behaviors. An **altruistic behavior** is one that helps ensure the success or survival of the rest of a social group, possibly at the expense of the success or survival of the individual. For example, the ground squirrel, a social mammal that lives in dens underground, will sound an alarm call if it sees a predator near the group. The alarm call does two things: first, it alerts the rest of the group to danger, and second, it calls the predator's attention to the particular squirrel that makes the noise. Therefore, in many instances, alerting the group results in the demise of the individual that sounded the alarm. Even though the alerter has not survived to reproduce, it has helped promote the survival of the rest of the clan, many of whom are probably close genetic relatives. In this way, the altruistic behavior of the ground squirrel has increased its own inclusive fitness by ensuring the survival of its siblings and other genetic relatives.

Chapter 22
Personality, Motivation, Attitudes, and Psychological Disorders

22.1 PERSONALITY

Theories of Personality

Personality, while very hard to precisely define, is essentially the unique pattern of thinking, feeling, and behavior associated with each person. Personalities are nuanced and complex. Various theories and perspectives on personality have evolved to help explain this fundamental aspect of individuality, including the psychoanalytic perspective, the humanistic perspective, the behaviorist perspective, the social cognitive perspective, the trait perspective, and the biological perspective. Therapies to treat personality disorders are based on the first four perspectives (psychoanalytic therapy, humanistic, or person-based therapy, and cognitive behavioral therapy).

Psychoanalytic Perspective

According to **psychoanalytic theory**, personality (made up of patterns of thoughts, feelings, and behaviors) is shaped by a person's unconscious thoughts, feelings, and memories. These unconscious elements are derived from his or her past experiences, particularly interactions with primary early caregivers. What a person is conscious of is quite limited compared with his or her vast unconscious stores of experiences, memories, needs, and motivations below the surface.

According to psychoanalytic theory, psychic energy is distributed among three personality components that function together: id, ego, and superego.

1) The largely unconscious **id** is the source of energy and instincts. Ruled by the **pleasure principle**, the id seeks to avoid pain and gain pleasure. It does not use logical or moral reasoning, and it does not distinguish mental images from external objects. According to Freud, young children function almost entirely from the id.

2) The **ego**, ruled by the **reality principle**, uses logical thinking and planning to control consciousness and the id. The ego tries to find realistic ways to satisfy the id's desire for pleasure.

3) The **superego** inhibits the id and influences the ego to follow moralistic and idealistic goals rather than just realistic goals; the superego strives for a "higher purpose." Based on societal values as learned from one's caregivers, the superego makes judgments of right and wrong and strives for perfection. The superego seeks to gain psychological rewards, such as feelings of pride and self-love, and to avoid psychological punishment such as feelings of guilt and inferiority.

According to psychoanalytic theory, at each developmental stage throughout the lifespan, certain needs and tasks must be satisfied. When these needs and tasks are not met, a person harbors unresolved unconscious conflicts that lead to psychological dysfunction. There are two different theories of developmental stages.

Psychosexual Stages (Freud)	Age	Psychosocial Stages (Erikson)
Oral • Sensual pleasure in mouth area	Birth to 1 year	Infancy • Trust vs. mistrust • Physical & emotional needs met
Anal • Sensual pleasure in controlling elimination	1–3 years	Early childhood • Autonomy vs. shame and doubts • Explore, make mistakes, test limits
Phallic • Sensual pleasure in genital area • Incestuous desire for the opposite-sex parent	3–6 years	Preschool age • Initiative vs. guilt • Make decisions
Latency • Sexual interests subside • Pursue school, friends, sports	6–12 years	School age • Industry vs. inferiority • Gender-role identity, school success, attain personal goals, understand the world
Genital • Sensual pleasure in genital area • Life/sexual energy fuels friendships, art, sports, careers	12–18 years	Adolescence • Identity vs. role confusion • Identity, goals, life meaning, limit-testing
	Young adulthood	Young adulthood • Intimacy vs. isolation • Form intimate relationships
	Middle adulthood	Middle age • Generativity vs. stagnation • Help next generation and resolve the difference between dreams and accomplishments
	Late adulthood	Later life • Integrity vs. despair • Look back with no regrets and feel personal worth

Table 1   Freud's and Erikson's Developmental Stages

According to **Sigmund Freud**, adult personality is largely determined during the first three psychosexual stages. If parents either frustrate or overindulge the child's expression of sensual pleasure at a certain stage so that the child does not resolve that stage's developmental conflicts, the child becomes **psychologically fixated** at that stage, and will, as an adult, continue to seek sensual pleasure through behaviors related to that stage.

Erik Erikson extended Freud's theory of developmental stages in two ways. Erikson added social and interpersonal factors, to supplement Freud's focus on unconscious conflicts and sexual urges within a person. And Erikson delineated eight developmental stages and conflicts in adolescence and adulthood, to supplement Freud's focus on early childhood. Note that for Erikson's stages, the age range is not strictly defined and can vary from individual to individual. For example, Erikson observed that many highly successful or influential people needed more time to discover their own identity, and the fourth stage of development for these individuals could extend well into their twenties and thirties. Stages could also overlap; for example, a child in the later part of the industry stage would likely still be working out conflicts related to initiative, and in the early phases of thinking about his identity.

Humanistic Perspective

In contrast to classical psychoanalytic theory, which tends to focus on conflicts and psychopathology, the **humanistic theory** focuses more on healthy personality development. According to this theory, humans are seen as inherently good and as having free will, rather than having their behavior determined by their early relationships. In humanistic theory, the most basic motive of all people is the **actualizing tendency**, which is an innate drive to maintain and enhance the organism. Like a child learning to walk, a person will grow toward **self-actualization**, or realizing his or her human potential, as long as no obstacle intervenes.

According to humanistic theory, as developed by **Carl Rogers**, when a child receives disapproval from a care-giver for certain behavior, he or she senses that the caregiver's positive regard is conditional. In order to win the caregiver's approval and still see both self and caregiver as good, the child introjects the caregiver's values, taking them on as part of his or her own self-concept. The **self-concept** is made up of the child's conscious, subjective perceptions and beliefs about him- or herself. The child's true values remain but are unconscious, as the child pursues experiences consistent with the introjected values rather than true values. The discrepancy between conscious introjected values and unconscious true values is the root of psychopathology. This discrepancy between the conscious and unconscious leads to tension, not knowing oneself, and a feeling that something is wrong. Rogers' solution was to for the parent (or therapist in treatment) to provide unconditional positive regard, which would allow the individual to pursue their own, unique and differentiated, self-concept.

People choose behavior consistent with their self-concepts. If they encounter experiences in life that contradict their self-concepts, they feel uncomfortable **incongruence**. By paying attention to his or her emotional reactions to experiences, a person in an incongruent state can learn what his or her true values are, and then become healthy again by modifying the introjected values and self-concept and growing toward fulfillment and completeness of self. However, people usually find it easier to deny or distort such experiences than to modify their self-concepts.

Behaviorist Perspective

According to the **behaviorist perspective**, personality is a result of learned behavior patterns based on a person's environment. Behaviorism is **deterministic**, proposing that people begin as blank slates, and environmental reinforcement and punishment completely determine and individual's subsequent behavior and personalities. This process begins in childhood and continues throughout the lifespan.

According to behaviorism, learning (and thus the development of personality) occurs through two forms of conditioning, classical conditioning, or operant conditioning. In classical conditioning, a person acquires a certain response to a stimulus after that stimulus is repeatedly paired with a second, different stimulus that already produces the desired response.

Social Cognitive Perspective

According to the **social cognitive perspective**, personality is formed by a reciprocal interaction among behavioral, cognitive, and environmental factors. The behavioral component includes patterns of behavior learned through classical and operant conditioning, as well as **observational learning**. Observational, or **vicarious**, learning occurs when a person watches another person's behavior and its consequences, thereby learning rules, strategies, and expected outcomes in different situations. For example, studies have found that children who watched aggressive and violent behavior in a video subsequently behaved with more aggression and violence toward a doll[1]. People are more likely to imitate models whom they like or admire, or who seem similar to themselves.

The cognitive component of personality includes the covert mental processes involved in observational or vicarious learning, as well as conscious cognitive processes such as self-efficacy beliefs (beliefs about one's own abilities). The environmental component includes situational influences, such as opportunities, rewards, and punishments.

Trait Perspective

A **personality trait** is a generally stable predisposition toward a certain behavior. Trait theories of personality focus on identifying, describing, measuring, and comparing individual differences and similarities with respect to such traits.

Trait theorists distinguish between surface and source traits. **Surface traits** are evident from a person's behavior. For example, a person might be described as talkative or exuberant. There are as many surface traits as there are adjectives for describing human behavior. Conversely, **source traits** are the factors underlying human personality and behavior; source traits are fewer and more abstract. Each trait is not binary but rather a continuum ranging between two or more extremes, such as extroversion and introversion. Trait theorists also differentiate among cardinal traits, which dominate a person's whole life and are very rare, central traits, which are stable characteristics used to describe a person, and secondary traits, which are abundant but more likely to vary based on situation.

The Five-Factor Model described by McCrae and Costa is one of the most popular trait theories of personality. The five factors in their model are extroversion, neuroticism, openness to experience, agreeableness, and conscientiousness. An individual can vary along each factor, and these traits have been shown through research to be predictive of an individual's behavior, and stable across the life span.

The **person-situation controversy** (also known and the **trait versus state controversy**) considers the degree to which a person's reaction in a given situation is due to their personality (trait) or is due to the situation itself (state). **Traits** are considered to be internal, stable, and enduring aspects of personality that should be consistent across most situations. **States** are situational; they are unstable, temporary, and variable aspects of personality that are influenced by the external environment. For example, extroversion is a trait, stress is a state. The primary question is whether personality is consistent over time and across situations and contexts. A fair amount of research suggests that while people's personality *traits* are fairly stable, their *behavior* in specific situations can be variable. In other words, people do not act with predictable consistency, even if their personality traits are predictably consistent. In unfamiliar situations, people tend to modify their behavior based on **social cues** (verbal or nonverbal hints that guide social interactions); therefore, specific traits may remain hidden. For example, a person who is normally quite extroverted may seem quiet and reserved in an unfamiliar formal situation. In familiar situations, people may "act more like themselves" (the same extroverted person may be considerably more talkative in a familiar situation with friends). Averaging behavior over many situations is the best way to reveal distinct personality traits.

---

[1] The infamous "Bobo doll" experiments conducted by Albert Bandura in the early 1960s; see Chapter 23.

Example 22-1: Which five factor model trait is most likely to be compromised due to unsuccessful resolution of Erikson's 4th stage?

- A) Openness
- B) Agreeableness
- C) Neuroticism
- D) Conscientiousness

Solution: Erikson's 4th stage is the industry vs. inferiority stage, which is concerned with learning about success and the drive to accomplish goals. Conscientiousness, or being careful, diligent, attentive, and aware, is most closely related to this resolution, and therefore most likely to be compromised (choice D is correct). Openness to experience is not necessarily compromised by lower industry (choice A is wrong). Agreeableness is related to how easy it is to get along with someone, how cooperative and kind they are. This is also not directly related to industry (choice B is wrong). Neuroticism is related to the amount of negative emotion someone experiences, and this is not necessarily compromised with unsuccessful resolution of industry vs. inferiority (choice C is wrong).

22.2 MOTIVATION

Factors that Influence Motivation

Instincts

There are several factors that are understood to influence motivation. The first is **instinct**: behaviors that are unlearned and present in fixed patterns throughout a species. In humans, instincts in babies include sucking behaviors, naturally holding the breath under water, and demonstrating fear when approaching drops in elevation. Instincts represent the contribution of genes, which predispose species to particular behaviors.

Drives / Negative Feedback Systems

Physiological drives can also push organisms to act in certain ways, as is the case when we are thirsty. A **drive** is an urge originating from a physiological discomfort such as hunger, thirst, or sleepiness. Drives can be useful for alerting an organism that it is no longer in a state of homeostasis, an internal state of equilibrium. They suggest that something is lacking: food, water, or sleep, for example. Drives often work through negative feedback systems, which are abundant in human physiology. The process of **negative feedback** works by maintaining stability or homeostasis; a system produces a product or end result, which feeds back to stop the system and maintain the product or end result within tightly controlled boundaries.

Arousal

However, instincts and drives cannot explain some of the artistic accomplishments of humans or the exploratory behavior of infants and animals. Even a toddler whose needs have all seemingly been met will wander around the room, putting objects in his or her mouth. This suggests that some behaviors are motivated by a desire to achieve an optimum level of arousal. Different people may have different optimal levels of arousal.

Needs

While including basic biological needs like the need for food, water, and shelter (the absence of which would produce physiological drives), this category also includes higher-level needs than those previously discussed. These include the need for belonging, positive affirmation, and love, which were elaborated by the humanist psychologist Abraham Maslow (see below).

Theories that Explain How Motivation Affects Human Behavior

Drive Reduction Theory

Since drives are physiological states of discomfort, it follows that we are motivated to reduce these drives through behaviors such as eating and drinking. Drive-reduction theory suggests that a physiological need creates an aroused state that drives the organism to reduce that need be engaging in some behavior. If your blood glucose drops, you feel hungry (or light-headed), and have a drive to eat. The greater the physiological need, the greater the physiological drive, an aroused, motivated state.

Incentive Theory

While drives are internal physiological needs, **incentives** are external stimuli, objects, and events in the environment that either help induce or discourage certain behaviors. Incentives can be positive and drive us to do something, or they can be negative and repel us from doing something. For example, if you were offered a new job accompanied by a large increase in salary, the salary might serve as a positive incentive. If the job also involved an increase in work hours, the increased workload might serve as a negative incentive. In general, behaviors are most strongly motivated when there are physiological needs, strong positive incentives, and a lack of negative incentives.

Maslow's Hierarchy of Needs

Abraham Maslow sought to explain human behavior by creating a hierarchy of needs (Figure 1). At the base of this pyramid are physiological needs discussed earlier, the basic elements necessary to sustain human life. If these needs are met, we will seek safety; if the need for safety is met, we will seek love, and so on. His pyramid suggests that some needs take priority over others. For example, an individual who is struggling every day to work and put food on the table will likely not be able to focus on fulfilling a cognitive need for belongingness by joining a community organization. The inclusion of higher-level needs, such as self-actualization and the need for recognition and respect from others also explains behaviors that the previous theories of motivation did not.

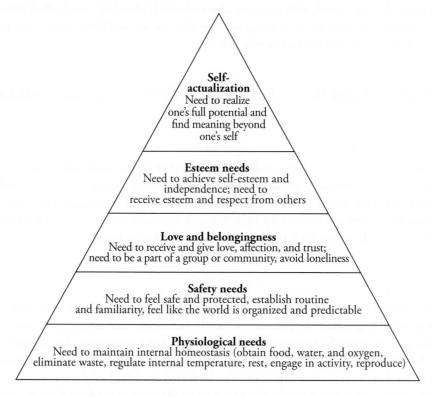

Figure 1 Maslow's Hierarchy of Needs

22.3 PSYCHOLOGICAL DISORDERS

It is estimated that in America, roughly 18% of adults (ages 18 and over) suffer from diagnosable mental illness, also known as a psychological disorder, each year. Roughly one in every six Americans has a diagnosable mental illness at any given time. Therefore, mental illness is an important part of our culture, and it is a significant component of our healthcare system. Psychological disorders, particularly when they go untreated, also affect our economy by impacting our social welfare and criminal justice systems.

Understanding Psychological Disorders

A **psychological disorder** is a set of behavioral and/or psychological symptoms that are not in keeping with cultural norms and that are severe enough to cause significant personal distress and/or significant impairment to social, occupational, or personal functioning. The presence of dysfunction is an important element of a psychological disorder.

Biopsychosocial Approach to Mental Health

Today, psychopathology recognizes the role of both nature (genetic predisposition) and nurture (environmental factors) on mental illness. Culture also influences the prevalence of various mental illnesses. For example, while not exclusive to Western cultures, eating disorders appear to be far more common in wealthier countries that espouse a thin ideal (like America) than they are in other parts of the world. It is possible that the underlying dynamic for various mental illnesses is similar, but that the manifestation of the illness is influenced by cultural or social factors. The following are the most common classes of disorders that are tested on the MCAT.

Broad Category	Description	Specific Psychological Disorders
Anxiety Disorders	Anxiety disorders are characterized by excessive fear (of specific real things or more generally) and/or anxiety (of real or imagined *future* things or events) with both physiological and psychological symptoms.	• Separation Anxiety Disorder • Specific Phobia(s) • Social Anxiety Disorder • Panic Disorder • Generalized Anxiety Disorder
Obsessive-Compulsive and Related Disorders	Disorders in this category are distinct from Anxiety Disorders in that they involve a pattern of obsessive thoughts or urges that are coupled with maladaptive behavioral compulsions; the compulsions are experienced as a necessary/urgent response to the obsessive thoughts/urges, creating rigid, anxiety-filled routines.	• Obsessive-Compulsive Disorder • Body Dysmorphic Disorder • Hoarding Disorder

22.3

Broad Category	Description	Specific Psychological Disorders
Trauma- and Stressor-Related Disorders	Traumas and stressors are central to the definition of these disorders, which involve unhealthy or pathological responses to one or more harmful or life-threatening events, including witnessing such an event. Subsequent symptoms include patterns of anxiety, depression, depersonalization, nightmares, insomnia, and/or a heightened startle response.	• Posttraumatic Stress Disorder • Acute Stress Disorder • Adjustment Disorders
Somatic Symptom Disorders	Somatic Symptom Disorders are characterized by symptoms that cannot be explained by a medical condition or substance use, and are not attributable to another psychological disorder, but that nonetheless cause emotional distress.	• Somatic Symptom Disorder • Illness Anxiety Disorder • Conversion Disorder • Factitious Disorder (imposed on self or another)
Bipolar and Related Disorders	Separate now from Mood Disorders, Bipolar and Related Disorders involve mood swings or cycles (called episodes) ranging from manic to depressive, in which manic episodes tend to be followed by depressive episodes and vice versa.	• Bipolar I Disorder • Bipolar II Disorder • Cyclothymic Disorder
Depressive Disorders	Depressive Disorders are characterized by a disturbance in mood or affect. Specific symptoms include difficulties in sleep, concentration, and/or appetite; fatigue; and inability to experience pleasure (anhedonia).	• Major Depressive Disorder • Persistent Depressive Disorder (dysthymia) • Premenstrual Dysphoric Disorder
Schizophrenia Spectrum and Other Psychotic Disorders	Psychotic disorders are characterized by a general "loss of contact with reality" that can include "positive" symptoms such as delusions and hallucinations and/or "negative" symptoms such as flattened affect (e.g., monotone vocal expression).	• Delusional Disorder • Brief Psychotic Disorder • Schizophreniform Disorder • Schizophrenia • Schizoaffective Disorder
Dissociative Disorders	Dissociative Disorders are characterized by disruptions in memory, awareness, identity, or perception. Many dissociative orders are thought to be caused by psychological trauma.	• Dissociative Identity Disorder • Dissociative Amnesia • Depersonalization/Derealization Disorder

Broad Category	Description	Specific Psychological Disorders
Personality Disorders	Personality Disorders are characterized by enduring maladaptive patterns of behavior and cognition that depart from social norms, present across a variety of contexts, and cause significant dysfunction and distress. These patterns permeate the broader personality of the person and typically solidify during late adolescence or early adulthood.	Cluster A: • Paranoid Personality Disorder • Schizoid Personality Disorder • Schizotypal Personality Disorder Cluster B: • Antisocial Personality Disorder • Borderline Personality Disorder • Histrionic Personality Disorder • Narcissistic Personality Disorder Cluster C: • Avoidant Personality Disorder • Dependent Personality Disorder • Obsessive-compulsive Personality Disorder

Table 2 Categories of Psychological Disorders

Alzheimer's Disease

Dementia is a term for a severe loss of cognitive ability beyond what would be expected from normal aging. Alzheimer's disease is the most prevalent form of dementia. It is a disease that is characterized behaviorally by an inability to form new memories, known as **anterograde amnesia**. Alzheimer's patients may be able to recall events from decades earlier but may forget people and events that were encountered recently. Their visual memory will be impaired as well, so they may often be lost and confused with regard to orientation. Needless to say, living with Alzheimer's disease can be very confusing and frustrating both for the patient and for family members.

Alzheimer's disease is a cortical disease, meaning that it affects the cortex, the outermost tissue of the brain. It is caused by the formation of **neuritic plaques,** hard formations of beta-amyloid protein and **neurofibrillary tangles** (clumps of tau protein).

There is some evidence of abnormalities in the activity of the neurotransmitter acetylcholine in the hippocampus. It should be no surprise that the hippocampus is involved, because this is the area of the brain that plays a major role in the formation of new memories. The disease tends to progress in a predictable pattern. As it progresses, the patient may lose older memories, language function, and spatial coordination. Eventually, patients are not able to perform daily functions without assistance.

Parkinson's Disease

Parkinson's disease is a movement disorder caused by the death of cells that generate dopamine in the **basal ganglia** and **substantia nigra**, two subcortical structures in the brain. Among the symptoms are a resting tremor (shaking), slowed movement, rigidity of movements of the face, and a shuffling gait. As the disease progresses, language is typically spared. However, depression and visual-spatial problems may arise. It is estimated that 50–80 percent of Parkinson's patients eventually experience dementia as their disease progresses. In order to treat Parkinson's, patients are given L-dopa treatments. L-dopa is a precursor to dopamine and is used because it is able to pass the blood–brain barrier and get into the brain's blood supply from the bloodstream in the body (dopamine is not able to cross the blood-brain barrier).

Example 22-2: Which symptom is most characteristic of a schizophrenia spectrum disorder?

A) Beliefs in uncanny physical powers
B) Persistent difficulty with sadness and feelings of worthlessness
C) Severe need for orderliness and discomfort with change in routine
D) Frequent oscillation among multiple split identities or personalities

Solution: One of the known symptoms of schizophrenia is delusional beliefs not grounded in reality, including delusions of grandeur (choice A is correct). Persistent sadness is more characteristic of depressive disorders, and although these may be comorbid with schizophrenia, feelings of sadness do not comprise part of the diagnostic criteria for schizophrenia disorders (choice B is wrong). Need for orderliness is most characteristic of obsessive-compulsive disorder (choice C is wrong). Dissociative identity disorders are characterized by fragmentation of a core identity into dissociative states (choice D is wrong).

Example 22-3: An individual calls a hotline reporting feelings of despair and sadness, coupled with inability to get out of bed, a complete lack of motivation, and suicidal ideations. They had not experienced a recent death in the family. Which of the following is the least likely explanation for these symptoms?

A) Borderline personality disorder
B) Histrionic personality disorder
C) Bipolar II disorder
D) Major depressive disorder

Solution: Histrionic personality disorder is characterized by need for the approval of others, need for constant attention and constantly "putting on a show." The symptoms described in the question stem are not consistent with the symptomology of Histrionic PD (choice B is correct). Borderline personality disorder is characterized by emotional instability and severe abandonment issues. It has high prevalence of suicidality and feelings of worthlessness, due to the severe emotional instability (choice A is wrong). Bipolar disorders (both I and II) include potentially severe depressive episodes that mirror the symptoms of major depressive disorders, such as the symptoms described in the question stem (choice C is wrong). The diagnostic criteria for major depressive disorder include each of the symptoms listed in the question stem, and is a likely explanation for the clinical presentation (choice D is wrong).

22.4 ATTITUDES

When psychologists refer to a person's **attitude**, they are referring to a person's feelings and beliefs about other people or events around them, and their tendency to react behaviorally based on those underlying evaluations. Attitudes are useful in that they provide a quick way to size things up and make decisions. However, they can also lead us astray when they lead to inaccurate snap judgments or when they remain fixed beliefs in the face of disconfirming evidence. Attitudes are considered to have three main components (the ABCs): affect (emotion), behavior tendencies, and cognition (thought).

The Link Between Attitudes and Behavior

Social psychologists have found that there are some situations in which attitudes better predict behavior. Those are as follows:

1) *When social influences are reduced.* Compared to attitudes, which are more internal, external behavior is much more susceptible to social influences. People are much more likely to be honest in a secret ballot process than if they must overtly express their opinions. This is in large part due to fear of criticism and the powerful influence of factors such as conformity and groupthink (discussed earlier).

2) *When general patterns of behavior, rather than specific behaviors, are observed.* Our attitudes are better at predicting overall decision-making rather than specific behaviors. For example, one who believes in a healthy lifestyle will tend to make healthier decisions than someone who does not, yet this attitude does not necessarily prevent someone from occasionally reaching for a slice of cheesecake. This is known as the **principle of aggregation**: an attitude affects a person's aggregate or average behavior, but not necessarily each isolated act.

3) *When specific, rather than general, attitudes are considered.* Belief in a healthy lifestyle can be a poor predictor of a specific behavior, such as eating properly. It would be wiser to compare the specific attitude that the individual has toward eating properly, because it will be a better predictor of this particular behavior. Thus, it is most accurate to consider specific attitudes closely related to the specific behavior of interest.

4) *When attitudes are made more powerful through self-reflection.* People are more likely to behave in accordance with their attitudes if they are given some time to prepare themselves to do so. When people act automatically, they may be impulsive and act in ways that do not match expressed beliefs. However, when given more time to deliberate over actions, they are more likely to act in ways that match.

Processes by Which Behavior Influences Attitudes

What is perhaps more interesting is the notion that behavior sometimes precedes and affects our attitudes. There are several situations in which behaviors are likely to influence attitudes.

1) *Role-playing.* The most notable influence of behavior on attitudes is **role-playing**. Consider how social roles such as "soldier" and "slave" may have affected how people have acted over the course of history. In wartime, soldiers' beliefs about the enemy become dramatically altered over time, with feelings of ambivalence giving way to perceiving the enemy as "evil."

2) *Public Declarations.* In order to please others, people may feel a pressure to adapt what they say. What's interesting is that saying something publicly—a **public declaration**—can become believing it in the absence of bribery, coercion, or some other blatant external motive. As we continue to express ourselves over time, we become more and more entrenched in believing what we say, a habit that is even stronger for statements made publicly.

3) *Justification of Effort.* Just as people may modify their attitudes to match their language, they may also modify them to match their behaviors. This is often referred to as **justification of effort**. For example, consider a student who works hard to study for the MCAT and earns a fantastic score, only to feel a calling toward becoming an actor rather than going to medical school at the end of the process. In order to justify the effort already put into the process, the student will feel a pressure to go to medical school.

Elaboration Likelihood Model

Persuasion is one method of attitude and behavior change. When you change your beliefs about something there are a few factors that likely come into play. The **elaboration likelihood model** explains when people will be influenced by the content of the speech (or the logic of the arguments), and when people will be influenced by other, more superficial characteristics like the appearance of the orator or the length of the speech.

Since persuasion can be such a powerful means for influencing what people think and do, much research has gone into studying the various elements of a message that might have an impact on its persuasiveness. The three key elements are message characteristics, source characteristics, and target characteristics.

1) The **message characteristics** are the features of the message itself, such as the logic and number of key points in the argument. Message characteristics also include more superficial things, such as the length of the speech or article and its grammatical complexity.
2) The **source characteristics** of the person or venue delivering the message, such as expertise, knowledge, and trustworthiness, are also of importance.
3) Finally, the **target characteristics** of the person receiving the message, such as self-esteem, intelligence, mood, and other such personal characteristics, have an important influence on whether a message will be perceived as persuasive.

The two **cognitive routes** that persuasion follows under this model are the central route and the peripheral route. Under the **central route,** people are persuaded by the content of the argument. They ruminate over the key features of the argument and allow those features to influence their decision to change their point of view. The **peripheral route** functions when people focus on superficial or secondary characteristics of the speech or the orator. Under these circumstances, people are persuaded by the attractiveness of the orator, the length of the speech, whether the orator is considered an expert in his field, and other features. The elaboration likelihood model then argues that people will choose the central route only when they are both motivated to listen to the logic of the argument (they are interested in the topic), and they are not distracted, thus focusing their attention on the argument. If those conditions are not met, individuals will choose the peripheral route, and they will be persuaded by more superficial factors. Messages processed via the central route are more likely to have longer-lasting persuasive outcomes than messages processed via the peripheral route.

Cognitive Dissonance Theory

When considering how behaviors can shape attitudes, self-justification plays an important part. In role-playing, public declarations, and justification of effort scenarios, individuals justify their actions (including language) through beliefs. The theory that seeks to explain why self-justification is such a powerful influence on attitude modification is cognitive dissonance theory.

Cognitive dissonance theory explains that we feel tension ("dissonance") whenever we hold two thoughts or beliefs ("cognitions") that are incompatible, or when attitudes and behaviors don't match. When this occurs, we may feel like hypocrites or feel confused as to where we stand. The theory explains that in order to reduce this unpleasant feeling of tension, we make our views of the world match how we feel or what we've done.

Example 22-4: How is the mere exposure effect likely to impact attitude, aggression, impression management (from end of Chapter 21)?

- A) An increase in the influence of behavior on attitude due to role-playing
- B) An increase in the influence of attitude on behavior due to increased social influences
- C) An increase in the influence of behavior on attitude due to justification of effort
- D) An increase in the influence of behavior on attitude due to the principle of aggregation

22.4

Solution: Mere exposure suggests that we have higher regard for people, things, and experiences that we come into contact with frequently. It is possible that due to repeated exposure, an individual might view time and energy spent as a type of effort and justify this effort by viewing the other person, thing, or experience in a more positive light. In this way, there could be a link between mere exposure and justification of effort. Note that not all correct answers on the MCAT are perfectly justified, and this is a classic example of a "least bad" answer being correct and requires POE to check all answer choices (choice C is correct). Mere exposure suggests simply coming into contact with someone or something, and although role-playing could be involved, there is no direct link between exposure and assuming roles (choice A is wrong). The influence of attitude on behavior is increased when social influences are reduced, so this answer choice reverses the relationship (choice B is wrong). This is also the case for choice D, because the principle of aggregation increases the influence of attitude on behavior, not the other way around (choice D is wrong).

Chapter 23
Learning, Memory, and Behavior

23.1 TYPES OF LEARNING

Nonassociative Learning

Nonassociative learning occurs when an organism is repeatedly exposed to one type of stimulus. Two important types of nonassociative learning are habituation and sensitization. A **habit** is an action that is performed repeatedly until it becomes automatic, and **habituation** follows a very similar process. Essentially, a person learns to "tune out" the stimulus. For example, suppose you live near train tracks and trains pass by your house on a regular basis. An example of habituation would be when you are able to tune out the sounds of the trains that pass by your house regularly.

Dishabituation occurs when the previously habituated stimulus is removed. After a person has been habituated to a given stimulus, the person is no longer accustomed to the stimulus. If the stimulus is then presented again, the person will react to it as if it was a new stimulus, and he or she is likely to respond even more strongly to it than before.

Sensitization is, in many ways, the opposite of habituation. During sensitization, there is an increase in the responsiveness due to either a repeated application of a stimulus or a particularly aversive or noxious stimulus. Instead of being able to "tune out" or ignore the stimulus and avoid reacting at all (as in habituation), the stimulus actually produces a more exaggerated response. Sensitization may also cause you to respond more vigorously to other similar stimuli. Sensitization is usually temporary and may not result in any type of long-term behavior change.

Associative Learning

Associative learning describes a process of learning in which one event, object, or action is directly connected with another. There are two general categories of associative learning: classical conditioning and operant conditioning.

Classical Conditioning

Classical conditioning is a process in which two stimuli are paired in such a way that the response to one of the stimuli changes. The archetypal example of this is Pavlov's dogs. **Ivan Pavlov**, who first named and described the process of classical conditioning, did so by training his dogs to salivate at the sound of a ringing bell. Dogs naturally salivate at the sight and smell of food; it is a biological response that prepares the dogs for food consumption. The stimulus (food) naturally produces this response (salivating), however, dogs do not intrinsically react to the sound of a bell in any particular way. Pavlov's famous experiment paired the sound of a bell (an auditory stimulus) with the presentation of food to the dogs, and after a while, the dogs began to salivate to the sound of a bell even in the absence of food. The process of pairing the two initially unrelated stimuli changed the dogs' response to the sound of the bell over time; they became conditioned to salivate when they heard it. The dogs effectively learned that the sound of the bell was meant to announce food.

This example demonstrates a few key concepts about classical conditioning. This type of learning relies on specific stimuli and responses.

- A **neutral stimulus** is a stimulus that initially does not elicit any intrinsic response. For Pavlov's dogs, this was the sound of the bell prior to the experiment.
- An **unconditioned stimulus** (US) is a stimulus that elicits an **unconditioned response** (UR). Think of this response like a reflex. It is not a learned reaction, but a biological one: in this case, the presentation of food is the unconditioned stimulus and the salivation is the unconditioned response. Dogs automatically salivate when food is presented.
- A **conditioned stimulus** (CS) is an originally neutral stimulus (bell) that is paired with an unconditioned stimulus (food) until it can produce the conditioned response (salivation) without the unconditioned stimulus (food).
- Finally, the **conditioned response** (CR) is the learned response to the conditioned stimulus. It is the same as the unconditioned response, but now it occurs without the unconditioned stimulus. For the dogs, salivating at the sound of the bell is the conditioned response.

Acquisition, extinction, spontaneous recovery, generalization, and discrimination are the processes by which classically conditioned responses are developed and maintained.

1) **Acquisition** refers to the process of learning the conditioned response. This is the time during the experiment when the bell and food are always paired.
2) **Extinction**, in classical conditioning, occurs when the conditioned and unconditioned stimuli are no longer paired, so the conditioned response eventually stops occurring. After the dogs have been conditioned to salivate at the sound of bell, if the sound is presented to the dogs over and over without being paired with the food, then after some period of time the dogs will eventually stop salivating at the sound of the bell.
3) **Spontaneous recovery** is when an extinct conditioned response occurs again when the conditioned stimulus is presented after some period of time. For example, if the behavior of salivating to the sound of the bell becomes extinct in a dog, and is then presented to the dog again after some amount of lapsed time and the dog salivates, the conditioned response was spontaneously recovered.
4) **Generalization** refers to the process by which stimuli other than the original conditioned stimulus elicit the conditioned response. So, if the dogs salivate to the sound of a chime or a doorbell, even though those were not the same sounds as the conditioned stimulus, the behavior has been generalized.
5) **Discrimination** is the opposite of generalization, and it occurs when the conditioned stimulus is differentiated from other stimuli; thus, the conditioned response only occurs for conditioned stimuli. If the dogs do not salivate at the sound of a buzzer or a horn, they have differentiated those stimuli from the sound of a bell.

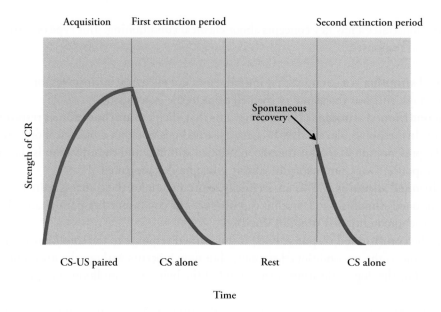

Figure 1 Curve of Acquisition, Extinction, and Spontaneous Recovery in Classical Conditioning

Organisms seem predisposed to learn associations that are adaptive in nature. One powerful and very long-lasting association in most animals (including humans) is **taste-aversion** caused by nausea and/or vomiting. An organism that eats a specific food and becomes ill a few hours later will generally develop a strong aversion to that food. Most organisms develop the aversion specifically to the smell or taste of the food (occurs in most mammals), but it is also possible to develop an aversion to the sight of the food (occurs in birds). The function of this quickly-learned response is to prevent an organism from consuming something that might be toxic or poisonous in the future. This response happens to be one that does not need a long acquisition phase (it is typically acquired after one exposure) and has a very long extinction phase; in fact for most organisms, it never extinguishes.

Operant Conditioning

The other category of associative learning is **operant** (or instrumental) **conditioning.** Whereas classical conditioning connects unconditioned and neutral stimuli to create conditioned responses, operant conditioning uses reinforcement (pleasurable consequences) and punishment (unpleasant consequences) to mold behavior and eventually cause associative learning. However, just as with classical conditioning, timing is everything. In classical conditioning, it was important for the neutral stimulus to be paired with the unconditioned stimulus (that is, for them to occur together or very close together in time), in order for the neutral stimulus to become conditioned. In operant conditioning, it is just as important for the reinforcement or the punishment to occur around the same time as the behavior in order for learning to occur, in this case just after.

One of the most famous people to conduct research in the area of operant conditioning was **B.F. Skinner**. Skinner worked with animals and designed an operant conditioning chamber (later called a "Skinner box") that he used in a series of experiments to shape animal behavior. For example, in one series of experiments, a hungry rat would be placed inside a Skinner box that contained a lever. If the rat pressed the lever, a food pellet would drop into the box. Often the rat would first touch the lever by mistake, but after discovering that food would appear in response to pushing the lever, the rat would continue to do so until it was sated. In another series of experiments, the Skinner box would be wired to deliver a painful electric shock until a lever was pushed. In this example, the rat would run around trying to avoid the shock at first, until accidentally hitting the lever and causing the shock to stop. On repeated trials, the rat would quickly push the lever to end the painful shock.

These examples demonstrate a few key concepts about operant conditioning.

1) **Reinforcement** is anything that will increase the likelihood that a preceding behavior will be repeated; the behavior is supported by a reinforcement. There are two major types of reinforcement: positive and negative.
   - **Positive reinforcement** is some sort of positive stimulus that occurs immediately following a behavior. In the above experiments, the food pellet was a positive reinforcer for the hungry rat because it causes the rat to repeat the desired behavior (push the lever).
   - **Negative reinforcement** is some sort of negative stimulus that is *removed* immediately following a behavior. In the above experiments, the electric shock is a negative reinforcer for the rat because it causes the rat to repeat the desired behavior (again, push the lever) to remove the undesirable stimulus (the painful shock).

Anything that *increases* a desired behavior is a reinforcer; both positive and negative reinforcements increase the desired behavior, but the process by which they do so is different. Positive reinforcement does it by adding something desirable; negative reinforcement does it by removing something undesirable). Positive in this context refers to something that is added to the environment, and negative refers to something that is taken away.

Another key distinction for reinforcement is between primary and secondary or unconditioned and conditioned reinforcers.

1) **Primary** (or unconditioned) **reinforcers** are somehow innately satisfying or desirable. These are reinforcers that we do not need to learn to see as reinforcers because they are integral to our survival. Food is a primary positive reinforcer for all organisms because it is required for survival. Avoiding pain and danger are primary negative reinforcers for the same reason; avoidance is important for survival.

2) **Secondary** (or conditioned) **reinforcers** are those that are learned to be reinforcers. These are neutral stimuli that are paired with primary reinforcers to make them conditioned. For example, suppose that every time a child reads a book, she receives a stamp. After accruing ten stamps, she can exchange these for a small pizza. The pizza, being food, is the primary reinforcer, and the stamps are secondary reinforcer.

Operant conditioning relies on a **reinforcement schedule**. This schedule can be **continuous**, in which every occurrence of the behavior is reinforced, or it can be **intermittent**, in which occurrences are sometimes reinforced and sometimes not. Continuous reinforcement will result in rapid behavior **acquisition** (or rapid learning), but it will also result in rapid **extinction** when the reinforcement ceases. Intermittent reinforcement typically results in slower acquisition of behavior, but great persistence (or resistance to extinction) of that behavior over time. Therefore, it is possible to initially condition a behavior using a continuous reinforcement schedule, then **maintain** that behavior using an intermittent reinforcement schedule. For instance, a dog can be trained to sit in response to a hand motion in a continuous reinforcement schedule where a treat is given every time the dog sits; once the dog has sufficiently mastered this behavior, you can switch to an intermittent reinforcement schedule, where the dog receives a treat only occasionally when it sits in response to the hand motion.

There are four important intermittent reinforcement schedules: fixed-ratio, variable-ratio, fixed-interval, and variable-interval. Ratio schedules are based on the number of instances of a desired behavior, and interval schedules are based on time.

1) A **fixed-ratio schedule** provides the reinforcement after a set number of instances of the behavior. Returning to the example of a hungry rat in a Skinner box, if the rat receives a food pellet every 10 times it pushes the lever, after it has been conditioned, the rat will demonstrate a high rate of response (in other words, it will push the lever rapidly, many times to get the food).

2) A **variable-ratio schedule** provides the reinforcement after an unpredictable number of occurrences. A classic example of reinforcement provided on a variable-ratio schedule is gambling; the reinforcement may be unpredictable, but the behavior will be repeated with the hope of a reinforcement. Both fixed-ratio schedules and variable-ratio schedules produce high response rates; the chances that a behavior will produce the desired outcome (a treat or a jackpot or some other reinforcement) increases with the number responses (times the behavior is performed).

3) A **fixed-interval schedule** provides the reinforcement after a set period of time that is constant. The behavior will increase as the reinforcement interval comes to an end. For example, if an employee is reinforced by attention from the boss, the employee might work hard all the time, thinking the boss will walk by at any second and notice the hard work (and provide the positive reinforcement, attention). Once the employee learns that the boss only walks by at the top of the hour every hour, the employee may become an ineffective worker throughout the day, but be more effective as the top of the hour approaches.

4) A **variable-interval schedule** provides the reinforcement after an inconsistent amount of time. This schedule produces a slow, steady behavior response rate, because the amount of time it will take to get the reinforcement is unknown. In the employee-boss example, if the boss walks by at unpredictable times each day, the employee does not know when they might receive the desired reinforcement (attention). Thus, the employee will work in a steady, efficient manner throughout the day, but not very quickly. The employee knows it doesn't matter how quickly he works at any given time, because the potential reinforcement is tied to an unpredictable time schedule.

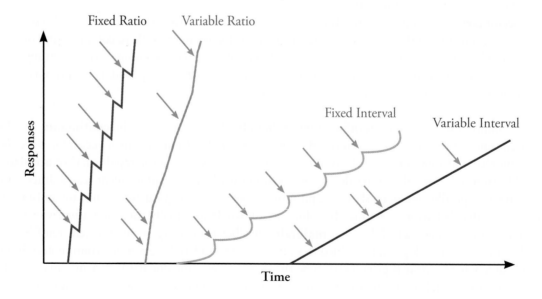

Figure 2   Behavior Response Patterns to Each of the Four Reinforcement Schedules

Like reinforcement, punishment is also an important element of operant conditioning, but the effect is the opposite: reinforcement *increases* behavior, while punishment *decreases* it. **Punishment** is the process by which a behavior is followed by a consequence that decreases the likelihood that the behavior will be repeated. Like reinforcement, punishment can be both positive AND negative. **Positive punishment** involves the application, or pairing, of an undesirable stimulus with the behavior. For example, if cadets speak out of turn in military boot camp, the drill sergeant makes them do twenty pushups. On the contrary, **negative punishment** involves the removal of a desirable stimulus after the behavior has occurred. For example, if a child breaks a window while throwing a baseball in the house, they lose TV privileges for a week. Positive punishment *adds* and negative punishment *subtracts*. Commonly, reinforcement and punishment are used in conjunction when shaping behaviors; however, it is uncommon for punishment to have as much of a lasting effect as reinforcement. Once the punishment has been removed, then it is no longer effective. Furthermore, punishment only instructs what *not* to do, whereas reinforcement instructs what *to* do. Reinforcement is therefore a better alternative to encourage behavior change and learning. Additionally, the processes described for classical conditioning (acquisition, extinction, spontaneous recovery, generalization, and discrimination) occur in operant conditioning as well.

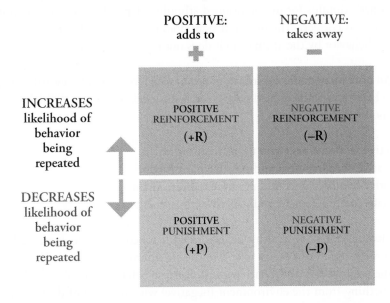

Figure 3   Schematic of Positive and Negative Reinforcements and Punishments

In conclusion, let's examine two specific types of operant learning: escape and avoidance. In **escape,** an individual learns how to get away from an aversive stimulus by engaging in a particular behavior. This helps reinforce the behavior so they will be willing to engage in it again. For example, a child does not want to eat her vegetables (aversive stimulus) so she throws a temper tantrum. If the parents respond by not making the child eat the vegetables, then she will learn that behaving in that specific way will help her escape that particular aversive stimulus. On the other hand, **avoidance** occurs when a person performs a behavior to ensure an aversive stimulus is not presented. For example, a child notices Mom cooking vegetables for dinner and fakes an illness so Mom will send him to bed with ginger ale and crackers. The child has effectively avoided confronting the aversive stimulus (the offensive vegetables) altogether. As long as either of these techniques work (meaning the parents do not force the child to eat the vegetables), the child is reinforced to perform the escape and/or avoidance behaviors.

Example 23-1: A bell has been used in conditioning paradigms to both indicate to organisms that a shock will occur, which can be preempted with pressing a lever, and to signal that food is on its way. What is the correct terminology to describe the use of the bell in each of these two instances, respectively?

- A) Avoidance and positive reinforcement
- B) Escape and unconditioned stimulus
- C) Positive reinforcement and spontaneous recovery
- D) Negative reinforcement and conditioned stimulus

Solution: If a bell is used to indicate that a shock will subsequently be initiated, and the organism can avoid the shock by pressing a lever, this is an example of avoidance. Note that avoidance is also a type of negative reinforcement, since pain from shock is removed from the environment (negative = taken away) and the behavior of pressing the lever is increased (increase in behavior = reinforcement). This eliminates choices B and C. In the second part, the food is used to signal that food will be presented, not in response to any behavior by the organism. Therefore, this indicates a classical conditioning paradigm, and the bell could be a conditioned stimulus (or unconditioned stimulus, depending on the amount of training that has occurred; choice D is correct). The question stem does not indicate that the presentation of the food is dependent on any behavior by the animal, so it does not represent reinforcement (choice A is wrong).

Example 23-2: An outpatient addiction rehab program uses a redeemable reward program to encourage alternative healthy behaviors while earned tokens are lost for relapse events. Which of the following best describes this methodology?

- A) Positive reinforcement and negative punishment
- B) Negative reinforcement and positive punishment
- C) Positive reinforcement and negative reinforcement
- D) Negative reinforcement and negative punishment

Solution: The encouragement of healthy behaviors with tokens seeks to increase behavior (reinforcement) by adding something, in this case a token, to the environment (positive). Therefore, this is a type of positive reinforcement (choices B and D are wrong). Relapse behaviors involve the loss of tokens. This is the removal of something from the environment (negative) with the goal of decreasing relapse behaviors (punishment). Therefore, it is a type of negative punishment (choice A is correct, and choice C is wrong).

Observational Learning

More advanced organisms, particularly humans, do not learn only through direct experience. **Observational learning,** also known as **social learning** or **vicarious learning**, is learning through watching and imitating others.

Modeling

Modeling is one of the most basic mechanisms behind observational learning. In modeling, an observer sees the behavior being performed by another person. Later, with the model in mind, the observer **imitates** the behavior he observed.

Typically, the likelihood of imitating a modeled behavior is based on how successful someone finds that behavior to be, or the type of reinforcement that the model received for his behavior. However, individuals may choose to imitate behaviors even if they do not observe the consequences of the model's behavior. For instance, **Albert Bandura** conducted a series of experiments using a Bobo doll. Bandura showed children videos of adults either behaving aggressively towards the Bobo doll (punching, kicking, and shouting at the doll) or ignoring him all together. Even when children did not see the consequences of the adult's behavior, they tended to imitate the behavior they saw. Later studies conducted by others support that humans are prone to imitation and modeling, and we are particularly likely to imitate those that we perceive as similar to ourselves, as successful, or as admirable in some way. Therefore, modeling, and social learning in general, is a very powerful influence on individuals' behaviors.

Social Cognitive Theory

The social cognitive perspective incorporates elements of cognition, learning, and social influence. **Social Cognitive Theory** is a theory of behavior change that emphasizes the interactions between people and their environment. However, unlike behaviorism (where the environment controls us), cognition (how we process our environment) is also important in determining our behavior. Social cognitive theory focuses on how we interpret and respond to external events, and how our past experiences, memories, and expectations influence our behavior. According to social cognitive theory, **social factors**, observational learning, and environmental factors can also influence a person's attitude change. The opinions and attitudes of your friends, family members, and other peer groups often have a major influence on your beliefs. Social cognition was discussed in Chapter 21.

Reciprocal determinism is the interaction between a person's behaviors (conscious actions), personal factors (individual motivational forces or cognitions; personality differences that drive a person to act), and environment (situational factors). There are three different ways that individuals and environments interact:

1) People choose their environments which in turn shape them. For example, the college that you chose to attend had some sort of a unique impact on you.
2) Personality shapes how people interpret and respond to their environment. For example, people prone to depression are more likely to view their jobs as pointless.
3) A person's personality influences the situation to which she then reacts. Experiments have demonstrated that how you treat someone else influences how they will treat you. For example, if you call customer service because you are furious about something, you are more likely to receive a defensive or aggressive response on the phone.

23.2 HUMAN DEVELOPMENT

Developmental psychology is the study of how humans develop physically, cognitively, and socially, throughout their lifetime. As previously discussed, genetics and environment play an important role in human development.

Early Brain Development

During prenatal development, the brain actually produces more neurons than needed. At birth, humans have the highest number of neurons at any point in their life, and these are pruned throughout the ensuing lifetime. However, the immature brain does not have many **neural networks**, or codified routes for information processing (the types that are generated in response to learning and experience throughout a lifetime). During infancy and early childhood development, these neurons form neural networks, and networks are reinforced by learning and behavior. From ages 3 to 6, the most rapid growth occurs in the frontal lobes, corresponding to an increase in rational planning and attention. The association areas, linked with thinking, memory, and language, are the last cortical areas to develop. (For more information on cognitive development, see Jean Piaget in Chapter 24.)

Maturation is the sequence of biological growth processes in human development. Maturation, while largely genetic, is still influenced by environment. For example, while humans are programmed to learn how to speak, first using one-word utterances, then developing progressively more complex speech, severe deprivation can significantly delay this process, while an incredibly nurturing environment might speed it up. The developing brain allows for motor development; as the nervous system and muscles mature, more and more complex physical skills develop. The sequence of motor development is almost entirely universal. Babies learn to roll over, then sit, then crawl, then stand, then walk (see rudimentary movements above). The development of the cerebellum is a necessary precursor to walking, and most humans learn to walk around age one.

Social Development and Attachment

From approximately 8–12 months of age, young children display **stranger anxiety** (crying and clinging to caregiver). Around this time, infants have developed schemas for familiar faces, and when new faces do not fit an already developed schema, the infant becomes distressed. Infant-parent attachment bonds are an important survival impulse. Stranger anxiety seems to peek around 13 months for children and then gradually declines. For many years it was assumed that infants attached to their parents because they provided nourishment, but an accidental experiment actually countered this assumption.

In the 1950s, two psychologists (**Harry Harlow** and **Margaret Harlow**) bred monkeys for experiments. To control for environment and to reduce the incidence of disease, infant monkeys were separated from their mothers at birth (maternal deprivation) and provided with a baby blanket. When the blankets were removed for laundering, the baby monkeys became very distressed because they had formed an intense attachment to the object. This physical attachment seemed to contradict the idea that attachment was formed based on nourishment, so the Harlows designed a series of experiments to further investigate. In one experiment, the Harlows fashioned two artificial mothers—one nourishing (a wire frame with a wooden head and a bottle) and the other cloth (wire frame with a wooden head and a cloth blanket wrapped around it). They found that the baby monkeys preferred the cloth mother, clinging to her and spending the majority of their time with her, visiting the other mother only to feed. Harlow concluded that "contact comfort" was an essential element of infant/mother bonding and essential to psychological development.

Mary Ainsworth conducted a series of experiments called the "strange situation experiments," where mothers would leave their infants in an unfamiliar environment (usually a laboratory playroom) to see how the infants would react. These studies suggested that attachment styles vary among infants. **Securely attached** infants in the presence of their mother (or primary caregiver) will play and explore; when the mother leaves the room, the infant is distressed, and when the mother returns, the infant will seek contact with her and is easily consoled. **Insecurely attached** infants in the presence of their mother (or primary caregiver) are less likely to explore their surroundings and may cling to their mother; when the mother leaves they will either cry loudly and remain upset or will demonstrate indifference to her departure and return. Observations indicate that securely attached infants have sensitive and responsive mothers (or primary caregivers) who are quick to attend to their child's needs in a consistent fashion. Insecurely attached infants have mothers (or primary caregivers) who are insensitive and unresponsive, attending to their child's needs inconsistently or sometimes even ignoring their children. In the Harlow's monkeys experiments described above, the cloth mother would be considered rather insensitive and unresponsive; when these monkeys were put in situations without their artificial mothers they became terrified[1].

23.3 MEMORY

Encoding

Process of Encoding Information

Encoding is the process of transferring sensory information into our memory system. Working memory—where information is maintained temporarily as part of a particular mental activity (learning, solving a problem)—is thought to include a phonological loop, visuospatial sketchpad, central executive, and episodic buffer (Chapter 24). Working memory is quite limited, and this model helps to explain the **serial position effect**. This effect occurs when someone attempts to memorize a series, such as a list of words. In an immediate recall condition (shortly after the information is first presented), the individual is more likely to recall the first and last items on the list. These phenomena are called the **primacy effect** and the **recency effect**. It is hypothesized that first items are more easily recalled because they have had the most time to be encoded and transferred to long-term memory. Last items may be more easily recalled because they may still be in the phonological loop and so may be readily available. When the individual is asked to recall the list at a later point, the individual tends to remember only the first items well. This may be because that was the only information that was transferred to long-term memory, whereas recent information from the phonological loop would quickly decay and be lost.

---

[1] Note: this type of extreme deprivation experiment would no longer be considered ethical or humane today; research animals in captivity are treated much better.

Processes That Aid in Encoding Memories

A **mnemonic** is any technique for improving retention and retrieval of information from memory. One simple process that aids memory is use of the phonological loop through **rehearsal**. If someone were to give you a phone number and you didn't have any way to record the information, you might repeat the digits over and over in your head until you were able to write them down. In some cases, repeated rehearsal can lead to encoding into long-term memory.

Chunking is a strategy in which information to be remembered is organized into discrete groups of data. For example, with phone numbers, one might memorize the area code, the first three digits, and the last four digits as discrete chunks. Thus, the number of "things" being remembered is decreased—in the case of a phone number, there are now three "things" to memorize instead of 10 individual digits. This is an important strategy because the limit of working memory is generally understood to be about seven digits. Even the process of remembering that a group of letters makes a particular word involves chunking.

There is some evidence that **depth of processing** is important for encoding memories. Information that is thought about at a deeper level is better remembered. For example, it is easier to remember the general plot of a book than it is the exact words, meaning that semantic information (meaning) is more easily remembered than grammatical information (form) when the goal is to learn a concept.

The **dual coding hypothesis** indicates that it is easier to remember words with associated images than either words or images alone. By encoding both a visual mental representation and an associated word, there are more connections made to the memory and an opportunity to process the information at a deeper level. For this reason, imagery is a useful mnemonic device. One aid for memory is to use the **method of loci**. This involves imagining moving through a familiar place, such as your home, and in each place, leaving a visual representation of a topic to be remembered. For recall, then, the images of the places could be called upon to bring into awareness the associated topics.

Memory Storage

Types of Memory Storage

Different stores of memory include sensory memory, short-term memory, and long-term memory. **Sensory memory,** the initial recording of sensory information in the memory system, is a very brief snapshot that quickly decays. Two types of sensory memory are iconic memory and echoic memory. **Iconic memory** is brief photographic memory for visual information, which decays in a few tenths of a second. **Echoic memory** is memory for sound, which lasts for about 3–4 seconds. This is why sometimes in a conversation, you might ask what someone said if you had trouble hearing him or her, only to hear and make sense of the words yourself a second later. Information from sensory memory decays rapidly if it is not passed through Broadbent's filter into short-term memory. **Short-term memory** is also limited in duration and in capacity. Recall capacity for an adult is typically around seven items, plus or minus two. This is why phone numbers with seven digits (excluding area code) are conveniently remembered. As discussed earlier, although chunking increases the amount of information remembered by putting more information into each chunk, it is still subject to this limit of about seven chunks. Information in short-term memory is retained only for about 20 seconds, unless it is actively processed so that it can be transferred into long-term memory. **Long-term memory** is information that is retained sometimes indefinitely; it is believed to have an infinite capacity.

Implicit or **procedural memory** refers to conditioned associations and knowledge of how to do something, while **explicit** or **declarative memory** involves being able to "declare" or voice what is known. For example, one could read a book on how to develop a great shot in basketball from cover to cover and be able to explain in great detail the necessary steps. However, this book knowledge would not likely translate into being able to execute the shot on the court without practice. Explaining the concept involves explicit or declarative memory, while not having practiced it indicates a lack of implicit or procedural memory. Semantic and episodic memory are two subdivisions of explicit memory. **Semantic memory** is memory for factual information, such as the capital of England. **Episodic memory** is autobiographical memory for information of personal importance, such as the situation surrounding a first kiss. Typically, semantic memory deteriorates before episodic memory does.

The distinction between explicit and implicit memory is supported by neurological evidence. Brain structures involved in memory include the hippocampus, cerebellum, and amygdala. The hippocampus is necessary for the encoding of new explicit memories. The cerebellum is involved in learning skills and conditioned associations (implicit memory). The amygdala is involved in associating emotion with memories, particularly negative memories. Interestingly, the implicit memories that infants make are retained indefinitely, but the explicit memories that infants make are largely not retained beyond about age four—a phenomenon known as **infantile amnesia**. It is only later, after the hippocampus has fully developed, that explicit memories are retained long-term.

Retrieval

Recall, Recognition, and Relearning

Retrieval is the process of finding information stored in memory. When most people think of retrieval, they think of **recall**, the ability to retrieve information. **Free recall** involves retrieving the item "out of thin air," while **cued recall** involves retrieving the information when provided with a cue. For example, a test of free recall would be to ask a student to name all of the capital cities of the world. A test of cued recall would be to provide the student with a list of countries and then ask him or her to name all of the capital cities of the world. Another type of retrieval is **recognition,** which involves identifying specific information from a set of information that is presented. One recognition task would be a multiple-choice question. Finally, **relearning** involves the process of learning material that was originally learned. Once we have learned and forgotten something, we are able to relearn it more quickly than when it was originally learned, which suggests that the information was in the memory system to be retrieved.

Retrieval Cues

Retrieval cues provide reminders of information. Within the network model of memory, we have already discussed how hints may activate a closely related node, making it easier to retrieve the node being searched for. Prior activation of these nodes and associations is called **priming**. Often, this process occurs without our awareness. For example, if you are shown several red items and then asked to name a fruit, you will be more likely to name a red fruit. The best retrieval cues are often contextual cues that had associations formed at the time that the memory was encoding, such as tastes, smells, and sights. Almost everyone has had the experience of not recognizing someone familiar because of seeing the person in another context.

The Role of Emotion in Retrieving Memories

In addition to words, events, and sensory input serving as retrieval cues, emotion can also serve as a retrieval cue. What we learn in one state is most easily recalled when we are once again in that emotional state, a phenomenon known as **mood-dependent memory**. Thus, when someone is depressed, events in the past that were sad are more likely to emerge to the forefront of his or her mind. This plays a role in maintaining the cycle of depression. When we are happy, we tend to remember past times that were also happy. In addition, emotion can bias the recall of memories. If someone is angry at a friend, the person is more likely to feel that the friendship has always been rotten, whereas in a moment when the friendship feels joyful, the person is more likely to perceive the relationship as having always been a joyful one.

Memory Dysfunctions

The hippocampus plays a role in the encoding of new explicit memories, the cerebellum in encoding implicit memories, and the amygdala helps to tie emotion to memories. Once information is in long-term memory, it is stored in various areas spread throughout the brain. Damage to parts of the brain by strokes, brain tumors, alcoholism, traumatic brain injuries, and other events can cause memory impairment. Patients with damage to the hippocampus could develop **anterograde amnesia**, an inability to encode new memories, or **retrograde amnesia**, an inability to recall information that was previously encoded (or both types of amnesia). In addition, neurological damage involving neurotransmitters can also cause memory dysfunction. One theory about the cause of Alzheimer's disease, for example, involves an inability to manufacture enough of the neurotransmitter acetylcholine, which results in, among other things, neuronal death in the hippocampus.

Decay

Memory decay results in a failure to retain stored information. Even if information is successfully encoded into memory, it can decay from our memory storage and be forgotten. However, decay does not happen in a linear fashion. Rather, the "forgetting curve" indicates that the longer the **retention interval**, or the time since the information was learned, the more information will be forgotten, with the most forgetting occurring rapidly in the first few days before leveling off. It is unclear why memories fade or erode with the passage of time. It is possible that the brain cells involved in the memory may die off, or perhaps that the associations among memories need to be refreshed in order not to weaken.

Interference

Interference can result in a failure to retrieve information that is in storage. The passage of time may create more opportunity for newer learning to interfere with older learning, which is especially common if the learned information is similar. **Proactive interference** happens when information previously learned interferes with the ability to recall information learned later. For example, remembering where you had parked your car in a parking garage will be more difficult once you have parked in that parking garage for months in different locations. **Retroactive interference** happens when newly learned information interferes with the recall of information learned previously. For example, someone who has moved frequently may find that learning new addresses and directions interferes with his or her ability to remember old addresses and directions. Of course, old and new information do not always interfere. Sometimes, old information facilitates the learning of new information through **positive transfer**. For example, knowing how to play American football may make it easier for someone to learn how to play rugby.

Memory Construction and Source Monitoring

Our memories are far from being snapshots of actual experience. We already know that when memories are encoded, they pass through a "lens"; the mood and selective attention of the observer influence how they are encoded. Memory is once again altered when passing through the "lens" of retrieval. When we remember something, we do not pull from a mental photo album, but rather, we draw a picture, *constructing* the recalled memory from information that is stored. This process is not foolproof.

Sometimes the information that we retrieve is based more on a **schema** than on reality. A schema is a mental blueprint containing common aspects of some part of the world. For example, if asked to describe what your 4th grade classroom looked like, you might "remember" a chalkboard, chalk, desks, posters encouraging reading, and books, based on your schema for such a classroom, even though the actual room may not have had posters. In this way, when we construct a memory, we tend to "fill in the blanks" by adding details that may not have been present at the time. We may also unknowingly alter details. For example, in eyewitness testimony, leading questions often cause witnesses to misestimate or misremember. When participants in an experiment were asked how fast cars were going when they *smashed* into each other, instead of just *hit* each other, they indicated higher speeds. Individuals in the first group also reported seeing broken glass and car parts, when there actually were none. After people are exposed to subtle misinformation, they are usually susceptible to the **misinformation effect**, a tendency to misremember.

Individuals may also misremember when asked to repeatedly imagine nonexistent actions and events. Simply repeatedly imagining that one did something can create **false memories** for an event. False memories are inaccurate recollections for an event and may be the result of the implanting of ideas. For example, if one repeatedly imagined being lost as a child in a shopping mall, this imagined occurrence would begin to feel familiar, and as it felt more familiar, it would take on the flavor of a real memory. In fact, it can be very difficult for people to distinguish between real memories and false memories by feeling, because both can be accompanied by emotional reactions and the sense of familiarity. For this reason, an individual's confidence in the validity of a memory has not been found to be a good indication of how valid it actually is.

When recalling information people are also susceptible to forgetting one particular fact—the information's source. This is an error in **source monitoring**. For example, you may recognize someone, but have no idea where you have seen the person before.

Example 23-3: Biology has been Matthew's favorite subject since high school. To help him remember metabolic pathways, he would imagine each step in the pathway located in a spot in his home, then when tested, he would visualize himself walking through his home and be able to "see" which step came next. This retrieval strategy utilizes:

- A) the method of loci.
- B) chunking.
- C) procedural memory.
- D) cued recall.

Solution: The question stem precisely describes the method of loci strategy, which involves visualizing objects to be remembered in a familiar location (choice A is correct). There is no indication that the strategy involved breaking items into smaller groups (choice B is wrong). Procedural memory is knowing how to do a process through muscle memory or repetition. The strategy involves are more conscious component of calling forth specific images (choice C is wrong). Cued recall refers to how material is tested, and whether there is a hint or clue to assist in recall. Since the question stem does not describe how the subject matter was tested, this is not the best choice (choice D is wrong).

23.3

Example 23-4: While studying for the MCAT, Katie notices that she could not remember the Organic Chemistry functional groups she had learned earlier that day, and that the Physics equations she memorized afterwards were "getting in the way." This best describes:

    A) proactive interference
    B) retroactive interference
    C) source monitoring errors
    D) reconstructive memory

Solution: Retroactive interference occurs when information learned more recently goes back in time and interferes with information learned prior. This fits the description in the question stem (choice B is correct). Proactive interference occurs when information learned earlier goes forward in time and interferes with information learned later (choice A is wrong). Source monitoring errors refer to mistakes in the attribution of where information was learned, not forgetting of that information (choice C is wrong). Reconstructive memory refers to the fact that many recollections are formed imperfectly with missing details, which are often filled in later to form a complete picture, but one that is only a partially accurate representation of the original event (choice D is wrong).

Chapter 24
Interacting with the Environment

24.1 ATTENTION

Selective Attention

Selective attention is the process by which one input is attended to and the rest are tuned out. This is necessary because we do not have the capacity to pay attention to everything in our environment. A resource model suggests that we only have a limited capacity to pay attention and so must devote our resources carefully.

One way that selective attention has been studied is using a dichotic listening setup. A person wears headphones and each ear hears a different dialogue. The individual is instructed to listen to information coming into one ear, called the **attended channel**, and to ignore input to the other ear, the **unattended channel**. When people do this, they are able to remember some of the message from the attended ear but lose almost everything from the unattended ear. The same observation has been made with visual stimuli; when people are told to focus on one visual aspect, they may miss other visual details.

The **Broadbent Filter Model of Selective Attention** (Figure 1) theorizes that inputs from the environment first enter a sensory buffer. One of these inputs is then selected and filtered based on physical characteristics of the input (for example, sensory modality). This theoretical filter is designed to keep our brains from being overloaded. Other sensory information stays in the sensory buffer briefly, but then quickly decays. At this point in the process, the information is still raw data that has just been filtered—it has not yet been transformed. It is in the next step, when the information enters short-term memory storage, where semantic (meaning-making) processes occur.

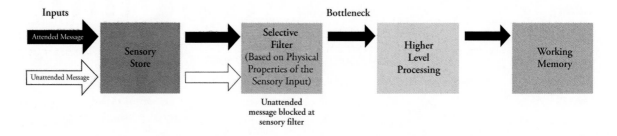

Figure 1   Broadbent Filter Model of Selective Attention

In the dichotic listening task described above, only information from the attended ear is allowed to pass through the filter. If an input in the sensory buffer does not go through the filter, the theory proposes that it remains briefly but then quickly decays and disappears.

To make matters more complicated, it seems that some unattended inputs are still detected. Imagine you are in a conversation with someone at a party in a room full of people. You are not aware of the content of any of the other conversations until suddenly you hear the name of your best friend mentioned in a conversation behind you. This phenomenon is known as the **cocktail party effect**. It happens when information of personal importance from previously unattended channels catches our attention. This observation cannot be well accounted for by the filter model of attention. Later adaptations of the original model have thus suggested that information from the unattended ear is not completely filtered out, but rather dampened, like turning the volume down on a television. Information from the unattended ear can still be processed at some level.

Anne Treisman's Attentuation Model tried to account for the cocktail party effect. Treisman believed that rather than a filter, the mind has an attenuator, which works like a volume knob—it "turns down" the unattended sensory input, rather than eliminating it.

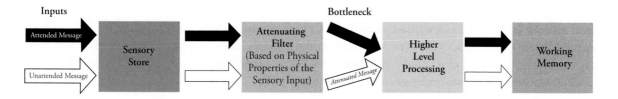

Figure 2   Treisman Attenuation Model of Selective Attention

The cocktail party effect has also been explained through the concept of **selective priming**. This idea suggests that people can be selectively primed to observe something, either by encountering it frequently or by having an expectation. If one is primed to observe something, one is more likely to notice it when it occurs.

Divided Attention

Divided attention concerns when and if we are able to perform multiple tasks simultaneously. It turns out that this depends on the characteristics of the activities one is trying to multitask. The **resource model of attention** says that we have a limited pool of resources on which to draw when performing tasks, both modality-specific resources and general resources. In general, if the resources required to perform multiple tasks simultaneously exceeds the available resources to do so, then the tasks cannot be accomplished at the same time. Three factors are associated with performance on multi-tasking: task similarity, task difficulty, and task practice.

Imagine listening to a talk radio program while trying to write a paper. It is likely that these two activities would be very difficult to pay attention to at the same time. They would interfere with each other because of their task similarity. One activity requires verbal input, while the other requires verbal output. However, if instead you were listening to classical music, you might be able to write a paper at the same time because you would be doing two dissimilar tasks; one requires auditory input resources, while the other requires verbal output.

Task difficulty also plays a role. If a task is more difficult, it requires more resources in general and would be hard to do simultaneously with another task without passing resource capacity. Imagine driving a car while conversing with your passengers. When driving through familiar neighborhoods in a single lane (an easy task), you may have no trouble carrying on a conversation. However, if you are about to enter a complicated intersection involving a lane change and a quick turn, attention to the conversation may have to stop and the you may become silent or miss what was said during that time. Alternatively, while deep in conversation, it is easy to miss a turn!

Finally, practice helps. That is, practice diminishes task resource demand so that we may free up those resources to allow for multitasking. For example, a new driver may have a hard time changing the radio station while driving, while an experienced driver may not find this difficult. This suggests that tasks tend to become automatic with practice, and they no longer need mechanisms of control to oversee them [which brain area is responsible for "muscle memory," or the ability to perform motor tasks unconsciously?[1]]. These tasks are well-learned routines that require fewer resources. On the other hand, novel, **controlled tasks** require flexibility and drain more resources, thus are typically not multitasked.

Example 24-1: Research shows that studying with background stimuli such as music or TV can have vastly different consequences for later performance. For example, certain types of instrumental and ambient music have actually been shown to improve retention, while lyrical music and television sitcoms or news are detrimental. These findings are most consistent with:

    A) state dependency.
    B) dual-coding.
    C) selective filtering.
    D) attenuation.

Solution: The question stem suggests that the type of stimulus is important for determining how distracting or detrimental it is. Some environmental stimuli are tuned out, while others seem to interfere with concentration. This is consistent with attenuation (choice D is correct). State dependency relates to the similarity between two environments: where something was learned, and where it was tested. The question stem does not describe the testing environment (choice A is wrong). Dual coding suggests that material is learned better when visual and acoustic stimuli are combined (choice B is wrong). Selective filtering would imply that individuals would be able to focus under each condition. The dependence on the type of background stimulus suggests that the filter does not respond to all types of distracting stimuli in the same way (choice C is wrong).

24.2 COGNITION

Information-Processing Models

With the advent of computers, psychologists were influenced to think about the human mind as if it were a computer processor. **Information-processing models** assume that information is taken in from the environment and processed through a series of steps including **attention**, **perception**, and **storage** into memory. Along the way, information is systematically transformed. Thus, our minds are like mental computer programs that change, store, use, and retrieve information.

---

[1] The cerebellum

Two theories of attention and perception were described above (the Broadbent Filter Model of Selective Attention and the Treisman Attenuation Model of Selective Attention). **Baddeley's Model of Working Memory** sought to better define short-term memory, which is renamed **working memory**. In his model, working memory consists of four components—a phonological loop, a visuospatial sketchpad, an episodic buffer, and a central executive. The **phonological loop** allows us to repeat verbal information to help us remember it. This may be what you use to remember a phone number that someone tells you when you have nothing with which to write it down. The **visuospatial sketchpad** serves a similar purpose for visuospatial information through the use of mental images. The **episodic buffer** is where information in the working memory can interact with information in long-term memory. For example, if a man sees a station wagon much like the one his father used to drive, he is able to make this connection through the interaction between his memory of his father's car and his current visual experience in the episodic buffer. The **central executive** is the overseer of the entire process, and orchestrates the process by shifting and dividing attention.

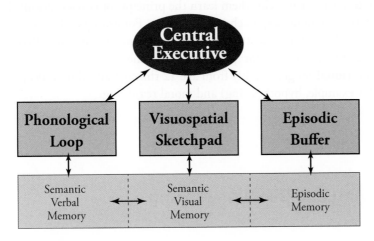

Figure 3   Baddeley Model of Working Memory

Cognitive Development

Piaget's Stages of Cognitive Development

Jean Piaget was one of the first developmental psychologists who studied cognitive development in children and fought against the notion that children were much like miniature adults in their abilities. He thought that the process of cognitive development involved forming **schemas**, or mental frameworks that shape and are shaped by our experience. As we encounter new experiences, Piaget believed that we either **assimilate** those experiences by conforming them into our existing schemas or we **accommodate** by adjusting our schemas to take into account the new experiences. For example, if a young girl believes that there is a monster under the bed but her parent turns on the light to reveal that there is nothing there, the girl can take two paths. She can assimilate this experience by believing that the monster still exists but runs away from light, or accommodate her schema by agreeing that there must be no monster.

Piaget's theory included four developmental stages. They are as follows:

1) **Sensorimotor Stage:** from birth to roughly age 2. Babies and young infants experience the world through their senses and movement, such as looking, touching, mouthing, and grasping. During this time, they learn about **object permanence**—the understanding that things continue to exist when they are out of sight. They also demonstrate stranger anxiety: distress when confronted with an unfamiliar person.

2) **Preoperational Stage:** roughly from ages 2 to 7. During this time, children learn that things can be represented through symbols such as words and images. This accompanies their learning during pretend play and development of language, but they still lack logical reasoning. They also are egocentric, meaning they do not understand that others have different perspectives.

3) **Concrete Operational Stage:** roughly from age 7 to 11. Children learn to think logically about concrete events. This helps them learn the principle of **conservation**: the idea that quantity remains the same despite changes in shape. For example, if water from a wide bowl is poured into a thin cylinder, it still has the same volume despite the difference in height. They also grasp mathematical concepts during this time.

4) **Formal Operational Stage:** roughly from age 12 through adulthood. People learn abstract reasoning (for example, hypothesizing) and moral reasoning.

Problem Solving and Decision Making

Problem Solving Approaches

For some problems, we may use a strategy of **trial and error**. For others, we may rely on following an **algorithm**, a step-by-step procedure. For others, we may use mental shortcuts, called **heuristics**. At times, we may use a combination of these strategies. For example, when changing a tire, an algorithm may be followed until it is discovered that a wrench is missing. At this point, other tools may be pulled out and experimented with through trial and error, until an appropriate one for the bolts is found. Sometimes we use problem-solving strategies consciously, while at other times this is an unconscious process. For example, we may not be actively thinking about a problem, but may be struck later in the shower with a sudden flash of inspiration, called **insight**.

Barriers to Effective Problem Solving

Confirmation bias is a tendency to search only for information that confirms our preconceived thinking, rather than information that might not support it. This can prevent you from approaching a problem from multiple perspectives, because you are more likely to view it from one way—your way. As a result, this bias can lead to faulty decision making; one-sided information may leave you without a complete picture of the situation.

A second obstacle to problem solving is **fixation**, an inability to see the problem from a fresh perspective. At times, this fixation results from the existence of a **mental set**, a tendency to fixate on solutions that worked in the past though they may not apply to the current situation. Another type of fixation is **functional fixedness**, a tendency to perceive the functions of objects as fixed and unchanging.

Heuristics, Biases, Intuition, and Emotion

Mental shortcuts, or heuristics, can increase efficiency in decision-making but can also lead to errors in judgment. The **representativeness heuristic** is a tendency to judge the likelihoods of an event occurring based on our typical mental representations of those events. For example, we may think that one is more likely to die from a shark attack than from being crushed by a vending machine because an animal attack is more representative of a cause of death in our schema. However, although both are extremely unlikely events, the odds of dying from getting crushed by a vending machine (1 in 176 million) is about 1.5 times higher than the odds of dying from a shark attack (1 in 264 million). The **availability heuristic** is a tendency to make judgments based on how readily available information is in our memories. If a memory is readily available, we may think the idea is more common than it actually is. For example, watching news programs about the spread of violent crime in inner city neighborhoods may lead to an overprediction of the likelihood of violent crime in one's own neighborhood.

Another susceptibility is **belief bias**, which is the tendency to judge arguments based on what one believes about their conclusions rather than on whether they use sound logic. For example, consider the statements "There are more drugs sold in poor communities" and "There is more violent crime in poor communities." Drawing a conclusion that drugs cause violent crime in poor communities, while it may seem like a valid conclusion, does not logically follow from the two statements. One may, however, draw this conclusion because it follows a preexisting belief. Once these preexisting beliefs are formed, they become resistant to change through a phenomenon known as **belief perseverance**, a tendency to cling to beliefs despite the presence of contrary evidence.

Overconfidence and Belief Perseverance

The use of intuitive heuristics and a tendency to confirm preconceived beliefs combine to lead to **overconfidence**, an overestimation of the accuracy of knowledge and judgments. For example, after hearing that a classmate completed an assignment quickly, along with their belief that a particular class is easy, students can be overconfident in how much time it would take to complete assignments or write papers, estimating that they would take less time than they actually do. People can also be influenced by how information is **framed**. For example, one study found that consumers are more likely to buy meat advertised as 75% lean than that labeled 25% fat. Similarly, rather than informing customers that they will be charged a "fee" for using a credit card, a company may choose to offer those who use cash a "discount" to make the same situation more palatable.

Example 24-2: Which of the following is NOT needed to apply a memory storage strategy that incorporates dual coding theory?

- A) Central executive
- B) Episodic buffer
- C) Visuospatial sketchpad
- D) Phonological loop

Solution: The dual coding theory involves combining visual and acoustic information. Therefore, the visuospatial sketchpad and phonological loop are both needed (choices C and D are wrong). The central executive coordinates between tasks and determine which of the subordinate systems is used. Therefore, it is also needed (choice A is wrong). The episodic buffer connects with previous experiences and events. It is possible to incorporate dual coding without using personal experiences as the visual or acoustic information; for example, studying the sound of a word in a foreign language together with an image of the object it represents (choice B is correct).

24.3   CONSCIOUSNESS

Consciousness is defined as the awareness that we have of ourselves, our internal states, and the environment. It is also important for reflection and exerts control by directing our attention. Thus, consciousness is always needed to complete novel and complex tasks, however, we may complete practiced and simple tasks, such as driving a familiar path, with little conscious awareness. We may also be influenced by subconscious cues without them entering our consciousness. These subconscious cues can be a basis for first impressions of others and even for prejudice.

States of Consciousness

Alertness and Sleep

Alertness and arousal involve the ability to remain attentive to what is going on. It is not possible to maintain a heightened state of alertness indefinitely, and alertness varies over a 24-hour cycle. Alertness and arousal are controlled by structures within the brainstem. These structures are known as the **reticular formation** (also known as the reticular activating system, or RAS).

Stages of Sleep

The best way to explain the stages of sleep is to put them in context of how they are measured and distinguished. **Polysomnography** (PSG) is a multimodal technique to measure physiological processes during sleep. PSG includes electroencephalogram (EEG—measures of electrical impulses in the brain), electromyogram (EMG—measures of skeletal muscle movements), electrooculogram (EOG—measures of eye movement), and other physiological indicators of sleep. Through experiments using PSG, research has shown there are four stages of sleep.

When a person is awake, but sleepy and relaxed, the individual's EEG changes from when they are alert. In this relaxed state, the EEG shows **alpha waves**, which have low amplitudes and high frequencies (8–12 Hz; Figure 4). These waves are the first indicator that a person is ready to drift off to sleep: the body relaxes; the person feels drowsy and closes his or her eyes.

When sleep begins, the first stage of non-REM (**Rapid Eye Movement**) sleep is entered. This is called **Stage 1 sleep**. During this stage, the EEG is dominated by **theta waves**: waves of low to moderate intensity and intermediate frequency (3–7 Hz; Figure 4). Further, EOG measures slow rolling eye movements and EMG measures moderate activity. The person becomes less responsive to stimuli and has fleeting thoughts.

Stage 2 sleep is denoted by a change to two distinct wave patterns on the EEG. Although a person still experiences theta waves, these waves are intermixed with these two patterns: K-complexes and sleep spindles. A **K-complex** typically has a duration of a half second and is large and slow. These each occur as a single wave amongst the theta waves. **Sleep spindles** are bursts of waves. They have a frequency of 12–14 Hz and are moderately intense. Like K-complexes, these spindles do not last long: only a half to one and a half seconds. During stage 2, there is no eye movement and EMG measures moderate activity. This stage brings increased relaxation in the body that is characteristic of sleep, such as decreased heart rate, respiration, and temperature.

During **Stage 3 sleep**, a person transitions into slow wave sleep (SWS). Stage 3 is characterized by **delta waves**, which are high amplitude, low frequency waves (0.5–3 Hz) and signify the deepest level of sleep. Initially, delta waves are mixed with higher-frequency waves, but as Stage 3 progresses, delta waves come to dominate. During SWS, a person continues to show no eye movement and moderate muscle movement. The heart rate and digestion slow, and growth hormones are secreted.

The final stage of sleep is **REM sleep**, which is characterized by bursts of quick eye movements. Also unique to REM sleep, the EEG measures waves that most resemble the beta waves seen in individuals when awake. Unlike the conscious state, REM sleep is characterized by low (almost no) skeletal muscle movement: hence the name "**paradoxical sleep**." Although the person physiologically appears to be awake, their muscle movement does not corroborate, as the individual is nearly paralyzed except for sudden bursts or twitches. REM sleep is generally when dreams occur.

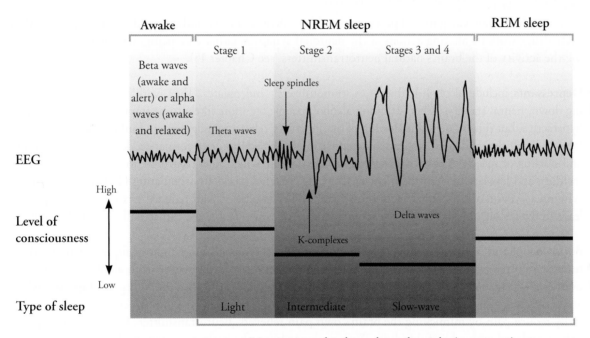

Figure 4　EEG Wave Forms During Wakefulness and Sleep

Sleep Disorders

Dyssomnias are abnormalities in the amount, quality, or timing of sleep, and include insomnia, narcolepsy, and sleep apnea. **Insomnia** is the most common sleep disorder and is characterized by difficulty falling or staying asleep. Insomnia is not the occasional inability to fall asleep due to anxiety or excitement, but rather is a persistent problem that can stem from chronic stress. Those with **narcolepsy** experience periodic, overwhelming sleepiness during waking periods that usually last less than 5 minutes. They can occur without warning at dangerous times, such as while driving or walking down stairs. **Sleep apnea** is a disorder that causes people to intermittently stop breathing during sleep, which results in awakening after a minute or so without air. This process can repeat hundreds of times a night, and it can deprive sufferers of deep sleep. Those with sleep apnea may not even be aware that they have it; sleep apnea is associated with obesity.

Parasomnias are abnormal behaviors that occur during sleep and include somnambulism and night terrors. **Somnambulism** (or sleepwalking) tends to occur during slow wave sleep (Stage 3), usually during the first third of the night. There may be genetic predispositions for sleepwalking and sleeptalking. **Night terrors** also usually occur during Stage 3 (unlike nightmares, which occur during REM sleep toward morning). A person experiencing a night terror may sit up or walk around, babble, and appear terrified, although none of this is recalled the next morning. Typically, when we sleep, the pons (located in the brainstem) serves to paralyze the body so that dreams are not acted out. Obviously, this does not occur during night terrors and somnambulism. Both of these disorders are more likely to appear in children.

Consciousness-Altering Drugs

There are three main categories of psychoactive drugs: depressants, stimulants, and hallucinogenics. All of these drugs work by altering actions at the neuronal synapses, either enhancing, dampening, or mimicking the activity of the brain's natural neurotransmitters (see Chapter 15).

Depressants include alcohol, barbiturates (tranquilizers), and opiates. They work by depressing, or slowing down, neural activity. When drinking alcohol, people are more likely to be impulsive and may appear hyperactive, but this is due to the slowing of brain activity related to judgment and inhibition in the frontal lobe. In larger doses, alcohol can lead to deterioration in skilled motor performance, decreased reaction time, and slurring of speech. Alcohol also suppresses REM sleep, which may contribute to the loss of short-term memory and less restful sleep the night of drinking. Alcohol works by stimulating GABA and dopamine systems. GABA is an inhibitory neurotransmitter and is associated with reduced anxiety, while dopamine leads to the feeling of minor euphoria. Prolonged and excessive alcohol use can actually shrink the brain.

Both alcohol and **barbiturates** depress the sympathetic nervous system ("fight or flight") activity. Barbiturates are often prescribed as sleep aids. They are dangerous in combination with alcohol and prone to overdose—too much of a depressive effect can actually shut down life-sustaining organs. **Opiates**, which are derivatives of opium (including morphine and heroin), also depress neural functioning. They temporarily reduce pain by mimicking the brain's own pain relievers, neurotransmitters known as endorphins; pain is replaced with a blissful feeling. With prolonged use, the brain may stop producing its own endorphins, leading to a painful withdrawal from the drug.

Stimulants include caffeine, nicotine, cocaine, and amphetamines ("speed"). They typically work by either increasing the release of neurotransmitter, reducing the reuptake of neurotransmitter, or both. Their overall effect is to speed up body functions, resulting in increased energy, respiratory rate, heart rate, and pupil dilation. People use stimulants to stay awake, enhance physical performance, and boost mood. Cocaine works by causing a "rush," a release of the brain's supply of neurotransmitters including dopamine, serotonin, and norepinephrine. While this creates a brief period of intense pleasure, it is followed by a depressive crash. MDMA, also known as ecstasy, is a stimulant and a mild hallucinogen. It works by triggering the release of dopamine and serotonin, as well as by blocking the reabsorption of serotonin so that it stays in the synapse longer. It causes emotional elevation, but long-term effects include damage to serotonin-producing neurons. The resulting reduction in serotonin levels can cause a depressed mood.

Hallucinogens, including LSD and marijuana, distort perceptions in the absence of any sensory input, creating hallucinations. After taking LSD, a user may see vivid images and colors. The experience may peak with a feeling of being separated from one's body or experiencing imagined scenes as if they were reality.

Emotions related to LSD can vary from euphoria to panic, depending on the person's mood and the context. Marijuana's active ingredient is THC, which affects functioning by stimulating cannabinoid receptors in the brain. It relaxes and disinhibits like alcohol, but also acts as a hallucinogen by amplifying sensory perceptions including colors, sounds, tastes, and smells. Marijuana can also impair motor skills, reaction time, and judgment. Marijuana has been used medically to help with nausea and pain.

Drug Addiction and the Reward Pathway in the Brain

The defining feature of drug addiction is a compulsion to use a drug repeatedly. Users can have psychological and/or physical dependence on drugs. A **psychological dependence** is often associated with the use of a drug in response to painful emotions related to depression, anxiety, or trauma. **Physical dependence** is evidenced by withdrawal. Withdrawal is an uncomfortable and often physically painful experience without the use of a drug. This discomfort is alleviated when the user takes the drug, reinforcing the addiction. Alcohol withdrawal is especially dangerous—excessive users must be slowly detoxified, as stopping suddenly is life-threatening. Even caffeine addiction can cause withdrawal, with the user experiencing headache, fogginess, and irritability that end when more caffeine is taken.

Addiction is biologically based.[2] Enjoyable behaviors produce activity in dopamine circuits in the brainstem, most notably in the **nucleus accumbens**, the "pleasure center" of the brain. This dopaminergic pathway is a natural pathway to a feeling of reward and pleasure. Many addictive drugs share the characteristic of stimulating the release of dopamine in the nucleus accumbens.

24.4   EMOTION

Three Components of Emotion

Emotion is complex and consists of three components: a physiological (body) component, a behavioral (action) component, and a cognitive (mind) component. The physical aspect of emotion is one of **physiological arousal**, or an excitation of the body's internal state. For example, when being startled at a surprise party, you may feel your heart pounding, your breathing becoming shallow and rapid, and your palms becoming sweaty. These are the sensations that accompany emotion (in this instance, surprise). The behavioral aspect of emotion includes some kind of expressive behavior; for example, spontaneously screaming and bringing your hands over your mouth. The cognitive aspect of emotion involves an appraisal or interpretation of the situation. Initially upon being startled, the thought "dangerous situation" or "fear" may arise, only to be reassessed as "surprise" and "excitement" after recognizing the circumstances as a surprise party. This describes how the situation is interpreted or labeled. Interestingly, many emotions share the same or very similar physiological and behavioral responses; it is the mind that interprets one situation that evokes a quickened heart rate and tears as "joyful" and another with the same responses as "fearful."

---

[2]   While some have argued that addiction should be viewed as a disease, this view is still controversial due to disagreement over the implications it could have for addicts, such as disempowerment.

24.4

Universal Emotions

Darwin assumed that emotions had a strong biological basis. If this is true, then emotions should be experienced and expressed in similar ways across cultures, and in fact, this has been found to be the case. There are six major universal emotions: happiness, sadness, surprise, fear, disgust, and anger. Regardless of culture, most people can readily identify these emotions simply by observing facial expressions. Further supporting the idea that emotions have an innate basis is the finding that children's capacities for emotional expression and recognition appear to develop along similar timelines, regardless of their environment. However, environmental factors like culture do play a role in how emotion is expressed.

Adaptive Role of Emotion

The relationship between performance and emotional arousal is a U-shaped correlation: People perform best when they are moderately aroused. This is known as the **Yerkes-Dodson Law**. A student will perform best when neither too complacent nor too overwhelmed, but rather in a "sweet spot" of optimum arousal (though this "sweet spot" can vary greatly from person to person and from task to task).

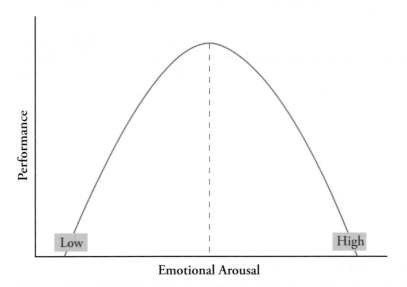

Figure 5 Yerkes-Dodson Law Regarding the Relationship Between Arousal and Performance

Theories of Emotion

There are three predominant theories that attempt to explain how the components of emotion—the physiological, the behavioral, and the cognitive—are interconnected.

James-Lange Theory

Don't look now, but there's a bear in the room. It's standing right behind you and it looks hungry. According to the **James-Lange Theory** of emotion, your physiological and behavioral responses to the bear lead to the cognitive aspect of emotion. That is, your likely physiological reaction—an increased heart rate and the behavioral reaction of running out of the house screaming—will be *followed by* the cognitive aspect—the conscious awareness and labeling of the experience as "fear." This may seem counterintuitive; it implies you feel afraid *because* you run away from the bear. This theory suggests that the emotional experience (the brain labeling the situation as fear-inducing) is *the result of the physiological and behavioral actions.*

Cannon-Bard Theory

According to the **Cannon-Bard Theory** of emotion, the physiological and the cognitive occur *simultaneously* and independently. They then lead to a behavioral reaction. Therefore, the sight of the bear would trigger a cognitive labeling ("There's a bear! Fear!") and the physiological response of sweating and a racing heart rate. Because these are independent, the sweaty palms and racing heart are unnecessary for identifying emotions. With this information in hand, you may then choose to escape the bear by running out of the house screaming. The Cannon-Bard Theory is able to explain the overlap in physiological states between emotions like fear and sexual arousal, because the cognitive labeling is independent from the physiological, rather than directly caused by it. However, it struggles to explain phenomena in which the behavioral response influences the physical and cognitive aspects of emotion (for example, smiling leads to a slightly increased feeling of happiness).

Schachter-Singer Theory

According to the **Schachter-Singer Theory** of emotion, once we experience physiological arousal, we make a conscious cognitive interpretation based on our circumstances, which allows us to identify the emotion that we are experiencing. Thus, like the James-Lange Theory, this suggests that each emotional experience begins with an assessment of our physiological reactions. Unlike James-Lange, however, it suggests that the cognitive label is given based on the situation, rather than being a one-to-one correlate of the physiological experience. Therefore, as in the Cannon-Bard Theory, physiological states can be similar but cognitively labeled differently (for example, fear and sexual arousal). Therefore, the sight of the bear would cause the physiological change of an increased heart rate, which would be interpreted as the result of fearing the bear because of the situation. This would then inform a behavioral response (running out of the house). This theory accounts for several situations, but suffers from the same shortcoming as the Cannon-Bard Theory in that it does not explain how behavioral responses influence physical and cognitive aspects of emotion.

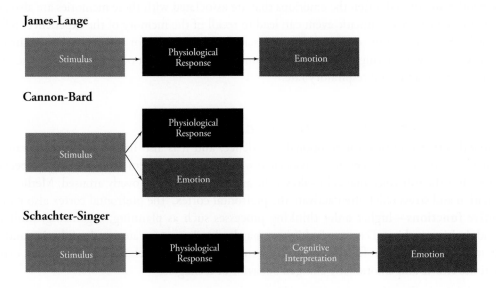

Figure 6   Schematic Comparison of the Theories of Emotion

The Role of the Limbic System in Emotion

The limbic[3] system is a collection of brain structures that lies on both sides of the thalamus; together, these structures appear to be primarily responsible for emotional experiences. The main structure involved in emotion in the limbic system is the **amygdala**, an almond-shaped structure deep within the brain. The amygdala serves as the conductor of the orchestra of our emotional experiences. It can communicate with the **hypothalamus**, a brain structure that controls the physiological aspects of emotion, such as sweating and a racing heart. It also communicates with the **prefrontal cortex**, located at the front of the brain, which controls approach and avoidance behaviors—the behavioral aspects of emotion. The amygdala plays a key role in the identification and expression of fear and aggression.

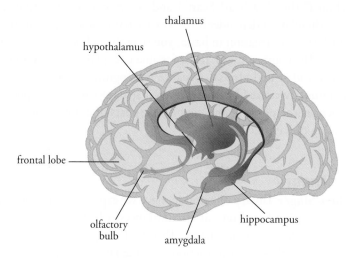

Figure 7 The Limbic System

Emotion and Memory

Emotional experiences can be stored as memories that can be recalled by similar circumstances. The limbic system also includes the **hippocampus**, a brain structure that plays a key role in forming memories. When memories are formed, often the emotions that are associated with these memories are also encoded. Similar circumstances to a traumatic event can lead to recall of the memory of the experience, referred to as "flashback." Sometimes this recall isn't even conscious; for example, for someone who was involved in a traumatic car accident, driving past the intersection where the incident occurred might cause increased muscle tension, heart rate, and respiratory rate.

Emotions, Temperament, and Decision Making

The prefrontal cortex is critical for emotional experience, and it is also important in temperament and decision making. The prefrontal cortex is associated with a reduction in emotional feelings, especially fear and anxiety. It is the soft voice that calms down the amygdala when it is overly aroused. Methods of emotion regulation and stress relief often activate the prefrontal cortex. The prefrontal cortex also plays a role in **executive functions**—higher order thinking processes such as planning, organizing, inhibiting behavior, and decision making. Damage to this area may lead to inappropriateness, impulsivity, and trouble with initiation. This area is not fully developed in humans until they reach their mid-twenties, explaining the sometimes erratic and emotionally charged behavior of teenagers.

---

[3]   In Latin, limbus is the term for "border" or "edge," or, particularly in medical terminology, a border of an anatomical component.

24.5   STRESS

Different Types of Stressors

There are three main types of stressors, which differ in terms of their severity: catastrophes, significant life changes, and daily hassles.

1) Catastrophes are unpredictable, large-scale events that include natural disasters and wartime events. They are events that almost everyone would appraise as dangerous and stress-inducing. The repercussions of a catastrophic event are often felt for years after the event. In the months following 9/11, many people developed psychological disorders including anxiety, depression, and Post-traumatic Stress Disorder (PTSD). Health consequences can also follow prolonged periods of stress, as may be common in refugee camps or shelters.

2) Significant life changes include events such as moving, leaving home, losing a job, marriage, divorce, death of a loved one, and other such changes. The frequency of these events during young adulthood may explain the high degree of stress during this time. These events can be risk factors for disease and death, with several concurrent events creating greater risk than single stressful events would.

3) Daily hassles are the everyday irritations in life including bills, traffic jams, misplacing belongings, and scheduling activities. These things are fairly universal events, but some people take them lightly, while others may become overwhelmed. These little stressors can accumulate and lead to health problems such as hypertension and immunosuppression.

24.6   LANGUAGE

Theories of Language Development

Language acquisition is the term used by psychologists to mean the way infants learn to understand and speak their native language (usually the language used by their parents), not the process of language learning in school or that of learning a foreign language. These other forms of language acquisition seem to work much differently.

B.F. Skinner's **behaviorist** model of language acquisition holds that infants are trained in language by operant conditioning (see Chapters 22 and 23 for more on behaviorism). Skinner argued that language use, though complex, is a form of behavior like any other, and so it is as subject to conditioning just as a rat pulling a lever to receive a food pellet.

Linguist **Noam Chomsky** pointed out several major flaws with the application of behaviorism to language acquisition, and he proposed an alternative to Skinner's model. Chomsky proposed that humans have an innate feature unique to the human mind that allows people to gain mastery of language from limited exposure during the sensitive developmental years in early childhood, a timeframe known as the **critical period**.

Language is a symbolic system that is codified for communication. Letters in an alphabet (or characters in other cultures) have specific meaning, and they are combined to form words (which also have agreed-upon meaning) and words combine for sentences. Language evolves constantly, and it is vital for shaping ideas about who we are relative to each other in society. The **Sapir-Whorf hypothesis** asserts that people understand their world through language and that language, in turn, shapes how we experience our world.

Different Brain Areas Control Language and Speech

Broca's area, located in the left hemisphere of the frontal lobe of the brain, is involved in the complicated process of speech production. Broca's area was discovered when several people who had injury to this area lost the ability to speak; a disorder now termed **Broca's aphasia**[4]. People with Broca's aphasia (also known as *expressive aphasia*) know what they want to say, but are unable to communicate it. **Wernicke's area**, located in the posterior section of the temporal lobe in the dominant hemisphere of the brain (the left for most people), is involved in the comprehension of speech and written language. Wernicke's area was also discovered with the help of people with injury to this area; in these individuals, speech production retains a natural sounding rhythm and syntax, but it is completely meaningless. In other words, people with **Wernicke's aphasia** (also known as *receptive aphasia*) do not have a problem producing speech, but are incapable of producing intelligible, meaningful language.

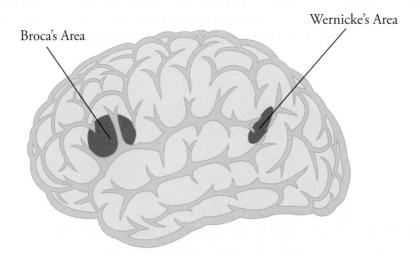

Figure 8   Approximate Location of Broca's Area and Wernicke's Area in the Brain

---

4   From the Greek word *aphatos* meaning "speechlessness"

Example 24-3: An adolescent progressing through Piaget's stage theory attends a peer leadership workshop and learns to manage his emotions by using a breathing technique to down-regulate stress hormone production. Which of the following theories best explains his ability to modulate emotions in this way?

    A) Concrete operations applied within a James-Lange paradigm
    B) Formal operations applied within a Schacter-Singer paradigm
    C) Concrete operations applied within a Canon-Bard paradigm
    D) Formal operations applied within a James-Lange paradigm

Solution: An adolescent would be in Piaget's formal operations stage, and hypothetical reasoning, which includes moral reasoning and emotional regulation, would develop during the formal operations stage (choices A and C are wrong). Emotional regulation and down-regulation of a physiological response requires a cognitive component, which is part of Schacter-Singer Theory but is not included in James-Lange or Canon-Bard theories (choice B is correct, and choice D is wrong).

24.7 MEASUREMENT TOOLS FOR STUDYING THE BRAIN

Behavioral Neuroscience is the area of psychology that looks for the neurophysiological correlates of behavior. This search can be broken down to answering two questions: "What parts of the brain are active during specific behaviors?" and "How do neurotransmitters and other chemicals affect behavior?" In fact, there is probably no area of psychology that today does not fall within the purview of neuroscience and exploration of brain-behavior correlates. First, it is important to understand what tools researchers have at their disposal for exploring the brain. There are three general categories: molecular methods, brain lesions, and neuroimaging. (Molecular methods are beyond the scope of the MCAT Psychology/Sociology section and some of these methods are covered in the Biology and Organic Chemistry sections of this book). Let's take a closer look at the other two methods: the clinical study of brain lesions and neuroimaging.

Brain Lesions

A landmark case in the history of neuroscience was the case of Phineas Gage. In the 1800s, Phineas Gage, a 25-year-old railroad worker, suffered an accident in which a railroad tie blasted through his head, entering under his cheekbone and exiting through the top of his skull. Gage survived, but after the accident, he was described by friends and associates as "no longer himself," prone to impulsivity, unable to stick to plans, and seemingly unable to demonstrate empathy. People who knew him said he was like a completely different person. The accident had severely damaged his **prefrontal cortex**, an area of the brain that is now known to be involved in reflection, planning, emotional regulation, and **theory of mind**—the ability to understand the perspectives of others.

Psychologists had also stumbled on an important methodology for mapping the brain: by observing the clinical changes in behavior that occurred after a lesion or accident, they could infer the role that the damaged area played in behavior and personality. The case study method has been critical to the study of behavioral neuroscience and discovering brain-behavior correlates. Throughout the 20th century, psychologists continued to study and document traumatic brain injuries such as Phineas Gage's as well as the effect of acute strokes. The rationale was simple: if damage to an area of the brain resulted in a change in behavior, then that area must be directly involved in, or part of a network of regions that is involved in, the functioning of that behavior.

Of course, this method offered limitations because scientists could not conduct double blind, randomized experimental studies, so researchers had to wait for a stroke or accident to occur, which could then only be studied one incident at a time. Later in the 20th century and continuing into the present, technological innovations have allowed neuroscientists to use various imaging techniques to study the brain in a more controlled fashion, and design studies—many of them experimental—to address specific hypotheses, rather than waiting for the data to come to them.

24.7

Neuroimaging Techniques

Neuroimaging techniques are either structural or functional. **Structural imaging** techniques provide a picture of the brain; they show anatomical regions, and where they are located with respect to each other. They do not, however, offer any insight into which regions are active at any given time. For this, neuroscientists use **functional imaging** techniques, which demonstrate which parts of the brain are active, and to what extent, as experimental participants manifest a behavior. Let's look first at the two important types of structural techniques, Computerized Tomography (CT) and Magnetic Resonance Imaging (MRI).

Computerized Tomography (CT) scans, also known as CAT (computerized axial tomography) scans, use a computer to combine many cross-sectional (tomographic) images generated from the differential absorption of X-rays of an anatomical part, in this case the human brain, or a subsection of it. These differential absorptions are used to create a three-dimensional structural "snapshot" that appears as a series of cross-sectional images.

Magnetic Resonance Imaging (MRI) uses strong magnets which cause protons to align, spin, and generate a detectable radio-frequency signal that is measured by antennas close to the anatomy being examined. Regular MRI (in contrast to "functional" MRI, see below) provides only structural data, high quality "snapshots" that provide three-dimensional views of the target tissue. Structural MRI cannot be used to analyze the function of the brain across time.

When comparing CT scans and MRIs, advantages of CT scans include a very rapid acquisition of images of a large portion of the body, generally lower cost, more open and less noisy machinery, subjects do not have to remain completely motionless, and there is no prohibition on implanted medical devices. For brain imaging, CT scans are preferred when speed is important, such as during a suspected stroke. Advantages of MRIs include higher resolution and therefore a more detailed image. MRI provides much more detail about soft tissues. Also, MRIs do not use X-rays, and do not include significant exposure to ionizing radiation, which make MRIs safer in most instances.

The other important types of imaging techniques are functional: they provide insight into which brain regions are active during any time. We'll look at four types of functional imaging: EEG, MEG, fMRI, and PET.

Electroencephalography (EEG) is a relatively noninvasive method of gathering functional information about brain activity. Electrodes are placed on the scalp to measure voltage fluctuations in the ionic currents of brain neurons. The resulting traces are known as electroencephalograms (EEGs), and each trace represents the net electrical signal of a large number of neurons. EEGs provide functional data of the brain's electrical neural oscillations (often referred to as "brain waves") that have extremely precise temporal resolution.

To prepare a subject for an EEG, a number of electrodes are placed on the subject's face and scalp, which allows the electrical potential of each electrode to be measured. Depending on a person's state of consciousness (awake, REM sleep. N1 sleep, N2 sleep, N3 sleep, etc.); the frequency, amplitude, and waveforms of the measured EEG traces differ. EEGs are useful in the diagnosis of seizures, sleep disorders, and other conditions that involve activity imbalances in certain parts of the brain.

Advantages of EEG compared to fMRI and PET (below) include less hardware bulk, lower hardware costs, relative tolerance of movement, much higher temporal resolution, non-aggravation of claustrophobia, and silence. However, disadvantages of EEG include far lower spatial resolution, poor measurement of neural activity that occurs below the cortex, poor signal to noise ratio, and significant additional preparation time.

Magnetoencephalography (MEG) is a functional neuroimaging technique for mapping brain activity that records the magnetic fields produced by the brain's electrical currents. MEG uses very sensitive magnetometers, typically using an array of SQUIDs (superconducting quantum interference devices).

MEG has more or less the same advantages and disadvantages as EEG compared to fMRI and PET. Compared to EEG, MEG has better spatial resolution of the brain activity it can detect, while EEG can detect activity in more areas of the brain. In addition, MEG requires expensive bulky machinery as well as a magnetically shielded room.

Functional magnetic resonance imaging (fMRI) uses a computer to combine a series of magnetic resonance images (see MRI, above) taken less than a second apart to provide a functional picture of how brain activity changes over time. FMRI can display changes in oxygen levels (which indicate blood flow) in various regions of the brain in real time and can be used to produce activation maps that indicate the areas of the brain involved in particular mental processes.

FMRI technology has several advantages over other methods of measuring brain structure (regular MRI) or real-time activity (fMRI). FMRI is also considered safer than PET (below) because PET requires subjects to be injected with radioactive substances. The locational precision of fMRI data is more precise than PET and far more precise than EEG. fMRI is also generally more cost effective than PET. The major disadvantage of fMRI (as with MRI, above) is that the subject has to remain completely still in a noisy, cramped space while the imaging is performed. For example, it is not possible to query a subject to answer simple questions during the fMRI of the brain.

Positron emission tomography (PET) is a nuclear medicine imaging technique that produces a three-dimensional image of functional metabolic processes across time. PET scans require the subject to be injected with a positron-emitting radionuclide tracer, which is introduced into the body on a biologically active molecule, such as glucose. Three-dimensional images of the tracer concentration within the body are then constructed by computer analysis that allow the movement of and changes in the tracer concentration to be displayed in real time.

24.7

In modern PET-CT scanners, three-dimensional PET imaging is often augmented with a CT X-ray scan performed on the patient during the same session, in the same machine. This combination (as well as the less common PET/MRI combination) can provide a detailed structural image of the brain together with functional data. PET is a valuable technique for some diseases and disorders because it is possible to image specific radio-chemicals used for particular bodily functions. For example, if a patient is injected with a radioactive glucose analog, a PET scan can be used to image and then analyze the uptake of this specific glucose analog in the brain.

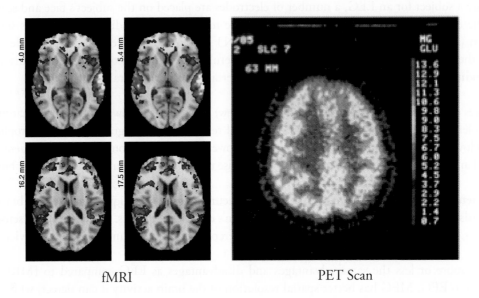

fMRI   PET Scan

Figure 9   fMRI versus PET

These are the primary methods of observing the brain itself, however, often researchers are also interested in understanding how the rest of the body is responding by measuring physiological markers that are associated with personality or behavior. For example, if a researcher was investigating the stress response, they would likely take data on electrical skin conductance, cortisol levels, heart rate, blood pressure, pupil dilation, etc. These indicators are also frequently used in Behavioral Neuroscience studies, especially research into stress and stress management.

Example 24-4: A lab mouse has a part of its cortex removed. Researchers are interested in the mouse's cognitive performance in the absence of this region. Which of the following techniques would be most effective for determining the organism's overall state of alertness and consciousness?

  A) fMRI
  B) CT scan
  C) PET
  D) EEG

Solution: EEGs are used to study diffuse neural activity and general state of consciousness (awake, alert, about to sleep, sleep stage, etc.). This would provide the most information about the organism's general state of consciousness (choice D is correct). fMRI and PET, although they are techniques that can be used to study the functional activity within certain regions of the brain, provide less information about the overall state of an organism's consciousness (choices A and C are wrong). CT Scan is a structural technique, and does not provide information about the functionality of the brain at the specific or general level (choice B is wrong).

Part 5

MCAT
General Chemistry

MCAT
General Chemistry

Chapter 25
Chemistry Fundamentals

25.1 METRIC UNITS

Before we begin our study of chemistry, we will briefly go over metric units. Scientists use the *Système International d'Unitès* (the International System of Units), abbreviated SI, to express measurements of physical quantities. The six MCAT-relevant **base units** of SI are given below:

SI Base Unit	Abbreviation	Measures
meter	m	length
kilogram	kg	mass
second	s	time
mole	mol	amount of substance
kelvin	K	temperature
ampere	A	electric current

The units of any physical quantity can be written in terms of the SI base units. For example, the SI unit of energy (the joule) is kilograms times meters^2 per second^2 (kg $\cdot$ m^2/s^2).

Multiples of the base units that are powers of ten are often abbreviated and precede the symbol for the unit. For example, m is the symbol for milli-, which means 10^{-3} (one thousandth). So, one thousandth of a second, 1 millisecond, would be written as 1 ms. Some of the most common power-of-ten prefixes are given in the list below:

Prefix	Symbol	Multiple
nano-	n	10^{-9}
micro-	μ	10^{-6}
milli-	m	10^{-3}
centi-	c	10^{-2}
kilo-	k	10^{3}
mega-	M	10^{6}

Two other units, ones that are common in chemistry, are the liter and the angstrom. The liter (abbreviated L) is a unit of volume equal to 1/1000 of a cubic meter:

$$1000 \text{ L} = 1 \text{ m}^3$$

$$1 \text{ L} = 1000 \text{ cm}^3$$

The most common way of expressing solution concentrations, **molarity (M)**, uses the liter in its definition: M = moles of solute per liter of solution. In addition, you will see the milliliter (mL) as often as you will see the liter. A simple consequence of the definition of a liter is the fact that one milliliter is the same volume as one cubic centimeter:

$$1 \text{ mL} = 1 \text{ cm}^3 = 1 \text{ cc}$$

The **angstrom**, abbreviated Å, is a unit of length equal to 10^{-10} m. The angstrom is convenient because atomic radii and bond lengths are typically around 1 to 3 Å.

25.2 DENSITY

The **density** of a substance is its mass per volume:

$$\text{Density: } \rho = \frac{\text{mass}}{\text{volume}} = \frac{m}{V}$$

In chemistry, densities are usually expressed in grams per cubic centimeter (g/cm^3). This unit of density is convenient because most liquids and solids have a density of around 1 to 20 g/cm^3.

For example, water has a density of 1 g/cm^3 (it varies slightly with temperature, but this is the value the MCAT will expect you to use).

25.3 MOLECULAR FORMULAS

When two or more atoms form a covalent bond they create a **molecule**. For example, when two atoms of hydrogen (H) bond with one atom of oxygen (O), the resulting molecule is H_2O, water. A compound's **molecular formula** gives the identities and numbers of the atoms in the molecule. For example, the formula $C_4H_4N_2$ tells us that this molecule contains four carbon atoms, four hydrogen atoms, and two nitrogen atoms.

Example 25-1: What is the molecular formula of acetaminophen, given the structural formula below?

Solution: There are 8 carbon atoms, 9 hydrogen atoms, 1 nitrogen atom, and 2 oxygen atoms. The molecular formula is $C_8H_9NO_2$.

25.4 EMPIRICAL FORMULAS

Let's look again at the molecule $C_4H_4N_2$. There are four atoms each of carbon and hydrogen and half as many (two) nitrogen atoms. Therefore, the smallest whole numbers that give the same *ratio* of atoms (carbon to hydrogen to nitrogen) in this molecule are 2:2:1. If we use *these* numbers for the atoms, we get the molecule's **empirical formula**: C_2H_2N. In general, to reduce a molecular formula to the empirical formula, divide all the subscripts by their greatest common factor. Here are a few more examples:

Molecular Formula	Empirical Formula
$C_6H_{12}O_6$	CH_2O
$K_2S_2O_8$	KSO_4
$C_{30}H_{27}N_3O_{15}$	$C_{10}H_9NO_5$

Example 25-2: What is the empirical formula of sodium dithionate, $Na_2S_2O_6$? Of sodium thiosulfate, $Na_2S_2O_3$?

Solution: The greatest common factor of 2, 2, and 6 is 2, so the empirical formula of sodium dithionate is $NaSO_3$. The greatest common factor of 2, 2, and 3 is 1, so the empirical formula of sodium thiosulfate is the same as its molecular formula, $Na_2S_2O_3$.

25.5 POLYATOMIC IONS

You should also be familiar with a handful of common polyatomic ions for the MCAT. Those in the table below are the ones you're most likely to come across.

Acetate (AcO⁻)	$CH_3CO_2^-$
Bicarbonate	HCO_3^-
Cyanide	CN^-
Hydroxide	OH^-
Nitrate	NO_3^-
Nitrite	NO_2^-
Perchlorate	ClO_4^-
Carbonate	CO_3^{2-}
Sulfate	SO_4^{2-}
Sulfite	SO_3^{2-}
Phosphate	PO_4^{3-}
Ammonium	NH_4^+
Hydronium	H_3O^+

25.6 FORMULA AND MOLECULAR WEIGHT

If we know the chemical formula, we can figure out the **formula weight**, which is the sum of the atomic weights of all the atoms in the molecule. The unit for atomic weight is the **atomic mass unit**, abbreviated **amu**. (Note: Although *weight* is the popular term, it should really be *mass*.) One atomic mass unit is, by definition, equal to exactly 1/12 the mass of an atom of carbon-12 (^{12}C), the most abundant naturally occurring form of carbon. The periodic table lists the atomic mass of each element, which is actually a weighted average of the atomic masses of all its naturally occurring forms (isotopes) based on their relative abundance. To calculate the formula weight of the compound in question, refer to the periodic table. The atomic mass of carbon is 12.0 amu, that of hydrogen is 1.0 amu, and that of nitrogen as 14.0 amu. Therefore, the formula weight for $C_4H_4N_2$ is

$$4(12) + 4(1) + 2(14) = 80$$

(The unit *amu* may not be explicitly included.) When a compound exists as discrete molecules, the term **molecular weight** (**MW**) is usually used instead of formula weight. For example, the molecular weight of water, H_2O, is $2(1) + 16 = 18$. The term formula weight is usually used for *ionic* compounds, such as NaCl. The formula weight of NaCl is $23 + 35.5 = 58.5$.

Example 25-3: What is the formula weight of cerium carbonate, $Ce_2(CO_3)_3$?

    A) 340 amu
    B) 400 amu
    C) 460 amu
    D) 520 amu

Solution: The masses of the elements are Ce = 140 amu, C = 12 amu, and O = 16 amu. The formula weight of $Ce_2(CO_3)_3$ is $2(140 \text{ amu}) + 3(12 \text{ amu}) + 9(16 \text{ amu}) = 460 \text{ amu}$.

25.7 THE MOLE

A **mole** is simply a particular number of things, like a dozen is any group of 12 things. One mole of anything contains 6.02×10^{23} entities. A mole of atoms is a collection of 6.02×10^{23} atoms; a mole of molecules contains 6.02×10^{23} molecules, and so on. This number, 6.02×10^{23}, is called **Avogadro's number**, denoted by N_A. What is so special about 6.02×10^{23}? The answer is based on the atomic mass unit, which is defined so that the mass of a carbon-12 atom is exactly 12 amu. *The number of carbon-12 atoms in a sample of mass of 12 grams is 6.02×10^{23}.* Avogadro's number is the link between atomic mass units and grams. For example, the periodic table lists the mass of sodium (Na, atomic number 11) as 23.0. This means that 1 atom of sodium has a mass of 23 atomic mass units, or that 1 *mole* of sodium atoms has a mass of 23 *grams*.

Since 1 mole of a substance has a mass in grams equal to the mass in amus of 1 formula unit of the substance, we have the following formula:

$$\# \text{ moles} = \frac{\text{mass in grams}}{\text{molecular weight (MW)}}$$

Example 25-4: Which has the greater formula weight: potassium dichromate ($K_2Cr_2O_7$) or lead azide $Pb(N_3)_2$?

Solution: The formula weight of potassium dichromate is

$$2(39.1) + 2(52) + 7(16) = 294.2$$

and the formula weight of lead azide is

$$207.2 + 6(14) = 291.2$$

Therefore, potassium dichromate has the greater formula weight.

Example 25-5: How many moles does a 96 gram sample of hydrazine, N_2H_4, contain?

Solution: The molecular weight of hydrazine is 2(14 g/mol) + 4(1 g/mol) = 32 g/mol. Using the formula above, we can see that

$$\# \text{ moles } = \frac{96 \text{ g}}{32 \text{ g/mol}} = 3 \text{ moles}$$

25.8   PERCENTAGE COMPOSITION BY MASS

A molecule's molecular or empirical formula can be used to determine the molecule's percent mass composition. For example, let's find the mass composition of carbon, hydrogen, and nitrogen in $C_4H_4N_2$. Using the compound's empirical formula, C_2H_2N, will give us the same answer, but the calculations will be easier because we'll have smaller numbers to work with. The empirical molecular weight is 2(12) + 2(1) + 14 = 40, so each element's contribution to the total mass is

$$\%C = \frac{2(12)}{40} = \frac{12}{20} = \frac{60}{100} = 60\%, \quad \%H = \frac{2(1)}{40} = \frac{1}{20} = \frac{5}{100} = 5\%, \quad \%N = \frac{14}{40} = \frac{7}{20} = \frac{35}{100} = 35\%$$

We can also use information about the percentage composition to determine a compound's empirical formula. Suppose a substance is analyzed and found to consist, by mass, of 70% iron and 30% oxygen. To find the empirical formula for this compound, the trick is to start with 100 grams of the substance. We choose 100 grams since percentages are based on parts in 100. One hundred grams of this substance would then contain 70 g of Fe and 30 g of O. Now, how many *moles* of Fe and O are present in this 100-gram substance? Since the atomic weight of Fe is 55.8 and that of O is 16, we can use the formula given above in Section 25.7 and find

$$\# \text{ moles of Fe} = \frac{70 \text{ g}}{55.8 \text{ g/mol}} \approx \frac{70}{56} = \frac{5}{4} \quad \text{and} \quad \# \text{ moles of O} = \frac{30 \text{ g}}{16 \text{ g/mol}} = \frac{15}{8}$$

Because the empirical formula involves the ratio of the numbers of atoms, let's find the ratio of the amount of Fe to the amount of O:

$$\text{Ratio of Fe to O} = \frac{5/4 \text{ mol}}{15/8 \text{ mol}} = \frac{5}{4} \cdot \frac{8}{15} = \frac{2}{3}$$

Since the ratio of Fe to O is 2:3, the empirical formula of the substance is Fe_2O_3.

Example 25-6: What is the empirical formula of a compound that is, by mass, 90 percent carbon and 10 percent hydrogen?

    A) CH_2
    B) C_2H_3
    C) C_3H_4
    D) C_4H_5

Solution: A 100-gram sample of this compound would contain 90 g of C and 10 g of H. Since the atomic weight of C is 12 and that of H is 1, we have

$$\text{\# moles of C} = \frac{90 \text{ g}}{12 \text{ g/mol}} = \frac{15}{2} \quad \text{and} \quad \text{\# moles of H} = \frac{10 \text{ g}}{1 \text{ g/mol}} = 10$$

Therefore, the ratio of the amount of C to the amount of H is

$$\frac{15/2 \text{ mol}}{10 \text{ mol}} = \frac{3}{4}$$

Because the ratio of C to H is 3:4, the empirical formula of the compound is C_3H_4, and choice C is the answer.

Example 25-7: What is the percent, by mass of water, in the hydrate $MgCl_2 \cdot 5H_2O$?

    A) 27%
    B) 36%
    C) 49%
    D) 52%

Solution: The formula weight for this hydrate is $24.3 + 2(35.5) + 5[2(1) + 16] = 185.3$. Since water's total molecular weight in this compound is $5[2(1) + 16] = 90$, we see that water's contribution to the total mass is $\%H_2O = 90/185.3$, which is a little *less* than one half (50 percent). Therefore, the answer is choice C.

25.8

25.9 CONCENTRATION

Molarity (*M*) expresses the concentration of a solution in terms of moles of solute per liter of solution:

$$\text{Molarity } (M) = \frac{\#\text{ moles of solute}}{\#\text{ liters of solution}}$$

Concentration is denoted by enclosing the solute in brackets. For instance, "$[Na^+] = 1.0\ M$" indicates a solution in which the concentration is equivalent to 1 mole of sodium ions per liter of solution.

Mole fraction simply expresses the fraction of moles of a given substance (which we'll denote here by S) relative to the total moles in a solution:

$$\text{mole fraction of S} = X_S = \frac{\#\text{ moles of substance S}}{\text{total }\#\text{ moles in solution}}$$

Mole fraction is a useful way to express concentration when more than one solute is present, and it is often used when discussing the composition of a mixture of gases.

25.10 CHEMICAL EQUATIONS AND STOICHIOMETRIC COEFFICIENTS

The equation

$$2\ Al + 6\ HCl \rightarrow 2\ AlCl_3 + 3\ H_2$$

describes the reaction of aluminum metal (Al) with hydrochloric acid (HCl) to produce aluminum chloride ($AlCl_3$) and hydrogen gas (H_2). The **reactants** are on the left side of the arrow, and the **products** are on the right side. A chemical equation is **balanced** if, for every element represented, the number of atoms on the left side of the arrow is equal to the number of atoms on the right side. This illustrates the **Law of Conservation of Mass** (or of **Matter**), which says that the amount of matter (and thus mass) does not change in a chemical reaction. For a *balanced* reaction such as the one above, the coefficients (2, 6, 2, and 3) preceding each compound—which are known as **stoichiometric coefficients**—tell us in what proportion the reactants react and in what proportion the products are formed. For this reaction, 2 atoms of Al react with 6 molecules of HCl to form 2 formula units of $AlCl_3$ and 3 molecules of H_2. The equation also means that 2 *moles* of Al react with 6 *moles* of HCl to form 2 *moles* of $AlCl_3$ and 3 *moles* of H_2.

The stoichiometric coefficients give the ratios of the number of molecules (or moles) that apply to the combination of reactants and the formation of products. They do *not* give the ratios by mass.

Balancing Equations

Balancing most chemical equations is simply a matter of trial and error. It's a good idea to start with the most complex species in the reaction. For example, let's look at the reaction above:

$$Al + HCl \rightarrow AlCl_3 + H_2 \text{ (unbalanced)}$$

Start with the most complex molecule, $AlCl_3$. The total number of atoms is calculated by multiplying the coefficient in front of a compound times the subscript within the formula. To get 3 atoms of Cl on the product side, we need to have 3 atoms of Cl on the reactant side; therefore, put a 3 in front of HCl:

$$Al + 3 HCl \rightarrow AlCl_3 + H_2 \text{ (unbalanced)}$$

We've now balanced the Cl's, but the H's are still unbalanced. Since we have 3 H's on the left, we need 3 H's on the right to accomplish this, so we put a coefficient of 3/2 in front of the H_2:

$$Al + 3 HCl \rightarrow AlCl_3 + 3/2 H_2$$

Notice that we put a 3/2 (*not* a 3) in front of the H_2, because a hydrogen molecule contains 2 hydrogen atoms. All the atoms are now balanced—we see 1 Al, 3 H's, and 3 Cl's on each side. Because it's customary to write coefficients as whole numbers, we multiply through by 2 to get rid of the fraction and write

$$2 Al + 6 HCl \rightarrow 2 AlCl_3 + 3 H_2$$

Example 25-8: Balance each of these equations:

a) $NH_3 + O_2 \rightarrow NO + H_2O$
b) $C_8H_{18} + O_2 \rightarrow CO_2 + H_2O$

Solution:

a) $4 NH_3 + 5 O_2 \rightarrow 4 NO + 6 H_2O$
b) $2 C_8H_{18} + 25 O_2 \rightarrow 16 CO_2 + 18 H_2O$

25.11

25.11 STOICHIOMETRIC RELATIONSHIPS IN REACTIONS

Once the equation for a chemical reaction is balanced, the stoichiometric coefficients tell us the relative amounts of the reactant species that combine and the relative amounts of the product species that are formed. For example, recall that the reaction

$$2 Al + 6 HCl \rightarrow 2 AlCl_3 + 3 H_2$$

tells us that 2 moles of Al react with 6 moles of HCl to form 2 moles of $AlCl_3$ and 3 moles of H_2.

Example 25-9: If 108 grams of aluminum metal are consumed, how many grams of hydrogen gas will be produced?

Solution: Because the stoichiometric coefficients give the ratios of the number of moles that apply to the combination of reactants and the formation of products—not the ratios by mass—we first need to determine how many *moles* of Al react. Since the molecular weight of Al is 27, we know that 27 grams of Al is equivalent to 1 mole. Therefore, 108 grams of Al is 4 moles. Now we use the stoichiometry of the balanced equation: for every 2 moles of Al that react, 3 moles of H_2 are produced. So, if 4 moles of Al react, we'll get 6 moles of H_2. Finally, we convert the number of moles of H_2 produced to grams. The molecular weight of H_2 is 2(1) = 2. This means that 1 mole of H_2 has a mass of 2 grams. Therefore, 6 moles of H_2 will have a mass of 6(2 g) = 12 grams.

Example 25-10: How many grams of HCl are required to produce 534 grams of aluminum chloride?

Solution: First, we'll convert the desired mass of $AlCl_3$ into moles. The molecular weight of $AlCl_3$ is 27 + 3(35.5) = 133.5. This means that 1 mole of $AlCl_3$ has a mass of 133.5 grams. Therefore, 534 grams of $AlCl_3$ is equivalent to 534/133.5 = 4 moles. Next, we use the stoichiometry of the balanced equation. For every 2 moles of $AlCl_3$ that are produced, 6 moles of HCl are consumed. So, if we want to produce 4 moles of $AlCl_3$, we'll need 12 moles of HCl. Finally, we convert the number of moles of HCl consumed to grams. The molecular weight of HCl is 1 + 35.5 = 36.5. This means that 1 mole of HCl has a mass of 36.5 grams. Therefore, 12 moles of HCl will have a mass of 12(36.5 g) = 438 grams.

Example 25-11: Consider the following reaction:

$$CS_2 + 3 O_2 \rightarrow CO_2 + 2 SO_2$$

How much carbon disulfide must be used to produce 64 grams of SO_2?

A) 38 g
B) 57 g
C) 76 g
D) 114 g

Solution: Since the molecular weight of SO_2 is 32.1 + 2(16) = 64, we know that 64 grams of SO_2 is equivalent to 1 mole. From the stoichiometry of the balanced equation, we see that for every 1 mole of CS_2 that reacts, 2 moles of SO_2 are produced. Therefore, to produce just 1 mole of SO_2, we need 1/2 mole of CS_2. The molecular weight of CS_2 is 12 + 2(32.1) ≈ 76, so 1/2 mole of CS_2 has a mass of 38 grams. The answer is choice A.

25.12   THE LIMITING REAGENT

Let's look again at the reaction of aluminum with hydrochloric acid:

$$2\ Al + 6\ HCl \rightarrow 2\ AlCl_3 + 3\ H_2$$

Suppose that this reaction starts with 4 moles of Al and 18 moles of HCl. We have enough HCl to make 6 moles of $AlCl_3$ and 9 moles of H_2. *However,* there's only enough Al to make 4 moles of $AlCl_3$ and 6 moles of H_2. This means that aluminum is the **limiting reagent** here, because we run out of this reactant *first*, so it limits how much product the reaction can produce.

Now suppose that the reaction begins with 4 moles of Al and 9 moles of HCl. There's enough Al metal to produce 4 moles of $AlCl_3$ and 6 moles of H_2. But there's only enough HCl to make 3 moles of $AlCl_3$ and 4.5 moles of H_2. In this situation, HCl is the limiting reagent. Notice that we had more moles of HCl than we had of Al and the initial mass of the HCl was greater than the initial mass of Al. Nevertheless, the limiting reagent in this case was the HCl. The limiting reagent is the reactant that is consumed first, not necessarily the reactant that's initially present in the smallest amount.

Example 25-12:   Consider the following reaction:

$$2\ ZnS + 3\ O_2 \rightarrow 2\ ZnO + 2\ SO_2$$

If 97.5 grams of zinc sulfide undergoes this reaction with 32 grams of oxygen gas, what will be the limiting reagent?

    A) ZnS
    B) O_2
    C) ZnO
    D) SO_2

Solution: Since the molecular weight of ZnS is $65.4 + 32.1 = 97.5$ and the molecular weight of O_2 is $2(16)$ $= 32$, this reaction begins with 1 mole of ZnS and 1 mole of O_2. From the stoichiometry of the balanced equation, we see that 1 mole of ZnS would react completely with $\frac{3}{2} = 1.5$ moles of O_2. Because we have only 1 mole of O_2, the O_2 will be consumed first; it is the limiting reagent, and the answer is choice B. Note that choices C and D can be eliminated immediately, because a limiting reagent is always a reactant.

25.13

25.13   SOME NOTATION USED IN CHEMICAL EQUATIONS

In addition to specifying what atoms or molecules are involved in a chemical reaction, an equation may contain additional information. One type of additional information that can be written right into the equation specifies the **phases** of the substances in the reaction, meaning, is the substance a solid, liquid, or gas? Another common condition is that a substance may be dissolved in water when the reaction proceeds. In this case, we'd say the substance is in aqueous solution. These four "states" are abbreviated and written in parentheses as follows: solid = (*s*), liquid = (*l*), gas = (*g*), and aqueous = (*aq*).

These immediately follow the chemical symbol for the reactant or product in the equation. For example, the reaction of sodium metal with water, which produces sodium hydroxide and hydrogen gas, could be written like this:

$$2 \, Na(s) + 2 \, H_2O(l) \rightarrow 2 \, NaOH(aq) + H_2(g)$$

In some cases, the reactants are heated to produce the desired reaction. To indicate this, we write a "Δ"—or the word "heat"—above (or below) the reaction arrow. For example, heating potassium nitrate produces potassium nitrite and oxygen gas:

$$2 \, KNO_3(s) \xrightarrow{\Delta} 2 \, KNO_2(aq) + O_2(g)$$

25.14   OXIDATION STATES

An atom's **oxidation state** (or **oxidation number**) is meant to indicate how the atom's "ownership" of its valence electrons changes when it forms a compound. For example, consider the formula unit NaCl. The sodium atom will transfer its valence electron to the chlorine atom, so the sodium's "ownership" of its valence electron has certainly changed. To indicate this, we'd say that the oxidation state of sodium is now +1 (or 1 *less* electron than it started with). On the other hand, chlorine accepts ownership of that 1 electron, so its oxidation state is –1 (that is, 1 *more* electron than it started with). Giving up ownership results in a more positive oxidation state; accepting ownership results in a more negative oxidation state.

This example of NaCl is rather special (and easy) since the compound is **ionic**, and we consider ionic compounds to involve the complete transfer of electrons. But what about a non-ionic (that is, a **covalent)** compound? *The oxidation state of an atom is the "charge" it would have if the compound were ionic.* Here's another way of saying this: the oxidation state of an atom in a molecule is the charge it would have if all the shared electrons were completely transferred to the more electronegative element. Note that for covalent compounds, this is not a real charge, just a bookkeeping trick.

The following list gives the rules for assigning oxidation states to the atoms in a molecule. If following one rule in the list causes the violation of another rule, the rule that is higher in the list takes precedence.

Rules for Assigning Oxidation States
1) The oxidation state of any element in its standard state is 0.
2) The sum of the oxidation states of the atoms in a neutral molecule must always be 0, and the sum of the oxidation states of the atoms in an ion must always equal the ion's charge.
3) Group 1 metals have a +1 oxidation state, and Group 2 metals have a +2 oxidation state.
4) Fluorine has a –1 oxidation state.
5) Hydrogen has a +1 oxidation state when bonded to something more electronegative than carbon, a –1 oxidation state when bonded to an atom less electronegative than carbon, and a 0 oxidation state when bonded to carbon.
6) Oxygen has a –2 oxidation state.
7) The rest of the halogens have a –1 oxidation state, and the atoms of the oxygen family have a –2 oxidation state.

It's worth noting a common exception to Rule 6: In peroxides (such as H_2O_2 or Na_2O_2), oxygen is in a -1 oxidation state (which is consistent with Rules 3 and 5 having a higher priority than Rule 6).

As we will discuss later, the order of electronegativities of some elements can be remembered with the mnemonic FONClBrISCH (pronounced "fawn-cull-brish"). This lists the elements in order from the most electronegative (F) to the least electronegative (H). Hence, bonds from H to anything before C in FONClBrISCH will give hydrogen a $+1$ oxidation state, and bonds from H to anything *not* found in the list will give H a -1 oxidation state.

Let's find the oxidation number of manganese in $KMnO_4$. By Rule 3, K is $+1$, and by Rule 6, O is -2. Therefore, the oxidation state of Mn must be $+7$ in order for the sum of all the oxidation numbers in this electrically-neutral molecule to be zero (the unbreakable Rule 2).

Like many other elements, transition metals can assume different oxidation states, depending on the compound they're in. (Note, however, that a metal will never assume a negative oxidation state!) The oxidation number of a transition metal is given as a Roman numeral in the name of the compound. Therefore, $FeCl_2$ is iron(II) chloride, and $FeCl_3$ is iron(III) chloride.

Example 25-13: Determine the oxidation state of each of the atoms in the following ions and compounds.

a) AlH_4^-
b) $Ca(BrO_3)_2$
c) CS_2

Solution:

a) By Rule 5, hydrogen has an oxidation state of -1 because aluminum is less electronegative than carbon; by Rule 2, aluminum must therefore have an oxidation state of $+3$.
b) By Rules 3 and 6, calcium has an oxidation state of $+2$ and oxygen has an oxidation state of -2; by Rule 2, bromine must therefore have an oxidation state of $+5$.
c) By Rule 7, sulfur has an oxidation state of -2; so by Rule 2, carbon must therefore have an oxidation state of $+4$.

25.14

Chapter 26
Atomic and Molecular Structure and Properties

1																	2
H 1.0																	**He** 4.0
3 **Li** 6.9	4 **Be** 9.0											5 **B** 10.8	6 **C** 12.0	7 **N** 14.0	8 **O** 16.0	9 **F** 19.0	10 **Ne** 20.2
11 **Na** 23.0	12 **Mg** 24.3											13 **Al** 27.0	14 **Si** 28.1	15 **P** 31.0	16 **S** 32.1	17 **Cl** 35.5	18 **Ar** 39.9
19 **K** 39.1	20 **Ca** 40.1	21 **Sc** 45.0	22 **Ti** 47.9	23 **V** 50.9	24 **Cr** 52.0	25 **Mn** 54.9	26 **Fe** 55.8	27 **Co** 58.9	28 **Ni** 58.7	29 **Cu** 63.5	30 **Zn** 65.4	31 **Ga** 69.7	32 **Ge** 72.6	33 **As** 74.9	34 **Se** 79.0	35 **Br** 79.9	36 **Kr** 83.8
37 **Rb** 85.5	38 **Sr** 87.6	39 **Y** 88.9	40 **Zr** 91.2	41 **Nb** 92.9	42 **Mo** 95.9	43 **Tc** (98)	44 **Ru** 101.1	45 **Rh** 102.9	46 **Pd** 106.4	47 **Ag** 107.9	48 **Cd** 112.4	49 **In** 114.8	50 **Sn** 118.7	51 **Sb** 121.8	52 **Te** 127.6	53 **I** 126.9	54 **Xe** 131.3
55 **Cs** 132.9	56 **Ba** 137.3	57 *****La** 138.9	72 **Hf** 178.5	73 **Ta** 180.9	74 **W** 183.9	75 **Re** 186.2	76 **Os** 190.2	77 **Ir** 192.2	78 **Pt** 195.1	79 **Au** 197.0	80 **Hg** 200.6	81 **Tl** 204.4	82 **Pb** 207.2	83 **Bi** 209.0	84 **Po** (209)	85 **At** (210)	86 **Rn** (222)
87 **Fr** (223)	88 **Ra** 226.0	89 †**Ac** 227.0	104 **Rf** (261)	105 **Db** (262)	106 **Sg** (266)	107 **Bh** (264)	108 **Hs** (277)	109 **Mt** (268)	110 **Ds** (281)	111 **Rg** (272)	112 **Cn** (285)	113 **Uut** (286)	114 **Fl** (289)	115 **Uup** (288)	116 **Lv** (293)	117 **Uus** (294)	118 **Uuo** (294)

*Lanthanide Series:

58 **Ce** 140.1	59 **Pr** 140.9	60 **Nd** 144.2	61 **Pm** (145)	62 **Sm** 150.4	63 **Eu** 152.0	64 **Gd** 157.3	65 **Tb** 158.9	66 **Dy** 162.5	67 **Ho** 164.9	68 **Er** 167.3	69 **Tm** 168.9	70 **Yb** 173.0	71 **Lu** 175.0

†Actinide Series:

90 **Th** 232.0	91 **Pa** (231)	92 **U** 238.0	93 **Np** (237)	94 **Pu** (244)	95 **Am** (243)	96 **Cm** (247)	97 **Bk** (247)	98 **Cf** (251)	99 **Es** (252)	100 **Fm** (257)	101 **Md** (258)	102 **No** (259)	103 **Lr** (260)

Periodic Table of the Elements

26.1   ATOMS

The smallest unit of any element is one **atom** of the element. All atoms have a central **nucleus**, which contains **protons** and **neutrons**, known collectively as **nucleons**. Each proton has an electric charge of +1 elementary unit; neutrons have no charge. Outside the nucleus, an atom contains electrons, and each **electron** has a charge of –1 elementary unit.

In every neutral atom, the number of electrons outside the nucleus is equal to the number of protons inside the nucleus. The electrons are held in the atom by the electrostatic attraction of the positively charged nucleus.

The number of protons in the nucleus of an atom is called its **atomic number**, Z. The atomic number of an atom uniquely determines what element the atom is, and Z may be shown explicitly by a subscript before the symbol of the element. For example, every beryllium atom contains exactly four protons, and we can write this as $_4$Be.

A proton and a neutron each have a mass slightly more than one atomic mass unit ($1 \text{ amu} = 1.66 \times 10^{-27} \text{ kg}$), and an electron has a mass that's only about 0.05 percent the mass of either a proton or a neutron. So, virtually all the mass of an atom is due to the mass of the nucleus.

The number of protons plus the number of neutrons in the nucleus of an atom gives the atom's **mass number**, A. If we let N stand for the number of neutrons, then $A = Z + N$.

In designating a particular atom of an element, we refer to its mass number. One way to do this is to write A as a superscript. For example, if a beryllium atom contains 5 neutrons, then its mass number is $4 + 5 = 9$, and we would write this as $_4^9$Be or simply as ^{9}Be. Another way is simply to write the mass number after the name of the elements, with a hyphen; ^{9}Be is beryllium-9.

26.2 ISOTOPES

If two atoms of the same element differ in their numbers of neutrons, then they are called **isotopes**. The atoms shown below are two different isotopes of the element beryllium. The atom on the left has 4 protons and 3 neutrons, so its mass number is 7; it's ^{7}Be (or beryllium-7). The atom on the right has 4 protons and 5 neutrons, so it's ^{9}Be (beryllium-9).

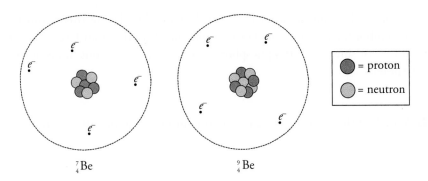

= proton	
= neutron	

$^7_4$Be $^9_4$Be

(These figures are definitely not to scale. If they were, each dashed circle showing the "outer edge" of the atom would literally be about 1500 m—almost a mile across! The nucleus occupies only the *tiniest* fraction of an atom's volume, which is mostly empty space.) Notice that these atoms—like all isotopes of a given element—*have the same atomic number but different mass numbers*.

Example 26-1: Which element has an isotope with a mass number of 84 that contains 46 neutrons in its nucleus?

   A) Krypton
   B) Rubidium
   C) Strontium
   D) Palladium

Solution: Since $A = 84$, $N = 46$, and $Z = A − N$, $Z = 84 − 46 = 38$. The element with an atomic number of 38 is Sr. Choice C is the correct answer.

Atomic Weight

Elements exist naturally as a collection of their isotopes. The **atomic weight of an element** is a *weighted average* of the masses of its naturally occurring isotopes. For example, boron has two naturally occurring isotopes: boron-10, with an atomic mass of 10.013 amu, and boron-11, with an atomic mass of 11.009 amu. Since boron-10 accounts for 20 percent of all naturally occurring boron, and boron-11 accounts for the other 80 percent, the atomic weight of boron is

$$(20\%)(10.013 \text{ amu}) + (80\%)(11.009 \text{ amu}) = 10.810 \text{ amu}$$

and this is the value listed in the periodic table. (Recall that the atomic mass unit is defined so that the most abundant isotope of carbon, carbon-12, has a mass of precisely 12 amu.)

26.3   IONS

When a neutral atom gains or loses electrons, it becomes charged, and the resulting atom is called an **ion**. For each electron it gains, an atom acquires a charge of –1 unit, and for each electron it loses, an atom acquires a charge of +1 unit. A negatively charged ion is called an **anion**, while a positively charged ion is called a **cation**.

We designate how many electrons an atom has gained or lost by placing this number as a superscript after the chemical symbol for the element. For example, if a lithium atom loses 1 electron, it becomes the lithium cation Li^{1+}, or simply Li^+. If a phosphorus atom gains 3 electrons, it becomes the phosphorus anion P^{3-}, or phosphide.

Example 26-2: Which of the following species contains 14 neutrons and 10 electrons?

> A) ^{26}Mg
> B) ^{22}Mg
> C) $^{26}Mg^{2+}$
> D) $^{22}Mg^{2+}$

Solution: Magnesium has $Z = 12$, and since there are only 10 electrons the correct answer must have a charge of +2. Choices A and B can be eliminated. The mass number, $A = Z + N$, is $12 + 14 = 26$, so choice C is the correct answer.

26.4   NUCLEAR STABILITY AND RADIOACTIVITY

The protons and neutrons in a nucleus are held together by a force called the **strong nuclear force**. It's stronger than the electrical force between charged particles, since for all atoms besides hydrogen, the strong nuclear force must overcome the electrical repulsion between the protons. In fact, of the four fundamental forces of nature, the strong nuclear force is the most powerful even though it only works over extremely short distances, as seen in the nucleus.

radioactive
beryllium
nucleus

stable
beryllium
nucleus

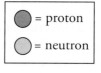
= proton
= neutron

Unstable nuclei are said to be **radioactive**, and they undergo a transformation to make them more stable, altering the number and ratio of protons and neutrons or just lowering their energy. Such a process is called **radioactive decay**, and we'll look at three types: **alpha**, **beta**, and **gamma**. The nucleus that undergoes radioactive decay is known as the **parent**, and the resulting more stable nucleus is known as the **daughter**.

Alpha (α) decay—nuclear emission of an **a particle** ($_2^4\alpha$) containing two protons and two neutrons. The a particle is equivalent to a helium nucleus ($_2^4$He), quickly loses energy traveling through the air, and can be stopped by the outer layers of human skin.

Beta (β) decay—involves the conversion of protons to neutrons or vice versa. β particles are more dangerous than α particles, and while they possess significantly greater penetrating ability, they can be stopped by aluminum foil or by a centimeter of plastic or glass.

- β⁻ decay occurs when an unstable nucleus contains too many neutrons and converts a neutron into a proton and an electron (also known as a β–**particle**, or $_{-1}^{0}\beta$). The resulting daughter nucleus has no change in mass number, but its atomic number increases by one. When the MCAT mentions "β decay" without any further qualification, it means β⁻ decay.
- β⁺ decay (**positron emission**) occurs when an unstable nucleus contains too few neutrons and converts a proton to a neutron and a **positron** (a particle identical to an electron but with a positive charge, or $_{+1}^{0}\beta$). The resulting daughter nucleus has no change in mass number, but its atomic number decreases by one.
- **Electron capture** is another way for an unstable nucleus to convert a proton into a neutron through capture of an electron ($_{-1}^{0}e$) from the closest electron shell ($n = 1$). Just like β⁺ decay, the resulting daughter nucleus has no change in mass number, but its atomic number decreases by one.

Gamma (γ) decay—the loss of one or more gamma photons ($_0^0\gamma$) from an excited state nucleus. This high frequency and energy form of electromagnetic radiation changes neither the atomic number nor mass number of the nucleus and can be stopped by a few inches of lead or a meter of concrete. Gamma decay often accompanies the other forms of nuclear decay described above.

Example 26-3: ^{90}Y, which undergoes β decay, is used in the treatment of non-Hodgkin lymphoma. Which of the following is the daughter nucleus of ^{90}Y?

    A) ^{89}Sr
    B) ^{90}Sr
    C) ^{90}Zr
    D) ^{91}Zr

Solution: β⁻ decay converts a neutron to a proton and does not affect the mass number, A, so choices A and D can be eliminated. According to the following equation, β⁻ decay increases the atomic number, Z, by one, so choice C is correct.

$$_{39}^{90}\text{Y} \rightarrow {}_{40}^{90}\text{Zr} + {}_{-1}^{0}\beta$$

26.4

Example 26-4: A certain radioisotope used in the treatment of bone cancers undergoes α-decay. Its daughter nucleus is ^{219}Rn. What is the identity of the radioisotope?

A) ^{215}Po
B) ^{217}Pb
C) ^{221}Th
D) ^{223}Ra

Solution: α-Particles contain two protons and two neutrons. To determine the parent nucleus in an alpha decay, we need to add two protons and two neutrons to the daughter nucleus. Choice D is correct, as shown in the following decay equation:

$$^{223}_{88}\text{Ra} \rightarrow {}^{219}_{86}\text{Rn} + {}^{4}_{2}\alpha$$

Example 26-5: Vitamin B$_{12}$ can be prepared with *radioactive* cobalt (^{58}Co), a known β$^+$ emitter, and administered orally as a diagnostic tool to test for defects in intestinal vitamin B$_{12}$ absorption. What is the daughter nucleus of ^{58}Co?

A) ^{57}Fe
B) ^{58}Fe
C) ^{59}Co
D) ^{59}Ni

Solution: All types of β$^+$ decay leave the mass of the daughter and parent elements the same, thus the mass must be 58, making choice B the only option. The β$^+$ decay of ^{58}Co is described by this nuclear reaction:

$$^{58}_{27}\text{Co} \rightarrow {}^{58}_{26}\text{Fe} + {}^{0}_{+1}\beta$$

Example 26-6: Decay chains occur when both parent and daughter nuclei can undergo radioactive decay. One potential series, starting with ^{237}Np, is comprised of the following sequential decays: alpha, beta, alpha, alpha, beta, alpha, alpha, alpha, beta, alpha, beta, alpha. Several nuclei in this chain also emit γ-rays. Which of the following is the final product of this decay chain?

A) ^{205}Ta
B) ^{205}Tl
C) ^{207}Ta
D) ^{207}Tl

Solution: There are 8 α-decays, 4 β-decays, and some γ-decays in this chain. The order of decays doesn't matter; the net reaction is given by

$$^{237}_{93}\text{Np} \rightarrow {}^{A}_{Z}X + 8\,{}^{4}_{2}\alpha + 4\,{}^{0}_{-1}\beta^- + {}^{0}_{0}\gamma$$

Each α-decay *decreases* A by 4 and Z by 2. Each β-decay *increases* Z by 1, and has no effect on A. The mass number of the final product is given by $A = 237 - 8(4) - 4(0) = 205$, so choices C and D can be eliminated. The atomic number of the final product is given by $Z = 93 - 8(2) - 4(-1) = 81$, so choice A ($Z = 73$) can be eliminated; choice B is correct. γ-decays don't change the identity of the isotope, so they can be ignored.

Half-Life

Different radioactive nuclei decay at different rates. The **half-life**, which is denoted by $t_{1/2}$, of a radioactive substance is the time it takes for one-half of some sample of the substance to decay. Thus, the shorter the half-life, the faster the decay. The amount of a radioactive substance decreases exponentially with time, as illustrated in the following graph.

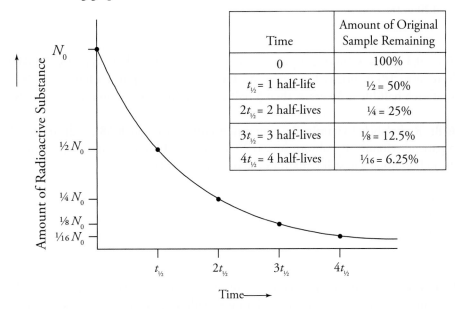

Time	Amount of Original Sample Remaining
0	100%
$t_{1/2}$ = 1 half-life	½ = 50%
$2t_{1/2}$ = 2 half-lives	¼ = 25%
$3t_{1/2}$ = 3 half-lives	⅛ = 12.5%
$4t_{1/2}$ = 4 half-lives	¹⁄₁₆ = 6.25%

For example, a radioactive sample with an initial mass of 80 grams and a half-life of 6 years will decay as follows:

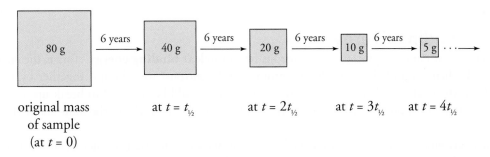

The equation for the exponential decay curve shown above is often written as $N = N_0 e^{-kt}$, but a simpler—and much more intuitive way—is

$$N = N_0 (1/2)^{T/t_{1/2}}$$

where $t_{1/2}$ is the half-life and T is the total time the sample has decayed. For example, when $T = 3t_{1/2}$, the number of radioactive nuclei remaining, N, is $N_0(1/2)^3 = 1/8\ N_0$, just what we expect. If the form $N_0 e^{-kt}$ is used, the value of k (known as the **decay constant**) is inversely proportional to the half-life: $k = (\ln 2)/t_{1/2}$. The shorter the half-life, the greater the decay constant, and the more rapidly the sample decays.

Example 26-7: Cesium-137 has a half-life of 30 years. How long will it take for only 0.3 g to remain from a sample that had an original mass of 2.4 g?

26.4

A) 60 years
B) 90 years
C) 120 years
D) 240 years

Solution: Since 0.3 grams is 1/8 of 2.4 grams, the question is asking how long it will take for the radioisotope to decrease to 1/8 its original amount. We know that this requires 3 half-lives, since $1/2 \times 1/2 \times 1/2 = 1/8$. So, if each half-life is 30 years, then 3 half-lives will be $3(30) = 90$ years, choice B.

Example 26-8: Radiolabeled vitamin B_{12} containing radioactive cobalt-58 is administered to diagnose a defect in a patient's vitamin-B_{12} absorption. If ^{58}Co has a half-life of 72 days, approximately what percentage of the radioisotope will still remain in the patient a year later?

A) 3%
B) 5%
C) 8%
D) 10%

Solution: One year is approximately equal to 5 half-lives of this radioisotope, since $5 \times 72 = 360$ days = 1 year. After 5 half-lives, the amount of the radioisotope will drop to $(1/2)^5 = 1/32$ of the original amount administered. Because $1/32 = 3/100 = 3\%$, the best answer is choice A.

Nuclear Binding Energy

Every nucleus that contains protons *and* neutrons has a **nuclear binding energy**. This is the energy that was released when the individual nucleons (protons and neutrons) were bound together by the strong force to form the nucleus. It's also equal to the energy that would be required to break up the intact nucleus into its individual nucleons. The greater the binding energy per nucleon, the more stable the nucleus.

When nucleons bind together to form a nucleus, some mass is converted to energy, so the mass of the combined nucleus is *less* than the sum of the masses of all its nucleons individually. The difference, Δm, is called the **mass defect**, and its energy equivalent *is* the nuclear binding energy. For a stable nucleus, the mass defect,

$$\Delta m = \text{(total mass of separate nucleons)} - \text{(mass of nucleus)}$$

will always be positive.

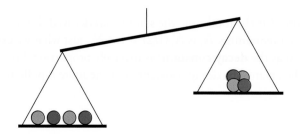

The nuclear binding energy, E_B, can be found from the mass defect using **Einstein's equations for mass-energy equivalence**: $E_B = (\Delta m)c^2$, where c is the speed of light (3×10^8 m/s). If mass is measured in kilograms and energy in Joules, then $1 \text{ kg} \leftrightarrow 9 \times 10^{16}$ J. But in the nuclear domain, masses are often expressed in atomic mass units ($1 \text{ amu} \approx 1.66 \times 10^{-27}$ kg), and energy is expressed in **electronvolts** ($1 \text{ eV} \approx 1.6 \times 10^{-19}$ J). In terms of these units, the equations for the nuclear binding energy, $E_B = (\Delta m)c^2$, can be written as $E_B \text{ (in eV)} = [\Delta m \text{(in amu)}] \times 931.5$ MeV.

Example 26-9: The mass defect of a tritium atom, ^3_1H, is about 0.009 amu. What is its nuclear binding energy, in electronvolts?

Solution: In terms of amus and electronvolts, the equation for the nuclear binding energy is $E_B\text{(in eV)} = [\Delta m\text{(in amu)}] \times 931.5$ MeV. Therefore, for the tritium nucleus, we have

$$E_B = (0.009) \times (931.5 \text{ MeV}) \approx 8.4 \text{ MeV}$$

26.5 ATOMIC STRUCTURE

Emission Spectra

Imagine a glass tube filled with a small sample of an element in gaseous form. When electric current is passed through the tube, the gas begins to glow with a color characteristic of that particular element. If this light emitted by the gas is then passed through a prism—which will separate the light into its component wavelengths—the result is the element's **emission spectrum**.

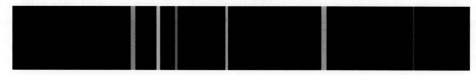

An atom's emission spectrum gives an energetic "fingerprint" of that element because it consists of a unique sequence of *bright* lines that correspond to specific wavelengths and energies. The energies of the photons, or particles of light that are emitted, are related to their frequencies, f, and wavelengths, λ, by the equation

$$E_{photon} = hf = h\frac{c}{\lambda}$$

where h is a universal constant called **Planck's constant** (6.63×10^{-34} J·s) and c is the speed of light. For the following discussion, a general understanding of the electromagnetic spectrum will be useful.

The Bohr Model of the Atom

In 1913 the Danish physicist Niels Bohr realized that the model of atomic structure of his time was inconsistent with emission spectral data. In order to account for the limited numbers of lines that are observed in the emission spectra of elements, Bohr described a new model of the atom. In this model that would later take his name, he proposed that the electrons in an atom orbited the nucleus in circular paths, much as the planets orbit the Sun in the solar system. Distance from the nucleus was related to the energy of the electrons; electrons with greater amounts of energy orbited the nucleus at greater distances. However, the electrons in the atom cannot assume any arbitrary energy, but they have *quantized* energy states, and thereby only orbit at certain allowed distances from the nucleus.

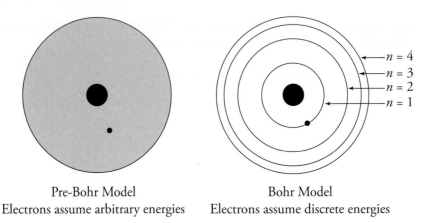

Pre-Bohr Model
Electrons assume arbitrary energies

Bohr Model
Electrons assume discrete energies

If an electron absorbs energy that's exactly equal to the difference in energy between its current level and that of an available higher lever, it "jumps" to that higher level. The electron can then "drop" to a lower energy level, emitting a photon with an energy exactly equal to the difference between the levels. This model predicted that elements would have line spectra instead of continuous spectra, as would be the case if transitions between all possible energies could be expected. An electron could only gain or lose very specific amounts of energy due to the quantized nature of the energy levels. Therefore, only photons with certain energies are observed. These specific energies corresponded to very specific wavelengths, as seen in the emission line spectra.

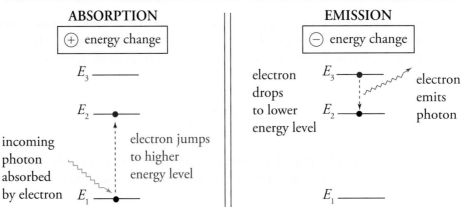

In the transition depicted below, an electron is initially in its **ground state** ($n = 1$), or its lowest possible energy level. When this electron absorbs a photon it jumps to a higher energy level, known as an **excited state** (in this case $n = 3$). Electrons excited to high energy don't always relax to the ground state in large jumps, rather they can relax in a series of smaller jumps, gradually coming back to the ground state. From this excited state the electron can relax in one of two ways, either dropping into the $n = 2$ level, or directly back to the $n = 1$ ground state. In the first scenario, we can expect to detect a photon with energy corresponding to the difference between $n = 3$ and $n = 2$. In the latter case we'd detect a more energetic photon of energy corresponding to the difference between $n = 3$ and $n = 1$.

Note: Distances between energy levels are not drawn to scale.

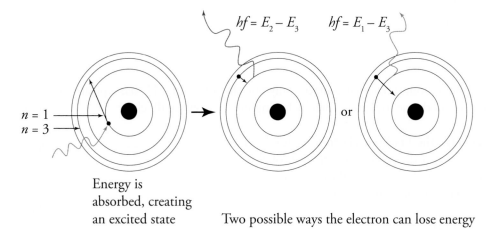

Energy is absorbed, creating an excited state

Two possible ways the electron can lose energy

The energies of these discrete energy levels were given by Bohr in the following equation, which only accurately predicted the behavior of atoms or ions containing one electron, now known as Bohr atoms. The value n in this case represents the energy level of the electron.

$$E_n = \frac{(-2.178 \times 10^{-18}\,\text{J})}{n^2}$$

Since we can calculate the energies of the levels of a Bohr atom, we can predict the wavelengths of photons emitted or absorbed when electrons transition between any two energy levels. To do this, we calculate the energy differences between discrete levels by subtracting the initial energy of the electron from the final energy of the electron. We can find the energies of the two possible emitted photons shown above as follows:

$$\Delta E_{3 \to 2} = \frac{(-2.178 \times 10^{-18}\,\text{J})}{(2)^2} - \frac{(-2.178 \times 10^{-18}\,\text{J})}{(3)^2}$$

$$\Delta E_{3 \to 2} = -3.025 \times 10^{-19}\,\text{J}$$

$$\Delta E_{3 \to 1} = \frac{(-2.178 \times 10^{-18}\,\text{J})}{(1)^2} - \frac{(-2.178 \times 10^{-18}\,\text{J})}{(3)^2}$$

$$\Delta E_{3 \to 2} = -1.936 \times 10^{-18}\,\text{J}$$

Note that both energies calculated above are negative, indicating that energy is being released by the electron as it falls from its excited state to a lower energy level. For electron transitions from the ground state to an excited state, the ΔE values will be positive, indicating energy is absorbed by the electron.

Once the energy is calculated, the wavelength of the photon can be found by employing the relation $\Delta E = h\dfrac{c}{\lambda}$. Not all electron transitions produce photons we can see with the naked eye, but all transitions in an atom will produce photons either in the ultraviolet, visible, or infrared region of the electromagnetic spectrum.

Example 26-10: Which of the following is NOT an example of a Bohr atom?

A) H
B) He⁺
C) Li²⁺
D) H⁺

Solution: A Bohr atom is one that contains only one electron. Since H⁺ has a positive charge from losing the one electron in the neutral atom thereby having no electrons at all, choice D is the answer.

Example 26-11: The first four electron energy levels of an atom are shown at the right, given in terms of electron volts. Which of the following gives the energy of a photon that could NOT be emitted by this atom?

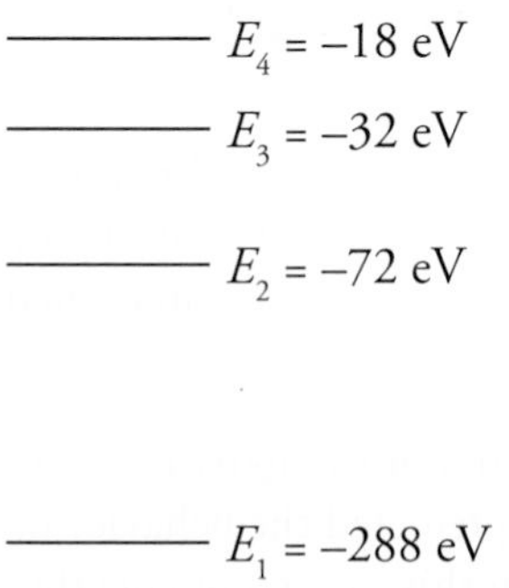

A) 14 eV
B) 40 eV
C) 44 eV
D) 54 eV

———— $E_4 = -18$ eV

———— $E_3 = -32$ eV

———— $E_2 = -72$ eV

———— $E_1 = -288$ eV

Solution: The difference between E_4 and E_3 is 14 eV, so a photon of 14 eV would be emitted if an electron were to drop from level 4 to level 3; this eliminates choice A. Similarly, the difference between E_3 and E_2 is 40 eV, so choice B is eliminated, and the difference between E_4 and E_2 is 54 eV, so choice D is eliminated. The answer must be choice C; no two energy levels in this atom are separated by 44 eV.

The Quantum Model of the Atom

While one-electron atoms produce easily predicted atomic spectra, the Bohr model does not do a good job of predicting the atomic spectra of many-electron atoms. This shows that the Bohr model cannot describe the electron-electron interactions that exist in many-electron atoms. The quantum model of the atom was developed to account for these differences. Bohr's model suggested, and we still hold to be true, that electrons held by an atom can exist only at discrete energy levels—that is, electron energy levels are quantized. This quantization is described by a unique "address" for each electron, consisting of four quantum numbers designating the shell, subshell, orbital, and spin. While the details of quantum numbers are beyond the scope of the MCAT, it is still useful to understand the conceptual basis of the quantum model.

The Energy Shell

The energy shell (n) of an electron in the quantum model of the atom is analogous to the circular orbits in the Bohr model of the atom. An electron in a higher shell has a greater amount of energy and a greater average distance from the nucleus. For example, an electron in the 3rd shell ($n = 3$) has a higher energy than an electron in the 2nd shell (where $n = 2$), which has more energy than an electron in the 1st shell ($n = 1$).

The Energy Subshell

In the quantum model of the atom, however, we no longer describe the path of electrons around the nucleus as circular orbits, but focus on the probability of finding an electron somewhere in the atom. Loosely speaking, an **orbital** describes a three-dimensional region around the nucleus in which the electron is most likely to be found.

A subshell in an atom is comprised of one or more orbitals, and it is denoted by a letter (*s*, *p*, *d*, or *f*) that describes the shape and energy of the orbital(s). The orbitals in the subshells get progressively more complex and higher in energy in the order listed above. Each energy shell has one or more subshells, and each higher energy shell contains one additional subshell. For example, the first energy shell contains the *s* subshell, while the second energy shell contains both the *s* and *p* subshell, etc.

26.5

The Orbital Orientation

Each subshell contains one or more orbitals of the same energy (also called degenerate orbitals), and these orbitals have different three-dimensional orientations in space. The number of orientations increases by two in each successive subshell. For example, the *s* subshell contains one orientation and the *p* subshell contains three orientations.

You should be able to recognize the shapes of the orbitals in the *s* and *p* subshells. Each *s* subshell has just one spherically symmetrical orbital. Each *p* subshell has three orbitals, each depicted as a dumbbell, with different spatial orientations.

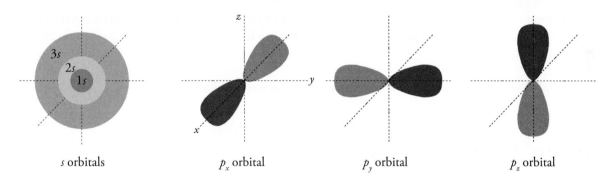

s orbitals p_x orbital p_y orbital p_z orbital

The Electron Spin

Every electron has two possible spin states, which can be considered the electron's intrinsic magnetism. Because of this every orbital can accommodate a maximum of two electrons, one spin-up and one spin-down. If an orbital is full, we say that the electrons it holds are "spin-paired."

26.6 ELECTRON CONFIGURATIONS

Now that we've described the modern quantum model of the atom, let's see how this is represented as an electron configuration. There are three basic rules:

1) *Electrons occupy the lowest energy orbitals available.* (This is the **Aufbau principle**.) Electron subshells are filled in order of increasing energy. The periodic table is logically constructed to reflect this fact, and therefore one can easily determine shell filling for specific atoms based on where they appear on the table. We will detail this in a future section on "Blocks."

2) *Electrons in the same subshell occupy available orbitals singly, before pairing up.* (This is known as **Hund's Rule**.)

3) *There can be no more than two electrons in any given orbital.* (This is the **Pauli exclusion principle**.)

For example, let's describe the locations for all the electrons in an oxygen atom, which contains eight electrons. Beginning with the first, lowest energy shell, there is only one subshell (s) and only one orientation in that subshell, and there can only be two electrons in that one orbital. Therefore, these two electrons fill the only orbital in the $1s$ subshell. We write this as $1s^2$, to indicate that there are two electrons in the $1s$ subshell.

We still have six electrons left, so let's move on to the second, next highest, energy shell. There are two subshells (s and p). Since the s subshell is lower in energy than the p subshell, the next two electrons go in the $2s$ subshell, that is, $2s^2$.

For the remaining four electrons, there would be three orientations of orbitals in the p subshell. According to Hund's Rule, we place one spin up electron in each of these three orbitals. The eighth electron now pairs up with an electron in one of the $2p$ orbitals. So, the last four electrons go in the $2p$ subshell: $2p^4$ (or more explicitly, $2p_x^2 2p_y^1 2p_z^1$).

The complete electron configuration for oxygen can now be written like this:

$$\text{Oxygen} = 1s^2 2s^2 2p^4$$

Here are the electron configurations for the first ten elements:

Z			1*s*	2*s*	2*p*		
1	H	$1s^1$	↑				
2	He	$1s^2$	↑↓				
3	Li	$1s^2 2s^1$	↑↓	↑			
4	Be	$1s^2 2s^2$	↑↓	↑↓			
5	B	$1s^2 2s^2 2p^1$	↑↓	↑↓	↑		
6	C	$1s^2 2s^2 2p^2$	↑↓	↑↓	↑	↑	
7	N	$1s^2 2s^2 2p^3$	↑↓	↑↓	↑	↑	↑
8	O	$1s^2 2s^2 2p^4$	↑↓	↑↓	↑↓	↑	↑
9	F	$1s^2 2s^2 2p^5$	↑↓	↑↓	↑↓	↑↓	↑
10	Ne	$1s^2 2s^2 2p^6$	↑↓	↑↓	↑↓	↑↓	↑↓

Example 26-12: What's the maximum number of electrons that can go into any *s* subshell? Any *p* subshell? Any *d*? Any *f*?

Solution: An *s* subshell has only one possible orbital orientation. Since only two electrons can fill any given orbital, an *s* subshell can hold no more than 1 × 2 = 2 electrons.

A *p* subshell has three possible orbital orientations (two more than an *s* subshell). Since again only two electrons can fill any given orbital, a *p* subshell can hold no more than 3 × 2 = 6 electrons.

A *d* subshell has five possible orbital orientations (two more than a *p* subshell). Since there are two electrons per orbital, a *d* subshell can hold no more than 5 × 2 = 10 electrons.

Finally, an *f* subshell has seven possible orbital orientations (two more than a *d* subshell). Since there are two electrons per orbital, an *f* subshell can hold no more than 7 × 2 = 14 electrons.

Example 26-13: Write down—and comment on—the electron configuration of argon (Ar, atomic number 18).

Solution: We have 18 electrons to successively place in the proper subshells, as follows: 1*s*: 2 electrons; 2*s*: 2 electrons; 2*p*: 6 electrons; 3*s*: 2 electrons; 3*p*: 6 electrons.

Therefore,

$$[\text{Ar}] = 1s^2 2s^2 2p^6 3s^2 3p^6$$

Notice that 3*s* and 3*p* subshells have their full complement of electrons. In fact, the **noble gases** (those elements in the last column of the periodic table) all have their outer 8 electrons in filled subshells: 2 in the *ns* subshell plus 6 in the *np*. (The lone exception, of course, is helium; but its one and only subshell, the 1*s*, is filled—with 2 electrons.) Because their 8 valence electrons are in filled subshells, we say that these atoms—Ne, Ar, Kr, Xe, and Rn—have a complete **octet**, which accounts for their remarkable chemical stability, and lack of reactivity.

Diamagnetic and Paramagnetic Atoms

An atom that has all of its electrons spin-paired is referred to as **diamagnetic**. For example, helium, beryllium, and neon are diamagnetic. A diamagnetic atom must contain an even number of electrons and have all of its occupied subshells filled. Since all the electrons in a diamagnetic atom are spin-paired, the individual magnetic fields that they create cancel, leaving no net magnetic field. Such an atom will be *repelled* by an externally produced magnetic field.

If an atom's electrons are not all spin-paired, it is said to be **paramagnetic**. Paramagnetic atoms are *attracted* into externally produced magnetic fields.

26.6

$\uparrow$ = spin-up electron
$\downarrow$ = spin-down electron

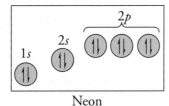

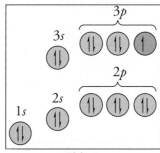

Neon
all electrons spin-paired
∴ diamagnetic
repelled from a magnetic field

Chlorine
not all electrons spin-paired
∴ paramagnetic
attracted into a magnetic field

Example 26-14: Which of the following elements is diamagnetic?

A) Sodium
B) Sulfur
C) Potassium
D) Calcium

Solution: First, a diamagnetic atom must contain an *even* number of electrons, because they all must be spin-*paired*. So, we can eliminate choices A and C, since sodium and potassium each contain an odd number of electrons (11 and 19, respectively). The electron configuration of sulfur is [Ne] $3s^2 3p^4$; by Hund's Rule, the 4 electrons in the $3p$ subshell will look like this:

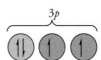

They're not all spin-paired, so sulfur is not diamagnetic. The answer must be choice D, calcium, because its configuration is [Ar] $4s^2$, and all of its electrons are spin-paired.

Blocks in the Periodic Table

s block →

——— *p* block ———→

——— *d* block ———→

	I	II											III	IV	V	VI	VII	VIII
1	1 **H** 1.0																	2 **He** 4.0
2	3 **Li** 6.9	4 **Be** 9.0											5 **B** 10.8	6 **C** 12.0	7 **N** 14.0	8 **O** 16.0	9 **F** 19.0	10 **Ne** 20.2
3	11 **Na** 23.0	12 **Mg** 24.3											13 **Al** 27.0	14 **Si** 28.1	15 **P** 31.0	16 **S** 32.1	17 **Cl** 35.5	18 **Ar** 39.9
4	19 **K** 39.1	20 **Ca** 40.1	21 **Sc** 45.0	22 **Ti** 47.9	23 **V** 50.9	24 **Cr** 52.0	25 **Mn** 54.9	26 **Fe** 55.8	27 **Co** 58.9	28 **Ni** 58.7	29 **Cu** 63.5	30 **Zn** 65.4	31 **Ga** 69.7	32 **Ge** 72.6	33 **As** 74.9	34 **Se** 79.0	35 **Br** 79.9	36 **Kr** 83.8
5	37 **Rb** 85.5	38 **Sr** 87.6	39 **Y** 88.9	40 **Zr** 91.2	41 **Nb** 92.9	42 **Mo** 95.9	43 **Tc** (98)	44 **Ru** 101.1	45 **Rh** 102.9	46 **Pd** 106.4	47 **Ag** 107.9	48 **Cd** 112.4	49 **In** 114.8	50 **Sn** 118.7	51 **Sb** 121.8	52 **Te** 127.6	53 **I** 126.9	54 **Xe** 131.3
6	55 **Cs** 132.9	56 **Ba** 137.3	57 ***La** 138.9	72 **Hf** 178.5	73 **Ta** 180.9	74 **W** 183.9	75 **Re** 186.2	76 **Os** 190.2	77 **Ir** 192.2	78 **Pt** 195.1	79 **Au** 197.0	80 **Hg** 200.6	81 **Tl** 204.4	82 **Pb** 207.2	83 **Bi** 209.0	84 **Po** (209)	85 **At** (210)	86 **Rn** (222)
7	87 **Fr** (223)	88 **Ra** 226.0	89 **†Ac** 227.0	104 **Rf** (261)	105 **Db** (262)	106 **Sg** (266)	107 **Bh** (264)	108 **Hs** (277)	109 **Mt** (268)	110 **Ds** (281)	111 **Rg** (272)	112 **Cp** (285)	113 **Uut** (286)	114 **Fl** (289)	115 **Uup** (288)	116 **Lv** (293)	117 **Uus** (294)	118 **Uuo** (294)

——— *f* block ———→

*Lanthanide Series:	58 **Ce** 140.1	59 **Pr** 140.9	60 **Nd** 144.2	61 **Pm** (145)	62 **Sm** 150.4	63 **Eu** 152.0	64 **Gd** 157.3	65 **Tb** 158.9	66 **Dy** 162.5	67 **Ho** 164.9	68 **Er** 167.3	69 **Tm** 168.9	70 **Yb** 173.0	71 **Lu** 175.0
†Actinide Series:	90 **Th** 232.0	91 **Pa** (231)	92 **U** 238.0	93 **Np** (237)	94 **Pu** (244)	95 **Am** (243)	96 **Cm** (247)	97 **Bk** (247)	98 **Cf** (251)	99 **Es** (252)	100 **Fm** (257)	101 **Md** (258)	102 **No** (259)	103 **Lr** (260)

The periodic table can be divided into blocks, as shown above. The name of the block (*s, p, d,* or *f*) indicates the highest-energy subshell containing electrons in the ground-state of an atom within that block. For example, carbon is in the *p* block, and its electron configuration is $1s^22s^22p^2$; the highest-energy subshell that contains electrons (the $2p$) is a *p* subshell. In addition, each horizontal row in the periodic table is called a **period**, and each vertical column is called a **group** (or **family**). The bold numbers next to the rows on the left indicate the period number; for example, potassium (K, atomic number 19) is in Period 4.

How do we use this block diagram to write electron configurations? To illustrate, let's say we want to write the configuration for chlorine ($Z = 17$). To get to $Z = 17$, imagine starting at $Z = 1$ (hydrogen) and filling up the subshells as we move along through the rows to $Z = 17$. (Notice that helium has been moved over next to hydrogen for purposes of this block diagram.) We'll first have $1s^2$ for the 2 atoms in Period 1, *s* block ($Z = 1$ and $Z = 2$); the $2s^2$ for the next 2 atoms, which are in Period 2, *s* block ($Z = 3$ and $Z = 4$); then $2p^6$ for the next 6 atoms, which are in Period 2, *p* block ($Z = 5$ through $Z = 10$); the $3s^2$ for the next 2 atoms, which are in Period 3, *s* block ($Z = 11$ and $Z = 12$); then, finally, $3p^5$ for the atoms starting with aluminum, Al, in Period 3, *p* block and counting through to chlorine, Cl. So, we've gone through the rows and blocks from the beginning and stopped once we hit the atom we wanted, and along the way we obtained $1s^22s^22p^63s^23p^5$. This is the electron configuration of chlorine.

The noble gases are often used as starting points, because they are at the end of the rows and represent a shell being completely filled; all that's left is to count over in the next row until the desired atom is reached. We find the closest noble gas that has an atomic number less than that of the atom for which we want to find an electron configuration. In the case of chlorine ($Z = 17$), the closest noble gas with a smaller atomic number is neon ($Z = 10$). Starting with neon, we have 7 additional electrons to take care of. To get to $Z = 17$, we go through the 2 atoms in the *s* block of Period 3 ($3s^2$), then notice that Cl is the fifth element in the *p* block, giving us $3p^5$. Therefore, the electron configuration of chlorine is the same as that of neon plus $3s^23p^5$, which we can write like this: Cl = [Ne] $3s^23p^5$.

The simple counting through the rows and blocks works as long as you remember this simple rule: whenever you're in the *d* block, *subtract 1 from the period number*. For example, the first row of the *d* block ($Z = 21$ through $Z = 30$) is in Period 4, but instead of saying that these elements have their outermost (or **valence**) electrons in the $4d$ subshell, we subtract 1 from the period number and say that these elements put their valence electrons in the $3d$ subshell.

In summary, the block in the table tells us in which subshell the outermost (valence) electrons of the atom will be. The period (row) gives the shell, *n*, as long as we remember the following fact about the atoms in the *d* block: electrons for an atom in the *d* block of Period *n* go into the subshell $(n − 1)d$. For example, the electron configuration for scandium (Sc, atomic number 21) is $[Ar]4s^2 3d^1$. (Note: if you ever need to write the electron configuration for an element in the *f* block, the rule is: *In the f block, subtract 2 from the period number.*)

Example 26-15: What is the correct ground-state electron configuration of a cobalt atom?

A) $[Ar]\ 4s^2\ 3d^6$
B) $[Ar]\ 4s^2\ 4d^7$
C) $[Ar]\ 4s^1\ 3d^8$
D) $[Ar]\ 4s^2\ 3d^7$

Solution: Co has an atomic number of 27, so the answer must contain 27 electrons; choice A can be eliminated. Choice B is incorrect because it has the $4d$ subshell, rather than the $3d$ subshell, being filled directly after the $4s$ orbital. Choice C violates the Aufbau principle by populating the $3d$ subshell before filling the $4s$ orbital, and is incorrect. The correct answer, choice D, has the correct number of electrons appropriately distributed in the correct orbitals.

Example 26-16: What is the maximum number of electrons that can be present in the $n = 3$ shell?

A) 6
B) 9
C) 12
D) 18

Solution: Every new energy level (*n*) adds a new subshell. That means that in the first energy level we have only the *s* subshell, while when $n = 2$ we have both *s* and *p* subshells, and when $n = 3$, there are *s*, *p*, and *d* subshells. Since there are 1, 3, and 5 *s*, *p*, and *d* orbitals, respectively, for a total of 9 orbitals, and since the maximum number of electrons in an orbital is 2, there can be a maximum of 18 electrons in the $n = 3$ shell.

Some Anomalous Electron Configurations

The process described above (reading across the periodic table, from top to bottom and left to right, using the blocks as a tool for the order of filling of subshells) to determine an atom's electron configuration works quite well for a large percentage of the elements, but there are a few atoms for which the anticipated electron configuration is not the actual configuration observed.

In a few instances, atoms can achieve a lower energy state (or a higher degree of stability) *by having a filled or half-filled, d subshell*. For example, consider chromium (Cr, $Z = 24$). On the basis of the block diagram, we'd expect its electron configuration to be [Ar] $4s^2 3d^4$. Recalling that a d subshell can hold a maximum of 10 electrons, it turns out that chromium achieves a more stable state by filling its d subshell with 5 electrons (*half-filled*) rather than leaving it with 4. This is accomplished by promoting one of its $4s$ electrons to the $3d$ subshell, yielding the electron configuration [Ar]$4s^1 3d^5$. As another example, copper (Cu, $Z = 29$) has an expected electron configuration of [Ar] $4s^2 3d^9$. However, a copper atom obtains a more stable, lower-energy state by promoting one of its $4s$ electrons into the $3d$ subshell, yielding [Ar] $4s^1 3d^{10}$ to give a *filled d* subshell.

Other atoms that display the same type of behavior with regard to their electron configuration as do chromium and copper include molybdenum (Mo, $Z = 42$, in the same family as chromium), as well as silver and gold (Ag and Au, $Z = 47$ and $Z = 79$, respectively, which are in the same family as copper).

Example 26-17: What is the electron configuration of an atom of silver?

Solution: As mentioned above, silver is one of the handful of elements with atoms that actually achieve greater overall stability by promoting one of its electrons into a higher subshell in order to make it filled. We'd expect the electron configuration for silver to be [Kr]$5s^2 4d^9$. But, by analogy with copper, we'd predict (correctly) that the actual configuration of silver is [Kr] $5s^1 4d^{10}$, where the atom obtains a more stable state by promoting one of its $5s$ electrons into the $4d$ subshell, to give a *filled d* subshell.

Electron Configurations of Ions

Recall that an ion is an atom that has acquired a nonzero electric charge. An atom with more electrons than protons is negatively charged and is called an anion; an atom with fewer electrons than protons is positively charged and is called a cation.

Atoms that gain electrons (anions) accommodate them in the first available orbital, the one with the lowest available energy. For example, fluorine (F, $Z = 9$) has the electron configuration $1s^2 2s^2 2p^5$. When a fluorine atom gains an electron to become the fluoride ion, F^-, the additional electron goes into the $2p$ subshell, giving the electron configuration $1s^2 2s^2 2p^6$, which is the same as the configuration of neon. For this reason, F^- and Ne are said to be **isoelectronic**.

In order to write the electron configuration of an ion for an element in the s or p blocks, we can use the blocks in the periodic table as follows. If an atom becomes an anion—that is, if it acquires one or more additional electrons—then we move to the *right* within the table by a number of squares equal to the number of electrons added in order to find the atom with the same configuration as the ion.

If an atom becomes a cation—that is, if it loses one or more electrons—then we move to the *left* within the table by a number of squares equal to the number of electrons lost in order to find the atom with the same configuration as the ion.

26.6

Example 26-18: What is the correct ground-state electron configuration of Te^{2-}? Of As^{3+}?

Solution: Both can be found from the periodic table. Finding tellurium ($Z = 52$), we move two places to the *right* because the atom has *gained* two electrons to become an anion. This means that Te^{2-} has the same electron configuration as Xe: $[Kr]\ 5s^2\ 4d^{10}\ 5p^6$.

Starting at arsenic ($Z = 33$) on the periodic table, we move three places to the *left* because the atom has *lost* three electrons to become a cation. As^{3+} has the same electron configuration as Zn: $[Ar]4s^2\ 3d^{10}$.

Electrons that are removed (*ionized*) from an atom always come from the valence shell (the highest n level), and the highest energy orbital within that level. For example, an atom of lithium, Li ($1s^2 2s^1$), becomes Li^+ ($1s^2$) when it absorbs enough energy for an electron to escape. However, recall from our discussion above that **transition metals** (which are the elements in the d block) have both ns and $(n-1)d$ electrons. To form a cation, atoms will always lose their valence electrons first, and since $n > n-1$, transition metals lose s electrons *before* they lose d electrons. Only after *all* s electrons are lost do d electrons get ionized. For example, the electron configuration for the transition metal titanium (Ti, $Z = 22$) is $[Ar]\ 4s^2 3d^2$. We might expect that the electron configuration of the ion Ti^+ to be $[Ar]\ 4s^2 3d^1$ since the d electrons are slightly higher in energy. However, the *actual* configuration is $[Ar]\ 4s^1 3d^2$, and the valence electrons (the ones from the highest n level) are ALWAYS lost first. Similarly, the electron configuration of Ti^{2+} is not $[Ar]\ 4s^2$—it's actually $[Ar]\ 3d^2$.

Example 26-19: What's the electron configuration of Cu^+? Of Cu^{2+}? Of Fe^{3+}?

Solution: Copper (Cu, $Z = 29$) is a transition metal, so it will lose its valence s electrons before losing any d electrons. Recall the anomalous electron configuration of Cu (to give it a filled $3d$ subshell): $[Ar]\ 4s^1 3d^{10}$. Therefore, the configuration of Cu^+ (the *cuprous* ion, Cu(I)) is $[Ar]\ 3d^{10}$, and that of Cu^{2+} (the *cupric* ion, Cu(II)) is $[Ar]\ 3d^9$. Since the electron configuration of iron (Fe, $Z = 26$) is $[Ar]\ 4s^2 3d^6$, the configuration of Fe^{3+} (the *ferric* ion, Fe(III)) is $[Ar]\ 3d^5$, since the transition metal atom Fe first loses both of its valence s electrons, then once they're ionized, one of its d electrons.

Excited State vs. Ground State

Assigning electron configurations as we've just discussed is aimed at constructing the *most probable* location of electrons, following the Aufbau principle. These configurations are the most probable because they are the lowest in energy, or as they are often termed, the ground state.

Any electron configuration of an atom that is *not* as we would assign it, provided it doesn't break any physical rules (no more than 2 e^- per orbital, no assigning non-existent shells such as $2d$, etc.) is an excited state. The atom has absorbed energy, so the electrons now inhabit states we wouldn't predict as the most probable ones.

Example 26-20: An atom of silicon absorbs a photon and transitions to an excited state. Which of the following could be the electron configuration of that excited state?

   A) $1s^2 2s^2 2p^5 3s^3 3p^2$
   B) $1s^2 2s^2 2p^6 3s^1 3p^3$
   C) $1s^2 2s^2 2p^6 3s^2 3p^2$
   D) $1s^2 2s^2 2p^6 3s^2 3p^3$

Solution: Each s subshell consists of one orbital that can hold two electrons. Choice A is eliminated because it's impossible to have a $3s^3$ configuration. Choice B is correct; one of the valence $3s$ electrons in the ground state is now in the higher energy $3p$ orbital. Choice C is the ground state configuration of a silicon atom, not an excited state configuration, and thus is incorrect. Choice D is incorrect as it has 15 electrons, but a neutral atom of silicon has only 14.

26.7 GROUPS OF THE PERIODIC TABLE AND THEIR CHARACTERISTICS

26.7

We will use the electron configurations of the atoms to predict their chemical properties, including their reactivity and bonding patterns with other atoms.

Recall that each horizontal row in the periodic table is called a **period**, and each vertical column is called a **group** (or **family**). Within any group in the periodic table, all of the elements have the same number of electrons in their outermost shell. For instance, the elements in Group II all have two electrons in their outermost shell. Electrons in an atom's outermost shell are called **valence** electrons, and it's the valence electrons that are primarily responsible for an atom's properties and chemical behavior.

Some groups (families) have special names.

Group	Name	Valence-Shell Configuration
Group I	*Alkali metals*	ns^1
Group II	*Alkaline earth metals*	ns^2
Group VII	*Halogens*	ns^2np^5
Group VIII	*Noble gases*	ns^2np^6
The d Block	*Transition metals*	
The s and p Blocks	*Representative elements*	
The f Block	*Rare earth metals*	

The valence-shell electron configuration determines the chemical reactivity of each group in the table. For example, in the noble gas family each element has eight electrons in its outermost shell (ns^2np^6). Such a closed-shell (fully-filled valence shell) configuration is called an octet and results in great stability (and therefore low reactivity) for an atom. For this reason, noble gases do not generally undergo chemical reactions, so most group VIII elements are inert. Helium is inert as well, but it has a closed shell with a stable duet ($1s^2$) of electrons.

Other elements experience similar increases in stability upon reaching this stable octet electron configuration, and most chemical reactions can be regarded as the quest for atoms to achieve such closed-shell stability. The alkali metals and alkaline earth metals, for instance, possess one (ns^1) or two (ns^2) electrons in their valence shells, respectively, and they behave as reducing agents (that is, lose valence electrons) in redox reactions in order to obtain a stable octet, generally as an M^+ or M^{2+} cation.

Similarly, the halogens (ns^2np^5) require only a single electron to achieve a stable octet. To achieve this state in their elemental form, halogens naturally exist as diatomic molecules (for example, F_2) where one electron from each atom is shared in a covalent bond. When combined with other elements, the halogens behave as powerful oxidizing agents (that is, gain electrons); they can become stable either as X^- anions or by sharing electrons with other nonmetals.

Reactions between elements on opposite sides of the periodic table can be quite violent. This occurs due to the great degree of stability gained for both elements when the valence electrons are transferred from the metal to the nonmetal. The relative reactivities within these and all other groups can be further explained by the periodic trends detailed in the next section.

Example 26-21: Which of the following elements has a closed valence shell, but not an octet?

    A) He
    B) Ne
    C) Br
    D) Rn

Solution: Choice A, He, is the correct choice because He, along with H^- and Li^+, has a completed $n = 1$ shell with only 2 electrons, since the $n = 1$ shell can fit only 2 electrons.

Example 26-22: Of the following, the element that possesses properties of both metals and nonmetals is:

    A) Si
    B) Al
    C) Zn
    D) Hg

Solution: Elements that possess qualities of both metals and nonmetals are called *metalloids*. These elements are B, Si, Ge, As, Sb, Te, and Po. Thus, choice A is the correct answer; the other choices are metals.

26.8 PERIODIC TRENDS

Shielding

Each filled shell between the nucleus and the valence electrons shields—or "protects"—the valence electrons from the full effect of the positively charged protons in the nucleus. This is called **nuclear shielding** or the **shielding effect**. As far as the valence electrons are concerned, the electrical pull by the protons in the nucleus is reduced by the negative charges of the electrons in the filled shells in between; the result is an effective reduction in the positive elementary charge, from Z to a smaller amount denoted by Z_{eff} (for *effective nuclear charge*).

Example 26-23: The electrons in a solitary He atom are under the influence of two forces, one attractive and one repulsive. What are these forces?

  A) Electrostatic attraction between the electrons and the nuclear protons and electrostatic repulsion between the electrons and nuclear neutrons
  B) Electrostatic attraction between the electrons and the nuclear protons and electrostatic repulsion between the electrons
  C) Gravitational attraction between the electrons and the nuclear protons and frictional repulsion between the electrons
  D) Gravitational attraction between the electrons and the entire nucleus and frictional repulsion between the electrons

Solution: Compared with the magnitude of electrostatic forces in an atom, gravitational forces between the electrons and nucleons of an atom are negligible, so choices C and D are eliminated. Furthermore, neutrons have no charge and thus do not participate in electrostatic forces, so choice A is eliminated. Remember that opposite charges attract and like charges repel. The best answer is choice B.

26.8

Atomic and Ionic Radius

With progression across any period in the table, the number of protons increases, and hence their total pull on the outermost electrons increases too. New shells are initiated only at the beginning of a period. So, as we go across a period, electrons are being added, but new shells are not; therefore, the valence electrons are more and more tightly bound to the atom because they feel a greater effective nuclear charge. Therefore, as we move from left to right across a period, **atomic radius** *decreases*.

However, with progression down a group, as new shells are added with each period, the valence electrons experience increased shielding. The valence electrons are less tightly bound since they feel a smaller effective nuclear charge. Therefore, as we go down a group, atomic radius *increases* due to the increased shielding.

If we form an ion, the radius will decrease as electrons are removed (because the ones that are left are drawn in more closely to the nucleus), and the radius will increase as electrons are added. So, in terms of radius, we have $X^+ < X < X^-$; that is, cation radius < neutral-atom radius < anion radius.

Ionization Energy

Because the atom's positively charged nucleus is attracted to the electrons in the atom, it takes energy to remove an electron. The amount of energy necessary to remove the least tightly bound electron from an isolated atom is called the atom's (**first**) **ionization energy** (often abbreviated **IE** or IE_1). As we move from left to right across a period, or up a group, the ionization energy *increases* since the valence electrons are more tightly bound. The ionization energy of any atom with a noble-gas configuration will always be very large. (For example, the ionization energy of neon is 4 times greater than that of lithium.) The **second ionization energy** (IE_2) of an atom, X, is the energy required to remove the least tightly bound electron from the cation X^+. Note that IE_2 will always be greater than IE_1.

Electron Affinity

The energy associated with the addition of an electron to an isolated atom is known as the atom's **electron affinity** (often abbreviated **EA**). If energy is *released* when the electron is added, the usual convention is to say that the electron affinity is negative; if energy is *required* in order to add the electron, the electron affinity is positive. The halogens have large negative electron affinity values, since the addition of an electron would give them the much desired octet configuration. So they readily accept an electron to become an anion; the increase in stability causes energy to be released. On the other hand, the noble gases and alkaline earth metals have positive electron affinities, because the added electron begins to fill a new level or sublevel and destabilizes the electron configuration. Therefore, anions of these atoms are unstable. Electron affinities typically become more negative as we move to the right across a row or up a group (noble gases excepted), but there are anomalies in this trend.

Electronegativity

Electronegativity is a measure of an atom's ability to pull electrons to itself when it forms a covalent bond; the greater this tendency to attract electrons, the greater the atom's electronegativity. Electronegativity generally behaves as does ionization energy; that is, as we move from left to right across a period, electronegativity increases. As we go down a group, electronegativity decreases. You should know the order of electronegativity for the nine most electronegative elements:

$$F > O > N \approx Cl > Br > I > S > C \approx H$$

Acidity

Acidity is a measure of how well a compound donates protons, accepts electrons, or lowers pH in a chemical system. A binary acid has the structure HX, and it can dissociate in water in the following manner: $HX \rightarrow H^+ + X^-$. Stronger acids have resulting X^- anions that are likely to separate from H^+ because they are stable once they do. Generally speaking, the ease with which an acid (HX) donates its H^+ is directly related to the stability of the conjugate base (X^-). With respect to the *horizontal* periodic trend for acidity, the more electronegative the element bearing the negative charge is, the more stable the anion will be. Therefore, acidity increases from left to right across a period. However, the *vertical* trend for acidity depends on the size of the anion. The larger the anion, the more the negative charge can be delocalized and stabilized. Therefore, acidity increases down a group or family in the periodic table.

Summary of Periodic Trends

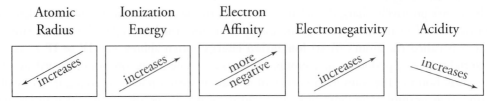

Example 26-24: Compared to calcium, beryllium is expected to have:

A) greater electronegativity and ionization energy.
B) smaller electronegativity and ionization energy.
C) greater electronegativity and smaller ionization energy.
D) smaller electronegativity and larger ionization energy

Solution: Beryllium and calcium are in the same group, but beryllium is higher in the column. We therefore expect beryllium to have greater ionization energy and a greater electronegativity than calcium (choice A), since both of these periodic trends tend to increase as we go up within a group.

Example 26-25: Which of the following will have a greater value for phosphorus than for magnesium?

I. Atomic radius
II. Ionization energy
III. Electronegativity

A) I only
B) I and II only
C) II and III only
D) I, II, and III

Solution: Magnesium and phosphorus are in the same period (row), but phosphorus is farther to the right. We therefore expect phosphorus to have a smaller atomic radius, making Roman numeral I false. This allows us to eliminate choices A, B, and D, leaving choice C as the correct answer. This is also consistent as we expect phosphorus to have a greater ionization energy and a greater electronegativity than magnesium, since both of these periodic trends tend to increase as we move to the right across a row. However, we expect the atomic radius of phosphorus to be smaller than that of magnesium, since atomic radii tend to *decrease* as we move to the right across a row. Therefore, the answer is choice C.

Example 26-26: Which of the following has the smallest atomic radius?

A) Beryllium
B) Potassium
C) Neon
D) Bromine

Solution: Atomic radius increases to the left and towards the bottom of the periodic table. Beryllium and potassium are in the same periods as neon and bromine, respectively. However, Be and K are on the far left of the periodic table, so they should be larger than Ne and Br, and choices A and B should be eliminated. Neon appears above and to the right of bromine in the periodic table, so choice C is correct, and choice D is incorrect.

26.8

Example 26-27: Which of the following is the most strongly acidic?

    A) CH_4
    B) PH_3
    C) H_2S
    D) H_2Se

Solution: The strongest acid will have the most stable conjugate base. This is reflected in the periodic trend, in which X–H bonds increase in acidity the further right and further down X is on the periodic table. Carbon is furthest up and furthest left on the periodic table, and would form the least stable conjugate base, so choice A is incorrect. When comparing atoms in the same row of the periodic table, as phosphorus and sulfur are, the more electronegative atom can better stabilize the negative charge in the conjugate base, so choice B is incorrect. Sulfur and selenium are in the same column of the periodic table. In this case, the larger atom will be better able to stabilize the negative charge on the conjugate base. Choice C is eliminated, and choice D is correct.

The physical properties of a substance are determined at the molecular level, and the chemistry of molecules is dominated by the reactivity of covalent and ionic bonds. An understanding of the fundamentals of bonding can provide the intuitive grasp necessary to answer a wide range of questions in both general and organic chemistry. This section will briefly outline some basic principles, that when mastered, will help lay a strong foundation for many chemistry concepts you will encounter on the MCAT.

26.9 LEWIS DOT STRUCTURES

Each dot in the picture below represents one of fluorine's valence electrons. Fluorine is a halogen, with a general valence-shell configuration of ns^2np^5, so there are $2 + 5 = 7$ electrons in its valence shell. We simply place the dots around the symbol for the element, one on each side, and, if there are more than 4 valence electrons, we just start pairing them up. So, for fluorine, we'd have:

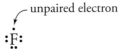

unpaired electron

This is known as a **Lewis dot symbol**. (*Note:* Electrons in *d* subshells are not considered valence electrons for transition metals since valence electrons are in the highest *n* level.) Here are some others:

$$K\cdot \quad \cdot Mg\cdot \quad \cdot \overset{\cdot}{B}\cdot \quad \cdot \overset{\cdot}{Si}\cdot \quad :\overset{\cdot}{P}\cdot \quad :\overset{\cdot}{O}: \quad :\overset{\cdot}{Cl}: \quad :\overset{\cdot\cdot}{Ne}:$$

Lewis dot structures are one type of model we use to represent what compounds look like at the molecular level. Since it's the valence electrons that are responsible for creating bonds in molecules, a Lewis dot structure that accounts for the number and location of all valence electrons gives us a sense of how molecules are held together and helps us understand their reactivity.

To create a Lewis dot structure for a molecule, we begin to pair up electrons from two separate atoms since two electrons are required to form a single bond. By sharing a pair of electrons to form a bond, each atom may acquire an octet configuration, thereby stabilizing both atoms. For example, each of the fluorine atoms below can donate its unpaired valence electron to form a bond and give the molecule F_2. The shared electrons are attracted by the nuclei of *both* atoms in the bond, which hold the atoms together.

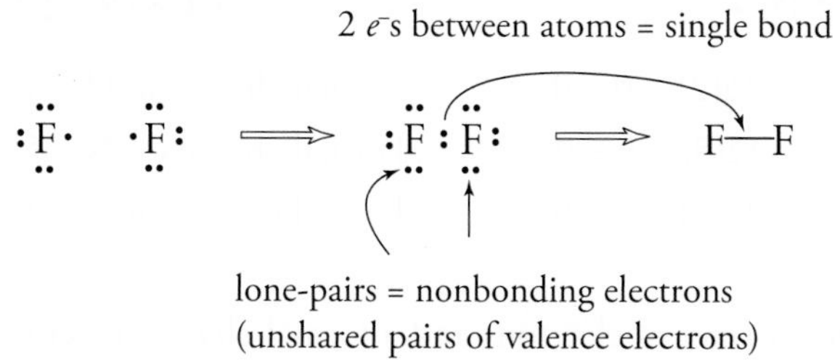

2 e^-s between atoms = single bond

:F· ·F: ⟹ :F:F: ⟹ F—F

lone-pairs = nonbonding electrons
(unshared pairs of valence electrons)

Note that in addition to the **single bond** (a bond formed from two electrons) between the fluorine atoms, each fluorine atom has three pairs of electrons that are not part of a bond. They help satisfy the octets of the F atoms and are known as "lone pairs" of electrons. We'll see in a bit how these lone pairs are important for determining physical properties of compounds, so don't forget to write these out too.

We can also use Lewis dot structures to show atoms that form multiple bonds—**double bonds** use four electrons while **triple bonds** require six. Here are a couple of examples:

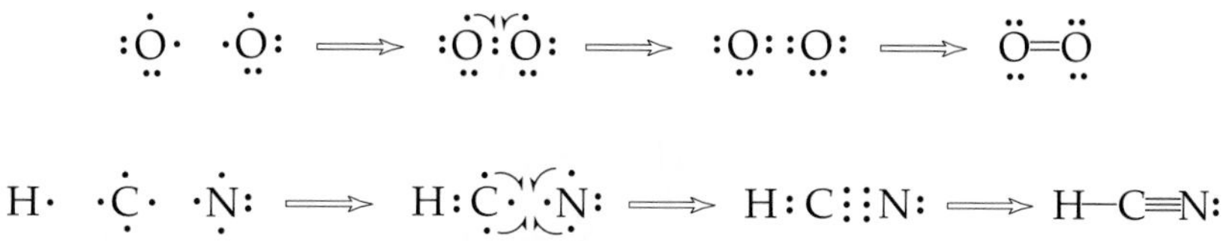

:Ö· ·Ö: ⟹ :Ö:Ö: ⟹ :O::O: ⟹ Ö=Ö

H· ·C· ·N: ⟹ H:C:N: ⟹ H:C::N: ⟹ H—C≡N:

Formal Charge

The last Lewis dot structure shown above for the molecule consisting of 1 atom each of hydrogen, carbon, and nitrogen was drawn with C as the central atom. However, it could have been drawn with N as the central atom, and we could have still achieved closed-shell configurations for all the atoms:

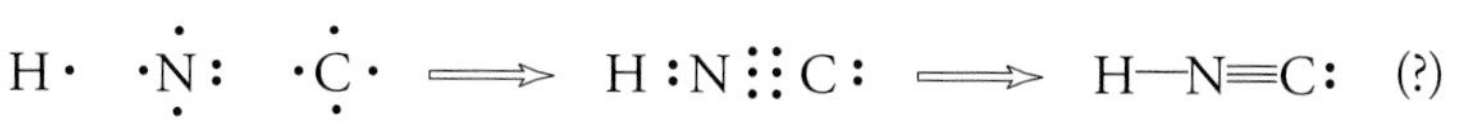

H· ·N: ·C· ⟹ H:N::C: ⟹ H—N≡C: (?)

The problem is that this doesn't give the correct structure for this molecule. The nitrogen atom is not actually bonded to the hydrogen. A helpful way to evaluate a proposed Lewis structure is to calculate the **formal charge** of each atom in the structure. These formal charges won't give the actual charges on the atoms; they'll simply tell us if the atoms are sharing their valence electrons in the "best" way possible, which will happen when the formal charges are all zero (or at least as small as possible). The formula for calculating the formal charge of an atom in a covalent compound is

$$\text{Formal charge (FC)} = V - \frac{1}{2}B - L$$

where V is the number of valence electrons, B is the number of bonding electrons, and L is the number of lone-paired (non-bonding) electrons. We'll show the calculations of the formal charges for each atom in both Lewis structures:

Formal charges

$$\text{H} \!:\! \text{C} \!:\!\!:\! \text{N} \!:$$

Formal charge on H = $1 - \frac{1}{2}(2) - 0 = 0$
Formal charge on C = $4 - \frac{1}{2}(8) - 0 = 0$
Formal charge on N = $5 - \frac{1}{2}(6) - 2 = 0$

$$\text{H} \!:\! \text{N} \!:\!\!:\! \text{C} \!:$$

Formal charge on H = $1 - \frac{1}{2}(2) - 0 = 0$
Formal charge on N = $5 - \frac{1}{2}(8) - 0 = +1$
Formal charge on C = $4 - \frac{1}{2}(6) - 2 = -1$

The best Lewis structures have an octet of electrons and a formal charge of zero on all the atoms. (Sometimes, this simply isn't possible, and then the best structure is the one that *minimizes* the magnitudes of the formal charges.) The fact that the HCN structure has formal charges of zero for all the atoms, but the HNC structure does not, tells us right away that the HCN structure is the better one. For dot structures that must contain formal charges on one or more atoms, the best structures have negative formal charges on the more electronegative element.

Example 26-28: What is the formal charge on each atom, excluding hydrogen, in nitromethane (CH_3NO_2)?

Solution:

$$FC = 6 - \frac{1}{2}(4) - 4 = 0$$

$$FC = 4 - \frac{1}{2}(8) - 0 = 0$$

$$FC = 5 - \frac{1}{2}(8) - 0 = +1$$

$$FC = 6 - \frac{1}{2}(2) - 6 = -1$$

Resonance

Recall that Lewis dot structures are a model that we use to help us understand where the valence electrons are in a molecule. All models, being simplifications of reality, have limitations, and Lewis dot structures are no exception. Sometimes it is impossible for one structure to accurately represent the reality of a molecule's electron distribution. To account for this complexity, we need two or more structures, called **resonance structures**, to accurately depict the bonding in a molecule. These structures are often needed when there are double or triple bonds in molecules along with one or more lone pairs of electrons.

Let's draw the Lewis structure for sulfur dioxide.

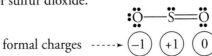

formal charges -----> (-1) $(+1)$ (0)

We could also draw the structure like this:

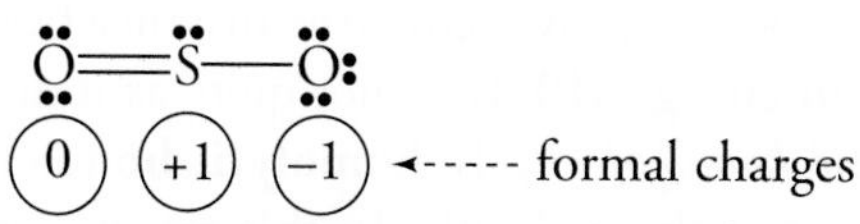

In either case, there's one S—O single bond and one S=O double bond. This would imply that the double-bonded O would be closer to the S atom than the single-bonded O (see Section 26.10, Bond Length and Bond Dissociation Energy). Experiment, however, reveals that the bond lengths are the same. Therefore, to describe this molecule, we say that it's an "average" (or, technically, a **resonance hybrid**) of the equivalent Lewis structures shown:

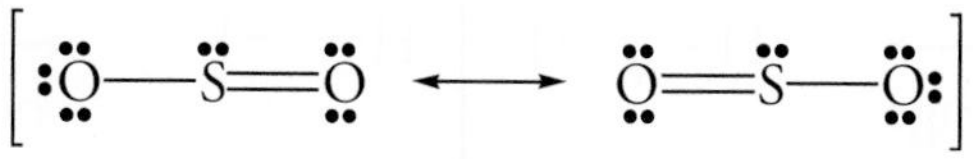

We can also symbolize the resonance hybrid with a single picture, like this:

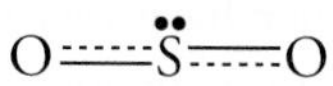

The dotted lines in the structure above indicate some double bond character for both S—O bonds, more of a "bond and a half."

In addition, a molecule may have two or more non-equivalent resonance structures, and the resonance hybrid is then a weighted average of them, as shown with formaldehyde below:

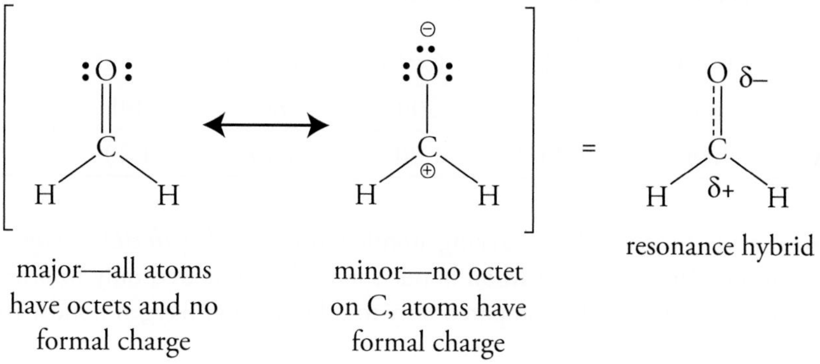

major—all atoms have octets and no formal charge

minor—no octet on C, atoms have formal charge

resonance hybrid

Example 26-29: Resonance structures are two or more structures where:

A) only atoms may move around.
B) only bonding electrons may move around.
C) only nonbonding electrons may move around.
D) only nonbonding electrons, and double and triple bonds may move around.

Solution: Choice D is the correct answer. (This definition is particularly important in organic chemistry.)

26.10 BOND LENGTH AND BOND DISSOCIATION ENERGY

While the term *bond length* makes good intuitive sense (the distance between two nuclei that are bonded to one another), **bond dissociation energy (BDE)** is not quite as intuitive. Bond dissociation energy is the energy required to break a bond *homolytically*. In **homolytic bond cleavage**, one electron of the bond being broken goes to each fragment of the molecule. In this process, two radicals form. This is *not* the same thing as **heterolytic bond cleavage** (also known as *dissociation*). In heterolytic bond cleavage, both electrons of the electron pair that make up the bond end up on the same atom; this forms both a cation and an anion.

These two processes are very different and hence have very different energies associated with them. Here, we will only consider homolytic bond dissociation energies.

When one examines the relationship between bond length and bond dissociation energy for a series of similar bonds, an important trend emerges: for similar bonds, *the higher the bond order, the shorter and stronger the bond*. Bond order is defined as the number of bonds between adjacent atoms, so a single bond has a bond order of 1, while a triple bond has a bond order of 3. The following table, which lists the bond dissociation energies (BDE, in kcal/mol) and the bond lengths (*r*, in angstroms, where 1 Å = 10^{-10} m) for carbon-carbon and carbon-oxygen bonds, illustrates this trend:

	C—C	C=C	C≡C	C—O	C=O	C≡O
BDE	83	144	200	86	191	256
r (in Å)	1.54	1.34	1.20	1.43	1.20	1.13

An important caveat arises because of the varying atomic radii: *bond length/BDE comparisons should only be made for <u>similar</u> bonds*. Thus, carbon-carbon bonds should be compared only to other carbon-carbon bonds; carbon-oxygen bonds should be compared only to other carbon-oxygen bonds, and so on.

Recall the shapes of atomic orbitals: *s* orbitals are spherical about the atomic nucleus, while *p* orbitals are elongated "dumbbell"-shaped about the atomic nucleus.

When comparing the same type of bonds, the greater the *s* character in the hybrid orbitals, the shorter the bond (because *s*-orbitals are closer to the nucleus than *p*-orbitals). A greater percentage of *p* character in the hybrid orbital also leads to a more directional hybrid orbital that is farther from the nucleus and thus a longer bond (see section 26.13 for all the details on hybridization). In addition, when comparing the same types of bonds, *the longer the bond, the weaker it is; the shorter the bond, the stronger it is*. In the following diagram, compare all the C—C bonds and all the C—H bonds:

$$1.06 \text{ Å} \qquad 1.46 \text{ Å}$$

H—C≡C—C‖‖‖‖‖H

sp   sp   sp³

s

1.21 Å

1.10 Å   s

Bond	Bond length	Bond	Bond length
C—C ($sp - sp$)	1.21 Å	C–H ($sp - s$)	1.06 Å
C—C ($sp - sp^3$)	1.46 Å	C–H ($sp^3 - s$)	1.10 Å

26.11 TYPES OF BONDS

Covalent Bonds

A **covalent bond** is formed between atoms when each contributes one or more of its unpaired valence electrons. The electrons are *shared* by both atoms to help complete both octets. There are minor variations in how the electrons are shared, however, so there are several classes of covalent bonds.

Polarity of Covalent Bonds

Recall that electronegativity refers to an atom's ability to attract another atom's valence electrons when it forms a bond. Electronegativity, in other words, is a measure of how much an atom will "hog" the electrons that it's sharing with another atom.

Consider hydrogen fluoride (HF) and molecular fluorine (F_2). Fluorine is more electronegative than hydrogen (remember the order of electronegativity?), so the electron density will be greater near the fluorine than near the hydrogen in HF. That means that the H—F molecule is partially negative (denoted by δ^-) on the fluorine side and partially positive (denoted by δ^+) on the hydrogen side. We refer to this as **polarity** and say that the molecule has a **dipole moment**. A bond is **polar** if the electron density between the two nuclei is uneven. This occurs if there is a difference in electronegativity of the bonding atoms, and the greater the difference, the more uneven the electron density and the greater the dipole moment.

A bond is **nonpolar** if the electron density between the two nuclei is even. This occurs when there is little to no difference in electronegativity between the bonded atoms, generally when two atoms of the same element are bonded to each other, as we see in F_2.

electron density

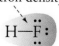

$\delta^+ \quad \overset{+}{\longrightarrow} \quad \delta^-$

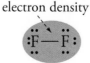 POLAR

electron density

:F̈—F̈: NONPOLAR

Coordinate Covalent Bonds

Sometimes, one atom will donate *both* of the shared electrons in a bond. That is called a **coordinate covalent bond**. For example, the nitrogen atom in NH_3 donates both electrons in its lone pair to form a bond to the boron atom in the molecule BF_3 to give the coordinate covalent compound F_3BNH_3:

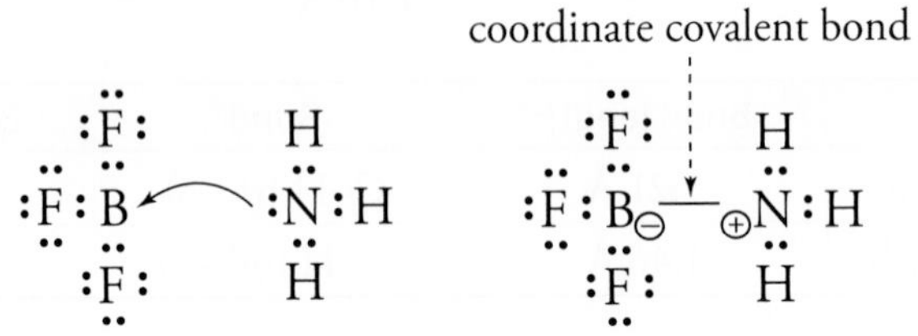

coordinate covalent bond

Since the NH_3 molecule donates a pair of electrons, it is known as a **Lewis base.** A Lewis base can act as a ligand, or a nucleophile (nucleus loving), and so all three terms are synonymous. Since the BF_3 molecule accepts a pair of electrons, it's known as a **Lewis acid** or **electrophile** (electron loving). When a coordinate covalent bond breaks, the electrons that come from the ligand will leave *with* that ligand.

Example 26-30: Identify the Lewis acid and the Lewis base in the following reaction, which forms a coordination complex:

$$4\ NH_3 + Zn^{2+} \rightarrow Zn(NH_3)_4{}^{2+}$$

Solution: Each of the NH_3 molecules donates its lone pair to the zinc atom, thus forming four coordinate covalent bonds. Since the zinc ion accepts these electron pairs, it's the Lewis acid; since each ammonia molecule donates an electron pair, they are Lewis bases (or ligands):

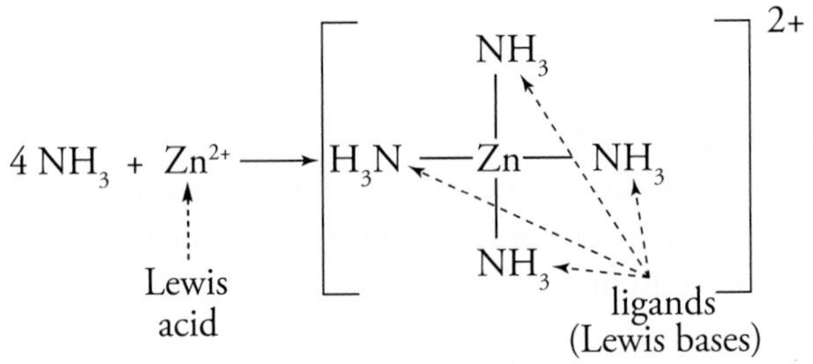

Ionic Bonds

While sharing valence electrons is one way atoms can achieve the stable octet configuration, the octet may also be obtained by gaining or losing electrons. For example, a sodium atom will give its valence electron to an atom of chlorine. This results in a sodium cation (Na^+) and a chloride anion (Cl^-), which form sodium chloride. They're held together by the electrostatic attraction between a cation and anion; this is an **ionic bond**.

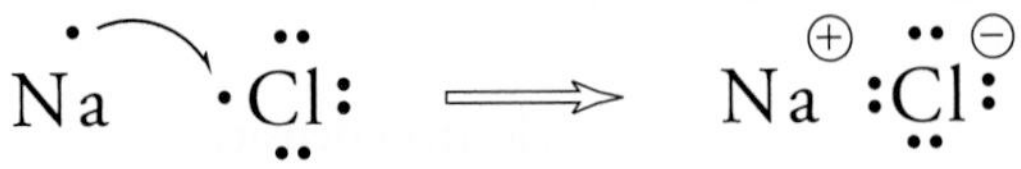

For an ionic bond to form between a metal and a non-metal, there has to be a big difference in electro-negativity between the two elements. Generally speaking, the strength of the bond is proportional to the charges on the ions, and it decreases as the ions get farther apart, or as the ionic radii increase. We can use this to estimate the relative strength of ionic systems. For example, consider MgS and NaCl. For MgS, the magnesium ion has a +2 charge and sulfide ion has a –2 charge, while for NaCl, the charges are +1 for sodium and –1 for chloride. Therefore, the MgS "bond" is expected to be about four times stronger than the NaCl "bond," assuming the sizes of the ions are very nearly the same.

Example 26-31: Which of the following is most likely an ionic compound?

    A) NO
    B) HI
    C) ClF
    D) KBr

Solution: A diatomic compound is ionic if the electronegativities of the atoms are very different. Of the atoms listed in the choices, those in choice D have the greatest electronegativity difference (K is an alkali metal, and Br is a halogen); K will give up its lone valence electron to Br, forming an ionic bond.

26.12 VSEPR THEORY

The shapes of simple molecules are predicted by **valence shell electron-pair repulsion (VSEPR) theory**. There's one rule: since electrons repel one another, electron pairs, whether bonding or nonbonding, attempt to move as far apart as possible.

For example, the bonding electrons in beryllium hydride, BeH_2, repel one another and attempt to move as far apart as possible. In this molecule, two pairs of electrons point in opposite directions:

The angle between the bonds is 180°. A molecule with this shape is said to be linear.

As the BeH_2 example shows, the total number of electron groups on the central atom of a molecule deter-mines its bond angles and *orbital geometry*. Electron groups are defined as any type of bond (single, double, triple) and lone pairs of electrons. Double and triple bonds count only as one electron group, even though they involve two and three pairs of electrons, respectively. To illustrate, the number of electron groups and orbital geometries of the central atom are shown for some example molecules:

| 2 electron groups | 3 electron groups | 4 electron groups |

The shape of a molecule (also referred to as the **molecular geometry**) is also a function of the location of the nuclei of its constituent atoms. Therefore, when lone electron pairs are present on the central atom of a molecule, as in NH_3 above, the shape is not the same as the orbital geometry. The table below shows how the presence of lone pairs determines the shape of a molecule:

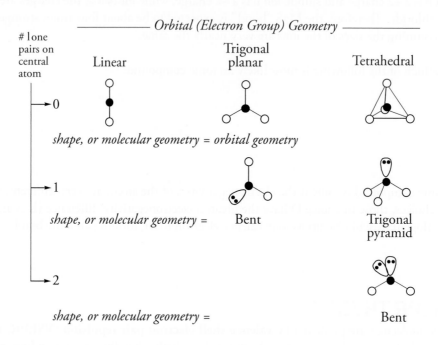

——————— *Orbital (Electron Group) Geometry* ———————

Example 26-32: Determine the orbital geometry and predict the shape of each of the following molecules or ions:

a) H_2O
b) SO_2
c) NH_4^+
d) PCl_3

Solution:

a)

orbital geometry: *tetrahedral*
shape: *bent*

b)

orbital geometry: *trigonal planar*
shape: *bent*

c)

orbital geometry: *tetrahedral*
shape: *tetrahedral*

d)

orbital geometry: *tetrahedral*
shape: *trigonal pyramid*

26.13 HYBRIDIZATION

In order to rationalize observed chemical and structural trends, chemists developed the concept of orbital hybridization. In this model, one imagines a mathematical combination of atomic orbitals centered on the same atom to produce a set of composite, **hybrid** orbitals. For example, consider an *s* and a *p* orbital on an atom.

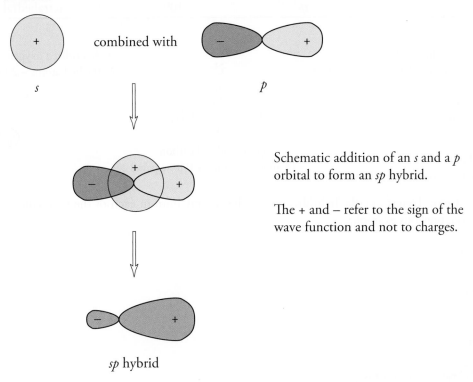

Schematic addition of an *s* and a *p* orbital to form an *sp* hybrid.

The + and – refer to the sign of the wave function and not to charges.

Notice that the new orbital is highly directional; this allows for better overlap when bonding.

There will be two such *sp* hybrid orbitals formed because two orbitals (the *s* and the *p*) were originally combined; that is, the total number of orbitals is conserved in the formation of hybrid orbitals. For this reason, the number of hybrid orbitals on a given atom of hybridization sp^x is $1 + x$ (1 for the *s*, *x* for the *p*'s), where *x* may be either 1, 2, or 3.

The percentages of the *s* character and *p* character in a given sp^x hybrid orbital are listed below:

sp^x hybrid orbital	s character	p character
sp	50%	50%
sp^2	33%	67%
sp^3	25%	75%

To determine the hybridization for most atoms in simple molecules, add the number of attached atoms to the number of non-bonding electron pairs (localized) and use the brief table below (which also gives the ideal bond angles and orbital geometry). The number of attached atoms plus the number of lone pairs is equal to the number of orbitals combined to make the new hybridized orbitals.

Electron Groups (# atoms + # lone pairs)	Hybridization	Bond Angles (ideal)	Orbital Geometry
2	sp	180°	linear
3	sp^2	120°	trigonal planar
4	sp^3	109.5°	tetrahedral

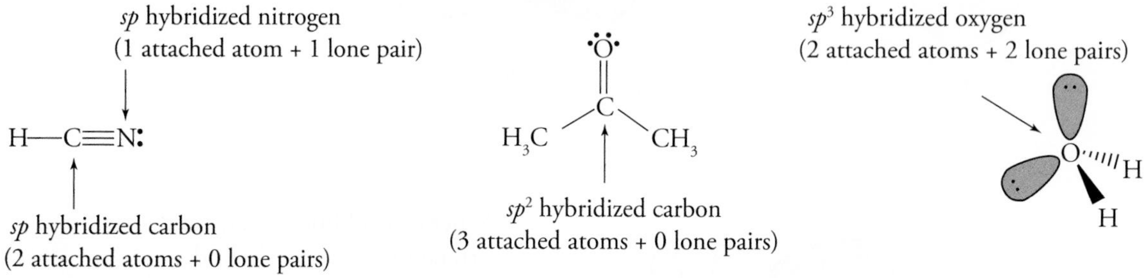

sp hybridized nitrogen
(1 attached atom + 1 lone pair)

$H\!-\!C\!\equiv\!N\!:$

sp hybridized carbon
(2 attached atoms + 0 lone pairs)

$H_3C \qquad CH_3$

sp² hybridized carbon
(3 attached atoms + 0 lone pairs)

sp³ hybridized oxygen
(2 attached atoms + 2 lone pairs)

Example 26-33: Determine the hybridization of the central atom in each of the following molecules or ions from the previous example:

a) H_2O
b) SO_2
c) NH_4^+
d) PCl_3

Solution:

a) Hybridization of O is sp^3.
b) Hybridization of S is sp^2.
c) Hybridization of N is sp^3.
d) Hybridization of P is sp^3.

26.13

Sigma (σ) Bonds

A σ **bond** consists of two electrons that are localized between two nuclei. It is formed by the end-to-end overlap of one hybridized orbital (or an *s* orbital in the case of hydrogen) from each of the two atoms participating in the bond. Below, we show the σ bonds in ethane, C_2H_6:

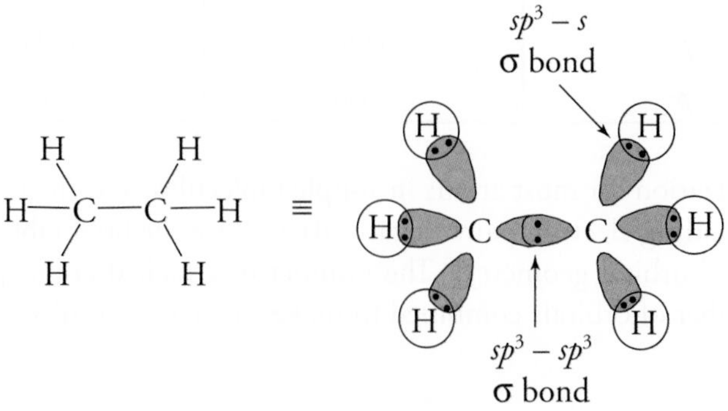

$sp^3 - s$
σ bond

$H\!-\!C\!-\!C\!-\!H$

$sp^3 - sp^3$
σ bond

Remember that an sp^3 carbon atom has 4 sp^3 hybrid orbitals, which are derived from one s orbital and three p orbitals.

Example 26-34: Label the hybridization of the orbitals comprising the σ bonds in the molecules shown below:

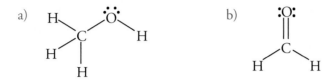

Solution:

a) Bonds to H are sp^3-s σ bonds. The C—O bond is an sp^3-sp^3 σ bond.
b) The bonds to H are sp^2-s σ bonds. The C=O bond contains an sp^2-sp^2 σ bond. (It's also composed of a π bond, which we'll discuss in the next section.)

Pi (π) Bonds

A π **bond** is composed of two electrons that are localized to the region that lies on opposite sides of the plane formed by the two bonded nuclei and immediately adjacent atoms, not directly between the two nuclei as with a σ bond. A π bond is formed by the proper, parallel, side-to-side alignment of two unhybridized p orbitals on adjacent atoms. (An sp^2 hybridized atom has three sp^2 orbitals—which come from one s and two p orbitals—plus one p orbital that remains unhybridized.) Below, we show the π bonds in ethene, C_2H_4:

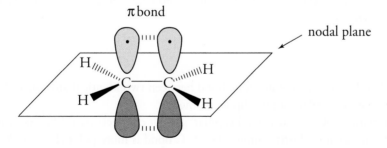

In any multiple bond, *there is only one σ bond; the remainder are π bonds.* Therefore,

a single bond: composed of 1 σ bond
a double bond: composed of 1 σ bond and 1 π bond
a triple bond: composed of 1 σ bond and 2 π bonds

Example 26-35: Count the number of σ– and π–bonds in each of the following molecules, including C—H bonds.

a)

b)

c)

d)

Solution:

a) 9 C—C σ, 3 C—C π, 16 C—H σ
b) 4 C—C σ, 2 C—C π, 1 C—N σ, 2 C—O σ, 1 C—O π, 4 C—H σ, 2 σ—H σ, 1 O—H σ
c) 6 C—C σ, 3 C—C π, 2 C—Br σ, 4 C—H σ
d) 1 C—C σ, 1 C—C π, 4 C—N σ, 1 C—N π, 3 C—H σ, 1 N—H σ

26.14 MOLECULAR POLARITY

A molecule as a whole may also be polar or nonpolar. If a molecule contains no polar bonds, it cannot be polar. In addition, if a molecule contains two or more symmetrically oriented polar bonds, the bond dipoles effectively cancel each other out, evenly distributing the electron density over the entire molecule. However, if the polar bonds in a molecule are not symmetrically oriented around the central atom (generally, though not always due to the presence of a lone pair of electrons on the central atom), the individual bond dipoles will not cancel. Therefore, there will be an uneven distribution of electron density over the entire molecule, and this results in a polar molecule.

Example 26-36: For each of the molecules N_2, OCS, and CCl_4, describe the polarity of each bond and of the molecule as a whole.

Solution:

- The N≡N bond is nonpolar (since it's a bond between two identical atoms), and since this *is* the molecule, it's nonpolar too; no dipole moment.
- For the molecule O=C=S, each bond is polar, since it connects two different atoms of unequal electronegativities. Furthermore, the O=C bond is more polar that then C=S bond, because the difference between the electronegativities of O and C is greater than the difference between the electronegativities of C and S. Therefore, the molecule as a whole is polar (that is, it has a dipole moment):

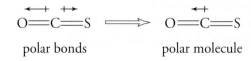

polar bonds   polar molecule

- For the molecule CCl_4, each bond is polar, since it connects two different atoms of unequal electronegativities. However, the bonds are symmetrically arranged around the central C atom, leaving the molecule as a whole nonpolar, with no dipole moment:

polar bonds   non-polar molecule

26.15   INTERMOLECULAR FORCES

Liquids and solids are held together by intermolecular forces, such as dipole-dipole forces and London dispersion forces. **Intermolecular forces** are the relatively weak interactions that take place between neutral molecules.

Polar molecules are attracted to ions, producing **ion-dipole** forces. **Dipole-dipole forces** are the attractions between the positive end of one polar molecule and the negative end of another polar molecule. (Hydrogen bonding [which we will look at more closely below] is the strongest dipole-dipole force.) A permanent dipole in one molecule may induce a dipole in a neighboring nonpolar molecule, producing a momentary **dipole-induced dipole force**.

Finally, an instantaneous dipole in a nonpolar molecule may induce a dipole in a neighboring nonpolar molecule. The resulting attractions are known as **London dispersion forces**, which are very weak and transient interactions between the instantaneous dipoles in nonpolar molecules. They are the weakest of all intermolecular interactions, and they're the "default" force; all an atom or molecule needs to experience them is electrons. In addition, as the size (molecular weight) of the molecule increases, so does its number of electrons, which increases its polarizability. As a result, the partial charges of the induced dipoles get larger, so the strength of the dispersion forces increases.

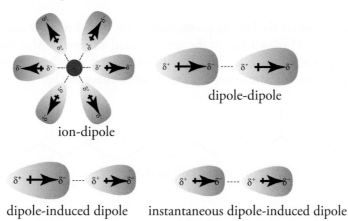

ion-dipole

dipole-dipole

dipole-induced dipole

instantaneous dipole-induced dipole
(London dispersion force)

26.15

For hydrocarbons, branching tends to inhibit London dispersion forces by reducing the surface area available for intermolecular interaction. Thus, branching tends to reduce attractive forces between molecules. Consider the following two constitutional isomers:

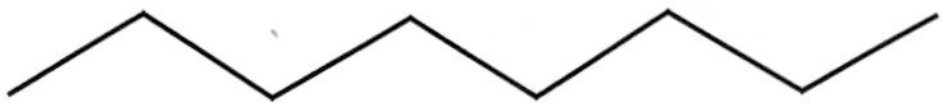

n-octane 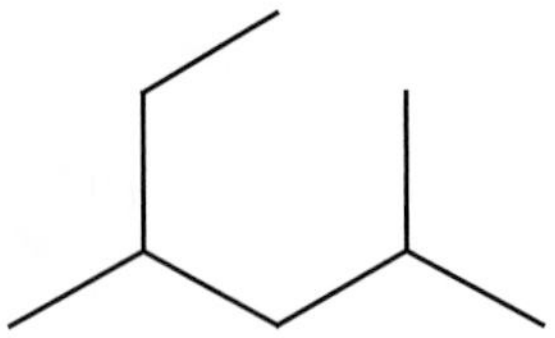   2,4-dimethylhexane

2,4-Dimethylhexane is a branched isomer of *n*-octane. Although each compound has the same molecular formula, C_8H_{18}, these two constitutional isomers have dramatically different physical properties. *n*-Octane requires much more energy to melt or boil, because unbranched, it experiences greater London dispersion forces than does the branched isomer 2,4-dimethylhexane. Therefore, *n*-octane has both a higher melting point and a higher boiling point than does 2,4-dimethylhexane, as well as a lower vapor pressure.

To summarize, substances with stronger intermolecular forces will exhibit greater melting points, greater boiling points, greater viscosities, and lower vapor pressures (more on this below) than similar compounds with weaker intermolecular forces. For example, many substances that experience only dispersion forces, such as fluorine (F_2) and chlorine (Cl_2), exist as gases under standard conditions (1 atm and 25°C). However, bromine (Br_2) is a liquid and iodine (I_2) is a solid because the strength of the dispersion forces increase as atomic size increases.

Example 26-37: Rank the following six hydrocarbons in order of increasing boiling point:

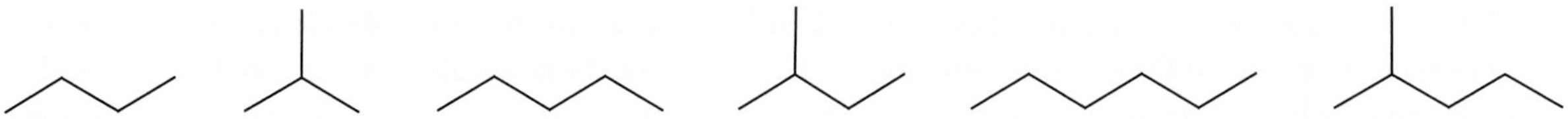

Solution: Since branching lowers the boiling point, each of the branched hydrocarbons has a lower boiling point than the unbranched hydrocarbon of the same molecular formula. Also, the larger the molecule, the greater the surface area over which van der Waals forces can act, so heavier molecules have higher boiling points. We can now put the whole sequence in order of increasing bp:

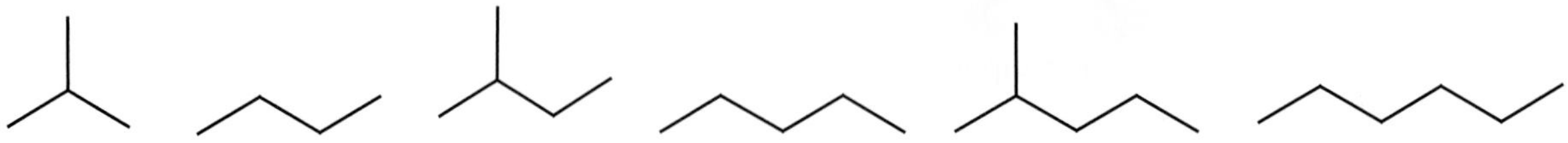

Increasing Boiling Point

Hydrogen Bonding

It's important to remember that a hydrogen bond is not a covalent bond, but an intermolecular force—and importantly—the strongest type of intermolecular force between neutral molecules. In order for a hydrogen bond to form, two very specific criteria must be fulfilled: 1) a molecule must have a covalent bond between H and either N, O, or F, and 2) another molecule must have a lone pair of electrons on an N, O, or F atom. Since these three elements have very different electronegativities than hydrogen, a very polarized bond is formed, creating notable dipoles in the molecules. A very common example of a substance that experiences hydrogen bonding is water:

4-nitrophenol
Intermolecular hydrogen bonding

2-nitrophenol
Intramolecular hydrogen bonding

One of the consequences of hydrogen bonding is the high boiling points of compounds such as NH_3, H_2O, and HF. The boiling points of these hydrogen-containing compounds are higher than those of the hydrogen-containing compounds of other elements from Groups V, VI, and VII (the groups where N, O, and F reside). For example, the boiling point of H_2S is approximately –50°C, while that of H_2O is (of course) 100°C.

Some molecules with both hydrogen-bond donation sites (the H atoms) and hydrogen-bond acceptor sites (the lone pairs) can participate in intramolecular hydrogen bonding. 2-Nitrophenol is one such example since the H of the hydroxyl group is close enough to the O of the nitro group. Intramolecular hydrogen bonding often reduces the amount of intermolecular interactions these molecules exhibit, thereby decreasing their boiling points.

Example 26-38: Identify the mixture of compounds that *cannot* experience hydrogen bonding with each other:

A) NH_3 / H_2O
B) H_2O / HF
C) HF / CO_2
D) H_2S / HCl

Solution: Hydrogen bonding occurs when an H covalently bonded to an F, O, or N electrostatically interacts with another F, O, or N (which doesn't need to have an H). Therefore, choices A, B, and C can all experience hydrogen bonding. Choice D, however, cannot, and this is the answer.

A final note: Dipole forces, hydrogen bonding, and London dispersion forces are all collectively known as van der Waals forces. However, you may sometimes see the term "van der Waals forces" used to mean only London dispersion forces.

26.15

Physical Properties of Compounds

One of the physical properties determined by the strength of the intermolecular forces of a substance is its vapor pressure. **Vapor pressure** is the pressure exerted by the gaseous phase of a liquid that evaporated from the exposed surface of the liquid. The weaker a substance's intermolecular forces, the higher its vapor pressure and the more easily it evaporates. For example, if we compare diethyl ether ($H_5C_2OC_2H_5$) and water, we notice that while water undergoes hydrogen bonding, diethyl ether does not, so despite its greater molecular mass, diethyl ether will vaporize more easily and have a higher vapor pressure than water. Easily vaporized liquids—liquids with *high* vapor pressures—like diethyl ether are said to be **volatile**.

While a substance's vapor pressure is determined in part by its intermolecular forces, vapor pressure is also temperature dependent and increases with the temperature of the substance. Increasing the average kinetic energy of the particles (which is proportional to temperature), allows them to overcome the intermolecular forces holding them together and increases the proportion of particles that can move into the gas phase. As a result, the vapor pressure of a substance is indirectly related to its boiling point.

Melting point (mp) and boiling point (bp) are also indicators of how well identical molecules interact with (attract) each other. Intermolecular forces must be overcome to melt (solid → liquid) or to boil (liquid → gas) any compound. The greater the attractive forces between molecules, the more energy will be required to get the compound to change phase. The weaker these forces, the lower the melting or boiling point.

Example 26-39: For each of the following pairs, predict which compound has the higher melting and boiling points.

a) CF_4 or CHF_3

b) 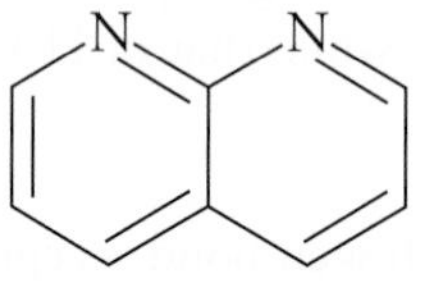   or

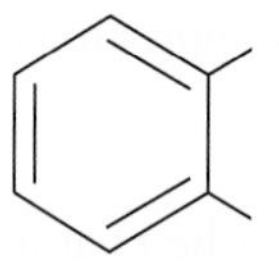

c) 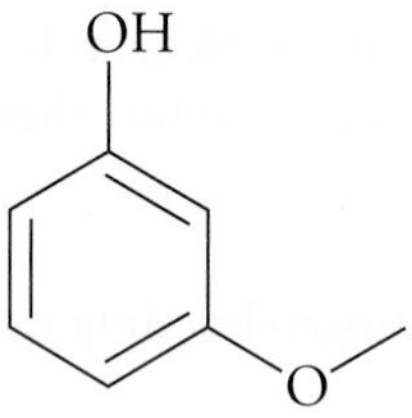   or

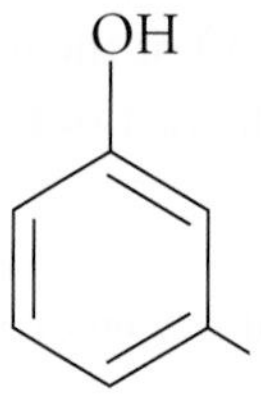

26.15

Solution:

a) CHF_3. CF_4 has 4 polar C—F bonds arranged symmetrically, so the molecule is nonpolar and experiences only London dispersion forces. CHF_3 is not symmetric. It has a net dipole moment, so it experiences dipole-dipole interactions. These are stronger interactions than London dispersion forces, so CHF_3 has a higher melting and boiling point.

b) Both molecules contain bond dipoles that do not completely cancel out due to symmetry, so both molecules experience dipole-dipole interactions. The two nitrogen atoms in the first molecule attract more electron density than the single nitrogen atom in the second, so the first molecule is more polar. As a result of these larger partial charge magnitudes, the first molecule experiences stronger intermolecular forces and has a higher melting and boiling point.

c) OH Both molecules experience hydrogen bonding. The first molecule has a methoxy group in place of a hydroxy group that is present in the second. Since the hydroxy group is a hydrogen bond donor and the methoxy group is not, the second molecule can participate in more hydrogen bonds, so it has a higher melting and boiling point.

26.16 TYPES OF SOLIDS

An **ionic solid** is held together by the electrostatic attraction between cations and anions in a **lattice** structure. Given the strength of these attractive forces, ionic solids are solids at room temperature.

In a **network solid**, atoms are connected in a lattice of covalent bonds. Like in an ionic solid, in a network solid the intermolecular forces are identical to the intramolecular forces resulting in a very hard solid at room temperature.

A metal, or a **metallic solid**, can be thought of as a covalently bound lattice of nuclei and their inner shell electrons, surrounded by a "sea" or "cloud" of electrons. At least one valence electron per atom is not bound to any one particular atom and is free to move throughout the lattice. These freely roaming valence electrons give metals their properties, namely making them malleable, ductile, and excellent conductors of electricity and heat.

The particles at the lattice points of a crystal of a **molecular solid** are molecules held together by the intermolecular interactions discussed above. Since these forces are *significantly* weaker than ionic, covalent, or metallic bonds, molecular compounds typically have much lower melting and boiling points than the other types of solids above and are commonly liquids or gases at room temperature.

26.16

Example 26-40: Which of the following has the lowest melting point?

A) $AlPO_4$
B) $(CH_3CH_2)_2O$
C) $(CH_3CH_2)_2NH$
D) Na

Solution: The correct answer should have the weakest attractive forces between molecules. Choice A can be eliminated because it is the only ionic solid given, and the electrostatic forces found within ionic solids are very strong. Both choices B and C would be molecular solids, so they can be compared to one another. Choice B, diethyl ether, experiences only dipole-dipole interactions. By contrast, choice C, diethylamine, can both donate and accept hydrogen bonds, which are generally stronger than dipole-dipole interactions: choice C can be eliminated. Choice D is held together by metallic bonding, which is significantly stronger than intermolecular forces. Choice D is eliminated, and choice B is correct.

26.16

Chapter 27
Thermodynamics

27.1   SYSTEM AND SURROUNDINGS

Why does anything happen? Why does a creek flow downhill, a puddle of water evaporate after it rains, a chemical reaction proceed? It's all **thermodynamics:** the transformation of energy from one form to another. The laws of thermodynamics underlie any event in which energy is transformed.

The Zeroth Law of Thermodynamics

The Zeroth Law is often conceptually described as follows: if two systems are both in thermal equilibrium with a third system, then the two initial systems are in thermal equilibrium with one another.

Thus, the Zeroth Law establishes a definition of thermal equilibrium. When systems are in thermal equilibrium with one another, their temperatures must be the same. When bodies of different temperatures are brought into contact with one another, heat will flow from the body with the higher temperature into the body with lower temperature in order to achieve equilibrium at the same temperature value.

The First Law of Thermodynamics

The first law states that *the total energy of the universe is constant.* Energy may be transformed from one form to another, but it cannot be created or destroyed.

An important result of the first law is that an isolated system has a constant energy—no transformation of the energy is possible. When systems are in contact, however, energy is allowed to flow, and thermal equilibrium can be attained. In addition, the first law also establishes that work can be put into a system to increase its overall energy. This may or may not occur with a corresponding change in temperature.

Conventions Used in Thermodynamics

In thermodynamics we have to designate a "starting line" and a "finish line" to be able to describe how energy flows in chemical reactions and physical changes. To do this we use three distinct designations to describe energy flow: the system, the surroundings, and the thermodynamic universe (or just universe).

The system is the thing we're looking at: a melting ice cube, a solid dissolving into water, a beating heart, anything we want to study. Everything else: the table the ice cube sits on and the surrounding air, the beaker that holds the solid and the water, the chest cavity holding the heart, is known collectively as the surroundings. The system and the surroundings taken together form the thermodynamic universe.

We need to define these terms so that we can assign a direction—and therefore a sign, either (+) or (–)—to energy flow. For chemistry (and for physics), we define everything in terms of what's happening to the *system.*

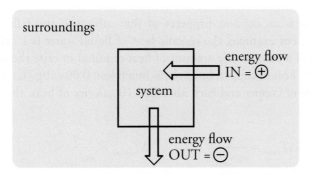

Consider energy flowing from the surroundings into the system, like the heat flowing from the table to the ice cube that's sitting on it. What is happening in the system? As energy flows in (here it's heat), the molecules in the system absorb it and start to jiggle faster. Eventually enough energy is absorbed to cause the ice to melt. Overall, the energy of the system *increased*, and we therefore give it a (+) sign. What about water when it freezes? Here, energy (once again, heat) leaves the water (our system), and the jiggling of the water molecules slows down. The energy of the system has *decreased*, and we therefore assign a (−) sign to energy flow. Finally, energy that flows into the system flows out of the surroundings, and energy that flows out of the system flows into the surroundings. Therefore, we can make these statements:

1) When energy flows into a system from the surroundings, the energy of the system increases and the energy of the surroundings decreases.
2) When energy flows out of a system into the surroundings, the energy of the system decreases and the energy of the surroundings increases.

Keep this duality in mind when dealing with energy.

27.2   CALORIMETRY

The amount of heat absorbed or released by a sample of a substance that is not changing phase is proportional to its change in temperature. The constant of proportionality is called the substance's **heat capacity, C**, which is the product of its **specific heat, c**, and its mass, m; that is, $C = mc$. We can write the equation $q = C\Delta T$ in this more explicit form:

$$q = mc\Delta T$$

where

> q = heat added to (or released by) a sample
> m = mass of the sample
> c = specific heat of the substance
> ΔT = temperature change

A substance's specific heat is an *intrinsic* property of that substance and tells us how resistant it is to changing its temperature. For example, the specific heat of liquid water is 1 calorie per gram-°C. (This is actually the definition of a **calorie**: the amount of heat required to raise the temperature of 1 gram of water by 1°C.) The specific heat of copper, however, is much less: 0.09 cal/g-°C. So, if we had a 1 g sample of water and a 1 g sample of copper and each absorbed 10 calories of heat, the resulting changes in the temperatures would be

$$\Delta T_{water} = \frac{q}{mc_{water}} \qquad\qquad \Delta T_{copper} = \frac{q}{mc_{copper}}$$

$$= \frac{10 \text{ cal}}{(1 \text{ g})(1\frac{\text{cal}}{\text{g-}^\circ\text{C}})} \qquad\qquad = \frac{10 \text{ cal}}{(1 \text{ g})(0.09\frac{\text{cal}}{\text{g-}^\circ\text{C}})}$$

$$= 10^\circ\text{C} \qquad\qquad = 111^\circ\text{C}$$

That's a big difference! So, while it's true that the temperature change is proportional to the heat absorbed, it's *inversely* proportional to the substance's heat capacity. A substance like water, with a relatively high specific heat, will undergo a smaller change in temperature than a substance (like copper) with a lower specific heat.

A few notes:

1) The specific heat of a substance also depends upon phase. For example, the specific heat of ice is different from that of liquid water.

2) The SI unit for energy is the joule, not the calorie. You may see specific heats (and heat capacities) given in terms of joules rather than calories. Remember, the conversion between joules and calories is: $1 \text{ cal} \approx 4.2 \text{ J}$.

3) Specific heats may also be given in terms of kelvins rather than degrees Celsius; that is, you may see the specific heat of water, say, given as $4.2 \text{ J/g} \cdot \text{K}$ rather than $4.2 \text{ J/g} \cdot \text{C}$. However, since the size of a Celsius degree is the same as a kelvin (that is, if two temperatures differ by 1°C, they also differ by 1K), the numerical value of the specific heat won't be any different if kelvins are used.

Example 27-1: Equal amounts of heat are absorbed by 10 g solid samples of four different metals, aluminum, lead, tin, and iron. Of the four, which will exhibit the *smallest* change in temperature?

A) Aluminum (specific heat = 0.9 J/g · K)
B) Lead (specific heat = 0.13 J/g · K)
C) Tin (specific heat = 0.23 J/g · K)
D) Iron (specific heat = 0.45 J/g · K)

Solution: Since q and m are constant, ΔT is inversely proportional to c. So, the substance with the greatest specific heat will undergo the smallest change in temperature. Of the metals listed, aluminum (choice A) has the greatest specific heat.

27.3 ENTHALPY

Enthalpy is a measure of the heat energy that is released or absorbed when bonds are broken and formed during a reaction that's run at constant pressure. The symbol for enthalpy is **H**. Some general principles about enthalpy prevail over all reactions:

- When a bond is formed, energy is released: $\Delta H < 0$.
- Energy must be put into a bond in order to break it: $\Delta H > 0$.

In a chemical reaction, energy must be put into the reactants to break their bonds. Once the reactant bonds are broken, the atoms rearrange to form products. As the product bonds form, energy is released. The enthalpy of a reaction is given by the difference between the enthalpy of the products and the enthalpy of the reactants.

$$\Delta H = H_{products} - H_{reactants}$$

The enthalpy change, ΔH, is also known as the **heat of reaction**.

If the products of a chemical reaction have stronger bonds than the reactants, then more energy is released in the making of product bonds than was put in to break the reactant bonds. In this case, energy is released overall from the system, and the reaction is **exothermic**. The products are in a lower energy state than the reactants, and the change in enthalpy, ΔH, is negative, since heat flows out of the system. If the products of a chemical reaction have weaker bonds than the reactants, then more energy is put in during the breaking of reactant bonds than is released in the making of product bonds. In this case, energy is absorbed overall and the reaction is **endothermic**. The products are in a higher energy state than the reactants, and the change in enthalpy, ΔH, is positive, since heat had to be added to the system from the surroundings.

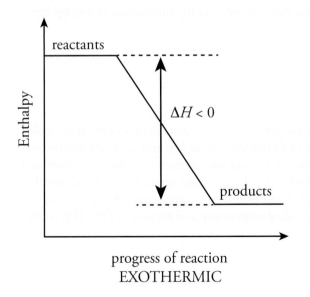

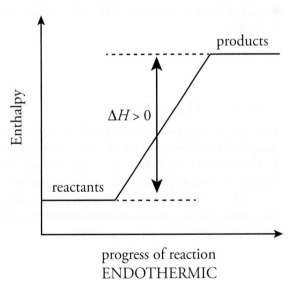

Example 27-2: The chemical synthesis of urea is given by the following reaction:

$$CO_2(aq) + 2\ NH_3(aq) \rightarrow CO(NH_2)_2(aq) + H_2O(l) \qquad\qquad \Delta H = -24.3\ kJ$$

a) How much heat is produced if 4 g of ammonia are allowed to react with excess carbon dioxide?

b) Is the reaction exothermic or endothermic?

c) How much urea was produced from a reaction that released 121 kJ of heat?

Solution:

a) The formula weight of ammonia is 17 g/mol, and (4 g)/(17g/mol) ≈ 0.25 mol. For every 2 mol of ammonia that react, 24.3 kJ of heat are produced. 0.25 mol is 1/8 of 2 mol, so the reaction will produce (1/8)(24.3kJ) ≈ 3 kJ of heat.

b) $\Delta H_{rxn} = H_{final} - H_{initial}$. Since the value of ΔH_{rxn} is negative, the final products have less enthalpy than the starting materials. Heat is released, and the reaction is exothermic.

c) One mole of urea is produced if 24.3 kJ of heat are released. A reaction that releases 121 kJ has released about five times as much heat, so approximately five moles of urea were produced.

27.4 CALCULATION OF ΔH_{rxn}

The heat of reaction (ΔH_{rxn}) can be calculated in a number of ways. Each of these will lead to the same answer given accurate starting values. The three most important methods to be familiar with are the use of standard heats of formation ($\Delta H°_f$), Hess's Law of Heat Summation, and the summation of average bond enthalpies.

Standard Conditions

Essentially every process is affected by temperature and pressure, so scientists have a convention called **standard conditions** for which most constants, heats of formation, enthalpies, and so on are determined. Under standard conditions, the temperature is 298 K (25°C) and the pressure is 1 atm. All solids and liquids are assumed to be pure, and solutions are considered to be at a concentration of 1 *M*. Values that have been determined under standard conditions are designated by a ° superscript: $\Delta H°$, for example. Be careful not to confuse *standard conditions* with *standard temperature and pressure* (STP). STP is 0°C, while standard conditions means 25°C.

Heat of Formation

The **standard heat of formation**, $\Delta H°_f$, is the energy change associated with making one mole of a compound *from its constituent elements in their natural or standard state,* which is the way the element exists under standard conditions. The convention is to assign elements in their standard state forms a $\Delta H°_f$ of zero. For example, the $\Delta H°_f$ of C(s) (as graphite) is zero. Diatomic elements, such as O_2, H_2, Cl_2 and so on are also defined as zero, rather than their atomic forms (such as O, Cl, etc.), because the diatomic state is the *natural* state for these elements at standard conditions. For example, $\Delta H°_f = 0$ for O_2, but for O, $\Delta H°_f$ = 249 kJ/mol at standard conditions, because it takes energy to break the O=O double bond.

When the $\Delta H°_f$ of a compound is positive, then an input of heat is required to make that compound from its constituent elements. When $\Delta H°_f$ is negative, making the compound from its elements gives off energy.

You can calculate the $\Delta H°$ of a reaction if you know the heats of formation of the reactants and products:

$$\Delta H°_{rxn} = (\Sigma n \times \Delta H°_{f,\ products}) - (\Sigma n \times \Delta H°_{f,\ reactants})$$

In the above equation "n" denotes the stoichiometric coefficient applied to each species in a chemical reaction as written. $\Delta H°_f$ of a given compound is the heat needed to form one mole, and as such, if two moles of a molecule are needed to balance a reaction, one must double the corresponding $\Delta H°_f$ in the enthalpy equation. If only half a mole is required, one must divide the $\Delta H°_f$ by 2.

Example 27-3: What is $\Delta H°$ for the following reaction under standard conditions if the $\Delta H°_f$ of $CH_4(g)$ = –75 kJ/mol, $\Delta H°_f$ of $CO_2(g)$ = –393 kJ/mol, and $\Delta H°_f$ of $H_2O(l)$ = –286 kJ/mol?

$$CH_4(g) + 2\ O_2(g) \rightarrow CO_2(g) + 2\ H_2O(l)$$

Solution: Using the equation for $\Delta H°_{rxn}$, we find that

$$\Delta H°_{rxn} = (\Delta H°_f CO_2 + 2\ \Delta H°_f H_2O) - (\Delta H°_f CH_4 + 2\ \Delta H°_f O_2)$$

$$= (-393\ kJ/mol + 2(-286)\ kJ/mol) - (-75\ kJ/mol + 0\ kJ/mol)$$

$$= -890\ kJ/mol$$

Hess's Law of Heat Summation

Hess's Law states that if a reaction occurs in several steps, then the sum of the energies absorbed or given off in all the steps will be the same as that for the overall reaction. This is due to the fact that enthalpy is a state function, which means that changes are independent of the pathway of the reaction. Therefore, ΔH is independent of the pathway of the reaction.

For example, we can consider the combustion of carbon to form carbon monoxide to proceed by a two-step process:

1) $C(s) + O_2(g) \rightarrow CO_2(g)$ $\quad\quad \Delta H_1 = -394$ kJ
2) $CO_2(g) \rightarrow CO(g) + 1/2\ O_2(g)$ $\quad\quad \Delta H_2 = +283$ kJ

To get the overall reaction, we add the two steps:

$$C(s) +\ 1/2\ O_2(g) \rightarrow CO(g)$$

So, to find ΔH for the overall reaction, we just add the enthalpies of each of the steps:

$$\Delta H_{rxn} = \Delta H_1 + \Delta H_2 = -394 \text{ kJ} + 283 \text{ kJ} = -111 \text{ kJ}$$

It's important to remember the following two rules when using Hess's Law:

1) *If a reaction is reversed, the sign of ΔH is reversed too.*
   For example, for the reaction $CO_2(g) \rightarrow C(s) + O_2(g)$, we'd have $\Delta H = +394 \text{ kJ}$.

2) *If an equation is multiplied by a coefficient, then ΔH must be multiplied by that same value.*
   For example, for $1/2 \ C(s) + 1/2 \ O_2(g) \rightarrow 1/2 \ CO_2(g)$, we'd have $\Delta H = -197 \text{ kJ}$.

Example 27-4: Data for the combustion reactions of glucose ($C_{12}H_6O_6$) and ethanol (C_2H_5OH) are given below:

a) $3 \ C_6H_{12}O_6(s) + 18 \ O_2(g) \rightarrow 18 \ CO_2(g) + 18 \ H2O(l)$ $\Delta H = -8424 \text{ kJ}$
b) $C_2H_5OH(l) + 3 \ O_2(g) \rightarrow 2 \ CO_2(g) + 3 \ H_2O(l)$ $\Delta H = -1370 \text{ kJ}$

Calculate the ΔH_{rxn} for the complete fermentation of glucose to ethanol and carbon dioxide:

$$\text{Net) } C_6H_{12}O_6(s) \rightarrow 2 \ C_2H_5OH(l) + 2 \ CO_2(g)$$

Solution: Reaction A has glucose as a starting material with a stoichiometric coefficient of 3. The net reaction has glucose as a starting material with a coefficient of 1, so reaction A must be divided by 3. Ethanol is a product in the net reaction; we need to reverse reaction B and multiply it by 2 to get the correct coefficient on ethanol. After these manipulations, reactions A and B will sum to give the net reaction, and by Hess's Law:

$$\Delta H_{net} = (1/3)\Delta H_A + (-1)(2)\Delta H_B = (1/3)(-8424 \text{ kJ}) + (-1)(2)(-1370 \text{ kJ})$$
$$\Delta H \text{net} \approx -2800 \text{ kJ} + 2740 \text{ kJ} = -70 \text{ kJ}$$

Summation of Average Bond Enthalpies

Enthalpy itself can be viewed as the energy stored in the chemical bonds of a compound. Bonds have characteristic enthalpies that denote how much energy is required to break them homolytically (often called the bond dissociation energy, or BDE; see Section 26.10).

As indicated at the start of this section, an important distinction should be made here in the difference in sign of ΔH for making a bond versus breaking a bond. One must, necessarily, infuse energy into a system to break a chemical bond. As such, the ΔH for this process is positive, making it endothermic. On the other hand, creating a bond between two atoms must have a negative value of ΔH. It therefore gives off heat and is exothermic. If this weren't the case, it would indicate that the bonded atoms were higher in energy than they were when unbound; such a bond would be unstable and immediately dissociate.

Therefore, we have a very important relation that can help you on the MCAT:

> Energy is needed to break a bond.
>
> Energy is released in making a bond.

From this we come to the third method of determining ΔH_{rxn}. If a question provides a list of bond enthalpies, ΔH_{rxn} can be determined through the following equation:

$$\Delta H_{rxn} = \Sigma \text{ (BDE bonds broken)} - \Sigma \text{ (BDE bonds formed)}$$

One can see that if stronger bonds are being formed than those being broken, then ΔH_{rxn} will be negative. More energy is released than supplied and the reaction is exothermic. If the opposite is true and breaking strong bonds takes more energy than is regained through the making of weaker product bonds, then the reaction is endothermic.

Example 27-5: Given the table of average bond dissociation energies below, calculate ΔH_{rxn} for the combustion of methane given in Example 27-3.

Bond	Average Bond Dissociation Energy (kJ/mol)
C—H	413
O—H	467
C=O	799
O=O	495

A) 824 kJ/mol
B) 110 kJ/mol
C) –824 kJ/mol
D) –110 kJ/mol

Solution: First, determine how many of each type of bond are broken in the reactants and formed in the products based on the stoichiometry of the balanced equation. Then, using the bond dissociation energies, we can calculate the enthalpy change:

$$\Delta H_{rxn} = \Sigma \text{ (BDE bonds broken)} - \Sigma \text{ (BDE bonds formed)}$$

$$\Delta H_{rxn} = (4(\text{C—H}) + 2(\text{O=O})) - (2(\text{C=O}) + 4(\text{O—H}))$$

$$= (4(413) + 2(495)) - (2(799) + 4(467))$$

$$= -824 \text{ kJ/mol}$$

The correct answer is choice C. You may notice that the two methods of calculating the reaction enthalpy for the same reaction did not produce exactly the same answer. This is due to the fact that bond energies are reported as the average of many examples of that type of bond, whereas heats of formation are determined for each individual chemical compound. The exact energy of a bond will be dependent not only on the two atoms bonded together but also the chemical environment in which they reside. The average bond energy gives an approximation of the strength of an individual bond, and as such, the summation of bond energies give an approximation of ΔH_{rxn}.

27.5 HEATS OF PHASE CHANGES

When matter undergoes a phase transition, energy is either absorbed or released. The amount of energy required to complete a transition is called the **heat of transition,** symbolized ΔH. For example, the amount of heat that must be absorbed to change a solid into liquid is called the **heat of fusion**, and the energy absorbed when a liquid changes to gas is the **heat of vaporization**. Each substance has a specific heat of transition for each phase change, and the magnitude is directly related to the strength and number of the intermolecular forces that substance experiences.

The amount of heat required to cause a change of phase depends on two things: the type of substance and the amount of substance. For example, the heat of fusion for H_2O is 6.0 kJ/mol. So, if we wanted to melt a 2 mol sample of ice (at 0°C), 12 kJ of heat would need to be supplied. The heat of vaporization for H_2O is about 41 kJ/mol, so vaporizing a 2 mol sample of liquid water (at 100°C) would require 82 kJ of heat. If that 2 mol sample of steam (at 100°C) condensed back to liquid, 82 kJ of heat would be released. In general, the amount of heat, q, accompanying a phase transition is given by

$$q = n \times \Delta H_{\text{phase change}}$$

where n is the number of moles of the substance. If ΔH and q are positive, heat is absorbed; if ΔH and q are negative, heat is released.

Example 27-6: The heat of crystallization of the saturated fatty acid myristic acid ($C_{14}H_{28}O_2$) is −45.4 kJ/mol and its melting point is 54°C. What is the change in heat needed to completely melt 580 g of myristic acid whose initial temperature is 54°C?

    A) −115 kJ
    B) −135 kJ
    C) 115 kJ
    D) 135 kJ

Solution: Since melting is an endothermic process, the heat needed should be a positive value, so we can eliminate choices A and B. The formula weight of myristic acid is 14(12 g/mol) + 28(1 g/mol) + 2(16 g/mol) ≈ 230 g/mol, so the sample contains (580 g)/(230 g/mol) ≈ 2.5 moles of myristic acid. Because the sample is being melted, the heat of fusion (which has the opposite sign, but the same magnitude, of the given heat of crystallization) must be used. Choice C is correct according to the following equation:

$$q = n \times \Delta H_{\text{fusion}} = 2.5 \text{ mol} \times 45.4 \text{ kJ/mol} \approx 115 \text{ kJ}$$

27.6 ENTROPY

The Second Law of Thermodynamics

There are several different ways to state the **Second Law of Thermodynamics**, each appropriate to the particular system under study, but they're all equivalent. One way to state this law is that the disorder of the universe increases in a spontaneous process. For this to make sense, let's examine what we mean by the term *spontaneous*. For example, water will spontaneously splash and flow down a waterfall, but it will not spontaneously collect itself at the bottom and flow up the cliff. A bouncing ball will come to rest, but a ball at rest will not suddenly start bouncing. If the ball is warm enough, it's got the energy to start moving, but heat—the disorganized, random kinetic energy of the constituent atoms—will not spontaneously organize itself and give the ball an overall kinetic energy to start it moving. From another perspective, heat will spontaneously flow from a plate of hot food to its cooler surroundings, but thermal energy in the cool surroundings will not spontaneously concentrate itself and flow into the food. None of these processes would violate the first law, but they do violate the second law.

Nature has a tendency to become increasingly disorganized, and another way to state the second law is that *all processes tend to run in a direction that leads to maximum disorder*. Think about spilling milk from a glass. Does the milk ever collect itself together and refill the glass? No, it spreads out randomly over the table and floor. In fact, it needed the glass in the first place just to have any shape at all. Likewise, think about the helium in a balloon: it expands to fill its container, and if we empty the balloon, the helium diffuses randomly throughout the room. The reverse doesn't happen. Helium atoms don't collect themselves from the atmosphere and move into a closed container. The natural tendency of *all* things is to increase their disorder.

We measure disorder or randomness as **entropy**. The greater the disorder of a system, the greater is its entropy. Entropy is represented by the symbol S, and the change in entropy during a reaction is represented by the symbol ΔS. The change in entropy is determined by the equation

$$\Delta S = S_{products} - S_{reactants}$$

If randomness increases—or order decreases—during the reaction, then ΔS is positive for the reaction. If randomness decreases—or order increases—then ΔS is negative. For example, let's look at the decomposition reaction for carbonic acid:

$$H_2CO_3 \rightleftharpoons H_2O + CO_2$$

In this case, one molecule breaks into two molecules, and disorder is increased. That is, the atoms are less organized in the water and carbon dioxide molecules than they are in the carbonic acid molecule. The entropy is increasing for the forward reaction. Let's look at the reverse process: if CO_2 and H_2O come together to form H_2CO_3, we've decreased entropy because the atoms in two molecules have become more organized by forming one molecule.

In general, entropy is predictable in many cases.

- Liquids have more entropy than solids.
- Gases have more entropy than solids or liquids.
- Particles in solution have more entropy than undissolved solids.
- Two moles of a substance have more entropy than one mole.
- The value of ΔS for a reverse reaction has the same magnitude as that of the forward reaction, but with opposite sign: $\Delta S_{reverse} = -\Delta S_{forward}$.

27.6

While the overall drive of nature is to increase entropy, reactions can occur in which entropy decreases, but we must either put in energy or gain energy from making more stable bonds. (We'll explore this further when we discuss Gibbs free energy.)

Example 27-8: Which of these processes would result in the greatest positive entropy change?

    A) $NaCl(aq) + CO_2(g) + NH_3(g) + H_2O(l) \rightarrow NaHCO3(s) + NH_4Cl(aq)$
    B) $CO(g) + H_2O(g) \rightarrow CO_2(g) + H_2(g)$
    C) $NaHCO_3(s) + CH_3COOH(aq) \rightarrow CH_3COONa(aq) + H_2O(l) + CO_2(g)$
    D) $2\,NH_4Cl(aq) + Pb(NO_3)_2(aq) \rightarrow 2\,NH_4NO_3(aq) + PbCl_2(s)$

Solution: The reaction in choice A converts two moles of gas and one mole of liquid to one mole of solid, so $\Delta S < 0$. The reaction in choice B has no change in number of moles or phase, so is unlikely to have a large value for ΔS. In choice C, one mole of solid is converted to one mole of a liquid and one mole of a gas, so $\Delta S > 0$, and this is the correct answer. In choice D, a solid precipitates from aqueous reactants, so $\Delta S < 0$.

Example 27-9: For the endothermic reaction

$$2\,CO_2(g) \rightarrow 2\,CO(g) + O_2(g)$$

which of the following is true?

    A) ΔH is positive, and ΔS is positive.
    B) ΔH is positive, and ΔS is negative.
    C) ΔH is negative, and ΔS is positive.
    D) ΔH is negative, and ΔS is negative.

Solution: Since we're told that the reaction is endothermic, we know that ΔH is positive. This eliminates choices C and D. Now, what about ΔS? Has the disorder increased or decreased? On the reactant side, we have one type of gas molecule, while on the right we have two. The reaction increases the numbers of gas molecules, so this describes an increase in disorder. ΔS is positive, and the answer is choice A.

The Third Law of Thermodynamics

The third law defines absolute zero to be a state of zero-entropy. At absolute zero, thermal energy is absent and only the least energetic thermodynamic state is available to the system in question. If only one state is possible, then there is no randomness to the system and $S = 0$. In this way, the third law describes the least thermally energetic state, and therefore the lowest achievable temperature. Kelvin defined the temperature at this state as 0 on his temperature scale.

27.7 GIBBS FREE ENERGY

The magnitude of the change in **Gibbs free energy**, ΔG, is the energy that's available (free) to do useful work from a chemical reaction. The spontaneity of a reaction is determined by changes in enthalpy and in entropy, and G includes both of these quantities. Now we have a way to determine whether a given reaction will be spontaneous. In some cases—namely, when ΔH and ΔS have different signs—it's easy. For example, if ΔH is negative and ΔS is positive, then the reaction will certainly be spontaneous (because the products have less energy and more disorder than the reactants; there are two tendencies for a spontaneous reaction: to decrease enthalpy and/or to increase entropy). If ΔH is positive and ΔS is negative, then the reaction will certainly be nonspontaneous (because the products would have more energy and less disorder than the reactants).

But what happens when ΔH and ΔS have the *same* sign? Which factor—enthalpy or entropy—will dominate and determine the spontaneity of the reaction? The sign of the single quantity ΔG will dictate whether or not a process is spontaneous, and we calculate ΔG from this equation:

> ### Change in Gibbs Free Energy
> $$\Delta G = \Delta H - T\Delta S$$

where T is the absolute temperature (in kelvins). And now, we can then say the following:

- $\Delta G < 0 \;\rightarrow\;$ spontaneous in the forward direction
- $\Delta G = 0 \;\rightarrow\;$ reaction is at equilibrium
- $\Delta G > 0 \;\rightarrow\;$ nonspontaneous in the forward direction

If ΔG for a reaction is positive, then the value of ΔG for the *reverse* reaction has the same magnitude but is negative. Therefore, the reverse reaction is spontaneous.

ΔG and Temperature

The equation for ΔG shows us that the entropy ($T\Delta S$) term depends directly on temperature. At low temperatures, the entropy doesn't have much influence on the free energy, and ΔH is the dominant factor in determining spontaneity. But as the temperature increases, the entropy term becomes more significant relative to ΔH and can dominate the value for ΔG. In general, the universe tends towards increasing disorder (positive ΔS) and stable bonds (negative ΔH), and a favorable combination of these will make a process spontaneous. The following chart summarizes the combinations of ΔH and ΔS that determine ΔG and spontaneity.

ΔH	ΔS	ΔG	Reaction is...?
–	+	–	spontaneous
+	+	– at sufficiently high T + at low T	spontaneous nonspontaneous
–	–	+ at high T – at sufficiently low T	nonspontaneous spontaneous
+	–	+	nonspontaneous

Important note: While values of ΔH are usually reported in terms of kJ, values of ΔS are usually given in terms of J. When using the equation $\Delta G = \Delta H - T\Delta S$, make sure that your ΔH and ΔS are expressed *both* in kJ or *both* in J.

Example 27-10: If it's discovered that a certain nonspontaneous reaction becomes spontaneous if the temperature is lowered, then which of the following must be true?

        A) ΔS is negative, and ΔH is positive.
        B) ΔS is negative, and ΔH is negative.
        C) ΔS is positive, and ΔH is positive.
        D) ΔS is positive, and ΔH is negative.

Solution: If the temperature at which the reaction takes place has an impact on the spontaneity of the reaction, that means that the signs of ΔH and ΔS must both be either positive or negative (eliminate choices A and D). Lowering the temperature term makes the $T\Delta S$ term a smaller value in magnitude, and it changes the sign of ΔG from positive to negative. That must mean that the ΔH is a negative value, as its impact is now more obvious at the new lower temperature, making choice B the correct answer.

27.8 REACTION ENERGY DIAGRAMS

A chemical reaction can be graphed as it progresses in a reaction energy diagram. True to its name, a reaction energy diagram plots the free energy of the total reactions versus the conversion of reactants to products.

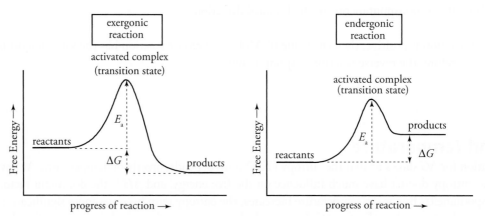

The ΔG of the overall reaction is the difference between the energy of the products and the energy of the reactants: $\Delta G_{rxn} = G_{products} - G_{reactants}$. When the value of $T\Delta S$ is very small, then ΔG can approximate ΔH, with the difference between the energy of products and reactants being very close to the heat of reaction, ΔH.

The activation energy, E_a, is the extra energy the reactants required to overcome the activation barrier, and it determines the kinetics of the reaction. The higher the barrier, the slower the reaction proceeds toward equilibrium; the lower the barrier, the faster the reaction proceeds toward equilibrium. However, E_a does *not* determine the equilibrium, and an eternally slow reaction (very big E_a) can have a very favorable (large) K_{eq}.

27.8

Kinetics vs. Thermodynamics

Just because a reaction is thermodynamically favorable (i.e., *spontaneous*), does not automatically mean that it will be taking place rapidly. **Do not confuse kinetics with thermodynamics** (this is something the MCAT will *try* to get you to do many times!). They are separate realms. *Thermodynamics predicts the spontaneity (and the equilibrium) of reactions, not their rates.* If you had a starting line and a finish line, thermodynamics tells you how far you will go, while kinetics tells you how quickly you will get there. A classic example to illustrate this is the formation of graphite from diamond. Graphite and diamond are two of the several different forms (**allotropes**) of carbon, and the value of ΔG° for the reaction $C_{(diamond)} \rightarrow C_{(graphite)}$ is about –2900 J/mol. Because ΔG° is negative, the formation of graphite is favored under standard conditions, but it's *extremely* slow. Even diamond heirlooms passed down through many generations are still in diamond form.

Reversibility

Reactions follow the principle of microscopic reversibility: the reverse reaction has the same magnitude for all thermodynamic values (ΔG, ΔH, and ΔS) but of the opposite sign, and the same reaction pathway, but in reverse. This means that the reaction energy diagram for the reverse reaction can be drawn by simply using the mirror image of the forward reaction. The incongruity you should notice is that E_a is different for the forward and reverse reactions. Coming from the products side towards the reactants, the energy barrier will be the difference between $G_{products}$ and the energy of the activated complex.

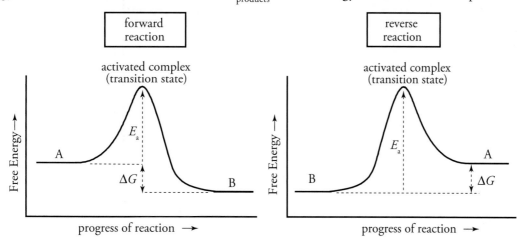

Kinetics vs. Thermodynamics

Reversibility

Chapter 28
Phases and Gases

28.1 PHYSICAL CHANGES

Matter can undergo physical changes as well as chemical changes. Melting, freezing, and boiling are all examples of physical changes. A key property of a physical change is that no *intra*molecular bonds are made or broken; a physical change affects only the *inter*molecular forces between molecules or atoms. For example, ice melting to become liquid water does not change the molecules of H_2O into something else. Melting reflects the disruption of the attractive interactions between the molecules.

Every type of matter experiences intermolecular forces such as dispersion forces, dipole interactions, and hydrogen bonding. All molecules have some degree of attraction towards each other (dispersion forces at least), and it's the intermolecular interactions that hold matter together as solids or liquids. The strength and the type of intermolecular forces depend on the identity of the atoms and molecules of a substance and vary greatly. For example, $NaCl(s)$, $H_2O(l)$, and $N_2(g)$ all have different kinds and strengths of intermolecular forces, and these differences give rise to their widely varying melting and boiling points.

Phase Transitions

Physical changes are closely related to temperature. What does temperature tell us about matter? Temperature is a measure of the amount of internal kinetic energy (the energy of motion) that molecules have. The average kinetic energy of the molecules of a substance directly affects its **state** or **phase**: whether it's a **solid, liquid,** or **gas.** Kinetic energy is also related to the degree of disorder, or **entropy.** In general, the higher the average kinetic energy of the molecules of a substance, the greater its entropy.

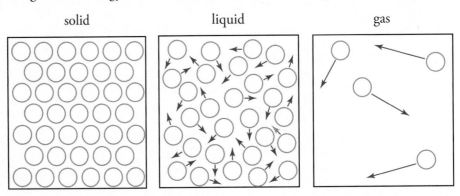

If we increase the temperature at a given pressure, a solid typically transforms into liquid and then into gas. What causes the phase transitions as the temperature increases? Phase changes are simply the result of breaking (or forming) intermolecular interactions. At low temperatures, matter tends to exist as a solid and is held together by intermolecular interactions. The molecules in a solid may jiggle a bit, but they're restricted to relatively fixed positions and form an orderly array, because the molecules don't have enough kinetic energy to overcome the intermolecular forces. Solids are the most ordered and least energetic of the phases. As a solid absorbs heat its temperature increases, meaning the average kinetic energy of the molecules increases. This causes the molecules to move around more, loosening the intermolecular interactions and increasing the entropy. When enough energy is absorbed for the molecules to move freely around one another, the solid melts and becomes liquid. At the molecular level, the molecules in a liquid are still in contact and interact with each other, but they have enough kinetic energy to escape fixed positions. Liquids have more internal kinetic energy and greater entropy than solids. If enough heat is absorbed by the liquid, the kinetic energy increases until the molecules have enough speed to escape intermolecular forces and vaporize into the gas phase. Molecules in the gas phase move freely of one another and experience very little, if any, intermolecular forces. Gases are the most energetic and least ordered of the phases.

To illustrate these phase transitions, let's follow ice through the transitions from solid to liquid to gas. Ice is composed of highly organized H_2O molecules held rigidly by hydrogen bonds. The molecules have limited motion. If we increase the temperature of the ice, the molecules will eventually absorb enough heat to move around, and the organized structure of the molecules will break down as fixed hydrogen bonds are replaced with hydrogen bonds in which the molecules are *not* in fixed positions. We observe the transition as ice melting into liquid water. If we continue to increase the temperature, the kinetic energy of the molecules eventually becomes great enough for the individual molecules to overcome all hydrogen bonding and move freely. This appears to us as vaporization, or boiling of the liquid into gas. At this point, the H_2O molecules zip around randomly, forming a high-entropy, chaotic swarm. All the phase transitions are summarized here.

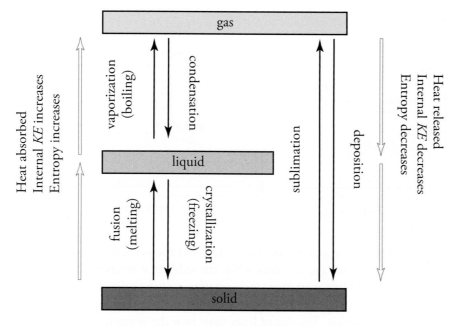

Example 28-1: Which of these phase changes is exothermic?

A) Boiling
B) Vaporization
C) Crystallization
D) Sublimation

Solution: Phase changes that bring molecules together (*freezing, condensation, deposition*) release heat: such processes are exothermic. Conversely, phase changes that spread molecules out (*melting/fusion, vaporization, sublimation*) absorb heat: such processes are endothermic. Choice C is the correct answer. (Note also that choices A and B are identical, so you know they must be wrong, no matter what.)

28.2 PHASE TRANSITION DIAGRAM/HEATING CURVE

Let's consider the complete range of phase changes from solid to liquid to gas. The process in this direction requires the input of heat. As heat is added to the solid, its temperature increases until it reaches its melting point. At that point, absorbed heat is used to change the phase to liquid, *not to increase the temperature.* One of the most important facts about physical changes of matter is that when a substance absorbs or releases heat, one of two things can happen: either its temperature changes or its phase will change, but not both at the same time. Once the sample has been completely melted, additional heat again causes its temperature to rise, until the boiling point is reached. At that point, absorbed heat is used to change the phase to gas, not to increase the temperature. Once the sample has been completely vaporized, additional heat again causes its temperature to rise. We can summarize all this with a **phase transition diagram** also known as a **heating curve**, which plots the temperature of the sample versus the amount of heat absorbed. The figure below is a typical heating curve.

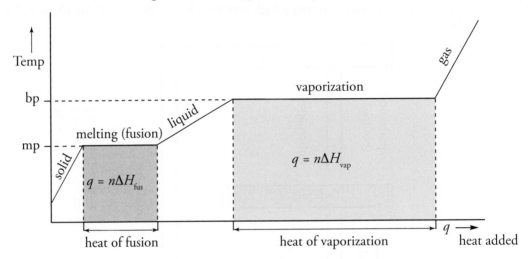

The horizontal axis represents the amount of heat added, and the vertical axis is the corresponding temperature of the substance. Notice the flat lines when the substance reaches its melting point (mp) and boiling point (bp). *During a phase transition, the temperature of the substance does not change.* Also, the greater the value for the heat of transition, the longer the flat line. A substance's heat of vaporization is always greater than its heat of fusion. The sloped lines show how the temperature changes (within a phase) as heat is added. Since $\Delta T = q/C$, the slopes of the non-flat lines are equal to $1/C$, the reciprocal of the substance's heat capacity in that phase.

Example 28-2: How much heat is needed to completely convert 5 g of water, initially at 60°C, to steam? ($\Delta H_{vap} = 2300$ J/g and $c_{water} = 4$ J/g-°C)

    A)   0.80 kJ
    B)   2.3 kJ
    C)   11.5 kJ
    D)   12.3 kJ

Solution: There are two steps here: (1) heat the water from 60°C to 100°C (i.e., the boiling point of water) and (2) vaporize the liquid water at 100°C to steam at 100°C.

$$
\begin{aligned}
q_{total} \quad &= q_1 + q_2 \\
&= mc_{water}\Delta T + m\Delta H_{vap} \\
&= (5\ g)(4\ J/g\text{-}°C)(100°C - 60°C) + (5\ g)(2300\ J/g) \\
&= 800\ J + 11{,}500\ J \\
&= 12{,}300\ J = 12.3\ kJ
\end{aligned}
$$

Phase Diagrams

The phase of a substance doesn't depend just on the temperature, it also depends on the pressure. For example, even at high temperatures, a substance can be squeezed into the liquid phase if the pressure is high enough, and at low temperature, a substance can enter the gas phase if that pressure is low enough. A substance's **phase diagram** shows how its phases are determined by temperature and pressure. The figure below is a generic example of a phase diagram.

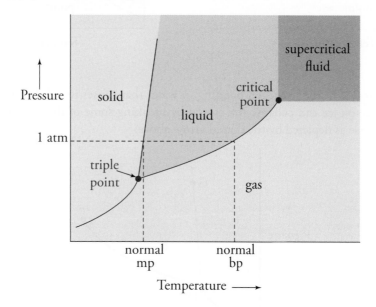

There are several important parts of the phase diagram.

- Boundary lines represent phase changes where two phases are at equilibrium.
- Drawing a horizontal line at 1 atm gives the **normal melting point** at the temperature it intersects the solid/liquid phase line.
- Drawing a horizontal line at 1 atm gives the **normal boiling point** at the temperature it intersects the gas/liquid phase line.
- The **triple point** occurs that the temperature and pressure where all lines intersect. Under these conditions, all three phases exist simultaneously at equilibrium, and therefore all phase changes are happening simultaneously.
- The end of the liquid/gas boundary is called the **critical point** and defines the beginning of the supercritical fluid phase where the gas and liquid phases have coalesced.

The Phase Diagram for Water

Water is the most common of a handful of substances that are denser in the liquid phase than in the solid phase. As a result, the solid-liquid boundary line in the phase diagram for water has a slightly *negative* slope, as opposed to the usual positive slope for most other substances. Compare these diagrams:

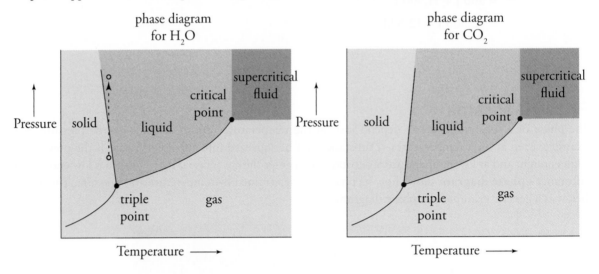

The negative slope is due to the hydrogen bonding in water that causes its solid phase to expand. Therefore, placing pressure on ice can collapse the crystal by breaking some of the hydrogen bonds, forming the mobile liquid phase as depicted by the dotted arrow above.

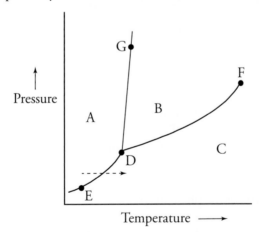

Example 28-3: The dashed arrow in the diagram indicates what type of phase transition?

A) Evaporation
B) Crystallization
C) Deposition
D) Sublimation

Solution: The arrow shows a substance in the solid phase (region A) moving directly to the gaseous phase (region C) without melting first. The phase transition from solid to gas is called sublimation, choice D.

28.3   GASES AND THE KINETIC-MOLECULAR THEORY

Unlike the condensed phases of matter (solids and liquids), **gases** have no fixed volume. A gas will fill all the available space in a container. Gases are *far* more compressible than solids or liquids, and their densities are very low (roughly 1 kg/m³ at standard temperature and pressure), about three to four orders of magnitude less than solids and liquids. But the most striking difference between a gas and a solid or liquid is that the molecules of a gas are free to move over large distances.

The most important properties of a gas are its **pressure**, **volume**, and **temperature**. How these macroscopic properties are related to each other can be derived from some basic assumptions concerning the *microscopic* behavior of gas molecules. These assumptions are the foundation of the **kinetic-molecular theory**.

Kinetic-molecular theory, a model for describing the behavior of gases, is based on the following assumptions:

1) The molecules of a gas are so small compared to the average spacing between them that the molecules themselves take up essentially no volume.

2) The molecules of a gas are in constant motion, moving in straight lines at constant speeds and in random directions between collisions. The collisions of the molecules with the walls of the container define the **pressure** of the gas (the average force exerted per unit area), and all collisions—molecules striking the walls and each other—are *elastic* (that is, the total kinetic energy is the same after the collision as it was before).

3) Since each molecule moves at a constant speed between collisions and the collisions are elastic, the molecules of a gas experience no intermolecular forces.

4) The molecules of a gas span a distribution of speeds, and the average kinetic energy of the molecules is directly proportional to the absolute temperature (the temperature in kelvins) of the sample: $KE_{avg} \propto T$.

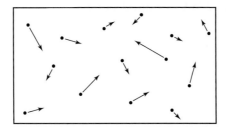

A gas that satisfies all these requirements is said to be an **ideal gas.** Most real gases behave like ideal gases under ordinary conditions, so the results that follow from the kinetic-molecular theory can be applied to real gases.

Units of Volume, Temperature, and Pressure

Volume

The SI unit for volume is the cubic meter (m³), but in chemistry, the **cubic centimeter** (**cm³** or **cc**) and **liter** (**L**) are commonly used. One cubic meter is equal to one thousand liters.

$$1 \text{ cm}^3 = 1 \text{ cc} = 1 \text{ mL} \quad \text{and} \quad 1 \text{ m}^3 = 1000 \text{ L}$$

Temperature

Temperature may be expressed in degrees Fahrenheit, degrees Celsius, or in kelvins (not degrees Kelvin). The relationship between kelvins and degrees Celsius is simple:

$$T \text{ (in K)} = T \text{ (in °C)} + 273.15$$

When dealing with gases, the best unit for expressing temperature is the kelvin (K). This is an absolute temperature scale whereby zero kelvin (0 K) defines a point of zero entropy where molecular motion is at a minimum. From a practical perspective, this avoids the issue of calculations involving negative temperatures, so all of the gas laws equations on the MCAT require the use of absolute temperatures.

Pressure

Since pressure is defined as force per unit area, the SI unit for pressure is the **pascal** (abbreviated **Pa**), where 1 Pa = 1 N/m². The unit is inconveniently small for normal calculations involving gases (for example, a nickel sitting on a table exerts about 140 Pa of pressure), so several alternative units for pressure are usually used.

The alternative units relationships are summarized below:

$$1 \text{ atm} = 760 \text{ torr} = 760 \text{ mm Hg} = 101.3 \text{ kPa}$$

Standard Temperature and Pressure

Standard Temperature and Pressure (STP) means a temperature of 0°C (273.15 K) and a pressure of 1 atm.

Example 28-4: A temperature of 273°C is equivalent to:

A) –100 K
B) 0 K
C) 100 K
D) 546 K

Solution: Choice A is eliminated, because negative values are not permitted when using the Kelvin temperature scale. Since $T \text{ (in K)} = T \text{ (in °C)} + 273$, we have

$$T \text{ (in K)} = 273 + 273 = 546 \text{ K}$$

Therefore, choice D is the answer.

28.4 THE IDEAL GAS LAW

The volume, temperature, and pressure of an ideal gas are related by a simple equation called the **Ideal Gas Law**. Most real gases under ordinary conditions act very much like ideal gases, so the Ideal Gas Law applies to most gas behavior:

Ideal Gas Law

$$PV = nRT$$

---

where

P = the pressure of the gas in atmospheres
V = the volume of the container in liters
n = the number of moles of the gas
R = the universal gas constant, 0.0821 L-atm/K-mol
T = the absolute temperature of the gas (that is, T in kelvins)

Questions on gas behavior typically take one of two forms. The first type of question simply gives you some facts, and you use $PV = nRT$ to determine a missing variable. In the second type, "before" and "after" scenarios are presented for which you determine the effect of changing the volume, temperature, or pressure. In this case, you apply the ideal gas law twice, once for each scenario.

1. If two moles of helium at 27°C fill a 3 L balloon, what is the pressure?

Take the ideal gas law, solve it for P, then plug in the numbers (and don't forget to convert the temperature in °C to kelvin!):

$$PV = nRT$$

$$P = \frac{nRT}{V}$$

$$P = \frac{(2 \text{ mol})(0.082 \text{ L-atm/K-mol})(300 \text{ K})}{3 \text{ L}}$$

$$P = 16 \text{ atm}$$

2. Argon, at a pressure of 2 atm, fills a 100 mL vial at a temperature of 0°C. What would the pressure of the argon be if we increase the volume to 500 mL, and the temperature is 100°C?

We're not told how much argon (the number of moles, n) is in the vial, but it doesn't matter since it doesn't change. Since R is also a constant, the ratio of PV/T, which is equal to nR, remains constant. Therefore,

$$\frac{P_1 V_1}{T_1} = \frac{P_2 V_2}{T_2} \quad \Rightarrow \quad P_2 = P_1 \frac{V_1}{V_2} \frac{T_2}{T_1}$$

$$P_2 = (2 \text{ atm}) \left(\frac{0.1 \text{ L}}{0.5 \text{ L}} \right) \left(\frac{373 \text{ K}}{273 \text{ K}} \right)$$

$$P_2 = 0.55 \text{ atm}$$

P-V-T Gas Laws in Systems Where n Is Constant

The general equation of $P_1 V_1 / T_1 = P_2 V_2 / T_2$ used above can be simplified whenever both the number of moles, n, and any one of the other variables (P, V, or T) are held constant. Each of these scenarios is associated with a named law with characteristics shown in the table below:

Law	Variables	Relationship	Constant	Equations
Boyle's Law	P, V	Inverse	T	$PV = k$; $P_1 V_1 = P_2 V_2$
Charles's Law	V, T	Direct	P	$V/T = k$; $V_1/T_1 = V_2/T_2$
Gay-Lussac's Law	P, T	Direct	V	$P/T = k$; $P_1/T_1 = P_2/T_2$

Consider a kinetic molecular theory analysis of the gas laws:

For **Charles's Law**, if the pressure is to remain constant, then a gas will expand when heated and contract when cooled. If the temperature of the gas is increased, the molecules will move faster, hitting the walls of the container with more force; in order to keep the pressure the same, the frequency of the collisions would need to be reduced. This is accomplished by expanding the volume. With more available space, the molecules strike the walls less often in order to compensate for hitting them harder.

- If the temperature is constant, $PV = k$ (where k is a constant). Therefore, the pressure is inversely proportional to the volume: $P \propto 1/V$

For **Boyle's Law**, if the volume decreases, the molecules have less space to move around in. As a result, they'll collide with the walls of the container more often, and the pressure increases. On the other hand, if the volume of the container increases, the gas molecules have more available space and collide with the wall less often, resulting in a lower pressure.

For **Gay-Lussac's Law**, if the temperature goes up, so does the pressure. As the temperature increases, the molecules move faster. As a result, they strike the walls of the container surface more often and with greater speed.

If only n (which tells us the amount of gas) stays constant, we can combine Boyle's Law and Charles's Law to get the three-variable **Combined Gas Law** (which we used to answer Question 2 above):

Combined Gas Law (constant n)

$$\frac{P_1 V_1}{T_1} = \frac{P_2 V_2}{T_2}$$

Example 28-5: Helium, at a pressure of 3 atm, occupies a 16 L container at a temperature of 30°C. What would be the volume of the gas if the pressure were increased to 5 atm and the temperature lowered to –20°C?

Solution: We use the Combined Gas Law after remembering to convert the given temperatures to kelvin:

$$\frac{P_1 V_1}{T_1} = \frac{P_2 V_2}{T_2} \quad \Rightarrow \quad V_2 = V_1 \frac{P_1}{P_2} \frac{T_2}{T_1} = (16\ \text{L})\left(\frac{3\ \text{atm}}{5\ \text{atm}}\right)\left(\frac{253\ \text{K}}{303\ \text{K}}\right) \approx (16\ \text{L})\left(\frac{3}{5}\right)\left(\frac{250\ \text{K}}{300\ \text{K}}\right) = 8\ \text{L}$$

All of these laws follow from the ideal gas law and can be derived easily from it. They tell us what happens when n and P are constant, when n and T are constant, when n and V are constant, and in the case of the combined gas law, when n alone is constant. But what about n when P, V, and T are constant? That law of gases was proposed by Avogadro:

- If two equal-volume containers hold gas at the same pressure and temperature, then they contain the same number of particles (regardless of the identity of the gas).

Avogadro's Law can be restated more broadly as $V/n = k$ (where k is a constant). We can also determine the **standard molar volume** of an ideal gas at STP, which is the volume that one mole of a gas—any *ideal* gas—would occupy at 0°C and 1 atm of pressure:

$$V = \frac{nRT}{P} = \frac{(1\ \text{mol})(0.0821\ \frac{\text{L·atm}}{\text{K·mol}})(273\ \text{K})}{1\ \text{atm}} = 22.4\ \text{L}$$

To give you an idea of how much this is, 22.4 L is equal to the total volume of three basketballs.

Avogadro's Law and the **standard molar volume** of a gas can be used to simplify some gas law problems. Consider the following questions:

3. Given the Haber process, $3\ H_2(g) + N_2(g) \rightarrow 2\ NH_3(g)$, if you start with 5 L of $H_2(g)$ and 4 L of $N_2(g)$ at STP, what will the volume of the three gases be when the reaction is complete?

We can answer this question by using the ideal gas law, or we can recognize that the only thing changing is n (the number of moles of each gas) and use the standard molar volume. If we further recognize that the standard molar volume is the same for all three gases, and it is this value that we'd use to convert each given volume into moles (and then vice versa), we can use the balanced equation to quickly determine the answer.

Since we need 3 L of H_2 for every 1 L of N_2, and we have 4 L of N_2 but only 5 L of H_2, H_2 will be the limiting reagent, and its volume will be zero at the end of the reaction. Since 1 L of N_2 is needed for every 3 L of H_2, we get

$$5 \text{ L of } H_2 \times \frac{1 \text{ L of } N_2}{3 \text{ L of } H_2} = 1.7 \text{ L of } N_2$$

So the amount of N_2 remaining will be $4 - 1.7 = 2.3$ L. The volume of NH_3 produced is

$$5 \text{ L of } H_2 \times \frac{2 \text{ L of } NH_3}{3 \text{ L of } H_2} = 3.3 \text{ L of } NH_3$$

Example 28-6: An ideal gas at 1.5 atm occupies a tank whose volume is controlled by a piston. The tank's initial volume is 8.0 L. If temperature is held constant throughout, to what volume does the gas need to be compressed to achieve a pressure of 6.0 atm?

Solution: Since n and T are constants, we can use Boyle's Law to find V_2:

$$P_1 V_1 = P_2 V_2 \Rightarrow V_2 = \frac{P_1 V_1}{P_2} = \frac{(1.5 \text{ atm})(8.0 \text{ atm})}{(6.0 \text{ atm})} = 2.0 \text{ L}$$

Note that since the pressure of the gas increases by a factor of four, the volume must decrease by the same factor.

Example 28-7: How many atoms are present in a 44.8 L sample of oxygen gas at $P = 1$ atm and $T = 273$ K?

    A) 6.02×10^{23}
    B) 1.20×10^{24}
    C) 2.41×10^{24}
    D) 4.82×10^{24}

Solution: The temperature and pressure conditions are the definition of STP, so 1 mole of an ideal gas would occupy 22.4 L. A volume of 44.8 L is exactly double this, so it must correspond to a 2 mole sample of O_2 gas. Since oxygen is a diatomic gas, each mole of O_2 contains 1.20×10^{24} atoms of O, so two moles must contain 2.41×10^{24} atoms of O (choice C).

28.5 DEVIATIONS FROM IDEAL-GAS BEHAVIOR

Let's review two of the assumptions that were listed for the kinetic-molecular theory:

1) The particles of an ideal gas experience no intermolecular forces.
2) The volume of the individual particles of an ideal gas is negligible compared to the volume of the gas container.

Under some conditions, namely high pressures and low temperatures, these assumptions don't hold up very well, and the laws for ideal gases don't rigorously apply to real gases.

To determine the effect of non-ideality on gases on a macroscopic level, work though the following thought experiments, which examine each assumption above independently:

1) *No intermolecular forces:*

    If a container has a fixed volume and we allow the gas to behave as a real gas with strongly attractive intermolecular forces (for example, like water vapor would have), the pressure of the container will decrease. The number of collisions that gas particles have with the container walls (which determines pressure) will lessen because the gas is pulled toward the other gas molecules. In addition, the collisions that do occur will involve a smaller transfer of momentum than if the gas were ideal. The resulting pressure of the real gas is therefore smaller than the ideal gas pressure, or $P_{real} < P_{ideal}$.

2) *Volumeless particles:*

    Now, instead of the ideal volumeless particles, give the individual gas particles finite volumes. The tricky part here is that the volume of a gas is defined as the free space the particles have in which to move around. For an ideal gas, this volume is simply the volume of the container, since there is no volume taken up by individual particles. However, at high pressures, the volume occupied by each gas particle becomes a greater proportion of the gas sample, so it is no longer negligible, and it reduces the free space available for particle movement. The overall effect is to decrease the volume, making $V_{real} < V_{ideal}$.

From these two thought experiments we see that the attractive forces between particles cause a decrease in pressure if the volume of the container is fixed, and accounting for particle volume causes a decrease in free space (system volume) if the pressure is fixed. As these two variables interact with many others in a real system, we can sometimes see deviations from the general principles outlined here.

To make accurate predictions about the deviations real gases show from ideal-gas behavior, the Ideal Gas Law must be altered. The **van der Waals equation** includes terms to account for the differences in the observed behavior of real gases and calculated properties of ideal gases, while maintaining the same form as the Ideal Gas Law:

van der Waals Equation

$$\left(P + \frac{an^2}{V^2}\right)(V - nb) = nRT$$

The an^2/V^2 term serves as a correction for the intermolecular forces that generally result in lower pressures for real gases, while the nb term corrects for the physical volume that the individual particles occupy in a real gas. Both a and b are known as van der Waals constants and are generally larger for gases that experience greater intermolecular forces (a) and have larger molecular weights, and therefore volumes (b).

To illustrate the impact of intermolecular forces on real gas pressure, let's compare the pressures of two moles of oxygen and two moles of water, each in separate 5 L containers at a moderate temperature (500 K). Using the Ideal Gas Law, we predict the following:

$$P_{ideal} = \frac{nRT}{V} = \frac{2\,\text{moles} \times 0.0821 \dfrac{\text{L·atm}}{\text{mol·K}} \times 500\,\text{K}}{5\,\text{L}} = 16.4\,\text{atm}$$

To use the van der Waals equation to predict the actual pressures, we can rearrange and solve for P.

$$P = \left(\frac{nRT}{V-nb}\right) - \left(\frac{an^2}{V^2}\right)$$

Therefore, for oxygen (where a = 1.34 atm·L^2/mol^2 and b = 0.0318 L/mol):

$$P_{O_2} = \left(\frac{2\text{ mol} \times 0.0821\text{ L·atm/mol·K} \times 500\,\text{K}}{5\text{ L} - 2\text{ mol} \times 0.0318\text{ L/mol}}\right) - \left(\frac{1.34\text{ atm·L}^2/\text{mol}^2 \times (2\text{ mol})^2}{(5\text{ L})^2}\right)$$

$$= 16.6\text{ atm} - 0.2\text{ atm} = 16.4\text{ atm}$$

Notice that the pressure, due to oxygen's lack of substantial intermolecular forces, is effectively the same as was predicted by the Ideal Gas Law. If we select a gas with significantly stronger intermolecular forces, the deviation from ideal gas behavior becomes more pronounced. For instance, the van der Waals "a" constant for water is significantly higher than that of oxygen due to water's ability to hydrogen bond (a = 5.47 atm·L^2/mol^2 and b = 0.0305 L/mol).

$$P_{H_2O} = \left(\frac{2\text{ mol} \times 0.0821\text{ L·atm/mol·K} \times 500\text{ K}}{5\text{ L} - 2\text{ mol} \times 0.0305\text{ L/mol}}\right) - \left(\frac{5.47\text{ atm·L}^2/\text{mol}^2 \times (2\text{ mol})^2}{(5\text{ L})^2}\right)$$

$$= 16.6\text{ atm} - 0.9\text{ atm} = 15.7\text{ atm}$$

This represents a 4% decrease in pressure from that predicted by the Ideal Gas Law.

To underscore the concept that gases behave more ideally at higher temperatures, if we increase the temperature of the system for any gas, the first term in the van der Waals equation approaches the pressure of the ideal gas while the second term remains unchanged. For example, if the temperature of our systems above is increased by 100 K (to 600 K), two moles of an ideal gas would exert 19.7 atm of pressure, while the van der Waals equation predicts pressures of 19.7 atm and 19.1 atm for oxygen and water, respectively. herefore, we can see that at increased temperature the real gas (H_2O) behaves more ideally since it now deviates by only 3% from the pressure predicted by the Ideal Gas Law.

So conceptually, why do higher pressures and lower temperatures cause larger deviations from ideal behavior? As pressure increases, gas particles become closer to one another. This accentuates the effects of attractive intermolecular forces, causing a decrease in observed pressure ($P_{real} < P_{ideal}$). Similarly, at low temperatures intermolecular forces become more important, and when taken to an extreme, cause condensation to occur. Liquids aren't very ideal gases. In addition, when gas particles are packed closer to one another at high pressures, particle volume of the gas itself begins to limit the free space in which the gas particles can move ($V_{real} < V_{ideal}$). However, under extremely high pressure, these particles can begin to repel one another leading to an increase in volume.

To summarize and focus on MCAT-relevance, those gases that behave most ideally have the weakest intermolecular forces and the smallest molecular weights (and volumes). Furthermore, by maintaining conditions of high temperature and low pressure, the potential interactions between particles are minimized and particle volume remains insignificant compared to the container size, helping to favor more ideal behavior for all gases.

Example 28-8: Of the following, which gas would likely *deviate* the most from ideal behavior at high pressure and low temperature?

    A) $He(g)$
    B) $H_2(g)$
    C) $O_2(g)$
    D) $H_2O(g)$

Solution: Since H_2O molecules will experience hydrogen bonding, they feel significantly stronger intermolecular forces than the other gases do. Therefore, of the choices given, $H_2O(g)$ will deviate the most from ideal behavior at high pressure and low temperature.

Example 28-9: Of the following, which gas would behave most like an ideal gas if all were at the same temperature and pressure?

    A) $O_2(g)$
    B) $CH_4(g)$
    C) $Ar(g)$
    D) $Cl_2(g)$

Solution: The molecules of a perfect (ideal) gas take up zero volume, so the gas in this list that will behave most like an ideal gas will be the one that takes up the smallest volume. O_2, CH_4, and Cl_2 are all polyatomic molecules that occupy more space than atomic argon. Therefore, choice C is the answer.

Example 28-10: Under which of the following conditions does the Ideal Gas Law give the most accurate results for a real gas?

    A) Low T and low P
    B) Low T and high P
    C) High T and low P
    D) High T and high P

Solution: Real gases can never behave as true ideal gases because 1) their molecules occupy space, and 2) their molecules experience attractive intermolecular forces. However, when gas molecules are spread out, these violations are minimized. The physical conditions that allow for gases to spread out are high temperature and low pressure, choice C.

28.6 DALTON'S LAW OF PARTIAL PRESSURES

Consider a mixture of, say, three gases in a single container.

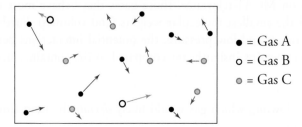

The total pressure is due to the collisions of all three types of molecules with the container walls. The pressure that the molecules of Gas A alone exert is called the **partial pressure** of Gas A, denoted by p_A. Similarly, the pressure exerted by the molecules of Gas B alone and the pressure exerted by the molecules of Gas C alone are p_B and p_C.

Dalton's law of partial pressures says that the total pressure is simply the sum of the partial pressures of all the constituent gases. In this case, then, we'd have

Dalton's Law
$$P_{tot} = p_A + p_B + p_C$$

So, if we know the partial pressures, we can determine the total pressure. We can also work backward. Knowing the total pressure, we can figure out the individual partial pressures. All that is required is the mole fraction. For example, in the diagram above, there are a total of 16 molecules: 8 of Gas A, 2 of Gas B, and 6 of Gas C. Therefore, the mole fraction of Gas A is $X_A = 8/16 = 1/2$, the mole fraction of Gas B is $X_B = 2/16 = 1/8$, and the mole fraction of Gas C is $X_C = 6/16 = 3/8$. *The partial pressure of a gas is equal to its mole fraction times the total pressure.* For example, if the total pressure in the container above is 8 atm, then

$$p_A = X_A P_{tot} = \frac{1}{2}P_{tot} = \frac{1}{2}(8\text{ atm}) = 4\text{ atm}$$

$$p_B = X_B P_{tot} = \frac{1}{8}P_{tot} = \frac{1}{8}(8\text{ atm}) = 1\text{ atm}$$

$$p_C = X_C P_{tot} = \frac{3}{8}P_{tot} = \frac{3}{8}(8\text{ atm}) = 3\text{ atm}$$

Example 28-11: Heliox refers to any gaseous mixture of helium and oxygen. It was previously used to treat asthma patients. One type of heliox contains 40% oxygen by volume. Calculate the total pressure of such a heliox mixture if the partial pressure of the helium is 3.0 atm.

A) 0.6 atm
B) 2.5 atm
C) 5.0 atm
D) 7.5 atm

Solution: If the heliox mixture contains 40% oxygen by volume, then its mol fraction is also 40% since $V \propto n$. Thus, $X_{O_2} = 0.4$, and the mol fraction of helium (X_{He}) in the mixture is 0.6.

Then, by Dalton's Law:

$$p_{He} = X_{He} P_{total}$$

$$P_{total} = \frac{p_{He}}{X_{He}} = \frac{3.0 \text{ atm}}{0.6} = 5.0 \text{ atm}$$

28.7 GRAHAM'S LAW OF EFFUSION

The escape of a gas molecule through a very tiny hole (comparable in size to the molecules themselves) into an evacuated region is called **effusion**:

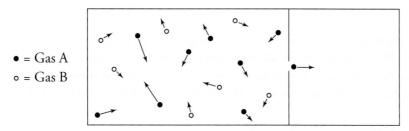

The gases in the left-hand container are at the same temperature, so their average kinetic energies are the same. If Gas A and Gas B have different molar masses, the heavier molecules will move, on average, slower than the lighter ones will. We can be even more precise. The average kinetic energy of a molecule of Gas A is $\frac{1}{2} m_A (v_A^2)_{avg}$, and the average kinetic energy of a molecule of Gas B is $\frac{1}{2} m_B (v_B^2)_{avg}$. Setting these equal to each other, we get

$$\frac{1}{2} m_A (v_A^2)_{avg} = \frac{1}{2} m_B (v_B^2)_{avg} \quad \Rightarrow \quad \frac{(v_A^2)_{avg}}{(v_B^2)_{avg}} = \frac{m_B}{m_A} \quad \Rightarrow \quad \frac{\text{rms } v_A}{\text{rms } v_B} = \sqrt{\frac{m_B}{m_A}}$$

(The abbreviation **rms** stands for *root-mean-square*; it's the square root of the mean [average] of the square of speed. Therefore, rms v is a convenient measure of the average speed of the molecules.) For example, if Gas A is hydrogen gas (H_2, molecular weight = 2) and Gas B is oxygen gas (O_2, molecular weight = 32), the hydrogen molecules will move, on average,

$$\sqrt{\frac{m_B}{m_A}} = \sqrt{\frac{32}{2}} = \sqrt{16} = 4$$

times faster than the oxygen molecules.

This result—which follows from one of the assumptions of the kinetic-molecular theory (namely that the average kinetic energy of the molecules of a gas is proportional to the temperature)—can be confirmed experimentally by performing an effusion experiment. Which gas should escape faster? The rate at which a gas effuses should depend directly on how fast its molecules move; the faster they travel, the more often they'd "collide" with the hole and escape. So we'd expect that if we compared the effusion rates for Gases A and B, we'd get a ratio equal to the ratio of their average speeds (if the molecules of Gas A travel 4 times faster than those of Gas B, then Gas A should effuse 4 times faster). Since we just figured out that the ratio of their average speeds is equal to the reciprocal of the square root of the ratio of their masses, we'd expect the ratio of their effusion rates to be the same. This result is known as **Graham's Law of Effusion**:

Graham's Law of Effusion

$$\frac{\text{rate of effusion of Gas A}}{\text{rate of effusion of Gas B}} = \sqrt{\frac{\text{molar mass of Gas B}}{\text{molar mass of Gas A}}}$$

Let's emphasize the distinction between the relationships of temperature to the kinetic energy and to the speed of the gas. The molecules of two different gases at the same temperature have the same average kinetic energy. But the molecules of two different gases at the same temperature don't have the same average *speed*. Lighter molecules travel faster, because the kinetic energy depends on both the mass and the speed of the molecules.

Also, it's important to remember that not all the molecules of the gas in a container—even if there's only one type of molecule—travel at the same speed. The figure below shows the distribution of molecular speeds for a gas at three different temperatures. Notice that the rms speeds increase as the temperature is increased.

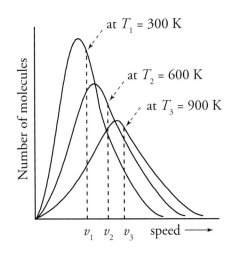

Example 28-12: A container holds methane (CH_4) and sulfur dioxide (SO_2), at a temperature of 227°C. Let v_M denote the rms speed of the methane molecules and v_S the rms speed of the sulfur dioxide molecules. Which of the following best describes the relationship between these speeds?

A) $v_S = 16\, v_M$
B) $v_S = 2\, v_M$
C) $v_M = 2\, v_S$
D) $v_M = 16\, v_S$

Solution: The molecular weight of methane is $12 + 4(1) = 16$, and the molecular weight of sulfur dioxide is $32 + 2(16) = 64$. Therefore,

$$\frac{v_M}{v_S} = \sqrt{\frac{m_S}{m_M}} = \sqrt{\frac{64}{16}} = \sqrt{4} = 2 \quad \Rightarrow \quad v_M = 2v_S$$

So, choice C is the answer.

Example 28-13: A container holds methane (CH_4) and sulfur dioxide (SO_2) at a temperature of 227°C. Let KE_M denote the average kinetic energy of the methane molecules and KE_S the average kinetic energy of the sulfur dioxide molecules. Which of the following best describes the relationship between these energies?

A) $KE_S = 4\, KE_M$
B) $KE_S = 3\, KE_M$
C) $KE_M = KE_S$
D) $KE_M = 4\, KE_S$

Solution: Since both gases are at the same temperature, the average kinetic energies of their molecules will be the *same* (remember: $KE_{avg} \propto T$). Thus, the answer is choice C.

Chapter 29
Kinetics

29.1   REACTION MECHANISM: AN ANALOGY

Chemical **kinetics** is the study of how reactions take place and how fast they occur. (Kinetics tells us nothing about the *spontaneity* of a reaction, however! We'll study that a little later.)

Consider this scenario: A group of people are washing a pile of dirty dishes and stacking them up as clean, dry dishes. Our "reaction" has dirty dishes as starting material, and clean, dry dishes as the product:

$$\text{dirty dish} \rightarrow \text{clean-and-dry dish}$$

But what about a *soapy* dish? We know it's part of the process, but the equation doesn't include it. When we break down the pathway of a dirty dish to a clean-and-dry dish, we realize that the reaction happens in several steps, a sequence of **elementary** steps that show us the reaction **mechanism:**

1) dirty dish $\rightarrow$ soapy dish
2) soapy dish $\rightarrow$ rinsed dish
3) rinsed dish $\rightarrow$ clean-and-dry dish

The soapy and rinsed dishes are reaction **intermediates**. They are necessary for the conversion of dirty dishes to clean-and-dry dishes, but they don't appear either in the starting material or products. If you add up all the reactants and products, the intermediates cancel out, and you'll have the overall equation.

In the same way, we write chemical reactions as if they occur in a single step:

$$2\,NO + O_2 \rightarrow 2\,NO_2$$

But in reality, things are a little more complicated, and reactions often proceed through intermediates that we don't show in the chemical equation. The truth for the reaction above is that it occurs in two steps:

1) $2\,NO \rightarrow N_2O_2$
2) $N_2O_2 + O_2 \rightarrow 2\,NO_2$

The N_2O_2 comes and goes during the reaction, but isn't part of the starting material or products. N_2O_2 is a reaction intermediate.

Just as the soapy dishes and rinsed dishes are produced and then consumed, we can identify an **intermediate** in a series of elementary steps as a substance that is produced in one elementary step and then consumed in a subsequent step. Although the two elementary steps don't need to be sequential, they often are. As above, note that intermediates will not be part of the overall balanced chemical reaction. Depending on the rate of the elementary step that consumes the intermediate, the concentration of the intermediate will vary in solution. As the consuming elementary step becomes faster, the steady-state concentration of the intermediate becomes smaller, and it becomes harder to detect the intermediate.

Rate-Determining Step

What determines the rate of a reaction? Consider our friends doing the dishes.

1) dirty dish → soapy dish   Bingo washes at 5 dishes per minute.

2) soapy dish → rinsed dish   Ringo rinses at 8 dishes per minute.

3) rinsed dish → clean-and-dry dish   Dingo dries at 3 dishes per minute.

What will be the rate of the overall reaction? Thanks to Dingo, the dishes move from dirty to clean-and-dry at only 3 dishes a minute. It doesn't matter how fast Bingo and Ringo wash and rinse; the dishes will pile up behind Dingo. The **rate-determining step** is Dingo's drying step, and true to its name, it determines the overall rate of reaction.

The slowest step in a process determines the overall reaction rate.

This applies to chemical reactions as well. For our chemical reaction given above, we have

$$2 \, NO \rightarrow N_2O_2 \quad \text{(fast)}$$

$$N_2O_2 + O_2 \rightarrow 2 \, NO_2 \quad \text{(slow)}$$

The second step is the slowest, and it will determine the overall rate of reaction. No matter how fast the first step moves along, the intermediates will pile up in front of the second step as it plods along. The slow step dictates the rate of the overall reaction.

Once again, there's an important difference between our dishes analogy and a chemical reaction: while the dishes pile up behind Dingo, in a chemical reaction the intermediates will not pile up. Rather, they will shuttle back and forth between reactants and products until the slow step takes it forward. This would be like taking a rinsed dish and getting it soapy again, until Dingo is ready for it!

Example 29-1: Which of the following is the best example of a rate?

A)   rate = $\Delta[A]/\Delta t$
B)   rate = $\Delta[A]/\Delta[B]$
C)   rate = $\Delta[A]\,\Delta[B]$
D)   rate = $\Delta[A]^2$

Solution: Regardless of the topic, rate is always defined as change in something over change in time. Choice A is the answer.

29.2 REACTION RATE

Activation Energy

Every chemical reaction has an **activation energy** (E_a), or the minimum energy required of reactant molecules during a molecular collision in order for the reaction to proceed to products. If the reactant molecules don't possess this much energy, their collisions won't be able to produce the products and the reaction will not occur. If the reactants possess the necessary activation energy, they can reach a high-energy (and short-lived!) **transition state**, also known as the **activated complex**. For example, if the reaction is $A_2 + B_2 \rightarrow 2\,AB$, say, the activated complex might look something like this:

$$
\begin{array}{ccccc}
\begin{matrix} A \\ | \\ A \end{matrix} & + & \begin{matrix} B \\ | \\ B \end{matrix} & \longrightarrow & \begin{matrix} A\text{-}\text{-}\text{-}B \\ \vdots \quad \vdots \\ A\text{-}\text{-}\text{-}B \end{matrix} & \longrightarrow & \begin{matrix} A\!-\!B \\ \\ A\!-\!B \end{matrix}
\end{array}
$$

reactants   activated   products
complex

Now that we have introduced all species that might appear throughout the course of a chemical reaction, we can illustrate the energy changes that occur as a reaction occurs in a **reaction coordinate diagram**. Consider the following two-step process and its reaction coordinate graph below:

Step 1:   A → X

Step 2:   X → B
_____

Overall reaction: A → B

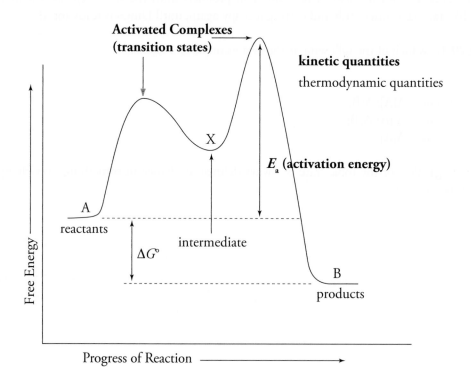

Notice that the transition state is always an energy maximum, and is therefore distinct from an intermediate. Remember that reaction intermediates (shown as X in this case) are produced in an early step of the mechanism, and they are later used up so they do not appear as products of the overall reaction. The intermediate is shown here as a local minimum in terms of its energy, but it has more energy than either the reactants or products. The high energy intermediate is therefore highly reactive, making it difficult to isolate.

Since the progress of the reaction depends on the reactant molecules colliding with enough energy to generate the activated complex, we can make the following statements concerning the reaction rate:

1) *The lower the activation energy, the faster the reaction rate.* The reaction coordinate above suggests that the second step of the mechanism will therefore be the slow step, or the rate-determining step, since the second "hill" of the diagram is higher.
2) *The greater the concentrations of the reactants, the faster the reaction rate.* Favorable collisions are more likely as the concentrations of reactant molecules increase.
3) *The higher the temperature of the reaction mixture, the faster the reaction rate.* At higher temperatures, more reactant molecules have a sufficient energy to overcome the activation-energy barrier, and molecules collide at a higher frequency, so the reaction can proceed at a faster rate.

Notice in the reaction coordinate diagram above that the $\Delta G°$ of the reaction has no bearing on the rate of the reaction, and vice versa. Thermodynamic factors and kinetic factors *do not affect each other* (a concept the MCAT loves to ask about).

29.3   CATALYSTS

Catalysts provide reactants with a different route, usually a shortcut, to get to products. A **catalyst** will almost always make a reaction go faster by either speeding up the rate-determining step or providing an optimized route to products. A catalyst that accelerates a reaction does so *by lowering the activation energy* of the rate-determining step, and therefore the energy of the highest-energy transition state:

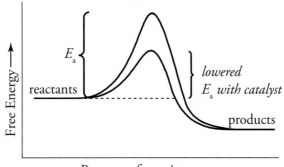

The key difference between a reactant and a catalyst is that the reactants are converted to products, but *a catalyst remains unchanged at the end of a reaction.* A catalyst can undergo a temporary change during a reaction, but it is always converted back to its original state. Like reaction intermediates, catalysts aren't included in the overall reaction equation.

Consider the decomposition of ozone:

$$O_3(g) + O(g) \rightarrow 2\,O_2(g)$$

This reaction actually takes place in two steps and is catalyzed by nitric oxide (NO):

1) **NO(g)** + $O_3(g) \rightarrow NO_2(g) + O_2(g)$
2) $NO_2(g) + O(g) \rightarrow$ **NO(g)** + $O_2(g)$

NO(g) is necessary for this reaction to proceed at a noticeable rate, and it even undergoes changes itself during the process. But NO(g) remains unchanged at the end of the reaction and makes the reaction occur much faster than it would in its absence. NO(g), a product of automobile exhaust, is a catalyst in ozone destruction.

It is important to note that the addition of a catalyst will affect the rate of a reaction, but not the equilibrium or the thermodynamics of the reaction. A catalyst provides a different pathway for the reactants to get to the products, and lowers the activation energy, E_a. But a catalyst does not change any of the thermodynamic quantities such as ΔG, ΔH, and ΔS of a reaction.

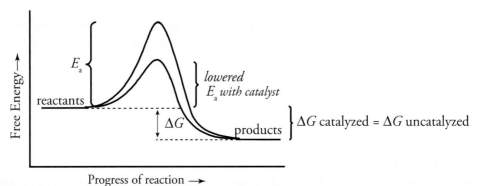

Example 29-2: Which of the following is true about the reaction mechanism shown below?

1) $H_3O^+ + H_2O_2 \rightarrow H_3O_2^+ + H_2O$ (fast)
2) $H_3O_2^+ + Br^- \rightarrow HOBr + H_2O$ (slow)
3) $HOBr + H_2O_2 \rightarrow H_3O^+ + O_2 + Br^-$ (fast)

    A) Br^- is a catalyst, and HOBr is an intermediate.
    B) Br^- is a catalyst, and H_2O is a transition state.
    C) H_3O^+ is a catalyst, and HOBr is a transition state.
    D) H_3O^+ is a catalyst, and Br^- is an intermediate.

Solution: Transition states are unstable, high-energy species, and generally do not appear in reaction mechanisms, so choices B and C are eliminated. Br^- is a catalyst, not an intermediate, so choice D can be eliminated. Choice A must be correct. Both Br^- and H_3O^+ act as catalysts in this mechanism; both are used up in one step and regenerated in a later step. HOBr fits the description of an intermediate: it is produced in Step 2, then consumed in Step 3.

Example 29-3: A reaction is run without a catalyst and is found to have an activation energy of 140 kJ/mol and a heat of reaction, ΔH, of 30 kJ/mol. In the presence of a catalyst, however, the activation energy is reduced to 120 kJ/mol. What will be the heat of reaction in the presence of the catalyst?

> A) −10 kJ/mol
> B) 10 kJ/mol
> C) 30 kJ/mol
> D) 50 kJ/mol

29.4

Solution: Catalysts affect only the kinetics of a reaction, not the thermodynamics. The heat of the reaction will be the same with or without a catalyst. The answer is choice C.

29.4 RATE LAWS

On the MCAT, you might be given data about the rate of a particular reaction and be asked to derive the **Rate Law**. The data for rate laws are determined by the *initial rates* of reaction and typically are given as the **rate at which the reactant disappears**. You'll rarely see products in a rate law expression, usually only reactants. What does a rate law tell us? Although a reaction needs all the reactants to proceed, *only those that are involved in the rate-determining step (the slow step) are part of the rate law expression.* Some reactants may not affect the reaction rate at all, and so they won't be a part of the rate law expression.

Let's look at a generic reaction, a A + b B → c C + d D, and its rate law:

$$\text{rate} = k\,[A]^x[B]^y$$

x = the **order** with respect to A

y = the **order** with respect to B

$(x + y)$ = the **overall order** of the reaction

k = the rate constant

The rate law can only be determined *experimentally*. You *can't* get the orders of the reactants, not to mention the rate constant k, just by looking at the balanced equation. The exception to this rule is for an *elementary step* in a reaction mechanism. The rate law is first order for a unimolecular elementary step and second order for a bimolecular elementary step. The individual order of the reactants in a rate law will follow from their stoichiometry in the rate-determining step (similar to the way they're included in an equilibrium constant).

Example 29-4: What is the order of reaction predicted by the mechanism below for the net reaction $2\,HI + H_2O_2 \rightarrow I_2 + 2\,H_2O$?

> 1) $HI + H_2O_2 \rightarrow HOI + H_2O$ (slow)
> 2) $HI + HOI \rightarrow I_2 + H_2O$ (fast)

Solution: Since each step in a reaction mechanism is an elementary step, the rate law for the slow, rate determining step is given by rate = $k[HI][H_2O_2]$. This rate law is first-order in each reactant, and second-order overall.

Let's look at a set of reaction rate data and see how to determine the rate law for the reaction

$$A + B + C \rightarrow D + E$$

Experiment	[A]	[B]	[C]	Initial reaction rate [M/s]
1	0.2 M	0.1 M	0.05 M	1×10^{-3}
2	0.4 M	0.1 M	0.05 M	2×10^{-3}
3	0.2 M	0.2 M	0.05 M	4×10^{-3}
4	0.2 M	0.1 M	0.10 M	1×10^{-3}

From the experimental data, we can determine the orders with respect to the reactants—that is, the exponents x, y, and z in the equation

$$\text{rate} = k[A]^x[B]^y[C]^z$$

and the overall order of the reaction, $x + y + z$.

Let's first find the order of the reaction with respect to Reactant A. As we go from Experiment 1 to Experiment 2, only [A] changes, so we can use the data to figure out the order of the reaction with respect to Reactant [A]. We notice that the value of [A] doubled, and the reaction rate doubled. Therefore, the reaction rate is proportional to [A], and $x = 1$.

Next, let's look at [B]. As we go from Experiment 1 to Experiment 3, only [B] changes. When [B] is doubled, the rate is quadrupled. Therefore, the rate is proportional to $[B]^2$, and $y = 2$.

Finally, let's look at [C]. As we go from Experiment 1 to Experiment 4, only [C] changes. When [C] is doubled, the rate is unaffected. This tells us that the reaction rate does not depend on [C], so $z = 0$.

Therefore, the rate law has the form: rate $= k[A][B]^2$

The reaction is first order with respect to [A], second order with respect to [B], zero order with respect to [C], and third order overall. In general, if a reaction rate increases by a factor f when the concentration of a reactant increases by a factor c, and $f = c^x$, then we can say that x is the order with respect to that reactant.

The Rate Constant

From the experimental data, you can also calculate the rate constant, k. For the reaction above, we found that the rate law is given by: rate $= k[A][B]^2$. Solve for k by using data from any experiment in the table. Experiment 1 gives:

$$k = \frac{\text{rate}}{[A][B]^2} = \frac{1 \times 10^{-3}}{(0.2)(0.1)^2} = 0.5$$

Any of the experiments will give you the same value for k because it's a constant for any given reaction at a given temperature. That is, each reaction has its own rate constant, which takes into account such factors as the frequency of collisions, the fraction of the collisions with the proper orientation to initiate the desired bond changes, and the activation energy. This can be expressed mathematically with the **Arrhenius equation**:

$$k = Ae^{-(E_a/RT)}$$

Here, A is the Arrhenius factor (which takes into account the orientation of the colliding molecules), E_a is the activation energy, R is the gas-law constant, and T is the temperature in kelvins. If we rewrite this equation in the form $\ln k = \ln A - (E_a/RT)$, we can more clearly see that *adding a catalyst* (thus decreasing E_a) or *increasing the temperature* will increase k. In either case, the expression E_a/RT decreases, and subtracting something smaller gives a greater result, so $\ln k$ (and thus k itself) will increase. (By the way, a rough rule of thumb is that the rate will increase by a factor of about 2 to 4 for every 10°C increase in temperature.)

The units of the rate constant are not necessarily uniform from one reaction to the next. Reactions of different orders will have rate constants bearing different units. In order to obtain the units of the rate constant, one must keep in mind that the rate, on the left side of the equation, must always have units of M/s as it measures the change in concentration of a species in the reaction over time. The units given to the rate constant must, when combined with the units of the concentrations in the rate equation, provide M/sec.

A generic second order rate equation takes the following form: Rate $= k[A][B]$

Assuming that the concentrations of both A and B are in molarity (M), then in order to give the left side of the equation units of M/s, the units of the rate constant must be $M^{-1}s^{-1}$. If the rate were third order, the units would be $M^{-2}s^{-1}$, or if first order then simply s^{-1}.

Experiment	[A]	[B]	Initial reaction rate [M/s]
1	0.1 M	0.2 M	2.0×10^{-5}
2	0.2 M	0.3 M	1.2×10^{-4}
3	0.1 M	0.4 M	4.0×10^{-5}
4	0.2 M	0.4 M	1.6×10^{-4}

Example 29-5: Using the data above, determine the value of the rate constant for the reaction A + B → C.

Solution: First, let's find the rate law. Comparing Experiments 3 and 4, we notice that when [A] doubled (and [B] remained unchanged), the reaction rate increased by a factor of 4. This means the reaction is second order with respect to [A]. Comparing Experiments 1 and 3, we notice that when [B] doubled (and [A] remained unchanged), the reaction rate increased by a factor of 2. This means the reaction is first order with respect to [B]. Therefore, the rate law is *rate* $= k[A]^2[B]$. Finally, using any of the experiments, we can solve for k; using the data in Experiment 1, say, we find that

$$k = \frac{\text{rate}}{[A]^2[B]} = \frac{2 \times 10^{-5}\, M/s}{2 \times 10^{-3}\, M^3} = 10^{-2}\, M^{-2}s^{-1} = 0.01\, M^{-2}s^{-1}$$

Chapter 30
Equilibrium

30.1 EQUILIBRIUM

Many reactions are reversible, and situations can occur in which the forward and reverse reactions come into a balance called **equilibrium**. How does equilibrium come about? Before any bonds are broken or made, the reaction flask contains only reactants and no products. As the reaction proceeds, products begin to form and eventually build up, and some of them begin to revert to reactants. That is, once products are formed, both the forward and reverse reactions will occur. Ultimately, the reaction will come to equilibrium, a state at which both the forward and reverse reactions occur at the same constant rate. At equilibrium, the overall concentration of reactants and products remains the same, but at the molecular level, they are continually interconverting. Because the forward and reverse processes balance one another perfectly, we don't observe any net change in concentrations.

> *When a reaction is at equilibrium (and only at equilibrium), the rate of the forward reaction is equal to the rate of the reverse reaction.*

Equilibria occur for *closed systems* (which means no new reactants, products, or other changes are imposed).

The Equilibrium Constant

Each reaction will tend towards its own equilibrium and, for a given temperature, will have an **equilibrium constant, K_{eq}**. For the generic, balanced reaction on the left, the equilibrium expression is shown at the right.

$$a\,A + b\,B \;\rightleftharpoons\; c\,C + d\,D \qquad\qquad K_{eq} = \frac{[C]^c\,[D]^d}{[A]^a\,[B]^b}$$

The constant K is often given a subscript to indicate the type of reaction it represents. For example, K_a (for acids), K_b (for bases), and K_{sp} (for solubility product) are all equilibrium constants. The equilibrium expression is derived from the ratio of the concentration of products to reactants at equilibrium, as follows:

1) Products are in the numerator, and reactants are in the denominator. They are in brackets because the equilibrium expression comes from the *concentrations* (at equilibrium) of the species in the reaction. For two or more reactants or products, multiply the concentrations of each species together.
2) The coefficient of each species in the reaction becomes an exponent on its concentration in the equilibrium expression.
3) Solids and pure liquids are *not* included, because their concentrations don't change. (A substance that's a solid or pure liquid in the reaction is often indicated by an "(s)" or "(l)" subscript, respectively. We're also allowed to omit solvents in dilute solutions because the solvents are in vast excess and their concentrations do not change.)
4) Aqueous dissolved particles are included.
5) If the reaction is gaseous, we can use the partial pressure of each gas as its concentration. The value of the equilibrium constant determined with pressures will be different than with molar concentrations because of their different units. The constant using partial pressures is often termed K_p.

The value of K_{eq} is constant at a given temperature for a particular reaction, no matter what ratio of reactants and products are given at the beginning of the reaction. That is, any closed system will proceed towards its equilibrium ratio of products and reactants even if you start with all products, or a mixture of some reactants and some products. You can even open the flask and add more of any reactant or product, and the system will change until it has reached the K_{eq} ratio. We'll discuss this idea in detail in just a moment, but right now focus on this:

The value of K_{eq} for a given reaction is a constant at a given temperature.

If the temperature changes, then a reaction's K_{eq} value will change.

The value of K_{eq} tells you the direction the reaction favors:

$K_{eq} < 1 \rightarrow$ reaction favors the reactants (more reactants than products at equilibrium)
$K_{eq} = 1 \rightarrow$ reaction has roughly equal amounts of reactants and products
$K_{eq} > 1 \rightarrow$ reaction favors the products (more products than reactants at equilibrium)

Example 30-1: Which of the following expressions gives the equilibrium constant for this reaction:

$$N_2O_5 + H_2O \rightleftharpoons 2\ HNO_3$$

A) $[N_2O_5][H_2O]/[2\ HNO_3]$
B) $[2\ HNO_3]/[N_2O_5][H_2O]$
C) $[N_2O_5][H_2O]/[HNO_3]^2$
D) $[HNO_3]^2/[N_2O_5][H_2O]$

Solution: The equilibrium constant is always written as products over reactants, so we can eliminate choices A and C immediately. Stoichiometric coefficients become exponents in the equilibrium constant expression, not coefficients inside the square brackets. Therefore, the coefficient of 2 for the product HNO_3 means the numerator must be $[HNO_3]^2$, so the answer is choice D.

Example 30-2: When the reaction $Zn^{2+} + 4\ Cl^- \rightleftharpoons [ZnCl_4]^{2-}$ reaches equilibrium, $[Zn^{2+}] = 0.5\ M$ and $[Cl^-] = 0.1\ M$. If the value of K_{eq} for this reaction is 1.6, what is the concentration of $[ZnCl_4]^{2-}$ at equilibrium?

A) $8 \times 10^{-2}\ M$
B) $8 \times 10^{-3}\ M$
C) $8 \times 10^{-5}\ M$
D) $8 \times 10^{-8}\ M$

Solution: The expression for K_{eq} is $\dfrac{[[ZnCl_4]^{2-}]}{[Zn^{2+}][Cl^-]^4}$. So, rearrange to solve for $[[ZnCl_4]^{2-}]$, and then substitute known values:

$$\left[[ZnCl_4]^{2-}\right] = (K_{eq})\left([Zn^{2+}]\right)\left([Cl^-]\right)^4 = (1.6)(0.5)(0.1)^4 = 0.8 \times 10^{-4} = 8 \times 10^{-5}$$

Choice C is the correct answer.

Example 30-3: The term *chemical equilibrium* applies to a system:

- A) where the forward and reverse reaction have stopped.
- B) whose rate law is of zero order.
- C) where individual molecules are still reacting, but there is no net change in the system.
- D) in which all components are in the same phase.

Solution: A *chemical equilibrium* is a dynamic equilibrium, which means that molecules are still reacting, but there is no net change in the composition of the system. Choice C is the best choice. Choice A describes a static equilibrium, but all chemical equilibria are dynamic. Choice B refers to rate, but all closed reactions may come to equilibrium, regardless of the order of the reaction. Finally, the term describing choice D is *homogeneous*, not *equilibrium*.

30.2   THE REACTION QUOTIENT

The equilibrium constant expression is a ratio: the concentration of the products divided by those of the reactants, each raised to the power equal to its stoichiometric coefficient in the balanced equation. If the reaction is not at equilibrium, the same expression is known simply as the **reaction quotient, Q**. For the generic, balanced reaction on the left, the reaction quotient is given on the right:

$$a \, A + b \, B \rightleftharpoons c \, C + d \, D \qquad\qquad Q = \frac{[C]^c \, [D]^d}{[A]^a \, [B]^b}$$

where the square brackets represent the molar concentrations of the species. The point now is that the concentrations in the expression Q do *not* have to be the concentrations at equilibrium. (If the concentrations are the equilibrium concentrations, the Q will equal K_{eq}.)

Comparing the value of Q to K_{eq} tells us in what direction the reaction will proceed. The reaction will strive to reach a state in which $Q = K_{eq}$. So, if Q is less than K_{eq}, then the reaction will proceed in the forward direction (in order to increase the concentration of the products and decrease the concentration of the reactants) to increase Q to the K_{eq} value. On the other hand, if Q is greater than K_{eq}, then the reaction will proceed in the reverse direction (in order to increase the concentrations of the reactants and decrease the concentrations of the products) to reduce Q to K_{eq}.

K_{eq} is the condition the reaction will try to achieve.

If $Q = K_{eq}$, the reaction is at equilibrium.

$$Q \implies K_{eq} \impliedby Q$$

If $Q < K_{eq}$,
reaction proceeds in
the **forward** direction
so Q gets closer to K_{eq}.

If $Q > K_{eq}$,
reaction proceeds in
the **reverse** direction
so Q gets closer to K_{eq}.

Example 30-4: The value of the equilibrium constant for the reaction

$$2\ COF_2(g) \rightleftharpoons CO_2(g) + CF_4(g)$$

is $K_{eq} = 2$. If a 1 L reaction container currently holds 1 mole each of CO_2 and CF_4 and 0.5 mole of COF_2, then:

A) the reaction is at equilibrium.
B) the forward reaction will be favored.
C) the reverse reaction will be favored.
D) no prediction can be made without knowing the pressure of the container.

Solution: The expression for Q is $\dfrac{[CO_2][CF_4]}{[COF_2]^2}$. Therefore, the value of Q is $(1)(1)/(0.5)^2 = 4$.

Since $Q > K_{eq}$, the reverse reaction will be favored (choice C).

30.3   LE CHÂTELIER'S PRINCIPLE

Le Châtelier's principle states that a system at equilibrium will try to neutralize any imposed change (or stress) in order to reestablish equilibrium. For example, if you add more reactant to a system that is at equilibrium, the system will react by favoring the forward reaction in order to consume that reactant and reestablish equilibrium.

To illustrate, let's look at the Haber process for making ammonia:

$$N_2(g) + 3\ H_2(g) \rightleftharpoons 2\ NH_3(g) + heat$$

Let's assume the reaction is at equilibrium; see how it reacts to disturbances to the equilibrium by changing the concentration of the species, the pressure, or the temperature.

Adding Ammonia

If we add ammonia, the system is no longer at equilibrium, and there is an excess of product. How can the reaction reestablish equilibrium? By consuming some of the added ammonia, the ratio of products to reactant would decrease towards the equilibrium ratio, so the reverse reaction will be favored (we say the system "shifts to the left"), converting ammonia into nitrogen and hydrogen, until equilibrium is restored.

You can see how this follows from comparing the reaction quotient of the disturbed system to the equilibrium constant. If we add ammonia to the reaction mixture, then $[NH_3]$ increases, and the reaction quotient, Q, becomes greater than K_{eq}. As a result, the reaction will proceed in the reverse direction in order to reduce Q to K_{eq}.

Removing Ammonia

If we remove the product, ammonia, then the forward reaction will be favored—the reaction "shifts to the right"—in order to reach equilibrium again. Again, you can see how this follows from comparing the reaction quotient of the disturbed system to the equilibrium constant. If we remove ammonia from the reaction mixture, then $[NH_3]$ decreases, and the reaction quotient, Q, becomes smaller than K_{eq}. As a result, the reaction will proceed in the forward direction in order to increase Q to K_{eq}.

Adding Hydrogen

If we add some reactant, say $H_2(g)$, then the forward reaction will be favored—the reaction "shifts to the right"—in order to reach equilibrium again. This follows from comparing the reaction quotient of the disturbed system to the equilibrium constant. If we add hydrogen to the reaction mixture, the $[H_2]$ increases, and the reaction quotient, Q, becomes smaller than K_{eq}. As a result, the reaction will proceed in the forward direction in order to increase Q to K_{eq}.

Removing Nitrogen

If we remove some reactant, say $N_2(g)$, then the reverse reaction will be favored—the reaction "shifts to the left"—in order to reach equilibrium again. Again, this follows from comparing the reaction quotient of the disturbed system to the equilibrium constant. If we remove nitrogen from the reaction mixture, then $[N_2]$ decreases, and the reaction quotient, Q, becomes larger than K_{eq}. As a result, the reaction will proceed in the reverse direction in order to decrease Q to K_{eq}.

Changing the Volume of the Reaction Container

The Haber process is a gaseous reaction, so a change in volume will cause the partial pressures of the gases to change. Specifically, a decrease in volume of the reaction container will cause the partial pressures of the gases to increase; an increase in volume reduces the partial pressures of the gases in the mixture. If the number of moles of gas on the left side of the reaction does not equal the number of moles of gas on the right, then a change in pressure due to a change in volume will disrupt the equilibrium ratio, and the system will react to reestablish equilibrium.

How does the system react? Let's first assume the volume is reduced so that the pressure increases. Look back at the equation for the Haber process: there are 4 moles of gas on the reactant side (3 of H_2 plus 1 of N_2) for every 2 moles of NH_3 gas formed. If the reaction shifts to the right, four moles of gas can be condensed into 2 moles, reducing the pressure to reestablish equilibrium. On the other hand, if the volume is increased so that the pressure decreases, the reaction will shift to the left, increasing the pressure to reestablish equilibrium.

To summarize, consider a gaseous reaction (at equilibrium) with unequal numbers of moles of gas of reactants and products. If the volume is reduced, increasing the pressure, a net reaction occurs favoring the side with the smaller total number of moles of gas. If the volume is expanded, decreasing the pressure, a net reaction occurs favoring the side with the greater total number of moles of gas. (This is only true for reactions involving gases.)

Changing the Temperature of the Reaction Mixture

Heat can be treated as a reactant or a product just like all the chemical reactants and products. Adding or removing heat (by increasing or decreasing the temperature) is like adding or removing any other reagent. Exothermic reactions release heat (which we note on the right side of the equation like a product), and the ΔH will be negative. Endothermic reactions consume heat (which we note on the left side of the equation like a reactant), and the ΔH will be positive.

The Haber process is an exothermic reaction. So, if you increase the temperature at which the reaction takes place once it's reached equilibrium, the reaction will shift to the left in order to consume the extra heat, thereby producing more reactants. If you decrease the temperature at which the reaction takes place once it's reached equilibrium, the reaction will shift to the right in order to produce extra heat, thereby producing more product.

Since the reverse of an exothermic reaction is an endothermic one (and vice versa), every equilibrium reaction involves an exothermic reaction and an endothermic reaction. We can then say this: *lowering* the temperature favors the *exothermic* reaction, while *raising* the temperature favors the *endothermic* one. Keep in mind that, unlike changes in concentration or pressure, changes in temperature *will* affect the reaction's K_{eq} value, depending on the direction the reaction shifts to reestablish equilibrium.

Note that the above changes are specific to the system *once it is at equilibrium*. The kinetics of the reaction are a different matter. Remember, all reactions proceed faster when the temperature is increased, and this is true for the Haber process. Indeed, in industry this reaction is typically run at around 500°C, despite the fact that the reaction is exothermic. The reason is that a fast reaction with a 10 percent yield of ammonia may end up being better overall than a painfully slow reaction with a 90 percent yield of ammonia. Heating a reaction gets it to equilibrium faster. Once it's there, adding or taking away heat will affect the equilibrium as predicted by Le Châtelier's principle.

Adding an Inert (or Non-Reactive) Gas

What if we injected some helium into a constant volume reaction container? This inert gas doesn't participate in the reaction (and for the MCAT, inert gases don't participate in *any* reaction), so it will change neither the partial pressure nor the concentration of the products or reactants. If neither of these values change, then there is no change in equilibrium.

However, if we inject some helium into a constant pressure container, like one with a movable piston, the extra gas particles will push against the piston, raising it to increase the volume and equilibrate the internal pressure of the gases with external pressure. Since the volume increases, the partial pressures of the gases involved in the reversible reaction will change, thereby causing a shift in the equilibrium as described above for volume changes.

Adding a Catalyst

Adding a catalyst to a reaction that's already at equilibrium has no effect. Because it increases the rate of both the forward and reverse reactions equally, the equilibrium amounts of the species are unchanged. So, the introduction of a catalyst would cause no disturbance. Remember that a catalyst increases the reaction rate but does *not* affect the equilibrium.

Example 30-5: Nitrogen dioxide gas can be formed by the endothermic reaction shown below. Which of the following changes to the equilibrium would *not* increase the formation of NO_2?

$$N_2O_4(g) \rightleftharpoons 2\, NO_2(g) \qquad \Delta H = +58\ kJ$$

A) An increase in the temperature
B) A decrease in the volume of the container
C) Adding additional N_2O_4
D) Removing NO_2 as it is formed

Solution: Since ΔH is positive, this reaction is endothermic, and we can think of heat as a reactant. So if we increase the temperature (thereby "adding a reactant," namely heat), the equilibrium would shift to the right, thus increasing the formation of NO_2. This eliminates choice A. Adding reactant (choice C) or removing product (choice D) would also shift the equilibrium to the right. The answer must be choice B. A decrease in the volume of the container would increase the pressure of the gases, causing the equilibrium to shift in favor of the side with the fewer number of moles of gases; in this case, that would be to the left.

Example 30-6: If the reaction

$$2\, NH_3(g) + 4\, O_3(g) \rightleftharpoons NH_4NO_3(s) + 4\, O_2(g) + H_2O(g) \qquad \Delta H = -702\ kJ$$

is at equilibrium, which one of the following changes would cause the formation of additional NH_4NO_3?

A) Decreasing the temperature
B) Adding 0.5 mol argon at constant pressure
C) Adding a catalyst
D) Removing some $O_3(g)$ from the reaction

Solution: The correct answer causes a shift in the system towards products, and must be choice A. Based on the sign of ΔH, the reaction is exothermic (that is, we can consider heat to be a product). Therefore, decreasing the temperature would shift the equilibrium to the right, and increase the amount of NH_4NO_3 present. Choice B is incorrect. Adding an inert gas at constant pressure has the same effect as increasing the volume of the reaction container: it causes a shift to the side with a greater number of moles of gas. In this case, that means a shift towards the reactants. Choice C is incorrect, since adding a catalyst to a reaction already at equilibrium will have no effect on the system. Choice D can also be eliminated, since removing a reactant will cause the system to shift left, decreasing the yield of NH_4NO_3.

30.4 SOLUTIONS AND SOLUBILITY

Solutions

A **solution** forms when one substance **dissolves** into another, forming a *homogeneous* mixture. The process of dissolving is known as **dissolution**. For example, sugar dissolved into iced tea is a solution (though so is unsweetened tea). A substance present in a relatively smaller proportion is called a **solute**, and a substance present in a relatively greater proportion is called a **solvent**. The process that occurs when the solvent molecules surround the solute molecules is known as **solvation**; if the solvent is water, the process is called **hydration**.

Solutions can involve any of the three phases of matter. For example, you can have a solution of two gases, of a gas in a liquid, of a solid in a liquid, or of a solid in a solid (an **alloy**). However, most of the solutions with which you're familiar have a liquid as the solvent. Salt water has solid salt ($NaCl$) dissolved into water, seltzer water has carbon dioxide gas dissolved in water, and vinegar has liquid acetic acid dissolved in water. In fact, most of the solutions that you commonly see have water as the solvent: lemonade, tea, soda pop, and corn syrup are examples. When a solution has water as the solvent, it is called an **aqueous** solution.

How do we know which solutes are soluble in which solvents? Well, that's easy:

Like dissolves like.

Solutes will dissolve best in solvents where the intermolecular forces being broken in the solute are being replaced by equal (or stronger) intermolecular forces between the solvent and the solute.

Electrolytes

When ionic substances dissolve, they **dissociate** into ions. Free ions in a solution are called **electrolytes** because the solution can conduct electricity. Some salts dissociate completely into individual ions, while others only partially dissociate (that is, a certain percentage of the ions will remain paired, sticking close to each other rather than being independent and fully surrounded by solvent). Solutes that dissociate completely (like ionic substances) are called **strong electrolytes**, and those that remain ion-paired to some extent are called **weak electrolytes**. (Covalent compounds that don't dissociate into ions are **nonelectrolytes**.) Solutions of strong electrolytes are better conductors of electricity than those of weak electrolytes.

Different ionic compounds will dissociate into different numbers of particles. Some won't dissociate at all, and others will break up into several ions. The **van't Hoff** (or **ionizability**) **factor** (i) tells us how many ions one unit of a substance will produce in a solution. For example,

- $C_6H_{12}O_6$ is non-ionic, so it does not dissociate. Therefore, $i = 1$.
  (Note: The van't Hoff factor for almost all biomolecules—hormones, proteins, steroids—is 1.)
- $NaCl$ dissociates into Na^+ and Cl^-. Therefore, $i = 2$.
- $CaCl_2$ dissociates into Ca^{2+} and $2\ Cl^-$. Therefore, $i = 3$.

Example 30-7: Of the following, which is the *weakest* electrolyte?

A) NH_4I
B) LiF
C) AgBr
D) H_2O_2

Solution: All ionic compounds, whether soluble or not, are defined as strong electrolytes, so choices A, B, and C are eliminated. Choice D, hydrogen peroxide, is a covalent compound that does not produce an appreciable number of ions upon dissolution and thus is a weak electrolyte. Choice D is the best answer.

The **concentration** of a solution tells you how much solute is dissolved in the solvent (see Section 30.8). A **concentrated** solution has a greater amount of solute per unit volume than a solution that is **dilute**. A **saturated** solution is one in which no more solute will dissolve. At this point, we have reached the **molar solubility** of the solute for that particular solvent, and the reverse process of dissolution, called **precipitation**, occurs at the same rate as dissolving. Both the solid form and the dissolved form of the solute are said to be in **dynamic equilibrium**.

Solubility

Solubility refers to the amount of solute that will saturate a particular solvent. Solubility is specific for the type of solute and solvent. For example, 100 mL of water at 25°C becomes saturated with 40 g of dissolved NaCl, but it would take 150 g of KI to saturate the same volume of water at this temperature. And both of these salts behave differently in methanol than in water. Solubility also varies with temperature, increasing or decreasing with temperature depending upon the solute and solvent as outlined in the first set of solubility rules below.

There are two sets of solubility rules that show up time and time again on the MCAT. The first set governs the general solubility of solids and gases in liquids, as a function of the temperature and pressure. These rules below should be taken as just rules of thumb because they are only 95 percent reliable (still not bad). Memorize the following:

> **Phase Solubility Rules**
> 1. The solubility of solids in liquids tends to increase with increasing temperature.
> 2. The solubility of gases in liquids tends to decrease with increasing temperature.
> 3. The solubility of gases in liquids tends to increase with increasing pressure.

Keep in mind, the solubility of a gas in a liquid is also a function of the partial pressure of that gas above the liquid and the Henry's Law constant (Solubility = kP). As partial pressure increases, the quantity of dissolved gas necessarily increases as the equilibrium constant remains unchanged.

The second set governs the solubility of salts in water. Memorize the following too:

> **Salt Solubility Rules**
> 1. All Group I (Li^+, Na^+, K^+, Rb^+, Cs^+) and ammonium (NH_4^+) salts are *soluble*.
> 2. All nitrate (NO_3^-), perchlorate (ClO_4^-), and acetate ($C_2H_3O_2^-$) salts are *soluble*.
> 3. All silver (Ag^+), lead (Pb^{2+}/ Pb^{4+}), and mercury (Hg_2^{2+}/ Hg^{2+}) salts are *insoluble*, *except* for their nitrates, perchlorates, and acetates.

Example 30-8: Which of the following salts is expected to be *soluble* in water?

    A) $PbC_2H_3O_2$
    B) Ag_2SO_4
    C) Hg_2Cl_2
    D) $PbCO_3$

Solution: According to the solubility rules for salts in water, choices B, C, and D are all insoluble by Rule 3. Since all acetate salts are soluble (Rule 2), choice A is correct.

Example 30-9: Which of the following acids could be added to an unknown salt solution and NOT cause precipitation?

    A) HCl
    B) HI
    C) H_2SO_4
    D) HNO_3

Solution: According to the solubility rules for salts, all nitrate (NO_3^-) salts are soluble. Therefore, only the addition of nitric acid guarantees that any new ion combination would be soluble. Choice D is the correct answer.

Solubility Product Constant

All salts have characteristic solubilities in water. Some, like NaCl, are very soluble, while others, like AgCl, barely dissolve at all. The extent to which a salt will dissolve in water can be determined from its **solubility product constant, K_{sp}.** The solubility product is simply another equilibrium constant, one in which the reactants and products are just the undissolved and dissolved salts.

For example, let's look at the dissolution of magnesium hydroxide in water:

$$Mg(OH)_2(s) \rightleftharpoons Mg^{2+}(aq) + 2\,OH^-(aq)$$

At equilibrium, the solution is *saturated*; the rate at which ions go into solution is equal to the rate at which they precipitate out. The equilibrium expression is

$$K_{sp} = [Mg^{2+}][OH^-]^2$$

Notice that we leave the $Mg(OH)_2$ out of the equilibrium expression because it's a pure solid. (The "concentration of a solid" is meaningless when discussing the equilibrium between a solid and its ions in a saturated aqueous solution.)

Solubility Computations

Let's say you know the K_{sp} for a solid, and you're asked to find out just how much of it can dissolve into water; that is, you're asked to determine the salt's **molar solubility**, the number of moles of that salt that will saturate a liter of water.

To find the solubility of $Mg(OH)_2$, we begin by figuring out how much of each type of ion we'll have once we have x moles of the salt. Since each molecule dissociates into one magnesium ion and two hydroxide ions, if x moles of this salt have dissolved, the solution contains x moles of Mg^{2+} ions and $2x$ moles of OH^- ions:

$$Mg(OH)_2(s) \rightleftharpoons Mg^{2+}(aq) + 2OH^-(aq)$$

$$x \rightleftharpoons x + 2x$$

So, if x stands for the number of moles of $Mg(OH)_2$ that have dissolved per liter of saturated solution (which is what we're trying to find), then $[Mg^{2+}] = x$ and $[OH^-] = 2x$. Substituting these into the solubility product expression gives us

$$K_{sp} = [Mg^{2+}][OH^-]^2$$

$$= x\,(2x)^2 = x\,(4x^2) = 4x^3$$

It is known that K_{sp} for $Mg(OH)_2$ at 25°C is about 1.6×10^{-11}. So, if we set this equal to $4x^3$, we can solve for x. We get $x \approx 1.6 \times 10^{-4}$. This means that a solution of $Mg(OH)_2$ at 25°C will be saturated at a $Mg(OH)_2$ concentration of $1.6 \times 10^{-4}\,M$.

Example 30-10: The value of the solubility product for copper(I) chloride is $K_{sp} = 1.2 \times 10^{-6}$. Under normal conditions, the maximum concentration of an aqueous CuCl solution will be:

    A) less than $10^{-6}\,M$.
    B) greater than $10^{-6}\,M$ and less than $10^{-4}\,M$.
    C) greater than $10^{-4}\,M$ and less than $10^{\,2}\,M$.
    D) greater than $10^{-2}\,M$ and less than $10^{-1}\,M$.

Solution: The equilibrium is $CuCl(s) \rightleftharpoons Cu^+(aq) + Cl^-(aq)$. If we let x denote $[Cu^+]$, then we also have $x = [Cl^-]$. Therefore, $K_{sp} = x \times x = x^2$; setting this equal to 1.2×10^{-6}, we find that x is $1.1 \times 10^{-3}\,M$. Therefore, the answer is choice C.

30.5 ION PRODUCT

The **ion product** is the reaction quotient for a solubility reaction. That is, while K_{sp} is equal to the product of the concentrations of the ions in solution when the solution is saturated (that is, *at equilibrium*), the ion product—which we'll denote by Q_{sp}—has exactly the same form as the K_{sp} expression, but the concentrations don't have to be those at equilibrium. The reaction quotient allows us to make predictions about what the reaction will do:

$$Q_{sp} < K_{sp} \rightarrow \text{more salt can be dissolved}$$
$$Q_{sp} = K_{sp} \rightarrow \text{solution is saturated}$$
$$Q_{sp} > K_{sp} \rightarrow \text{excess salt will precipitate}$$

For example, let's say we had a liter of solution containing 10^{-4} mol of barium chloride and 10^{-3} mol of sodium sulfate, both of which are soluble salts:

$$BaCl_2(s) \rightarrow Ba^{2+}(aq) + 2Cl^-(aq)$$

$$Na_2SO_4(s) \rightarrow 2Na^+(aq) + SO_4^{2-}(aq)$$

When you mix two salts in solution, ions can recombine to form new salts, and you have to consider the new salt's K_{sp}. Barium sulfate, $BaSO_4$, is a slightly soluble salt, and at 25°C, its K_{sp} is 1.1×10^{-10}. Its dissolution equilibrium is

$$BaSO_4(s) \rightleftharpoons Ba^{2+}(aq) + SO_4^{2-}(aq)$$

Its ion product is $Q_{sp} = [Ba^{2+}][SO_4^{2-}]$, so in this solution, we have $Q_{sp} = (10^{-4})(10^{-3}) = 10^{-7}$, which is much greater than its K_{sp}. Since $Q_{sp} > K_{sp}$, the reverse reaction would be favored, and $BaSO_4$ would precipitate out of solution.

Example 30-11: Will a precipitate form when 50 mL of 0.20 M $AgNO_3$ and 50 mL of 0.10 M $CaCl_2$ are mixed? The K_{sp} of AgCl is 1.8×10^{-10}.

Solution: In order to determine if a precipitate will form, we need to calculate Q_{sp} for the following reaction:

$$AgCl(s) \rightleftharpoons Ag^+(aq) + Cl^-(aq)$$

We calculate the concentrations of the ions using the formula $C_1V_1 = C_2V_2$. Once the solutions are mixed,

$C_{2[Ag^+]} = \dfrac{(0.20)(50)}{(100)} = 0.10\,M$ and $C_{2[Cl^-]} = \dfrac{2(0.10)(50)}{(100)} = 0.10\,M$. (Recall that there are two Cl^- ions per

unit of $CaCl_2$.) Therefore, $Q_{sp} = [Ag^+][Cl^-] = (0.10)(0.10) = 1.0 \times 10^{-2}$. Since $Q_{sp} > K_{sp}$, the reaction needs

to proceed in the reverse direction to reach equilibrium, and a precipitate of AgCl will form when the

solutions are mixed.

30.6 THE COMMON-ION EFFECT

Let's consider again a saturated solution of magnesium hydroxide:

$$Mg(OH)_2(s) \rightleftharpoons Mg^{2+}(aq) + 2OH^-(aq)$$

What would happen if we now added some sodium hydroxide, NaOH, to this solution? Since NaOH is very soluble in water, it will dissociate completely:

$$NaOH(s) \rightarrow Na^+(aq) + OH^-(aq)$$

The addition of NaOH has caused the amount of hydroxide ion—the **common ion**—in the solution to increase. This disturbs the equilibrium of magnesium hydroxide; since the concentration of a product of that equilibrium is increased, Le Châtelier's principle tells us that the system will react by favoring the reverse reaction, producing solid $Mg(OH)_2$, which will precipitate. Therefore, the molar solubility of the slightly soluble salt [in this case, $Mg(OH)_2$] is decreased by the presence of another solute (in this case, NaOH) that supplies a common ion. This is the **common-ion effect**.

Example 30-12: Barium chromate solid ($K_{sp} = 1.2 \times 10^{-10}$) is at equilibrium with its dissociated ions in an aqueous solution. If calcium chromate ($K_{sp} = 7.1 \times 10^{-4}$) is introduced into the solution, it will cause the molar quantity of:

    A) solid barium chromate to increase and barium ion to decrease.
    B) solid barium chromate to increase and barium ion to increase.
    C) solid barium chromate to decrease and barium ion to decrease.
    D) solid barium chromate to decrease and barium ion to increase.

Solution: The answer is choice A. The introduction of additional chromate ion (CrO_4^{2-})—the common ion—will cause the amount of barium ion in solution to decrease (since the solubility equilibrium of $BaCrO_4$ will be shifted to the left, consuming Ba^{2+}). And, as a result, the amount of solid barium chromate will increase, because some will precipitate.

30.7 COMPLEX ION FORMATION AND SOLUBILITY

Complex ions consist of metallic ions surrounded by generally two, four, or six ligands, also known as Lewis bases. Complexed metal ions may have extremely different solubility properties than the "naked," hydrated metal ions. Therefore, the addition of ligands may substantially alter the solubility of simple metal salts. For example, as described by the solubility rules in Section 30.4 above, silver chloride (AgCl) is largely insoluble in water as is evident by its extremely low K_{sp} (1.7×10^{-10}). However, addition of AgCl to an aqueous solution containing ammonia (NH_3) results in greater solubility, owing to the formation of the complex ion $[Ag(NH_3)_2]^+$. The overall effect is described by the equations below:

$$AgCl(s) \; \rightleftharpoons \; Ag^+(aq) \; + \; Cl^-(aq) \qquad\qquad K_{sp} = 1.6 \times 10^{-10}$$

$$Ag^+(aq) \; + \; 2\,NH_3(aq) \; \rightleftharpoons \; [Ag(NH_3)_2]^+\,(aq) \qquad\qquad K_{eq} = 1.5 \times 10^7$$

Overall: $\quad AgCl(s) \; + \; 2\,NH_3(aq) \; \rightleftharpoons \; [Ag(NH_3)_2]^+\,(aq) \; + \; Cl^-(aq) \qquad K_{overall} \approx 10^{-3}$

The inclusion of ammonia in the system greatly increases the propensity of the AgCl(s) to exist as ions in solution. While the final value of K (10^{-3}) is still less than 1, it is several orders of magnitude greater than the initial K_{sp} of AgCl. The dissolution of the initial silver salt can be favored even more by taking advantage of Le Châtelier's Principle through the simple addition of excess ammonia.

30.8 THERMODYNAMICS AND EQUILIBRIUM

In Section 27.7 on Gibbs Free Energy, we saw that if ΔG was negative we could expect a reaction to proceed spontaneously in the forward direction, with the opposite being true for the case in which ΔG is positive. When a system proceeds in one direction or another, there is necessarily a change in the relative values of products and reactants that redefine ΔG, and the reaction proceeds until ΔG is equal to 0 and equilibrium is achieved. Therefore, there must be a relationship between ΔG and the reaction quotient Q, as well as the equilibrium constant K_{eq}. This relationship is given in the following equation.

$$\Delta G = \Delta G° + RT \ln Q$$

As the superscript denotes, $\Delta G°$ is the Gibbs free energy for a reaction under standard conditions. You may recall from Section 30.2 that when $Q = K$ the reaction is at equilibrium. Since ΔG is always equal to zero at equilibrium we can change the equation to

$$0 = \Delta G° + RT \ln K_{eq} \qquad \text{or} \qquad \Delta G° = -RT \ln K_{eq}$$

It is important to draw the distinction between ΔG and $\Delta G°$. Whereas ΔG is a statement of spontaneity of a reaction in one direction or another, $\Delta G°$ is, as seen in its relation to K_{eq}, a statement of the relative proportions of products and reactants present at equilibrium. The standard state $\Delta G°$ for a reaction only describes a reaction at one specific temperature, pressure, and set of concentrations, whereas ΔG changes with changing reaction composition until it reaches zero. From the above relationship, we can surmise the following:

$\Delta G° < 0$; $K_{eq} > 1$, products are favored at equilibrium
$\Delta G° = 0$; $K_{eq} = 1$, products and reactants are present in roughly equal amounts at equilibrium
$\Delta G° > 0$; $K_{eq} < 1$, reactants are favored at equilibrium

The difference between the heights of the reactants and products on any reaction coordinate diagram is $\Delta G°$. As we know from analyzing these plots if the reactants are higher than the products, we expect the products to be favored. This would give us the expected negative value of $\Delta G°$, and likewise a value of K_{eq} greater than 1.

Example 30-13: The $\Delta G°$ value for a certain reaction is −34.5 kJ/mol. Which of the following statements is true about the reaction when it is at standard conditions?

A) $Q > K_{eq}$ and $K_{eq} > 1$
B) $Q = 1$ and $K_{eq} > 1$
C) $Q < K_{eq}$ and $K_{eq} < 1$
D) $Q = 1$ and $K_{eq} < 1$

Solution: Since the sign of $\Delta G°$ is negative, K must be greater than 1, according to the equation $\Delta G° = -RT \ln K$. Choices C and D are incorrect. At standard conditions, all reactants and products have concentrations of 1 M or partial pressures of 1 atm by definition, so Q must be equal to 1. Choice B is the correct answer.

Chapter 31
Acids and Bases

31.1 DEFINITIONS

There are two important definitions of acids and bases that you should be familiar with for the MCAT.

Brønsted-Lowry Acids and Bases

Brønsted and Lowry offered the following definitions:

Acids are proton (H⁺) donors.
Bases are proton (H⁺) acceptors.

While the often seen hydroxide ions qualify as Brønsted-Lowry bases, many other compounds fit this definition as well. Since a Brønsted-Lowry base is any substance that is capable of accepting a proton, any anion or any neutral species with a lone pair of electrons can function as a base.

If we consider the reversible reaction below:

$$H_2CO_3 + H_2O \rightleftharpoons H_3O^+ + HCO_3^-$$

then according to the Brønsted-Lowry definition, H_2CO_3 and H_3O^+ are acids and HCO_3^- and H_2O are bases. The Brønsted-Lowry definitions of acid and bases are the most important ones for MCAT General Chemistry.

Lewis Acids and Bases

Lewis's definitions of acids and bases are broader:

Lewis acids are electron-pair acceptors.
Lewis bases are electron-pair donors.

If we consider the reversible reaction below:

$$AlCl_3 + H_2O \rightleftharpoons (AlCl_3OH)^- + H^+$$

then according to the Lewis definition, $AlCl_3$ and H^+ are acids because they accept electron pairs; H_2O and $(AlCl_3OH)^-$ are bases because they donate electron pairs. Lewis acid/base reactions frequently result in the formation of coordinate covalent bonds, as discussed earlier. For example, in the reaction above, water acts as a Lewis base since it donates both of the electrons involved in the coordinate covalent bond between OH^- and $AlCl_3$. $AlCl_3$ acts as a Lewis acid, since it accepts the electrons involved in this bond.

31.2 CONJUGATE ACIDS AND BASES

When a Brønsted-Lowry acid donates an H^+, the remaining structure is called the **conjugate base** of the acid. Likewise, when a Brønsted-Lowry base bonds with an H^+ in solution, this new species is called the **conjugate acid** of the base. To illustrate these definitions, consider this reaction:

$$NH_3 + H_2O \rightleftharpoons NH_4^+ + OH^-$$

acid–base conjugates (top bracket over NH_3 and NH_4^+)

acid–base conjugates (bottom bracket over H_2O and OH^-)

Considering only the forward direction, NH_3 is the base and H_2O is the acid. The products are the conjugate acid and conjugate base of the reactants: NH_4^+ is the conjugate acid of NH_3, and OH^- is the conjugate base of H_2O:

acid $\dashrightarrow$ conjugate base

$$NH_3 + H_2O \rightleftharpoons NH_4^+ + OH^-$$

base $\dashrightarrow$ conjugate acid

Now consider the reverse reaction in which NH_4^+ is the acid and OH^- is the base. The conjugates are the same as for the forward reaction: NH_3 is the conjugate base of NH_4^+, and H_2O is the conjugate acid of OH^-:

conjugate base $\dashleftarrow$ acid

$$NH_3 + H_2O \rightleftharpoons NH_4^+ + OH^-$$

conjugate acid $\dashleftarrow$ base

The difference between a Brønsted-Lowry acid and its conjugate base is that the base is missing an H^+. The difference between a Brønsted-Lowry base and its conjugate acid is that the acid has an extra H^+.

Example 31-1: Which one of the following can behave as a Brønsted-Lowry acid but not a Lewis acid?

- A) CF_4
- B) $NaAlCl_4$
- C) HF
- D) Br_2

Solution: A Brønsted-Lowry acid donates an H^+, while a Lewis acid accepts a pair of electrons. Since a Brønsted-Lowry acid must have an H in the first place, only choice C can be the answer.

Example 31-2: What is the conjugate base of HCO_3^-?

    A) H_2CO_3
    B) HCO_2^-
    C) CO_3^{2-}
    D) CO_2

Solution: The conjugate base has one fewer H^+ than the acid. Of the four answer choices, only choice C fits this description. Note that choice A has one more H^+ than the HCO_3^- ion; that makes H_2CO_3 the conjugate *acid* of HCO_3^-.

31.3 THE STRENGTHS OF ACIDS AND BASES

Brønsted-Lowry acids can be placed into two big categories: *strong* and *weak*. Whether an acid is strong or weak depends on how completely it ionizes in water. A **strong** acid is one that dissociates completely (or very nearly so) in water; hydrochloric acid, HCl, is an example:

$$HCl(aq) + H_2O(l) \rightarrow H_3O^+(aq) + Cl^-(aq)$$

This reaction goes essentially to completion.

On the other hand, hydrofluoric acid, HF, is an example of a **weak** acid, since its dissociation in water,

$$HF(aq) + H_2O(l) \rightleftharpoons H_3O^+(aq) + F^-(aq)$$

does not go to completion; most of the HF remains undissociated.

If we use HA to denote a generic acid, its dissociation in water has the form

$$HA(aq) + H_2O(l) \rightleftharpoons H_3O^+(aq) + A^-(aq)$$

The strength of the acid is directly related to how much the products are favored over the reactants. The equilibrium expression for this reaction is

$$K_a = \frac{[H_3O^+][A^-]}{[HA]}$$

This is written as K_a, rather than K_{eq}, to emphasize that this is the equilibrium expression for an acid-dissociation reaction. In fact, K_a is known as the **acid-ionization** (or **acid-dissociation**) **constant** of the acid (HA). If $K_a > 1$, then the products are favored, and we say the acid is strong; if $K_a < 1$, then the reactants are favored and the acid is weak. We can also rank the relative strengths of acids by comparing their K_a values: The larger the K_a value, the stronger the acid; the smaller the K_a value, the weaker the acid.

The acids for which $K_a > 1$—the strong acids—are so few that you should memorize them.

$$HI, HBr, HCl, HClO_4, H_2SO_4, HNO_3.$$

The values of K_a for these acids are so large that most tables of acid ionization constants don't even list them. On the MCAT, you may assume that any acid that's not in this list is a weak acid. (Other acids that fit the definition of *strong* are so uncommon that it's very unlikely they'd appear on the test. For example, $HClO_3$ has a K_a of 10, and could be considered strong, but it is definitely one of the weaker strong acids and is not likely to appear on the MCAT.)

Example 31-3: In a 1 M aqueous solution of boric acid (H_3BO_3, $K_a = 5.8 \times 10^{-10}$), which of the following species will be present in solution in the greatest quantity?

    A) H_3BO_3
    B) $H_2BO_3^-$
    C) HBO_3^{2-}
    D) H_3O^+

Solution: The equilibrium here is $H_3BO_3(aq) + H_2O(l) \rightleftharpoons H_3O^+(aq) + H_2BO_3^-(aq)$. Boric acid is a weak acid (it's not on the list of strong acids), so the equilibrium lies to the left (also, notice how small its K_a value is). So, there'll be very few H_3O^+ or $H_2BO_3^-$ ions in solution but plenty of undissociated H_3BO_3. The answer is choice A.

Example 31-4: Of the following acids, which one would dissociate to the least extent in water?

    A) Chlorous acid, $HClO_2$ ($K_a = 1.1 \times 10^{-2}$)
    B) Lactic acid, $CH_3CH(OH)COOH$ ($K_a = 1.4 \times 10^{-4}$)
    C) Ammonium ion, NH_4^+ ($K_a = 5.6 \times 10^{-10}$)
    D) Pyridinium ion, $C_5H_4NH^+$ ($K_a = 5.6 \times 10^{-6}$)

Solution: The acid that dissociates to the least extent in water is the weakest acid, which has the smallest K_a value. Of the choices given, NH_4^+ (choice C) has the smallest K_a value.

We can apply the same ideas as above to identify strong and weak *bases*. If we use B to denote a generic base, its dissolution in water has the form

$$B(aq) + H_2O(l) \rightleftharpoons HB^+(aq) + OH^-(aq)$$

The strength of the base is directly related to how much the products are favored over the reactants. If we write the equilibrium constant for this reaction, we get

$$K_b = \frac{[HB^+][OH^-]}{[B]}$$

This is written as K_b, rather than K_{eq}, to emphasize that this is the equilibrium expression for a base-dissociation reaction. In fact, K_b is known as the **base-ionization** (or **base-dissociation**) **constant**. We can rank the relative strengths of bases by comparing their K_b values: The larger the K_b value, the stronger the base; the smaller the K_b value, the weaker the base.

31.3

For the MCAT and general chemistry, you should know about the following strong bases that may be used in aqueous solutions:

Common Strong Bases	
Group 1 hydroxides (For example, NaOH)	
Group 1 oxides (For example, Li_2O)	
Some group 2 hydroxides ($Ba(OH)_2$, $Sr(OH)_2$, $Ca(OH)_2$)	
Metal amides (For example, $NaNH_2$)	

Weak bases include ammonia (NH_3) and amines, as well as the conjugate bases of many weak acids, as we'll discuss below.

The Relative Strengths of Conjugate Acid-Base Pairs

Let's once again look at the dissociation of HCl in water:

$$HCl(aq) + H_2O(l) \rightarrow H_3O^+(aq) + Cl^-(aq)$$

no basic properties

The chloride ion (Cl^-) is the conjugate base of HCl. Since this reaction goes to completion, there must be no reverse reaction. Therefore, Cl^- has no tendency to accept a proton and thus does not act as a base. The conjugate base of a strong acid has no basic properties in water.

On the other hand, hydrofluoric acid, HF, is a weak acid since its dissociation is not complete:

$$HF(aq) + H_2O(l) \rightleftharpoons H_3O^+(aq) + F^-(aq)$$

Since the reverse reaction does take place to a significant extent, the conjugate base of HF, the fluoride ion, F^-, *does* have some tendency to accept a proton, and so behaves as a weak base. The conjugate base of a weak acid is a weak base.

In fact, the weaker the acid, the more the reverse reaction is favored, and the stronger its conjugate base. For example, hydrocyanic acid (HCN) has a K_a value of about 5×10^{-10}, which is much smaller than that of hydrofluoric acid ($K_a \approx 7 \times 10^{-4}$). Therefore, the conjugate base of HCN, the cyanide ion, CN^-, is a stronger base than F^-.

The same ideas can be applied to bases:

1) The conjugate acid of a strong base has no acidic properties in water. For example, the conjugate acid of LiOH is Li^+, which does not act as an acid in water.
2) The conjugate acid of a weak base is a weak acid (and the weaker the base, the stronger the conjugate acid). For example, the conjugate acid of NH_3 is NH_4^+, which is a weak acid.

Example 31-5: Of the following anions, which is the strongest base?

- A) I^-
- B) CN^-
- C) NO_3^-
- D) Br^-

Solution: Here's another way to ask the same question: Which of the following anions has the weakest conjugate acid? Since HI, HNO_3, and HBr are all strong acids, while HCN is a weak acid, CN^- (choice B) has the weakest conjugate acid, and is thus the strongest base.

Amphoteric Substances

Take a look at the dissociation of carbonic acid (H_2CO_3), a weak acid, and how its conjugate base dissociates:

$$H_2CO_3(aq) + H_2O(l) \rightleftharpoons H_3O^+(aq) + HCO_3^-(aq) \quad (K_a = 4.5 \times 10^{-7})$$

$$HCO_3^-(aq) + H_2O(l) \rightleftharpoons H_3O^+(aq) + CO_3^{2-}(aq) \quad (K_a = 4.8 \times 10^{-11})$$

The conjugate base of carbonic acid is HCO_3^-, which also has an ionizable proton. Carbonic acid is said to be **polyprotic**, because it has more than one proton to donate.

In the first reaction, HCO_3^- acts as a base, but in the second reaction it acts as an acid. Whenever a substance can act as either an acid or a base, we say that it is **amphoteric**. The conjugate base of a weak polyprotic acid is always amphoteric, because it can either donate or accept another proton. Also notice that HCO_3^- is a weaker acid than H_2CO_3; in general, every time a polyprotic acid donates a proton, the resulting species will be a weaker acid than its predecessor.

31.4 THE ION-PRODUCT CONSTANT OF WATER

Water is amphoteric. It reacts with itself in a Brønsted-Lowry acid-base reaction, one molecule acting as the acid, the other as the base:

$$H_2O(l) + H_2O(l) \rightleftharpoons H_3O^+(aq) + OH^-(aq)$$

This is called the autoionization (or self-ionization) of water. The equilibrium expression is

$$K_w = [H_3O^+][OH^-]$$

This is written as K_w, rather than K_{eq}, to emphasize that this is the equilibrium expression for the autoionization of water; K_w is known as the ion-product constant of water. Only a very small fraction of the water molecules will undergo this reaction, and it's known that at 25°C,

$$K_w = 1.0 \times 10^{-14}$$

(Like all other equilibrium constants, K_w varies with temperature; it increases as the temperature increases. However, because 25°C is so common, this is the value you should memorize.) Since the number of H_3O^+ ions in pure water will be equal to the number of OH^- ions, if we call each of their concentrations x, then $x^2 = K_w$, which gives $x = 1 \times 10^{-7}$. That is, the concentration of both types of ions in pure water is 1×10^{-7} M. (In addition, K_w is constant at a given temperature, regardless of the H_3O^+ concentration.)

If the introduction of an acid increases the concentration of H_3O^+ ions, then the equilibrium is disturbed, and the reverse reaction is favored, decreasing the concentration of OH^- ions. Similarly, if the introduction of a base increases the concentration of OH^- ions, then the equilibrium is again disturbed; the reverse reaction is favored, decreasing the concentration of H_3O^+ ions. However, in either case, the product of $[H_3O^+]$ and $[OH^-]$ will remain equal to K_w.

For example, suppose we add 0.002 moles of HCl to water to create a 1-liter solution. Since the dissociation of HCl goes to completion (it's a strong acid), it will create 0.002 moles of H_3O^+ ions, so $[H_3O^+] = 0.002$ M. Since H_3O^+ concentration has been increased, we expect the OH^- concentration to decrease, which it does:

$$[OH^-] = \frac{K_w}{[H_3O^+]} = \frac{1 \times 10^{-14}}{2 \times 10^{-3}} = 5 \times 10^{-12} \, M$$

31.5   pH

The pH scale measures the concentration of H^+ (or H_3O^+) ions in a solution. Because the molarity of H^+ tends to be quite small and can vary over many orders of magnitude, the pH scale is logarithmic:

$$pH = -\log[H^+]$$

This formula implies that $[H^+] = 10^{-pH}$. Since $[H^+] = 10^{-7}$ M in pure water, the pH of water is 7. At 25°C, this defines a pH neutral solution. If $[H^+]$ is greater than 10^{-7} M, then the pH will be less than 7, and the solution is said to be acidic. If $[H^+]$ is less than 10^{-7} M, the pH will be greater than 7, and the solution is basic (or alkaline). Notice that a *low* pH means a *high* $[H^+]$ and the solution is *acidic*; a *high* pH means a *low* $[H^+]$ and the solution is basic.

The range of the pH scale for most solutions falls between 0 and 14, but some strong acids and bases extend the scale past this range. For example, a 10 M solution of HCl will fully dissociate into H^+ and Cl^-. Therefore, the $[H^+] = 10$ M, and the pH = –1.

An alternate measurement expresses the acidity or basicity in terms of the hydroxide ion concentration, $[OH^-]$, by using pOH. The same formula applies for hydroxide ions as for hydrogen ions.

$$pOH = -\log[OH^-]$$

This formula implies that $[OH^-] = 10^{-pOH}$.

Acids and bases are inversely related: the greater the concentration of H^+ ions, the lower the concentration of OH^- ions, and vice versa. Since $[H^+][OH^-] = 10^{-14}$ at 25°C, the values of pH and pOH satisfy a special relationship at 25°C:

$$pH + pOH = 14$$

So, if you know the pOH of a solution, you can find the pH, and vice versa. For example, if the pH of a solution is 5, then the pOH must be 9. If the pOH of a solution is 2, then the pH must be 12.

On the MCAT, it will be helpful to be able to figure out the pH even in cases where the H^+ concentration isn't exactly equal to the whole-number power of 10. In general, if y is a number between 1 and 10, and you're told that $[H^+] = y \times 10^{-n}$ (where n is a whole number), then the pH will be between $(n-1)$ and n. For example, if $[H^+] = 6.2 \times 10^{-5}$, then the pH is between 4 and 5.

Relationships Between Conjugates

pK_a and pK_b

The definitions of pH and pOH both involved a negative logarithm. In general, "p" of something is equal to the $-\log$ of that something. Therefore, the following definitions won't be surprising:

$$pK_a = -\log K_a$$

$$pK_b = -\log K_b$$

Because H^+ concentrations are generally very small and can vary over such a wide range, the pH scale gives us more convenient numbers to work with. The same is true for pK_a and pK_b. Remember that the larger the K_a value, the stronger the acid. Since "p" means "take the negative log of…," the *lower* the pK_a value, the stronger the acid. For example, acetic acid (CH_3COOH) has a K_a of 1.75×10^{-5}, and hypochlorous acid (HClO) has a K_a of 2.9×10^{-8}. Since the K_a of acetic acid is larger than that of hypochlorous acid, we know this means that more molecules of acetic acid than hypochlorous acid will dissociate into ions in aqueous solution. In other words, acetic acid is stronger than hypochlorous acid. The pK_a of acetic acid is 4.8, and the pK_a of hypochlorous acid is 7.5. The acid with the lower pK_a value is the stronger acid. The same logic applies to pK_b: the lower the pK_b value, the stronger the base.

K_a and K_b

Let's now look at the relationship between the K_a and the K_b for an acid-base conjugate pair by working through an example question. Let K_a be the acid-dissociation constant for formic acid (HCOOH) and let K_b stand for the base-dissociation constant of its conjugate base (the formate ion, $HCOO^-$). If K_a is equal to 5.6×10^{-11}, what is $K_a \times K_b$?

The equilibrium for the dissociation of HCOOH is

$$HCOOH(aq) + H_2O(l) \rightleftharpoons H_3O^+(aq) + HCOO^-(aq) \qquad K_a = \frac{[H_3O^+][HCOO^-]}{[HCOOH]}$$

and the equilibrium for the dissociation of $HCOO^-$ is

$$HCOO^-(aq) + H_2O(l) \rightleftharpoons HCOOH(aq) + OH^-(aq) \qquad K_b = \frac{[HCOOH][OH^-]}{[HCOO^-]}$$

Therefore,

$$K_a K_b = \frac{[H_3O^+][HCOO^-]}{[HCOOH]} \times \frac{[HCOOH][OH^-]}{[HCOO^-]} = [H_3O^+][OH^-]$$

We now immediately recognize this product as K_w, the ion-product constant of water, whose value (at 25°C) is 1×10^{-14}.

This calculation wasn't special for HCOOH; we can see that the same thing will happen for any acid and its conjugate base. So, for any acid-base conjugate pair, we'll have

$$K_a K_b = K_w = 1 \times 10^{-14}$$

This gives us a way to quantitatively relate the strength of an acid and its conjugate base. For example, the value of K_a for HF is about 7×10^{-4}; therefore, the value of K_b for its conjugate base, F^-, is about 1.4×10^{-11}. For HCN, $K_a \approx 5 \times 10^{-10}$, so K_b for CN^- is 2×10^{-5}.

It also follows from our definitions and logarithm algebra that for an acid-base conjugate pair at 25°C, we'll have

$$pK_a + pK_b = 14$$

Example 31-6: Of the following liquids, which one contains the lowest concentration of H_3O^+ ions?

    A) Lemon juice (pH = 2.3)
    B) Blood (pH = 7.4)
    C) Seawater (pH = 8.5)
    D) Coffee (pH = 5.1)

Solution: Since $pH = -\log [H_3O^+]$, we know that $[H_3O^+] = 1/10^{pH}$. This fraction is smallest when the pH is greatest. Of the choices given, seawater (choice C) has the highest pH.

Example 31-7: What is the pH of a solution at 25°C whose hydroxide ion concentration is 1×10^{-4} M?

Solution: Since $pOH = -\log[OH^-]$, we know that $pOH = 4$. Therefore, the pH is 10.

Example 31-8: If 99% of the H_3O^+ ions are removed from a solution whose pH was originally 3, what will be its new pH?

Solution: If 99% of the H_3O^+ ions are removed, then only 1% remain. This means that the number of H_3O^+ ions is now only 1/100 of the original. If $[H_3O^+]$ is decreased by a factor of 100, then the pH is *increased* by 2—to pH 5 in this case—since $\log 100 = 2$.

pH Calculations

For Strong Acids

Strong acids dissociate completely, so the hydrogen ion concentration will be the same as the concentration of the acid. That means that you can calculate the pH directly from the molarity of the solution. For example, a 0.01 M solution of HCl will have $[H^+] = 0.01$ M and pH = 2.

For Weak Acids

Weak acids come to equilibrium with their dissociated ions. In fact, for a weak acid at equilibrium, the concentration of undissociated acid will be much greater than the concentration of hydrogen ion. To get the pH of a weak acid solution, you need to use the equilibrium expression.

Let's say you add 0.2 mol of HCN (hydrocyanic acid, a weak acid) to water to create a 1-liter solution, and you want to find the pH. Initially, $[HCN] = 0.2$ M, and none of it has dissociated. If x moles of HCN are dissociated at equilibrium, then the equilibrium concentration of HCN is $0.2 - x$. Now, since each molecule of HCN dissociates into one H^+ ion and one CN^- ion, if x moles of HCN have dissociated, there'll be x moles of H^+ and x moles of CN^-:

	HCN	$\rightleftharpoons$	H^+	+	CN^-
initial:	0.2 M		0 M		0 M
at equilibrium:	$(0.2 - x)$ M		x M		x M

(Actually, the initial concentration of H^+ is 10^{-7} M, but it's so small that it can be neglected for this calculation.) Our goal is to find x, because once we know $[H^+]$, we'll know the pH. So, we set up the equilibrium expression:

$$K_a = \frac{[H^+][CN^-]}{[HCN]} = \frac{x^2}{0.2 - x}$$

It's known that the value of K_a for HCN is 4.9×10^{-10}. Because the K_a is so small, not that much of the HCN is going to dissociate. (This assumption, that x added to or subtracted from a number is negligible, is always a good one when $K < 10^{-4}$ [the usual case found on the MCAT].) That is, we can assume that x is going to be a very small number, insignificant compared to 0.2; therefore, the value $(0.2 - x)$ is almost exactly the same as 0.2. By substituting 0.2 for $(0.2 - x)$, we can solve the equation above for x:

$$\frac{x^2}{0.2} \approx 4.9 \times 10^{-10}$$
$$x^2 \approx 1 \times 10^{-10}$$
$$\therefore x \approx 1 \times 10^{-5}$$

Since $[H^+]$ is approximately 1×10^{-5} M, the pH is about 5.

We simplified the computation by assuming that the concentration of hydrogen ion [H⁺] was insignificant compared to the concentration of undissociated acid [HCN]. Since it turned out that $[H^+] \approx 10^{-5}\ M$, which is much less than $[HCN] = 0.2\ M$, our assumption was valid. On the MCAT, you should always simplify the math wherever possible.

Example 31-9: What is pH of a solution made by dissolving 0.3 mol of lactic acid ($CH_3CH(OH)COOH$, $K_a = 1.4 \times 10^{-4}$) in 1 L of solution?

Solution: Before any lactic acid has dissociated, $[CH_3CH(OH)COOH] = 0.3\ M$. If x moles of $CH_3CH(OH)COOH$ are dissociated at equilibrium, then the equilibrium concentration of $CH_3CH(OH)COOH$ in a 1-L solution is $(0.3 - x)\ M$. Now, since each molecule of $CH_3CH(OH)COOH$ dissociates into one H^+ ion and one $CH_3CH(OH)COO^-$ ion, if x moles of $CH_3CH(OH)COOH$ have dissociated, there'll be x moles of H^+ and x moles of $CH_3CH(OH)COO^-$:

	$CH_3CH(OH)COOH(aq)$	$\rightleftharpoons$	$H^+(aq)$ + $CH_3CH(OH)COO^-(aq)$	
initial:	0.3		0	0
change:	$-x$		$+x$	$+x$
equilibrium:	$0.3 - x$		x	x

(We neglect the initial concentration of H^+ produced from the autoionization of water, $10^{-7}\ M$, because it is so small compared to the concentrations of the other species.) Our goal is to find $[H^+]$ so that we can calculate the pH. Assuming that x is much smaller than $0.3\ M$, so that $0.3 - x \approx 0.3 \approx [CH_3CH(OH)COOH]$, we can set up the equilibrium expression:

$$K_a = \frac{\left[H^+\right]\left[CH_3CH(OH)COO^-\right]}{\left[CH_3CH(OH)COOH\right]} \approx \frac{x^2}{0.3}$$

and then solve the expression for x:

$$\frac{x^2}{0.3} \approx 1.4 \times 10^{-4}$$

$$x^2 \approx 4.2 \times 10^{-5} = 42 \times 10^{-6}$$

$$x \approx 6.5 \times 10^{-3}$$

Since $[H^+]$ is approximately $6 \times 10^{-3}\ M$, which rounds to $1 \times 10^{-2}\ M$, the pH will be between 2 and 3.

31.6 NEUTRALIZATION REACTIONS

When an acid and a base are combined, they will react in what is called a **neutralization reaction**. Oftentimes this reaction will produce a salt and water. Here's an example:

$$HCl \quad + \quad NaOH \quad \rightarrow \quad NaCl \quad + \quad H_2O$$

$$\text{acid} \qquad \text{base} \qquad\qquad \text{salt} \qquad \text{water}$$

This type of reaction takes place when, for example, you take an antacid to relieve excess stomach acid. The antacid is a weak base, usually carbonate, that reacts in the stomach to neutralize acid.

If equimolar amounts of a strong acid and strong base react (as in the example above), the resulting solution will be pH neutral. However, if the reaction involves a weak acid or weak base, the resulting solution will not be pH neutral.

No matter how weak an acid or base is, when mixed with an equimolar amount of a strong base or acid, we can expect complete neutralization. It has been found experimentally that all neutralizations have the same exothermic "heat of neutralization," the energy released from the reaction that is the same for all neutralizations: $H^+ + OH^- \rightarrow H_2O$.

As you can see from the reaction above, equal molar amounts of HCl and NaOH are needed to complete the neutralization. To determine just how much base (B) to add to an acidic solution (or how much acid (A) to add to a basic solution) in order to cause complete neutralization, we just use the following formula:

$$a \times [A] \times V_A = b \times [B] \times V_B$$

where a is the number of acidic hydrogens per formula unit and b is a constant that tells us how many H^+ ions the base can accept.

For example, let's calculate how much 0.1 M NaOH solution is needed to neutralize 40 mL of a 0.3 M HCl solution:

$$V_B = \frac{a \times [A] \times V_A}{b \times [B]} = \frac{1 \times (0.3M) \times (40\text{mL})}{1 \times (0.1M)} = 120 \text{ mL}$$

Example 31-10: Binary mixtures of equal moles of which of the following acid-base combinations will lead to a complete (99+%) neutralization reaction?

> I. HCl and NaOH
> II. HF and NH_3
> III. HNO_3 and $NaHCO_3$

> A) I only
> B) I and II only
> C) II and III only
> D) I, II, and III

Solution: Remember, regardless of the strengths of the acids and bases, all neutralization reactions go to completion. Choice D is the correct answer.

31.7 HYDROLYSIS OF SALTS

A **salt** is an ionic compound, consisting of a cation and an anion. In water, the salt dissociates into ions, and depending on how these ions react with water, the resulting solution will be either acidic, basic, or pH neutral. To make the prediction, we notice that there are essentially two possibilities for both the cation and the anion in a salt:

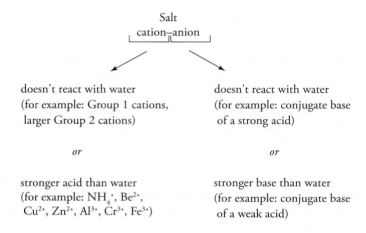

Whether the salt solution will be acidic, basic, or pH neutral depends on which combination of possibilities (four total) from the diagram above applies. The reaction of a substance—such as a salt or an ion—with water is called a hydrolysis reaction, a more general use of the term since the water molecule may not be split. Let's look at some examples.

If we dissolve NaCl in water, Na^+ and Cl^- ions go into solution. Na^+ ions are Group 1 ions and do not react with water. Since Cl^- is the conjugate base of a strong acid (HCl), it also doesn't react with water. These ions just become hydrated (surrounded by water molecules). Therefore, the solution will be pH neutral.

How about NH_4Cl? In solution it will break into NH_4^+ and Cl^-. The ammonium ion is a stronger acid than water (it's the conjugate acid of NH_3, a weak base), and Cl^- will not react with water. As a result, a solution of this salt will be acidic (note the formation of hydronium ions as products), and have a pH less than 7. NH_4Cl is called an acidic salt.

$$NH_4^+(aq) + H_2O(l) \rightleftharpoons NH_3(aq) + H_3O^+(aq)$$

Now let's consider sodium acetate, $Na(CH_3COO)$. In solution it will break into Na^+ and CH_3COO^-. Na^+ is a Group 1 cation and does not react with water. However, CH_3COO^- is a stronger base than water since it's the conjugate base of acetic acid (CH_3COOH), a weak acid. Therefore, a solution of the salt will be basic (note the formation of hydroxide ions as products) and have a pH greater than 7. $NaCH_3COO$ is a basic salt.

$$CH_3COO^-(aq) + H_2O(l) \rightleftharpoons CH_3COOH(aq) + OH^-(aq)$$

Example 31-11: Which of the following is an acidic salt?

    A) $FeCl_3$
    B) $CaBr_2$
    C) NaF
    D) $Sr(CH_3COO)_2$

Solution: To determine if a salt is acidic, it is only necessary to look at the cation. Choices B, C, and D all have cations from Group 1 or 2 which are neutral in solution; they are incorrect. The correct answer is choice A. It contains Fe^{3+}, a small, highly charged metal cation which is a stronger acid than water. (Choice B is a neutral salt, and choices C and D are basic salts.)

31.8 BUFFER SOLUTIONS

A **buffer** is a solution that resists changing pH when a small amount of acid or base is added. The buffering capacity comes from the presence of a weak acid and its conjugate base (or a weak base and its conjugate acid) in roughly equal concentrations.

One type of buffer is made from a weak acid and a salt of its conjugate base. To illustrate how a buffer works, let's look at a specific example and add 0.1 mol of acetic acid (CH_3COOH) and 0.1 mol of sodium acetate ($NaCH_3COO$) to water to obtain a 1-liter solution. Since acetic acid is a weak acid ($K_a = 1.75 \times 10^{-5}$), it will partially dissociate to give some acetate (CH_3COO^-) ions. However, the salt is soluble and will dissociate completely to give plenty of acetate ions. The addition of this common ion will shift the acid dissociation to the left, so the equilibrium concentrations of undissociated acetic acid molecules and acetate ions will be essentially equal to their initial concentrations, 0.1 M.

$$CH_3COOH + H_2O \rightleftharpoons H_3O^+ + CH_3COO^-$$

Since buffer solutions are designed to resist changes in pH, let's first figure out the pH of this solution. Writing the expression for the equilibrium constant gives

$$K_a = \frac{[H_3O^+][CH_3COO^-]}{[CH_3COOH]}, \text{ which we can solve for } [H_3O^+]: [H_3O^+] = \frac{K_a[CH_3COOH]}{[CH_3COO^-]}$$

Since the equilibrium concentrations of both CH_3COOH and CH_3COO^- are 0.1 M, this equation tells us that

$$[H_3O^+] = \frac{K_a[CH_3COOH]}{[CH_3COO^-]} = \frac{K_a(0.1M)}{0.1M} = 1.75 \times 10^{-5}$$

and pH $= -\log[H_3O^+]$, so pH $= -\log(1.75 \times 10^{-5})$, and pH $= 4.76$.

Okay, now let's see what happens if we add a little bit of strong acid—HCl, for example. If we add, say, 0.005 mol of HCl, it will dissociate completely in solution into 0.005 mol of H^+ ions and 0.005 mol of Cl^- ions. The Cl^- ions will have no effect on the equilibrium, but the added H^+ (or H_3O^+) ions will. Adding a product shifts the equilibrium to the left, and the acetate ions react with the additional H_3O^+ ions to produce additional acetic acid molecules. As a result, the concentration of acetate ions will drop by 0.005, from 0.1 M to 0.095 M; the concentration of acetic acid will increase by 0.005, from 0.1 M to 0.105 M.

Let's now use Equation (1) above to find the new pH:

$$[H_3O^+] = \frac{K_a[CH_3COOH]}{[CH_3COO^-]} = \frac{K_a(0.105\ M)}{0.095\ M} = 1.75 \times 10^{-5}(1.105) = 1.93 \times 10^{-5}$$

and pH $= -\log(1.93 \times 10^{-5})$, so pH $= 4.71$.

Notice that the pH dropped from 4.76 to 4.71, a decrease of just 0.05. If we had added this HCl to a liter of pure water, the pH would have dropped from 7 to 2.3, a *much* larger decrease! The buffer solution we created was effective at resisting a large drop in pH because it had enough base (in the form of acetate ions in this case) to neutralize the added acid.

Now let's see what happens if we add a little bit of strong base—KOH, for example. If we add, say, 0.005 mol of KOH, it will dissociate completely in solution into 0.005 mol of K^+ ions and 0.005 mol of OH^- ions. The K^+ ions will have no effect, but the added OH^- ions will shift the equilibrium to the right, since they'll react with acetic acid molecules to produce more acetate ions ($CH_3COOH + OH^- \rightarrow CH_3COO^- + H_2O$). As a result, the concentration of acetic acid will drop by 0.005, from 0.1 M to 0.095 M; the concentration of acetate ions will increase by 0.005, from 0.1 M to 0.105 M. Let's again use Equation (1) above to find the new pH:

$$[H_3O^+] = \frac{K_a[CH_3COOH]}{[CH_3COO^-]} = \frac{K_a(0.095\ M)}{0.105\ M} = 1.75 \times 10^{-5}(0.905) = 1.58 \times 10^{-5}$$

and pH $= -\log(1.58 \times 10^{-5})$, so pH $= 4.80$.

Notice that the pH increased from 4.76 to 4.80, an increase of just 0.04. If we had added this KOH to a liter of pure water, the pH would have increased from 7 to 11.7, a much larger increase! The buffer solution we created was effective at resisting a large rise in pH because it had enough acid to neutralize the added base.

If we generalize Equation (1) to any buffer solution containing a weak acid and a salt of its conjugate base, we get $[H_3O^+] = K_a([weak\ acid]/[conjugate\ base])$. Taking the –log of both sides give us the

> **Henderson-Hasselbalch Equation (for acid)**
>
> $$pH = pK_a + \log\left(\frac{[conjugate\ base]}{[weak\ acid]}\right)$$

To design a buffer solution, we choose a weak acid whose pK_a is as close to the desired pH as possible. An ideal buffer would have [weak acid] = [conjugate base], so pH = pK_a. If no weak acid has the exact pK_a needed, just adjust the initial concentrations of the weak acid and conjugate base accordingly.

We can also design a buffer solution by choosing a weak base (and a salt of its conjugate acid) such that the pK_b value of the base is as close to the desired pOH as possible. The version of the Henderson-Hasselbalch equation in this situation looks like this:

Henderson-Hasselbalch Equation (for base)

$$pOH = pK_b + \log\left(\frac{[\text{conjugate acid}]}{[\text{weak base}]}\right)$$

Example 31-12: As hydrogen ions are added to an acidic buffer solution, what happens to the concentrations of undissociated acid and conjugate base?

Solution: The conjugate base, A^-, reacts with the added H^+ to form HA, so the conjugate base decreases and the undissociated acid increases.

31.9   INDICATORS

An **indicator** is a weak acid that undergoes a color change when it's converted to its conjugate base. Let HA denote a generic indicator. In its non-ionized form, it has a particular color, which we'll call color #1. When it has donated a proton to become its conjugate base, A^-, it has a different color, which we'll call color #2.

Indicator

$$HA + H_2O \rightleftharpoons H_3O^+ + A^-$$

color #1   **color #2**

Under what conditions would an indicator change its color? What if an indicator were added to an acidic solution—that is, one whose pH were quite low due to a high concentration of H_3O^+ ions? Then, according to Le Châtelier, the indicator's equilibrium would shift to the left, and the indicator would display color #1. Conversely, if the indicator were added to a basic solution (that is, one with plenty of OH^- ions), the amount of H_3O^+ would decrease, and the indicator's equilibrium would be shifted to the right, causing it to display color #2. We can make this discussion a little more precise.

Take the expression for the indicator's equilibrium constant, $K_a = [H_3O^+][A^-]/[HA]$ and easily rearrange it into

$$\frac{[H_3O^+]}{K_a} = \frac{[HA]}{[A^-]}$$

Written this way, we can see that

- If $[H_3O^+] \gg K_a$, then $[HA] \gg [A^-]$, so we'd see color #1.
- If $[H_3O^+] \approx K_a$, then $[HA] \approx [A^-]$, so we'd see a mix of colors #1 & #2.
- If $[H_3O^+] \ll K_a$, then $[HA] \ll [A^-]$, so we'd see color #2.

Note that the indicator changes color within a fairly short pH range, about 2 units:

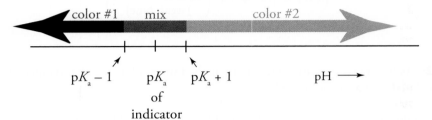

Therefore, if we want our indicator to be useful, we need to select one whose pK_a value is convenient for our purposes. For example, phenolphthalein is an indicator with a pK_a value of about 9.0. When added to a solution whose pH is less than 8, it remains colorless. However, if the solution's pH is above 10, it will turn a deep magenta. (For 8 < pH < 10, the solution will be a paler pink.) Thus, phenolphthalein can be used to differentiate between a solution whose pH is, say, 7 from one whose pH is 11. However, the indicator methyl orange could not distinguish between two such solutions: it would be yellow at pH 7 and yellow at pH 11. Methyl orange has a pK_a of about 3.8, so it changes color around pH 4.

Note: The $pK_a \pm 1$ range for an indicator's color change is convenient and typical, but it's not a hard-and-fast rule. Some indicators (like methyl orange) have a color-change range of only 1.2 (rather than 2) pH units. Also, some indicators have more than just two colors. Polyprotic indicators, like thymol blue and bromocesol green, can change color more than once, and can therefore exhibit more than two distinct colors.

31.10 ACID-BASE TITRATIONS

An **acid-base titration** is an experimental technique used to determine the identity of an unknown weak acid (or weak base) by determining its pK_a (or pK_b). Titrations can also be used to determine the concentration of *any* acid or base solution (whether it be known or unknown). The procedure consists of adding a strong acid (or a strong base) of *known* identity and concentration—the **titrant**—to a solution containing the unknown base (or acid). (One never titrates an acid with an acid or a base with a base.) While the titrant is added in small, discrete amounts, the pH of the solution is recorded (with a pH meter).

If we plot the data points (the pH value versus the volume of titrant added), we obtain a graph called a titration curve. Let's consider a specific example: the titration of HF (a weak acid) with NaOH (a strong base).

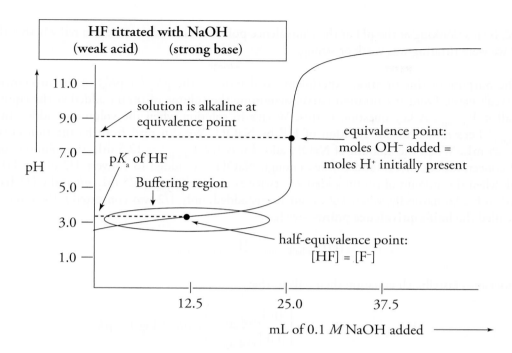

When the amount of titrant added is 0, the pH is of course just the pH of the original, pure solution of HF. Then, as NaOH is added, an equivalent amount of HF will be neutralized according to the reaction

$$NaOH + HF \rightarrow Na^+ + F^- + H_2O$$

As HF is neutralized, the pH will increase. But from the titration curve, we can see that the pH is certainly not increasing very rapidly as we add the first 20 or so mL of NaOH. This should tell you that at the beginning of this titration the solution is behaving as a buffer. As HF is being converted into F^-, we are forming a solution that contains a weak acid and its conjugate base. This section of the titration curve, where the pH changes very gradually, is called the **buffering domain** (or **buffering region**).

Now, as the experiment continues, the solution suddenly loses its buffering capability and the pH increases dramatically. At some point during this drastic increase, all HF is neutralized and no acid remains in solution. Every new ion of OH^- that is added remains in solution. Therefore, the pH continues to increase rapidly until the OH^- concentration in solution is not that much different from the NaOH concentration in the titrant. From here on, the pH doesn't change very much and the curve levels off.

There is a point during the drastic pH increase at which just enough NaOH has been added to completely neutralize all the HF. This is called the **acid-base equivalence point**. At this point, we simply have Na^+ ions and F^- ions in solution. Note that the solution should be *basic* here. In fact, from what we know about the behavior of conjugates, we can state the following facts about the equivalence point of different titrations:

- For a weak acid (titrated with a strong base), the equivalence point will occur at a pH > 7.
- For a weak base (titrated with a strong acid), the equivalence point will occur at a pH < 7.
- For a strong acid (titrated with a strong base) or for a strong base (titrated with a strong acid), the equivalence point will occur at pH = 7.

Therefore, by just looking at the pH at the equivalence point of our titration, we can tell whether the acid (or base) we were titrating was weak or strong.

Recall the purpose of this titration experiment: to determine the pK_a (or pK_b) of the unknown weak acid (or weak base). From the titration curve, determine the volume of titrant added at the equivalence point; call it $V_{at\ equiv}$. A key question is this: What's in solution when the volume of added titrant is $1/2\ V_{at\ equiv}$? Let's return to our titration of HF by NaOH. We can read from its titration curve that $V_{at\ equiv} = 25$ mL. When the amount of NaOH added was $1/2\ V_{at\ equiv} = 12.5$ mL, the solution consisted of equal concentrations of HF and F^-, i.e., enough NaOH was added to convert $1/2$ of the HF to F^-. (After all, when the amount of titrant added was twice as much, $V_{at\ equiv} = 25$ mL, *all* of the HF had been converted to F^-. So naturally, when $1/2$ as much was added, only $1/2$ was converted.) Therefore, at this point—called the **half-equivalence point**—we have

$$[HF]_{at\ half\text{-}equiv} = [F^-]_{at\ half\text{-}equiv}$$

The Henderson-Hasselbalch equation then tells us that

$$pH_{at\ half\text{-}equiv} = pK_a + \log\left(\frac{[F^-]_{at\ half\text{-}equiv}}{[HF]_{at\ half\text{-}equiv}}\right) = pK_a + \log 1 = pK_a$$

31.10

The pK_a of HF equals the pH at the half-equivalence point. For our curve, we see that this occurs around pH 3.2, so we conclude that the pK_a of HF is about 3.2.

Compare the sample titration curves for a weak base titrated with a strong acid to the one for a weak acid titrated with a strong base (like the one we just looked at). Note the pH at the equivalence point (relative to pH 7) for each curve.

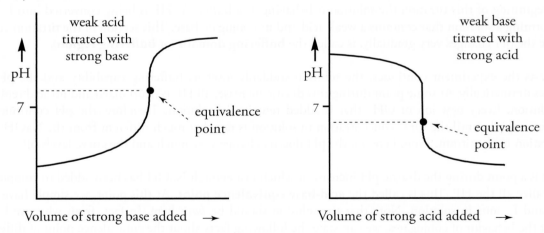

As mentioned above, the titration curve for a strong acid-strong base titration would have the equivalence point at a neutral pH of 7.

The titration curve for the titration of a polyprotic acid (like H_2CO_3 or an amino acid) will have more than one equivalence point. The number of equivalence points is equal to the number of ionizable hydrogens the acid can donate.

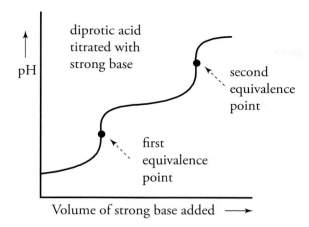

diprotic acid titrated with strong base

pH

second equivalence point

first equivalence point

Volume of strong base added

Example 31-13: A fifty mL solution of HCOOH (formic acid) is titrated with 0.2 M NaOH. The equivalence point is reached when 40 mL of the NaOH solution has been added. What was the original concentration of the formic acid solution?

Solution: Using our formula, $a \times [A] \times V_A = b \times [B] \times V_B$, we find that

$$[A] = \frac{b \times [B] \times V_B}{a \times V_A} = \frac{1 \times (0.2\ M) \times (40\ \text{mL})}{1 \times (50\ \text{mL})} = 0.16\ M$$

31.10

Example 31-14: Methyl red is an indicator that changes from red to yellow in the pH range 4.4–6.2. For which of the following titrations would methyl red be useful for indicating the equivalence point?

    A) HCN titrated with KOH
    B) NaOH titrated with HI
    C) C_6H_5COOH (benzoic acid) titrated with LiOH
    D) $C_6H_5NH_2$ (aniline) titrated with HNO_3

Solution: Since methyl red changes color in a range of *acidic* pH values, it would be an appropriate indicator for a titration whose equivalence point occurs at a pH less than 7. For a weak base titrated with a strong acid, the equivalence point occurs at a pH less than 7. Only choice D describes such a titration.

Chapter 32
Electrochemistry

32.1 OXIDATION-REDUCTION REACTIONS

Recall that the **oxidation number** (or **oxidation state**) of each atom in a molecule describes how many electrons it is donating or accepting in the overall bonding of the molecule. Many elements can assume different oxidation states depending on the bonds they make. A reaction in which the oxidation numbers of any of the reactants change is called an **oxidation-reduction** (or **redox**) reaction.

In a redox reaction, atoms gain or lose electrons as new bonds are formed. The total number of electrons does not change, of course; they're just redistributed among the atoms. When an atom loses electrons, its oxidation number increases; this is **oxidation**. When an atom gains electrons, the oxidation number decreases; this is **reduction**. A mnemonic device is helpful:

LEO the lion says GER

LEO: Lose Electrons = Oxidation

GER: Gain Electrons = Reduction

Another popular mnemonic is

OIL RIG

OIL: Oxidation Is electron Loss

RIG: Reduction Is electron Gain

An atom that is oxidized in a reaction loses electrons to another atom. We call the oxidized atom a **reducing agent** or **reductant**, because by giving up electrons, it reduces another atom that gains the electrons. On the other hand, the atom that gains the electrons has been **reduced**. We call the reduced atom an **oxidizing agent** or **oxidant**, because it oxidizes another atom that loses the electrons. (You may want to review Section 25.14 on Oxidation States.)

Take a look at this redox reaction:

$$Fe + 2\ HCl \rightarrow FeCl_2 + H_2$$

The oxidation state of iron changes from 0 to +2. The oxidation state of hydrogen changes from +1 to 0. (The oxidation state of chlorine remains at –1.) So, iron has lost two electrons, and two protons (H^+) have gained one electron each. Therefore, the iron has been oxidized, and the hydrogens have been reduced. In order to better see the exchange of electrons, a redox reaction can be broken down into a pair of **half-reactions** that show the oxidation and reduction separately. These **ion-electron** equations show only the actual oxidized or reduced species—and the electrons involved—in an electron-balanced reaction. For the redox reaction shown above, the ion-electron half-reactions are

oxidation: $\quad Fe \rightarrow Fe^{2+} + 2e^-$

reduction: $\quad 2\ H^+ + 2e^- \rightarrow H_2$

Example 32-1: For the redox reaction

$$Al_2O_3 + 3\,C \rightarrow 2\,Al + 3\,CO$$

which of the following shows the reduction half-reaction?

    A) $C + O^{2-} \rightarrow CO + e^-$
    B) $C + O^{2-} \rightarrow CO + 2\,e^-$
    C) $Al^{2+} + 2\,e^- \rightarrow Al$
    D) $Al^{3+} + 3\,e^- \rightarrow Al$

Solution: First, eliminate choices A and B; these are oxidation half-reactions. (Choice A is also not charge-balanced.) Aluminum has an oxidation number of +3 in Al_2O_3, so choice D is correct. Choice C has the wrong charge on Al.

32.2 GALVANIC CELLS

Because a redox reaction involves the transfer of electrons, and the flow of electrons constitutes an electric current that can do work, we can use a spontaneous redox reaction to generate an electric current.

One **electrode**, generally composed of a metal (labeled the **anode**) gets oxidized, and the electrons its atoms lose travel along the wire to a second metal electrode (labeled the **cathode**). It is at the cathode that reduction takes place. Electrons always flow through the conducting wire from the anode to the cathode. This electron flow is the electric current that is produced by the spontaneous redox reaction between the electrodes.

Let's look at a specific galvanic cell, with the anode made of zinc and the cathode made of copper. The anode is immersed in a $ZnSO_4$ solution, the cathode is immersed in a $CuSO_4$ solution, and the half cells are connected by a **salt bridge** containing an aqueous solution of KNO_3. When the electrodes are connected by a wire, zinc atoms in the anode are oxidized ($Zn \rightarrow Zn^{2+} + 2e^-$), and the electrons travel through the wire to the cathode. There, the Cu^{2+} ions in solution pick up these electrons and get reduced to copper metal ($Cu^{2+} + 2e^- \rightarrow Cu$), which accumulates on the copper cathode. The sulfate anions balance the charge on the Zn^{2+}, but do not participate in any redox reaction, and are therefore known as spectator ions.

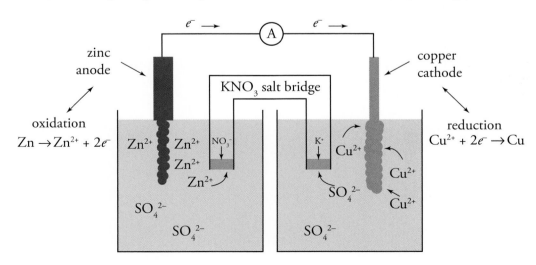

The Zn^{2+} ions that remain in the solution in the zinc half-cell attract NO_3^- ions from the salt bridge, and K^+ ions in the salt bridge are attracted into the copper half-cell. Notice that anions in solution travel from the right cell to the left cell—and cations travel in the opposite direction—using the salt bridge as a conduit. This movement of ions completes the circuit and allows the current in the wire to continue, until the zinc strip is consumed. Remember that anions from the salt bridge go to the anode and cations from the salt bridge go to the cathode.

Notice that the anode is always the site of oxidation, and the cathode is always the site of reduction. One way to help remember this is just to notice that "a" and "o" (anode and oxidation) are both vowels, while "c" and "r" (cathode and reduction) are both consonants. Another popular mnemonic is "an ox, red cat" for "anode = oxidation, reduction = cathode."

We often use a shorthand notation, called a **cell diagram**, to identify the species present in a galvanic cell. Cell diagrams are read as follows:

Anode | Anodic solution (concentration) || Cathodic solution (concentration) | Cathode

If the concentrations are not specified in the cell diagram, you should assume they are 1 M.

Example 32-2: In the electrochemical cell described by the following cell diagram, what reaction occurs at the cathode?

$$Ni(s) \mid Ni^{2+}(aq) \mid\mid H^+(aq) \mid H_2(g)$$

A) $Ni^{2+} + 2\,e^- \rightarrow Ni$
B) $Ni \rightarrow Ni^{2+} + 2\,e^-$
C) $2\,H^+ + e^- \rightarrow H_2$
D) $H_2 \rightarrow 2\,H^+ + e^-$

Solution: In a cell diagram, the cathode is always represented by the right-hand side, so choices A and B can be eliminated. In any electrochemical cell, reduction occurs at the cathode, so the answer is choice C.

32.3 STANDARD REDUCTION POTENTIALS

To determine whether the redox reaction of a cell is spontaneous and can produce an electric current, we need to figure out the cell voltage. Each half-reaction has a potential (E), which is the cell voltage it would have if the other electrode were the standard reference electrode. (*Note*: We usually consider cells at standard conditions: 25°C, 1 atm pressure, aqueous solutions at 1 M concentrations, and with substances in their standard states. To indicate standard conditions, we use a ° superscript on quantities such as E and ΔG.) By definition, the standard reference electrode is the site of the redox reaction $2\,H^+ + 2e^- \rightarrow H_2$, which is assigned a potential of 0.00 volts. By adding the half-reaction potential for a given pair of electrodes, we get the cell's overall voltage. Tables of half-reaction potentials are usually given for reductions only. Since each cell has a reduction half-reaction and an oxidation half-reaction, we get the potential of the oxidation by simply reversing the sign of the corresponding reduction potential.

For example, the standard reduction potential for the half-reaction $Cu^{2+} + 2e^- \rightarrow Cu$ is +0.34 V. The standard reduction potential for the half-reaction $Zn^{2+} + 2e^- \rightarrow Zn$ is –0.76 V. Reversing the zinc reduction to an oxidation, we get $Zn \rightarrow Zn^{2+} + 2e^-$, with a potential of +0.76 V. Therefore, the overall cell voltage for the zinc-copper cell is (+0.76 V) + (+0.34 V) = +1.10 V:

$$
\begin{array}{lll}
\text{oxidation:} & Zn \rightarrow Zn^{2+} + 2e^- & E° = +0.76\ V \\
\text{reduction:} & \underline{Cu^{2+} + 2e^- \rightarrow Cu} & \underline{E° = +0.34\ V} \\
& Zn + Cu^{2+} \rightarrow Zn^{2+} + Cu & E° = +1.10\ V
\end{array}
$$

The free-energy change, $\Delta G°$, for a redox reaction in which cell voltage is $E°$ is given by the equation

$$\Delta G° = -\,nFE°$$

where n is the number of moles of electrons transferred and F stands for a **faraday** (the magnitude of the charge of one mole of electrons, approximately 96,500 coulombs). Since a reaction is spontaneous if $\Delta G°$ is negative, this equation tells us that the redox reaction in a cell will be spontaneous if the cell voltage is positive.

> If the cell voltage is positive, then the reaction is spontaneous.
>
> If the cell voltage is negative, then the reaction is nonspontaneous.

Oxidizing and Reducing Agents

We can also use reduction potentials to determine whether reactants are good or poor oxidizing or reducing agents. For example, let's look again at the half-reactions in our original zinc-copper cell. The half-reaction $Zn^{2+} + 2e^- \rightarrow Zn$ has a standard potential of –0.76 V, and the half-reaction $Cu^{2+} + 2e^- \rightarrow Cu$ has a standard potential of +0.34 V. The fact that the reduction of Zn^{2+} is nonspontaneous means that the oxidation of Zn is spontaneous, so Zn would rather give up electrons. If it does, this means that Zn acts as a reducing agent because in giving up electrons it reduces something else. The fact that the reduction of Cu^{2+} has a positive potential tells us that this reaction would be spontaneous at standard conditions. In other words, Cu^{2+} is a good oxidizing agent because it's looking to accept electrons, thereby oxidizing something else.

32.3

> The more negative the reduction potential, the weaker the reactant is as an oxidizing agent, and the stronger the product is as a reducing agent.
>
> The more positive the reduction potential, the stronger the reactant is as an oxidizing agent, and the weaker the product is as a reducing agent.

For example, given that $Pb^{2+} + 2e^- \rightarrow Pb$ has a standard potential of –0.13 V, and $Al^{3+} + 3e^- \rightarrow Al$ has a standard potential of –1.67 V, what could we conclude? Well, since Al^{3+} has a large negative reduction potential, the product, aluminum metal, is a good reducing agent. In fact, because the reduction potential of Al^{3+} is more negative than that of Pb^{2+}, we'd say that aluminum is a stronger reducing agent than lead.

Example 32-3: A galvanic cell is set to operate at standard conditions. If one electrode is made of magnesium and the other is made of copper, then the magnesium electrode will serve as the:

- A) anode and be the site of oxidation.
- B) anode and be the site of reduction.
- C) cathode and be the site of oxidation.
- D) cathode and be the site of reduction.

Reaction	$E°$ (volts)
$Li^+ + e^- \rightarrow Li$	−3.05
$Mg^{2+} + 2e^- \rightarrow Mg$	−2.36
$Al^{3+} + 3e^- \rightarrow Al$	−1.67
$Zn^{2+} + 2e^- \rightarrow Zn$	−0.76
$Fe^{2+} + 2e^- \rightarrow Fe$	−0.44
$Pb^{2+} + 2e^- \rightarrow Pb$	−0.13
$2 H^+ + 2e^- \rightarrow H_2$	0.00
$Cu^{2+} + 2e^- \rightarrow Cu$	0.34
$Ag^+ + e^- \rightarrow Ag$	0.80
$Pd^{2+} + 2e^- \rightarrow Pd$	0.99
$Pt^{2+} + 2e^- \rightarrow Pt$	1.20
$Au^{3+} + 3e^- \rightarrow Au$	1.50
$F_2 + 2e^- \rightarrow 2 F^-$	2.87

Solution: First, eliminate choices B and C since the anode is always the site of oxidation and the cathode is always the site of reduction. From the table, we see that the reduction of Mg^{2+} is nonspontaneous, whereas the reduction of Cu^{2+} is spontaneous. Therefore, the copper electrode will serve as the cathode and be the site of reduction, and the magnesium electrode will serve as the anode and be the site of oxidation (choice A).

Example 32-4: What is the standard cell voltage for the oxidation of Li by Mg^{2+}?

Solution: The half-reactions are

$$Li \rightarrow Li^+ + e^- \qquad E° = +3.05 \text{ V}$$

$$Mg^{2+} + 2 e^- \rightarrow Mg \qquad E° = -2.36 \text{ V}$$

Note that since the half-reaction for lithium has been reversed, the sign of $E°$ has also been changed from its value in the table. Since the question only asks for the $E°$, we can simply add up the $E°$ for the reduction and oxidation half-reactions to get the $E°$ for the overall reaction: $E° = (+3.05) + (-2.36) = 0.69$ V. There is no need to multiply both sides of the first half-reaction by the stoichiometric coefficient 2 before adding it to the second one. We'd only need to do that if we wanted to get the balanced redox reaction.

Example 32-5: Of the following, which is the strongest reducing agent?

    A) Zn
    B) Fe
    C) Pd
    D) Pd^{2+}

Solution: Remember the rule: the more negative the reduction potential, the stronger the product is as a reducing agent. Zn (choice A) is the product of a redox half-reaction whose potential is −0.76 V. Fe (choice B) is the product of a redox half-reaction whose potential is −0.44 V. So, we know we can eliminate choice B. Pd (choice C) is the product of a redox half-reaction whose potential is +0.99 V, so choice C is eliminated. Finally, in order for Pd^{2+} to be a reducing agent, it would have to be oxidized—that is, lose more electrons. A cation getting further oxidized? Not likely, especially when there's a neutral metal (choice A) that is happier to do so.

Example 32-6: Which of the following best approximates the value of $\Delta G°$ for this reaction:

$$2\ Al + 3\ Cu^{2+} \rightarrow 2\ Al^{3+} + 3\ Cu?$$

    A) −(12)(96,500) J
    B) −(6)(96,500) J
    C) +(6)(96,500) J
    D) +(12)(96,500) J

Solution: The half-reactions are

$$2\ (Al \rightarrow Al^{3+} + 3e^-) \qquad E° = +1.67\ V$$
$$3\ (Cu^{2+} + 2e^- \rightarrow Cu) \qquad E° = 0.34\ V$$

so the overall cell voltage is $E° = 2.01\ V \approx 2\ V$. Because the number of electrons transferred is $n = 2 \times 3 = 6$, the equation $\Delta G° = -nFE°$ tells us that choice A is the answer:

$$\Delta G° = -\ (6)(96,500)(2)\ J = -\ (12)(96,500)\ J$$

32.4   NONSTANDARD CONDITIONS

All the previous discussion of potentials assumed the conditions to be standard state, meaning that all aqueous reactants in the mixture were 1 M in concentration. So long as this is true, the tabulated values for reduction potentials apply to each half reaction.

However, since conditions are not always standard we must have a way to alternatively, and more generally, describe the voltage of an electrochemical reaction. To do this we use the Nernst equation.

$$E = E° - \left(\frac{RT}{nF}\right) \ln Q$$

It describes how deviations in temperature and concentration of reactants can alter the voltage of a reaction under nonstandard conditions. As in the standard chemical systems previously discussed, the concentrations of product and reactants will change until $Q = K_{eq}$, and $E = 0$.

Concentration Cells

A **concentration cell** is a galvanic cell that has identical electrodes but which has half-cells with different ion concentrations. Since the electrodes and relevant ions in the two beakers have the same identities, the *standard* cell voltage, $E°$, would be zero. But, such a cell is *not* standard because both electrolytic solutions in the half-cells are not 1 M. So even though the electrodes are the same, in a concentration cell there *will* be a potential difference between them, and an electric current will be produced. For example, let's say both electrodes are made of zinc, and the $[Zn^{2+}]$ concentrations in the electrolytes were 0.1 M and 0.3 M, respectively. We'd expect electrons to be induced to flow through the conducting wire to the half-cell with the higher concentration of these positive ions. So, the zinc electrode in the 0.1 M solution would serve as the anode, with the liberated electrons flowing across the wire to the zinc electrode in the 0.3 M solution, which serves as the cathode. When the concentrations of the solutions become equal, the reaction will stop.

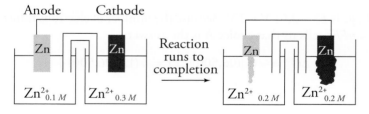

32.5   REDOX TITRATIONS

Just as the titration of an acid with a strong base of known concentration can provide information about the initial acid solution (most notably the concentration and pK_a), titration of a redox active species with a strong oxidant or reductant can be used to determine similar unknowns.

Most redox titrations involve the use of a redox indicator. Much like an indicator in acid/base chemistry, a redox indicator uses a change in color to determine the endpoint. However, in a redox reaction, this change in color is due to a change in oxidation state rather than loss or gain of a proton. One commonly used redox indicator is the Ce^{4+} ion, a strong oxidant according to the equation below:

$$Ce^{4+} \ + \ 1\,e^- \ \rightarrow \ Ce^{3+} \qquad E° \approx 1.5 \text{ V } (1\ M \text{ HCl solution})$$

The Ce^{4+} ion is bright yellow in solution, whereas the reduced Ce^{3+} is colorless. This color change, along with the comparatively high redox potential, make Ce^{4+} an ideal indicator for the determination of the concentration of solutions of oxidizable species.

For example, cerium is known to oxidize secondary alcohols to ketones in aqueous solution. As such, titration with Ce^{4+} is an appropriate method for the determination of alcohol concentration in solution, or for the determination of the number of secondary hydroxyl groups present in a chemical species. As long as the Ce^{4+} added to the solution is consumed, the solution will remain colorless. However, the solution will turn yellow immediately after all oxidizable hydroxyls have been consumed. Knowledge of the concentration of the Ce^{4+} titrant allows for the determination of initial alcohol concentration.

A redox titration curve, similar to an acid-base titration curve, can be plotted for any such redox titration. An example is given below where a generic reductant is titrated with Ce^{4+}.

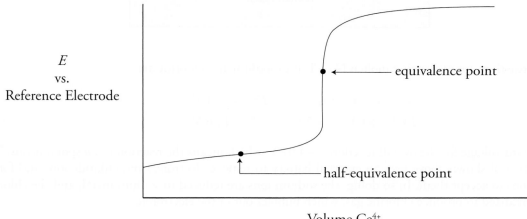

The equivalence point on the plot above will coincide with the solution turning yellow, indicating the completion of the redox reaction and the total consumption of the reductant as described by the system's balanced redox equation. The significance of the half-equivalence point can be seen in the Nernst equation:

$$E = E° - (RT/nF) \ln Q$$

In this case, Q refers to the ratio of oxidized and non-oxidized reactant. At the half-equivalence point, these two quantities are equal and $Q = 1$. Since $\ln(1) = 0$, at the half equivalence point, the value of E (measured against whichever reference electrode one chooses) is equal to the value of $E°$ for the redox couple being titrated.

32.6 ELECTROLYTIC CELLS

Unlike a galvanic cell, an **electrolytic cell** *uses* an external voltage source (such as a battery) to *create an electric current* that forces a nonspontaneous redox reaction to occur. This is known as **electrolysis**. A typical example of an electrolytic cell is one used to form sodium metal and chlorine gas from molten NaCl.

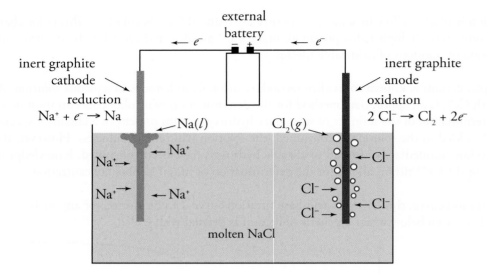

The half-reactions for converting molten Na^+Cl^- into sodium and chlorine are

$$Na^+ + e^- \rightarrow Na(l) \qquad E° = -2.71 \text{ V}$$
$$2\, Cl^- \rightarrow Cl_2(g) + 2e^- \qquad E° = -1.36 \text{ V}$$

The standard voltage for the overall reaction is −4.07 V, which means the reaction is *not* spontaneous. The electrolytic cell shown above uses an external battery to remove electrons from chloride ions and forces sodium ions to accept them. In so doing, the sodium ions are reduced to sodium metal, and the chloride ions are oxidized to produce chlorine gas, which bubbles out of the electrolyte.

Electrolytic cells are also used for plating a thin layer of metal on top of another material, a process known as **electroplating**. If a fork is used as the cathode in an electrolytic cell whose electrolyte contains silver ions, silver will precipitate onto the fork, producing a silver-plated fork. Other examples of metal plating include gold-plated jewelry, and plating tin or chromium onto steel (for tin cans and car bumpers).

Galvanic vs. Electrolytic Cells

Notice that in both galvanic cells and electrolytic cells, the anode is the site of oxidation and the cathode is the site of reduction. Furthermore, electrons in the external circuit always move from the anode to the cathode. The difference, of course, is that a galvanic cell uses a spontaneous redox reaction to create an electric current, whereas an electrolytic cell uses an electric current to force a nonspontaneous redox reaction to occur.

It follows that in a galvanic cell, the anode is negative and the cathode is positive since electrons are spontaneously moving from a negative to a positive charge. However, in an electrolytic cell the anode is positive and the cathode is negative since electrons are being forced to move where they don't want to go.

Galvanic	Electrolytic
Reduction at cathode	
Oxidation at anode	
Electrons flow from anode to cathode	
Anions migrate to anode	
Cations migrate to cathode	
Spontaneously generates electrical power ($\Delta G° < 0$)	Nonspontaneous, requires an external electric power source ($\Delta G° > 0$)
Total $E°$ of reaction is positive	Total $E°$ of reaction is negative
Anode is negative	Anode is positive
Cathode is positive	Cathode is negative

32.6

Example 32-7: The final products of the electrolysis of aqueous NaCl are most likely:

A) Na(*s*) and Cl$_2$(*g*)
B) HOCl(*aq*) and Na(*s*)
C) Na(*s*) and O$_2$(*g*)
D) NaOH(*aq*) and HOCl(*aq*)

Solution: This is a little tricky, but it provides a good example of using the process of elimination. We're not expected to be able to answer this question outright, since there is virtually no information provided. Instead, realize that choices A, B, and C list metallic sodium as a final product. That's a problem because we're in an aqueous medium, and we know that sodium metal reacts violently in water to form NaOH and hydrogen gas and fire. So after eliminating these choices, we're left with choice D.

Common Rechargeable Batteries

One particularly useful galvanic cell uses two different oxidations states of Pb for its constitutive electrodes and sulfuric acid as an electrolyte. Often referred to as lead-acid batteries, these cells constitute the oldest type of rechargeable batteries, and are perhaps most commonly employed as automobile batteries.

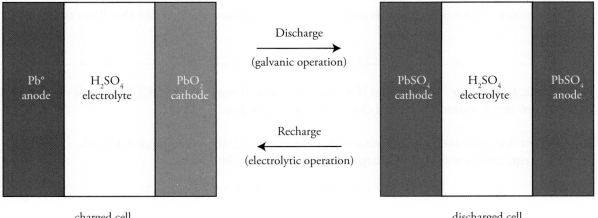

As depicted in the simplified figure on the previous page, fully charged lead acid batteries utilize $Pb°$ as an anodic electrode and a cathode consisting of PbO_2. As the battery discharges, $Pb°$ undergoes a two-electron oxidation to $PbSO_4$, while PbO_2 is reduced to the same species, as described by the following equations.

$$Pb° + HSO_4^- \rightarrow PbSO_4 + H^+ + 2\,e^-$$

$$PbO_2 + HSO_4^- + 3\,H^+ + 2\,e^- \rightarrow PbSO_4 + 2\,H_2O$$

Recharging the battery involves reversing the electron flow of discharge with applied voltage, as an electrolytic cell. The oxidation of $PbSO_4$ back to PbO_2, along with the regeneration of $Pb°$ by the reduction of $PbSO_4$ restores the initial potential of the cell.

32.7

Nickel-cadmium batteries, or NiCad batteries, are another common type of rechargeable battery. These cells utilize a metallic $Cd°$ anode and a nickel oxide hydroxide ($NiO(OH)$) cathode. The redox reactions involved in the discharge of the battery are given below. To facilitate these reactions, NiCad cells contain an alkaline KOH electrolyte.

$$Cd° + 2\,OH^- \rightarrow Cd(OH_2) + 2\,e^-$$

$$2\,NiO(OH) + 2\,H_2O + 2\,e^- \rightarrow 2\,Ni(OH)_2 + 2\,OH^-$$

Recharging spent NiCad batteries, as one might expect, involves applying a voltage to run these two reactions in reverse (typical electrolytic-cell behavior).

32.7 FARADAY'S LAW OF ELECTROLYSIS

We can determine the amounts of sodium metal and chlorine gas produced at the electrodes in the electrolytic cell shown in Section 32.6 using Faraday's Law of Electrolysis:

> **Faraday's Law of Electrolysis**
> The amount of chemical change is proportional to the amount of electricity that flows through the cell.

For example, let's answer this question: If 5 amps of current flowed in the NaCl electrolytic cell for 1930 seconds, how much sodium metal and chlorine gas would be produced?

Step 1: First determine the amount of electricity (in coulombs, C) that flowed through the cell.
We use the equation $Q = It$ (that is, charge = current × time) to find that

$$Q = (5\text{ amps})(1930\text{ sec}) = 9650\text{ coulombs}$$

Step 2: Use the faraday, F, to convert Q from Step 1 to moles of electrons.
The faraday is the magnitude of the charge on 1 mole of electrons; it's a constant equal to $(1.6 \times 10^{-19} \text{ C}/e^-)(6.02 \times 10^{23} \text{ } e^-/\text{mol}) \approx 96{,}500 \text{ C/mol}$. So, if 9650 C of charge flowed through the cell, this represents

$$9650 \text{ C} \times \frac{1 \text{ mol } e^-}{96{,}500 \text{ C}} = 0.1 \text{ mol } e^-$$

Step 3: Use the stoichiometry of the half-reactions to finish the calculation.

a)   From the stoichiometry of the reaction $Na^+ + e^- \rightarrow Na$, we see that 1 mole of electrons would give 1 mole of Na. Therefore, 0.1 mol of electrons gives 0.1 mol of Na. Since the molar mass of sodium is 23 g/mol, we'd get $(0.1)(23 \text{ g}) = 2.3$ g of sodium metal deposited onto the cathode.

b)   From the stoichiometry of the reaction $2 \text{ Cl}^- \rightarrow Cl_2(g) + 2e^-$, we see that for every 1 mole of electrons lost, we get $\frac{1}{2}$ mole of $Cl_2(g)$. Since Step 2 told us that 0.1 mol of electrons were liberated at the anode, 0.05 mol of $Cl_2(g)$ was produced. Because the molar mass of Cl_2 is $2(35.5 \text{ g/mol}) = 71 \text{ g/mol}$, we'd get $(0.05 \text{ mol})(71 \text{ g/mol}) = 3.55$ g of chlorine gas.

Example 32-8: A solution of $KAu(CN)_4$ is used in gold plating. Approximately 200 mg of gold are deposited onto the surface of an object. Approximately how much charge was applied to achieve this result? $(F = 96{,}500 \text{ C/mol } e^-)$

    A)   100 C
    B)   300 C
    C)   10,000 C
    D)   30,000 C

Solution: Start by figuring out the oxidation state of Au in $KAu(CN)_4$. Since K in a compound always has an oxidation number of +1, and each cyanide ion counts as −1, the Au atom must be in the +3 oxidation state. Thus, the reduction half-reaction is $Au^{3+} + 3 \text{ } e^- \rightarrow Au(s)$. The key is to use the stoichiometric ratio present in that reaction to bridge between moles of Au and moles of electrons. This is a Faraday's Law question that can be solved with unit analysis (and a bit of rounding):

$$\left(200 \text{ mg Au}\right)\left(\frac{1 \text{ g}}{1000 \text{ mg}}\right)\left(\frac{\text{mol Au}}{\sim 200 \text{ g}}\right)\left(\frac{3 \text{ mol } e^-}{\text{mol Au}}\right)\left(\frac{\sim 100{,}000 \text{ C}}{\text{mol } e^-}\right) = 300 \text{ C}$$

Choice B is correct.

Part 6

MCAT
Organic Chemistry

Chapter 33
Organic Chemistry
Fundamentals

33.1 NOMENCLATURE BASICS AND FUNCTIONAL GROUPS

This section covers the fundamentals of nomenclature in organic chemistry. Although this section will require memorization as your primary study technique, it is in your best interest to be comfortable reading, hearing, and using this terminology. Although most of the terminology that appears on the MCAT is IUPAC, some common nomenclature is also used.

Basic Nomenclature

Carbon Chain Prefixes and Alkane Names			
Number of carbon atoms in a row	Prefix	Alkane	Name
1	meth-	CH_4	methane
2	eth-	CH_3CH_3	ethane
3	prop-	$CH_3CH_2CH_3$	propane
4	but-	$CH_3CH_2CH_2CH_3$	butane
5	pent-	$CH_3(CH_2)_3CH_3$	pentane
6	hex-	$CH_3(CH_2)_4CH_3$	hexane
7	hept-	$CH_3(CH_2)_5CH_3$	heptane
8	oct-	$CH_3(CH_2)_6CH_3$	octane
9	non-	$CH_3(CH_2)_7CH_3$	nonane
10	dec-	$CH_3(CH_2)_8CH_3$	decane

In the case of an all-carbon containing ring, these are preceded by the prefix **cyclo-**. Hence, a six-membered ring containing all $-CH_2-$ units is called *cyclohexane*.

Nomenclature For Substituents			
Substituent	Name	Substituent	Name
$-CH_3$	methyl	$-CH_2CH_2CH_2CH_3$	butyl (or *n*-butyl)
$-CH_2CH_3$	ethyl	$CH_3CHCH_2CH_3$ (with bond down)	*sec*-butyl
$-CH_2CH_2CH_3$	propyl	$-C(CH_3)_2-CH_3$ with CH_3 above and CH_3 below	*tert*-butyl (or *t*-butyl)
$H_3C-\underset{|}{\overset{H}{C}}-CH_3$	isopropyl		

Common Functional Groups

R = alkyl group   X = halogen (F, Cl, Br, I)

R₃C—CR₃
alkane

R₂C=CR₂
alkene or olefin

RC≡CR
alkyne

R—X
alkyl halide

R—ÖH
alcohol

R—S̈H
thiol

R—Ö—R
ether

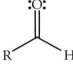
epoxide or oxirane

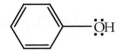
phenol

aldehyde

ketone

hemiacetal

acetal

cyanohydrin

amine

imine

enamine

carboxylic acid

acid halide

acid anhydride

ester

lactone

amide

lactam

33.2 ABBREVIATED LINE STRUCTURES

The prevalence of carbon-hydrogen (C—H) bonds in organic chemistry has led chemists to use an abbreviated drawing system, merely for convenience. Abbreviated line structures use only a few simple rules:

1. Carbons are represented simply as vertices.
2. C—H bonds are not drawn.
3. Hydrogens bonded to any atom *other* than carbon must be shown.

To illustrate rules 1 and 2, pentane can be represented using the full Lewis structure,

or using the abbreviated line structure.

Although C—H bonds are not drawn, the number of hydrogens required to complete carbon's valency are assumed. To clarify this, let's look more closely at the abbreviated line structure of pentane:

These three carbon atoms are each bonded to two other carbon atoms. In order to complete carbon's valency, we assume there are two hydrogens bonded to each of these carbons.

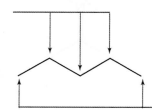

These two carbon atoms are each bonded to one other carbon atom. In order to complete carbon's valency, we assume there are three hydrogens bonded to each of these carbons.

This must be correct, because if we draw out all of the hydrogens in pentane, we get the full Lewis structure shown above.

To illustrate rule 3, consider dimethyl amine:

full Lewis structure

abbreviated line structure

Remember that hydrogens bonded to carbon can be assumed (the methyl groups in dimethyl amine, for example), but hydrogens bonded to any other atom must be shown. Lone pairs of electrons are often omitted.

Example 33-1: Translate each of the following Lewis structures into an abbreviated line structure:

(a)

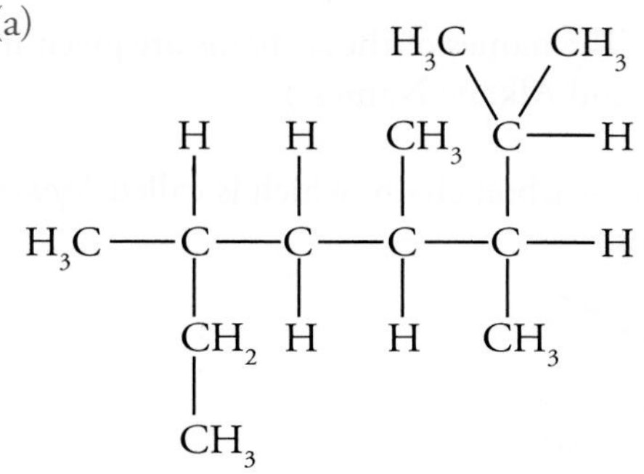

(b)

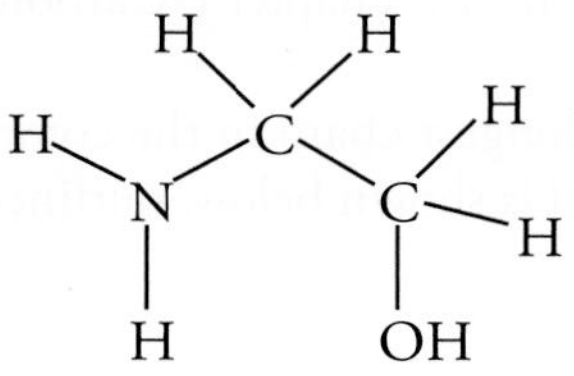

Solution:

(a)

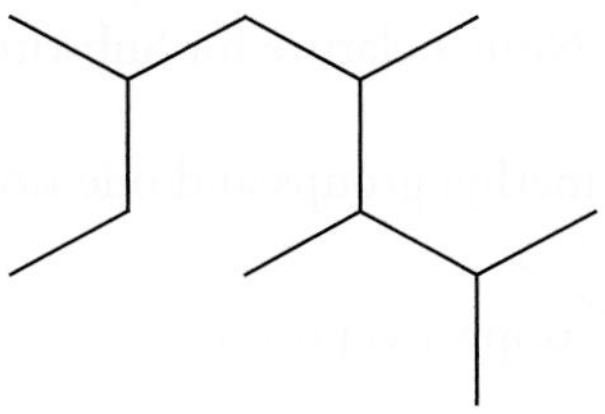

(b)

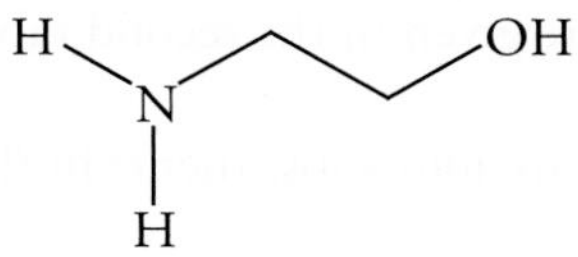

Example 33-2: Translate each of the following abbreviated line structures into a Lewis structure:

(a)

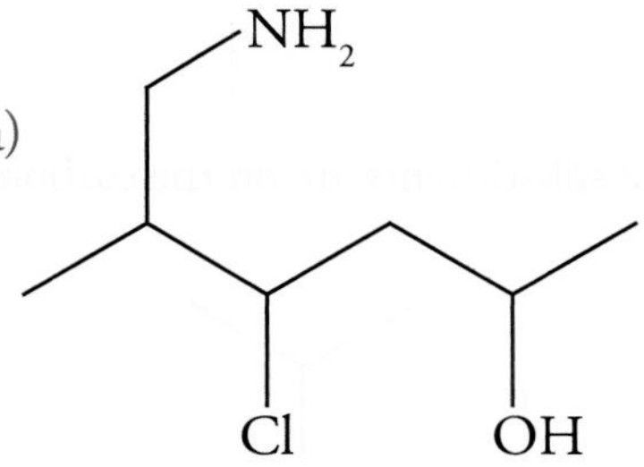

(b)

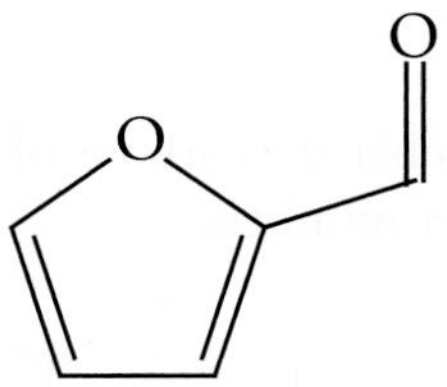

Solution:

(a)

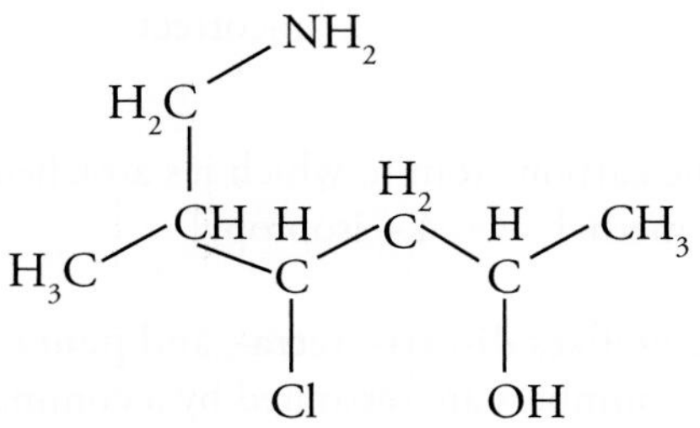

(b)

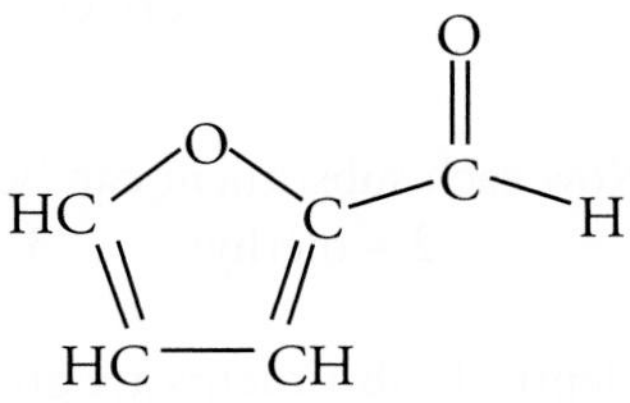

33.3 NOMENCLATURE OF ALKANES

33.3

Alkanes are named by a set of simple rules. One particular alkane (shown below) will be used to illustrate this process:

1. Identify the longest continuous carbon chain. The names of these chains are given in the first table in this chapter ("Carbon Chain Prefixes and Alkane Names").

   The longest chain in the compound above is a 7-carbon chain, which is called *heptane*. (This chain is shown below, outlined by dashed lines.)

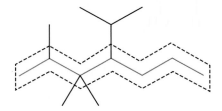

2. Identify any substituents on this chain. The names of some common hydrocarbon substituents are given in the second table in this chapter ("Nomenclature for Substituents").

   There are four substituents in this example: three methyl groups and one isopropyl group.

   methyl group   isopropyl group

   methyl groups

3. Number the carbons of the main chain such that the substituents are on the carbons with lower numbers.

   1 2 3 4 5 6 7   7 6 5 4 3 2 1
   correct   incorrect

   Now each substituent can be associated with the carbon atom to which it's attached:
   2 – methyl   3 – methyl   3 – methyl   4 – isopropyl

4. Identical substituents are grouped together; the prefixes **di-**, **tri-**, **tetra-**, and **penta-** are used to denote how many there are, and their carbon numbers are separated by a comma.

In this case, we have

$$\left.\begin{array}{l} 2-\text{methyl} \\ 3-\text{methyl} \\ 3-\text{methyl} \end{array}\right\} \longrightarrow 2,3,3\text{-trimethyl}$$

5. Alphabetize the substituents, ignoring the prefixes di-, tri-, et cetera and *n-*, *sec-*, *tert-*, and separate numbers from words by a hyphen and numbers from numbers by a comma. Note that "iso" is not a prefix but is part of the name of the substituent, so it is NOT ignored when alphabetizing.

The complete name for our molecule is therefore **4-isopropyl-2,3,3-trimethylheptane.**

Example 33-3: Name each of the following alkanes:

(a) (b) 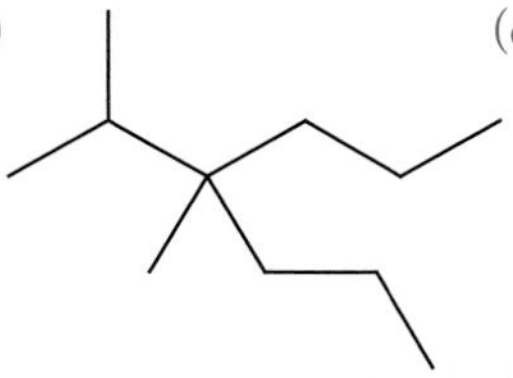 (c)

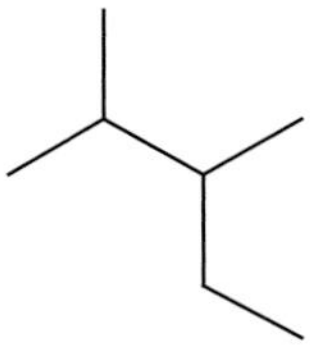

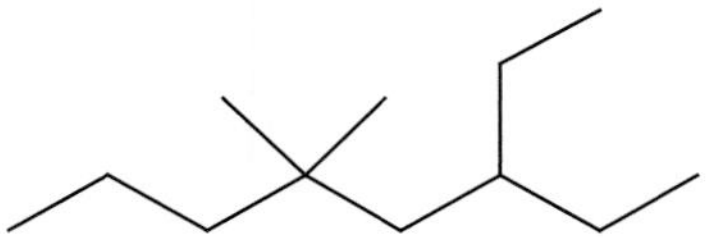

Solution:

(a) 2,3-dimethylpentane
(b) 4-isopropyl-4-methylheptane
(c) 3-ethyl-5,5-dimethyloctane

33.4 NOMENCLATURE OF HALOALKANES

Alkanes with halogen (F, Cl, Br, I) substituents follow the same set of rules as simple alkanes. Halogens are named using these prefixes:

Halogen	Prefix
fluorine	fluoro-
chlorine	chloro-
bromine	bromo-
iodine	iodo-

By applying the same rules as for naming simple alkanes, verify the following names:

Structure   Name

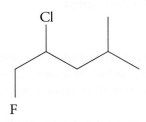

2-chloro-1-fluoro-4-methylpentane

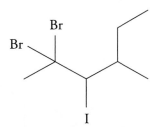

2,2-dibromo-3-iodo-4-methylhexane

Example 33-4: Name each of the following haloalkanes:

(a)   (b)

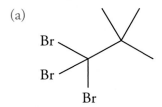

Solution:

(a)   1,1,1-tribromo-2,2-dimethylpropane
(b)   2-fluoro-2,3-dimethylpentane

Example 33-5: For each name, draw the structure:

(a)   3,4-difluoro-2,2,3-trimethylpentane
(b)   3-bromo-4-chloro-5,5-diethylnonane

Solution:

(a)   (b)

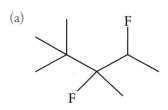
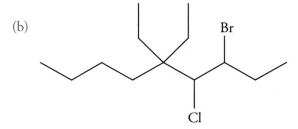

33.5   NOMENCLATURE OF ALCOHOLS

Alcohols also follow many of the same nomenclature rules as alkanes. Hydroxyl groups (–OH), however, are typically denoted by a suffix to the main alkyl chain. The table of straight-chain alcohols given below shows that to denote a hydroxyl group, the suffix **-ol** replaces the last **-e** in the name of the alkane.

Alkanes		Alcohols	
Structure	Name	Structure	Name
CH_4	methane	CH_3OH	methanol
CH_3CH_3	ethane	CH_3CH_2OH	ethanol
$CH_3CH_2CH_3$	propane	$CH_3CH_2CH_2OH$	propanol
$CH_3CH_2CH_2CH_3$	butane	$CH_3CH_2CH_2CH_2OH$	butanol

When the position of the hydroxyl group needs to be specified, the number is placed after the name of the longest carbon chain and before the -ol suffix, separated by hyphens. For example:

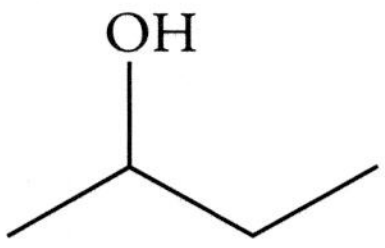

butan-2-ol
(or 2-butanol)
or *sec*-butanol

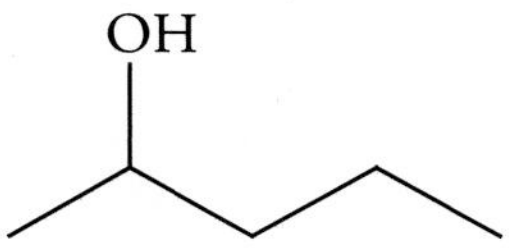

pentan-2-ol
(or 2-pentanol)

Priorities are assigned (the way the main carbon chain is numbered) to give the lowest number to the hydroxyl group. For example:

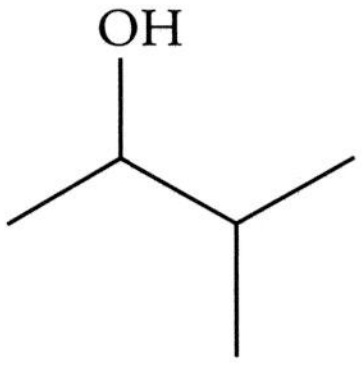

3-methylbutan-2-ol
not
2-methylbutan-3-ol

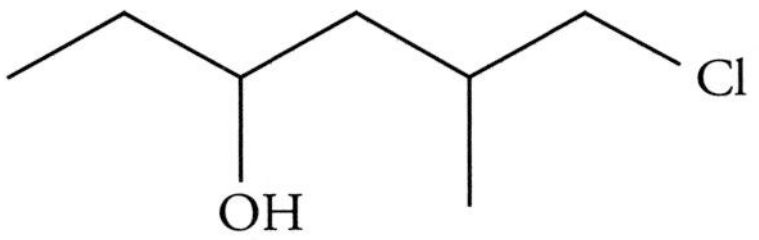

6-chloro-5-methylhexan-3-ol

Example 33-6: Name each of the following molecules:

(a)

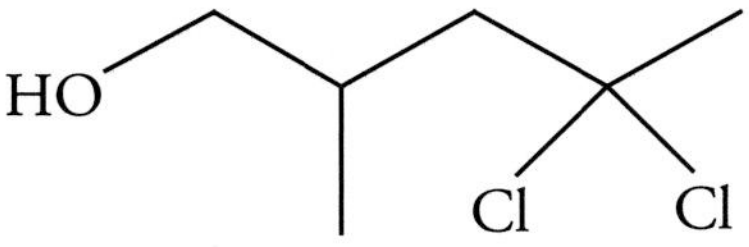

(b)

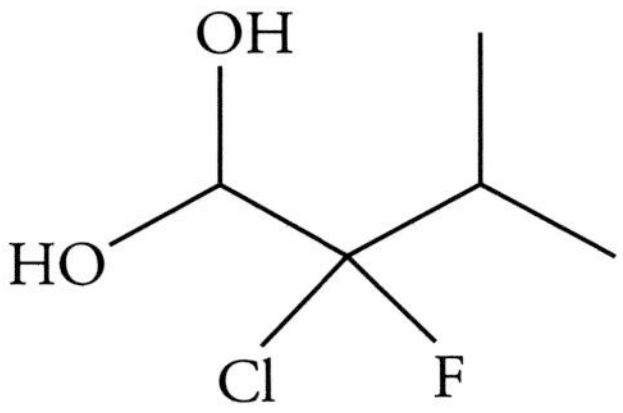

Solution:

(a)   4,4-dichloro-2-methylpentanol (the "-1-" is assumed if no number is given)
(b)   2-chloro-2-fluoro-3-methylbutane-1,1-diol

Chapter 34
Structure and Stability

34.1   THE ORGANIC CHEMIST'S TOOLBOX

Structural Formulas

By definition, an organic molecule is said to be **saturated** if it contains no π bonds and no rings; it is **unsaturated** if it has at least one π bond or a ring. A saturated compound with n carbon atoms has exactly $2n + 2$ hydrogen atoms, while an unsaturated compound with n carbon atoms has fewer than $2n + 2$ hydrogens.

The formula below is used to determine the **degree of unsaturation** (d) of simple organic molecules:

$$\text{degree of unsaturation} = \frac{(2n + 2) - x}{2}$$

n = number of carbons
x = number of hydrogens

One degree of unsaturation indicates the presence of one π bond or one ring; two degrees of unsaturation means there are two π bonds (two separate double bonds or one triple bond), or one π bond and one ring, or two rings, and so on. The presence of heteroatoms can also affect the degree of unsaturation in a molecule. This is best illustrated through a series of related molecules that all have one degree of unsaturation.

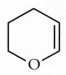

$d = [(2 \times 4 + 2) - 8]/2 = 1$
1-Butene has one degree of unsaturation—a double bond

$d = [(2 \times 5 + 2) - 8]/2 = 2$
Divalent atoms (e.g., O or S) can be ignored

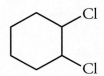

$d = [(2 \times 6 + 2) - 12]/2 = 1$
Each halogen is "replaced" by 1 H

$d = [(2 \times (3 + 1) + 2) - (7 + 1)]/2 = 1$
Trivalent atoms (e.g., N and P) are "replaced" by 1 C and 1 H

Example 34-1: Determine the degree of unsaturation of each of these molecules. Which, if any, are saturated?

    a) C_6H_8
    b) C_4H_6O
    c) C_3H_8O
    d) C_3H_5Br

Solution:

a) $d = [(2 \times 6 + 2) - 8]/2 = 3$.
b)   Ignore the O, and find that $d = [(2 \times 4 + 2) - 6]/2 = 2$.
c)   Ignore the O, and find that $d = [(2 \times 3 + 2) - 8]/2 = 0$. *This molecule is saturated.*
d)   Since Br is a halogen, we treat it like a hydrogen, so $d = [(2 \times 3 + 2) - (5 + 1)]/2 = 1$.

Hybridization

Every pair of electrons must be housed in an electronic orbital (either an *s*, *p*, *d*, or *f*). For example, the carbon atom in methane, CH_4, has *four* pairs of electrons surrounding it (four single covalent bonds and no lone pairs) so it must provide *four* orbitals to house these electrons. Orbitals always get "used" in the following order:

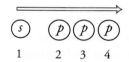

So, since the carbon atom in methane must provide *four* orbitals, we just count: 1…2…3…4.

Therefore, the hybridization of the carbon atom in methane is $s + p + p + p$, which is written as sp^3. The sum of the exponents in the hybridization nomenclature tells us how many orbitals of this type are used. So, in methane, there are $1 + 3 = 4$ hybrid orbitals. The following table gives the hybridization of the central atom for each of the orbital geometries:

Number of Electron Groups	Orbital Geometry	Hybridization of Central Atom
2	Linear	sp
3	Trigonal Planar	sp^2
4	Tetrahedral	sp^3

Reaction Intermediates

Carbocations, or **carbonium ions**, are positively charged species with a full positive charge on carbon. The reactivity of these species is determined by what type of carbon bears the positive charge. On the MCAT, carbocations will always be sp^2 hybridized with an empty p orbital.

Carbanions are negatively charged species with a full negative charge localized on carbon. The reactivity of these species is determined by what type of carbon bears the negative charge.

Stability Continuum				
Carbocations	3°	2°	1°	methyl
Carbanions	methyl	1°	2°	3°
	more stable	→		less stable
	less reactive	→		more reactive
	lower energy	→		higher energy

It's essential to understand the stabilities of reaction intermediates, because generally the reactivity of a molecule is inversely related to its stability. This means the molecules that are more stable are less reactive, while higher energy species will be more reactive. This theme will resurface over and over again in organic chemistry, and it is a useful rule of thumb to keep in mind when you need to predict how a reaction might proceed.

Inductive Effects

All substituent groups surrounding a reaction intermediate can be thought of as electron-withdrawing groups or electron-donating groups. **Electron-withdrawing** groups pull electrons toward themselves through σ bonds. **Electron-donating** groups donate (push) electron density away from themselves through σ bonds. Groups *more* electronegative than carbon tend to withdraw, while groups *less* electronegative than carbon tend to donate. On the MCAT, alkyl substituents are always electron-donating groups.

Electron
Withdrawal

Electron
Donation

Electron-donating groups tend to stabilize electron-deficient intermediates (carbocations), while electron-withdrawing groups tend to stabilize electron-rich intermediates (carbanions). The stabilization of reaction intermediates by the sharing of electrons through σ bonds is called the **inductive effect**.

Example 34-2: Inductive effects frequently alter the reactivity of molecules. Justify the fact that trichloroacetic acid (pK_a = 0.6) is a better acid than acetic acid (pK_a = 4.8).

Solution: The chlorine atoms in trichloroacetic acid are electron withdrawing. This decreases the amount of electron density elsewhere in the molecule, especially in the O–H bond. With less electron density, the O–H bond is weaker, making it more acidic than the O–H bond in acetic acid.

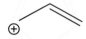

Resonance Stabilization

While induction works through σ bonds, resonance stabilization occurs in conjugated π systems. A **conjugated system** is one containing three or more atoms that each bear a p orbital. These orbitals are aligned so they are all parallel, creating the possibility of delocalized electrons.

Electrons that are confined to one orbital, either a bonding orbital between two atoms or a lone-pair orbital, are said to be **localized**. When electrons are allowed to interact with orbitals on adjacent atoms, they are no longer confined to their original "space" and so are termed **delocalized**. Consider the allyl cation:

The electrons in the π bond can interact with the empty p orbital on the carbon bearing the positive charge. This is illustrated by the following resonance structures:

delocalized picture, or resonance hybrid

The electron density is spread out—delocalized—over the entire 3-carbon framework in order to stabilize the carbocation. So, we might say of the allyl cation that both the electrons and the positive charge are delocalized.

As the allyl cation demonstrates, it often happens that a single Lewis structure for a molecule is not sufficient to most accurately represent the molecule's true structure. It is important to remember that resonance structures are just multiple representations of the actual structure. The molecule does not become one resonance structure or another; it exists as a combination of all resonance structures, although all may not contribute equally. All resonance structures must be drawn to give an accurate picture of the real nature of the molecule. In the case of the allyl cation, the two structures are equivalent and will have equivalent energy. They will also contribute equally to the delocalized picture of what the molecule really looks like. This average of all resonance contributors is called the **resonance hybrid**.

Benzene (C_6H_6) is another common molecule that exhibits resonance. Looking at a Lewis representation of benzene might lead one to believe that there are two distinct types of carbon-carbon bonds: single σ bonds (this structure of benzene has three such bonds) and double bonds (of which there are also three). Thus, one might expect two distinct carbon-carbon bond lengths: one for the single bonds and one for the double bonds. Yet experimental data clearly demonstrate that all the C—C bond lengths are identical in benzene. All the carbons of benzene are sp^2 hybridized, so they each have an unhybridized p orbital. Two structures can be drawn for benzene, which differ only in the location of the π bonds. The true structure of benzene is best pictured as a resonance hybrid of these structures. Perhaps a better representation of benzene shows both resonance contributors, like this:

benzene

Notice that these resonance structures differ only in the arrangement of their π electrons, not in the locations of the atoms. All six unhybridized p orbitals are aligned parallel with one another. This alignment of adjacent unhybridized p orbitals allows for delocalization of π electrons over the entire ring. Whenever we have a delocalized π system (aligned p orbitals), resonance structures can be drawn.

Delocalization of electrons is also observed in thiophene:

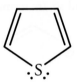

Here the sulfur atom has two pairs of non-bonding electrons. Notice that these electrons are one atom away from two π bonds. One pair of these electrons is actually in an unhybridized p orbital, such that it can be delocalized into the cyclic π system. Here are the representative resonance structures:

The other pair of electrons, however, is in a hybrid orbital and cannot delocalize into the π system. Here the delocalization of sulfur's electrons imparts aromatic stability to the molecule. The hybridization of the sulfur is therefore most correctly represented as sp^2.

Example 34-3: For the following molecules, indicate the hybridization and idealized bond angles for the indicated atoms.

a)

b)

c)

d)

Solution: Remember to always draw the electrons on nitrogen if they are not drawn in the structure.

a) i) sp^2, 120°   ii) sp^2, 120°   iii) sp^2, 120° (The lone pair is delocalized, so it's not counted.)
   iv) sp^3, 109°   v) sp^2, 120°   vi) sp^2, 120°
b) i) sp^3, 109°   ii) sp^3, 109°   iii) sp^3, 109°
c) i) sp^2, 120°   ii) sp^2, 120°   iii) sp^2, 120°   iv) sp^2, 120°
d) i) sp^3, 109°   ii) sp, 180°   iii) sp^3, 109°   iv) sp^3, 109°

So why all this focus on resonance? In general, the more stable a molecule is, the less reactive it will be. Since the delocalization of charge tends to stabilize molecules, resonance has a big impact on the reactivity of molecules.

Since it's important to recognize molecules that are stabilized by resonance, we'll next review the three basic principles of resonance delocalization.

1. Resonance structures can never be drawn through atoms that are truly sp^3 hybridized. Remember that an sp^3-hybridized atom is one with a total of four σ bonds and/or lone electron pairs.

No resonance
structures possible!

No resonance structures are
possible with these electrons.

No resonance structures are
possible with these electrons.

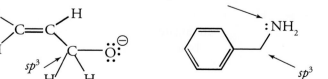

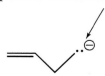

2. Resonance structures usually involve electrons that are adjacent to (one atom away from) a π bond or an unhybridized *p* orbital. Here are some examples of molecules that are resonance stabilized:

3. Resonance structures of lowest energy are the most important. Remember that the evaluation of resonance structure stability involves three main criteria:
   a. Resonance contributors in which the octet rule is satisfied for all atoms are more important than ones in which it is not. This is the most important of the three criteria listed here and takes priority over items b and c below.
   b. Resonance contributors that minimize separation of charge (formal charge) are better than those with a large separation of charge.
   c. In structures with formal charge(s), the more important resonance contributor has negative charges on the more electronegative atom(s) and positive charge(s) on the less electronegative atom(s).

Now that we can identify valid resonance structures of any given molecule and rank those resonance structures based on their relative energies, let's use this information to demonstrate the close relationship between stability and reactivity by examining acidity.

Acidity

Let's review the definition of a Brønsted-Lowry acid. Simply put, it's a molecule that can donate a proton (H⁺), and once the molecule has done so, it most commonly takes on a negative charge. This deprotonated structure is referred to as the conjugate base of the acid.

$$HCl \longrightarrow H^+ + Cl^-$$

acid   conjugate
                      base

The strength of an acid refers to the degree to which it dissociates (or donates its proton) in solution. The more the acid dissociates, the stronger the acid is said to be. Acids that dissociate completely are said to be strong. Most organic acids, and all organic acids you're likely to see on the MCAT, are said to be weak acids because they do NOT dissociate completely in solution.

The strength of the acid is determined by the extent to which the negative charge on the conjugate base is stabilized. This means all you need to rank the relative acidity of organic compounds on the MCAT is your background in ranking the stability of reactive intermediates.

Electronegativity Effects

Let's compare the acidity of an alcohol like propanol and an alkane like propane. If we compare the stability of each conjugate base, we find that the alkoxide ion is a relatively stable species compared to the carbanion since the negative charge is located on the very electronegative oxygen atom rather than on a carbon atom.

$$CH_3CH_2CH_2 \!-\! \overset{\cdot\cdot}{\underset{\cdot\cdot}{O}} \!-\! H$$

an alcohol

$$CH_3CH_2CH_2 \!-\! \overset{\cdot\cdot}{\underset{\cdot\cdot}{O}} {:}^{\ominus}$$

an alkoxide ion

$$CH_3CH_2CH_2 \!-\! H$$

an alkane

$$CH_3CH_2\overset{\cdot\cdot}{C}H_2{}^{\ominus}$$

a carbanion

Therefore, alcohols are considerably more acidic than hydrocarbons.

Resonance Effects

Let's next compare the relative acidities of propanol and propanoic acid.

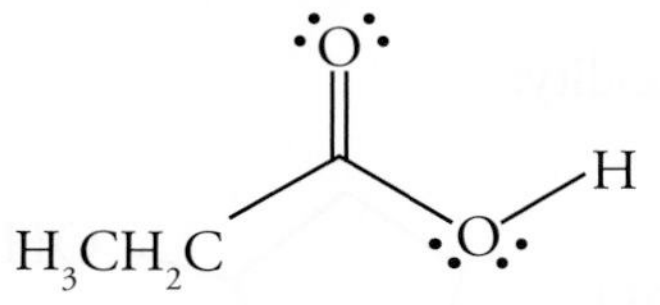

a carboxylic acid

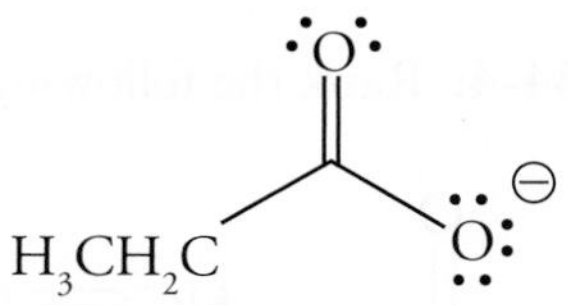

a carboxylate ion

In the carboxylate ion, the electrons on the negatively charged oxygen are adjacent to a π bond and can therefore be delocalized. This leads to greater stability of the carboxylate anion and thus to higher acidity of the conjugate acid.

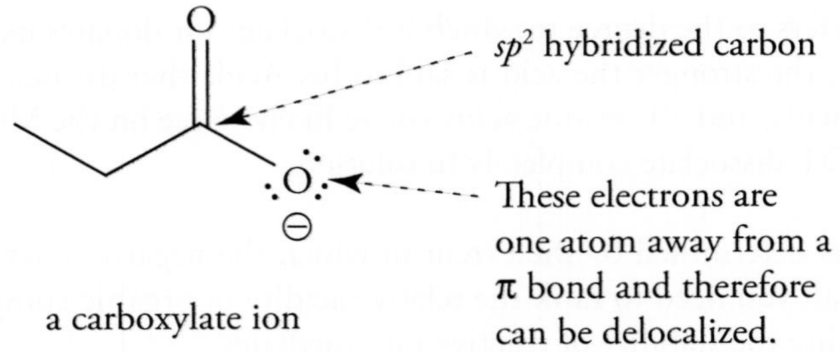

a carboxylate ion

Note that the two resonance structures of the carboxylate ion are equivalent, and are therefore of equal energy.

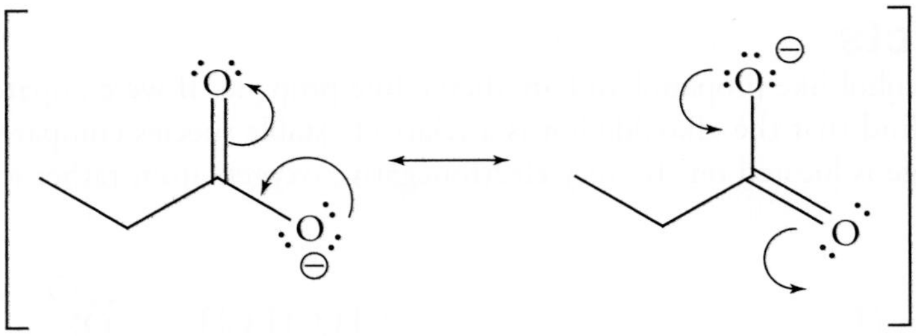

resonance structures for carboxylate ion

In contrast, the electrons on the oxygen of the propoxide ion below have no adjacent empty p orbital or π system. Therefore, they are localized and highly reactive, making an alkoxide ion a very strong base (much like OH^-) and the alcohol a weak acid.

an alkoxide ion

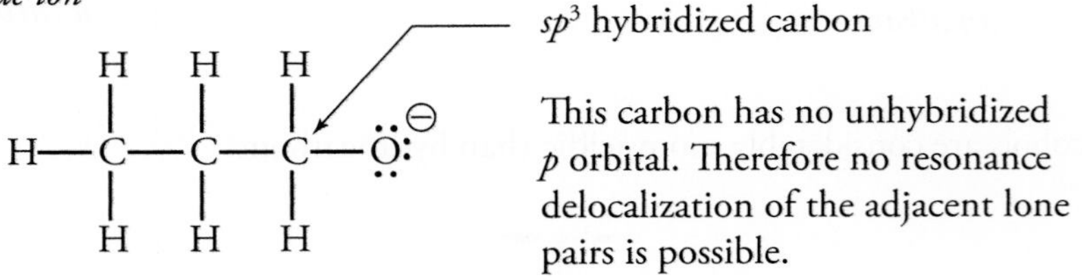

n-propoxide

This makes carboxylic acids, as their name suggests, much more acidic than alcohols.

Example 34-4: Rank the following acids in order of increasing acidity:

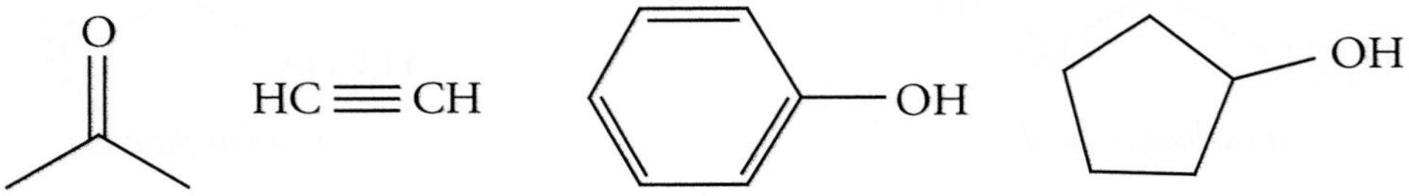

Solution: We examine the conjugate base of each acid in order to determine which one will have the more stabilized anion.

For the acetylene, there are no possible resonance structures for its conjugate base, and the negative charge is localized on carbon, an element with low electronegativity; **rank 1st** as the weakest acid.

In acetone, the hydrogens next to the carbonyl are acidic because there are two resonance structures for the conjugate base of a ketone. One is stable with the negative charge on oxygen, and one is higher in energy with the negative charge on carbon. Even though it has resonance, it is less acidic than cyclopentanol (see below) because some of the charge resides on the carbon; **rank 2nd**.

There are no possible resonance structures for this molecule, but the negative charge resides on an electronegative oxygen; **rank 3rd**.

Four resonance structures are possible for the phenoxide ion because the negative charge on the oxygen is adjacent to a benzene ring. However, they are not all of equivalent energy because the negative charge resides on the less electronegative C in three of the four structures. The delocalization of charge means that a phenol (–OH group attached to a benzene ring) is more acidic than an alkyl alcohol; **rank 4th** as the strongest acid.

Note that the phenol on the previous page would still be less acidic than a carboxylic acid since both resonance structures of a carboxylate ion have the negative charge on oxygen, rather than the less electronegative carbon in the phenoxide ion.

To summarize, here is a general ranking of the relative acidities of the most important organic functional groups you are likely to see on the MCAT:

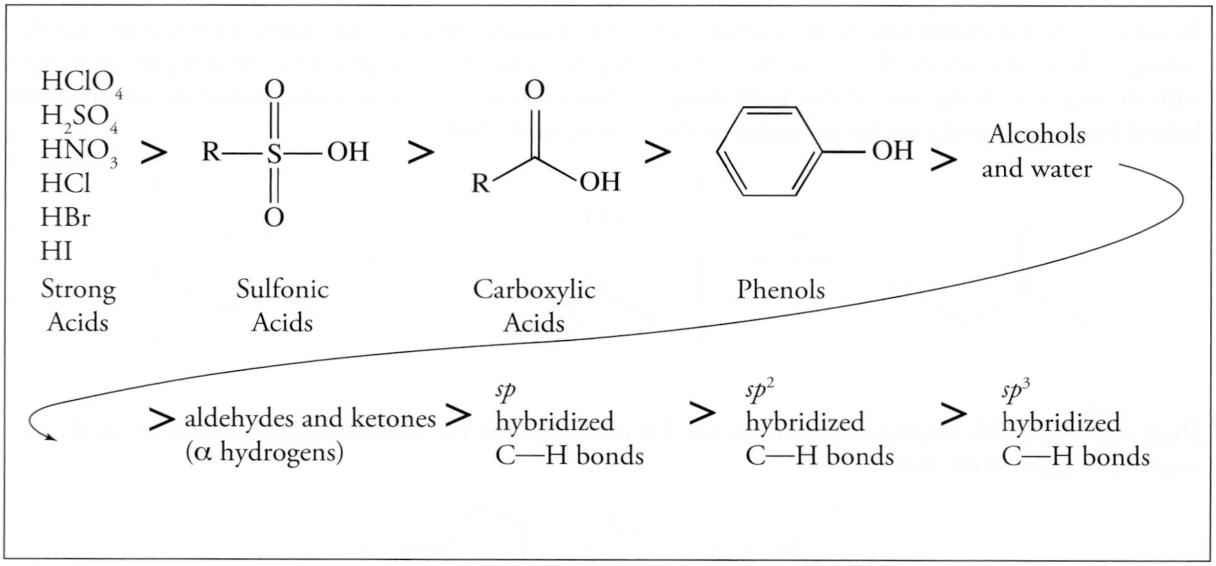

Figure 1 General Rule of Thumb for Organic Compound Acidity

Inductive Effects

As we've just learned, the acidity of carboxylic acids compared to alcohols results from the resonance stability of the carboxylate anion. In addition, Example 34-4 briefly illustrated how electron-withdrawing substituents next to the carboxylic acid group can increase the acidity of this (or any) functional group by increasing the stability of the negative charge on the anion. To expand upon this idea, inductive effects decrease with increasing distance; the closer the electron-withdrawing group is to the acidic proton (or the negative charge on the conjugate base), the greater the stabilizing effect. The following order of acidity for the isomers of fluorobutanoic acid should help clarify this point.

Order of Acidity

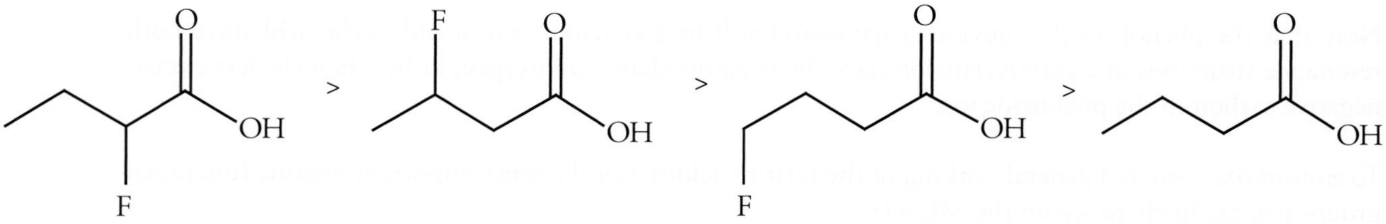

most acidic   least acidic

The magnitude of the effect is also dependent on the strength of the electron withdrawing substituent. In general, the more electronegative a substituent is, the greater its inductive effect will be. As shown below, while trifluoro-, trichloro-, and tribromoacetic acid all have substantially lower pK_a values than standard acetic acid ($pK_a = 4.76$); the trend in their acidities mirrors the electronegativity of their respective inductive group.

| pK_a = | 0.23 | 0.66 | 0.73 |

Example 34-5: Rank the following five compounds in order of decreasing acidity.

Solution:

c)	>	b)	>	a)	>	e)	>	d)
difluorinated carboxylic acid		monofluorinated carboxylic acid in α position		monofluorinated carboxylic acid in β position		phenol with electron withdrawing nitro group		diketone with 2 α protons adjacent to 2 carbonyls

Effects of Substituents on Acidity

Electron-withdrawing substituents on phenols increase their acidity. As an example, consider *para*-nitrophenol. The nitro group is strongly electron withdrawing and greatly stabilizes the phenoxide ion through resonance. Once the *para*-nitrophenol is deprotonated, it's easy to see how the nitro group can withdraw electrons through the delocalized π system such that the negative charge on the phenoxide oxygen can be delocalized all the way to an oxygen atom of the nitro group. This electron-withdrawing resonance stabilization of the nitro group increases the acidity of *para*-nitrophenol as compared to a phenol that does not have electron-withdrawing substituents.

On the other hand, consider a substituted phenol that has an electron-*donating* group rather than an electron-*withdrawing* group. A good example of this is *para*-methoxyphenol. Here, it is easy to see how once *para*-methoxyphenol is deprotonated, the negative charge on the oxygen can be destabilized by the donation of a lone pair of electrons from the methoxy oxygen so a negative charge is placed on a carbon that's adjacent to the negatively charged phenoxide oxygen. Electron-donating groups tend to destabilize a phenoxide ion and decrease the acidity of substituted phenols.

Example 34-6: For the following group of phenols, rank them in order of decreasing acidity.

Solution:

B > A > C. Due to the lone pair of electrons on the N, the NH_2 group is an electron-donating group. As such, it will decrease the acidity of the phenol, making it the least acidic of the three compounds.

Nucleophiles and Electrophiles

Most organic reactions occur between nucleophiles and electrophiles. **Nucleophiles** are species that have unshared pairs of electrons or π bonds and, frequently, a negative (or partial negative, δ^-) charge. As the name *nucleophile* implies, they are "nucleus-seeking" or "nucleus-loving" molecules. Since nucleophiles are electron pair donors, they are also known as **Lewis bases**. Here are some common examples of nucleophiles:

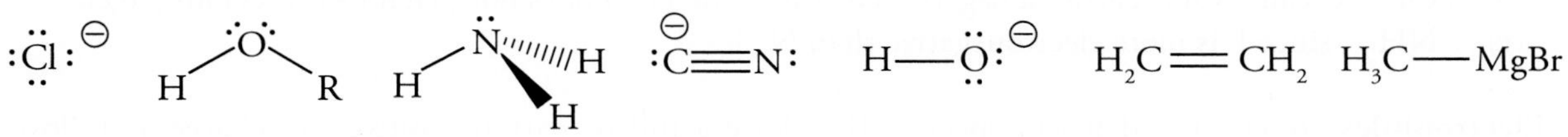

$$:\!\ddot{C}\!l\!:^{\ominus} \qquad \underset{H}{\overset{:\ddot{O}:}{\diagdown}}\!\!\underset{R}{\diagup} \qquad \underset{H}{\overset{:\ddot{N}''''''H}{\diagdown}}\!\!\underset{H}{\diagup} \qquad :C\!\equiv\!N\!:^{\ominus} \qquad H\!-\!\ddot{O}\!:^{\ominus} \qquad H_2C\!=\!CH_2 \quad H_3C\!-\!MgBr$$

Nucleophilicity is a measure of how "strong" a nucleophile is. There are general trends for relative nucleophilicities:

1. **Nucleophilicity increases as negative charge increases.** For example, NH_2^- is more nucleophilic than NH_3.
2. **Nucleophilicity increases going down the periodic table within a particular group.** For example, $F^- < Cl^- < Br^- < I^-$.
3. **Nucleophilicity increases going left in the periodic table across a particular period.** For example, NH_2^- is more nucleophilic than OH^-.

Trend #2 is directly related to a periodic trend introduced in general chemistry: **polarizability**. Polarizability is how easy it is for the electrons surrounding an atom to be distorted. As you go down any group in the periodic table, atoms become larger and generally more polarizable and more nucleophilic.

Trend #3 is related to the electronegativity of the nucleophilic atom. The more electronegative the atom is, the better it is able to support its negative charge. Therefore, the less electronegative an atom is, the higher its nucleophilicity.

You should note that Trend #2 should only be applied for atoms within a column of the periodic table, while Trend #3 should be applied for atoms across a row of the periodic table.

Example 34-7: In each of the following pairs of molecules, identify the one that is more nucleophilic.

a) $H-\ddot{\underset{..}{O}}:^{\ominus}$ or $H-\ddot{\underset{..}{S}}:^{\ominus}$

b) $H-\ddot{\underset{..}{O}}:^{\ominus}$ or $\overset{\displaystyle :\ddot{O}:}{\underset{\displaystyle H\qquad H}{}}$

c) $\underset{\displaystyle H\qquad H}{\overset{\displaystyle \ominus}{:\ddot{N}:}}$ or $:\ddot{\underset{..}{F}}:^{\ominus}$

Solution:

a) SH^-, since by Trend #2 on the previous page, S is more nucleophilic than O.
b) OH^-, because OH^- carries a negative charge, while H_2O does not (Trend #1, previous page).
c) NH_2^-, since F is more electronegative than N.

Electrophiles are electron-deficient species. They have a full or partial positive (δ^+) charge and "love electrons." Frequently, they have an incomplete octet. **Electrophilicity** is a measure of how strong an electrophile is. Since electrophiles are electron pair acceptors, they are also known as **Lewis acids**. Here are some common examples of electrophiles:

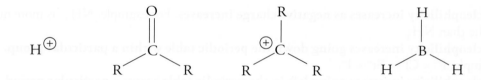

In all organic reactions (except free-radical and pericyclic reactions), nucleophiles are attracted—and donate a pair of electrons—to electrophiles. When the electrophile accepts the electron pair (a Lewis acid/Lewis base reaction), a new covalent bond forms between the two species, which we can represent symbolically like this:

$$\overset{\oplus}{E} \quad + \quad :\overset{\ominus}{Nu} \quad \longrightarrow \quad E-Nu$$

Leaving Groups

Generally speaking, the biggest take-home message about leaving groups is that they are more likely to dissociate from their substrate (that is, do their "leaving") if they are more stable in solution. Sound familiar? Our understanding of stability and reactivity is all we need to explain relative leaving group ability. For example, leaving groups that are resonance-stabilized (like tosylate, mesylate, and acetate) are some of the best ones out there.

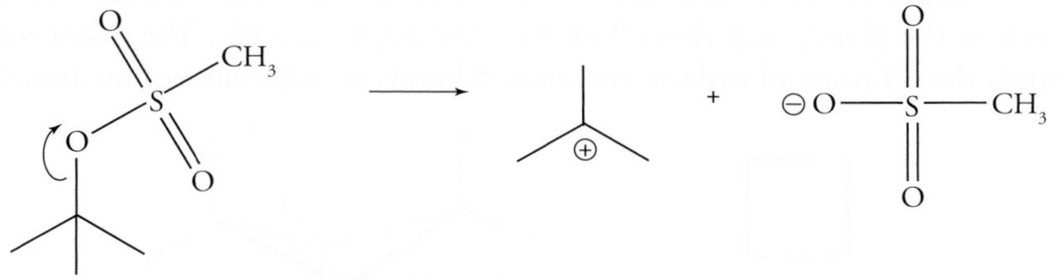

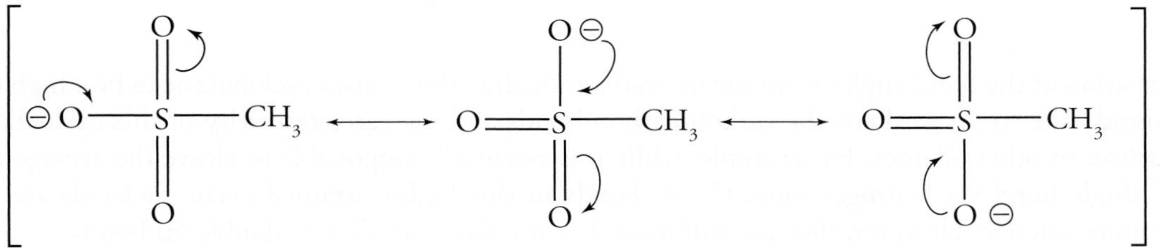

Figure 2   Resonance Structures of the Mesylate Leaving Group

In addition, weak bases (I⁻, Br⁻, Cl⁻, etc.) are good leaving groups because their negative charge is stabilized due to their large size. In fact, it's because basicity decreases down a family in the periodic table that leaving group ability increases. This periodic trend will be true for any family, though the halogens are the most common leaving groups you'll likely come across.

Strong bases (HO⁻, RO⁻, NH_2^-, etc.), on the other hand, are great electron donors because they cannot stabilize their negative charge very well, making them very reactive. As a result, these groups are more likely to stay bound to their substrate rather than dissociate in solution. As you might expect, strong bases are therefore bad leaving groups.

Now just because you're a bad leaving group one minute doesn't mean you can't be made better. For example, while the –OH group of an alcohol is unlikely to dissociate as OH⁻, treating the compound with acid protonates a lone pair of electrons on the oxygen, thereby making the –OH into $-OH_2^+$. The altered group can dissociate as a neutral water molecule, and *voila!*—no negative charge to stabilize. This trick will work for any of the strong bases listed above, and is the reason why many organic reactions are acid-catalyzed.

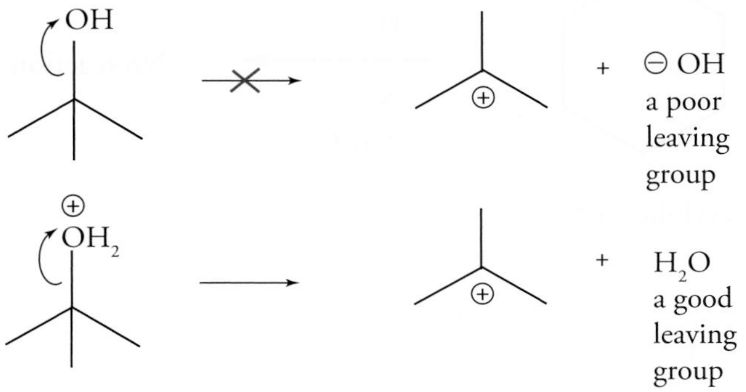

Ring Strain

The last item in our toolbox is a feature of organic molecules that, unlike inductive and resonance effects, contributes to instability in a molecule: **ring strain**. Ring strain arises when bond angles between ring atoms deviate from the ideal angle predicted by the hybridization of the atoms. compare two cycloalkanes to highlight these concepts.

Cyclobutane (C_4H_8) might be expected to have 90° bond angles due to its structure. However, one of the carbons is bent out of the plane, such that all of the bond angles are 88°. The distortion of the cyclobutane ring minimizes the eclipsing of carbon-hydrogen σ bonds on adjacent carbon atoms.

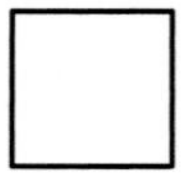

Cyclobutane

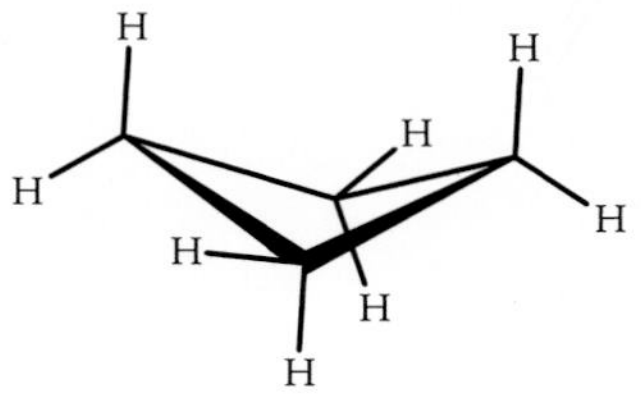

The deviation of the bond angles from the normal tetrahedral 109° causes cyclobutane to be a high energy compound. The strain weakens the carbon-carbon bonds and increases reactivity of this cycloalkane in comparison to other alkanes. For example, while it is essentially impossible to cleave the average alkane C—C single bond via hydrogenation, C—C bonds in this highly strained cyclic molecule are significantly more reactive. However, they are still much less reactive than C = C double (π) bonds.

Hydrogenation Reaction of Cyclobutane

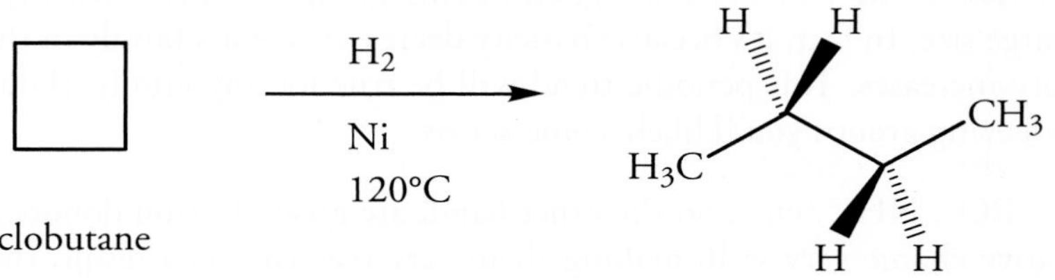

cyclobutane

butane

Unlike cyclobutane, cyclohexane is strain free because of the near-tetrahedral bond angles (109°) it has due to the conformation it adopts. Consequently, this compound does not undergo hydrogenation reactions under normal conditions, and reacts similarly to straight chain alkanes.

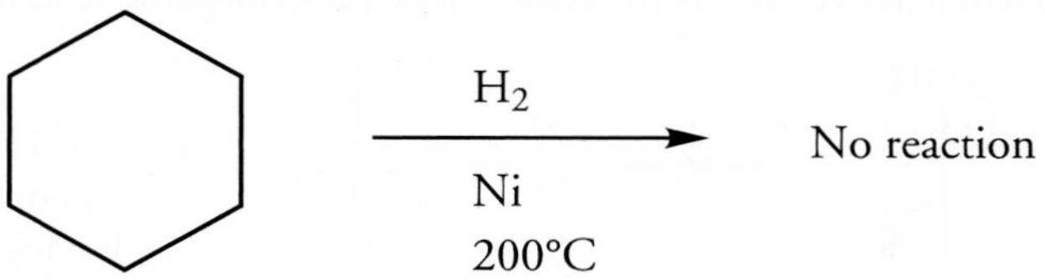

cyclohexane

34.2   ISOMERISM

Constitutional Isomerism

Constitutional (or, less precisely, *structural*) **isomers** are compounds that have the same molecular formula but have their atoms connected together differently. Take pentane (C_5H_{12}), for example. *n*-Pentane is a fully-saturated hydrocarbon that has two additional constitutional isomers:

| *n*-pentane | isopentane | neopentane |

Example 34-8: Draw (and name) all the constitutional isomers of hexane, C_6H_{14}. (*Hint*: There are five of them altogether.)

Solution:

| *n*-hexane | 2-methylpentane | 3-methylpentane |

| 2, 3-dimethylbutane | 2, 2-dimethylbutane |

Conformational Isomerism

Conformational isomers are compounds that have the same molecular formula and the same atomic connectivity, but differ from one another by rotation about a σ bond. In truth, they are the exact same molecule. For saturated hydrocarbons there are two orientations of σ bonds attached to adjacent sp^3 hybridized carbons on which we will concentrate. These are the **staggered** conformation and the **eclipsed** conformation. In staggered conformations, a σ bond on one carbon bisects the angle formed by two σ bonds on the adjacent carbon. In an eclipsed conformation, a σ bond on one carbon directly lines up with a σ bond on an adjacent carbon. Both conformations can be visualized using either the flagged bond notation, or the Newman projection, as shown with ethane (C_2H_6) below.

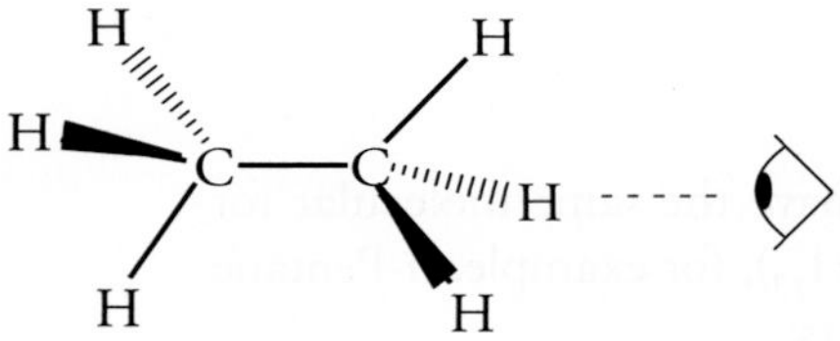

A staggered conformation

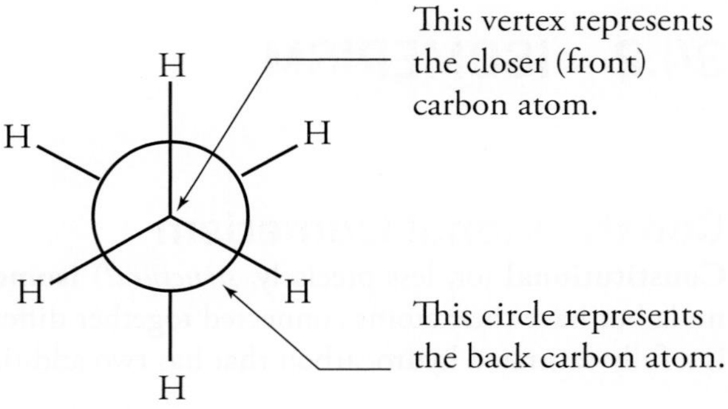

This vertex represents the closer (front) carbon atom.

This circle represents the back carbon atom.

A staggered conformation

If we were to look down the C–C bond, we would see:

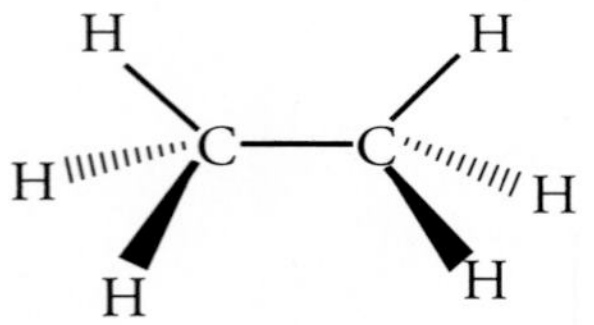

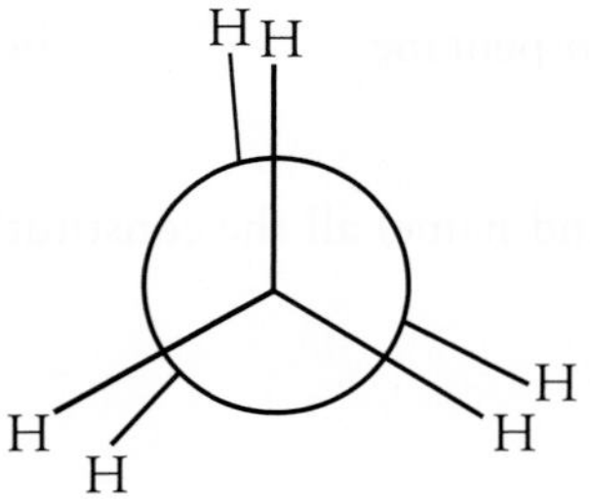

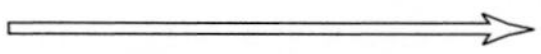

An eclipsed conformation

An eclipsed conformation

Example 34-9: For a), represent the flagged bond notation conformation as a Newman projection. For b), represent the Newman projection using flagged bond notation, and be sure to label which bond you are looking down when translating from the Newman projection.

a)

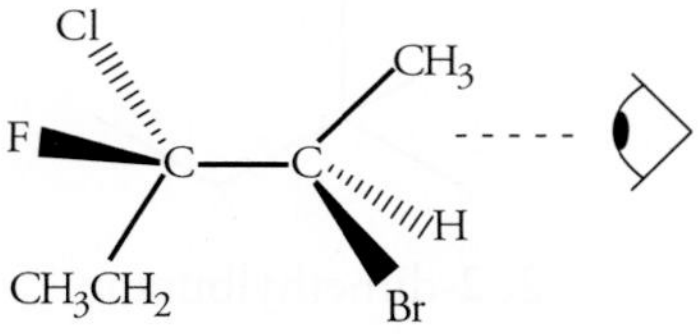

b)

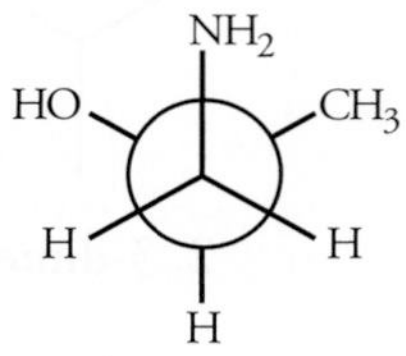

Solution:

a)

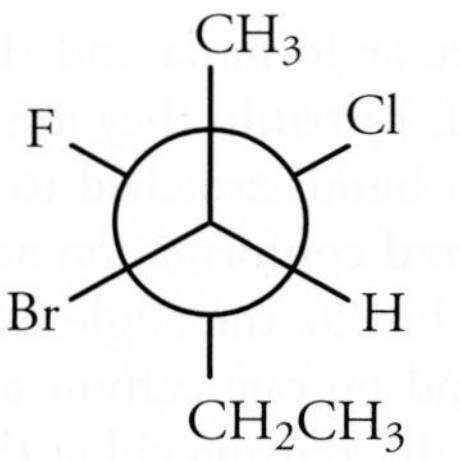

b)

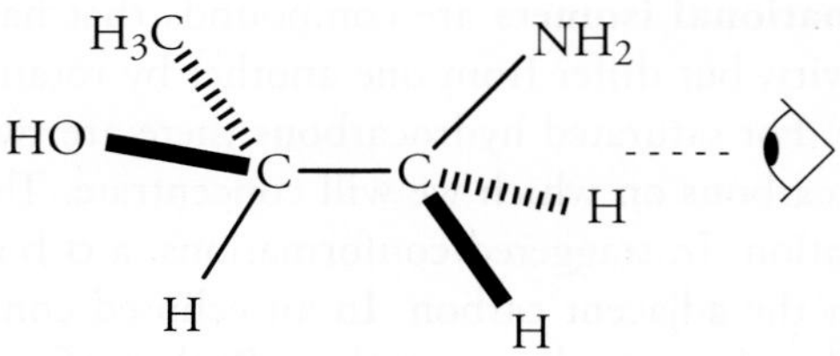

Using these notations, we turn our attention to the conformational analysis of hydrocarbons as demonstrated for *n*-butane.

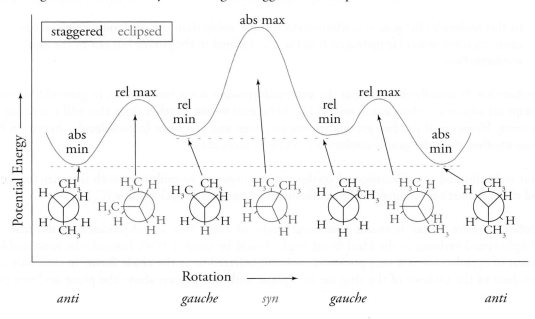

staggered conformation

less crowded
more stable

eclipsed conformation

more crowded
electronic repulsion
less stable

The σ bonds should actually directly line up with each other. For clarity here, they are not directly aligned.

It's important to note, however, that there are an infinite number of conformations for a molecule that has free rotation around a C—C bond, and that all of these other conformations are energetically related to the staggered and eclipsed conformations on which we will concentrate. For example, relative to the carbon atom in the rear of a Newman projection, the front carbon atom could be rotated *any number of degrees*. Any change in the rotation of one carbon, relative to its adjacent neighbor, is a change in molecular conformation.

A staggered conformation is more stable than an eclipsed conformation for two reasons. Covalent bonds repel one another simply because they are composed of (negatively charged) electrons. In the staggered conformation, the σ bonds are as far apart as possible, while in the eclipsed conformation they are directly aligned with one another. In addition, it is more favorable to have atoms attached to the σ bonds in the roomier staggered conformation where they are 60° apart, rather than the eclipsed conformation where they experience more steric repulsion. There are further aspects to consider in conformational analysis. Not all staggered conformations are of equal energy. Likewise, not all eclipsed conformations are of equal energy. The following demonstrates this by examining all staggered and eclipsed conformations for *n*-butane.

The most stable conformation of *n*-butane is referred to as the ***anti* conformation** and arises when the two largest groups attached to adjacent carbons are 180° apart. This produces the most sterically favorable, and hence the lowest energy conformation. Now we proceed through a series of 60° rotations around the C2–C3 σ bond until we return to the initial conformation (360°). In our first rotation, we go from the *anti* staggered to an eclipsed conformation and observe the relative energy maximum that results from the alignment of the methyls and hydrogens. Next, as we rotate another 60°, we fall again into a staggered conformation that resides in a relative energy minimum. Notice that this energy minimum is not as low as the *anti* conformation. In this structure, the methyl substituents are closer together (60° apart); this is referred to as a ***gauche* conformation**. In our next 60° rotation, we travel to the absolute maximum on our potential energy diagram. In this eclipsed conformation, the two methyl groups are directly aligned behind one another and are therefore in the most crowded and unfavorable environment. This conformation is referred to as the ***syn* conformation**. As we continue our rotation, we fall from the absolute energy maximum and go through the corresponding staggered and eclipsed conformations encountered before.

Example 34-10: Draw a Newman projection for the most stable conformation of each of these compounds:

a) 2,2,5,5-tetramethylhexane (about the C3—C4 bond)
b) 1,2-ethanediol

Solution:

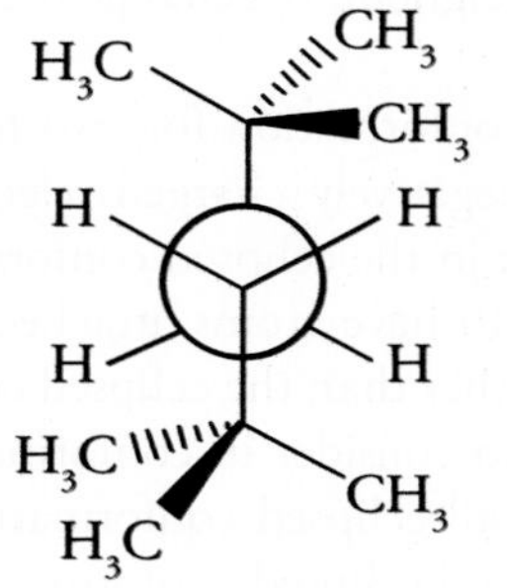

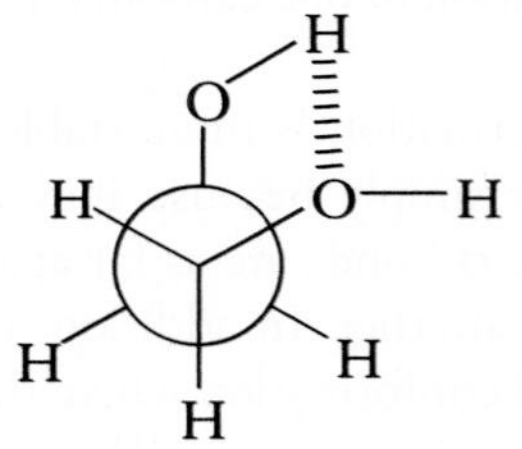

b)   In this molecule, the *gauche* conformation is more stable than the *anti* conformation, because an intramolecular hydrogen bond can be formed in the *gauche* but not in the *anti* conformation.

Remember that it's usually the case that the *anti* conformation is the more stable. In general, the two largest groups on adjacent carbon atoms would like to be *anti* to one another since this will minimize steric interactions. However, if the two groups are not too large and can form intramolecular hydrogen bonds with one another, then the *gauche* conformation can be more stable.

Thus far we've limited our discussion of conformational isomers to molecules with unrestricted rotation around σ bonds. Let's now consider the conformational analysis of cyclohexane (C_6H_{12}).

If cyclohexane were planar, it would have bond angles of 120°. This would produce considerable strain on sp^3 hybridized carbons as the ideal bond angle should be around 109°. Instead, the most stable conformation of cyclohexane is a very puckered molecule referred to as the **chair form**. In the chair conformation, four of the carbons of the ring are in a plane with one carbon above the plane and one carbon below the plane. There are two chair conformations for cyclohexane, and they easily interconvert at room temperature:

Chair representations of cyclohexane

As one chair conformation flips to the other chair conformation, it must pass through several other less stable conformations It is important to remember, however, that all of these high energy conformations do not play an important role in cyclohexane chemistry.

Notice that there are two distinct types of hydrogens in the chair forms of cyclohexane. Six of the hydrogens lie on the equator of the ring of carbons. These hydrogens are referred to as **equatorial hydrogens**. The other six hydrogens lie above or below the ring of carbons; these are called **axial hydrogens**.

At room temperature there is sufficient thermal energy to inter-convert the two chair conformations. Note that when a hydrogen (or any substituent group) is axial in one chair conformation, it becomes equatorial when cyclohexane flips to the other chair conformation. The same is also true for an equatorial hydrogen that flips to an axial position when the chair forms interconvert.

These factors become important when examining substituted cyclohexanes. Let's first consider methylcyclohexane. The methyl group can occupy either an equatorial or axial position:

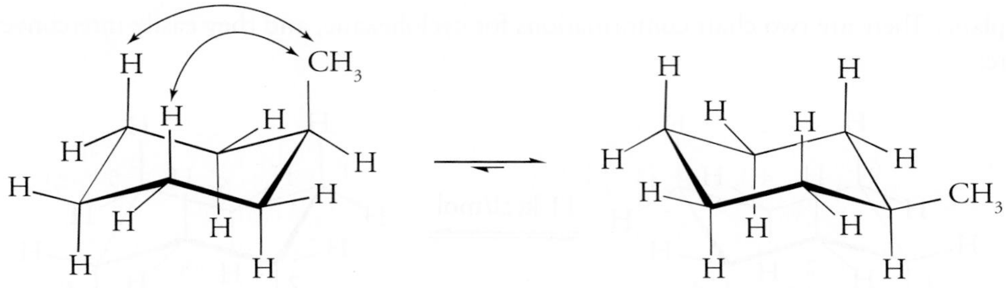

two 1, 3-diaxial CH₃–H
interactions

no 1, 3-diaxial CH₃–H
interactions

It is more favorable for large groups to occupy the equatorial position rather than a crowded axial position. This is because in the axial position, the methyl group is crowded by the other two hydrogens that are also occupying axial positions on the same side of the ring. This is referred to as a **1,3-diaxial interaction**.

Example 34-11: In each of the following pairs of substituted cyclohexanes, identify the more stable isomer:

a)

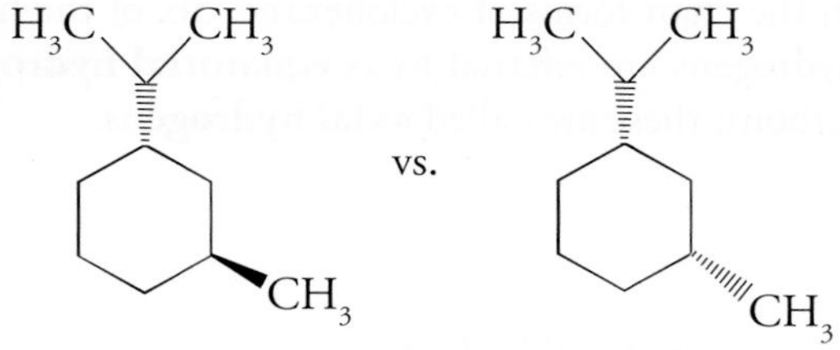

vs.

b)

vs.

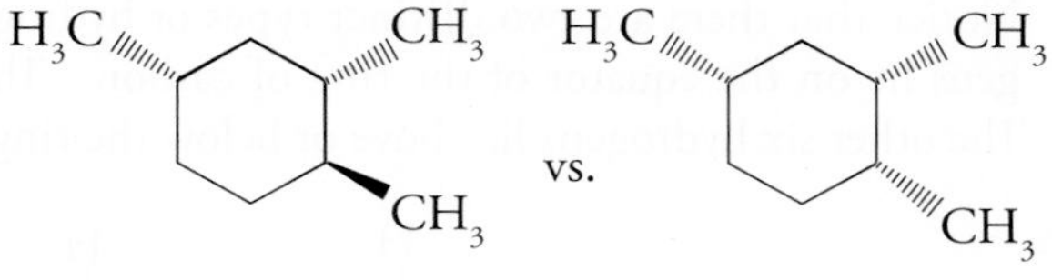

Solution: Draw chair conformations of each isomer and compare them to see which is more stable. As a good rule of thumb, it's best to first put the bulkier (that is, the larger) substituent in a roomier equatorial position and decide if it's the more stable of the two chair conformations; it usually is. (See figures below.)

a)

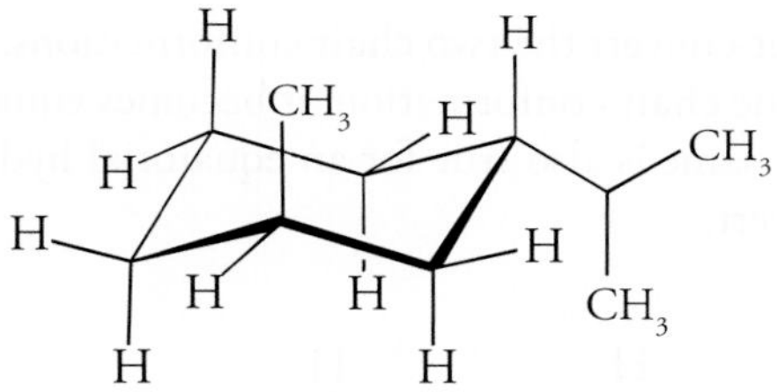

two 1, 3-diaxial CH₃–H
interactions

This is the more stable isomer.

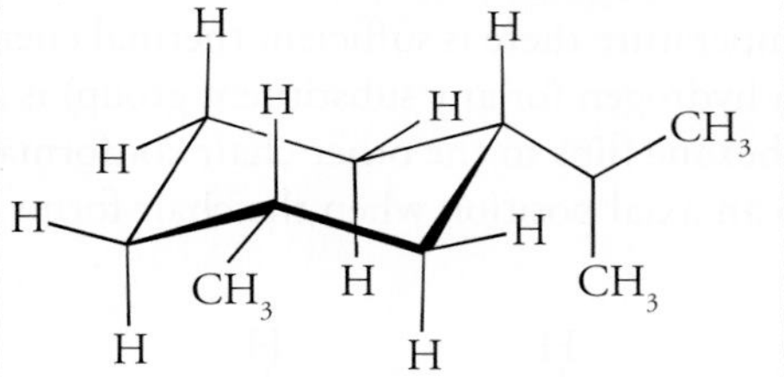

vs.

no 1, 3-diaxial CH₃–H
interactions

b)

This is the more stable isomer.

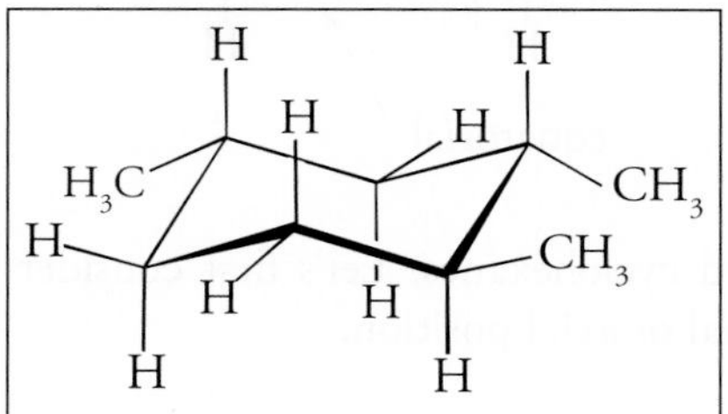

no 1, 3-diaxial CH₃–H
interactions

vs.

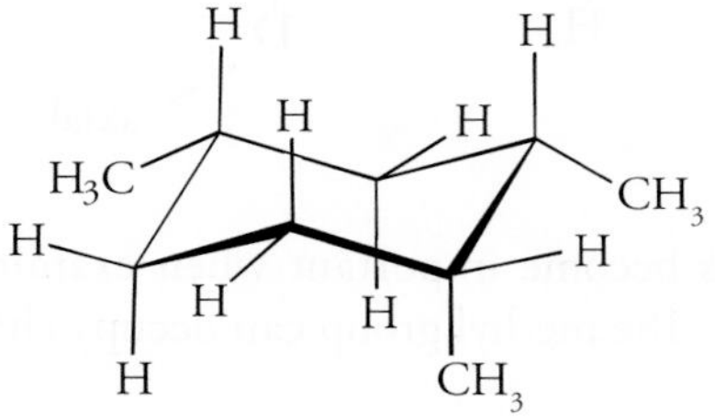

two 1, 3-diaxial CH₃–H
interactions

Stereoisomerism

Stereoisomerism is of major importance in organic chemistry, especially when looking at biological molecules, so several questions relating to stereochemistry routinely appear on the MCAT. **Stereoisomers** are molecules that have the same molecular formula and connectivity but differ from one another only in the spatial arrangement of the atoms. They cannot be interconverted by rotation of σ bonds. For example, consider the following two molecules:

Molecule I   Molecule II

Both molecules have the same molecular formula, C_2H_5ClO, with the same atoms bonded to each other. However, if one superimposes II onto I without any rotation, the result is

Note that while the $-CH_3$ and $-OH$ groups superimpose, the $-Cl$ and $-H$ do not. Likewise, if we rotate Molecule II so that the $-OH$ is pointing directly up (12 o'clock) and the $-CH_3$ is pointing at about 7 o'clock, and then attempt to superimpose II on I, the result is

While the $-Cl$ and the $-H$ groups are now superimposed, the $-CH_3$ and the $-OH$ are not. No matter how one rotates Molecules I and II, two of the substituent groups will be superimposed, while the other two will not. Hence, they are indeed different molecules: they are stereoisomers.

34.2

Chirality

Any molecule that cannot be superimposed on its mirror image is said to be **chiral**, while a molecule that *can* be superimposed on its mirror image has a plane of symmetry and is said to be **achiral**. It's important that you be able to identify **chiral centers**. For carbon, a chiral center will have four different groups bonded to it. Note that since a carbon atom has four different groups attached to it, it must be sp^3 hybridized with (approximately) 109° bond angles and tetrahedral geometry. Such a carbon atom is also sometimes referred to as a **stereocenter**, a **stereogenic center**, or an **asymmetric center**.

Example 34-12: Identify all the chiral centers in the following molecules and determine how many possible stereoisomers each compound has by placing a star next to each chiral center. (Note: the number of possible stereoisomers equals 2^n, where n is the number of chiral centers.)

a)

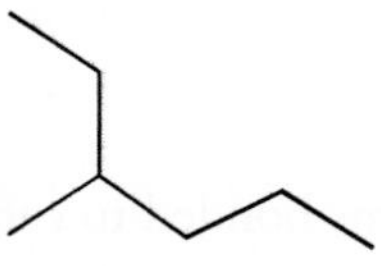

b)

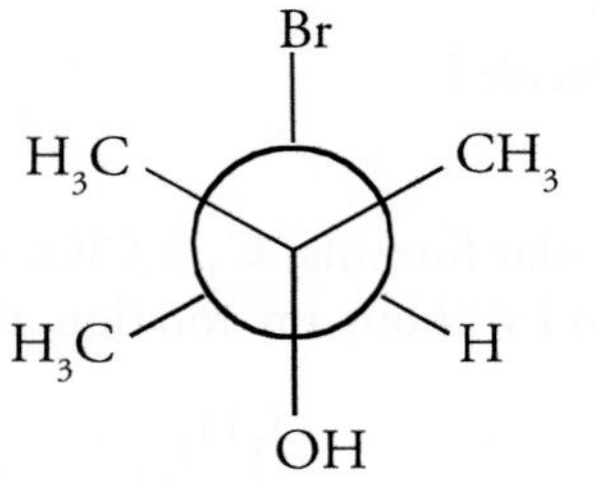

c)

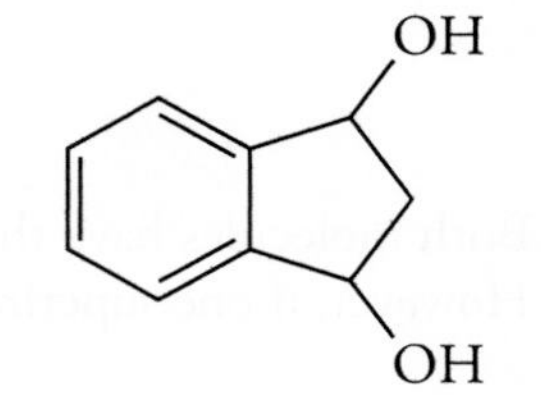

d)

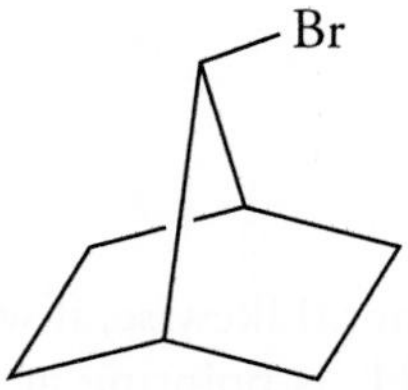

e)

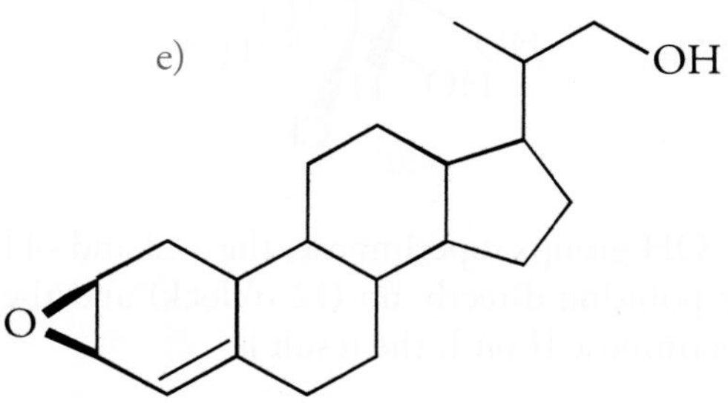

f)

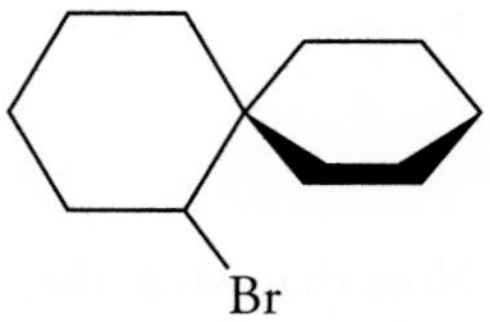

Solution:

a)   This molecule has 1 chiral center and, therefore, 2 possible stereoisomers:

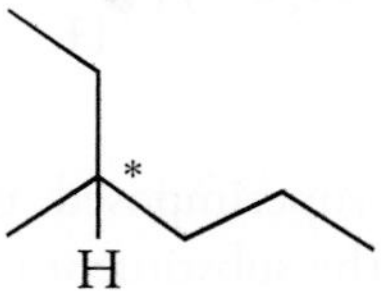

b)   This molecule has 1 chiral center and, therefore, 2 possible stereoisomers:

the back carbon

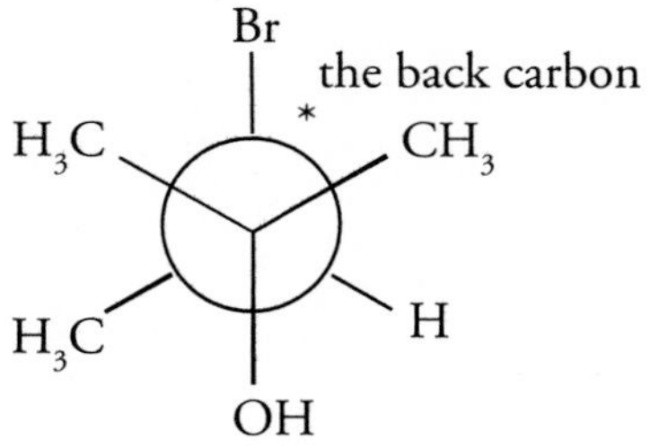

c) There are 2 chiral centers, which would seem to indicate 4 possible stereoisomers, however, there are only 3, because structures (iii) and (iv) are actually the same:

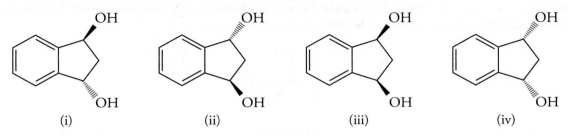

(i) (ii) (iii) (iv)

d) This molecule contains an internal plane of symmetry (pink) and thus has no chiral centers.

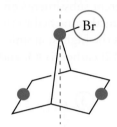

e) This molecule has 9 chiral centers and, therefore, $2^9 = 512$ possible stereoisomers:

f) This molecule has 1 chiral center and, therefore, 2 possible stereoisomers:

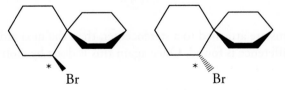

Absolute Configuration

Chiral centers (carbon atoms bearing four different substituents) can be assigned an **absolute configuration**. There is an arbitrary set of rules for assigning absolute configuration to a stereocenter (known as the Cahn-Ingold-Prelog rules), which can be illustrated using Molecule A:

Molecule A

1. Priority is assigned to the four different substituents on the chiral center according to increasing atomic number of the atoms directly attached to the chiral center. Going one atom out from the chiral center, bromine has the highest atomic number and is given highest priority, #1; oxygen is next and is therefore #2; carbon is #3; and the hydrogen is the lowest priority group, #4:

   If isotopes are present, then priority among these are assigned on the basis of atomic weight with the higher priority being assigned to the heavier isotope (since they are all of the same atomic number). For example, the isotopes of hydrogen are ^1H, ^2H = D (deuterium), and ^3H = T (tritium), and for the following molecule, we'd assign priorities as shown:

   If two identical atoms are attached to a stereocenter, then the next atoms in both chains are examined until a difference is found. Once again this is done by atomic number. Note the following example:

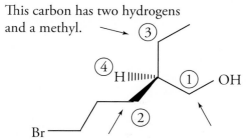

This carbon has two hydrogens and a methyl.

This carbon has two hydrogens followed by a –CH₂CH₂Br.

This carbon has two hydrogens and an –OH.

2.   A multiple bond is counted as two single bonds for both of the atoms involved. For example:

Carbon bonded to two oxygens and one hydrogen.

Carbon bonded to two hydrogens and only one oxygen.

3.   Once priorities have been assigned, the molecule is rotated so that the lowest priority group points directly away from the viewer. Then simply trace a path from the highest priority group to the lowest remaining priority group. If the path traveled is *clockwise*, then the absolute configuration is **R** (from the Latin *rectus*, right). Conversely, if the path traveled is *counterclockwise*, then the absolute configuration is **S** (from the Latin *sinister*, left).

Note: The two-dimensional representation (on the left) of the following hypothetical molecule is known as the "Fischer projection," named after famous organic chemist Emil Fischer.

The Fischer projection is a simplification of the actual three-dimensional structure. In the Fischer projection, as shown on the right, vertical lines are assumed to go back into the page, and horizontal lines are assumed to come out of the page.

The Fischer projection will be very important in our discussion of carbohydrates and will be covered extensively in future chapters.

Example 34-13: Assign absolute configurations to the following molecules.

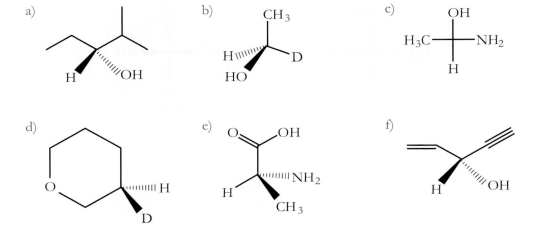

Solution:

a) *R.* Either rotate the molecule so the lowest priority group is in the back,

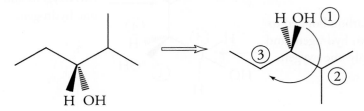

or simply trace it as it stands and invert the configuration (since the lowest priority group is coming toward you):

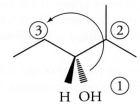

b) *R.* The lowest priority group is already pointing away from you and the trace is clockwise.

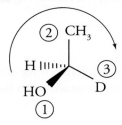

c) *R.* Recall Fischer notation for molecules, note that the lowest priority group is pointing away from you, and the trace is clockwise.

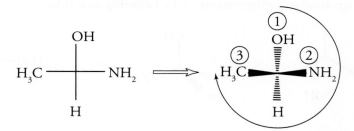

d) *R*. The lowest priority group is going into the plane of the page. Since the path is traveled clockwise, the configuration is *R*.

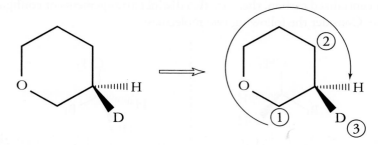

e) *S*. Rotate so the lowest priority group is in back,

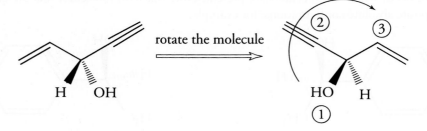

or exchange two groups, −H and −NH₂:

f) *R*. Rotate so the lowest priority group is in the back:

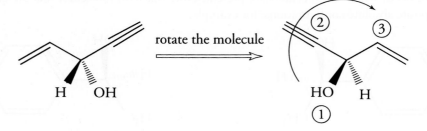

Enantiomers

It is important to be able to identify chiral centers because, as we have seen, when there are four different groups attached to a centralized carbon, there are two distinct arrangements or configurations possible for these groups in space. Consider the following two molecules:

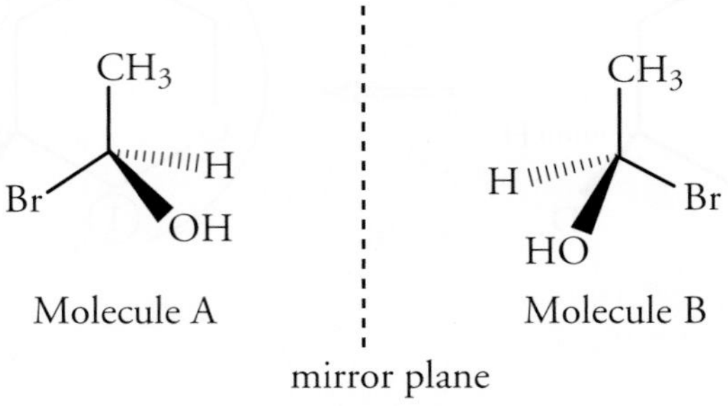

mirror plane

Molecule A has one chiral center with four different groups attached. Notice that Molecule B also has a chiral center and that the four groups attached to it are the same as those in Molecule A. Observe the mirror plane that has been drawn between Molecules A and B. Molecules A and B are mirror images of each other, but they are not superimposable; therefore, they are chiral.

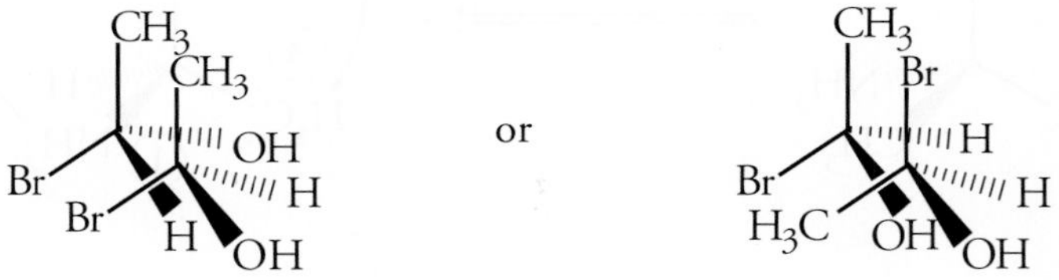

These molecules are **enantiomers**: non-superimposable mirror images.

Enantiomers can occur when chiral centers are present. Note that two molecules that are enantiomers will always have opposite absolute configurations; for example,

What are the properties of enantiomers? That is, how do they differ from one another? Most chemical properties such as melting point, boiling point, polarity, and solubility are the same for both pure enantiomers of an enantiomeric pair. That is, the pure enantiomers shown above will have many identical physical properties.

Optical Activity

One important property that differs between enantiomers is the manner in which they interact with plane-polarized light. A compound that rotates the plane of polarized light is said to be **optically active**. A compound that rotates plane-polarized light clockwise is said to be **dextrorotatory** (*d*), also denoted by (+), while a compound that rotates plane-polarized light in the counterclockwise direction is said to be **levorotatory** (*l*), also denoted by (−). The magnitude of rotation of plane-polarized light for any compound is called its **specific rotation**. This property is dependent on the structure of the molecule, the concentration of the sample, and the path length through which the light must travel.

A pair of enantiomers will rotate plane-polarized light with equal magnitude, but in opposite directions. For example, pure (+)-2-bromobutanoic acid has a specific rotation of +39.5°, while (−)-2-bromobutanoic acid has a specific rotation of −39.5°.

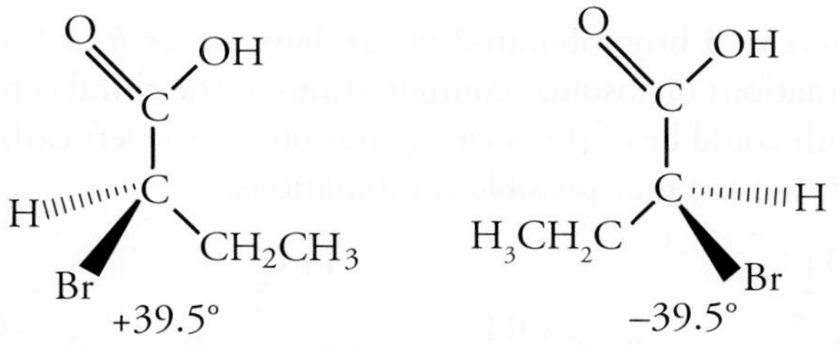

(+) and (−)-2-bromobutanoic acid

What do you think the specific rotation of an equimolar mixture of the two enantiomers above will be? Since one enantiomer will rotate plane-polarized light in one direction, while the other enantiomer will rotate light by the same magnitude in the opposite direction, the specific rotation of a 50/50 mixture of enantiomers —a **racemic mixture**—is 0°. Therefore, a racemic mixture of enantiomers, also known as a *racemate*, is not optically active.

Example 34-14: What is the specific rotation of the *R* enantiomer of 2-bromobutanoic acid? Of the *S* enantiomer?

Solution:

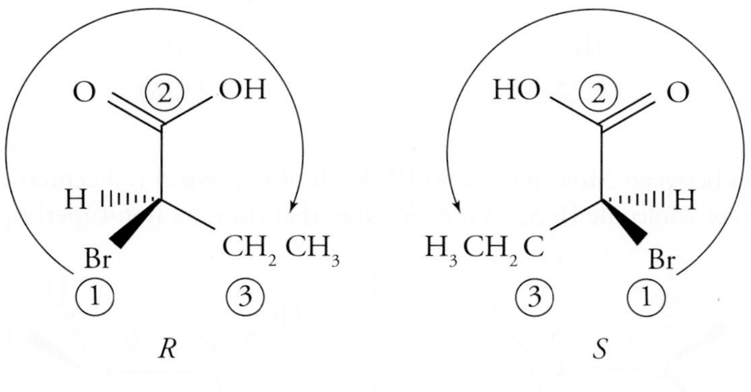

The magnitude of rotation cannot be predicted; it must be experimentally determined. It just so happens in this case that the *R* enantiomer has the (+) rotation [while the *S* enantiomer has the (−) rotation.] But be careful: ***This is only coincidental. (+) and (−) say nothing about whether the absolute configuration is R or S.*** There is no correlation between the sign of rotation and the absolute configuration.

34.2

Diastereomers

In the preceding discussions on stereoisomerism we have focused on molecules that have only one chiral center. What about molecules with multiple stereocenters? Remember that the number of possible stereoisomers is 2^n, where n is the number of chiral centers. If there is one chiral center, then there are two possible stereoisomers: the enantiomeric pair R and S. Two chiral centers means there are four possible stereoisomers. Consider the following molecule (3-bromobutan-2-ol), for example:

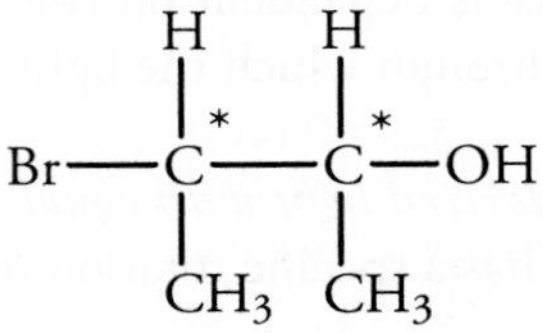

Each of the two chiral centers in 3-bromobutan-2-ol can have either R or S absolute configuration. This leads to four possible combinations of absolute configurations at the chiral centers. Both carbons could be of the S configuration or both could be of the R configuration; or, the left carbon could be R and the right carbon S, or vice versa. Here are the four possible combinations:

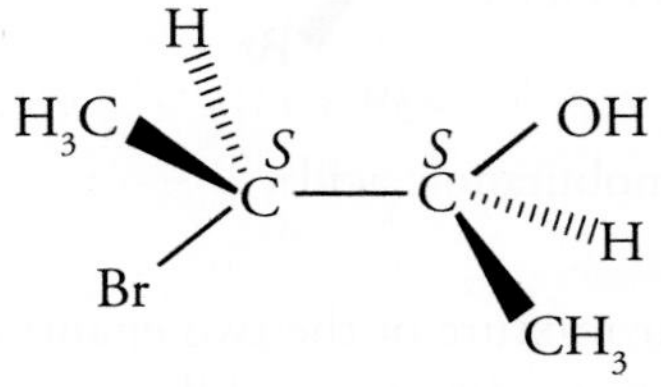

I
(S, S)

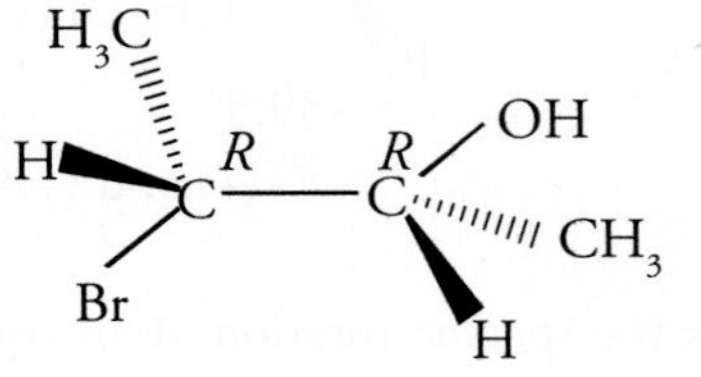

II
(R, R)

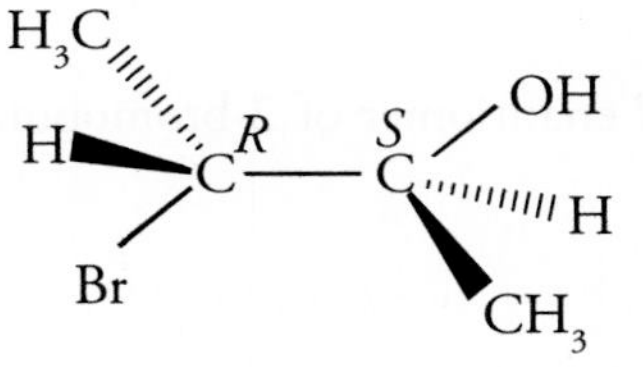

III
(R, S)

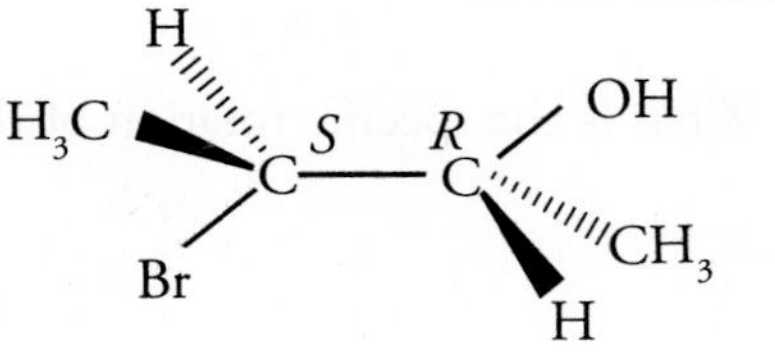

IV
(S, R)

What's the relationship between Molecules I and II? Each of the two chiral centers in Molecule I is of the opposite configuration of Molecule II: S, S vs. R, R. Note that they are non-superimposable mirror images:

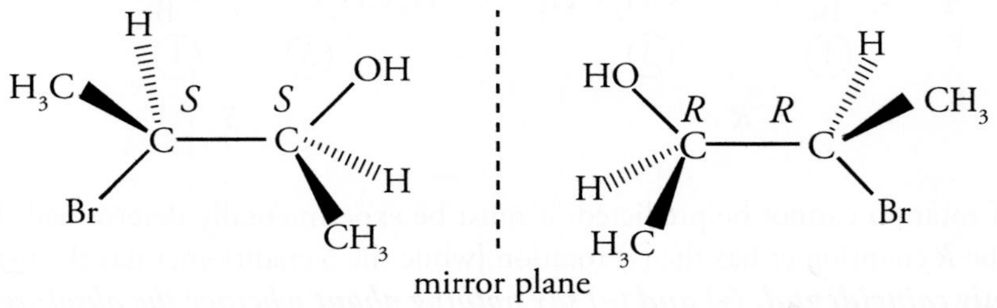

mirror plane

I

II

Therefore, these molecules are enantiomers. What about Molecules III and IV? Once again, each of the two chiral centers in Molecule III is of the opposite configuration of those in Molecule IV. This makes Molecules III and IV an enantiomer pair, just as we noted for Molecules I and II on the previous page. Is there a relationship between Molecules I and III?

By mentally moving Molecule III to the left and aligning it over Molecule I, we see that the right chiral centers of both molecules are directly superimposable (*S* superimposes onto *S*). Also note that no matter what we do, we cannot get the left chiral centers of Molecules I and III to superimpose (*S* does not superimpose onto *R*).

Molecules I and III are diastereomers. **Diastereomers** are stereoisomers that are not enantiomers. That is, diastereomers are stereoisomers that are non-superimposable, non-mirror images. The same is true for Molecules I and IV. One of the chiral centers is of the same absolute configuration, while the other chiral center is of the opposite configuration:

The figure below summarizes all possible stereochemical relationships between isomers containing two stereocenters. Inverting at least one, but not all, of the chiral centers within a molecule will form a diastereomer of that molecule. Enantiomers can be formed by inverting every stereocenter within the molecule.

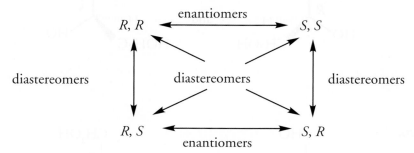

Example 34-15: For each pair of molecules below, state the relationship between them.

(a)

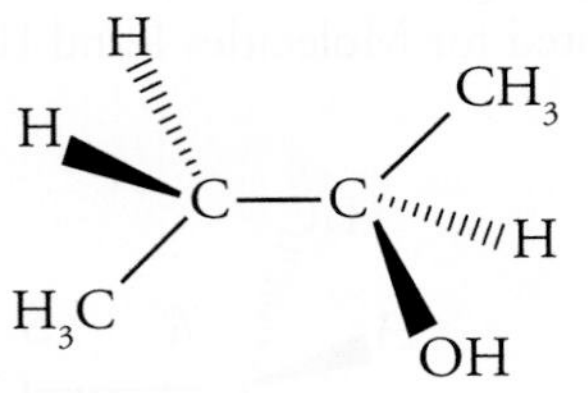

and

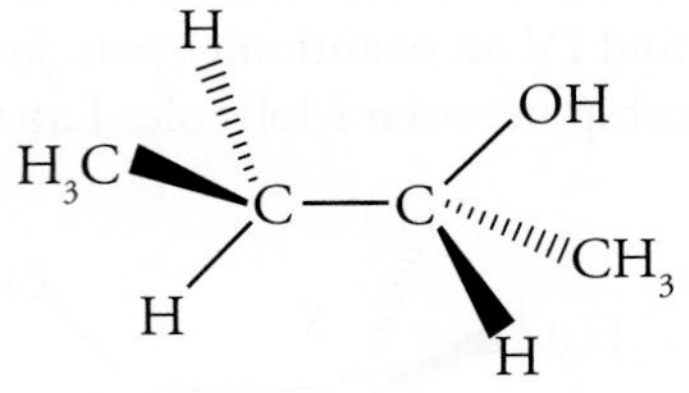

(b)

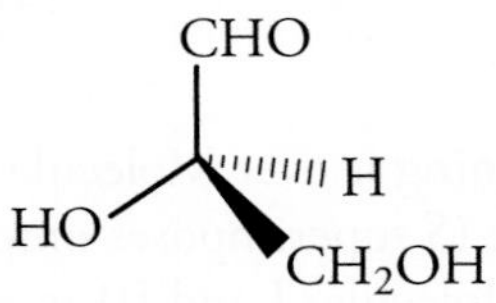

and

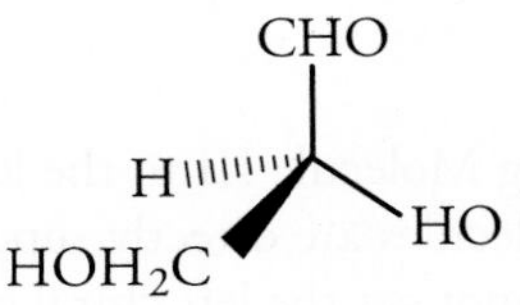

(c)

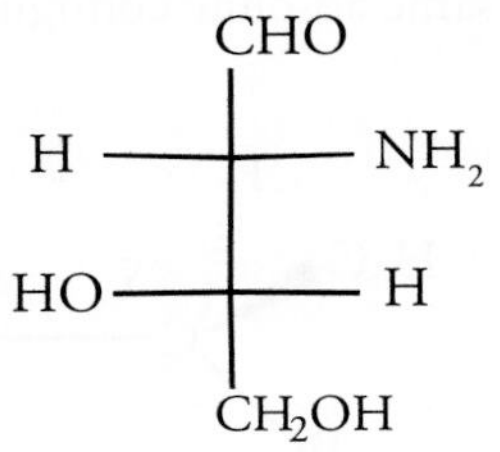

and

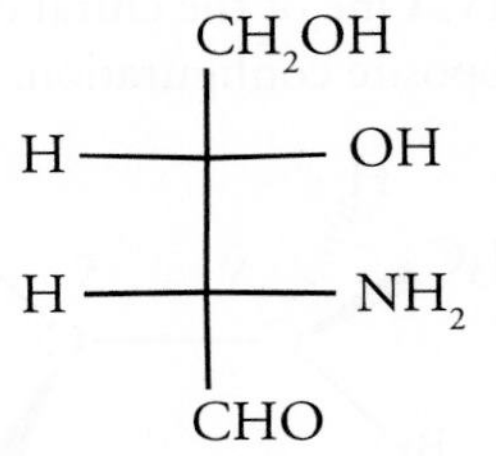

Solution:

a) The molecules are *identical*. (The left carbon is not a chiral center.)

b) *Enantiomers.*

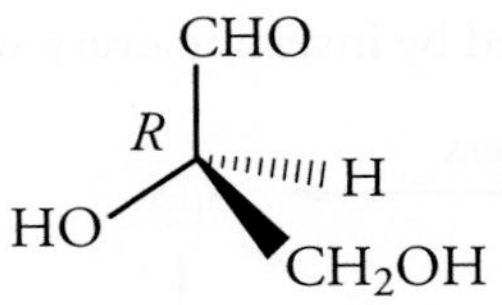

and

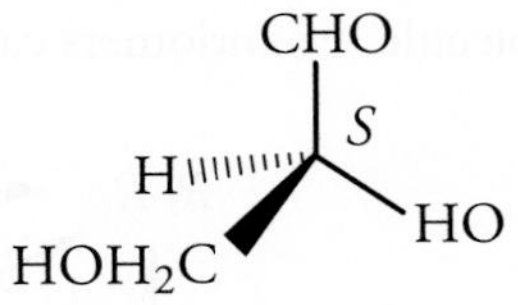

c) *Diastereomers.*

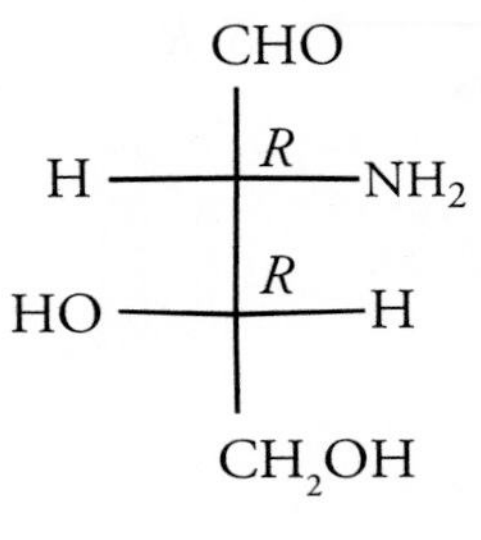

and

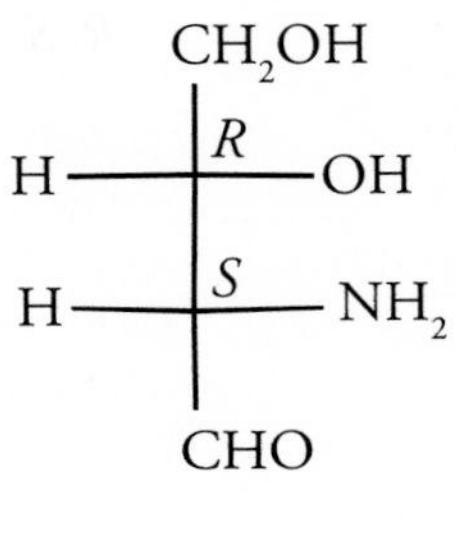

While the structures of diastereomers are similar, their physical and chemical properties can vary dramatically. They can have different melting points, boiling points, solubilities, dipole moments, specific rotations, etc. Most importantly for the MCAT, the specific rotation of diastereomers is also different, but *there is no relationship between the specific rotations of diastereomers as there is for enantiomers*. There is no way to predict the specific rotation of one diastereomer if you know the degree of rotation of another.

Resolution of Enantiomers

Nature has evolved intricate mechanisms for the bio-synthesis of enantiomerically pure, optically active compounds. For example, L-(+)-tartaric acid, D-(+)-fructose, and L-(+)-valine are all isolated as a single enantiomer from their respective biological sources.

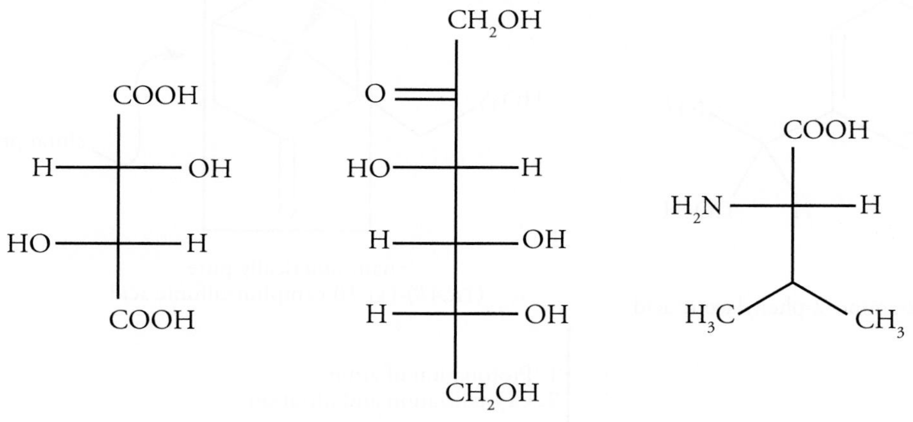

L-(+)-tartaric acid
(2R, 3R)-tartaric acid

D-(+)-fructose

L-(+)-valine

Unfortunately, the laboratory syntheses of enantiomerically pure compounds is often laborious and expensive. It is generally more time- and cost-effective to synthesize chiral targets as racemic mixtures. For example, the reduction of 2-butanone (achiral) to 2-butanol (chiral) yields both enantiomers.

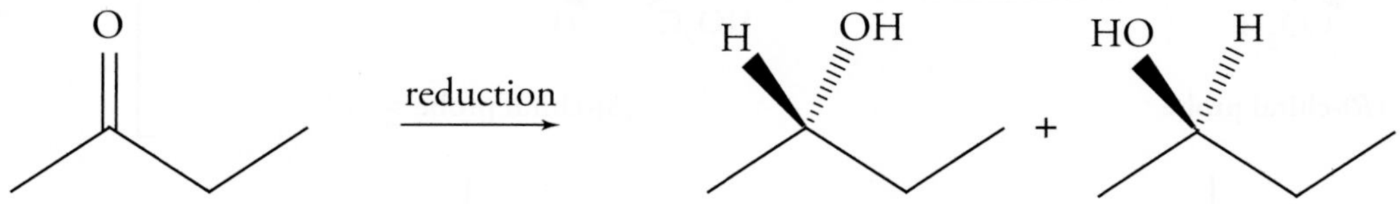

2-butanone

reduction

(S)-2-butanol

(R)-2-butanol

If only one enantiomer of 2-butanol is needed, the two alcohols must be separated. Since enantiomers have identical chemical and physical properties, separating a racemic mixture is a nontrivial process called **resolution**.

34.2

The traditional method for resolving a racemic mixture is through the use of an enantiomerically pure chiral probe, or resolving agent, that associates with the components of the mixture through either covalent bonds or intermolecular forces (like hydrogen bonds or salt interactions). The resulting products will be diastereomers, capable of separation due to their different physical properties.

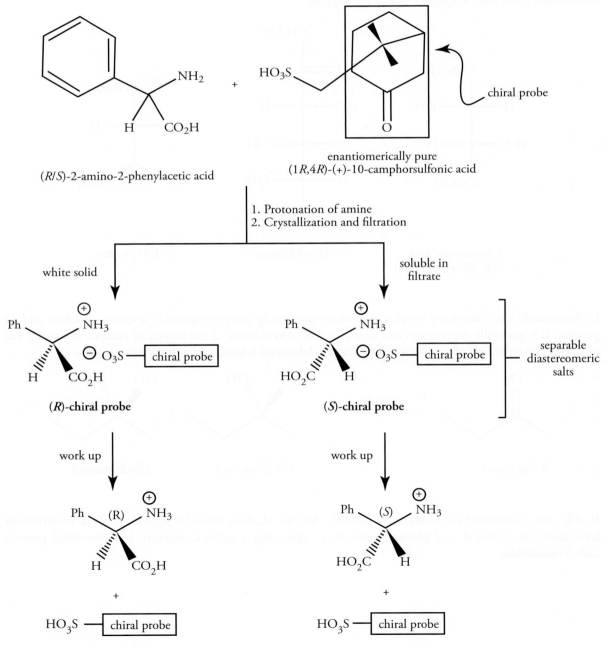

For example, racemic (±)-2-amino-2-phenylacetic acid can be resolved with enantiomerically pure (1R,4R)-(+)-10-camphorsulfonic acid, as shown in the figure below.

Protonation of the amine by the sulfonic acid produces two diastereomeric salts with different chemical and physical properties. In this particular instance, these salts have different solubilities; the *R* salt precipitates as a crystalline solid, while the *S* salt remains dissolved in the filtrate. A simple filtration process is used to separate the two, which can be released from the probe and isolated as enantiomerically pure material in a subsequent work-up step.

Epimers

Epimers are a subclass of diastereomers that differ in their absolute configuration at a single chiral center (only *one* stereocenter is inverted). To illustrate epimeric relationships, let's look at the Fischer projections of some sugars.

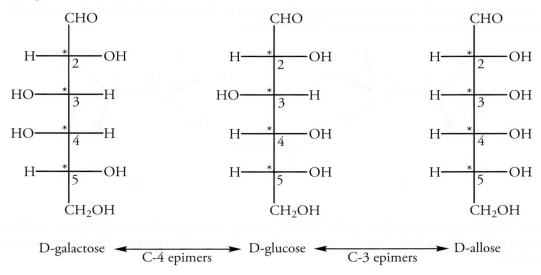

Concerning the three sugars above, we see that D-glucose and D-galactose differ in stereochemistry at only one chiral center (C-4). Thus, D-glucose and D-galactose are said to be C-4 epimers, and C-4 is called the **epimeric carbon**. Likewise, D-glucose and D-allose differ in structure at a single chiral center (C-3). D-Glucose and D-allose are C-3 epimers, with C-3 being the epimeric carbon. Cyclic forms of sugars have one more stereochemical relationship—they can be anomers.

What about D-galactose and D-allose? What is the relationship between these two molecules? We can see that these two sugars differ at two chiral centers (C-3 and C-4). At least one, but not all, of the stereocenters have been inverted. Therefore, they are diastereomers, but *NOT* epimers. Note that all epimers are diastereomers, but not all diastereomers are epimers.

Meso Compounds

Let's look at another molecule with more than one stereocenter. Consider 2,3-butanediol:

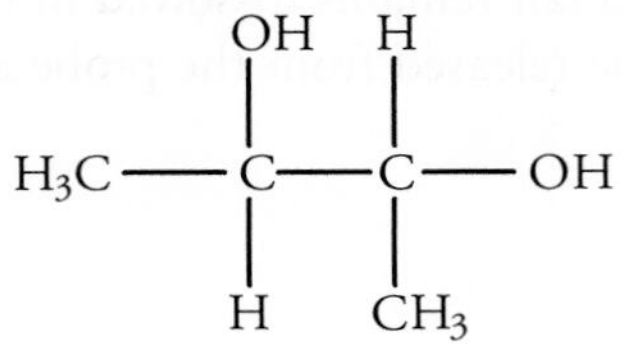

Upon inspection, we determine that there are two chiral centers and therefore four possible stereoisomers. Notice that both chiral centers have the same groups attached to them: –H, –CH$_3$, –OH, and –CH(OH)CH$_3$. When the same four groups are attached to two chiral centers, the molecule can have an internal plane of symmetry. Let's examine this a little more closely. We first consider the *R, R* stereoisomer and the *S, S* stereoisomer of 2,3-butanediol:

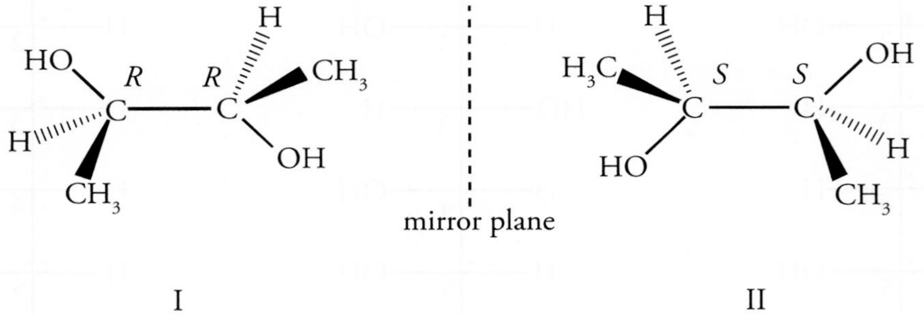

mirror plane

I   II

There are two things to notice here. First, I and II are non-superimposable mirror images and therefore enantiomers. Second, in both I and II there is no internal plane of symmetry. This is demonstrated for Molecule II:

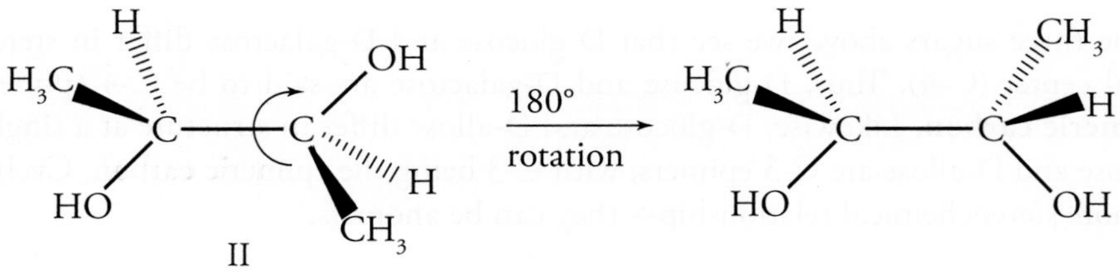

180° rotation

II

The –OH groups line up on the two chiral centers, but the –CH$_3$ groups and –H atoms do not. The optical rotation of a 50/50 mixture of molecules I and II would measure zero because this is a racemic mixture.

Now look at the *R*, *S* stereoisomer and its mirror image:

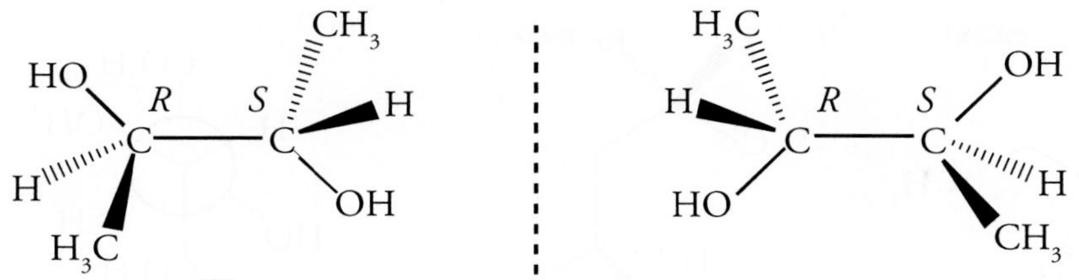

III and IV are actually
the same molecule.

Rotate the entire molecule
so that the two –OH groups
are as in III.

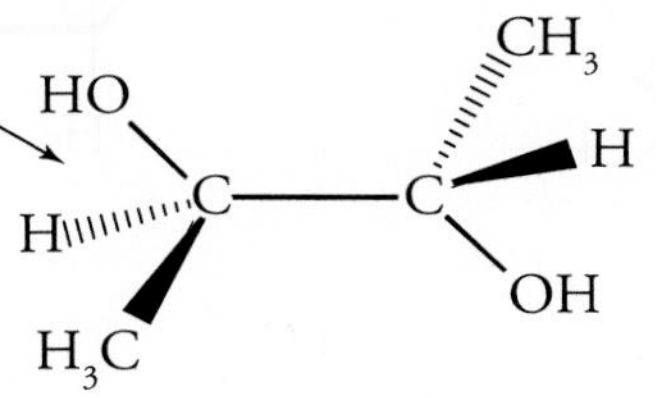

IV

It turns out that Molecules III and IV are directly superimposable and therefore identical. This is because there is an internal plane of symmetry within the molecule.

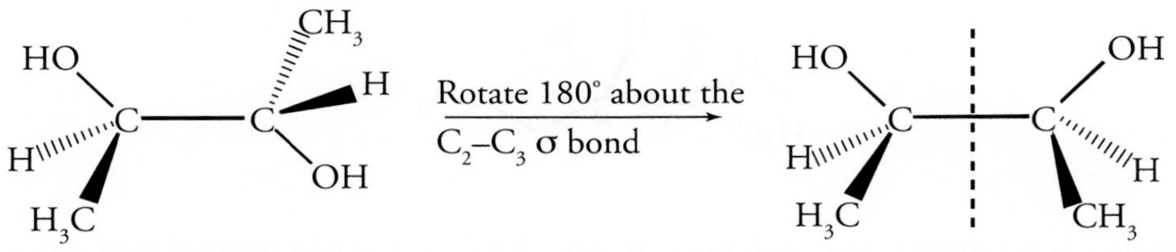

Rotate 180° about the
C_2–C_3 σ bond

III

One side of the molecule is the
mirror image of the other side.
This is a *meso* compound.

When there's an internal plane of symmetry in a molecule that contains chiral centers, the compound is called a **meso** compound. Actually then, 2,3-butanediol has only *three* stereoisomers, not four. Molecules I and II are enantiomers, while III and IV are the same molecule. Molecule III (or IV) is an example of a meso compound. Meso compounds have chiral centers but are not optically active (so they are achiral) because one side of the molecule is a mirror image of the other. In a sense, the optical activity imparted by one side of the molecule is canceled by its other side.

Example 34-16: Which of the following molecules are optically active?

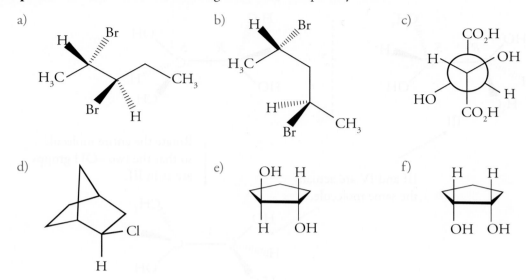

a)

b)

c)

d)

e)

f)

Solution:

a) This molecule is optically active. It has two chiral centers, but no internal mirror plane. Therefore, it is not a meso compound and will rotate plane-polarized light.

b) This molecule is a meso compound due to its two chiral centers and internal mirror plane. It will be optically inactive. Be sure to look for rotations around σ bonds in order to find the mirror planes of some molecules.

c) By rotating around the C-2 to C-3 bond to put the molecule into an eclipsed conformation, you can see that there is an internal mirror plane in the molecule. Since C-2 and C-3 are also chiral centers with four different substituents, this is a meso compound, and it will be optically inactive.

d)   This molecule has three chiral centers (the two bridgehead carbons are chiral), but no plane of symmetry. It is therefore chiral and optically active.

e)   There is no mirror image in this molecule even though it has two chiral centers (they have the same absolute configuration). It will therefore be optically active.

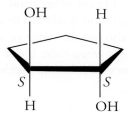

f)   This molecule does have an internal mirror plane, and its two chiral centers have opposite absolute configurations. It is therefore meso, and not optically active.

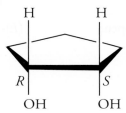

Geometric Isomers

Geometric isomers are diastereomers that differ in orientation of substituents around a ring or a double bond. Cyclic hydrocarbons and double bonds (alkenes) are constrained by their geometry, meaning they do not rotate freely about all bonds. So, there's a difference between having substituents on the same side of the ring (or double bond) and having substituents on opposite sides. For example, the following are geometric isomers of 1,2-dimethylcyclohexane:

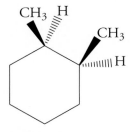

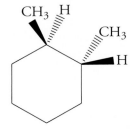

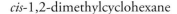

cis-1,2-dimethylcyclohexane   *trans*-1,2-dimethylcyclohexane

Priority of substituent groups is assigned the same way as for absolute configuration. On C-1, the methyl group is given higher priority than the H, and the same is true on C-2. The molecule in which the two higher-priority groups are on the same side is termed *cis*, and the molecule in which the two higher-priority groups are on opposite sides of the ring is termed *trans*.

34.2

The same-side/opposite-side substituent relativity also occurs with double bonds, but in this case the stereochemistry is officially designated by (Z) or e). The (Z)/e) notation is a completely unambiguous way to specify the appropriate stereochemistry at the double bond. In this system, a high and low priority group are assigned at each carbon of the double bond based on atomic number, just as with absolute configuration. If the two high priority groups are on the *same* side, the configuration at the double bond is Z (from the German *zusammen*, meaning *together*). On the other hand, if the two high priority groups are on opposite sides of the double bond, the configuration is referred to as E (from the German *entgegen*, meaning *opposite*). Be aware, that the MCAT may also use the terms *cis* and *trans* when referring to double bonds. However, this is usually reserved for the case when there is one H attached to each carbon of the double bond, as shown below. The geometric isomers of 2-bromo-1-chloropropene and of 1,2-dibromoethene are shown below:

Highest priority groups (Br and Cl) on same side, so Z.

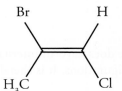

Highest priority groups (Br and Cl) on opposite side, so E.

(Z)-2-bromo-1-chloropropene

(E)-2-bromo-1-chloropropene

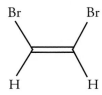

cis-1,2-dibromoethene

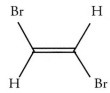

trans-1,2-dibromoethene

SUMMARY OF ISOMERS

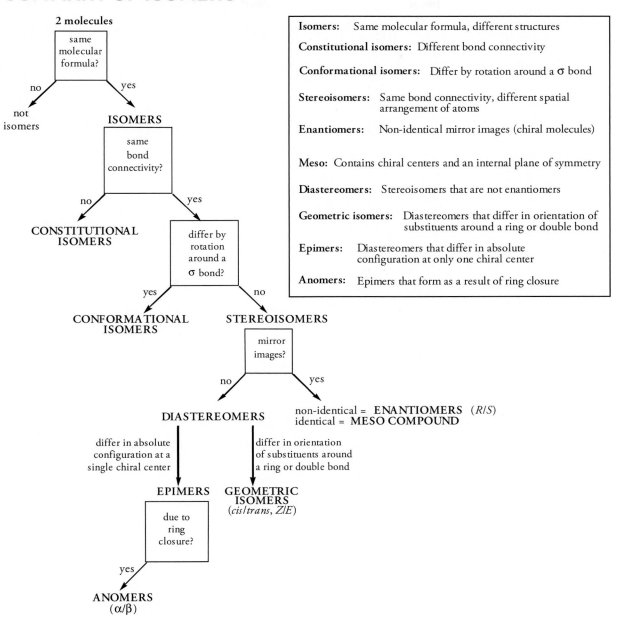

Isomers: Same molecular formula, different structures

Constitutional isomers: Different bond connectivity

Conformational isomers: Differ by rotation around a σ bond

Stereoisomers: Same bond connectivity, different spatial arrangement of atoms

Enantiomers: Non-identical mirror images (chiral molecules)

Meso: Contains chiral centers and an internal plane of symmetry

Diastereomers: Stereoisomers that are not enantiomers

Geometric isomers: Diastereomers that differ in orientation of substituents around a ring or double bond

Epimers: Diastereomers that differ in absolute configuration at only one chiral center

Anomers: Epimers that form as a result of ring closure

Chapter 35
Organic Chemistry
Reactions: Nucleophilic
Substitution and
Addition

35.1   NUCLEOPHILIC SUBSTITUTIONS

Nucleophilic substitution reactions replace a leaving group in an electrophilic substrate with a nucleophile. In this context, the bonds that break during the substitution will do so via a heterolytic cleavage where the leaving group takes both electrons from the bond that connected it to the electrophile. This also means you can recognize a substitution reaction by the fact that one σ bond is broken to the leaving group, while another is formed to the incoming nucleophile. Therefore, there is no net change in the number of σ bonds or π bonds over the course of the reaction.

The S$_N$2 Mechanism

The first nucleophilic mechanism we'll examine is the S$_N$2 mechanism. Typical electrophiles (also known as the substrates) for this type of reaction are alkyl halides. Alkyl halides are alkanes that contain at least one halogen (fluorine, chlorine, bromine, or iodine). Since halogen atoms are electronegative, are large in size, and are the conjugate bases of strong acids (except for F$^-$), most halides (Cl$^-$, Br$^-$, I$^-$) make good leaving groups.

For example, when 1-iodobutane is treated with a Br$^-$ nucleophile, an S$_N$2 reaction occurs in which bromide replaces the I$^-$ group (known as the leaving group) to yield 1-bromobutane.

1-iodobutane   1-bromobutane

In the first (and only) step of this reaction (see the mechanism below), because the nucleophilic bromide anion attacks the electrophilic carbon at the *same time* that the leaving group leaves, the attack must occur *from the backside* of the substrate. The bromine-carbon bond forms as the iodine-carbon bond is broken, *in a single step*, to yield bromobutane.

The Mechanism

Let's look at a chiral substrate in order to see the stereochemical implications of this concerted mechanism. When (*R*)-1-deutero-1-chloroethane is treated with iodide, the typical backside attack occurs. As the new C—I bond begins to form while the C—Cl bond breaks, the reaction proceeds through a *pentavalent transition state*. As you can see in the product below, there is complete *inversion of configuration* at the carbon being attacked by the nucleophile. This is always the case in an S$_N$2 reaction on a chiral substrate.

backside attack

pentavalent
transition state

inverted product

Furthermore, the rate of the reaction is a function of two variables—that is, **bimolecular**. The rate of the reaction depends on the concentrations of both the nucleophile and the electrophile, and is equal to the product of the rate constant (k), the concentration of the nucleophile ($[I^-]$), and the concentration of the electrophile ($[R\text{-}Cl]$).

$$\text{reaction rate} = k[\text{nucleophile}][\text{electrophile}]$$

We can now explain what we mean when we say that this reaction proceeds by an "S_N2" mechanism. The "S" indicates that it is a <u>s</u>ubstitution reaction mechanism, the subscript "N" indicates that it is <u>n</u>ucleophilic, and the "2" indicates that it is <u>b</u>imolecular.

The rate of the reaction depends not only on the concentration of the electrophile, but also on the degree of substitution of the electrophilic carbon. Since the transition state is sterically crowded with five groups attached, the more bulky those groups are, the harder it is for the nucleophile to gain access to the reactive site. Therefore, less substituted substrates react faster than more substituted ones via the S_N2 mechanism.

The last factor to consider in substitution reactions is the solvent. To favor an S_N2 mechanism, protic solvents such as water and alcohols should be avoided. Since these hydrogen bonding solvents are able to strongly solvate the nucleophile, they hinder the backside attack necessary for the concerted reaction. To prevent this interference, polar, *aprotic* solvents such as acetone, DMF (dimethylformamide), or DMSO (dimethylsulfoxide) should be used. Their polar nature allows the charged nucleophiles and leaving groups to remain dissolved, but they are not as efficient at completely solvating the nucleophile.

Key Features of an S_N2 Reaction

Reactivity of substrate:	$CH_3 > 1° > 2° \gg 3°$ (Because of steric hindrance)
Stereochemistry:	Complete stereochemical inversion of the carbon that is attacked by the nucleophile
Kinetics:	reaction rate = $k[\text{nucleophile}][\text{electrophile}]$
Solvent:	S_N2 reactions are favored by polar, aprotic (non-hydrogen bonding) solvents
Rearrangements:	Not possible due to concerted mechanism; no carbocations are present in solution
Favoring Conditions:	Strong, non-bulky nucleophile will favor S_N2 reactions over S_N1 (see next section)

The S$_N$1 Mechanism

In contrast to the concerted S$_N$2 mechanism, the course of S$_N$1 substitution reactions, a carbocation (carbonium ion) forms. Let's take a moment to review the relative stability of carbocations. Remember that the formation of charged species from neutral ones is generally an energetically disfavorable process; that is, it is energetically *uphill*. But some ions are more stable than others. For alkyl cations, the relative stabilities due to the inductive effect are given below.

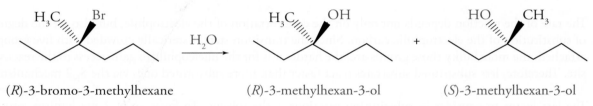

Now that we have reviewed the basics of carbocation stability, let's consider an example where a chiral halide undergoes an S$_N$1 substitution reaction. When (*R*)-3-bromo-3-methylhexane is treated with H$_2$O, a racemic mixture of 3-methylhexan-3-ol is formed:

S$_N$1 substitution occurs in *two distinct steps*, unlike S$_N$2 reactions that occur in one step. In the first step of the S$_N$1 reaction, a *planar carbocation* with 120° bond angles forms (see mechanism below). This occurs when the leaving group falls off (dissociates). This is the slow step of the mechanism, or the rate limiting step. In the final step of this reaction, *racemization* occurs as the nucleophile attacks equally *on either side* of the carbocation. The result is a racemic mixture.

The Mechanism

Unlike the S_N2 reaction explained above where the rate of the reaction was a function of two variables, the S_N1 reaction rate is a function of only one variable, that is, **unimolecular**. The rate of the S_N1 reaction depends only upon the concentration of the electrophile (the species that loses the leaving group over the course of the reaction). The rate of the reaction is equal to the product of the rate constant (k), and the electrophile concentration ([R-Br]):

$$\text{reaction rate} = k[\text{electrophile}]$$

As before, we can now explain what we mean when we say that this reaction proceeds by an "S_N1" mechanism. The "S" indicates that it is a <u>s</u>ubstitution reaction mechanism, the subscript "N" indicates that it is <u>n</u>ucleophic, and the "1" indicates that it is <u>uni</u>molecular.

The rate of the reaction depends not only on the concentration of the electrophile, but also on the degree of substitution of the electrophilic carbon. Since the dissociation of the leaving group is the slow step of the mechanism, anything that makes that step more favorable will speed up the reaction. As was just discussed, the more substituted the carbocation intermediate, the more stable it is. Therefore, more substituted substrates will dissociate to make more stable intermediates faster, speeding up the rate of the entire reaction.

To favor an S_N1 mechanism, protic solvents such as water and alcohols should be used. The role of the solvent is twofold. The protic solvent helps to stabilize the forming carbocation and solvate the leaving group, thereby facilitating the first, or slow step of the mechanism. Secondly, the solvent then behaves as the nucleophile in a **solvolysis** reaction, attacking the carbocation intermediate. This produces an alcohol product if water is used as the solvent and an ether if the reaction is run in an alcoholic solvent.

Key Features of an S$_N$1 Reaction

Reactivity of substrate: 3° > 2° >> 1° (Due to stabilization of the carbocation)

Stereochemistry: Almost complete racemization due to nucleophilic attack on either side of p orbital

Kinetics: reaction rate = k[electrophile]

Solvent: S$_N$1 reactions are favored by protic (hydrogen bonding) solvents. (This stabilizes the carbocation.)

Rearrangements: Carbocation rearrangement is possible; if the carbocation can rearrange to one that is more stable, it will

Favoring conditions: Non-basic, weaker nucleophiles favor unimolecular substitutions. Often the solvent acts as the nucleophile (solvolysis).

Alcohols undergo substitution reactions just as alkyl halides do. They can undergo either S$_N$1 or S$_N$2 substitution reactions depending upon the degree of substitution of the alcohol. Alcohols are treated with strong mineral acids to make their bad –OH leaving group into a good one (H$_2$O). In S$_N$2 reactions, the conjugate base of the mineral acid will attack while the leaving group leaves. In S$_N$1 reactions, the water will first dissociate, followed by nucleophilic attack of the halide ion on the carbocation intermediate.

Example 35-1: Predict whether the following substitution reactions will proceed via an S$_N$1 or an S$_N$2 mechanism.

a)

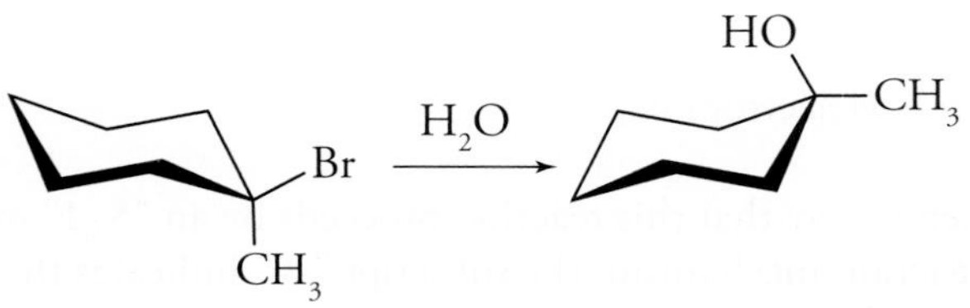

b)

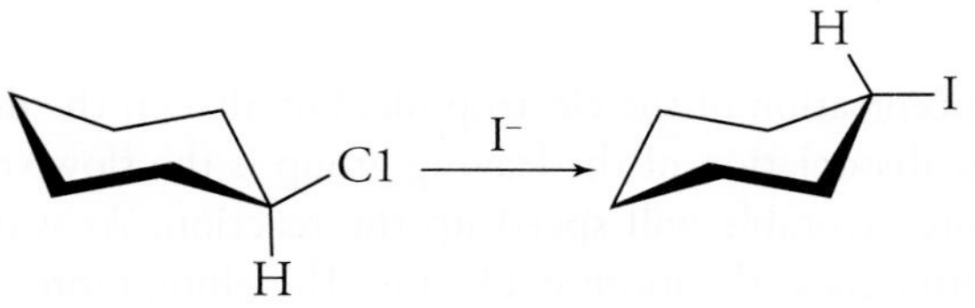

c)

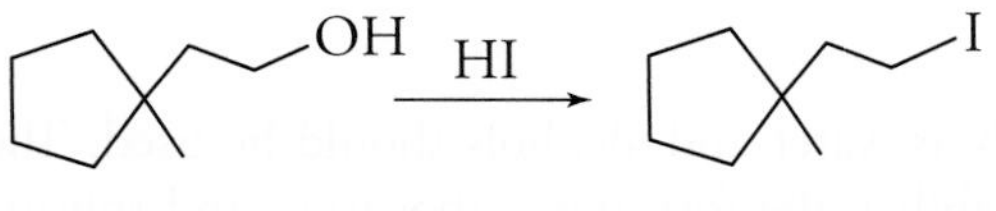

d)

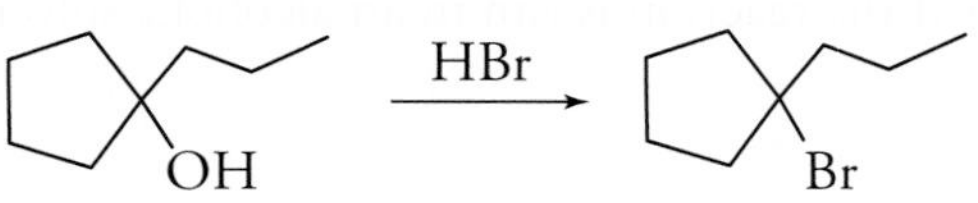

Solution:

a) 3° bromide, S_N1
b) 2° chloride, S_N2
c) 1° alcohol, S_N2
d) 3° alcohol, S_N1

35.2   ALDEHYDES AND KETONES

Two very important classes of oxygen-containing organic compounds are aldehydes and ketones. We begin the discussion of these functional groups by looking at a common way carbonyls are formed—the oxidation of an alcohol. Oxidizing agents are able to absorb electrons (and be reduced). Below are some common oxidizing agents that appear on the MCAT. Note that only the anhydrous oxidant (PCC) will NOT overoxidize the primary alcohol to the carboxylic acid (we'll talk more about this functional group later). All oxidizing agents shown can be used to form ketones from secondary alcohols. Tertiary alcohols cannot be oxidized to a carbonyl compound since the oxidizing agent must remove a H atom from the C bearing the –OH group.

Aqueous Oxidants	Anhydrous Oxidant
Chromic Acid (H_2CrO_4)	
Chromate Salts (CrO_4^{2-})	
Dichromate Salts ($Cr_2O_7^{2-}$)	Pyridinium Chlorochromate (PCC)
Permanganate (MnO_4^-)	
Chromium Trioxide (CrO_3)	

Now that we understand how aldehydes and ketones are formed, let's look at their reactivities. The key to understanding the chemistry of aldehydes and ketones is to understand the electronic structure and properties of the carbonyl group. The C=O double bond is very polarized because oxygen is much more electronegative than carbon, and so it is able to pull the π electrons of the C=O double bond toward itself and away from carbon. This is illustrated by the following resonance structures:

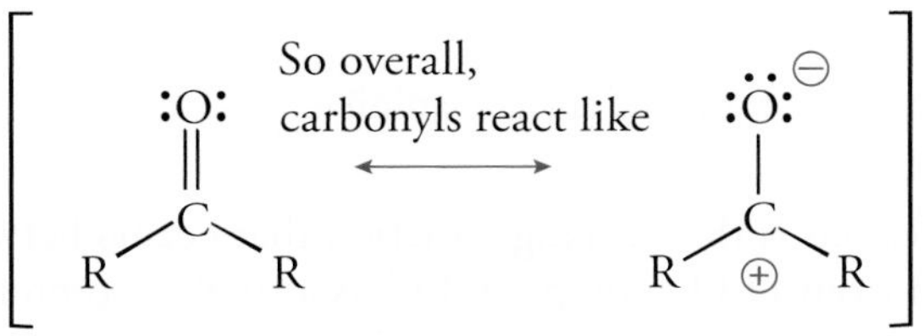

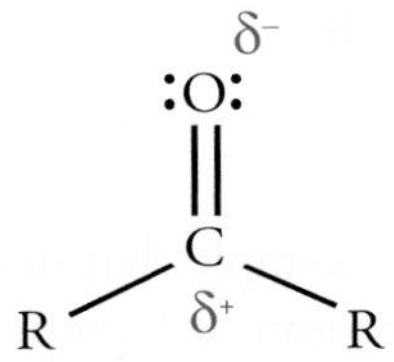

This bond polarization renders the carbon atom electrophilic (δ^+) and accounts for two kinds of reactions of aldehydes and ketones. First, these molecules have *acidic protons* α *to (i.e., next to) the carbonyl group.*

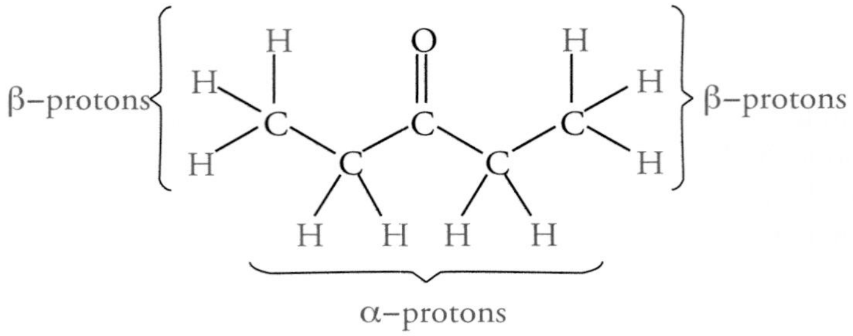

An α-proton is acidic because the electrons left behind upon deprotonation can delocalize into the π system of the carbonyl. Second, the electrophilic carbon of the carbonyl group makes aldehydes and ketones *susceptible to nucleophilic attack*. In the aldol condensation, which we will study in some detail, both of these types of reactivity are involved in a single reaction.

Acidity and Enolization

The first type of reaction that is commonly observed with aldehydes and ketones is the result of the relative acidity of protons that are α to the carbonyl group. These α-protons are sufficiently acidic that they can be removed by a strong base [such as hydroxide ion (OH⁻) or an alkoxide ion (OR⁻)] to yield a carbanion. This carbanion can be easily formed because the electrons that are left behind on the carbon can be delocalized into the carbonyl π system. In this way, the negative charge can be delocalized onto the electronegative oxygen atom. A resonance-stabilized carbanion of this type is referred to as an **enolate ion**. *An enolate ion is negatively charged and nucleophilic.* The nucleophilic character of an enolate ion lies predominantly at the carbon at which the proton was abstracted, *not* the oxygen atom of the carbonyl. This is why the α-carbon of enolates is the nucleophile in most common enolate reactions.

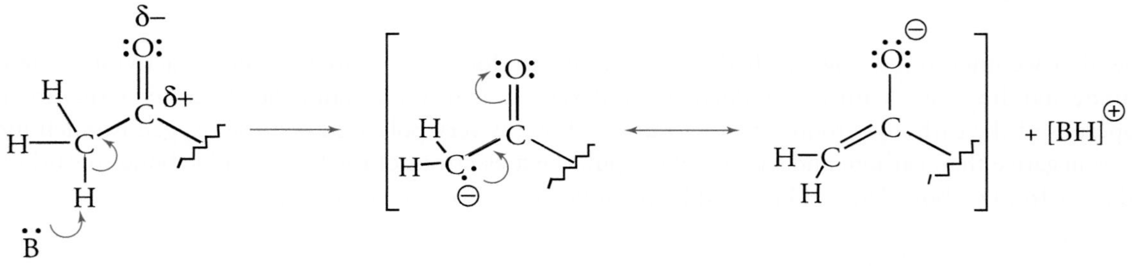

resonance forms of enolate anion

An example that demonstrates the acidity of α-protons is the exchange reaction that occurs between the α-proton of Compound I (below) and deuterium from D_2O. Compound I has a single α-proton that is α to *two* carbonyl groups in comparison to the six other α-protons in the molecule that are α to only *one* carbonyl group. It is this lone α-proton that exchanges with a deuterium of D_2O over the course of a couple of days, even in the absence of base. Being next to two carbonyl groups greatly enhances the acidity of this α-proton and allows it to exchange (although slowly) with a deuterium from D_2O. The mechanism of this exchange, which essentially consists of protonation of the intermediate enolate ion, is shown in the following figure:

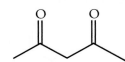

Compound I

$+ \quad D_2O \xrightarrow{\text{several days}}$ $+ \ HOD$

Example 35-2: As a review of acidity, for each of the following pairs of compounds, identify the one with the more acidic proton.

a) vs.

b) 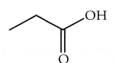 vs.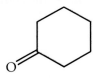

c) vs.

d) vs.

e) vs.

Solution:

a)

b)

c)

d)

e)

Keto-Enol Tautomerism

A ketone is converted into an enol by deprotonation of an α-carbon atom and subsequent protonation of the carbonyl oxygen. These two forms of the molecule are very similar to one another and differ only by the position of a proton and a double bond. This is referred to as **keto-enol tautomerism**. Two molecules are **tautomers** if they are readily interconvertible constitutional isomers in equilibrium with one another.

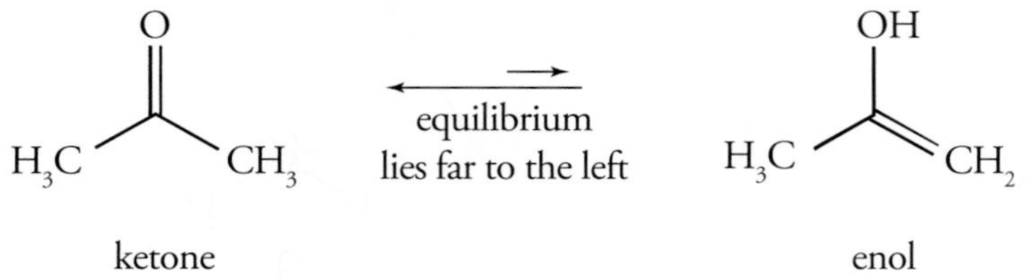

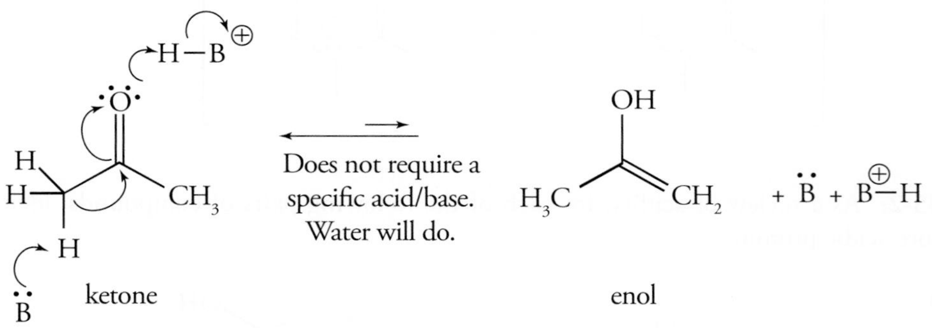

ketone   equilibrium   enol
lies far to the left

ketone   Does not require a   enol
specific acid/base.
Water will do.

Tautomerization has consequences for molecules with chiral α-carbons. Imagine an alcohol with a chiral center adjacent to the hydroxyl group (as shown below). If this stereochemically-defined alcohol were oxidized, the corresponding ketone would have racemic stereochemistry.

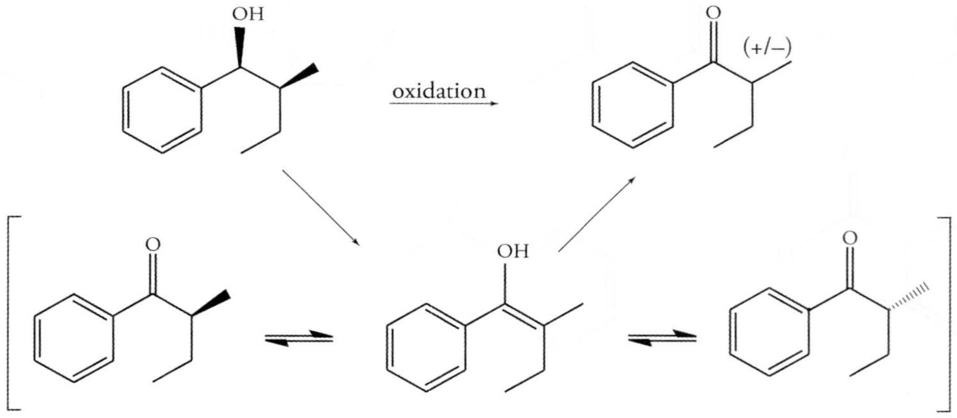

Because the α-carbon of the compound is sp^2 hybridized and planar in the enol tautomer, protonation to form the keto tautomer can occur from both the top and bottom faces of the double bond. This loss of defined stereochemistry, which results in a mixture of R and S configurations at the once chiral α-carbon, is termed **racemization**.

Nucleophilic Addition Reactions to Aldehydes and Ketones

Because of the polarized nature of the C=O double bond in aldehydes and ketones, the carbon of the carbonyl group is very electrophilic. This means that it will attract nucleophiles and can readily be reduced. The attack of a nucleophile upon the carbon of a carbonyl group, called a nucleophilic addition reaction, is shown below with a generic nucleophile (Nu:).

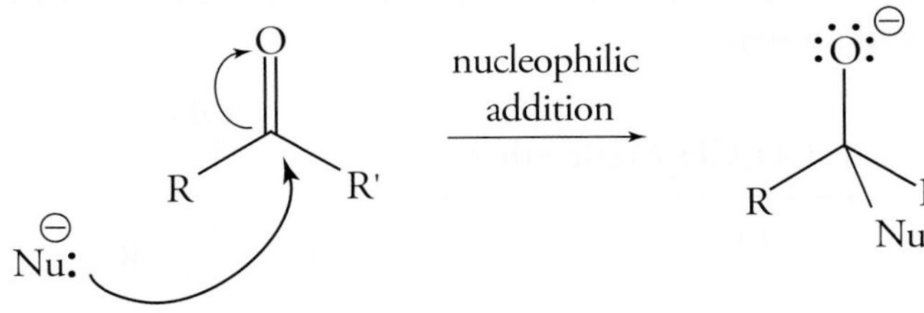

Nucleophilic addition reactions are defined by the bonding changes that occur over the course of the reaction. In these reactions, a π bond in the starting material is broken, and two σ bonds in the product result. This very general reaction allows for the conversion of aldehydes or ketones into a variety of other functional groups, such as alcohols, via hydride reduction:

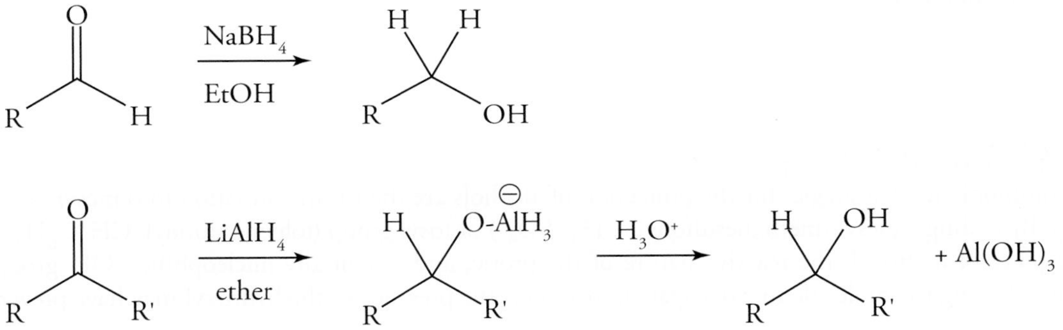

Note: Sodium borohydride ($NaBH_4$) and lithium aluminum hydride ($LiAlH_4$) are common reducing agents seen on the MCAT. In general, strong reducing agents easily lose electrons by adding hydride (a hydrogen atom and a pair of electrons) to the carbonyl. Reducing agents often have many hydrogens attached to other elements with low electronegativity.

Organometallic Reagents

Organometallic reagents are commonly used to perform nucleophilic addition to a carbonyl carbon. The basic structure of an organometallic reagent is $R^- M^+$. They act as electron rich, or anionic carbon atoms and therefore function as either strong bases or nucleophiles. Grignard and lithium reagents are the most common organometallic reagents.

Grignard reagents are generally made via the action of an alkyl or acyl halide on magnesium metal, as depicted below.

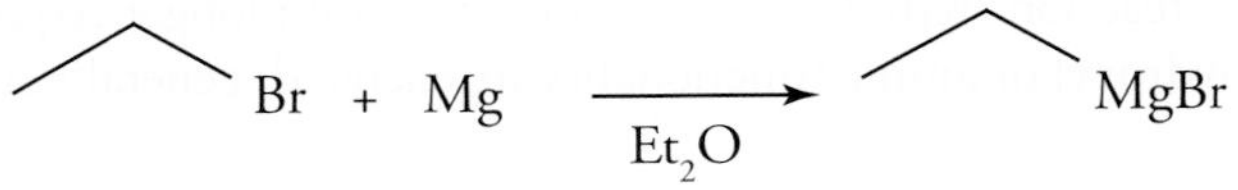

To avoid unwanted protonation of the very basic Grignard reagent, the reaction is carried out in an aprotic solvent such as diethyl ether.

The carbonyl containing compounds are then added to the Grignard reagents to yield alcohol products. In the reaction below, the methyl magnesium bromide acts as a nucleophile and adds to the electrophilic carbonyl carbon. An intermediate alkoxide ion is formed that is rapidly protonated to produce the alcohol during an aqueous acidic workup step.

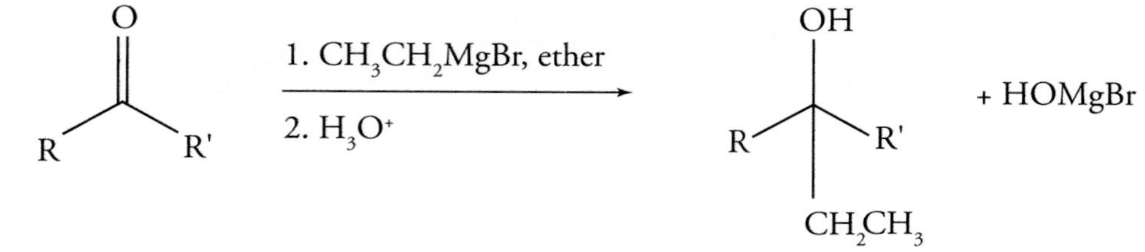

In addition to using an aprotic solvent, care must also be taken to avoid the presence of any other acidic hydrogens in the substrate molecule bearing the carbonyl. This means that alcohol groups or carboxylic acid groups must be absent, or else first be protected, before the Grignard reagent can be added to the carbonyl compound.

Mesylates and Tosylates

Two commonly used strategies for the protection of alcohols are their transformation into mesylates and tosylates. By adding a mesyl (methanesulfonyl, $CH_3-SO_3^-$) or tosyl group (toluenesulfonyl, $CH_3C_6H_4-SO_3^-$) in the place of hydroxyl, the reactive nature of the protic, and potentially nucleophilic −OH group is removed, allowing the molecule to participate in reactions the presence of the hydroxyl may have prevented.

The formation of mesylates and tosylates from alcohols are shown below. Reaction of a sulfonyl chloride, either mesyl chloride or tosyl chloride, with an alcohol in the presence of a base (generally triethylamine or pyridine) leads to nucleophilic attack at the sulfur, followed by expulsion of the chloride.

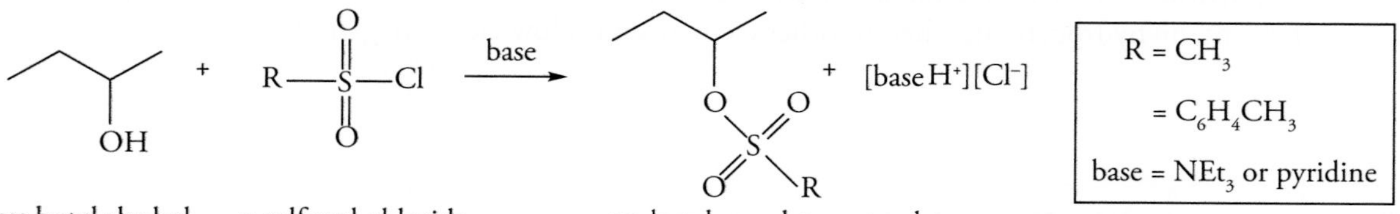

sec-butyl alcohol   a sulfonyl chloride   *sec*-butyl mesylate or tosylate

The base in each reaction is required to neutralize the HCl (consisting of the hydroxyl proton and the chloride from the sulfonyl group) and pull it out of solution as an ammonium or pyridinium chloride salt.

These groups, particularly the tosyl group, may be similarly utilized in the protection of amino (−NH₂) groups. In either case, hydroxyl or amino, the protected functionality is rendered sufficiently inert for the purposes of the subsequent reaction steps. Once the protection is no longer required, the protecting group may be removed and the hydroxyl or amine functionality regenerated, generally under reductive conditions.

In addition to their use as protecting groups, both mesylates and tosylates are good leaving groups in reactions featuring nucleophilic attack. Whereas hydroxyl is a poor leaving group requiring a very strong nucleophile for displacement, conversion of a hydroxyl into a mesylate or tosylate makes attack and displacement facile.

Acetals and Hemiacetals

Acetals and hemiacetals, which are of fundamental importance in biochemical reactions that occur in living organisms, can be synthesized from nucleophilic addition reactions to aldehydes or ketones. There are many examples of these molecules in common biochemical pathways. Before we learn the chemistry of these groups, we must be able to identify acetals and hemiacetals.

Note: The terms *ketal* and *hemiketal* refer to acetals and hemiacetals made from *ketones*, but this nomenclature appears infrequently.

General Formulas

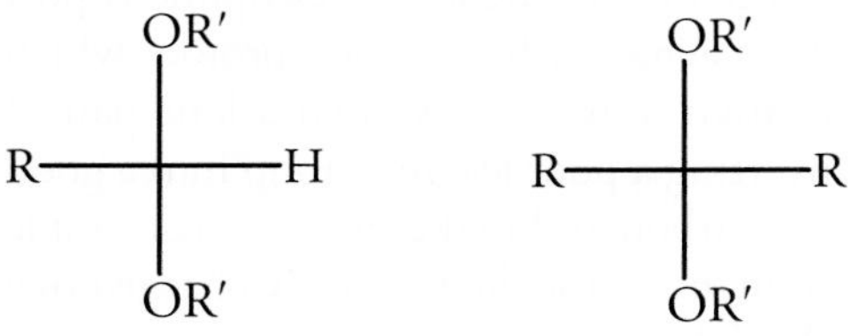

acetals 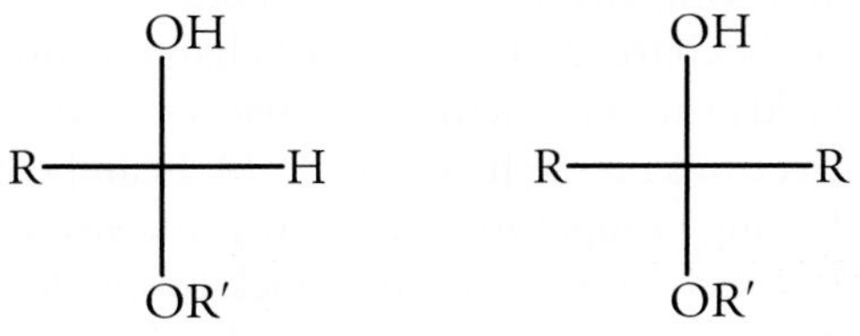   hemiacetals

Example 35-3: For each of the following compounds, identify whether it's an acetal, hemiacetal, or neither:

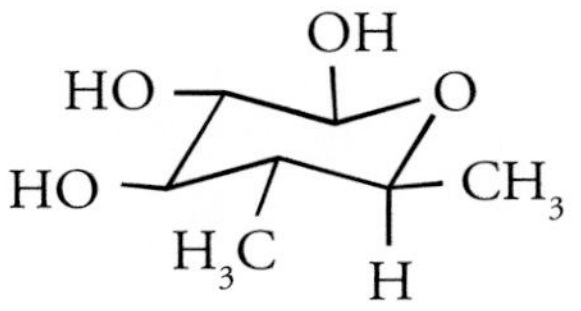

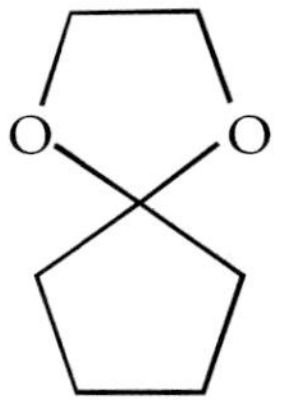

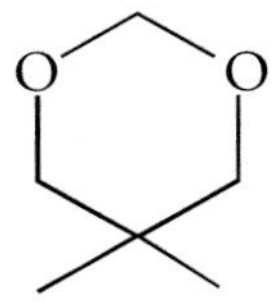

Solution:

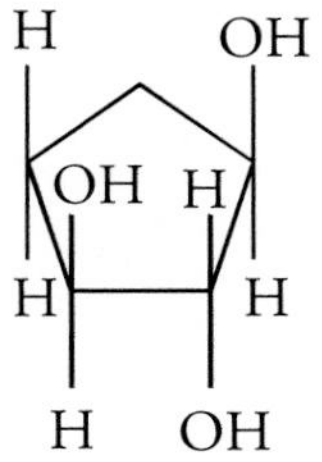

    a)   hemiacetal
    b)   acetal
    c)   neither
    d)   acetal

Acetals are formed when aldehydes or ketones react with alcohols in the presence of acid. This occurs by a nucleophilic addition mechanism. It is easy to predict the product of an acetal formation reaction. Notice that *hydrogens or carbons attached to the carbonyl carbon* of the aldehyde or ketone *remain attached* in the acetal product with the subsequent addition of two –OR groups from the alcohol. Also, note that an intermediate hemiacetal results from the addition of one –OR group to an aldehyde or ketone with subsequent protonation of the carbonyl oxygen. The aldehyde or ketone, the hemiacetal, and the acetal are all in equilibrium with one another. In order for the hemiacetal to form the acetal, a molecule of water must be lost.

Acetal Formation

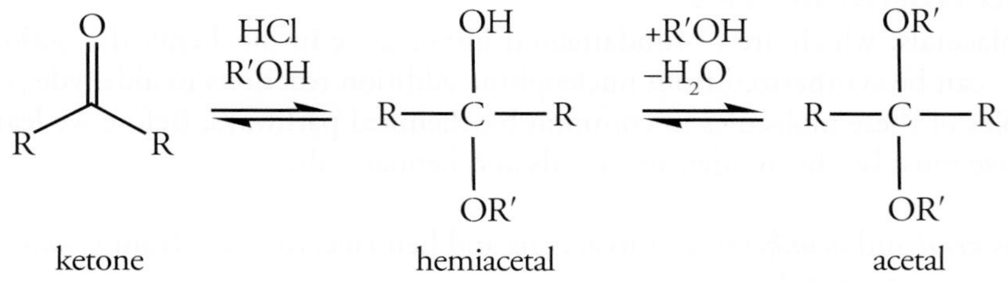

ketone   hemiacetal   acetal

The mechanism of this important reaction is shown below. In the first step, the carbonyl oxygen is protonated, making the carbonyl carbon even more susceptible to nucleophilic attack by the oxygen of the attacking alcohol molecule. Following nucleophilic attack, the oxygen of the alcohol nucleophile is positively charged. This positive charge is unfavorable, and neutrality is achieved by loss of a proton, which yields the intermediate hemiacetal. Remember that the reaction mixture is acidic so that a lone pair of electrons on the hemiacetal –OH can be protonated, thereby converting a poor leaving group into a good leaving group. Once again, this increases the electrophilicity of the carbon and makes it more susceptible to a second nucleophilic attack by an alcohol molecule. All that remains is for the positively charged oxygen from the attacking alcohol to lose a proton to yield the acetal product.

The Mechanism

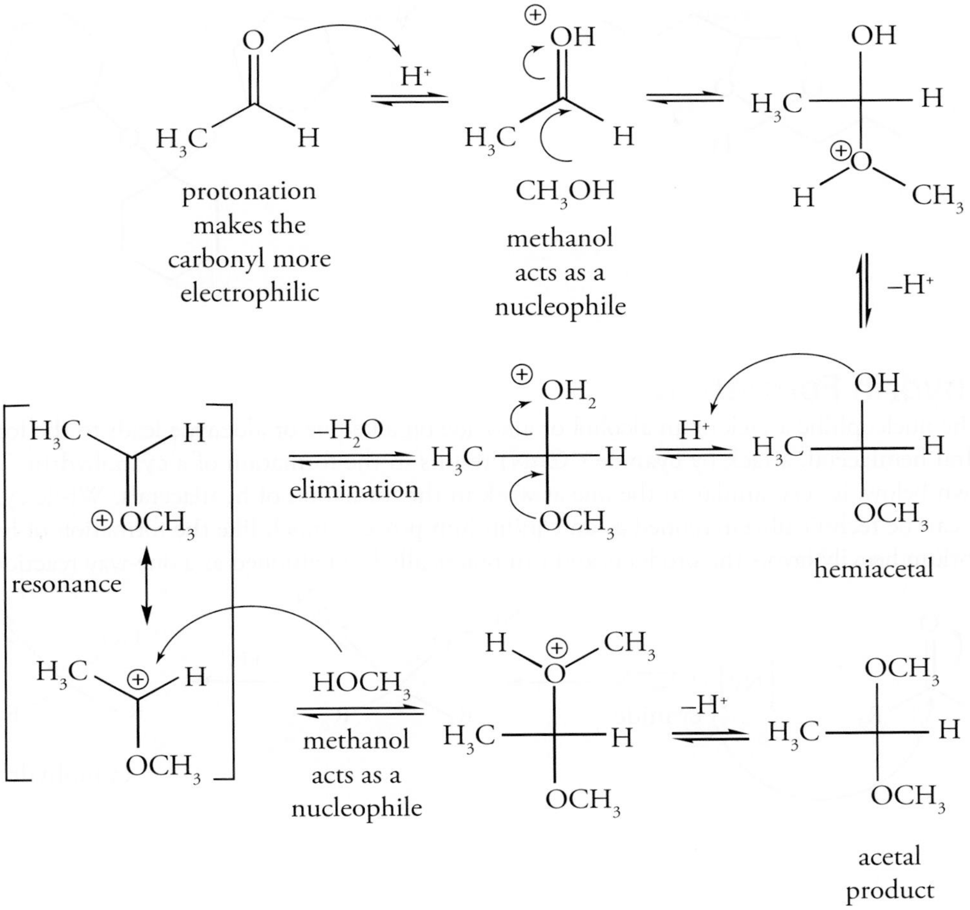

H+
protonation makes the carbonyl more electrophilic
CH3OH
methanol acts as a nucleophile
–H+
H+
hemiacetal
–H2O
elimination
resonance
HOCH3
methanol acts as a nucleophile
–H+
acetal product

Example 35-4: Predict the acetal product from the following reactions:

a)

b)

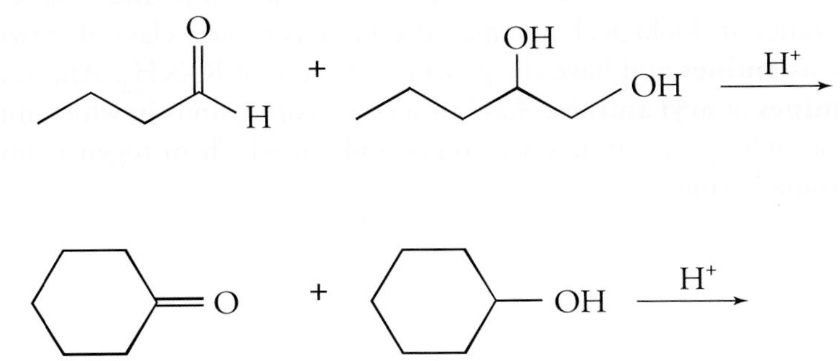

35.2

Solution:

a)

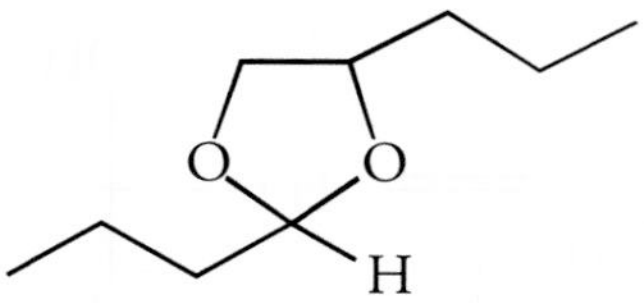

b)

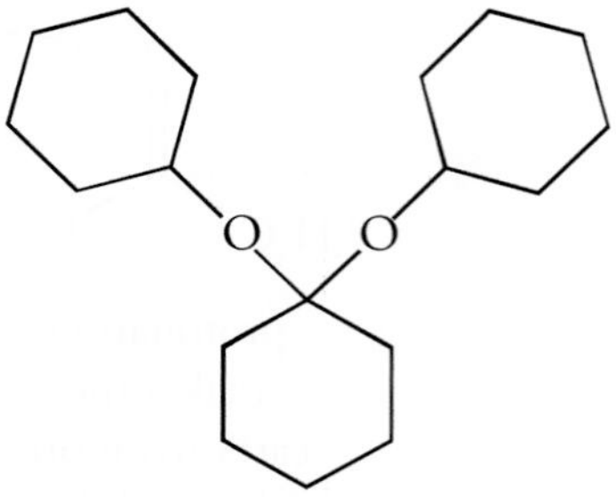

Cyanohydrin Formation

Whereas the nucleophilic attack of an alcohol or alkoxide on a ketone or aldehyde leads to the formation of a tetrahedral hemiacetal, attack by cyanide ($^-$C≡N) results in the formation of a cyanohydrin. The mechanism, shown below, is very similar to the one at work in the formation of hemiacetals. While cyanohydrin formation can be technically envisioned as an equilibrium process, much like the formation of hemiacetals, the equilibrium heavily favors the products and can practically be envisioned as a one-way reaction.

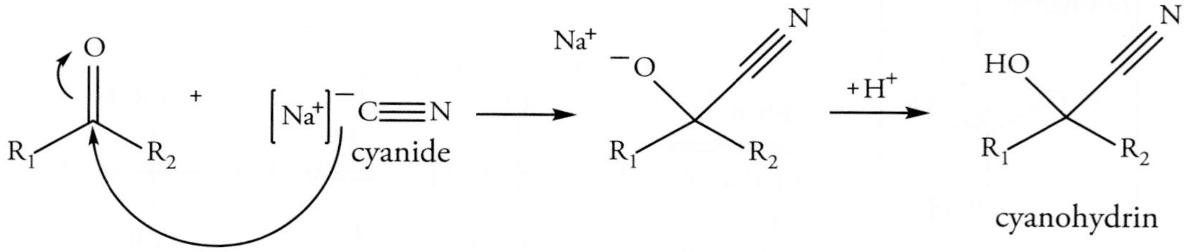

Amines

Before looking at the next few examples of nucleophilic addition reactions, we should first briefly discuss the nucleophile used in the reactions—namely amines. Organic compounds that contain nitrogen are of fundamental importance in biological systems. The most common class of nitrogen-containing compounds are referred to as **amines** and have the general structure of R–NH_2. Amines can be further classified as either **alkyl amines** or **aryl amines**. *Alkyl* amines are compounds in which nitrogen is bound to an sp^3-hybridized carbon, while *aryl* amines are compounds in which nitrogen is bonded to an sp^2-hybridized carbon of an aromatic ring.

Amines can be further categorized as primary amines, secondary amines, tertiary amines, and quaternary ammonium ions. Below are a few examples of common amines, one of each type.

$CH_3CH_2\ddot{N}H_2$
ethylamine
(primary)

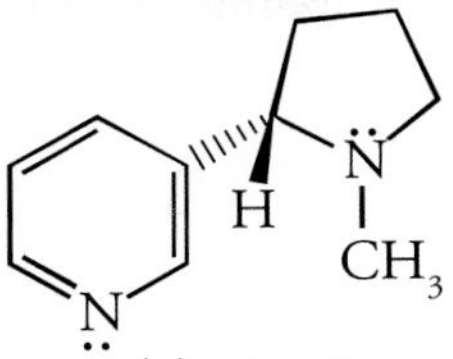

(–)-nicotine
(tertiary)

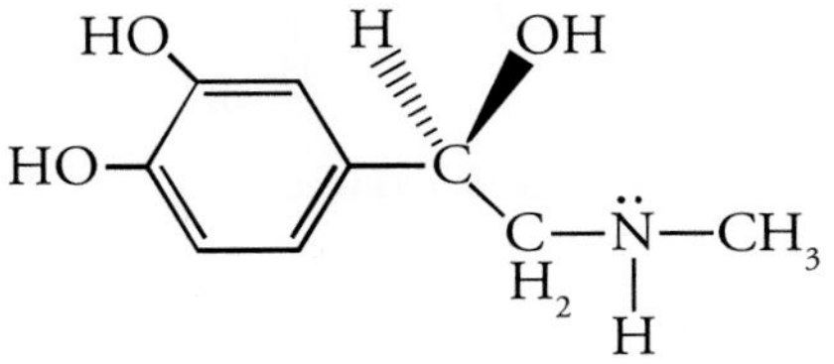

epinephrine
(secondary)

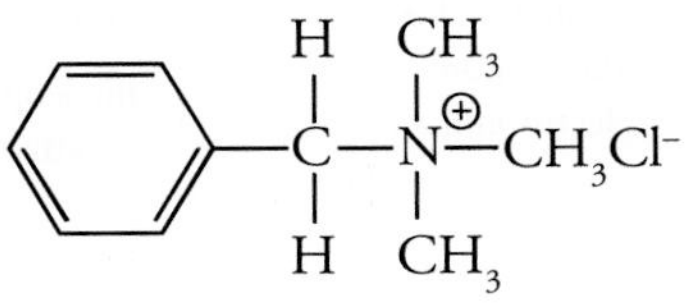

benzyltrimethyl-ammonium chloride
(quaternary)

In the simple methyl amine, CH_3NH_2, notice that the nitrogen has three σ bonds and one lone electron pair. Its hybridization is therefore sp^3 with approximately 109° bond angles. The molecular geometry of an alkyl amine is pyramidal.

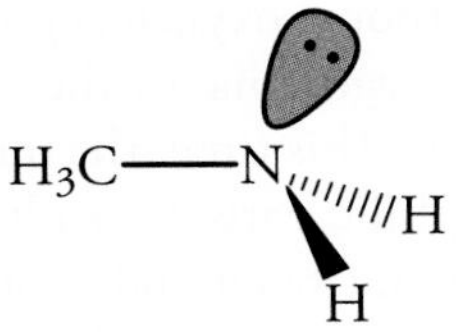

Nitrogen Hybridization	sp^3
Bond Angles	109°
Molecular Geometry	pyramidal

Methyl amine

Most importantly, because of the lone pair of electrons on the N, amines behave as either Brønsted-Lowry bases or as nucleophiles. Let's now look at a few reactions in which the nucleophile is an amine.

Imine Formation

A class of reactions that closely resembles acetal formation are the reactions of aldehydes or ketones with amines. These reactions are often catalyzed under weakly acidic conditions (pH about 4–5). When an aldehyde or ketone reacts with a primary amine (RNH_2), an imine will form.

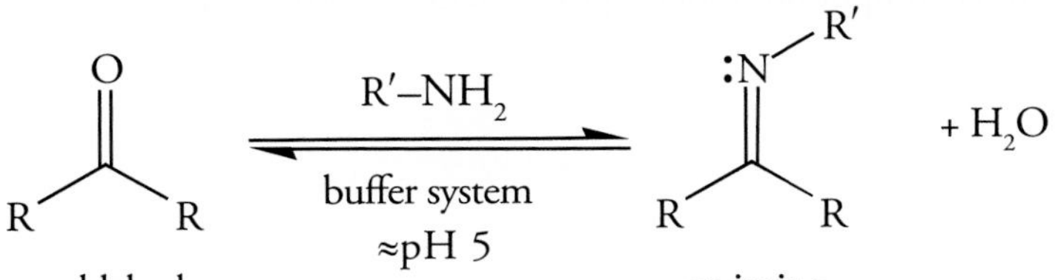

an aldehyde
or ketone

an imine

$R'–NH_2$

buffer system
≈pH 5

$+ H_2O$

As in the acetal formation reaction, whatever R groups are originally attached to the carbonyl carbon stay attached in the product, and a molecule of water is liberated as a byproduct. A brief examination of the reaction mechanism will help illustrate these common features.

Mechanism

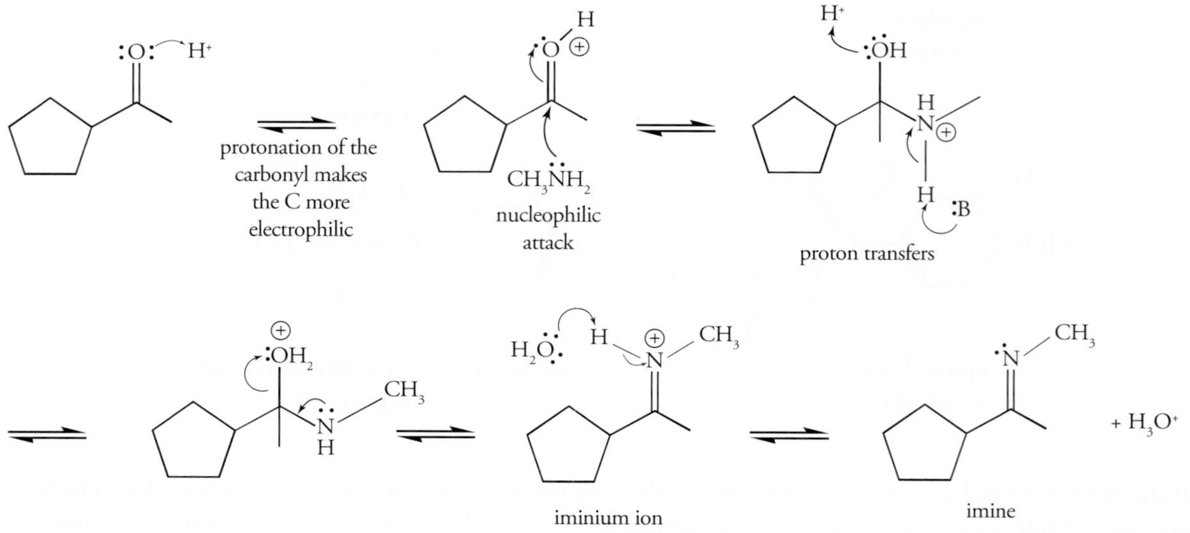

In the first step of this reaction, a lone pair of electrons on the carbonyl oxygen is protonated by the acidic medium. As in acetal formation, protonation of the carbonyl oxygen makes the carbonyl carbon more electrophilic and therefore more susceptible to nucleophilic attack. This time, the nucleophile is a primary amine, but attack by the nucleophilic nitrogen on the electrophilic carbon results in a similar tetrahedral intermediate. This intermediate is then deprotonated at the nitrogen and protonated at the oxygen, thereby converting a poor leaving group (–OH) into a good one (–OH$_2^+$). Next, the oxygen departs as a neutral water molecule, leaving behind a carbocation that is resonance-stabilized by the lone pair of electrons on nitrogen, reminiscent of the stabilization by the incoming oxygen during acetal formation. (*Note*: Only the more stable resonance form is shown in the mechanism above.) The similarities to acetal formation end here, as the final step of imine production is the deprotonation of the iminium ion to regenerate the acid catalyst.

Enamine Formation

While imines are derived from primary amines, if a secondary amine (R$_2$NH) is used under similar reaction conditions, the result is a functional group called an enamine. The overall reaction of a typical enamine synthesis is shown below. Note that this is another reversible reaction and that enamines can be hydrolyzed to the carbonyl compound under aqueous acidic conditions.

The mechanism of enamine formation is identical to imine formation until the final step. Since the in-coming amine is secondary rather than primary, the iminium ion cannot be deprotonated as in the imine mechanism. Instead, deprotonation of a hydrogen α to the double bond, now substantially more acidic on account of the positive charge on nitrogen, yields the enamine.

Enamines are a class of organic molecules resembling enols, in which the enol-oxygen of the aldehyde or ketone is replaced by a secondary amine. The chemistry of enamines is similar to enol chemistry in that it is largely governed by the resonance between the enamine and iminium structures. The partial double-bond character in the C—N bond, implied by the iminium resonance structure, results in the sp^2-hybridization of the enamine nitrogen and hindered rotation around the C—N bond (and the C—C$_\alpha$ bond in acyclic compounds).

As the iminium resonance form above suggests, the α-carbon of the enamine is nucleophilic and will readily react with electrophiles. The increased donor ability of nitrogen, as compared to oxygen, results in enamines being more nucleophilic than neutral enols, but less nucleophilic than charged enolates (as we'll see shortly). As shown below, attack by the nucleophilic α-carbon on the polarized carbon of an alkyl halide results in the expulsion of the halide leaving group. This generates an iminium ion, which, as mentioned above, will reform the carbonyl under acidic, aqueous workup conditions.

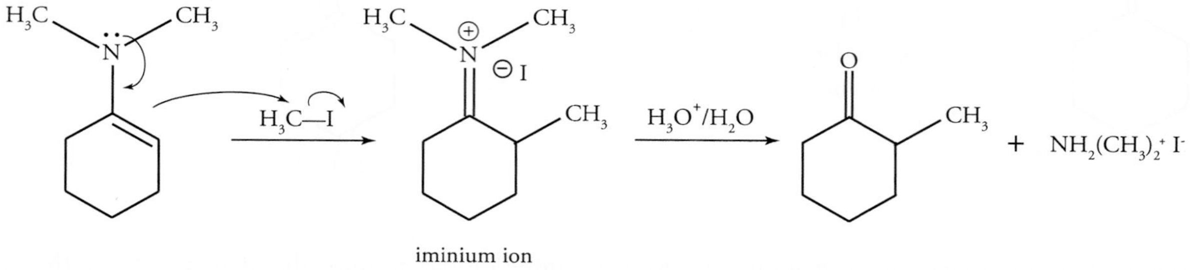

iminium ion

Example 35-5: Predict the major organic product of each of the following reactions:

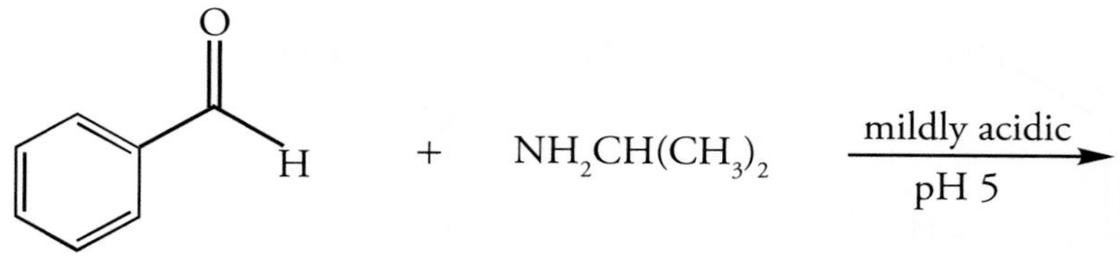

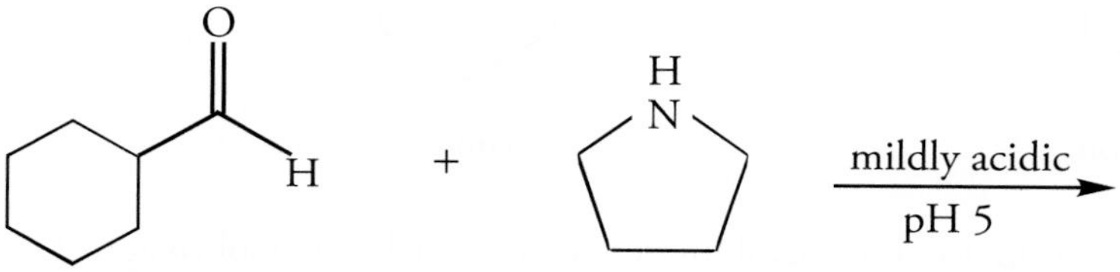

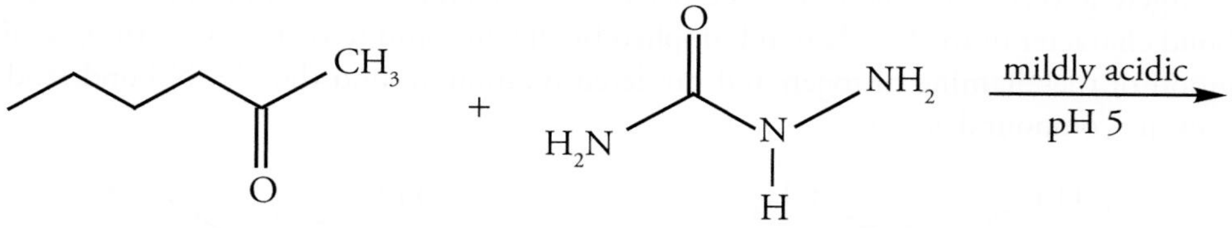

Solution:

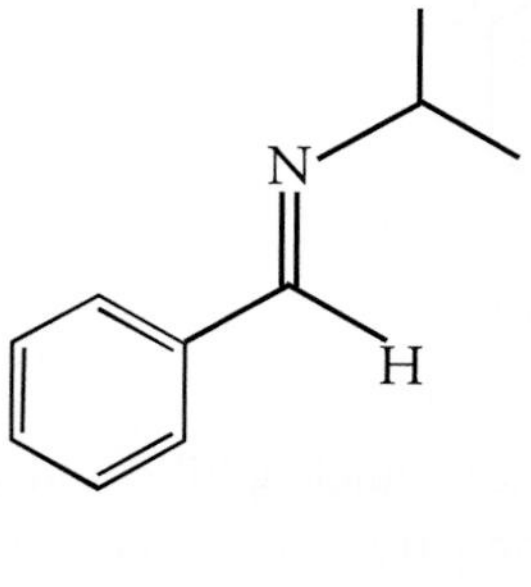

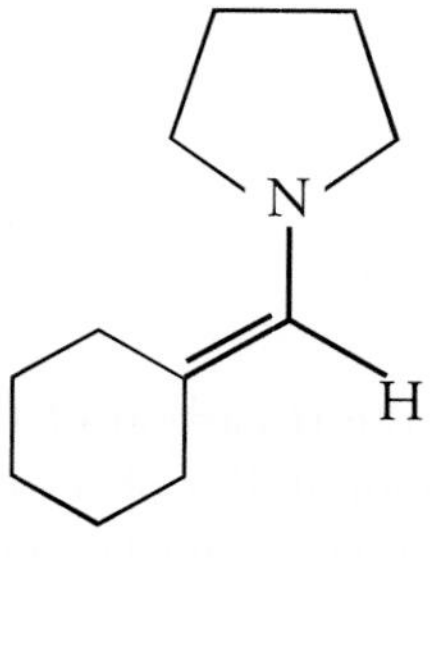

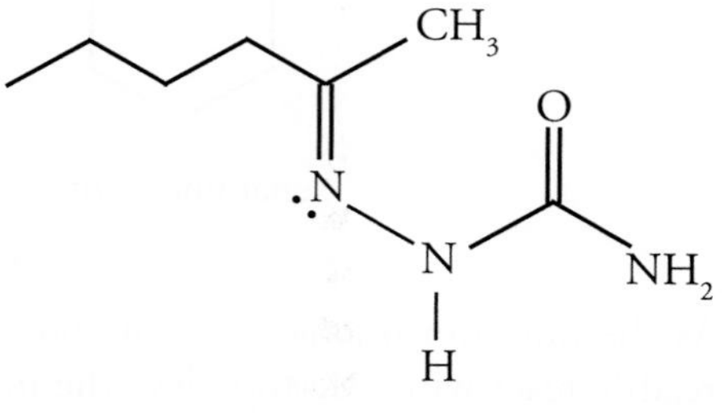

Aldol Condensation

A classic reaction in which the enolate anion of one carbonyl compound reacts with the carbonyl group of another carbonyl compound is called the aldol condensation. This reaction combines the two types of aldehyde/ketone reactivities: the acidity of the α-proton and the electrophilicity of the carbonyl carbon, and it forms a α-hydroxycarbonyl compound as the product.

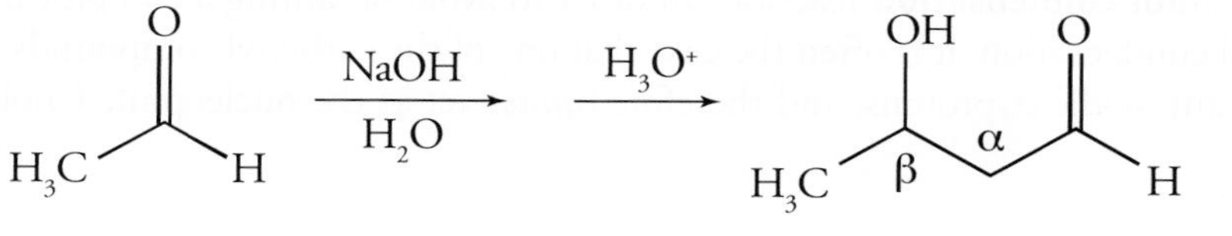

β–hydroxyaldehyde

As the mechanism below shows, in the first step of this reaction, a strong base removes an α-proton from the aldehyde or ketone, resulting in the formation of a resonance-stabilized enolate anion. (Remember, the enolate anion is nucleophilic and usually reacts at the carbon atom that was deprotonated.) Next, the α-carbon of the enolate anion attacks the carbonyl carbon of another aldehyde molecule, thereby generating an alkoxide ion that is subsequently protonated by a molecule of water. This results in the formation of a general class of molecules referred to as β-hydroxy carbonyl compounds.

The Mechanism

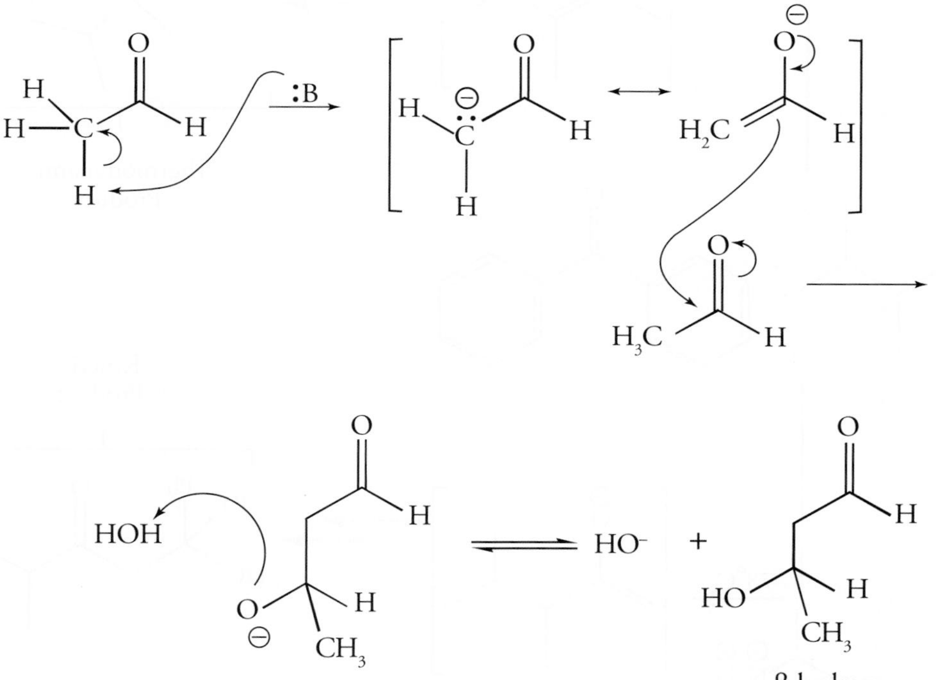

β-hydroxy aldehyde

There are three important points to note about this reaction. First, it requires a strong base (typically hydroxide, OH⁻ or an alkoxide ion RO⁻) to remove an α-proton adjacent to the carbonyl group. Second, one of the aldehydes or ketones must act as a source for the enolate ions while the other aldehyde or ketone will come under nucleophilic attack by the enolate carbanion. Third, the aldol condensation does not require the two carbonyl groups that participate in the reaction to be the same. When they are different, it is called a **crossed aldol condensation** reaction. In order to avoid obtaining a complex mixture of products in a crossed aldol condensation, it is often the case that one of the carbonyl compounds is chosen such that it does not have any acidic α-protons, and therefore *cannot* act as the nucleophile (enolate ion), it *must* be the electrophile.

Kinetic vs. Thermodynamic Control of the Aldol Reaction

When asymmetric ketones with more than one set of α-protons are treated with base, two different enolates are possible. When these ketones are used to perform aldol reactions, different products are formed depending on which enolate is used. Regiochemical control of such a reaction can be achieved through the choice of base and the reaction conditions, as depicted here.

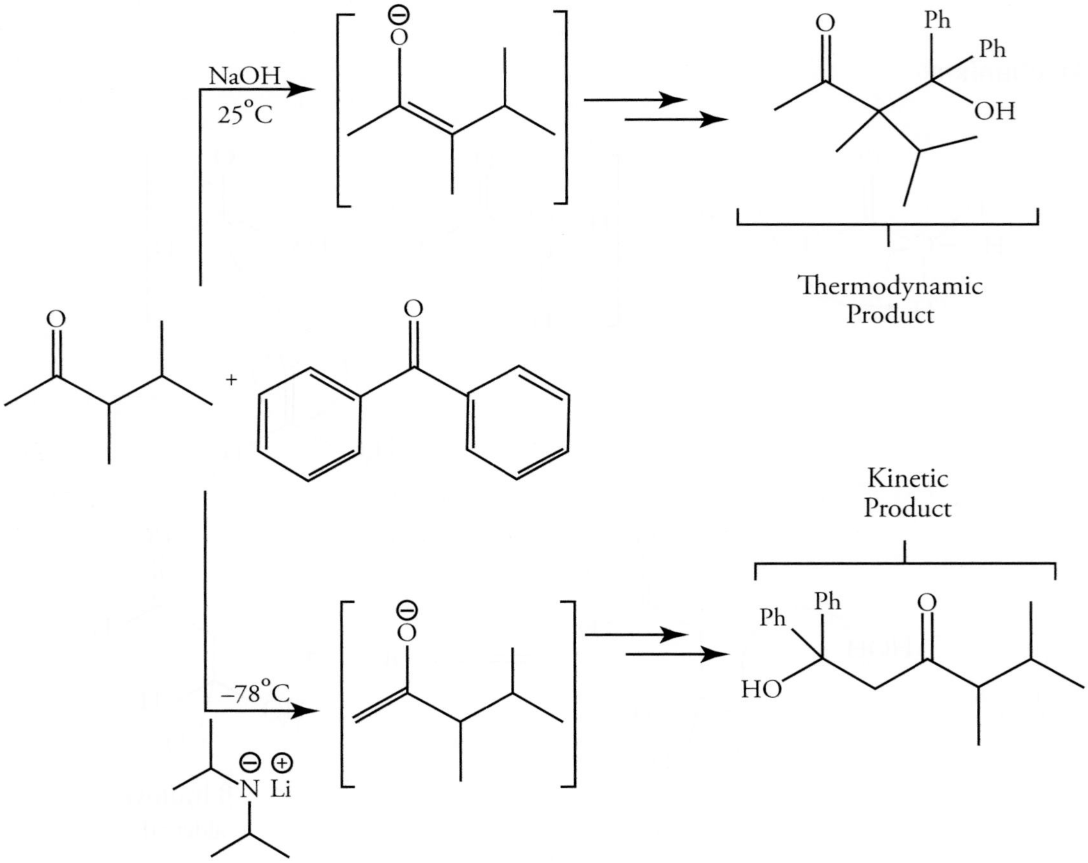

The upper-pathway, run at room temperature with an unencumbered base, is said to be under *thermodynamic* control. In general, double bonds with more carbon-substituents (fewer vinyl-hydrogens) are more thermodynamically stable than less-substituted alkenes. In the absence of other constraints, the enolate formed by removing protons from the more sterically crowded α-carbon will be favored.

Formation of the less-substituted enolate (the lower-pathway) may be achieved by denying the base access to the more sterically hindered α-carbon. Two ways to do this include using a bulky base that cannot fit into the area required to remove the sterically-shielded proton (in this case, lithium diisopropylamide, or LDA), or by doing the reaction at very low temperature. At a reduced temperature, there is not enough energy to overcome the activation barrier associated with the base approaching the more crowded α-carbon. Through use of these constraints, the base will deprotonate the less hindered, more kinetically accessible α-carbon. These reactions are said to be under **kinetic control**.

Retro-Aldol Reaction and Dehydration

Though stabilized by an intramolecular hydrogen bond between the hydroxyl and carbonyl groups, and hence generally thermodynamically stable at moderate temperatures and pH levels, β-hydroxy aldehydes and ketones are not immune to further transformations. When treated with strong bases, deprotonation of the free hydroxyl group may induce the reverse of the initial aldol condensation in a reaction known as a retro-aldol reaction. It is useful to note that the constitutive pieces of any β-hydroxy aldehyde or ketone synthesized via an aldol reaction may be determined by working through the mechanism of the retro-aldol.

If the β-hydroxyaldehyde or ketone products are heated, they will undergo an elimination reaction (dehydration) to form an α,β-**unsaturated carbonyl compound**. Notice that the newly formed carbon-carbon π bond is in conjugation with the carbonyl group; this stabilizes the molecule.

β-hydroxy carbonyl

α,β-unsaturated carbonyl compound
(some *Z* compound will also form)

Example 35-6: Predict the condensation products of each of the following reactions. Show both the β-hydroxy carbonyl product and the elimination product.

a)

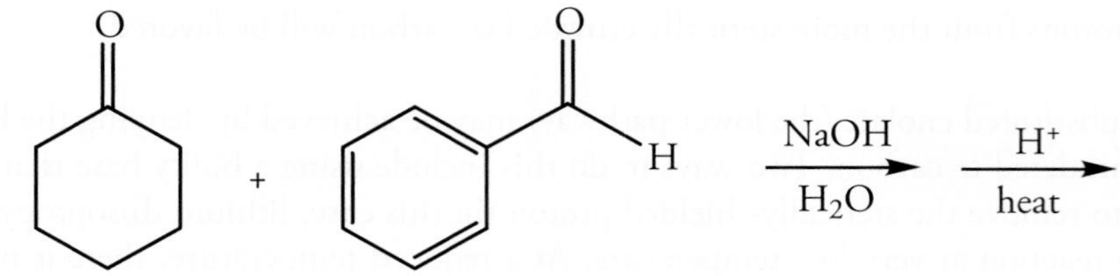

b)

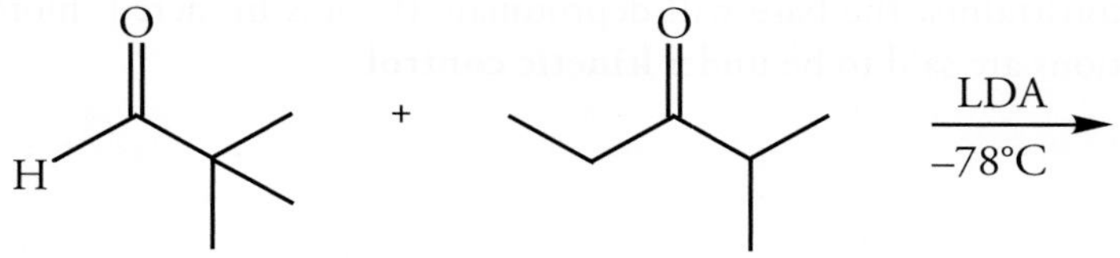

c)

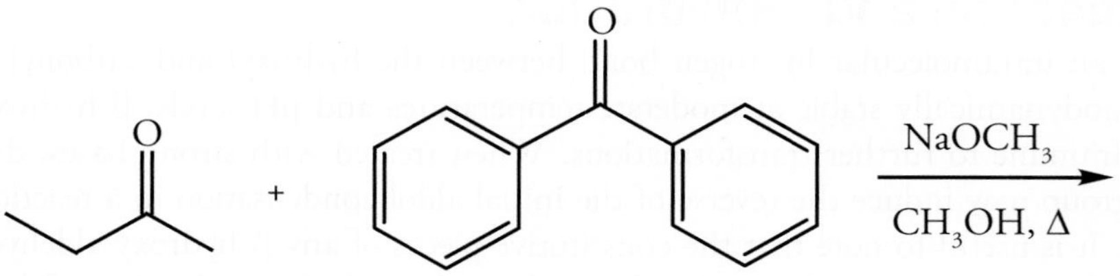

Solution:

a)

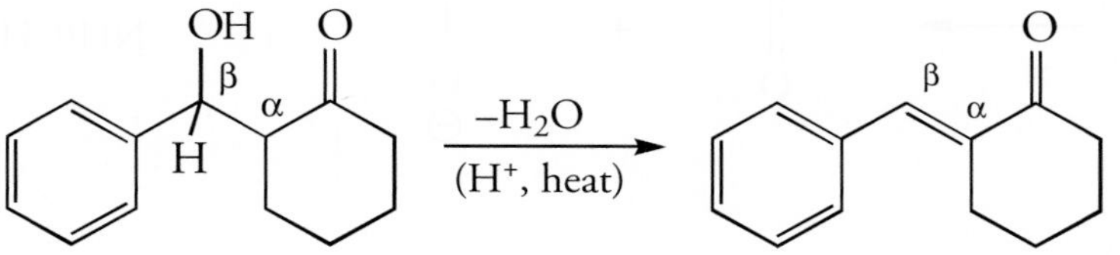

b)

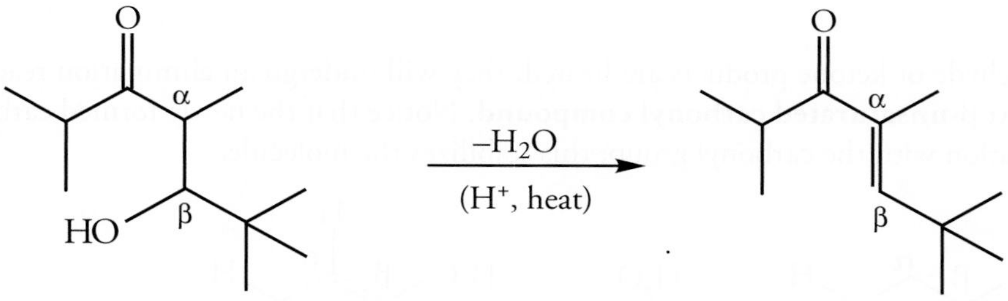

c)

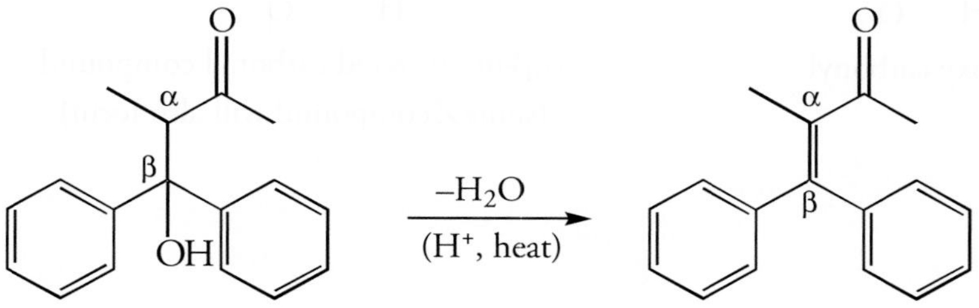

35.3 CARBOXYLIC ACIDS

Carboxylic acids are of fundamental importance in many biological systems. Fatty acids, for example, are long chain carboxylic acids that play important roles in both cellular structure and metabolism. In the following sections, we'll explore the basic physical properties and common chemical reactions of carboxylic acids and their derivatives.

Hydrogen Bonding

Carboxylic acids form strong hydrogen bonds because the carboxylate group contains both a hydrogen bond donor and a hydrogen bond acceptor. This can be seen in the intermolecular hydrogen bonding of acetic acid. Notice that the acidic proton is the hydrogen bond donor and a lone pair of electrons on the carbonyl oxygen is the hydrogen bond acceptor. For this reason, carboxylic acids can form stable hydrogen bonded dimers, giving them high melting and boiling points.

Reduction of Carboxylic Acids

Earlier in the chapter we discussed the use of boron and aluminum hydrides in the reduction of ketones and aldehydes to their respective alcohols. Carboxylic acids can similarly be reduced to primary alcohols, with one important difference: $LiAlH_4$ is effective, but $NaBH_4$ is not. As aluminum is slightly more electropositive than boron, the Al—H bond is more highly polarized, more reductive, and ultimately capable of performing these more challenging reductions.

Decarboxylation Reactions of β-Keto Acids

Carboxylic acids that have carbonyl groups β to the carboxylate are unstable because they are subject to decarboxylation. The reaction proceeds through a cyclic transition state and results in the loss of carbon dioxide from the β-keto acid.

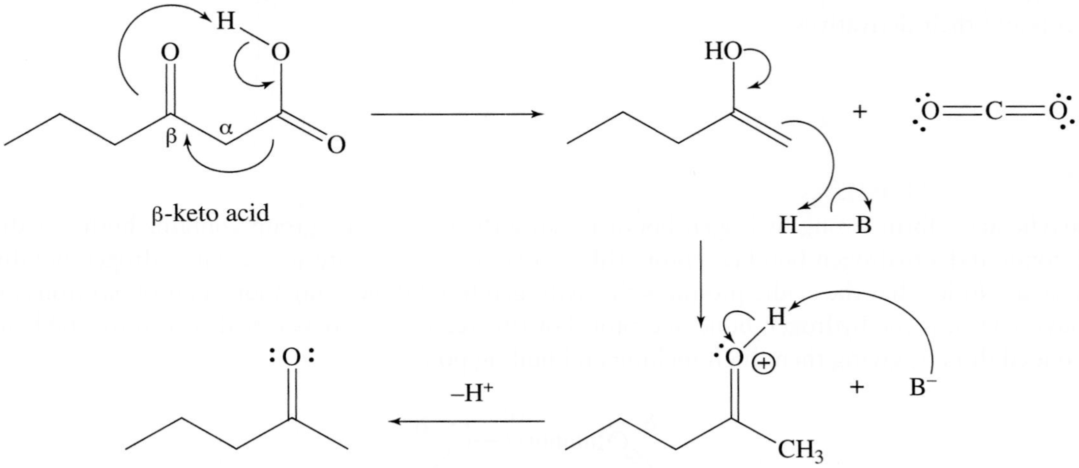

β-keto acid

35.4   CARBOXYLIC ACID DERIVATIVES

Carboxylic acid derivatives include acid chlorides, acid anhydrides, esters, and amides. The general chemical structures for these acid derivatives are

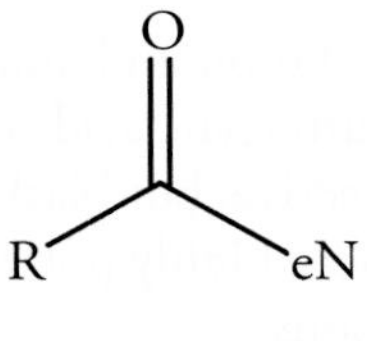

(eN = electronegative group)

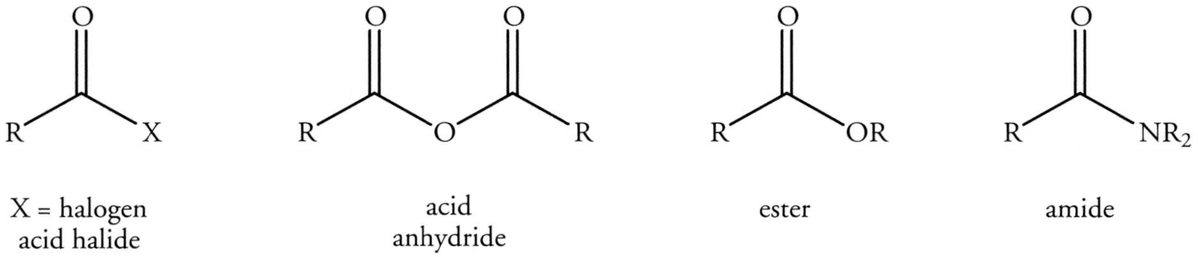

X = halogen
acid halide

acid
anhydride

ester

amide

As you might expect, the derivatives of carboxylic acids react similarly to aldehydes because they are also electrophilic at the carbonyl carbon atom. However, unlike reactions with aldehydes and ketones, nucleophilic additions to carboxylic acid derivatives are usually followed by elimination. (Note that additions and eliminations are opposites—while you can recognize an addition reaction because a π bond is broken and replaced by two new σ bonds, eliminations are the reverse. A new π bond is formed while two σ bonds break.) This is because the tetrahedral intermediate formed upon attack of the nucleophile on the carbonyl carbon has both a negatively charged oxygen atom (the former carbonyl oxygen) and a good leaving group (the eN-group of the carboxylic acid derivative). This elimination by the electrons on the oxygen atom regenerates the carbonyl, thereby displacing the leaving group (eN⁻). This is called a **nucleophilic addition-elimination reaction,** and it is sometimes referred to as an acyl substitution.

| Acid derivative | Tetrahedral intermediate | New acid derivative |

Esterification Reactions

An **esterification reaction** occurs when a carboxylic acid reacts with an alcohol in the presence of a catalytic amount of acid.

Esterification

a carboxylic acid   an alcohol   an ester

The following mechanism shows the formation of methyl benzoate from benzoic acid and methanol. We see that protonation of the carbonyl oxygen makes the carbonyl carbon more electrophilic, and nucleophilic attack by the oxygen of the alcohol results in a tetrahedral intermediate that is neutralized by deprotonation. An –OH group of the tetrahedral intermediate is then protonated, converting a poor leaving group (–OH) into a good one ($-OH_2^+$). As a result, a water molecule departs, leaving behind the protonated form of the ester. Deprotonation of the carbonyl oxygen yields the ester product and regenerates the acid catalyst.

The Acid-Catalyzed Mechanism

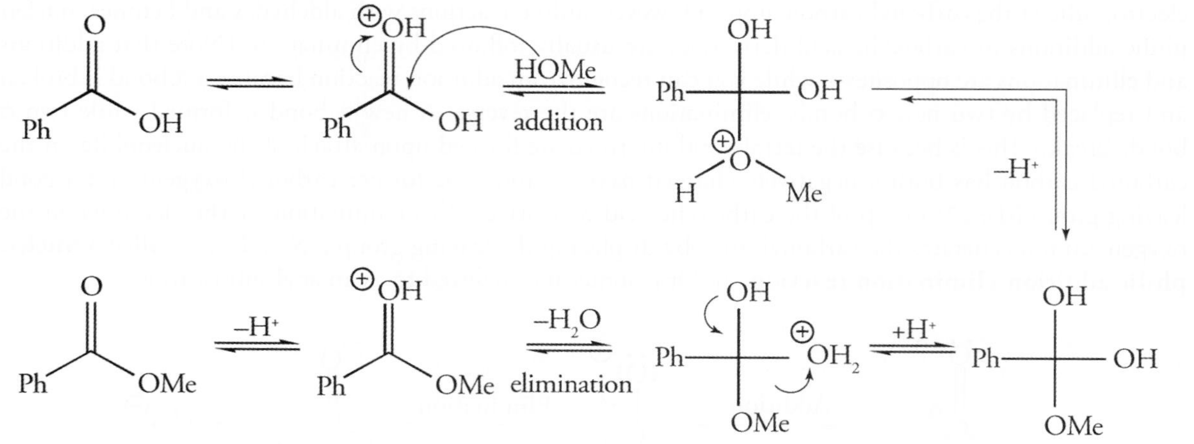

The hydrolysis of the ester formed above to form the carboxylic acid and alcohol can be achieved under acidic conditions, as it's just the reverse of the process shown. Note that each step of the mechanism above is an equilibrium step, so is therefore reversible.

Transesterification

Not only can esters be hydrolyzed to carboxylic acids, but treatment of esters with alcohols, generally with acid catalysis, results in a process known as transesterification. Following an equivalent mechanism as shown above for hydrolysis, the nucleophilic attack by an alcohol on the electrophilic carbonyl-carbon of the ester results in the replacement of the original –OR (below depicted as EtO–) with the incoming alcohol (depicted below as isobutanol).

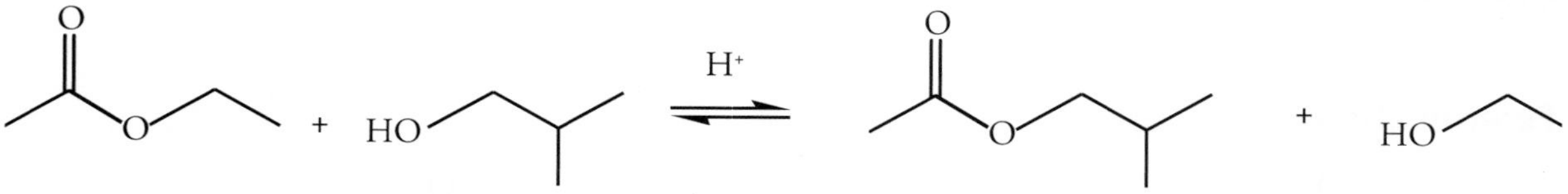

Like the esterification/hydrolysis reactions, the two esters exist in equilibrium, but there are a number of ways to favor the formation of the desired ester. One way is to employ conditions that remove by-products of the reaction from solution. For example, since ethanol is more volatile than isobutanol, mildly heating the reaction on the previous page will drive ethanol into the vapor phase and push the reaction to the right via Le Châtelier's principle. Similarly, using a large excess of the alcohol constituting the desired –OR in the product serves to shift the equilibrium in the desired direction. Such conditions are indicated as in the equation below.

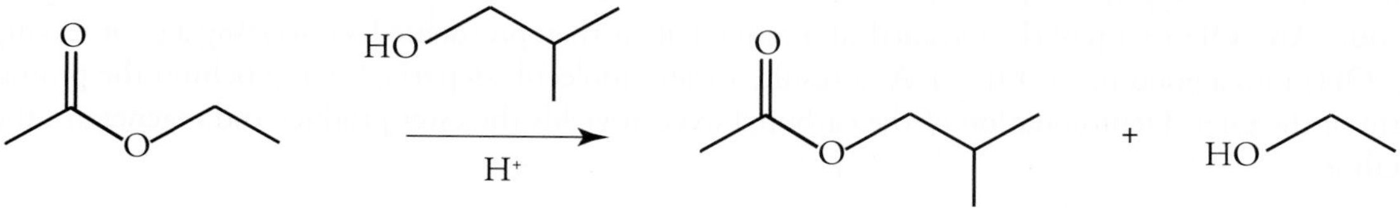

Placing isobutanol above or below the arrow denotes that it is used as the solvent, and is therefore in great excess. As a result, the equilibrium is essentially halted and the reaction is driven completely to the right. The reverse reaction is, of course, still possible if the isobutanol solvent is removed and replaced with ethanol.

Base-Mediated Ester Hydrolysis Mechanism

We now consider the corresponding *base*-mediated hydrolysis of methyl benzoate, commonly referred to as saponification. In the first step of the reaction, the strongly nucleophilic hydroxide ion directly attacks the electrophilic carbonyl carbon. The nucleophilic attack results in the formation of a tetrahedral intermediate.

The tetrahedral intermediate then undergoes an elimination reaction, reforming the carbonyl when a pair of electrons on the negatively charged oxygen regenerates the carbon-oxygen π bond. This eliminates the alkoxide ion as a leaving group. However, since the reaction is carried out under basic conditions and the alkoxide ion is a strong enough base to deprotonate the newly formed carboxylic acid, the final step of the mechanism is the acid-base reaction shown on the previous page. In order to recover the carboxylic acid from this process, the reaction must have a final aqueous acidic workup.

In summary, these two reactions, the acid-catalyzed hydrolysis of an ester and the base-mediated hydrolysis of an ester, display the most common reactivities of all of the carboxylic acid derivatives. Both of these reactions give the same products, but by different mechanisms. Most importantly, both of the mechanisms proceed through nucleophilic addition and elimination steps. A good understanding of these two reaction mechanisms leads to a solid understanding of all of the reactions of carboxylic acids and their derivatives.

Synthesis of the Carboxylic Acid Derivatives

Now that we understand how the electronic structure of the carboxylic acid derivatives relates to their reactivity, the synthesis of carboxylic acid derivatives should be straightforward. For the most part, we shall only be concerned with the interconversion of one derivative to another.

Acid Halides

Carboxylic acid halides are made from the corresponding carboxylic acid and either $SOCl_2$ or PX_3 (X = Cl, Br).

35.4

Acid Anhydrides

As their name implies, anhydrides (meaning "without water") can be prepared by the condensation of two carboxylic acids with the loss of water.

Acid anhydrides are also prepared from addition of the corresponding carboxylic acid (or carboxylate ion) to the corresponding acid halide.

Esters

Esters are most easily synthesized from the corresponding carboxylic acid and an alcohol, as we saw earlier. This reaction is referred to as **esterification**. Esters can also be prepared from an acid halide, an anhydride, or another ester and a corresponding alcohol.

Amides

Amides can be prepared from the corresponding acid halide, anhydride, or ester with the desired amine. They *cannot* be prepared from the carboxylic acid directly. This is because amines are very basic, and carboxylic acids are very acidic; an acid-base reaction occurs much faster than the desired addition-elimination reaction.

Carboxylic acids can be prepared from *any* of the derivatives merely by heating the derivative in acidic aqueous solutions.

Relative Reactivity of Carboxylic Acid Derivatives

Now that we are familiar with the general reactivity of carboxylic acid derivatives, we will examine how chemical *structure* affects the *relative* chemical reactivity of common acid derivatives. The order of reactivity in nucleophilic addition-elimination reactions for acid derivatives is

| Acid chlorides | Acid anhydrides | Esters | Amides |

If we examine the leaving groups of these acid derivatives, it is clear that the reactivity of acid derivatives in nucleophilic addition-elimination reactions decreases with increasing basicity of the leaving group.

Acid Derivative Reactivity

Acid Derivative	*Leaving Group*	
acid chloride	Cl⊖	Chloride anion is a very good leaving group. It is a very weak base since it is the conjugate base of the strong acid HCl ($pK_a = -7$).
acid anhydride	⊖O–C(=O)–R	This is a fairly good leaving group. It is the conjugate base of the weakly acidic carboxylic acid ($pK_a = 4–5$).
ester	⊖:Ö–R	An alkoxide ion is a rather poor leaving group. It is moderately basic since it is the conjugate base of alcohol, which is a fairly weak acid ($pK_a = 15–19$).
amide	⊖:N̈–R' / H	This is a horrible leaving group. It is strongly basic since it is the conjugate base of an amine, which is a terrible acid ($pK_a = 35–40$).

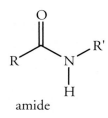
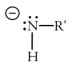

While acid chlorides and anhydrides are readily hydrolyzed in water, esters and amides are much more stable. Esters require either acidic or basic conditions and elevated temperatures in order to effect hydrolysis, and amides are generally only hydrolyzed under acidic conditions, high temperatures, and long reaction times.

35.4

Chapter 36
Biologically Important Molecules

Many of the details about the biologically important macromolecules are presented in the Biochemistry section of this book. In this chapter, we present some of the details from an Organic Chemistry perspective.

36.1 AMINO ACIDS

Proteins are biological macromolecules that act as enzymes, hormones, receptors, antibodies, and support structures inside and outside cells. Proteins are composed of twenty different amino acids linked together in polymers. The composition and sequence of amino acids in the polypeptide chain is what makes each protein unique and enables it to fulfill its special role in the cell.

Amino Acid Structure and Nomenclature

Understanding the structure of amino acids is key to understanding both their chemistry and the chemistry of proteins. The generic formula for all twenty amino acids is shown below.

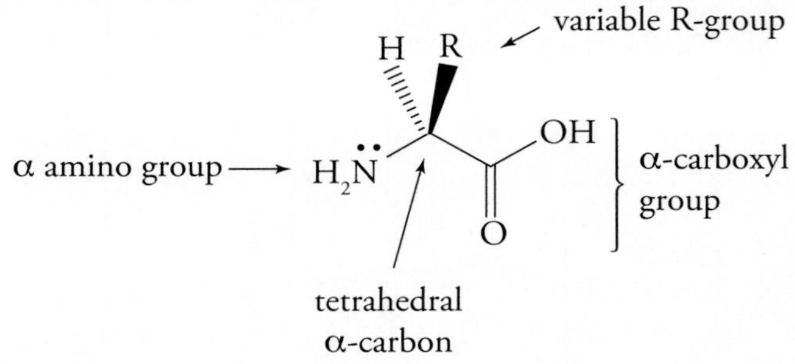

Figure 1   Generic Amino Acid Structure

All twenty amino acids share the same nitrogen-carbon-carbon backbone. The unique feature of each amino acid is its **side chain** (variable R-group), which gives it the physical and chemical properties that distinguish it from the other nineteen. Note that the α-carbon of each of the twenty amino acids is a stereocenter (has four different groups), except in the case of glycine, whose α-carbon is bonded to two hydrogen atoms. This means that all of the amino acids are chiral except for glycine.

L- and D-Amino Acids

Chemists often draw chiral molecules in their **Fischer projection** to illustrate stereochemistry. Let's review how Fischer projections denote the absolute stereochemistry of molecules. The conformation of a molecule that is shown in a Fischer projection happens to be the least stable, fully eclipsed form of the molecule. In Fischer projections the most oxidized carbon is at the top, and the structure is extended vertically until the final carbon atom is reached. This leaves the substituents on each carbon atom to occupy the horizontal positions of each carbon atom in the chain. This is illustrated below.

CHO group at top, with structures for L-amino acid and D-amino acid:

$$O=C-O^{\ominus}$$

$$H_3\overset{\oplus}{N}-\!\!\!\!-\!\!\!\!-H$$

$$R$$

L-amino acid

$$O=C-O^{\ominus}$$

$$H-\!\!\!\!-\!\!\!\!-\overset{\oplus}{N}H_3$$

$$R$$

D-amino acid

In the Fischer projection, it's understood that all horizontal lines are projecting from the plane of the page toward the viewer, and all vertical lines are projecting into the plane of the page, away from the viewer.

*All animal amino acids are of the L-configuration, with the amino group drawn on the **Left** in Fischer notation.* Some D-amino acids, with the amino group on the right, occur in a few specialized structures, such as bacterial cell walls. The L and D classification system can be a source of great confusion. For the MCAT, it is most important to remember that *all animal amino acids have the L configuration and that all naturally occurring carbohydrates have the D configuration.* (Carbohydrates are discussed in a later section of this chapter.) For completeness, though, we'll take the time to discuss the meaning of D and L now.

Assigning the Configuration to a Chiral Center

L- and D-amino acids and L- and D-carbohydrates are **enantiomeric stereoisomers**. The simplest (smallest) carbohydrate has only three carbons and only one chiral center. It is called **glyceraldehyde**. Since it has one chiral center, this molecule can exist in one of two enantiomeric forms, (+)-glyceraldehyde and (−)-glyceraldehyde. In reactions occurring in living organisms, CHOH groups are added to carbon #1 of glyceraldehyde to form larger carbohydrate molecules with more than one chiral center. In this synthetic process, the configuration at the original glyceraldehyde chiral carbon (#2) is not changed. So, if you start with (−)-glyceraldehyde and build a longer carbohydrate chain, that carbohydrate chain will have a penultimate (second-to-last) carbon atom with the same configuration as (−)-glyceraldehyde. So why not just call the new, larger carbohydrate "(−)?" You cannot refer to the new carbohydrate as (−) because you have added several new chiral centers, and now if you put the new molecule in solution and measure its optical rotation with a polarimeter, the optical activity may in fact be (+). What is needed is a way to name a carbohydrate that would specify that it had been built up from (−)- or (+)-glyceraldehyde without worrying about its actual optical activity.

$$CHO$$

$$HO-\!\!\!\!-\!\!\!\!-H$$

$$CH_2OH$$

L-(−)-Glyceraldehyde

$$CHO$$

$$H-\!\!\!\!-\!\!\!\!-OH$$

$$CH_2OH$$

D-(+)-Glyceraldehyde

The solution is to nickname (–)-glyceraldehyde as "L-glyceraldehyde" and to likewise refer to (+)-glyceraldehyde as "D-glyceraldehyde." Now we can refer to all carbohydrates built up from (–)-glyceraldehyde as "L" carbohydrates, without specifying whether they rotate plane-polarized light to the left (–) or to the right (+). All we have to do is look at the last chiral carbon in the chain and decide whether it looks like C2 from L- or D-glyceraldehyde.

Once again, the important thing to remember is that *all animal amino acids are derived from L-glyceraldehyde* (because they share the same basic structure at the penultimate carbon). Hence, they all have the L configuration. *Animal carbohydrates are chemically derived from D-glyceraldehyde*, and are thus all D.

There is another classification system, in which chiral centers are denoted either *R* or *S*. This system describes the *absolute configuration* of the chiral center; it refers to the actual three-dimensional arrangement of groups, as in a model or drawing; it says nothing about what the molecule will do to plane-polarized light.

In summary, you can see that three classification systems are used to organize amino acids and carbohydrates:

1. (+) and (–) describe optical activity, and mean the same thing as *d* and *l*, respectively;
2. *R* and *S* describe actual structure or absolute configuration; and
3. D and L tell us the basic precursor of a molecule (D- or L-glyceraldehyde).

You can also see that the three different classification systems don't describe each other in any way. A molecule that has the *R* configuration of its only stereocenter might rotate plane-polarized light *either* clockwise *or* counterclockwise, and hence be *either* (+) *or* (–). And a molecule that is experimentally determined to be (+) might be either D or L. However, two of the three classification systems go together for certain molecules. All D-sugars have the *R* configuration at the penultimate carbon atom because they are all derived from D-glyceraldehyde. Similarly, all L-sugars have the *S* configuration at the penultimate carbon atom. This is true only because carbohydrates are named according to the configuration of the last chiral center in the chain (which, remember, is synthetically derived from glyceraldehyde). By the same rationale, all L-amino acids are *S*, and all D-amino acids are *R*. (Note that the only exception is for cysteine, because the R group (CH_2SH) of this amino acid has a higher priority than the COOH group.)

- You crash-land on Mars without any food but notice that Mars is loaded with edible-looking plants. Martian life has evolved with all L-carbohydrates. Can you metabolize carbohydrates from Mars?[1]

---

[1] No. Enzyme activity depends on three-dimensional shape, and all animal digestive enzymes have active sites specific for substrate carbohydrates with the D configuration.

Synthesis of Amino Acids

Nature has developed complicated mechanisms for the syntheses of the amino acids it uses to build proteins. In the laboratory, synthetic chemists have developed their own set of tools with which to make these essential building blocks available. Two important synthetic methods for the production of amino acids are the Strecker and Gabriel syntheses.

Strecker Synthesis

The Strecker synthesis utilizes ammonium and cyanide salts to transform aldehydes into α-amino acids. While naturally occurring amino acids are stereochemically pure (L-enantiomers), those produced via this process are racemic. Despite this drawback, a variety of both naturally-occurring and non-natural amino acids may be easily synthesized, depending on the substitution of the aldehyde. An example of the Strecker synthesis applied to the production of (D,L)-valine is shown below:

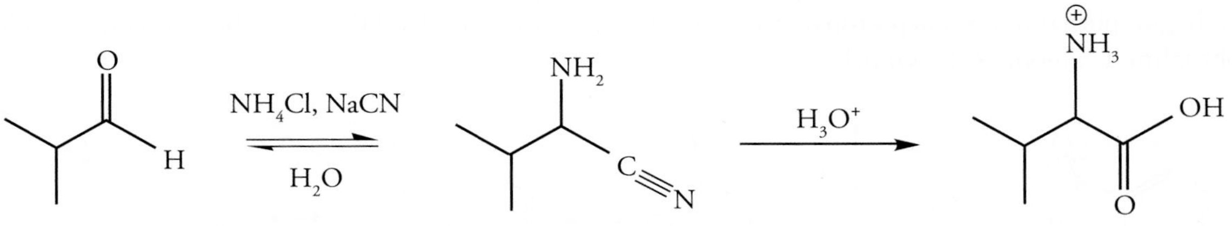

2-methylpropanal   (D,L)-valine

The combination of an ammonium halide and alkali cyanide results in the formation of alkali halide salts and the *in situ* production of the active species, NH_3 and HCN. In the first step of the reaction, the aldehyde reacts with ammonia to yield an imine.

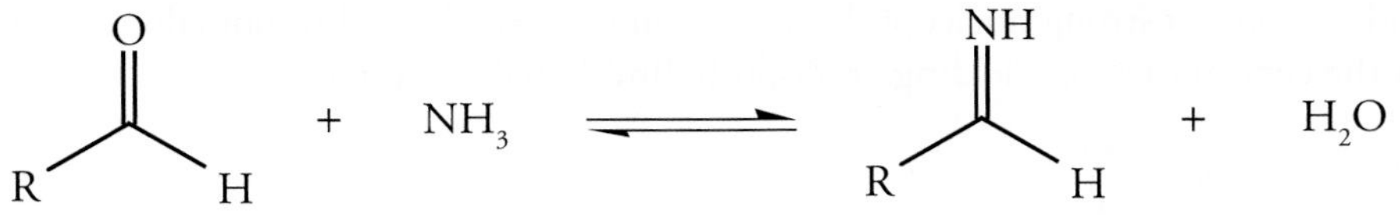

When protonated by HCN, the imine becomes more electrophilic, enabling attack by the remaining cyanide ion on the imine-carbon and concomitant formation of an α-amino nitrile. This attack by cyanide on an unsaturated carbon electrophile resembles the mechanism previously described for the formation of cyanohydrins. The difference is that the Strecker synthesis utilizes an imine (rather than a carbonyl) as substrate for the attack.

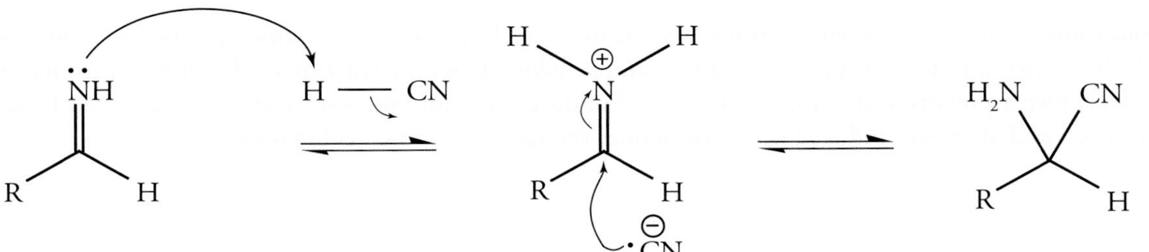

imine   α-amino nitrile

In a subsequent step, acid catalyzed hydrolysis of the α-amino nitrile gives the α-amino acid.

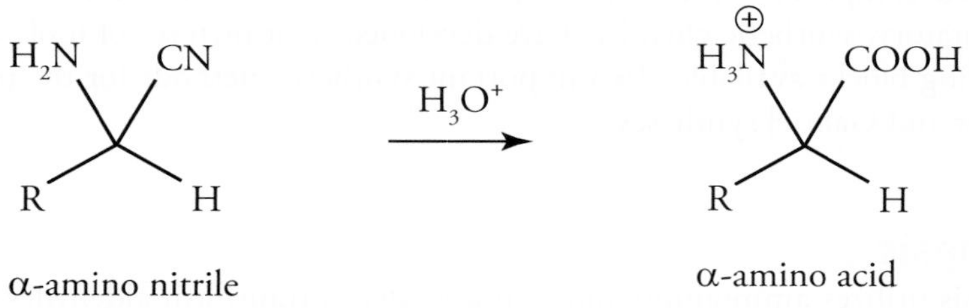

α-amino nitrile   α-amino acid

Gabriel-Malonic Ester Synthesis

The Gabriel-malonic ester synthesis is another useful method for the production of α-amino acids. Over the course of the reaction, the nitrogen in a molecule of phthalimide is converted into a primary amine. To begin, phthalimide is deprotonated with potassium hydroxide (KOH) to give the resonance-stabilized phthalimide anion, as shown below:

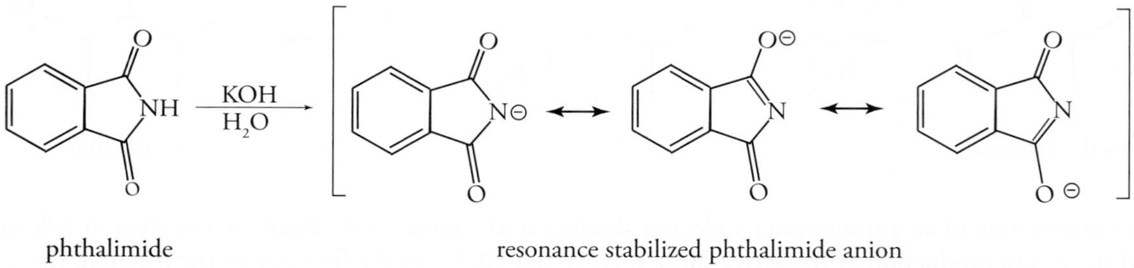

phthalimide   resonance stabilized phthalimide anion

The phthalimide anion is a strong nucleophile, and when treated with α-bromomalonic ester, it displaces bromide from the central carbon, yielding an *N*-phthalimidomalonic ester.

N-phthalimidomalonic ester

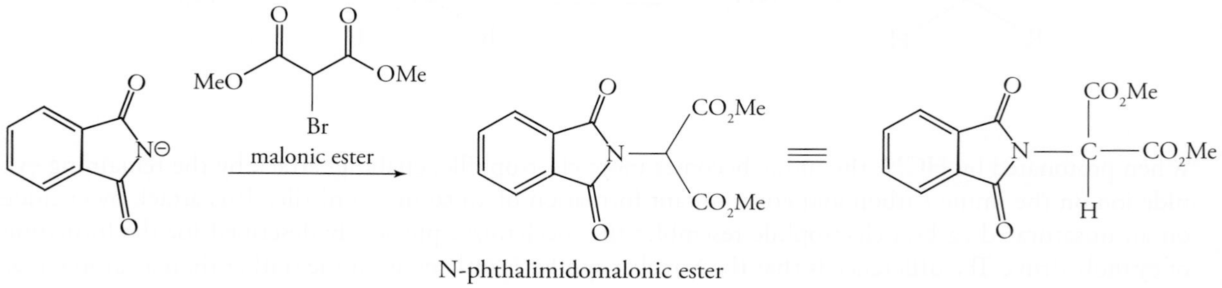

Enolization of the α-carbon with a strong base creates a nucleophilic carbon, which can be functionalized with the desired amino acid side-chain. The example below shows the reaction of the enolate with methyl iodide to give a precursor of alanine. The phthalimido group and both esters are then subjected to acid hydrolysis, and after heat-induced decarboxylation, the racemic amino acid may be isolated.

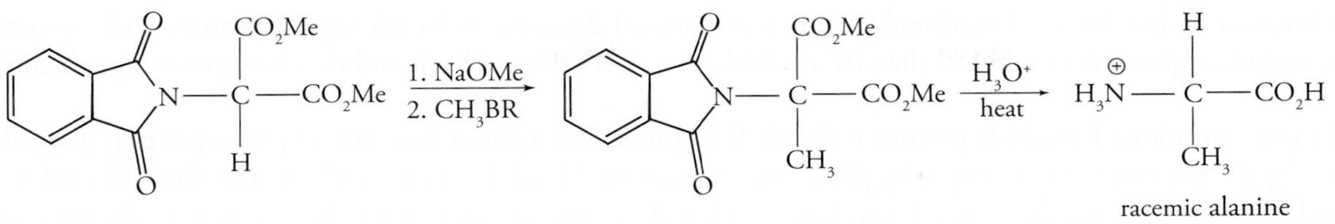

racemic alanine

Amino Acid Reactivity

Since amino acids are composed of an acidic group (the carboxylic acid) and a basic group (the amine), we must be sure to understand the acid/base chemistry of amino acids. Later, we will review amide bond formation by examining formation of the peptide bond in protein synthesis.

Reviewing the Fundamentals of Acid/Base Chemistry

Before we can discuss amino acids, we must be sure to understand the fundamentals of acid/base chemistry because each amino acid is **amphoteric**, which means it has both acidic and basic activity. This should make sense since an amino acid contains the acidic carboxylic acid group and the basic amino group.

Remember from general chemistry that acids can be defined as proton (H^+) donors, and bases can be defined as proton acceptors. Thus, in the case of the equation below, H_2A^+ is a proton donor (acid), and A^- is a proton acceptor (base); HA may act as either acid or base. The equations below also show how to calculate the equilibrium constant (K) for an acid dissociation reaction. The equilibrium constant for an acid dissociation reaction is given a special name: **acid dissociation constant**, abbreviated K_a. The equilibrium reactions for the first and second proton dissociation reactions are described by the equations for the acid dissociation constants K_{a1} and K_{a2}.

$$H_2A^+ \underset{(K_{a1})}{\rightleftharpoons} HA + H^+ \underset{(K_{a2})}{\rightleftharpoons} A^- + 2H^+$$

$$K_a = \frac{[\text{products}]}{[\text{reactants}]} \implies \boxed{K_{a1} = \frac{[HA][H^+]}{[H_2A^+]}} \boxed{K_{a2} = \frac{[A^-][H^+]}{[HA]}}$$

Figure 2   The Acid Dissociation Reaction

- In the equilibrium between H_2A^+, HA, and A^- above, which statement is true?[2]
  A) HA will act as a base by donating a proton.
  B) HA will act as an acid by accepting a proton.
  C) HA can act as either an acid or a base, depending on whether it accepts or donates a proton.
  D) HA is in chemical equilibrium with H_2A^+ and A^- and in that capacity cannot act as either an acid or a base.

---

[2] Choice **C** is correct: in the equilibrium shown, HA can either act as an acid by donating a proton (choice B is wrong) or as a base by accepting a proton (choice A is wrong). Remember also that equilibrium is not a fixed state. In other words, HA is not doomed to stay HA forever; it can move forward and back between the states shown (choice D is wrong).

Whether a molecule (or a functional group) is protonated depends on its affinity for protons and the concentration of protons in solution that are available to it. Let's discuss both and do a few practice problems.

The concentration of available protons is simply [H⁺] (moles/liter), but it is usually expressed as **pH**, defined as *–log [H⁺]*. If you're wondering why pH is used instead of [H⁺], it has to do with the fact that [H⁺] values tend to be clumsy numbers, so a logarithmic scale reduces the amount of writing we have to do; we use the *negative* logarithm simply to avoid writing an extra minus sign. For example, instead of writing [H⁺] = $10^{-3.46}$, we can write pH = 3.46. The pH inside cells is 7.4. This is often referred to as **physiological pH**, and it is carefully regulated by buffers in the blood because extremes of pH disrupt protein structure.

The affinity of a functional group (such as an amino or carboxyl group) for protons is given by the acid dissociation constant K_a for that functional group, which is simply the equilibrium constant for the dissociation of the acid form (HA) into a proton (H⁺) plus the conjugate base (A⁻). The equilibrium constant describes a reaction's tendency to move right or left as it moves toward equilibrium from some starting point. This affinity can also be expressed as pK_a, defined as $-\log K_a$. Carboxyl groups of amino acids generally have a pK_a of about 2 (stronger acid), while the ammonium groups generally have a pK_a of 9 or 10 (weaker acid).

The mathematical formula that describes the relationship between pH, pK_a, and the position of equilibrium in an acid-base reaction is known as the **Henderson–Hasselbalch** equation:

$$pH = pK_a + \log \frac{[A^-]}{[HA]} = pK_a + \log \frac{[\text{base form}]}{[\text{acid form}]}$$

Given the pH and the pK_a, we can calculate the ratio of the base and acid forms of a compound at equilibrium. Just remember these rules:

- Low pH means high [H⁺].
- Lower pK_a (same as higher K_a) describes a stronger acid that can donate a proton even when there are already excess protons (high [H⁺], low pH).

3) The text above states that physiological pH is 7.4. Is this more or less acidic—and are there more or fewer extra protons—than in pure water?[3]

4) Acetic acid (CH_3COOH) has pK_a = 4.7. Calculate the equilibrium ratio of [CH_3COO^-] to [CH_3COOH] at pH 4.7.[4]

5) Which functional group on amino acids has a stronger tendency to donate protons: carboxyl groups (pK_a = 2.0) or ammonium groups (pK_a = 9)? Which group will donate protons at the lowest pH?[5]

---

[3] Remember that a larger pH implies *fewer* extra protons, since pH = $-\log[H^+]$. A pH of 7.4 describes a solution with slightly fewer extra free protons, i.e., a slightly less acidic (more basic) solution, relative to a pH 7.0 solution.

[4] First, substitute into the equation: 4.7 = 4.7 + log [CH_3COO^-]/[CH_3COOH]. Then, solve: 0 = log [CH_3COO^-]/[CH_3COOH]. What has a log of 0? In other words, ten to the power of 0 is equal to what? 10^0 = [CH_3COO^-]/[CH_3COOH] = 1.0. So when the pH = pK_a, the ratio of base to acid is 1 to 1. That's a fact worth memorizing.

[5] A higher pK_a means that a higher proportion of the protonated form is present relative to the unprotonated form, according to the H-H equation. High pK_a indicates a weak acid. Acids with low pK_as, tend to deprotonate more easily. Therefore, ammonium groups have a stronger tendency to keep their protons and carboxyl groups will donate protons at the lowest pH (highest [H⁺]).

Application of Fundamental Acid/Base Chemistry to Amino Acids

With that review of acids and bases, we are now prepared to discuss amino acid reactivity. The review is important because all amino acids contain an amino group that acts as a base and a carboxyl group ($pK_a \approx 2$) that acts as an acid. In its protonated, or acidic form, the amine is called an **ammonium group**, and has a pK_a between 9–10. For example:

$$-NH_3^+ \rightleftharpoons -NH_2 + H^+ \qquad pK_a \approx 9$$

$$-COOH \rightleftharpoons -COO^- + H^+ \qquad pK_a \approx 2$$

6) Assuming a pK_a of 2, will a carboxylate group be protonated or deprotonated at pH 1.0?[6]
7) Will the amino group be protonated or deprotonated at pH 1.0?[7]
8) At pH 6.0, between the pK_as of the ammonium and carboxyl groups, what will be the net charge on a molecule of glycine?[8]

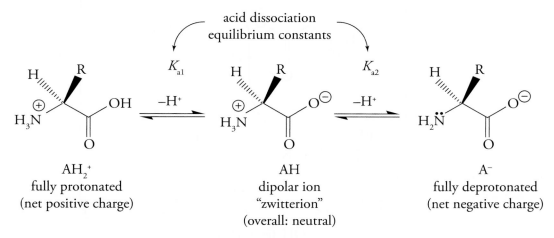

Figure 3 Important Amino Acid Conjugate Acid/Base Pairs

The Isoelectric Point of Amino Acids

There is a pH for every amino acid at which it has no overall net charge (the positive and negative charges cancel). A molecule with positive and negative charges that balance is referred to as a dipolar ion or **zwitterion**. The pH at which a molecule is uncharged (zwitterionic) is referred to as its **isoelectric point** (pI). "Zwitter" is German for "hybrid," implying that an amino acid at its pI has both (+) and (–) charges.

It is possible to calculate the pI of an amino acid—in other words, to figure out the pH value at which (+) and (–) charges balance (that's the definition of pI). For a molecule with two functional groups, such as glycine, the calculation is simple: just *average the pKₐs of the two functional groups*. The pI of more

---

[6] The pH is less than the pK_a here, so protonation wins over dissociation, and the group will be protonated. The correct answer is –COOH.

[7] The pH is much lower than the pK_a for the ammonium group, so the amino group is protonated: NH_3^+.

[8] The carboxyl group will be deprotonated (COO^-) with a charge of –1 and the amino group will be protonated (NH_3^+) with a charge of +1, creating a net charge of 0 per glycine molecule.

complex molecules can also be calculated, but for the MCAT, you should know how to calculate the pI of a molecule with two functional groups (with no acidic or basic functional groups in the side chain). Another important thing to know for the MCAT is how to compare the pH of a solution to the pK_a of a functional group of an amino acid and determine if a site is mostly protonated or deprotonated. If the pH is higher than the pK_a, the site is mostly deprotonated; if the pH is lower than the pK_a, the site is mostly protonated. This can be illustrated in the titration curve for glycine:

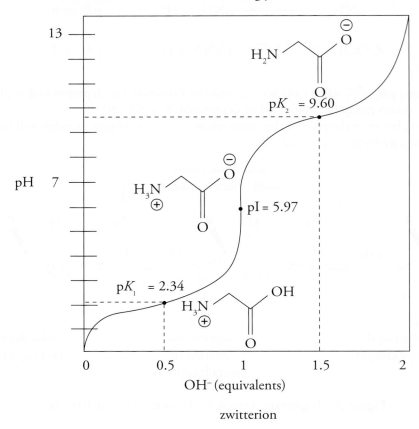

zwitterion

9) What is the pI of glycine?[9]

---

[9] To calculate the pI, just average the pK_as of the two functional groups: (9.60 + 2.34)/2 = 5.97, or roughly 6.

Amino Acid Separation—Gel Electrophoresis

Gel electrophoresis is a general separation technique that can be used to separate amino acids based on their charge. In general, when employing this technique, amino acids are loaded onto a gel that is held at a constant pH, then exposed to an electric field. When the pH of the gel is different than the pI of the amino acids, each amino acid will bear an overall charge because pI is specific to the unique structure of the side chain of each amino acid. The amino acids will therefore migrate through the gel based on their charge and the external electric field. The MCAT tends to ask about how specific amino acids will migrate relative to each other in these separation conditions. In order to answer these questions, an understanding of the relationship between pH, pK_a, and pI (as discussed previously) is required. See the table below, which summarizes how pH will determine the direction of amino acid migration during an electrophoresis separation:

pH	Charge on Amino Acid	Direction of Migration
greater than pI	negative	toward positive electrode
lower than pI	positive	toward negative electrode
equal to pI	neutral (zwitterion)	no migration

10) A sample of glycine is loaded on a gel in a pH = 6.0 solution with a (+) electrode at one end and a (−) electrode at the other end. Will the majority of the glycine migrate toward the negative terminal, migrate toward the positive terminal, or not migrate in either direction?[10]

11) pK_a values for the three functional groups in glutamic acid are 9.7 for the amino group, 2.2 for the α−carboxyl, and 4.2 for the side chain carboxyl. What pole (− or +) will glutamic acid migrate toward in an electric field at physiological pH (7.4)?[11]

12) What pole (− or +) would glutamic acid migrate toward in an electric field in a pH 1.0 solution?[12]

13) Which of these amino acids is most likely to be found on the interior of a protein at pH 7.0?[13]
   A. Alanine
   B. Aspartic acid
   C. Phenylalanine
   D. Glycine

14) Which of the following amino acids is most likely to be found on the exterior of a protein at pH 7.0?[14]
   A. Valine
   B. Alanine
   C. Threonine
   D. Isoleucine

---

[10] At this pH level, glycine has a net charge of zero. Hence, it will not move in an electric field.

[11] The amino group will be protonated ($-NH_3^+$), and both carboxyl groups deprotonated ($-CO_2^-$), producing an average charge per glutamic acid molecule of −1. Thus, glutamic acid will migrate toward the oppositely charged (+) pole at pH 7.4.

[12] Both carboxyl groups in glutamic acid would be protonated and uncharged ($-CO_2H$), and the amino group would be protonated and charged ($-NH_3^+$). The net charge is +1, so glutamic acid would migrate toward the (−) pole.

[13] Asp is incorrect, since this amino acid is charged at a pH of 7. Of the three remaining, phenylalanine has the largest hydrophobic group, and is therefore the most likely to be found on the interior of a protein. The answer is choice **C**.

[14] Valine, alanine, and isoleucine all contain hydrophobic residues and thus are more likely to be found on the interior. The answer is choice **C**.

36.2 PROTEINS

The Peptide Bond

Polypeptides are formed by linking amino acids together in peptide bonds. A **peptide bond** is formed between the carboxyl group of one amino acid and the α-amino group of another amino acid with the loss of water. This occurs by the same nucleophilic addition-elimination mechanism shown in Section 35.4 for formation of any one of the carboxylic acid derivatives from any other carboxylic acid derivative. Remember that a peptide bond is just an amide bond between two amino acids. The figure below shows the formation of a dipeptide from the amino acids glycine and alanine.

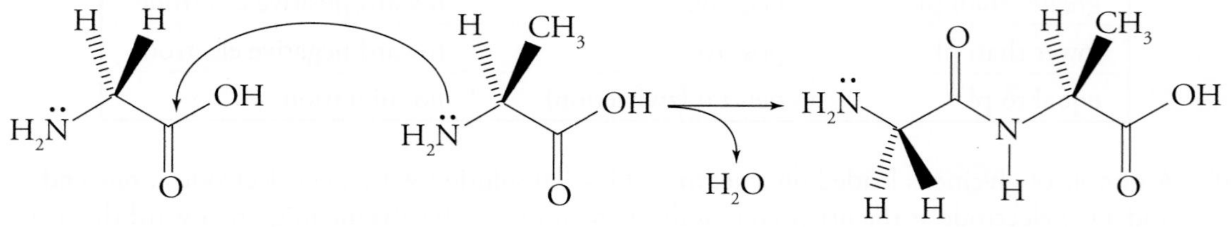

Figure 4 Peptide Bond (Amide Bond) Formation

DCC Coupling

In order to synthesize peptides artificially in the laboratory, **DCC coupling** is used. In the first step of the coupling process, DCC, or dicyclohexyl carbodiimide, converts the OH of the carboxylate group in an amino acid into a good leaving group. In the next step, the amino group of a second amino acid attacks the carbonyl carbon of the "activated" amino acid. Finally, the DCC leaves with the oxygen to which it is bonded. To assure that amino acids are added in a unidirectional manner and in the proper order for the desired peptide, the reaction is run using protecting groups so that only one of the carboxyl groups and one of the amino groups are available to react. See the example reaction that follows.

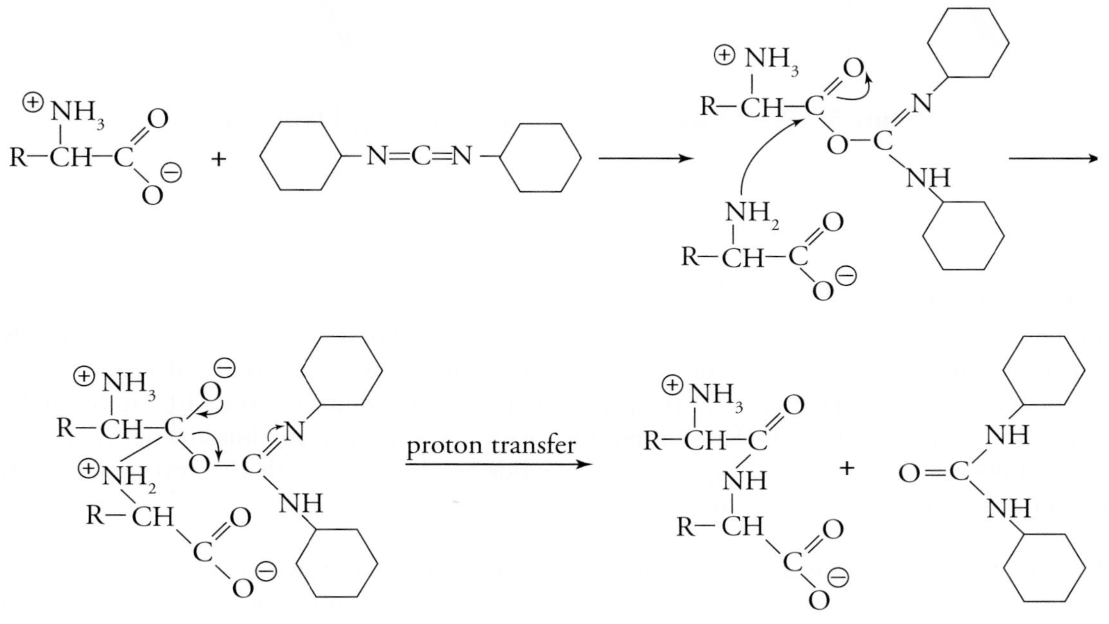

In a polypeptide chain, the N–C–C–N–C–C pattern formed from the amino acids is known as the **backbone** of the polypeptide. An individual amino acid is termed a **residue** when it is part of a poly-peptide chain. The amino terminus is the first end made during polypeptide synthesis, and the carboxy terminus is made last. Hence, by convention, the amino-terminal residue is also always written first.

15) In the oligopeptide Phe-Glu-Gly-Ser-Ala, state the number of acid and base functional groups, which residue has a free α-amino group, and which residue has a free α-carboxyl group. (Refer to the beginning of the chapter for structures.)[15]

16) Thermodynamics states that free energy must decrease for a reaction to proceed spontaneously and that such a reaction will spontaneously move toward equilibrium. The reaction coordinate diagram above shows the free energy changes during peptide bond formation. At equilibrium, which is thermodynamically favored: the dipeptide or the individual amino acids?[16]

17) In that case, how are peptide bonds formed and maintained inside cells?[17]

---

[15] As stated above, the amino end is always written first. Hence, the oligopeptide begins with an exposed Phe amino group and ends with an exposed Ala carboxyl; all the other backbone groups are hitched together in peptide bonds. Out of all the R-groups, there is only one acidic or basic functional group, the acidic glutamic acid R-group. This R-group plus the two terminal backbone groups gives a total of three acid/base functional groups.

[16] The dipeptide has a higher free energy, so its existence is less favorable. In other words, existence of the chain is less favorable than existence of the isolated amino acids.

[17] During protein synthesis, stored energy is used to force peptide bonds to form. Once the bond is formed, even though its destruction is thermodynamically favorable, it remains stable because the activation energy for the hydrolysis reaction is so high. In other words, hydrolysis is thermodynamically favorable but kinetically slow.

Planarity of the Peptide Bond

The peptide bond is planar and rigid because the resonance delocalization of the nitrogen's electrons to the carbonyl oxygen gives substantial double bond character to the bond between the carbonyl carbon and the nitrogen, as shown below. Hence, there can be no rotation around the peptide bond.

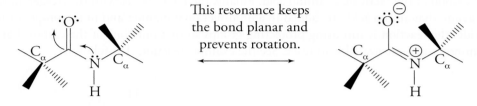

This resonance keeps the bond planar and prevents rotation.

Figure 5   Resonance Structure of the Planar, Rigid Peptide Bond

Hydrolysis of the Peptide Bond

Hydrolysis refers to any reaction in which water is inserted in a bond to cleave it. We have already discussed the details of hydrolysis reactions that covered the hydrolysis of an ester under both acidic and basic reaction conditions. Hydrolysis of the peptide bond (amide bond) to form a free amine and a carboxylic acid is thermodynamically favored (products have lower free energy), but kinetically slow. There are two common means of accelerating the rate of peptide bond hydrolysis (that is, two common ways to destroy proteins): strong acids and proteolytic enzymes.

Acid hydrolysis is the cleaving of a protein into its constituent amino acids with strong acid and heat. This is a non-specific means of cleaving peptide bonds. The amount of each amino acid present after hydrolysis can then be quantified to determine the overall amino acid content of the protein.

18)   If a tripeptide of Gly-Phe-Ala is subjected to acid hydrolysis, can the order of the residues in the tripeptide be determined afterward?[18]

---

[18]   No. After hydrolysis all amino acids are separate and have free amino and carboxyl groups.

36.3 CARBOHYDRATES

Carbohydrates are chains of hydrated carbon atoms with the molecular formula $C_nH_{2n}O_n$. The chain usually begins with an aldehyde or ketone and continues as a polyalcohol in which each carbon has a hydroxyl substituent. Carbohydrates are produced by photosynthesis in plants and by biochemical synthesis in animals. Carbohydrates can be broken down to CO_2 in a process called **oxidation**, which is also known as burning or combustion. Because this process releases large amounts of energy, carbohydrates serve as the principle energy source for cellular metabolism. Glucose in the form of the polymer cellulose is also the building block of wood and cotton. Understanding the nomenclature, structure, and chemistry of carbohydrates is essential to understanding cellular metabolism. This chapter will also help you understand key facts such as why we can eat potatoes and cotton candy but not wood and cotton T-shirts.

Structure and Nomenclature of Monosaccharides

A single carbohydrate molecule is a **monosaccharide** (meaning "single sweet unit"), also known as a **simple sugar**. Two monosaccharides bonded together form a **disaccharide**; several bonded together make an **oligosaccharide**, and many make a **polysaccharide**. If these polymers are subjected to strong acid, they are hydrolyzed to monosaccharides, which are not further hydrolyzed.

Classes of monosaccharides are given a two-part name. The first part is either "aldo" or "keto," depending on whether an aldehyde or a ketone is present. The second part reveals the number of carbon atoms in the chain: trioses are the smallest and have three carbons; tetroses have four, pentoses five, hexoses six, and heptoses seven. For example, the *polyhydroxy aldehyde glucose* is an *aldohexose* because it is a six-carbon chain beginning in an aldehyde. "Glucose" and "fructose" are examples of **common names**. IUPAC nomenclature is not usually used with individual carbohydrates because the systematic names are so long.

The carbons in monosaccharides are numbered beginning with carbon #1 at the *most oxidized end* of the carbon chain, which is the end with the aldehyde or ketone.

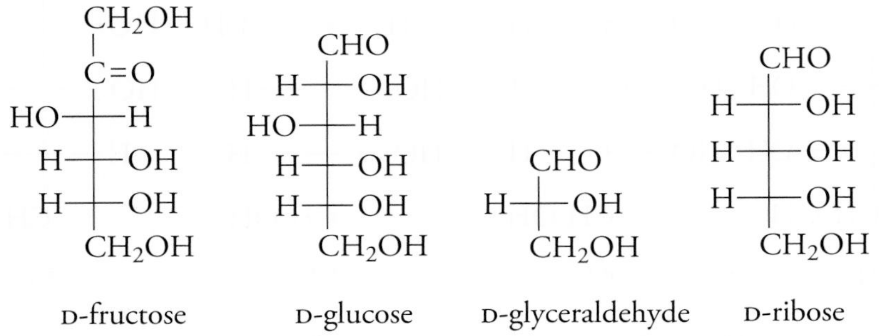

Figure 6 Some Metabolically Important Simple Sugars and Common Sugars on the MCAT

19) Which of the sugars in the figure above is a ketohexose?[19]
20) Which carbon (#?) is the most oxidized in D-fructose?[20]

---

[19] Fructose. It has six carbons, making it a hexose, and the carbonyl group is located on carbon #2, making it a ketose. Fructose is a polyhydroxy ketone, or a ketohexose.

[20] Carbon #2

Absolute Configuration of Monosaccharides

Because carbohydrates contain chiral carbons, it is also necessary to classify them according to stereochemistry. Like amino acids, carbohydrates are assigned one of two configurations, either D or L, based on the configuration of the last chiral carbon in the chain (farthest from the aldehyde or ketone). By convention, this configuration is determined by comparison with glyceraldehyde. If a monosaccharide's last chiral carbon matches the chiral carbon of D-glyceraldehyde, it will be assigned the "D" label. The sugars in our bodies have the D configuration. When you are drawing a Fischer projection of a monosaccharide, put the aldehyde or ketone on top and the CH_2OH group (last carbon) on the bottom. The last chiral carbon will have its OH on the **Left** for L monosaccharides. However, we have only D-sugars in our bodies. Remember that we have only L-amino acids and only D-sugars.

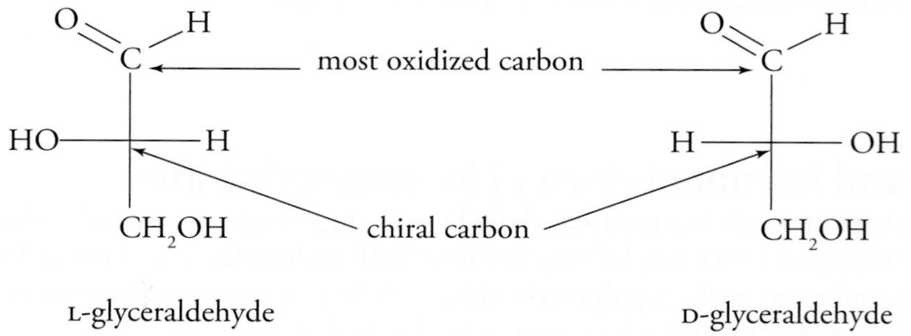

Figure 7   The Fischer Notation for Carbohydrates

For a given class of monosaccharide (like any other chiral molecule), there are 2^n different stereoisomers, where n is the number of chiral carbons.

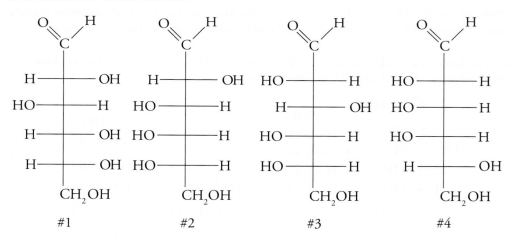

Figure 8   Four Monosaccharide Stereoisomers

21) Consider the four monosaccharides on the previous page. Which one of the following is correct?[21]

    A. Carbohydrate #2 is a D sugar and an enantiomer of #4.

    B. Carbohydrate #2 is an enantiomer of #3.

    C. Carbohydrates #1 and #3 are epimers and enantiomers.

    D. Carbohydrates #1 and #3 are enantiomers.

22) There are __ aldohexoses and __ D-aldohexoses (tough question but you *do* have all the information you need to figure it out).[22]

23) Is it possible to produce a diastereomer of D-glyceraldehyde? How about an epimer?[23]

Since we already discussed the relationships between the terms *isomer, stereoisomer, enantiomer, diastereomer,* and *epimer* in Chapter 34, we will not discuss them again here. The following Venn diagram represents a concise way of categorizing these terms. It shows which groups are subsets of which. *Isomers* have the same atoms but different bonds, unless they are also stereoisomers. Stereoisomers have the same atoms and the same bonds, but different bond geometries. All stereoisomers are either enantiomers or diastereomers. Some diastereomers are epimers.

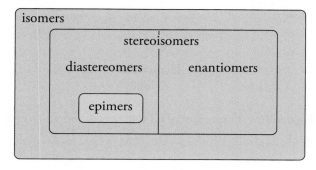

Figure 9   A Venn Diagram for Stereoisomers

Cyclic Structures of Monosaccharides

So far, we have represented the monosaccharides as straight chain structures. In solution, however, hexoses and pentoses spontaneously form five- and six-membered rings. In fact, the cyclic structures are thermodynamically favored so that only a small percentage usually exist in the open chain form. The six-membered ring structures are termed **pyranoses** due to their resemblance to pyran, and five-membered sugar rings are termed **furanoses** due to their resemblance to furan.

---

[21] Sugar #2 is an L sugar, since the last chiral OH is on the left (choice A is false and can be eliminated). Sugars #2 and #3 are not mirror images, so they cannot be enantiomers (choice B is false and can be eliminated). Since sugars #1 and #3 are non-superimposable images, the are enantiomers (choice **D** is the correct statement), and remember that epimers are never enantiomers (choice C is false and can be eliminated).

[22] There are 2^4 aldohexoses, because there are 4 chiral carbons (#2, 3, 4, and 5). There are only 2^3 D-aldohexoses, because when you specify the "D" configuration, you leave only 3 variable chiral centers.

[23] No, it is not possible to make a glyceraldehyde diastereomer, because the molecule has only one chiral carbon. The only stereoisomer of D-glyceraldehyde is L-glyceraldehyde, an enantiomer. You can't make an epimer because the word "epimer" is reserved for sugars with more than one chiral center.

Pyran   Furan

Let's take glucose as an example. The ring forms when the OH on C5 nucleophilically attacks the carbonyl carbon (C1), forming a **hemiacetal**. The reactions involved, in which an alcohol reacts with an aldehyde to produce a hemiacetal (one –OR group and one –OH group) and subsequently an acetal (two –OR groups), are shown below (see also Section 36.1). The difference between an acetal and a hemiacetal is that the hemiacetal is in constant equilibrium with the carbonyl form. The acetal form, in contrast, is quite stable, requiring an enzyme to react.

Aldehyde   Hemiacetal   Acetal
                             (labile)   (stable)

Figure 10   Formation of a Hemiacetal and an Acetal

The figure below shows the reaction for glucose. Note that two different ring structures are shown, α and β. The α or β ring is formed depending upon from which face of the carbonyl the C5-hydroxyl group attacks. If the attack comes from one face, the carbonyl oxygen will become an equatorial hydroxyl group; if the attack comes from the other face, the carbonyl oxygen will become an axial hydroxyl group. [To distinguish the forms, remember, "It's always better to βE up (happy)!" This will help you remember that in β-D-Glucose, the anomeric hydroxyl group is up.] The two forms are called **anomers**, and C1 (designated with an asterisk in the figures) is called the **anomeric carbon**. The anomeric carbon is always the carbonyl carbon, so in aldoses it is C1, but in ketoses it is C2. The interconversion between the two anomers is called **mutarotation**.

Also, remember that *axial* substituents on six-membered chair rings are those that point *straight up or down*. The *equatorial* substituents point *out* from the ring. Equatorial substituents have less steric hindrance with the ring and are thus thermodynamically more favorable.

(* = anomeric carbon)

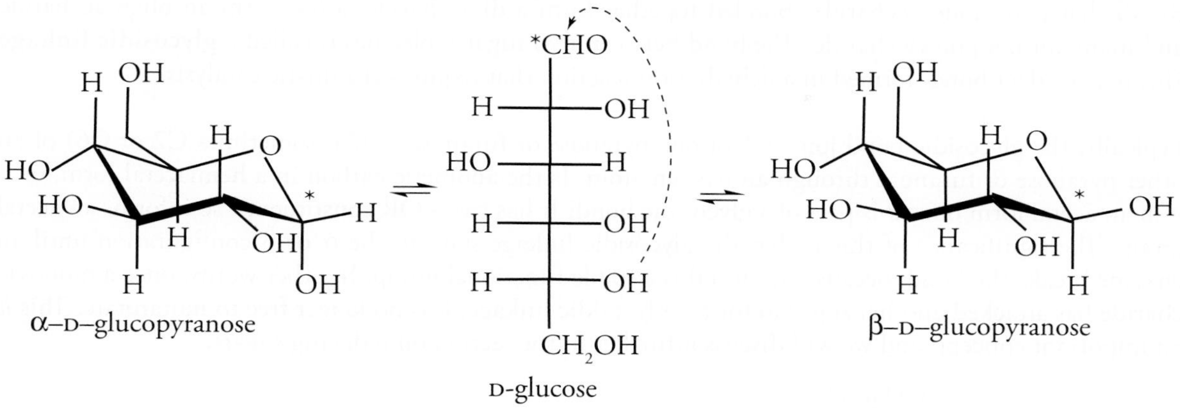

α–D–glucopyranose   D-glucose   β–D–glucopyranose

24) Why doesn't glucose cyclize into three- or four-membered rings?[24]
25) A solution of glucose may contain both furanose and pyranose rings. How can the same sugar exist in both forms?[25]

Another way to represent cyclic sugars is called Haworth notation. The groups on the *left* in Fischer notation are *above* the ring in Haworth notation (as in the chair form).

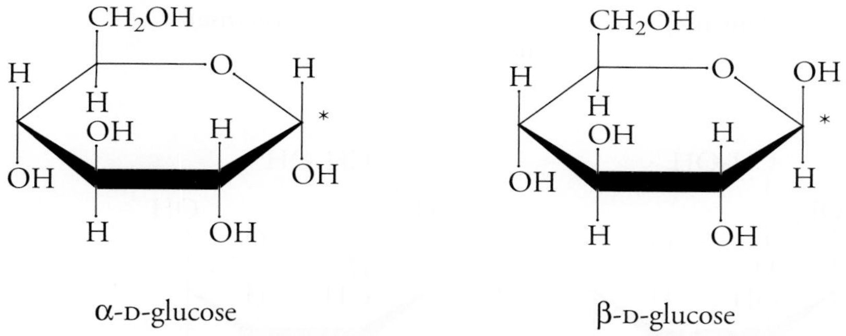

α-D-glucose   β-D-glucose

Figure 11   Haworth Representation of Glucopyranose

---

[24] Smaller rings necessitate bond angles that are much narrower than the normal tetrahedral angle. Strained bonds are unfavorable because they are high energy.

[25] The structure that forms depends on which OH attacks the carbonyl carbon (C#1). If OH_4 attacks the carbonyl, the result will be a five-membered ring. If OH_5 attacks, the result will be a six-membered ring. If you actually counted the structures in solution, you'd find more six-membered rings, since these are inherently more stable due to bond angles.

Structure and Nomenclature of Disaccharides

Recall that two monosaccharides bonded together form a disaccharide, a few form an oligosaccharide, and many form a polysaccharide. The bond between two sugar molecules is called a **glycosidic linkage**. This is a covalent bond, formed in a dehydration reaction that requires enzymatic catalysis.

Typically, the glycosidic bond joins C1 of one pyranose or furanose to C4 (sometimes C2 or C6) of another pyranose or furanose through an oxygen atom. Is the anomeric carbon in a hemiacetal form, or is it in an acetal form once it is part of a glycosidic bond? It has two –OR constituents, so it forms an acetal group. The significance of this is that the glycosidic linkage stays in the α or β configuration until an enzyme breaks the bond, because the acetal is a stable functional group. In other words, once a monosaccharide has attacked another sugar to form a glycosidic linkage, it is no longer free to mutarotate. This is an important concept, and we will discuss it further in the section on reducing sugars.

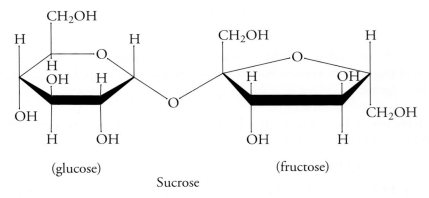

Sucrose

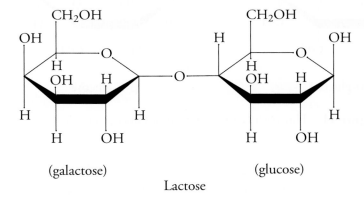

Lactose

Figure 12   Disaccharides and the α- or β-Glycosidic Bond

Glycosidic linkages are named according to which carbon in each sugar comprises the linkage. The configuration (α or β) of the linkage is also specified. For example, lactose (milk sugar) is a disaccharide joined in a galactose-β-1,4-glucose linkage (above). Sucrose (table sugar) is also shown above, with a glucose unit and a fructose unit.

26) Does sucrose contain an α- or β-glycosidic linkage?[26]

Some common disaccharides you might see on the MCAT are sucrose (Glc-α-1,2-Fru), lactose (Gal-β-1,4-Glc), and maltose (Glc-α-1,4-Glc). However, you should NOT try to memorize these linkages.

Polymers made from monosaccharides form important biological macromolecules. Glycogen serves as an energy storage carbohydrate in animals and is composed of thousands of glucose units joined in α-1,4 linkages; α-1,6 branches are also present. Starch is the same as glycogen (except that the branches are a little different), and it serves the same purpose in plants. Cellulose is also a polymer of glucose; the β-glycosidic bonds allow the polymer to assume a long, straight, fibrous shape. Wood and cotton are made of cellulose.

The hydrolysis of polysaccharides into monosaccharides is essential for monosaccharides to enter metabolic pathways (for example, glycolysis) and be used for energy by the cell. Different enzymes catalyze the hydrolysis of different linkages. The enzyme is named for the sugar it hydrolyzes. For example, the enzyme that catalyzes the hydrolysis of maltose into two glucose monosaccharides is called **maltase**. Each enzyme is highly specific for its linkage.

This specificity is a great example of the significance of stereochemistry. Consider cellulose. A cotton T-shirt is pure sugar. The only reason we can't digest it is that mammalian enzymes can't deal with the β-glycosidic linkages that make cellobiose from glucose. Cellulose is actually the energy source in grass and hay. Cows are mammals, and all mammals lack the enzymes necessary for cellobiose breakdown. To live on grass, cows depend on bacteria that live in an extra stomach called a rumen to digest cellulose for them. If you're really on the ball, you're next question is: Humans are mammals, so how can we digest lactose, which has a β linkage? The answer is that we have a specific enzyme, **lactase**, which can digest lactose. This is an exception to the rule that mammalian enzymes cannot hydrolyze β-glycosidic linkages. People without lactase are **lactose malabsorbers**, and any lactose they eat ends up in the colon. There it may cause gas and diarrhea, if certain bacteria are present; people with this problem are said to be **lactose intolerant**. People produce lactase as children so that they can digest mother's milk, but most adults naturally stop making this enzyme, and thus become lactose malabsorbers and sometimes intolerant.

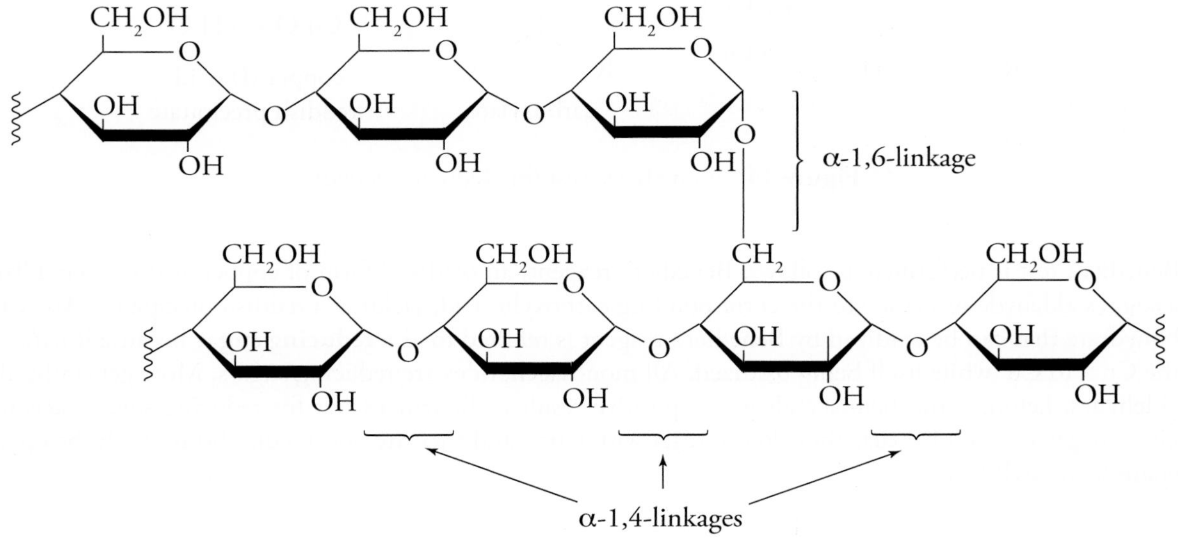

Figure 13 The Polysaccharide Glycogen

---

[26] The anomeric carbon of glucose is pointing down, which means the linkage is α-1,2. So, sucrose is Glc-α-1,2-Fru.

Hydrolysis of Glycosidic Linkages

Disaccharides and polysaccharides are broken down into their component monosaccharides by enzymatic hydrolysis. This just means water is the nucleophile, and one of the sugars is the leaving group (the one that was the attacker during bond formation). In other words, the cleavage reaction is precisely the reverse of the formation reaction.

Hydrolysis of polysaccharides into monosaccharides is favored thermodynamically. This means the hydrolysis of polysaccharides releases energy in the cell. However, it does not occur at a significant rate without enzymatic catalysis. As catalysts, enzymes increase reaction rates by lowering the activation energy but do not change final concentrations of reactants and products.

27) Which requires net energy input: polysaccharide synthesis or hydrolysis?[27]
28) If the activation energy of polysaccharide hydrolysis were so low that no enzyme was required for the reaction to occur, would this make polysaccharides better for energy storage?[28]

Reducing Sugars

Benedict's test is a chemical assay that detects the carbonyl units of sugars. It is useful because it distinguishes hemiacetals from acetals [only hemiacetals are in equilibrium with the carbonyl (open-chain) form]. For example, if you had a white powder that you knew to be composed of glucose, you would be able to say whether the glucose existed in the free monosaccharide form or was in the form of glycogen. How? Well, if it's in the monosaccharide form, there will be many hemiacetals, and Benedict's test will be strongly positive. However, if the powder consists of only relatively few glycogen molecules, Benedict's will be only weakly positive. This is because all the glucose units in a glycogen polymer are tied up in acetal linkages, except for the very first one in the chain (the one which was first attacked during polymerization).

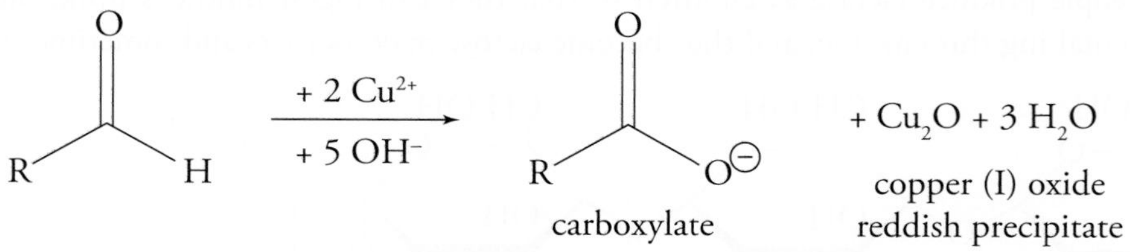

Figure 14 Benedict's Test for Reducing Sugars

Benedict's test is performed as follows: Benedict's reagent, an oxidized form of copper, is used to oxidize a sugar's aldehyde or ketone to the corresponding carboxylic acid, yielding a reddish precipitate. Any carbohydrate that can be oxidized by Benedict's reagent is referred to as a **reducing sugar** because it *reduces* the Cu^{2+} to Cu^+ while itself being oxidized. All monosaccharides are reducing sugars. More generally, all aldehydes, ketones, and hemiacetals give a positive result in Benedict's test for reducing sugars; acetals give a negative result because they do not react with Cu^{2+}, and they are not in equilibrium with the open-chain (carbonyl) form.

---

[27] Because hydrolysis of polysaccharides is thermodynamically favored, energy input is required to drive the reaction toward polysaccharide synthesis.

[28] No, because then polysaccharides would hydrolyze spontaneously (they'd be unstable). The high activation energy of polysaccharide hydrolysis allows us to use enzymes as gatekeepers—when we need energy from glucose, we open the gate of glycogen hydrolysis.

29) Which carbon of glucose can be oxidized by Benedict's reagent? What about fructose?[29]

Recall that we've said once a monosaccharide has attacked another sugar to form a glycosidic linkage, it is no longer free to mutarotate. Now we can expand this statement as follows: once a monosaccharide has attacked another sugar to form a glycosidic linkage, its anomeric carbon is in an acetal configuration and is thus no longer free to mutarotate *nor to reduce Benedict's reagent.*

30) If 98% of a monosaccharide is present as the ring form at equilibrium in solution, then how much of the sugar can be oxidized in Benedict's reaction?[30]

31) Is lactose a reducing sugar? What about sucrose? (You may refer back to the text and figures previously.)[31]

36.4 LIPIDS

Lipids are oily or fatty substances that play three physiological roles, summarized here and discussed below.

- In cellular membranes, phospholipids constitute a barrier between intracellular and extracellular environments.
- In adipose cells, triglycerides (fats) store energy.
- Finally, cholesterol is a special lipid that serves as the building block for the hydrophobic steroid hormones.

The cardinal characteristic of the lipid is its **hydrophobicity**. Hydrophobic means *water-fearing*. It is important to understand the significance of this. Since water is very polar, polar substances dissolve well in water; these are known as *water-loving*, or **hydrophilic** substances. Carbon-carbon bonds and carbon-hydrogen bonds are nonpolar. Hence, substances that contain only carbon and hydrogen will not dissolve well in water.

Fatty Acid Structure

Fatty acids are composed of long unsubstituted alkanes that end in a carboxylic acid. The chain is typically 14 to 18 carbons long, and because they are synthesized two carbons at a time from acetate, only *even-numbered* fatty acids are made in human cells. A fatty acid with no carbon-carbon double bonds is said to be **saturated** with hydrogen because every carbon atom in the chain is covalently bound to the maximum number of hydrogens. **Unsaturated** fatty acids have one or more double bonds in the tail.

---

[29] The anomeric carbon, which is #1 for aldoses like glucose and #2 for ketoses like fructose.

[30] 100% will be oxidized. In a monosaccharide, the ring form is in equilibrium with the open chain form. So when the open chain form is used up in the oxidation reaction, it will be replenished by other rings opening up (Le Châtelier's principle).

[31] Lactose (Gal-β-1-,4-Glc) is a reducing sugar. Although the attacking anomeric carbon becomes locked in an acetal, the anomeric carbon of the *attacked* monosaccharide is still free to mutarotate or react with Benedict's reagent. Sucrose (Glc-α-1-,2-Fru) is not a reducing sugar, because it is made of glucose and fructose, which are both joined at their anomeric carbons. Carbon #1 of glucose is the anomeric carbon, since glucose is an aldose; carbon #2 of fructose is the anomeric carbon, since fructose is a ketose.

These double bonds are almost always (*Z*) (or *cis*). The position of a double bond in the alkyl chain of a fatty acid is denoted by the symbol Δ and the number of the first carbon involved in the double bond. Carbons are numbered starting with the carboxylic acid carbon. For example, a (*Z*) double bond between carbons 3 and 4 in a fatty acid would be referred to as (*Z*)-Δ^3 (or *cis*-Δ^3).

Saturated fatty acid

Unsaturated fatty acid

32) What is the correct nomenclature for the double bond in the unsaturated fatty acid above?[32]

The drawing on the next page illustrates how free fatty acids interact in an aqueous solution; they form a structure called a **micelle**. The force that drives the tails into the center of the micelle is called the **hydrophobic interaction**. The hydrophobic interaction is a complex phenomenon. In general, it results from the fact that water molecules must form an orderly **solvation shell** around each hydrophobic substance. The reason is that H_2O has a dipole that "likes" to be able to share its charges with other polar molecules. A solvation shell allows for the most water-water interaction and the least water-lipid interaction. The problem is that forming a solvation shell is an increase in order and thus a decrease in entropy ($\Delta S < 0$), which is unfavorable according to the Second Law of Thermodynamics. In the case of the fatty acid micelle, water forms a shell around the spherical micelle with the result being that water interacts with polar carboxylic acid head groups while hydrophobic lipid tails hide inside the sphere.

Soaps are the sodium salts of fatty acids ($RCOO^-Na^+$). They are **amphipathic**, which means both hydrophilic and hydrophobic.

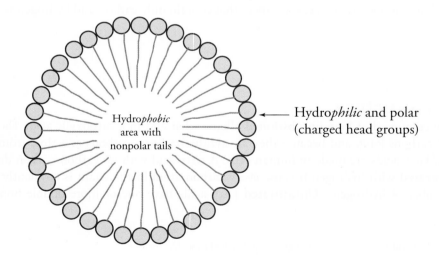

Hydrophobic area with nonpolar tails

← *Hydrophilic* and polar (charged head groups)

Figure 15 A Fatty Acid Micelle

---

[32] This double bond extends between carbons 7 and 8, and is *cis*. The bond therefore is *cis*-Δ^7.

Triacylglycerols (TG)

The storage form of the fatty acid is fat. The technical name for fat is **triacylglycerol** or **triglyceride** (shown below). The triglyceride is composed of three fatty acids esterified to a glycerol molecule. Glycerol is a three-carbon triol with the formula $HOCH_2–CHOH–CH_2OH$. As you can see, it has three hydroxyl groups that can be esterified to fatty acids. It is necessary to store fatty acids in the relatively inert form of fat because free fatty acids are reactive chemicals.

Figure 16   A Triglyceride (Fat)

Introduction to Lipid Bilayer Membranes

Membrane lipids are **phospholipids** derived from diacylglycerol phosphate or DG-P. For example, phosphatidyl choline is a phospholipid formed by the esterification of a choline molecule $[HO(CH_2)_2N^+(CH_3)_3]$ to the phosphate group of DG-P. Phospholipids are **detergents**, substances that efficiently solubilize oils while remaining highly water-soluble. Detergents are like soaps, but stronger.

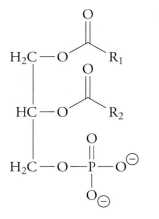

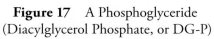

Figure 17   A Phosphoglyceride (Diacylglycerol Phosphate, or DG-P)

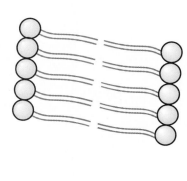

Figure 18   A Small Section of a Lipid Bilayer Membrane

We saw previously how fatty acids spontaneously form micelles. Phospholipids also minimize their interactions with water by forming an orderly structure—in this case, it is a **lipid bilayer** (below). Hydrophobic interactions drive the formation of the bilayer, and once formed, it is stabilized by van der Waals forces between the long tails.

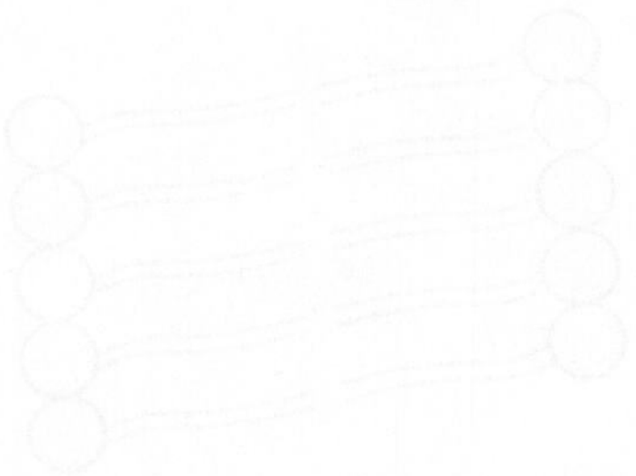

Part 7

MCAT Physics

Chapter 37
Kinematics and Dynamics

37.1   UNITS AND DIMENSIONS

Before we begin our study of physics, we'll briefly go over metric units. Scientists—and the MCAT—use the S̲ystème I̲nternational d'Unités (the International System of Units), abbreviated **SI**, to express the measurements of physical quantities. The **base units** of the SI that we'll be interested in (at least for most of our study of MCAT Physics) are listed below:

SI base unit	abbreviation	measures	dimension
meter	m	length	L
kilogram	kg	mass	M
second	s	time	T

This system of units is also referred to as the **mks system** (m̲ for meters, k̲ for kilograms, and s̲ for seconds). Each **dimension** is simply an abbreviation for the quantity that is being measured; it does not depend on the particular unit that's used. For example, we could measure a distance in miles, meters, or furlongs—to name a few—but in all cases, we're measuring a *length*. We say that distance has the dimensions of length, L. As another example, we could measure an object's speed in miles per hour, meters per second, or furlongs per fortnight; but regardless what units we use, we're always dividing a length by a time. Therefore, speed has dimensions of length per time (L/T).

Any physical quantity can be written in terms of the SI base units. Here are some examples:

quantity	symbol	units	dimensions
speed	v	m/s	L/T
density	ρ	kg/m^3	M/L^3
work	W	kg·m^2/s^2	ML^2/T^2

Multiples of the base units that are powers of ten are often abbreviated and precede the symbol for the unit. For example, "n" is the symbol for nano-, which means 10^{-9} (one billionth). Thus, one billionth of a second, 1 nanosecond, would be written as 1 ns. The letter "M" is the symbol for mega-, which means 10^6 (one million), so a distance of one million meters, 1 megameter, would be abbreviated as 1 Mm.

Some of the most common power-of-ten prefixes are given in the following list:

prefix	symbol	multiple
pico-	p	10^{-12}
nano-	n	10^{-9}
micro-	μ	10^{-6}
milli-	m	10^{-3}
centi-	c	10^{-2}
kilo-	k	10^3
mega-	M	10^6
giga-	G	10^9

You should memorize this list.

On the MCAT, you won't need to convert between the American system of units (which uses things like inches, feet, yards, and pounds) and the metric system, so don't bother memorizing conversions like 2.54 cm = 1 inch or 39.37 inches = 1 meter, etc. You will need to be able to convert within the metric system using the powers-of-ten prefixes.

Example 37-1: Express a density of 5500 kg/m³ in g/cm³.

Solution: All we want to do with this physical measurement is to change the units in which it's expressed. For that, we need conversion factors. A **conversion factor** is simply a fraction whose value is 1, that multiplies a measurement in one set of units to give the equivalent measurement in a different set of units. In this case, we'd write

$$\rho = 5.5 \times 10^3 \; \frac{kg}{m^3} \times \left(\frac{10^3 \; g}{1 \; kg} \right) \times \left(\frac{1 \; m}{10^2 \; cm} \right)^3 = 5.5 \frac{g}{cm^3}$$

Notice that each of these conversion factors is written so that the unit we want to change (that is, the unit we want to eliminate) cancels out. The fraction

$$\frac{1 \; kg}{10^3 \; g}$$

is also a conversion factor for mass, but writing it like this would not have been helpful in this particular problem because then the "kg" would not have canceled.

Example 37-2: If a ball is dropped from a great height, then the force of air resistance it feels at any point during its descent is given by the equation $F = KD^2v^2$, where D is the diameter of the ball and v is its speed. If the units of F are kg·m/s², what are the units of K?

Solution: If the equation $F = KD^2v^2$ is to be valid, then the units of the left-hand side must be the same as the units of the right-hand side. To specify the unit of a quantity, we put brackets around it; for example, $[F]$ denotes the units of F; that is, $[F] = $ kg·m/s². So we need to make sure that $[F] = [KD^2v^2]$, which means

$$[F] = [K][D]^2[v]^2$$
$$\frac{kg \cdot m}{s^2} = [K] \cdot m^2 \cdot \left(\frac{m}{s} \right)^2$$
$$= [K] \cdot \frac{m^4}{s^2}$$
$$kg \cdot m = [K] \cdot m^4$$
$$\therefore [K] = \frac{kg}{m^3}$$

37.2 KINEMATICS

Kinematics is the description of motion in terms of an object's position, velocity, and acceleration. The MCAT will expect not only that you can answer mathematical questions about these quantities but also that you know the definitions of these quantities.

Displacement

The **displacement** of an object is its change in position. It is a vector quantity, so it contains both length and direction. For motion in a line, direction is indicated by sign. For example, let's say we were measuring an object moving along a straight line by laying a meter stick along the object's line of motion. If the object starts at, say, the *10 cm* mark on the meter stick and moves to the *70 cm* mark, then its position changed by 70 cm − 10 cm = 60 cm, so we'd say its displacement is +60 cm. Note that we find displacement by subtracting the object's initial position from its final position: displacement = Δ(position) = position$_{final}$ − position$_{initial}$.

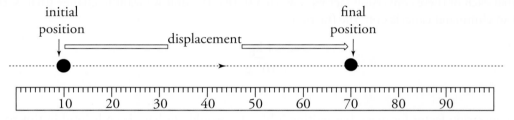

Now, what if the object moved from the *70 cm* mark on the meter stick to the *10 cm* mark? Then its displacement would be 10 cm − 70 cm = −60 cm.

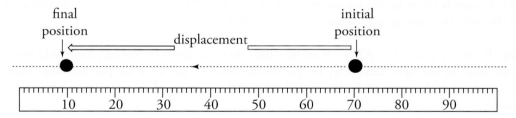

The motion of the object can be more complicated. For example, what if the object started at the *10 cm* mark, moved to the *50 cm* mark, back to the *40 cm* mark, and then over to the *70 cm* mark?

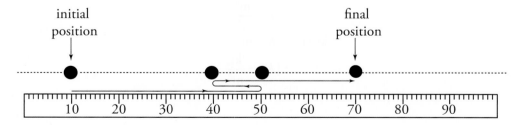

This example brings up a crucial point about displacement. The *total* distance that the object travels is (40 cm) + (10 cm) + (30 cm) = 80 cm, but the object's displacement is still Δ(position) = 70 cm − 10 cm = + 60 cm.

Displacement gives us the *net* distance traveled by the object, which may very well be less than the total distance. So, the displacement is a vector that always points from the object's initial position to its final position, *regardless of the path the object took*, and whose magnitude is the *net* distance traveled by the object. There are multiple different symbols that are used to represent the displacement vector, such as Δ**s**, but the most common one is the single letter **d** (sometimes Δ**s**). Sometimes, we use Δ**x** if we know the displacement is horizontal or Δ**y** if we know the displacement is vertical. Be aware that the MCAT also uses the word *displacement* to mean just the magnitude of the displacement vector (that is, just the net distance traveled by the object without regard for direction); the question will make it clear which meaning is intended.

Displacement

$$\mathbf{d} = \text{position}_{\text{final}} - \text{position}_{\text{initial}} = \text{net distance plus direction}$$

For example, if a sprinter runs 400 meters around a circular track and returns to her starting point, she has covered a *total* distance of 400 meters, but her *displacement* is zero. If a sprinter runs 300 meters north, then 400 meters east, he's covered a total distance of 700 m, but his displacement is only 500 meters.

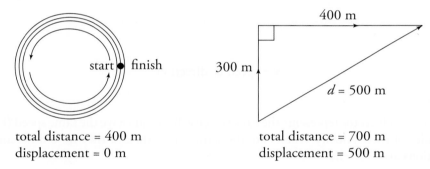

total distance = 400 m
displacement = 0 m

total distance = 700 m
displacement = 500 m

Example 37-3: Though the total length of all pathways of the human circulatory system is on the order of 10^8 m, a typical red blood cell may complete a circuit of about 3 meters in one minute.

a) What is the total distance traveled by a red blood cell in an hour?
b) What is its total displacement in that time?

Solution:

a) If 3 m are traveled in a minute, then 3 m/min × 60 min/hour = 180 m will be traveled in an hour.
b) Displacement is the net change in position. If a circuit is completed, regardless of the number of times, the displacement is 0 m.

Velocity

Displacement tells us how much an object's position changes. **Velocity** tells us how *fast* an object's position changes. If you're in a car traveling at 60 miles per hour along a long, straight highway, then this means your position changes by 60 miles every hour. To calculate velocity, simply divide how much the position has changed by how much time it took for it to change; in other words, divide displacement by time.

Average Velocity

$$\text{average velocity} = \frac{\text{displacement}}{\text{time}}$$

$$\overline{\mathbf{v}} = \frac{\Delta x}{\Delta t} = \frac{\mathbf{d}}{\Delta t}$$

This is actually the definition of **average velocity**, and we place a bar above the **v** to signify that it's an *average*. So, **v** is velocity and $\overline{\mathbf{v}}$ is average velocity. (If the velocity happens to be constant, then there's no distinction between *velocity* and *average velocity*, and we don't need the bar.) Notice right away that velocity is a vector; after all, we're dividing a vector (the displacement, **d**) by a number, so we're left with a vector. In fact, because Δt is always positive, $\overline{\mathbf{v}}$ always points in the same direction as **d**.

The magnitude of the velocity vector is called the **speed**. Speed is a scalar; it has no direction and can never be negative. (Notice that the speedometer in your car is well-named; it only tells you how fast the car is moving, not the direction of motion. It's not a "velocity-o-meter.") Velocity is a vector that specifies both speed and direction.

Velocity

$$\mathbf{v} = \text{speed \& direction}$$

In the figure below, each vector represents the car's velocity. Both cars have the same speed (let's say 20 m/s), so the magnitudes of their velocity vectors are the same. Nevertheless, they have different velocities, because the directions are different.

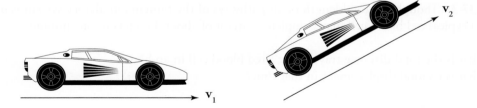

These two cars have the same speed but different velocities. Is it possible for two cars to have the same velocity but different speeds? No. Velocity is speed plus direction, so if the velocities are the same, then the speeds (and the directions) are the same.

Example 37-4: Though the total length of all pathways of the human circulatory system is on the order of 10^8 m, a typical red blood cell may complete a circuit of about 3 meters in one minute.

- a) What is the average velocity of this red blood cell?
- b) What is its average speed?

Solution:

- a) In Example 37-3(b) we determined that the displacement of the red blood cell was 0 m. Thus, by definition, the average velocity must be 0 m/s.
- b) Average speed is not the magnitude of average velocity. (Confusing, though this example should make clear why this must be the case.) Rather, it is by definition the total distance traveled divided by time. In this case, v = (3 m/min)(1/60 min/sec) = 1/20 m/s or 0.05 m/s.

Example 37-5: A sprinter runs 400 meters around a circular track and returns to her starting point, covering a total distance of 400 meters in 50 seconds. What was her average speed? What was her average velocity?

Solution: The sprinter's average speed was (400 m)/(50 s) = 8 m/s. However, because her displacement is 0, her average velocity was zero.

Example 37-6: A sprinter runs 300 meters north, then 400 meters east, which takes 100 seconds.

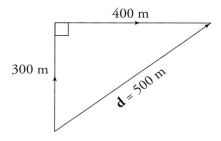

What was his average speed? What was the magnitude of his average velocity?

Solution: The sprinter's average speed was (700 m)/(100 s) = 7 m/s. However, because his displacement is 500 m, his average velocity has a magnitude of (500 m)/(100 s) = 5 m/s.

Acceleration

Velocity tells us how fast an object's position changes. **Acceleration** tells us how fast an object's *velocity* changes.

Average Acceleration

$$\text{average acceleration} = \frac{\text{change in velocity}}{\text{time}}$$

$$\overline{a} = \frac{\Delta v}{\Delta t}$$

Acceleration is a little trickier than velocity. Even though both involve how fast something changes, acceleration is how fast velocity changes, and an object's velocity changes if the speed *or* the direction changes. So, for example, an object can be accelerating even if its speed is constant. This is a very important point and a potential MCAT trap.

In everyday language, we use the word *acceleration* to describe what happens when we step on the gas pedal and go faster. Well, that's certainly an example of acceleration even from the "proper" physics perspective, but it isn't the only example of acceleration.

What happens when you step on the brake? You slow down. Is that acceleration? Yes, although we might also call it a *deceleration*, because our speed changes.

Now, imagine that you set the car on cruise control at, say, 60 miles per hour. Up ahead you see a curve in the road, so as you approach it, you slowly turn the wheel to stay on the road. Even though your speed remains constant, your direction of motion changes, which means your velocity vector changes. Thus, you experience an acceleration.

Let's try this one. Throw a baseball straight up into the air. It rises, gets to the top of its path, then falls back down. At the moment it's at the top of its path, its velocity is zero. What is the ball's acceleration at this point?

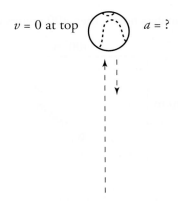

$v = 0$ at top $a = ?$

A common answer is, "If the velocity is 0, then the acceleration is 0 too." Let's see why this isn't the case here. What's happening to the baseball's velocity at the top of the path? Its direction is changing from up to *down*. The fact that the velocity is changing means there's an acceleration, so the acceleration can't be zero at the top of the path. Here's another way of looking at it: What if the acceleration *were* zero at the top? Zero acceleration means no change in velocity, so if $a = 0$ at a certain point, then whatever velocity there is at that point will stay constant. Does the velocity of the baseball remain zero? No, because the ball immediately starts to fall toward the ground (it doesn't just hover in the air!).

Example 37-7: The velocity of an object moving along a straight line changes from $\mathbf{v}_i = 4$ m/s at time $t_i = 0$ to $\mathbf{v}_f = 10$ m/s at time $t_f = 2$ sec.

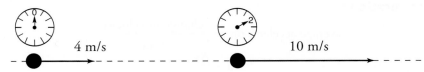

What was the object's average acceleration during this time interval?

Solution: By definition of average acceleration, we have

$$\bar{\mathbf{a}} = \frac{\Delta \mathbf{v}}{\Delta t} = \frac{\mathbf{v}_{fi} - \mathbf{v}}{t_{fi} - t} = \frac{10 \text{ m/s} - 4 \text{ m/s}}{(2 \text{ s}) - 0 \text{ s}} = 3 \text{ m/s}^2$$

Notice that $\bar{\mathbf{a}}$ is positive, which means that it points to the right, just like $\mathbf{v}_i$. If the acceleration points in the *same* direction as the initial velocity, then the object's speed is *increasing*.

Example 37-8: The velocity of an object moving along a straight line changes from $\mathbf{v}_i = 7$ m/s at time $t_i = 0$ to $\mathbf{v}_f = 1$ m/s at time $t_f = 3$ sec.

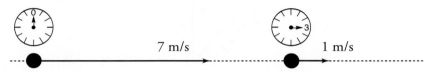

7 m/s   1 m/s

What was the object's average acceleration during this time interval?

Solution: By definition of average acceleration, we have

$$\bar{\mathbf{a}} = \frac{\Delta \mathbf{v}}{\Delta t} = \frac{\mathbf{v}_{fi} - \mathbf{v}}{t_{fi} - t} = \frac{1 \text{ m/s} - 7 \text{ m/s}}{(3 \text{ s}) - 0 \text{ s}} = -2 \text{ m/s}^2$$

Notice that $\bar{\mathbf{a}}$ is negative, which means that it points to the left, in the direction opposite to $\mathbf{v}_i$. If the acceleration points in the direction *opposite* to the initial velocity, then the object's speed is *decreasing*.

Example 37-9: The velocity of an object changes from $\mathbf{v}_1$ at time $t_i = 0$ to $\mathbf{v}_2$ at time $t_f = 2$ sec.

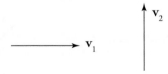

Which of the following best illustrates the object's average acceleration during this time interval?

A) ↑

B) ↘

C) ↗

D) ↘

Solution: By definition of average acceleration, we have

$$\overline{\mathbf{a}} = \frac{\Delta\mathbf{v}}{\Delta t} = \frac{\mathbf{v}_2 - \mathbf{v}_1}{t_{\mathrm{fi}} - t} = \frac{\mathbf{v}_2 - \mathbf{v}_1}{2\,\mathrm{s}}$$

The direction of $\overline{\mathbf{a}}$ is (always) the same as the direction of $\Delta\mathbf{v} = \mathbf{v}_2 - \mathbf{v}_1 = \mathbf{v}_2 + (-\mathbf{v}_1)$. The following diagram shows how we find $\mathbf{v}_2 + (-\mathbf{v}_1)$:

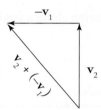

Therefore, choice B is the best answer.

The direction of **a** tells **v** how to change; the following diagrams summarize the possibilities:

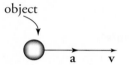

object

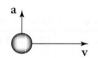

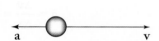

a in the same direction as **v** means object's speed is increasing.

a perpendicular to **v** means object's speed is constant.

a in the opposite direction from **v** means object's speed is decreasing.

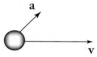

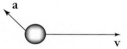

a at an angle between 0° and 90° to **v** means object's speed is increasing and direction of **v** is changing.

a at an angle between 90° and 180° to **v** means object's speed is decreasing and direction of **v** is changing.

37.3   UNIFORMLY ACCELERATED MOTION

In the last section, we defined the principal quantities of kinematics: displacement, velocity, and acceleration. In this section, we'll summarize the mathematical relationships between them in the special but important case of **uniformly accelerated motion**. This is motion in which the object's acceleration, **a**, is constant.

The definition of average velocity is $\bar{\mathbf{v}} = \Delta \mathbf{s} / \Delta t$. We can rewrite this equation without a fraction like this: $\Delta \mathbf{s} = \bar{\mathbf{v}} \Delta t$. To simplify the notation, let's agree to (1) use **d** for displacement, (2) use t, rather than Δt, for the time interval, and (3) abandon the bolding for vectors (although we'll still specify the direction of a vector by either a plus or a minus sign). With this change in notation, the equation reads simply $d = \bar{v}t$. In the case of uniformly accelerated motion (which means a is constant), the average velocity, $\bar{v}$ is just the average of the initial and final velocities: $\frac{1}{2}\left(v_i + v_f\right)$. Using t instead of Δt for the time interval means that we're setting the initial time, t_i, equal to 0 and that we're letting t stand for the final time, t_f (notice that $\Delta t = t_f - t_i = t - 0 = t$). The initial velocity is then the velocity at time 0, which we write as v_0 (pronounced "v zero" or "v naught") and the final velocity is v (dropping the subscript "f" on v_f just like we're dropping the subscript "f" on t_f). Therefore, the average velocity can be written as $\bar{v} = \frac{1}{2}\left(v_0 + v\right)$, and the equation for d becomes $d = \frac{1}{2}\left(v_0 + v\right)t$.

The definition of average acceleration is $\bar{a} = \Delta v / \Delta t$. We can rewrite this equation without a fraction like this: $\Delta v = \bar{a} \Delta t$. Now, since we are specifically looking at uniformly accelerated motion (motion in which the acceleration is constant), there's no need for the bar on the **a**. After all, if **acceleration** is a constant, there's no distinction between **a** and **ā** . So, removing the bar and using the simplified notation described in the last paragraph, the equation becomes $\Delta v = at$, or $v = v_0 + at$.

The two equations $d = \frac{1}{2}\left(v_0 + v\right)t$ and $v = v_0 + at$ follow directly from the definitions of average velocity and acceleration. There are three other equations that relate these quantities, but they would require more algebra to derive them. Instead of boring you with the details, we'll just state them. Since there are five equations, we call them **The Big Five**:

The Big Five

1.	$d = \frac{1}{2}(v_0 + v)t$	missing a
2.	$v = v_0 + at$	missing d
3.	$d = v_0 t + \frac{1}{2}at^2$	missing v
4.	$d = vt - \frac{1}{2}at^2$	missing v_0
5.	$v^2 = v_0^2 + 2ad$	missing t

Notice that these equations involve *five* quantities—d, v_0, v, a, and t—and there are *five* equations. Each equation has exactly one of those quantities missing, and this is how you decide which equation to use in a particular problem. A quantity is *missing* from the problem if it's *not given and not asked for*. For example, if a question does not give or ask for v, then use Big Five #3; if a question does not give or ask for t, then use Big Five #5. On the MCAT, the Big Five equations that are used most frequently are #2, #3, and #5.

Example 37-10: An object has an initial velocity of 3 m/s and a constant acceleration of 2 m/s^2 in the same direction. What will the object's velocity be at $t = 6$ s?

Solution: We're given v_0, a, and t, and asked for v. Since the displacement, d, is neither given nor asked for, we use Big Five #2:

$$v = v_0 + at = 3 \text{ m/s} + (2 \text{ m/s}^2)(6 \text{ s}) = 15 \text{ m/s}$$

Example 37-11: A particle has an initial velocity of 10 m/s and a constant acceleration of 3 m/s^2 in the same direction. How far will the particle travel in 4 seconds?

Solution: We're given v_0, a, and t, and asked for d. Since the final velocity, v, is missing, we use Big Five #3:

$$d = v_0 t + \tfrac{1}{2} at^2 = (10 \text{ m/s})(4 \text{ s}) + \tfrac{1}{2}(3 \text{ m/s}^2)(4 \text{ s})^2 = 64 \text{ m}$$

Example 37-12: An object starts from rest and travels in a straight line with a constant acceleration of 4 m/s^2 in the same direction until its final velocity is 20 m/s. How far does it travel during this time?

Solution: We're given v_0, a, and v, and asked for d. Since the time, t, is neither given nor asked for, we use Big Five #5. Because the object starts from rest, we know that $v_0 = 0$, so we get

$$v^2 = v_0^2 + 2ad \;\rightarrow\; v^2 = 2ad \;\rightarrow\; d = \frac{v^2}{2a} = \frac{(20 \text{ m/s})^2}{2(4 \text{ m/s}^2)} = 50 \text{ m}$$

Example 37-13: A particular red blood cell traveling through the aorta has a peak speed of 92 cm/s after accelerating for 98 ms at a rate of 470 cm/s^2. What was its speed before undergoing this acceleration?

Solution: We're given a, v, and t, and asked for v_0. Since the displacement, d, is neither given nor asked for, we use Big Five #2:

$$v = v_0 + at \rightarrow v_0 = v - at = (92 \text{ cm/s}) - (470 \text{ cm/s}^2)(0.098 \text{ s}) \approx 45 \text{ cm/s}$$

The MCAT will sometimes present information graphically. You probably won't see a kinematics graph on the exam (though you might), but you probably will have to interpret some kind of graph. This next example shows you how. Consider the following graph, which gives an object's velocity, v, as a function of time, t:

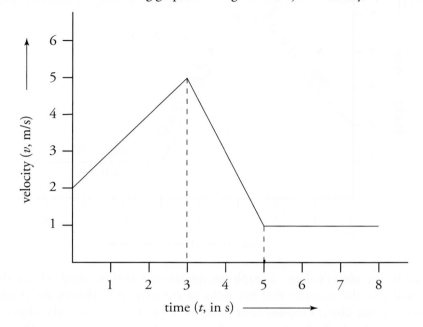

The object's velocity at $t = 0$ is $v = 2$ m/s, and it steadily increases to $v = 5$ m/s at time $t = 3$ s. From $t = 3$ s to $t = 5$ s, the velocity decreases to $v = 1$ m/s. Then, from $t = 5$ s to $t = 8$ s, the object's velocity remains constant at $v = 1$ m/s.

Let's figure out the object's acceleration during these time intervals. From $t = 0$ to $t = 3$ s, its acceleration is

$$a = \frac{\Delta v}{\Delta t} = \frac{v - v_0}{t} = \frac{(5 \text{ m/s}) - (2 \text{ m/s})}{3 \text{ s}} = 1 \text{ m/s}^2$$

Note that $\Delta\mathbf{v}$ is the vertical change in this graph and Δt is the horizontal change, from $t = 0$ to $t = 3$ s. Remember, slope is *rise over run*. That is, dividing a vertical change by the corresponding horizontal change gives the slope of a graph. In this case, then, the slope of the velocity versus time graph gives the acceleration.

From $t = 3$ s to $t = 5$ s, the acceleration is

$$a = \frac{\Delta v}{\Delta t} = \frac{v - v_0}{t_f - t_i} = \frac{(1 \text{ m/s}) - (5 \text{ m/s})}{5 \text{ s} - 3 \text{ s}} = -2 \text{ m/s}^2$$

This is the slope of the graph from $t = 3$ s to $t = 5$ s.

Finally, from $t = 5$ s to $t = 8$ s, the object's velocity remained constant at $v = 1$ m/s. Since the object's velocity didn't change, we expect its acceleration during this time interval to be zero. The graph is flat here, and the slope of a flat line is 0.

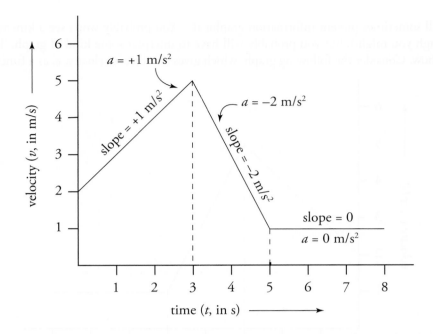

Besides asking about the object's slope, a graph-interpretation question could ask for the area under a curve. The area will give the quantity that has units of *rise times run*, that is, the product of the axes. For example, what was the object's *displacement* from $t = 5$ s to $t = 7$ s? Since the object's velocity was a constant $v = 1$ m/s, we just use the basic equation *distance = rate × time* (which is really just Big Five #1 in the case where v is constant) to find that $d = (1 \text{ m/s})(2 \text{ s}) = 2$ m.

But if we look at the graph, we realize that what we've just found is the *area* under the graph from $t = 5$ s to $t = 7$ s. After all, the area under the graph is comprised of rectangles whose height is a velocity and whose base is a time. The area of a rectangle is *base × height* (*bh*), so we're multiplying velocity × time, and that gives us displacement.

What is the object's displacement from $t = 0$ to $t = 3$ s? It will be the area under the velocity versus time graph from $t = 0$ to $t = 3$ s. The figure below shows that we can split this area into two pieces: a triangle whose area is $\frac{1}{2}bh = \frac{1}{2}(3\,\text{s})(3 \text{ m/s}) = \frac{9}{2}$ m and a rectangle whose area is $bh = (3\,\text{s})(2 \text{ m/s}) = 6$ m. Therefore, the object's displacement from $t = 0$ to $t = 3$ s, which is the *total* area under the graph between $t = 0$ and $t = 3$ s, is $\left(\frac{9}{2}\text{ m}\right) + (6\text{ m}) = 10.5$ m.

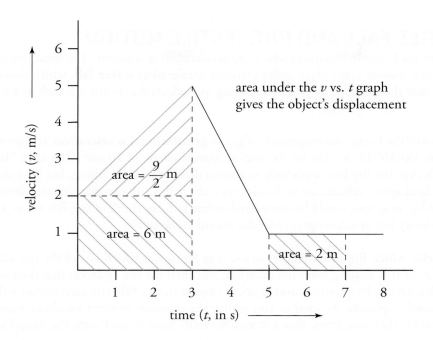

area under the *v* vs. *t* graph gives the object's displacement

We can check this result using Big Five #1:

$$d = \frac{1}{2}(v_0 + v)t = \frac{1}{2}(2 \text{ m/s} + 5 \text{ m/s})(3\text{ s}) = 10.5 \text{ m}$$

Example 37-14: For the object whose velocity versus time graph is shown below, what is its displacement from $t = 2$ s to $t = 5$ s?

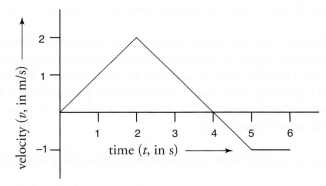

Solution: The area under the graph (or, more precisely, the area between the graph and the *t*-axis) gives the object's displacement. The area under the graph from $t = 2$ s to $t = 4$ s is $\frac{1}{2}bh = \frac{1}{2}(2 \text{ s})(2 \text{ m/s}) = 2$ m. After $t = 4$ s, the graph is *below* the *t*-axis, so any area here counts *negatively*. From $t = 4$ s to $t = 5$ s, the area is $\frac{1}{2}bh = \frac{1}{2}(1 \text{ s})(-1 \text{ m/s}) = -0.5$ m. Therefore, the total area between the graph and the *t*-axis, from $t = 2$ s to $t = 5$ s, is $(2 \text{ m}) + (-0.5 \text{ m}) = 1.5$ m.

37.4 FREE FALL AND PROJECTILE MOTION

The Big Five are used only in situations where the acceleration is constant. The most important "real life" situation in which motion takes place under constant acceleration is **free fall**, which describes an object moving only under the influence of gravity (ignoring any effects due to the air, such as air resistance and buoyancy).

Near the surface of the Earth, the magnitude of **g**, the **gravitational acceleration**, is approximately equal to 9.8 m/s². *For the MCAT, we can use the simpler approximation of 10 m/s².* The term "free fall" might make you think that The Big Five apply only to objects that are actually falling, but if we throw a baseball up into the air (and ignore effects due to the air), then the ball is still experiencing the downward acceleration due to gravity, so it, too, would be considered in free fall. So, think of free fall not as a description of a downward velocity but as a description of a downward *acceleration*.

The way we decide which Big Five equation to use is to figure out which one of the five kinematics quantities (d, v_0, v, a, or t) is missing from the question, and then use the equation that does not involve this missing quantity. Often, in questions asking about objects in free fall, the acceleration will not be given because it's known implicitly. As soon as you realize the question involves an object moving under the influence of gravity, then you know that a is automatically known; on Earth, the magnitude of this a is about 10 m/s².

However, there is one thing you will have to decide on once you've selected which Big Five equation to use. Gravitational acceleration, like any acceleration, is a vector, so it has magnitude and direction. We know the magnitude is 10 m/s² and the direction is downward, but is *down* the positive direction or the negative direction? The answer is, it's up to you. One possibility is to let the direction of the object's displacement be the positive direction in every problem (this is almost always the simplest, most intuitive, decision). If the object's displacement is *down*, then call *down* the positive direction, and use $a = +g = +10$ m/s² in whichever Big Five equation you've selected. If the object's displacement is *up*, call *up* the positive direction (and thus *down* is automatically the negative direction), and use $a = -g = -10$ m/s².

It's important to remember that once you make your decision about which direction, up or down, is the positive direction, your decision applies to all other vectors in that problem: namely, v_0, v, and d. Therefore, if *down* is positive, for example, then in addition to the downward acceleration being positive, a downward initial velocity is positive, a downward final velocity is positive, and a downward displacement is positive. (This would mean that an upward initial velocity is negative, an upward final velocity is negative, and an upward displacement is negative.)

Example 37-15: An object is dropped from a height of 80 m. How long will it take to strike the ground?

Solution: We're given v_0, a, and d, and asked for t. Since the final velocity, v, is neither given nor asked for, we use Big Five #3. Because the object is falling, its displacement is downward, so let's call *down* the positive direction; this means that $a = +g = +10$ m/s². Since the term *dropped* means that the object's initial velocity is 0 m/s, we find that

$$d = v_0 t + \tfrac{1}{2}at^2 \rightarrow d = \tfrac{1}{2}at^2 \rightarrow t = \sqrt{\frac{2d}{a}} = \sqrt{\frac{2d}{+g}} = \sqrt{\frac{2(80 \text{ m})}{+10 \text{ m/s}^2}} = 4 \text{ s}$$

Example 37-16: An object is dropped from a height of 80 m. What is its velocity as it strikes the ground?

Solution: Don't make the common mistake of thinking that the answer is 0 because once the object hits the ground, it stops. When an object strikes something, there will always be a change in acceleration from just gravity, so the assumption that $|a| = 10$ m/s² will no longer be valid. The question is really asking for the velocity of the object *as* it slams into the ground, and this won't be zero. We're given v_0, a, and d, and asked for v. Since the time, t, is neither given nor asked for, we use Big Five #5. Because the object is falling, its displacement is downward, so let's call *down* the positive direction. This means that $a = +g = +10$ m/s². Since the term *dropped* means that the object's initial velocity is 0, we find that

$$v^2 = v_0^2 + 2ad \rightarrow v^2 = 2ad \rightarrow v = \sqrt{2ad} = \sqrt{2(+g)d} = \sqrt{2(+10 \text{ m/s}^2)(80 \text{ m})} = 40 \text{ m/s}$$

Example 37-17: A ball is thrown straight upward with an initial speed of 30 m/s. How high will it go?

Solution: We're given v_0, a, and v, and asked for d. (We know v because the question is asking how high the ball will go; at the top of the ball's path, its velocity at this point is 0.) Since the time, t, is missing, we use Big Five #5. Since we're interested only in the object's upward motion, let's call *up* the positive direction. This means that $v_0 = +30$ m/s and $a = -g = -10$ m/s². Because the velocity of the ball is 0 at its highest point, we find that

$$v^2 = v_0^2 + 2ad \rightarrow 0 = v_0^2 + 2ad \rightarrow d = -\frac{v_0^2}{2a} = -\frac{v_0^2}{2(-g)} = -\frac{(+30 \text{ m/s})^2}{2(-10 \text{ m/s})} = 45 \text{ m}$$

Notice that the displacement, d, turned out to be positive; that's because we chose *up* to be our positive direction, and the ball moves *up* to its highest position.

The examples we've worked through so far have involved objects that move along a straight line, either horizontal or vertical. However, if we were to throw a baseball up at an angle to the ground, the path the ball would follow (its **trajectory**) would not be a straight line. If we neglect effects due to the air, the path will be a *parabola*.

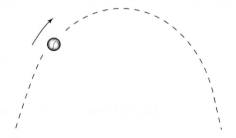

In this case, the motion of an object, experiencing only the constant, downward acceleration due to gravity (free fall), is called **projectile motion**. This is also a case of uniformly accelerated motion.

Because the projectile is experiencing both horizontal and vertical motion, we'll need to analyze both. But the trick is to analyze them *separately*. We'll use The Big Five to look at the horizontal motion, simply specializing the variables to horizontal motion; for example, we'll use x instead of d, we'll use v_{0x} and v_x instead of v_0 and v, and we'll use a_x instead of a. The same will be true for the vertical motion. We'll use

The Big Five to look at the vertical motion, too, and simply specialize the variables to vertical motion; we'll use y instead of d, v_{0y} and v_y instead of v_0 and v, and a_y instead of a. In this case, a_y will be equal to the gravitational acceleration.

In order to make an object follow a parabolic path, we'll need to launch the object at an angle to the horizontal. Therefore, the initial velocity vector $\mathbf{v}_0$ will have a nonzero horizontal component (v_{0x}) *and* a nonzero vertical component (v_{0y}). In terms of the **launch angle**, θ_0, which is the angle the initial velocity vector makes with the horizontal, we have $v_{0x} = v_0 \cos \theta_0$ and $v_{0y} = v_0 \sin \theta_0$.

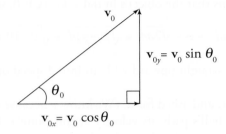

Let's first take care of the horizontal motion. This is the easier of the two for one important reason: once the projectile is launched, it no longer experiences a horizontal acceleration. That is, a_x will be zero throughout the projectile's flight. If the horizontal acceleration is zero throughout the projectile's flight, then *the horizontal velocity will be constant throughout the flight*. If the horizontal velocity does not change, then whatever it was initially is all it'll ever be; that is, the horizontal velocity of the projectile at any point during its flight will be equal to the initial horizontal velocity, v_{0x}. Finally, if a_x is always equal to 0, then by using Big Five #3, we have $x = v_{0x}t$ (this is just *distance = rate × time* in the case where the rate is constant).

For the vertical motion, we realize that there *is* an acceleration; after all, the gravitational acceleration is vertical. In order to write down the equations for the vertical motion, we need to make a decision about which direction is positive. Let's call *up* the positive direction, so that *down* is the negative direction; this will mean that $a_y = -g$. Big Five #2 now tells us that the vertical component of the velocity, v_y, will be $v_{0y} + a_y t = v_{0y} + (-g)t$ at time t. Big Five #3 tells us that the vertical displacement of the projectile, y, will be $v_{0y}t + \frac{1}{2}a_y t^2 = v_{0y}t + \frac{1}{2}(-g)t^2$.

Projectile Motion

	Horizontal Motion	Vertical Motion
displacement:	$x = v_{0x}t$	$y = v_{0y}t + \frac{1}{2}(-g)t^2$
velocity:	$v_x = v_{0x}$ (constant!)	$v_y = v_{0y} + (-g)t$
acceleration:	$a_x = 0$	$a_y = -g$
	$(v_{0x} = v_0 \cos\theta_0)$	$(v_{0y} = v_0 \sin\theta_0)$

In addition to these formulas (which are really nothing new, since they're just a few of the Big Five equations), there are a couple of other facts worth knowing. The first involves the projectile's velocity at the top of its trajectory. Since the top of the parabola is the parabola's turning point, and an object's velocity is always tangent to its path (whatever the shape of the trajectory), the projectile's velocity will be horizontal at the top of the parabola. This means that the vertical velocity is zero. (*Be careful* not to say that the velocity is zero at the top. For a projectile moving in a parabolic path, it's only the *vertical* velocity that's zero at the top; the horizontal velocity is still there!)

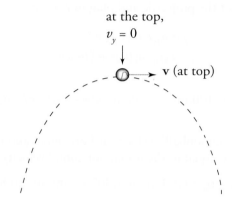

The second fact reflects the symmetry of the parabolic shape of the path. If we were to draw a vertical line up from the ground through the top point on the parabola, we'd notice that the left and right sides are just mirror images of each other. One of the consequences of this observation is that the time the projectile takes to reach the top will be the same as the time it takes to drop back down (to the same height from which it was launched). Therefore, *the projectile's total flight time will be twice the time required to reach the top*. So, for example, if the time it takes the projectile to reach the top of the parabola is 3 seconds, then the total flight time will be 6 seconds, because it'll take another 3 seconds to come back down.

Example 37-18: A cannonball is shot from ground level with an initial velocity of 100 m/s at an angle of 30° to the ground.

   a)   How high will the cannonball go?
   b)   What is the cannonball's velocity at the top of its path?
   c)   What will be the cannonball's total flight time?
   d)   How far will the cannonball travel horizontally?

Solution:

   a)   The maximum height reached by the projectile is the displacement y at the moment the cannonball is at the top of the parabola. What does it mean for the projectile to be at the top of the parabola? It means the vertical velocity is zero. So, we'll set the vertical velocity equal to zero:

$$v_y = v_{0y} + \left(-g\right)t \text{ with } v_y = 0 \ \rightarrow \ v_{0y} + \left(-g\right)t = 0 \ \rightarrow \ t = \frac{v_{0y}}{g} = \frac{v_0 \sin\theta_2}{g}$$

This is how long it'll take the projectile to reach the top. If we plug in $v_0 = 100$ m/s, $\theta_0 = 30°$, and $g = 10$ m/s^2, we find that

$$t = \frac{v_0 \sin \theta_0}{g} = \frac{(100 \text{ m/s}) \sin 30°}{10 \text{ m/s}^2} = 5 \text{ s}$$

So now the question is, "What is y when $t = 5$ s?" All we need to do is take the equation for the vertical displacement of the projectile and plug in $t = 5$ s:

$$y = v_{0y}t + \tfrac{1}{2}(-g)t^2$$
$$= (v_0 \sin \theta_0)t + \tfrac{1}{2}(-g)t^2$$

$$\therefore y \text{ (at } t = 5 \text{ s)} = (100 \text{ m/s} \cdot \sin 30°)(5 \text{ s}) + \tfrac{1}{2}(-10 \text{ m/s}^2)(5 \text{ s})^2 = 125 \text{ m}$$

b)   At the top of its path, the cannonball's velocity is horizontal, and the horizontal velocity is the same throughout the flight, equal to the initial horizontal velocity:

$$v_x = v_{0x} = v_0 \cos \theta_0 = (100 \text{ m/s}) \cos 30° \approx (100 \text{ m/s})(0.85) = 85 \text{ m/s}$$

c)   The projectile's total flight time is just equal to twice the time required for it to reach the top. Since we found in part (a) that it takes 5 seconds for the cannonball to reach the top, its total flight time will be $2 \times (5 \text{ s}) = 10$ s.

d)   The question is asking for the horizontal displacement at the time when the cannonball strikes the ground. We found in part (b) that the cannonball's horizontal velocity is a constant 85 m/s, and we found in part (c) that the cannonball's total flight time is 10 seconds. Therefore, the total horizontal displacement is

$$x = v_{0x}t = (85 \text{ m/s})(10 \text{ s}) = 850 \text{ m}$$

(The total horizontal displacement is called the **range** of the projectile.)

Example 37-19: A ball is kicked from ground level, travels as an ideal projectile in a parabolic path, and hits the ground 4 seconds after it was kicked. If its initial vertical speed was 20 m/s, how high did the ball go?

Solution: If the total flight time was 4 seconds, that means it took half that time, 2 seconds, to reach the top of the parabola (its highest point). Therefore, since we're given that $v_{0y} = 20$ m/s, the vertical displacement of the ball at $t = 2$ s was

$$y = v_{0y}t + \tfrac{1}{2}(-g)t^2$$
$$= (20 \text{ m/s})(2 \text{ s}) + \tfrac{1}{2}(-10 \text{ m/s}^2)(2 \text{ s})^2$$
$$= 20 \text{ m}$$

37.4

37.5 MASS, FORCE, AND NEWTON'S LAWS

So far we've studied kinematics, which is the description of motion in terms of an object's position, velocity, and acceleration. Now we'll begin our study of **dynamics**, which is the *explanation* of motion in terms of the forces that act on an object. On the MCAT, you will often encounter problems that require you to use both dynamics and kinematics.

Simply put, a **force** is a push or pull exerted by one object on another. If you pull on a rope attached to a crate, you create a *tension* in the rope that pulls the crate. When a sky diver is falling through the air, the Earth exerts a downward pull called the *gravitational force*, and the air exerts an upward force called *air resistance*. When you stand on the floor, the floor provides an upward, supporting force called the *normal force*. If you slide a book across a table, the table exerts a *frictional force* against the book, so the book slows down and eventually stops. Static cling provides a simple example of the *electrostatic force*. (In fact, all of the forces mentioned above, with the exception of gravity, are due ultimately to the electromagnetic force.)

Newton's First Law

An object's state of motion—its *velocity*—will not change unless a net force acts on the object.

That is, if no net force acts on an object, then:

if the object is at rest, it will remain at rest;

and

if the object is moving, then it will continue to move with constant velocity

(constant speed in a straight line).

Or, more simply: **no net force = no acceleration**.

How forces affect motion is described by three physical laws, known as **Newton's laws**. They form the foundation of mechanics, and you should memorize them.

The first law says that objects naturally resist changing their velocity. In other words, objects at rest don't just suddenly start moving all on their own. Some external source must exert a force to make them move. Also, an object that's already moving doesn't change its velocity. It doesn't go faster, or slower, or change direction all by itself; something must exert some force on it to make any of these changes happen. This property of objects, their natural resistance to change in their state of motion, is called **inertia**. In fact, the first law is often referred to as the *Law of Inertia*.

It's important to note that the first law applies when there is no *net* force on an object. This could mean there are no forces at all, though that couldn't happen in our universe; more commonly, it means the forces on an object balance out, in other words, the total of all the forces, in each dimension, is zero. We'll work examples of computing net force when we get to Newton's Second Law.

The **mass** of an object is the quantitative measure of its inertia; intuitively, mass measures how much matter is contained in an object. Mass is measured in *kilograms*, abbreviated kg. (Note: An object whose mass is 1 kg weighs a little more than 2 pounds on Earth, but be careful not to confuse mass with weight; they're different things.) Compared to an object whose mass is just 1 kg, an object whose mass is 100 kg has 100 times the inertia. Intuitively, we'd find it 100 times more difficult to cause the same change in its motion than we would with the 1 kg object. This point will be clearer after we state the second of Newton's laws.

37.5

Newton's Second Law

If $\mathbf{F}_{net}$ is the net—or total—force acting on an object of mass m, then the resulting acceleration of the object, $\mathbf{a}$, satisfies this simple equation:

$$\mathbf{F}_{net} = m\mathbf{a}$$

Forces are represented by vectors, because a force has a magnitude and a direction. If two different forces (let's call them $\mathbf{F}_1$ and $\mathbf{F}_2$) act on an object, then the total—or *net*—force on the object is the sum of these individual forces: $\mathbf{F}_{net} = \mathbf{F}_1 + \mathbf{F}_2$. Since forces are vectors, they must be added as vectors; that is, their directions must be taken into account. The following figures show some examples of obtaining $\mathbf{F}_{net}$ from the individual forces that act on an object:

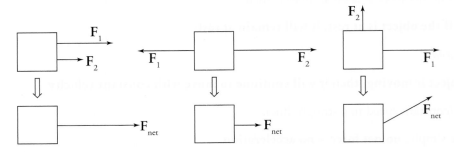

Note the following facts about the equation $\mathbf{F}_{net} = m\mathbf{a}$:

1. $\mathbf{F}_{net}$ is the sum of all the forces that act *on* the object; namely, the object whose mass, m, is on the other side of the equation. Any force exerted *by* the object is *not* included in $\mathbf{F}_{net}$.
2. Because m is a *positive* number, the direction of $\mathbf{a}$ is always the same as the direction of $\mathbf{F}_{net}$. Therefore, an object will accelerate in the direction of the net force it feels. This does not mean that an object will always *move* in the direction of $\mathbf{F}_{net}$. Be sure that this distinction makes sense, because it can be a source of confusion, and therefore a potential MCAT trap. Newton's Second Law tells us about the direction of an object's *acceleration* but does not define the direction of an object's velocity.
3. What if $\mathbf{F}_{net} = 0$? Then $\mathbf{a} = 0$. What does $\mathbf{a} = 0$ mean? It means that the object's velocity does not change, which is also what Newton's *First* Law says. But how about this question: Does $\mathbf{F}_{net} = 0$ mean that $\mathbf{v} = 0$? Not necessarily! $\mathbf{F}_{net} = 0$ means that an object won't *accelerate*, not that it won't move. This is a key point and another potential MCAT trap. If the object is already moving at, say, 100 m/s toward the north, then it will continue to move at 100 m/s toward the north as long as the net force on the object remains zero.
4. Because $\mathbf{F}_{net} = m\mathbf{a}$ is a vector equation, it automatically means that the components of both sides must be the same. In other words, $\mathbf{F}_{net}$ could be written as the sum of a force in the horizontal direction, $(\mathbf{F}_{net,\,x})$ plus a force in the vertical direction $(\mathbf{F}_{net,\,y})$; these would be the

horizontal and vertical components of $\mathbf{F}_{net}$. The equation $\mathbf{F}_{net} = m\mathbf{a}$ would then tell us that $\mathbf{F}_{net,\,x} = m\mathbf{a}_x$ and $\mathbf{F}_{net,\,y} = m\mathbf{a}_y$. So, dividing the horizontal component of the net force by m gives us the horizontal component of the object's acceleration, and dividing the vertical component of the net force by m gives us the vertical component of the object's acceleration.

5. The unit of force is equal to the unit of mass times the unit of acceleration:

$$[F] = [m][a] = \text{kg} \cdot \text{m/s}^2$$

A force of 1 kg·m/s² is called 1 **newton** (abbreviated N). A force of 1 N is about equal to a quarter of a pound, or about the weight of a medium-sized apple (on Earth).

Newton's Third Law

If Object 1 exerts a force, $\mathbf{F}_{1\text{-on-2}}$, on Object 2, then Object 2 exerts a force, $\mathbf{F}_{2\text{-on-1}}$, on Object 1. These forces, $\mathbf{F}_{1\text{-on-2}}$ and $\mathbf{F}_{2\text{-on-1}}$, have the same magnitude but act in opposite directions, so

$$\mathbf{F}_{1\text{-on-2}} = -\mathbf{F}_{2\text{-on-1}}$$

and they act on different objects. These two forces are said to form an **action–reaction pair**.

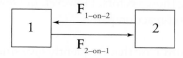

This is the law commonly stated as, "For every action, there is an equal but opposite reaction." Unfortunately, this popular version of Newton's Third Law can lead to confusion. Essentially, Newton's Third Law says that the *forces* in an action–reaction pair have the same magnitude and act in opposite directions (and on "opposite" objects). It does *not* say that the *effects* of these forces will be the same. For example, suppose that two skaters are next to and facing each other on a skating rink. Let's say that Skater 1 has a mass of 50 kg and Skater 2 has a mass of 100 kg. Now, what if Skater 1 pushes on Skater 2 with a force of 50 N? Then $\mathbf{F}_{1\text{-on-2}} = 50$ N and $\mathbf{F}_{2\text{-on-1}} = -50$ N, by Newton's Third Law.

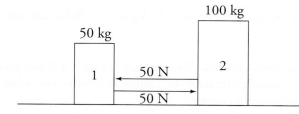

But will the *effects* of these equal-strength forces be the same? No, because the masses of the objects are different. The accelerations of the skaters will be

$$a_1 = \frac{F_{2\text{-on-1}}}{m_1} = \frac{-50\text{ N}}{50\text{ kg}} = -1\text{ m/s}^2 \quad \text{and} \quad a_2 = \frac{F_{1\text{-on-2}}}{m_2} = \frac{+50\text{ N}}{100\text{ kg}} = +0.5\text{ m/s}^2$$

So, Skater 2 will move away with an acceleration of 0.5 m/s², while Skater 1 moves away, in the opposite direction, with an acceleration of twice that magnitude, 1 m/s². (Note that this acceleration lasts only so long as the skaters are in contact: once contact is broken, net force and acceleration go to zero.)

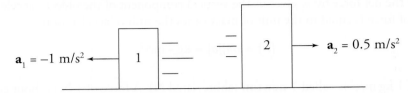

Therefore, while the forces are the same (in magnitude), the effects of these forces —that is, the resulting accelerations (and velocities)—are not the same, because the masses of the objects are different. Newton's Third Law says nothing about mass; it only tells us that the action and reaction forces will have the same magnitude. So, the point is not to interpret "equal but opposite reaction" as meaning "equal but opposite effect," because if the masses of the interacting objects are not the same, then the resulting accelerations (and velocities) of the objects will not be the same.

The key to distinguishing Newton's First Law from Newton's Third Law is to focus on the description of the forces. In Newton's First Law, all of the forces must be acting on a *single* object; thus, the net force on a single object is calculated by adding those vectors. However, in Newton's Third Law, each force must be acting on a *different* object in an action-reaction pair.

There are two aspects of Newton's Third Law that frequently give students trouble. First, just because two forces are equal and opposite does *not* mean they form an action-reaction pair; the forces also have to be from two objects acting on each other, not two objects acting on a third object. Second, the third law applies even when the objects are accelerating; even if one object is accelerating, the second object pushes or pulls just as hard on the first as the first pushes or pulls on the second.

Example 37-20: An object of mass 50 kg moves with a constant velocity of magnitude 1000 m/s. What is the net force on this object?

Solution: If the object moves with constant velocity, then the net force it feels must be zero, regardless of the object's mass or speed.

Example 37-21: The net force on an object of mass 10 kg is zero. What can you say about the speed of this object?

Solution: If the net force on an object is zero, all we can say is that it will not accelerate; its velocity may be zero, or it may not. Without more information, we cannot determine the object's speed; all we know is that whatever the speed is, it will remain constant.

Example 37-22: For 6 seconds, you push a 120 kg crate along a frictionless horizontal surface with a constant force of 60 N parallel to the surface. If the crate was initially at rest, what will its velocity be at the end of this 6-second time interval?

Solution: Answering this question requires starting with dynamics and ending with kinematics. Using Newton's Second Law, we find that the acceleration of the crate is $a = F/m = (60 \text{ N})/(120 \text{ kg}) = 0.5 \text{ m/s}^2$. Using Big Five #2, we now find that $v = v_0 + at = 0 + (0.5 \text{ m/s}^2)(6 \text{ s}) = 3 \text{ m/s}$.

Example 37-23: A 1000 kg car moving 20 m/s brakes to a stop in 20 m. What constant force the brakes apply during this process?

Solution: Answering this question requires starting with kinematics and ending with dynamics. We're given v^0, v, and d, and we're looking for a. Missing t, we use Big 5 #5:

$$v^2 = v_0^2 + 2ad = 0 + \left(2g \frac{h}{2} \right) = gh$$

Now we use Newton's Second Law: $F = ma = (1000 \text{ kg})(-10 \text{ m/s}^2) = -10^4$ N.

Example 37-24: For 6 seconds, you pull a 120 kg crate along a frictionless horizontal surface with a constant force of 60 N directed at an angle of 60° to the surface. If the crate was initially at rest, what will its horizontal velocity be at the end of this 6-second time interval?

Solution: To find the horizontal velocity, we need the horizontal acceleration.

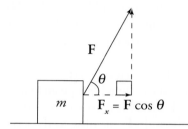

Using Newton's Second Law, we find that the horizontal acceleration of the crate is $a_x = F_x/m = (F \cos \theta)/m = (60 \text{ N})(\cos 60°)/(120 \text{ kg}) = (30 \text{ N})/(120 \text{ kg}) = 0.25 \text{ m/s}^2$. Using Big Five #2, we now find that $v_x = v_{0x} + a_x t = 0 + (0.25 \text{ m/s}^2)(6 \text{ s}) = 1.5 \text{ m/s}$.

Example 37-25: When a doctor injects someone with a hypodermic needle, she exerts about 15 N of force to pierce adult skin. Once the skin has been pierced, considerably less force is required to push the needle deeper. If a force of 5 N on the plunger is required to initiate the injection, how hard should one pull back on the barrel to minimize risk of hematoma to the patient once the needle is inserted into the vein?

Solution: According to Newton's Second Law, $\mathbf{F}_{net} = m\mathbf{a}$. Minimizing risk of hematoma implies that the acceleration of the stationary needle should be zero (so it won't move deeper in or out of the vein during the injection). Thus, $\mathbf{F}_{net} = 0$, and $F_{plunger} = F_{barrel}$, or $F_{barrel} = 5$ N.

Example 37-26: Two crates are moving along a frictionless horizontal surface. The first crate, of mass M = 100 kg, is being pushed by a force of 300 N. The first crate is in contact with a second crate, of mass m = 50 kg.

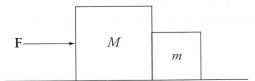

a) What's the acceleration of the crates?
b) What's the force exerted by the larger crate on the smaller one?
c) What's the force exerted by the smaller crate on the larger one?

Solution:

a) The force **F** is pushing on a combined mass of 100 kg + 50 kg = 150 kg, so by Newton's Second Law, the acceleration of both crates will be a = (300 N)/(150 kg) = 2 m/s².

b) Because M and m are in direct contact, each is pushing on the other with a certain force. Let **F$_2$** be the force that M exerts on m. Then we must have $F_2 = ma$, so F_2 = (50 kg)(2 m/s²) = 100 N.

c) By Newton's Third Law, if the force that M exerts on m is **F$_2$**, then the force that m exerts on M must be −**F$_2$**. So, if we call "to the right" our positive direction, then the force that m exerts on M is −100 N. We can check that this is correct by looking at all the forces acting on M. We have **F** pushing to the right and −**F$_2$** pushing to the left. The net force on M is therefore **F**$_{net on M}$ = **F** + (−**F$_2$**) = (300 N) + (−100 N) = 200 N. If this is correct, then $F_{net\ on\ M}$ should equal Ma. Since M = 100 kg and a = 2 m/s², we get Ma = 200 N, which does match what we found for $F_{net\ on\ M}$. (In effect, what's happening here is that M is using 200 N of the 300 N force from **F** for its own motion and passing the remaining 100 N along to m, so that both move together with the same acceleration.)

Example 37-27: The figure below shows all the forces acting on a 5 kg object. The magnitude of **F$_1$** is 50 N. If the acceleration of the object is 8 m/s², what's the magnitude of **F$_2$**?

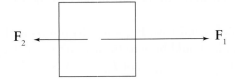

Solution: The net force on the block is just the sum of **F$_1$** and **F$_2$**, so **F**$_{net}$ = **F$_1$** + **F$_2$** = (+50 N) + **F$_2$**, if we call "to the right" our positive direction. The net force must be ma = (5 kg)(8 m/s²) = 40 N. Since (+50 N) + **F$_2$** must be 40 N, we know that **F$_2$** = −10 N; that is, **F$_2$** has magnitude 10 N (and points to the left).

Example 37-28: According to Newton's Third Law, every force is "accompanied by" an equal but opposite force. If this is true, shouldn't these forces cancel out to zero? How could we ever accelerate an object?

Solution: The answer does not involve the masses of the objects; Newton's Third Law says nothing about mass. The key is to remember what F_{net} means; it's the sum of all the forces that act *on* an object, not *by* the object. Let's say we have a pair of objects, 1 and 2, and an action–reaction pair of forces between them, and we wanted to find the acceleration of Object 2. We'd find all the forces that act on Object 2. One of these forces is F_{1-on-2}. The reaction force, F_{2-on-1}, is *not* included in $F_{net-on-2}$ because it doesn't act on Object 2; it's a force *by* Object 2. So, the reason why the two forces in an action–reaction pair don't cancel each other is that we'd never add them in the first place because they don't act on the same object.

37.6   NEWTON'S LAW OF GRAVITATION

The mass of an object is a measure of its inertia, its resistance to acceleration. We'll now look at the related concept of an object's weight.

Although in everyday language the terms *mass* and *weight* are sometimes used interchangeably, in physics they have very different technical meanings. The **weight** of an object is the gravitational force exerted on it by the earth (or by whatever planet it happens to be on or near). **Mass** is an intrinsic property of an object and does not change with location. Put a baseball in a rocket and send it to the Moon. The baseball's *weight* on the Moon is less than its weight here on Earth, but you'd have as much "baseball stuff" there as you would here; that is, the baseball's *mass* would *not* change.

Since weight is a force, we can use $F = ma$ to compute it. What acceleration would the gravitational force (which is what *weight* means) impose on an object? The gravitational acceleration, of course! Therefore, setting $a = g$, the equation $F = ma$ becomes

$$w = mg$$

This is the equation for the weight, w, of an object of mass m. (Weight is often symbolized by F_{grav}, rather than w; we'll use both notations.) Note that mass and weight are proportional but not identical. Furthermore, mass is measured in kilograms, while weight is measured in newtons.

Example 37-29:

a)   Find the weight of an object whose mass is 50 kg.
b)   Find the mass of an object whose weight is 50 N.

Solution:

a) To find an object's weight, we multiply its mass by g. Using $g = 10$ m/s^2 (or, equivalently, $g = 10$ N/kg), we find that $w = mg = (50$ kg$)(10$ N/kg$) = 500$ N.

b) To find an object's mass, we divide its weight by g. With $g = 10$ N/kg, we find that $m = w/g = (50$ N$)/(10$ N/kg$) = 5$ kg.

Most of the time, we'll use the formula $w = mg$ to find the weight of an object whose mass is m. However, the value of g can change, and if we're not near the surface of Earth (where we know that g is approximately 10 m/s^2), we may not know the value of g. In that case, we'll invoke another law discovered by Newton:

Newton's Law of Gravitation

Every object in the universe exerts a gravitational pull on every other object. The magnitude of this gravitational force is proportional to the product of the objects' masses and inversely proportional to the square of the distance between them. The constant of proportionality is denoted by G and known as Newton's universal gravitational constant.

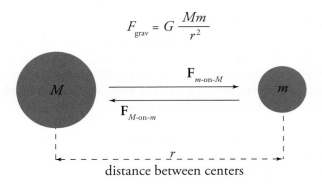

The value of G is roughly 6.7×10^{-11} N·m^2/kg^2, but don't bother memorizing this constant. The AAMC has removed gravitation from the list of topics subject to memory questions, so the main point of this section is to make connections between basic physics principles and to anticipate certain problem-solving techniques.

One of the most important features of Newton's Law of Gravitation is that it's an **Inverse-Square Law**. This means that the magnitude of the gravitational force is *inversely* proportional to the *square* of the distance between the centers of the objects. Another important physical law, Coulomb's Law (for the electrostatic force between two charges), which we'll see later, is also an inverse-square law.

Also notice that the forces illustrated in the box above form an action–reaction pair. Even if M and m are different, the gravitational force that M exerts on m has the same magnitude as the gravitational force that m exerts on M. (If the directions of the force vectors in the box above seem backward, remember that gravity is always a *pulling* force; therefore, in the figure above, $\mathbf{F}_{M\text{-on-}m}$ pulls to the left, toward M, while $\mathbf{F}_{m\text{-on-}M}$ pulls to the right, toward m.) Of course, the accelerations of the objects will have different magnitudes if the masses are different, as we discussed earlier when we studied Newton's Third Law.

Example 37-30: What will happen to the gravitational force between two objects if the distance between their centers is doubled? What if the distance is cut in half?

Solution: Since the gravitational force obeys an inverse-square law, if r increases by a factor of 2, then F_{grav} will *decrease* by a factor of $2^2 = 4$. On the other hand, if r decreases by a factor of 2, then F_{grav} will *increase* by a factor of $2^2 = 4$.

Notice that the two formulas given in this section, $w = mg$ and $F_{grav} = GMm/r^2$, are really formulas for the same thing. After all, weight *is* gravitational force. Therefore, we could set these expressions equal to each other:

$$mg = G\frac{Mm}{r^2}$$

Then, dividing both sides by m, we get

$$g = G\frac{M}{r^2}$$

This formula tells us how to find the value of the gravitational acceleration, g. On Earth, we know that $g \approx 10$ m/s². If we were to go to the top of a mountain, then the distance r to the center of the Earth would increase, but compared to the radius of the Earth, the increase would be very small. As a result, while the value of g *is* less at the top of a mountain than at the Earth's surface, the difference is small enough that it can usually be neglected. However, at the position of a satellite orbiting the Earth, for example, the distance to the center of the Earth has now increased dramatically (for example, many satellites have an orbit radius that's over 6.5 times the radius of the Earth), and the resulting decrease in g would definitely need to be taken into account.

This formula for g also shows us why g changes from planet (or moon) to planet. For example, on Earth's moon, the value of g is only about 1.6 m/s² (about a sixth of what it is on Earth) because the mass of the Moon is so much smaller than the mass of the Earth. It's true that the radius of the Moon is smaller than the radius of the Earth, which would, by itself, make g bigger, but M is *much* smaller, and this is why the value of g on the surface of the Moon is smaller than its value on the surface of the Earth. So, while big G is a universal gravitational constant, the value of little g depends on where you are.

Example 37-31: The radius of Earth is approximately 6.4×10^6 m. What's the mass of Earth?

Solution: We can use the formula $g = GM/r^2$ to solve for M:

$$M = \frac{gr^2}{G} = \frac{(10 \text{ m/s}^2)(6.4 \times 10^6 \text{ m})^2}{6.7 \times 10^{-11} \frac{\text{N} \cdot \text{m}^2}{\text{kg}^2}} \approx 6 \times 10^{24} \text{ kg}$$

Example 37-32: The mass of Mars is about 1/10 the mass of Earth, and the radius of Mars is about half that of Earth. Is the value of g on the surface of Mars less than, greater than, or equal to the value of g on Earth?

Solution: We'll use the formula $g = GM/r^2$ to compare the two values of g:

$$\frac{g_{\text{Mars}}}{g_{\text{Earth}}} = \frac{G\dfrac{M_{\text{Mars}}}{r_{\text{Mars}}^2}}{G\dfrac{M_{\text{Earth}}}{r_{\text{Earth}}^2}} = \frac{M_{\text{Mars}}}{M_{\text{Earth}}} \cdot \left(\frac{r_{\text{Earth}}}{r_{\text{Mars}}}\right)^2 = \frac{1}{10} \cdot 2^2 = 0.4$$

Therefore, the value of g on Mars is only about 40% of its value here.

Example 37-33: A long, flat, frictionless table is set up on the surface of the Moon (where $g = 1.6$ m/s^2). An object whose mass on Earth is 4 kg is also transported there.

  a) What is the object's mass on the Moon?
  b) What is the object's weight on the Moon?
  c) If we drop this object from a height of $h = 20$ m, with what speed will it strike the lunar surface?
  d) If we wish to push this object across the table to give it an acceleration of 3 m/s^2, how much force must we exert? Would this force be different if the table and object were back on Earth?

Solution:

  a) The mass is the same, 4 kg.
  b) The weight of the object on the Moon is $w = m \cdot g_{\text{moon}} = (4 \text{ kg})(1.6 \text{ m/s}^2) = 6.4$ N. Notice that the object's weight on the Moon is different from its weight on Earth.
  c) Calling *down* the positive direction and using Big Five #5 with $v_0 = 0$ and $a = g_{\text{moon}} = 1.6$ m/s^2, we find that

$$v^2 = v_0^2 + 2ad \rightarrow v^2 = 2gh \rightarrow v = \sqrt{2gh} = \sqrt{2(1.6 \text{ m/s}^2)(20 \text{ m})} = 8 \text{ m/s}$$

  d) Using $F = ma$, we get $F = (4 \text{ kg})(3 \text{ m/s}^2) = 12$ N. Since Newton's Second Law depends only on mass (not on weight, because there's no g in Newton's Second Law), we'd need this same force even if the object and table were back on Earth.

Example 37-34: The human body can only withstand a vertical *g-force* of about $5g$ before the body has difficulty pumping blood out of the feet and into the brain. Approximately how much upward force could be applied to a 60 kg person at sea level before that person risked fainting? (The phrase "g-force" is a misnomer, because it actually refers to acceleration: The real *force* involved is the normal force from the surface of contact. A person in free fall experiences "zero gees.")

Solution: A person standing motionless on flat ground experiences a normal force equal to his weight, *mg*. That corresponds to $1g$. Thus, the additional upward force from the surface should provide an additional $4g$ of acceleration. According to Newton's Second Law, $\mathbf{F}_{\text{net}} = m\mathbf{a} = 60 \text{ kg} \times 40 \text{ m/s}^2 = 2400$ N.

37.7 CONTACT FORCES: THE NORMAL FORCE, FRICTION, AND TENSION

In order to state the equations we'll use to figure out these frictional forces, we first need to discuss another contact force, the one known as the normal force.

Place a book on a flat table. Assuming that the book isn't too heavy and the tabletop isn't made of, say, tissue paper, the book will remain supported by the table. One force acting on the book is the downward gravitational force. If this were the only force acting on the book, then the book would fall through the table. Hence, there must be an upward force acting on the book that cancels out the book's weight. This supporting force, which acts perpendicular to the tabletop, is called the **normal force**. It's called the *normal* force because it is, by definition, perpendicular to the surface that exerts it. The word *normal* means *perpendicular*. We'll denote the normal force by **N** or by $\mathbf{F_N}$. [Don't confuse **N** (or its magnitude, N) with the abbreviation for the newton, N.] In the case of an object simply lying on a flat surface, the magnitude of the normal force is just equal to the object's weight. As a result, the book feels a downward force of magnitude $w = mg$ and an upward force of magnitude $F_N = mg$, so the net force on the book is 0.

37.7

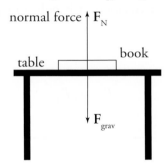

Example 37-35: Do the normal force and the gravitational force described in the preceding paragraph form an action–reaction pair?

Solution: No. While these forces *are* equal but opposite, they do not form an action–reaction pair, because they act on the same object (namely, the book). The forces in an action–reaction pair always act on different objects. So, while it's true that the forces in an action–reaction pair are always equal but opposite, it is not true that any pair of equal but opposite forces must always form an action–reaction pair. The reaction force to $\mathbf{F}_{\text{table-on-book}}$, which is the normal force, is $\mathbf{F}_{\text{book-on-table}}$. The reaction force to $\mathbf{F}_{\text{Earth-on-book}}$, which is the weight of the book, is $\mathbf{F}_{\text{book-on-Earth}}$. The force $\mathbf{F}_{\text{table-on-book}}$ is not the reaction to $\mathbf{F}_{\text{Earth-on-book}}$.

For an object on a horizontal surface that feels no other downward forces, the normal force will be equal to the weight of the object. However, there are many cases in which the normal force isn't equal to the weight of the object. For example, suppose we place a book against a vertical wall and push on the book with a horizontal force **F**. Then the magnitude of the normal force exerted by the wall will be equal to F, which may certainly be different from the weight of the book. Here's another example (which we'll look at in more detail in the next section): If we place a book on an inclined plane (e.g., a ramp), then the normal force exerted by the ramp on the book will not be equal to the weight of the book. What we can say is the general definition of the normal force: *The normal force is the perpendicular component of the contact force exerted by a surface on an object.*

There is often another force between the surface and the object parallel to the surface: **friction**. Some of the examples in the preceding sections described a frictionless surface. Of course, there's no such thing as a truly frictionless surface, but when a problem uses a term like *frictionless*, it simply means that friction is so weak that it can be neglected. Having frictionless surfaces also made those examples easier, so we could become comfortable with Newton's laws while first learning to apply them. However, there are cases in which friction cannot be ignored, so we need to learn how to handle such situations.

The force of friction exerted by a surface on an object in contact with is related to the normal force. In the case of sliding (kinetic) friction, the magnitude of the force of friction is directly proportional to the magnitude of the normal force. The constant of proportionality depends on what the surface is made of and what the object is made of; this constant is called the **coefficient of kinetic friction**, denoted by μ_k (the Greek letter *mu*, with subscript k), where the k denotes <u>k</u>inetic friction. For every pair of surfaces, the coefficient μ_k is an experimentally determined positive number with no units, and the greater its value, the greater the force of kinetic friction. For example, the value of μ_k for rubber-soled shoes on ice is only about 0.1, while for rubber-soled shoes on wood, the value of μ_k is much higher; it's about 0.7 for your sneakers, but could be greater than 1 if you walk around in rock-climbing shoes.

Notice carefully that this is *not* a vector equation. It is only an equation giving the *magnitude* of $\mathbf{F}_f$ in terms of the *magnitude* of $\mathbf{F}_N$.

37.7

Force of Kinetic Friction

$$F_f = \mu_k F_N$$

When two materials are in contact, there's an electrical attraction between the atoms of one surface with those of the other; this attraction will make it difficult to slide one object relative to the other. In addition, if the surfaces aren't perfectly smooth, the roughness will also increase the force required to slide the objects against each other. **Friction** is the term we use for the combination of these effects. Fortunately, the forces due to all those intermolecular forces and to the interactions of surface irregularities can be expressed by a single equation.

The MCAT will expect you to know about two big categories of friction; they're called **static friction** and **kinetic** (or **sliding**) **friction**. When there's no relative motion between the surfaces that are in contact (that is, when there's no sliding), we have static friction; when there *is* relative motion between the surfaces (that is, when there *is* sliding), we have kinetic friction.

The magnitude of the force of kinetic friction is given by the equation $F_f = \mu_k F_N$. The direction of the force of kinetic friction is always parallel to the surface and in the opposite direction to the object's velocity (relative to the surface).

Example 37-36: A book of mass $m = 2$ kg slides across a flat tabletop. If the coefficient of kinetic friction between the book and table is 0.4, what's the magnitude of the force of kinetic friction on the book?

Solution: Because the magnitude of the normal force is $F_N = mg = (2 \text{ kg})(10 \text{ m/s}^2) = 20$ N, the magnitude of the force of kinetic friction is $F_f = \mu_k F_N = (0.4)(20 \text{ N}) = 8$ N.

The formula for static friction is similar to the one for kinetic friction, but there are two important differences. First, given a pair of surfaces, there's a **coefficient of static friction** between them, μ_s (the subscript s now denotes static friction), and on the MCAT, it's always greater than the coefficient of kinetic friction. This is equivalent to saying that, in general, static friction is capable of being stronger than kinetic friction. To illustrate this, imagine there's a heavy crate sitting on the floor and you want to push the crate across the room. You walk up to the crate and push on it, harder and harder until, finally, it "gives" and starts sliding. Once the crate is sliding, it's easier to keep it sliding than it was to get it started in the first place. The friction that resisted your initial push to get the crate moving was static friction. Because it was easier to keep it sliding than it was to get it started sliding, kinetic friction must be weaker than the maximum static friction force.

The second difference between the formula for kinetic friction and the one for static friction is that there's actually no general equation for the force of static friction. All we have is an equation for the *maximum* force of static friction. It's important that you understand this distinction. Let's go back to that heavy crate sitting on the floor. Let's say you know by previous experience that it'll take 400 N of force on your part to get that crate sliding. So, what if you push with a force of 100 N? Well, obviously, the crate won't move. Therefore, there must be another 100 N acting on the crate, opposite to your push, to make the net force on the crate zero. Okay, what if you now push on the crate with a force of 200 N? The crate still won't move, so there must now be another 200 N acting on the crate, opposite to your push, to make the net force on the crate zero. Whatever force you exert on the crate, as long as it's less than 400 N, will cause the force of static friction to cancel you out. Static friction is capable of supplying any necessary force, but only up to a certain maximum. That's why we can't write down a general equation for the force of static friction, only an equation for the maximum force of static friction. The equation looks just like the one above, except we replace μ_k by μ_s, and add the word "max" to denote that all this equation gives is the maximum force of static friction.

Maximum Force of Static Friction

$$F_{f, \text{max}} = \mu_s F_N$$

The maximum magnitude of the force of static friction is given by the equation $F_{f, \text{max}} = \mu_s F_N$. The direction of the force of static friction (maximum or not) is always parallel to the surface and in the opposite direction to the direction it would slide if there were no friction. The magnitude of the force of static friction is whatever value, up to the maximum given by the equation, it takes to cancel out the force(s) that are trying to make the object slide.

Example 37-37: A crate that weighs 1000 N rests on a horizontal floor. The coefficient of static friction between the crate and the floor is 0.4. If you push on the crate with a force of 250 N, what is the magnitude of the force of static friction?

Solution: The answer is not 400 N. The *maximum* force of static friction that the floor could exert on the crate is $F_{f,\,max} = \mu_s F_N = (0.4)(1000\ N) = 400\ N$. However, if you exert a force of only 250 N on the crate, then static friction will only be 250 N. (Just imagine what would happen to the crate if you pushed on it with a force of 250 N and the floor pushed it back toward you with a force of 400 N!)

Example 37-38: You push a 50 kg block of wood across a flat concrete driveway, exerting a constant force of 300 N. If the coefficient of kinetic friction between the wood and concrete is 0.5, what will be the acceleration of the block?

Solution: The normal force acting on the block has a magnitude of $F_N = mg = (50\ kg)(10\ m/s^2) = 500\ N$. Therefore, the force of kinetic friction acting on the sliding block has a magnitude of $F_f = \mu_k F_N = (0.5)(500\ N) = 250\ N$. This means that the net force acting on the block (and parallel to the driveway) is equal to $F - F_f = (300\ N) - (250\ N) = 50\ N$. If $F_{net} = 50\ N$ and $m = 50\ kg$, then $a = F_{net}/m = (50\ N)/(50\ kg) = 1\ m/s^2$.

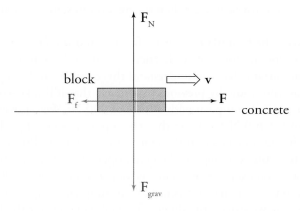

Example 37-39: Instead of pushing the block by a force that's parallel to the driveway, you wrap a rope around the block, sling the rope over your shoulder, and walk it across the driveway. If the rope makes an angle of 30° to the horizontal, and the tension in the rope is 300 N (the same force you exerted on the block in the last example), what will the block's acceleration be now?

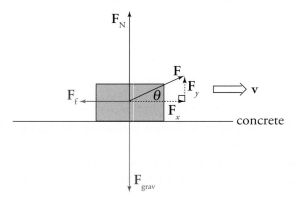

Solution: This is a tough question, but it uses a lot of the material we've covered so far. First, we'll need the normal force to find the friction force. The net vertical force on the block is 0 (because we're not lifting the block off the ground or watching it fall through the concrete). Therefore, $F_N + F_y = F_{grav}$, so $F_N = F_{grav} - F_y$. (Here's another example of the normal force not equaling the weight of the object.) Since

$F_y = F \sin \theta = F \sin 30° = (300 \text{ N})(0.5) = 150 \text{ N}$, we have $F_N = (500 \text{ N}) - (150 \text{ N}) = 350 \text{ N}$. (Intuitively, the normal force is less than the weight of the block because the vertical component of the tension in the rope is "taking some of the pressure" off the surface.) Therefore, $F_f = \mu_k F_N = (0.5)(350 \text{ N}) = 175 \text{ N}$. Now, the horizontal force that you provide is $F_x = F \cos \theta = F \cos 30° \approx (300 \text{ N})(0.85) = 255 \text{ N}$. Therefore, the net force acting on the block, parallel to the driveway, is equal to $F_x - F_f = (255 \text{ N}) - (175 \text{ N}) = 80 \text{ N}$. If $F_{net} = 80 \text{ N}$ and $m = 50 \text{ kg}$, then $a = F_{net}/m = (80 \text{ N})/(50 \text{ kg}) = 1.6 \text{ m/s}^2$. (Notice that you get the block moving faster—even exerting the same force—by doing it this way!)

So far, we've had practice problems where the object is moving along a flat, horizontal surface. However, the MCAT will also expect you to handle questions in which the object is on a ramp, or, in fancier language, an **inclined plane**.

The figure below shows an object of mass m on an inclined plane; the angle the plane makes with the horizontal (the **incline angle**) is labeled θ. If we draw the vector representing the weight of the object, we notice that it can be written in terms of two components: one parallel to the ramp and one perpendicular to it. The diagram on the left shows that the magnitudes of the components of the object's weight, $\mathbf{w} = m\mathbf{g}$, are $mg \sin \theta$ (parallel to the ramp) and $mg \cos \theta$ (perpendicular to the ramp).

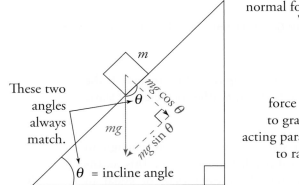
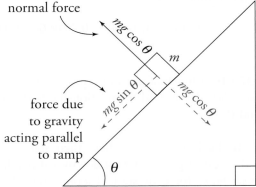

Therefore, as illustrated in the diagram on the right,

the force due to gravity acting parallel to the inclined plane = $mg \sin \theta$
and the normal force from the plane = $mg \cos \theta$,

where θ is measured between the incline and horizontal. **You should memorize both of these facts.**

Incidentally, any time we see an angle in an MCAT problem we'll probably be breaking a vector (say a force, a velocity, or an acceleration) into components. When we looked at projectile motion, we broke the projectile's initial velocity into horizontal and vertical components; here, we're breaking the force of gravity into a component parallel to and one perpendicular to the surface of the incline. Why the difference? In general, the components you'll use will be vertical and horizontal, *unless* the object can only move along one possible line; in that case, the components to use will be the direction of (possible) travel (in this case, parallel to the incline) and the direction perpendicular to that.

Example 37-40: A block of mass m slides down a ramp of incline angle 60°. If the coefficient of kinetic friction between the block and the surface of the ramp is 0.2, what's the block's acceleration down the ramp?

Solution: There are two forces acting parallel to the ramp: $mg \sin \theta$ (directed downward along the ramp) and F_f, the force of kinetic friction (directed upward along the ramp). Therefore, the net force down the ramp is $F_{net} = mg \sin \theta - F_f$. To find F_f, we multiply F_N by μ_k. Since $F_N = mg \cos \theta$, we have

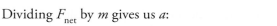

$$F_{net} = mg \sin \theta - \mu_k mg \cos \theta$$

37.7

Dividing F_{net} by m gives us a:

$$a = \frac{F_{net}}{m} = \frac{mg \sin \theta - \mu_k mg \cos \theta}{m} = g(\sin \theta - \mu_k \cos \theta)$$

Putting in the numbers, we get

$$a = (10 \text{ m/s}^2)(\sin 60° - 0.2 \cos 60°) \approx (10 \text{ m/s}^2)(0.85 - 0.2 \cdot \tfrac{1}{2}) = 7.5 \text{ m/s}^2$$

Example 37-41: A block of mass m is placed on a ramp of incline angle θ. If the block doesn't slide down, find the relationship between μ_s (the coefficient of static friction) and θ.

Solution: If the block doesn't slide, then static friction is strong enough to withstand the pull of gravity acting downward parallel to the ramp. This means that the *maximum* force of static friction must be greater than or equal to $mg \sin \theta$. Since $F_{f(static), max} = \mu_s F_N$, and $F_N = mg \cos \theta$, we have $F_{f(static), max} = \mu_s mg \cos \theta$. Therefore,

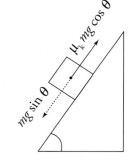

$$F_{f \, (static) \, max} \geq mg \sin \theta$$
$$\mu_s mg \cos \theta \geq mg \sin \theta$$
$$\mu_s g \cos \theta \geq g \sin \theta$$
$$\mu_s \geq \frac{\sin \theta}{\cos \theta}$$
$$\therefore \mu_s \geq \tan \theta$$

In addition to the two contact forces between an object and a surface, there is a third contact force associated with taut strings or ropes attached to objects. That force is tension. As with the normal force and static friction, tension has no general equation for determining its magnitude. Also like those other forces, though, there is a general rule for its direction: ropes don't push! This means that whenever you incorporate the tension forces in a diagram, you need to specify which object those forces act upon, an then draw the tension forces pointing away from (pulling on) the object under scrutiny.

A **pulley** is a device that changes the direction (but not the magnitude) of the tension because it changes the direction of the string or rope that passes over it. (We'll use $\mathbf{F_T}$ or $\mathbf{T}$ to denote a tension force.)

Pulleys can also be used to decrease the force necessary to lift an object. For example, consider the pulley system illustrated on the left below. If we pull down on the string on the right with a force of magnitude F_T, then we'll create a tension force of magnitude F_T throughout the entire string. As a result, there will be *two* tension forces, each of magnitude F_T, pulling up to lift the block (and the bottom pulley, too, but we assume that the pulleys are massless; that is, the mass of any pulley is small enough that it can be ignored). Therefore, we only need to exert half as much force to lift the block! This simple observation, that a pulley system (with massless, frictionless pulleys) causes a constant tension to exist through the entire string, which can lead to multiple tension forces pulling on an object, is the key to many MCAT problems on pulleys.

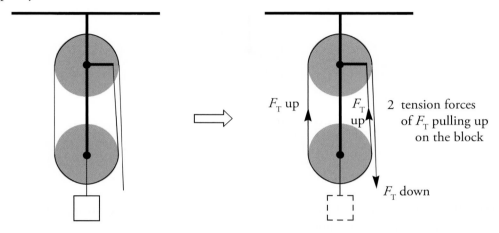

Pulley systems like this multiply our force by however many strings are pulling on the object.

Example 37-42: In the figure below, how much force would we need to exert on the free end of the cord in order to lift the plank (mass M = 300 kg) with constant velocity? (Ignore the masses of the pulleys.)

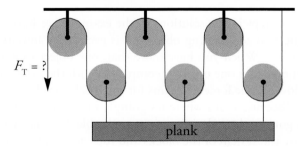

Solution: As a result of our pulling downward, there will be 6 tension forces pulling up on the plank:

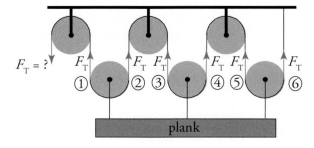

In order to lift with constant velocity (acceleration = zero), we require the net force on the plank to be zero. Therefore, the total of all the tension forces pulling up, $6F_T$, must balance the weight of the plank downward, Mg. This gives us

$$6F_T = Mg \rightarrow F_T = \frac{Mg}{6} = \frac{(300 \text{ kg})(10 \frac{\text{N}}{\text{kg}})}{6} = 500 \text{ N}$$

Example 37-43: Two blocks are connected by a cord that hangs over a pulley. One block has a mass, M, of 10 kg, and the other block has a mass, m, of 5 kg. What will be the magnitude of the acceleration of the system of blocks once they are released from rest?

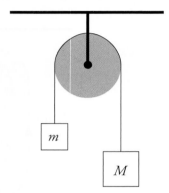

Solution: We'll solve this by a step-by-step approach using a **force diagram**. To apply Newton's Second Law, $\mathbf{F}_{net} = m\mathbf{a}$, to any problem, we follow these steps:

Step 1: Draw all the forces that act *on* the object. (That is, draw the force diagram.)
Step 2: Choose a direction to call *positive* (simply take the direction of the object's motion to be positive; it's almost always the easiest, most natural decision).
Step 3: Find $\mathbf{F}_{net}$ and set it equal to $m\mathbf{a}$.

We have effectively done these steps in the solutions to the examples we have seen already, but now that we have a situation involving two accelerating objects, it is even more important to make sure that we have a systematic plan of attack. When you have more than one object to worry about, just make sure that the Step-2 decision you make for one object is compatible with the Step-2 decision you make for the other one(s). On the left below are the force diagrams for the blocks on the pulley. Notice that we call *up* the positive direction for m (because that's where it's going), and we call *down* the positive direction for M (because that's where *it's* going); these decisions are compatible, because when m moves in its positive direction, so does M. Because the system of the blocks and rope accelerates as one, the positive directions for each block must be compatible (the blocks could not both accelerate upward or downward).

37.7

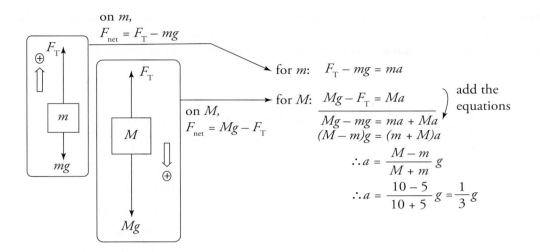

on m,
$F_{net} = F_T - mg$

for m: $\quad F_T - mg = ma$

for M: $\quad Mg - F_T = Ma$

on M,
$F_{net} = Mg - F_T$

add the equations

$$Mg - mg = ma + Ma$$
$$(M - m)g = (m + M)a$$

$$\therefore a = \frac{M - m}{M + m}\, g$$

$$\therefore a = \frac{10 - 5}{10 + 5}\, g = \frac{1}{3}\, g$$

Because *up* is the positive direction for little m, the force F_T on m is positive and the force mg is negative; therefore, for little m, we have $F_{net} = F_T + (-mg) = F_T - mg$. Since *down* is the positive direction for big M, the force Mg on M is positive and the force F_T is negative; therefore, for big M, we have $F_{net} = Mg + (-F_T) = Mg - F_T$. On the right above, we've written down F_{net} = mass × acceleration for each block. There are two equations, but we have two unknowns (F_T and a), so we *need* two equations. To solve the equations, the trick is simply to *add the equations*. Notice that this makes the F_T's drop out, so all we're left with is one unknown, a, which we can solve for immediately. The calculation shown above gives $a = g/3$, so we get $a = 3.3 \text{ m/s}^2$.

If the question had asked for the tension in the cord, we could now use the value we found for a and plug it back into either of our two equations (we'd get the same answer no matter which one we used). Using $F_T - mg = ma$, we'd find that

$$F_T = ma + mg = m(a + g) = m(\tfrac{1}{3}g + g) = \tfrac{4}{3}mg = \tfrac{4}{3}(5 \text{ kg})(10 \tfrac{\text{N}}{\text{kg}}) = 67 \text{ N}$$

Example 37-44: In the figure below, the block of mass m slides up a frictionless inclined plane, pulled by another block of mass M that is falling. If $\theta = 30°$, $m = 20$ kg, and $M = 40$ kg, what's the acceleration of the block on the ramp?

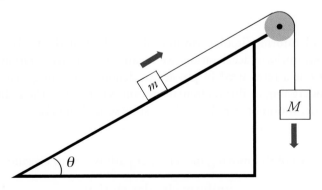

Solution: On the left below are the force diagrams for the blocks. Notice that we call *up the ramp* the positive direction for *m* (because that's where it's going), and we call *down* the positive direction for *M* (because that's where *it's* going); these decisions are compatible, because when *m* moves in its positive direction, so does *M*.

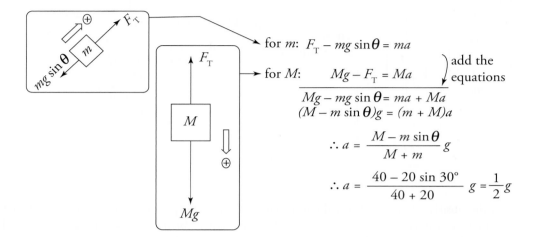

for *m*: $F_T - mg \sin\theta = ma$

for *M*: $Mg - F_T = Ma$ — add the equations

$Mg - mg \sin\theta = ma + Ma$

$(M - m \sin\theta)g = (m + M)a$

$\therefore a = \dfrac{M - m \sin\theta}{M + m} g$

$\therefore a = \dfrac{40 - 20 \sin 30°}{40 + 20} g = \dfrac{1}{2} g$

Because *up the ramp* is the positive direction for little *m*, the force F_T on *m* is positive and the force due to gravity along the ramp, $mg \sin\theta$, is negative; therefore, for little *m*, we have $F_{net} = F_T + (-mg \sin\theta) = F_T - mg \sin\theta$. Since *down* is the positive direction for big *M*, the force Mg on *M* is positive and the force F_T is negative; therefore, for big *M*, we have $F_{net} = Mg + (-F_T) = Mg - F_T$. On the right above, we've written down F_{net} = mass × acceleration for each block. As in the preceding example, there are two equations, (and two unknowns, F_T and *a*). Again using the trick of adding the equations, the F_T's drop out, and all we're left with is one unknown, *a*, to solve for. The calculation shown above gives $a = g/2$, so we get $a = 5$ m/s².

37.8 UNIFORM CIRCULAR MOTION

So far, we've analyzed motion that takes place along a straight line (horizontal, vertical, or slanted) or along a parabola. The MCAT will also require that you know how to analyze an object that moves in a circular path.

The title of this section is Uniform Circular Motion (often abbreviated UCM). What does *uniform* mean here? When we talk about uniform acceleration, we mean constant acceleration; uniform density means constant density; *uniform* is a term used in physics to denote something that remains constant. What property of an object undergoing uniform circular motion is constant? The radius of its path is constant, but that's already in the definition of *circular*, so it must be something else.

> An object moving in a circular path is said to execute
>
> **uniform circular motion**
>
> if its *speed* is constant.

The acceleration of an object undergoing uniform circular motion always points toward the center of the circle. The term **centripetal** (from the Latin, meaning *to seek the center*) is therefore used to describe the acceleration of an object undergoing UCM.

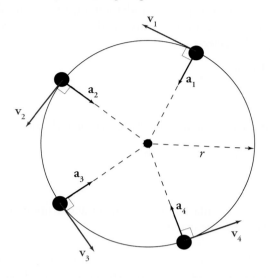

Since each **v** is tangent to the circle, and each **a** always points to the center of the circle, **v** and **a** are always perpendicular to each other at any position of the object.

Note that **a** is continually changing along with **v**. This differentiates uniform circular motion from projectile motion, where the parabolic trajectory is due to a constant acceleration (and force) pointing down.

We now know the *direction* of the centripetal acceleration at any point on the circle; what is its *magnitude*? If v is the speed of the object and r is the radius of the circular path, then the magnitude of the centripetal acceleration, a_c, is v^2/r.

Magnitude of Centripetal Acceleration

$$a_c = \frac{v^2}{r}$$

If an object is accelerating, then it must be feeling a force (after all, $\mathbf{F}_{net} = m\mathbf{a}$, so you can't have an acceleration without a force). Since $\mathbf{F}_{net}$ and **a** always point in the same direction, no matter what the path of the object, the net force on an object undergoing UCM must, like **a**, point toward the center. So, guess what we call it? **Centripetal force** (denoted $\mathbf{F}_c$). This is the *net* force directed toward the center that acts on an object to make it execute uniform circular motion. And since $F_{net} = ma$, we'll have $\mathbf{F}_c = m\mathbf{a}_c$ and $F_c = ma_c$, so the magnitude of the centripetal force is mv^2/r, where m is the mass of the object that's moving around the circle.

Magnitude of Centripetal Force

$$F_c = ma_c = \frac{mv^2}{r}$$

Example 37-45: An object of mass 3 kg moves at a constant speed of 4 m/s in a circular path of radius 0.5 m. What is the magnitude of its acceleration? What is the magnitude of the net force on the object?

Solution: An object moving in a circular path at constant speed is undergoing uniform circular motion. Although its speed is constant, the object is always accelerating, because its direction is constantly changing. The acceleration of the object is the centripetal acceleration,

$$a_c = \frac{v^2}{r} = \frac{(4 \text{ m/s}^2)^2}{0.5 \text{ m}} = 32 \text{ m/s}^2$$

From Newton's Second Law, we can now determine the magnitude of the net force the object feels:

$$F_c = ma_c = (3 \text{ kg})(32 \text{ m/s}^2) = 96 \text{ N}$$

Example 37-46: If an object undergoing uniform circular motion is being acted upon by a constant force toward the center, why doesn't the object fall into the center?

Solution: Actually, it *is* falling toward the center, but because of its speed, the object remains in a circular orbit around the center. Remember: the direction of **v** is not necessarily the same as the direction of $\mathbf{F}_{net}$. So, just because $\mathbf{F}_{net}$ points toward the center does not mean that **v** must point toward the center. It's the direction of the *acceleration*, not the velocity that always matches the direction of $\mathbf{F}_{net}$. Let's look at the motion of the object at a certain point in its circular path:

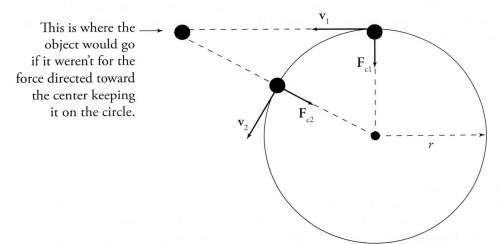

This is where the object would go if it weren't for the force directed toward the center keeping it on the circle.

In this figure, the net force on the object at Position 1 points downward (toward the center of the circle). Therefore, it's telling $\mathbf{v}_1$ to move downward a little, so that at the next moment, at Position 2, the velocity will point downward slightly. Notice that this is just what we want in order to keep the object traveling in a circle! If it weren't for this force pointing toward the center (that is, if the centripetal force were suddenly removed), then the object's velocity wouldn't change. It would not continue to move in a circle but would instead fly off in a straight line, tangent to the circle at the point where the force was removed.

Example 37-47: How would the net force on an object undergoing uniform circular motion have to change if the object's speed doubled?

Solution: Centripetal force, mv^2/r, is proportional to the *square* of the speed. So, if the object's speed increased by a factor of 2, then the magnitude of $\mathbf{F}_c$ would have to increase by a factor of $2^2 = 4$.

Solving circular motion problems often involves something more than simply using the formulas $a_c = v^2/r$ or $F_c = mv^2/r$. The key to solving such problems is to answer this question:

What provides the centripetal force?

In other words, what force(s) act in the dimension toward the center of the circle?

Centripetal force is not some new kind of force like gravity or tension. It's simply the name for the net force directed toward the center of the circular path. The vector sum of forces such as gravity and tension is what gets *called* centripetal force, when those forces, or components of them, are directed toward the center of the circle. When drawing a force diagram for an object undergoing UCM, here are a couple of tips:

1. Do not add a force called $\mathbf{F}_c$ in your picture; forces such as gravity, tension, normal force, etc. *do* go in your picture, but $\mathbf{F}_c$ doesn't. Remember, $\mathbf{F}_c$ is what the forces toward the center have to add up to.
2. Always call *toward the center* the positive direction. Any forces toward the center are then positive forces, and any forces directed away from the center are negative. You'll need this to find F_{net} and then set the result equal to F_c.

Example 37-48: A string is tied around a rock of mass 0.2 kg, and the rock is then whirled at a constant speed v in a horizontal circle of radius 0.4 m, as shown in the figure below. If $\sin\theta = 0.4$ and $\cos\theta = 0.9$, what's v?

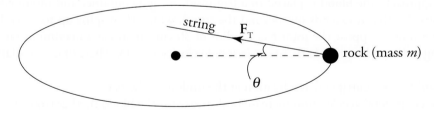

Solution: First, let's draw a bigger force diagram:

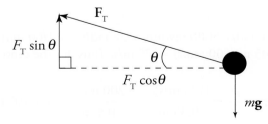

(This figure also shows why the end of the string is slightly above the center of the circle. The string has to point upward a little in order for there to be an upward component of the tension to cancel out the weight of the rock and allow the rock to revolve in a *horizontal* circle.) Because the rock is moving in a horizontal circle and not accelerating vertically, we know that the net vertical force must be zero. Therefore, the vertical component of the string's tension, $F_y = F_T \sin\theta$, must balance out the weight of the rock, *mg*:

$$F_T \sin\theta = mg$$

From this, we can figure out that

$$F_T = \frac{mg}{\sin\theta} = \frac{(0.2 \text{ kg})(10\frac{\text{N}}{\text{kg}})}{0.4} = 5 \text{ N}$$

Now, let's look at the circular motion: *What provides the centripetal force?* As the diagram shows, there's only one force directed toward the center of the circle (namely, the horizontal component of the tension, $F_x = F_T \cos\theta$) so this must be it:

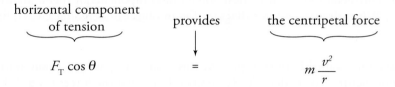

We now just plug in the value we found for F_T to get *v*:

$$F_T \cos\theta = m\frac{v^2}{r} \rightarrow v = \sqrt{\frac{rF_T \cos\theta}{m}} = \sqrt{\frac{(0.4 \text{ m})(5 \text{ N})(0.9)}{0.2 \text{ kg}}} = 3 \text{ m/s}$$

Example 37-49: Separating blood plasma from the solid bodies in blood (blood cells and platelets) by rapid sedimentation requires use of a *centrifuge* to produce the necessary accelerations on the order of 5000*g*. In one approach, the blood is placed in a bag inside a rigid container and mounted to the end of a horizontal rotor (so that it extends out beyond the rotor), which then spins up to several thousands of revolutions per minute. Suppose the rotor has a radius of 30 cm, rotates at a maximum rate of 5000 rpm, and that the bag is 10 cm long. Note that translational velocity $v = r\omega$, where ω is in radians/second.

a) What will be the centripetal acceleration at the middle of the bag?
b) Will the centripetal acceleration increase or decrease for the blood further from the axis of rotation?

Solution:

a) First we convert rpm to rad/s: 5000 rev/min × 2π rad/rev × 1/60 min/s ≈ 500 rad/s. Now $v = r\omega = (0.30 \text{ m} + 0.05 \text{ m})(500 \text{ rad/s}) = 175 \text{ m/s}$. Thus, for the centripetal acceleration we have

$$a_c = \frac{v^2}{r} = \frac{(175 \text{ m/s})^2}{0.35 \text{ m}} \approx \frac{(200 \text{ m/s})^2}{0.5 \text{ m}} = 8 \times 10^4 \text{ m/s}^2$$

This is 8000*g*, more than enough acceleration to achieve separation of blood.

b) Your first instinct upon reading this question might be to say, "I know that centripetal acceleration is inversely proportional to the radius, so increasing the distance from the central axis should decrease the acceleration." That would be wrong: Such reasoning implicitly (and falsely) assumes that speed is constant as radius increases, but for a *rigid rotator* like a centrifuge or a merry-go-round, translational speed is proportional to the radius according to the equation $v = r\omega$, (the constant is the angular speed ω). If you're having trouble picturing this, imagine what happens when you're on a merry-go-round: standing at the center, you are spinning in place and thus have a translational speed of zero (your position isn't changing with time). The further you get from the center, the faster you are moving. Thus, because of the v^2 term in the numerator, $a_c \propto r$, and centripetal acceleration increases for blood further from the axis of rotation.

Example 37-50: From the perspective of the blood cells in the bag as the centrifuge spins (or any other mass undergoing circular motion, such as passengers on a turning bus), a *centrifugal pseudo-force* acts on them pushing outward from the axis of rotation. This is called a pseudo-force because it does not exist as an additional force in the frame of reference of a lab worker using the centrifuge, but only exists within the accelerating frame of reference (such a reference frame is also called a *non-inertial frame* because Newton's First Law does not apply within it). The magnitude of the centrifugal pseudo-force on a mass m is given by $F_{centrifugal} = m\omega^2 r$, where ω and r are as previously defined. Suppose a red blood cell with a mass of 30 picograms lies at the outer edge of the blood bag described in example 37-49. What centrifugal pseudo-force does it experience as the centrifuge spins with a constant rotational speed of $\omega = 500$ rad/s?

37.8

Solution: Applying the equation for the centrifugal pseudo-force yields

$$F_{centrifugal} = m\omega^2 r = \left(30 \times 10^{-12} \text{ grams}\right)\left(\frac{1 \text{ kg}}{10^3 \text{ grams}}\right)\left(500 \frac{\text{rad}}{\text{s}}\right)^2 (40 \text{ cm})\left(\frac{1 \text{ m}}{10^2 \text{ cm}}\right) =$$

$$\left(3 \times 25 \times 4\right)\left(10^{-15} \times 10^4 \times 10^{-1}\right)\text{newtons} = 3 \times 10^{-10} \text{ N outward from the center}$$

37.9   CENTER OF MASS, TORQUE, AND EQUILIBRIUM

In the examples we have considered so far, objects were treated as though they were each a single particle. In fact, in the step-by-step solution to one of the pulley problems, we drew a force diagram showing all the forces acting on the objects in the system. To make that step go faster, we sometimes just represent each object by a dot and draw the force arrows on the dot. For example, the force diagram in the solution to Example 37-38 could have been drawn like this:

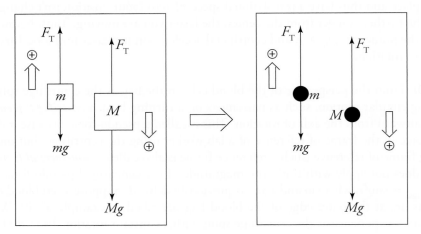

Each dot really denotes the *center of mass* (or gravity—the terms are interchangeable on the MCAT) of the object, the point at which we could consider all the mass of the object to be concentrated for force problems like the pulley example.

For a simple object such as a sphere, block, or cylinder, whose density is constant (that is, for an object that's *homogeneous*), the center of mass is where you'd expect it to be—at its geometric center.

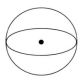 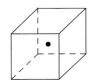 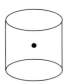

Note that in some cases, the center of mass isn't even located within the body of the object:

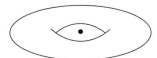

For a nonhomogeneous object, such as a hammer, whose density *does* vary from point to point, there's no single-step way mathematically to calculate the location of the center of mass.

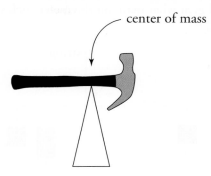

center of mass

However, there is a simpler type of problem on which the MCAT *will* expect you to locate the center of mass. The situation involves a series of masses arranged in a line. For example, imagine that you had a stick with several blocks hanging from it. Where should you attach a string to the stick so that this mobile would balance?

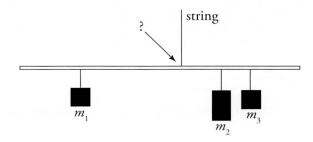

37.9

For a problem like this, in which each individual mass can be considered to be at a single point in space, here's the formula for the location of the center of mass:

Center of Mass for Point Masses

$$x_{CM} = \frac{m_1 x_1 + m_2 x_2 + m_3 x_3 \ldots}{m_1 + m_2 + m_3 \ldots}$$

(The location of the center of mass is often denoted by $\overline{x}$ as well. We'll use both notations.) To use this formula, follow these steps:

Step 1: Choose an origin (a reference point to call $x = 0$). The locations of the objects will be measured relative to this point. Often the easiest point to use will be at the location of the left-hand mass, but any point is fine; if a coordinate system is given in the problem, use it.

Step 2: Determine the locations (x_1, x_2, x_3, etc.) of the objects.

Step 3: Multiply each mass by its location ($m_1 x_1$, $m_2 x_2$, $m_3 x_3$, etc.) then add.

Step 4: Divide by the total mass ($m_1 + m_2 + m_3 + \ldots$).

Example 37-51: In the figure below, three blocks hang below a massless meter stick. Block m_1 hangs from the *20 cm* mark, block m_2 hangs from the *70 cm* mark, and block m_3 hangs from the *80 cm* mark. If m_1 = 2 kg, m_2 = 5 kg, and m_3 = 3 kg, at what mark on the meter stick should a string be attached so that this system would hang horizontally?

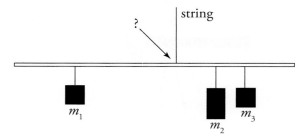

37.9

Solution: The first step is to choose an origin, a reference point to call $x = 0$. We are free to choose our zero mark anywhere we want, but the simplest choice here is the one implicitly mentioned in the question itself. The question wants to know at what mark on the meter stick we should attach the string; in other words, how far from the left end of the meter stick should we attach the string? Since the question asks essentially, "How far from the *left end…?*" the best place to choose our zero mark is at the *left end*. We now can write x_1 = 20 cm, x_2 = 70 cm, and x_3 = 80 cm. Using the formula above, we find that

$$x_{CM} = \frac{m_1 x_1 + m_2 x_2 + m_3 x_3}{m_1 + m_2 + m_3}$$

$$= \frac{(2 \text{ kg})(20 \text{ cm}) + (5 \text{ kg})(70 \text{ cm}) + (3 \text{ kg})(80 \text{ cm})}{(2 \text{ kg}) + (5 \text{ kg}) + (3 \text{ kg})}$$

$$= \frac{630 \text{ kg} \cdot \text{cm}}{10 \text{ kg}}$$

$$\therefore x_{CM} = 63 \text{ cm}$$

What if we had instead chosen the center of the meter stick (the *50 cm* mark) to be our origin? In that case, we would have found x_1 = −30 cm (because m_1 hangs from the *20 cm* mark, and *20 cm* is 30 cm to the *left*—hence the minus sign—of *50 cm*), x_2 = 20 cm, and x_3 = 30 cm. The formula would have told us that

$$x_{CM} = \frac{m_1 x_1 + m_2 x_2 + m_3 x_3}{m_1 + m_2 + m_3}$$

$$= \frac{(2 \text{ kg})(-30 \text{ cm}) + (5 \text{ kg})(20 \text{ cm}) + (3 \text{ kg})(30 \text{ cm})}{(2 \text{ kg}) + (5 \text{ kg}) + (3 \text{ kg})}$$

$$= \frac{130 \text{ kg} \cdot \text{cm}}{10 \text{ kg}}$$

$$\therefore x_{CM} = 13 \text{ cm}$$

Well, 13 cm to the *right* (because x_{CM} is *positive*) of the *50 cm* mark is the *63 cm* mark, the same answer we found before.

Example 37-52: Falls are one of the most serious medical issues among the elderly. Falls result when the center of mass of a person's body is not located over a base of support (determined largely by one's foot placement) and the person is unable to correct for the imbalance with sufficient speed and coordination. Center of mass when standing still is determined by body shape and weight distribution. It's important to keep in mind that when people move, they redistribute their body mass and thus change the location of their centers of mass. What are some likely physical (as opposed to physiological, neurological, or environmental) risk factors for falling, and some possible avoidance strategies?

Solution: One risk factor for falling is obesity: not only does this shift the center of mass while standing still, but because it can affect walking motion, the obese individual may be more likely to experience a shift of the center of mass outside the base of support while moving and be less able to prevent the fall once it begins. Another is posture. For example, people often develop a head protrusion and thoracic kyphosis (a hump in the upper back) as they age, shifting the center of mass forward.

Many ways of shifting the body's center of mass closer to the feet and thus making it more likely that the center of mass will remain above the base of support (at least while both feet are planted) are impractical: heavy shoes and pants, for example. However, apart from exercises and physical therapies to avoid or alleviate the risk factors mentioned above, one common risk avoidance strategy is to increase the size of the support base with a cane or a walker. Both of these have the effect of providing a larger total area that the center of mass can occupy without causing imbalance.

37.9

Torque

If forces act on a line through the center of mass, then the motion of the object will be just as previous examples have described using Newton's laws. However, what if we want an object to spin (or stop spinning), instead of or in addition to translating through space? Imagine a bucket. One way would be to grab the handle and then rotate our hand, or we could place our hands on opposite sides of the bucket and then, by moving our hands in opposite directions, rotate the bucket. In order to make an object *spin*, we need to exert a *torque*.

Torque is the measure of a force's effectiveness at making an object spin or rotate. (More precisely, it's the measure of a force's effectiveness at making an object *accelerate* rotationally.) If an object is initially at rest, and then it starts to spin, something must have exerted a torque. And if an object is already spinning, something would have to exert a torque to get it to stop spinning.

All systems that can spin or rotate have a "center" of turning. This is the point that does not move while the remainder of the object is rotating, effectively becoming the center of the circle. There are many terms used to describe this point, including **pivot point** and **fulcrum**.

Let's say we want to tighten a bolt with a wrench. The figure below illustrates the situation.

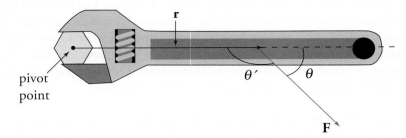

If we applied the force **F** to the wrench, would we make the wrench and the bolt rotate? Yes, because this force **F** has *torque*. (Notice: Torque is not a force; it's a property of a force.) To say how *much* torque **F** provides, we need a couple of preliminary definitions. First, the vector from the center of rotation (the **pivot point**) to the point of application of the force is called the **radius vector**, **r**. The angle between the vectors **r** and **F** is called θ. Now notice in the figure above that the angle between the vectors **r** and **F** at the point where they actually meet is denoted by θ'. This is because the angle between two vectors is actually the angle they make *when they start at the same point*. But in the figure, the vector **r** starts at the pivot point (which is where **r** always starts), and **F** starts at the *end* of **r** (which is where **F** always starts). One way to find the correct angle between these vectors is to imagine sliding **r** over so that it does start where **F** starts; the dashed line in the figure shows the line along which such a translated **r** vector would lie and the resulting correct angle θ. However, all this fuss about which angle is the correct one doesn't really matter, as you'll soon see.

The amount of torque a force **F** provides depends on three things: the magnitude of **F**, the length of **r**, and the angle θ.

Torque

$$\tau = rF \sin \theta$$

(The letter we use for torque is τ, the Greek letter *tau*.) From this equation, we can immediately figure out the unit of torque:

$$[\tau] = [r][F] = \text{m·N} = \text{N·m}$$

There's no special name for this unit; it's just a newton-meter.

For example, let's say that $F = 20$ N, $r = 10$ cm, and $\theta = 30°$. Then the torque provided by this force would be $\tau = rF \sin \theta = (0.1 \text{ m})(20 \text{ N}) \sin 30° = 1$ N·m. Notice that if we had instead used θ', we would have gotten the same answer, since $\theta' = 150°$ and $\sin 150° = \sin 30°$. This is why we don't have to worry about which angle, θ or θ', is the true angle between **r** and **F** when we calculate torque, because **r** and **F** will always be *supplements* (they'll add up to 180°) and the sine of an angle is always equal to the sine of its supplement. Therefore, $\tau = rF \sin \theta = rF \sin \theta'$.

Look at this force on the wrench:

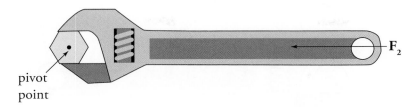

Our intuition tells us that this force would not make the wrench (or bolt) rotate. Therefore, we expect that this force has zero torque. Using the definition, we can see that this is true. If we were to draw the **r** vector from the pivot to the point where F_2 is applied, we'd see that the value of $\sin \theta$ is 0, so $\tau_2 = 0$. Forces with no torque (like this one) cannot increase (or decrease) the rotational speed of an object.

How about this force on the wrench?

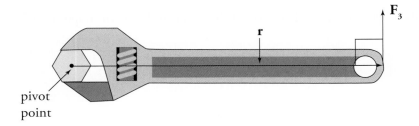

The force F_3 is perpendicular to its **r** vector, so $\theta = 90°$ and $\sin \theta = 1$, its maximum value. Therefore, when $r \perp F$, we get the maximum torque for a given r and F, and the equation for torque gives us simply $\tau_3 = rF_3$. (This situation is very common, by the way.)

$$\text{If } r \perp F, \text{ then } \tau = rF.$$

The force F_3 above would produce counterclockwise rotation, so we say that it produces a **counterclockwise (CCW)** torque. The force F_4 below would produce clockwise rotation, so we say it produces a **clockwise (CW)** torque.

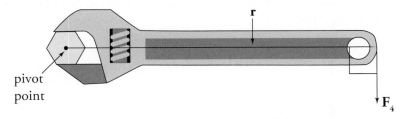

If $F_3 = F_4$, then these forces produce the same amount of torque, but one is clockwise and the other is counterclockwise. If we want to distinguish between them mathematically, we can say that $\tau_3 = +rF_3$ and $\tau_4 = -rF_4$, since it's customary to specify CCW rotation as positive and CW as negative.

The other method for calculating torque, which gives the same answer as the method we've just described, is based on the *lever arm* of a force. Let's look again at the first picture of our wrench:

37.9

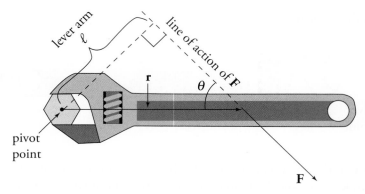

This time, however, rather than measuring the distance from the pivot to the *point* where the force is applied (the length *r*), we'll measure the shortest distance from the pivot to the *line* along which **F** is applied. This distance, which is always perpendicular to the line of action of F, is called the **lever arm** of **F**, written as ℓ or l.

Once we know the lever arm, ℓ, the definition of the torque of **F** is then simply $\tau = \ell F$.

Torque

$$\tau = \ell F$$

To see that this gives the same value for the torque as the formula $\tau = rF \sin \theta$, just notice that in the picture on the preceding page (bottom), the lever arm, ℓ, is the side opposite the angle θ in a right triangle whose hypotenuse is *r*; therefore, $\ell = r \sin \theta$. So, $\tau = \ell F$ is the same as $\tau = (r \sin \theta)F$. Because you can use either formula for calculating the torque, use whichever one is more convenient in a particular problem. In general, it's convenient to use the lever arm method if the length of the lever arm is obvious from the situation; otherwise, use $\tau = rF \sin \theta$.

For the force $\mathbf{F}_5$ shown on the next page, our intuition tells us that this force would not make the wrench (or bolt) rotate. Therefore, we expect that this force has zero torque. Using the definition of lever arm, we can see that this is true. The line of action of $\mathbf{F}_5$ passes right through the pivot point, so the level arm of the force is zero, and $\tau_5 = \ell_5 F_5 = (0)F_5 = 0$.

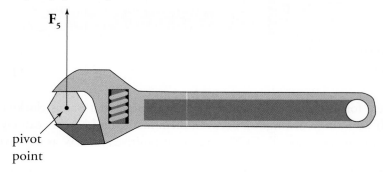

In general, if a force acts at the pivot or along a line through the pivot, then its torque is zero.

Example 37-53: A square metal plate (of side length s) rests on a flat table, and we exert a force **F** at one corner, parallel to one of the sides, as shown below. What is the torque of this force?

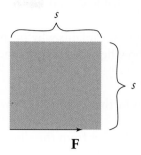

Solution: First note that any object that can rotate freely, meaning unconstrained to rotate about a particular pivot point (by a hinge or fastener, for example), will naturally rotate about its center of mass. We'll calculate the torque of **F** by two different methods: first using the formula $\tau = rF \sin\theta$, and then using the formula $\tau = \ell F$.

Method 1. We draw in the **r** vector, which points from the pivot to the point where the force is applied. The angle between **r** and **F** can be taken to be $\theta = 45°$. If s is the length of each side of the square, then the length of **r** is $\frac{1}{2}s\sqrt{2}$ (because r is the hypotenuse of a 45°-45° right triangle, it's $\sqrt{2}$ times the length of each leg).

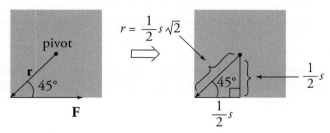

This gives $\tau = rF \sin\theta = \left(\frac{1}{2}s\sqrt{2}\right)(F)\sin 45° = \left(\frac{1}{2}s\sqrt{2}\right)(F)\left(\frac{\sqrt{2}}{2}\right) = \frac{1}{2}sF.$

Method 2. The line of action of the force **F** is simply the bottom side of the square. The perpendicular distance from the pivot to the side of the square is half the length of the square, $\frac{1}{2}s$, so this is the lever arm, ℓ.

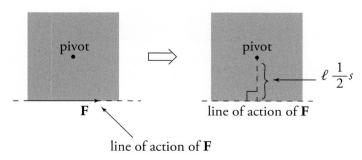

Therefore, $\tau = \ell F = \frac{1}{2}sF.$

In this situation, the formula using the lever arm is the easier way to calculate the torque. That's because you can look at the diagram and see the length of the lever arm right away. If you find yourself having to *calculate* the length of the lever arm, you probably should just be using $\tau = rF \sin \theta$.

Example 37-54: Which of the following best explains why people with bicep attachment points farther from their elbows tend to have greater elbow flexion strength, and thus an improved ability to perform a dumbbell curling exercise?

    A) An attachment point that is farther from the elbow increases the force provided by muscle contraction.

    B) An attachment point that is farther from the elbow decreases the force provided by muscle contraction.

    C) An attachment point that is farther from the elbow results in a greater torque produced by the bicep as it contracts.

    D) An attachment point that is closer to the hand results in a lesser torque produced by the bicep as it contracts.

Solution: The first two answer choices discuss a difference in the muscle's contraction force. This force is a function of the muscle fibers, not its point of attachment to the forearm, which eliminates choices A and B. An attachment point farther from the elbow increases r, the distance from the pivot point (elbow) to the where the force is applied (at the attachment), so according to the equation for torque, $\tau = rF \sin\theta$, this would increase the torque created by the biceps contraction, which makes choice C correct. The distance to the hand is a trap answer: there are two torques acting on someone curling a dumbbell or other mass, one provided by the contraction of the biceps muscle and an opposing one from the weight of the dumbbell acting downward at the hand. Both torques depend on the radial distance from the pivot point, which is the elbow.

Example 37-55: A homogeneous rectangular sheet of metal lies on a flat table and is able to rotate around an axis through its center, perpendicular to the table. Four forces, all of the same magnitude, are exerted on the sheet as shown below:

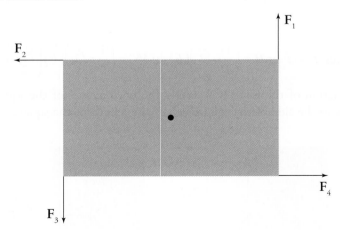

Which one of the following statements is true?

    A) The net force is zero, but the net torque is not.

    B) The net torque is zero, but the net force is not.

    C) Neither the net force nor the net torque is zero.

    D) Both the net force and the net torque equal zero.

Solution: There are two vertical forces that point in opposite directions (so they cancel), and two horizontal forces that point in opposite directions (so *they* cancel). Therefore, the net force, $\mathbf{F}_{net} = \mathbf{F}_1 + \mathbf{F}_2 + \mathbf{F}_3 + \mathbf{F}_4$, is zero. Eliminate choices B and C.

Now for the torques. In the figure below, each force has its corresponding lever arm. Notice that each force produces a counterclockwise (CCW) torque. As a result, the total, or net, torque cannot be zero. (The net torque is zero only when the total counterclockwise torque balances the total clockwise torque.) Therefore, the answer is choice A.

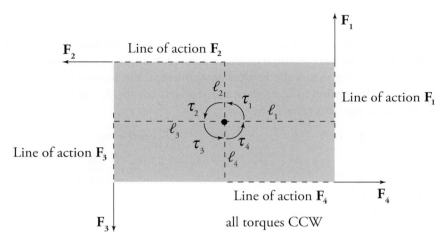

Now that we've covered force and torque, we finish by considering the special cases in which the net value of one or both of them is zero. (Cases in which some physical quantity equals zero are almost always interesting, so pay special attention to zeros as you prepare for the MCAT!) As it's used in physics, the term **equilibrium** indicates these zeros. Notice that equilibrium does not mean zero velocity. As long as the velocity of the system remains constant (no change in speed or direction), then we can say that the system is in equilibrium. If the velocity happens to be zero, then we say the system is in **static** equilibrium.

There are actually two kinds of equilibrium, because there are two kinds of acceleration. There's *translational* equilibrium and *rotational* equilibrium. A system is said to be in **translational equilibrium** if the forces cancel; if $F_{net} = 0$, then the translational acceleration (*a*) is zero. A system is in **rotational equilibrium** if the torques cancel; if $\tau_{net} = 0$, then the rotational acceleration (denoted by α, the Greek letter *alpha*) is zero. If the term *equilibrium* is used without specifying which type, then it's assumed that the system is in *both* translational and rotational equilibrium.

37.9

Example 37-56: In the figure below, a block of mass 40 kg is held in place by two ropes exerting equal tension forces. If cos θ = 2/3, what's the tension in each rope?

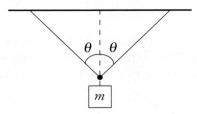

Solution: At the point where the mass is attached to the two ropes, we balance the forces. The horizontal forces automatically balance (we have $F_T \sin \theta$ pointing to the left and $F_T \sin \theta$ pointing to the right). For the vertical forces, we notice that there's the vertical component of the tension in the left-hand rope plus the vertical component of the tension in the right-hand rope ($F_T \cos \theta + F_T \cos \theta = 2F_T \cos \theta$), to balance out the weight of the block, mg. This gives us

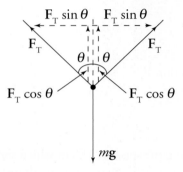

$$2F_T \cos \theta = mg$$

$$F_T = \frac{mg}{2 \cos \theta}$$

$$= \frac{(40 \text{ kg})(10 \frac{N}{kg})}{2\left(\frac{2}{3}\right)}$$

Chapter 38
Work and Energy

38.1   WORK

Imagine a constant force **F** pushing a crate through a displacement **d**, as shown below:

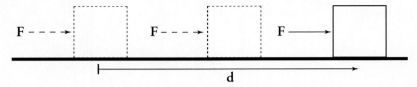

(Notice that the force **F** here doesn't just act momentarily at the initial position of the crate, with the crate then sliding across the floor with **F** removed; the force **F** is assumed to act constantly over the entire displacement.) We say that the **work** done by **F** is the product of F and d: Work $W = Fd$.

For example, if the magnitude of **F** is 20 N and the magnitude of **d** is 5 m, then the work done by the force **F** in the situation pictured above is (20 N)(5 m) = 100 N·m. When it's used to measure work, the newton-meter (N·m) is renamed the **joule**, abbreviated J. Therefore, we have $W = 100$ J.

The situation pictured above is quite special, however, because the vectors **F** and **d** point in the same direction. What if **F** and **d** do not point in the same direction? For example, what if we tie one end of a rope around the crate, sling the other end over our shoulder and pull the crate across the floor? Then our force **F** (which is actually the tension in the rope) will be at an angle to the displacement:

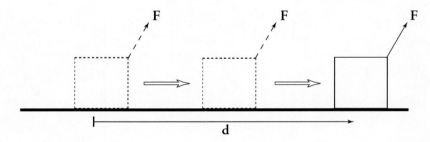

In this case, the work done by **F** is not the product of F and d. It's only the component of the force in the direction of **d** that does work. If θ is the angle between **F** and **d**, then the component of **F** that's parallel to **d** has magnitude $F \cos \theta$. Therefore, the work done by **F** is $(F \cos \theta)(d)$.

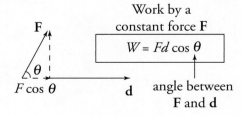

Work by a
constant force **F**

$$W = Fd \cos \theta$$

angle between
F and **d**

Work by a Constant Force, F

$$W = Fd \cos\theta$$

where θ = angle between **F** and **d**

Notice that the formula $W = Fd \cos \theta$ includes the formula $W = Fd$ as a special case. After all, if **F** and **d** do point in the same direction, then $\theta = 0°$, and $\cos \theta = \cos 0° = 1$, so $Fd \cos \theta$ becomes Fd. Therefore, the formula $W = Fd \cos \theta$ covers all cases of a constant force **F** acting through a displacement **d**.

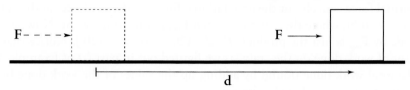

Example 38-1: In the situation pictured above, assume the mass of the crate, m, is 20 kg and the coefficient of kinetic friction between the crate and the floor is 0.4. If $F = 100$ N and $d = 6$ m,

a) How much work is done by **F**?
b) How much work is done by the normal force?
c) How much work is done by gravity?
d) How much work is done by the force of friction?
e) What is the total work done on the crate?

Solution:

a) Because **F** is parallel to **d**, the work done by **F** is simply $Fd = (100 \text{ N})(6 \text{ m}) = 600$ J.
b) The normal force is perpendicular to the floor, and to **d**. Since the angle between $\mathbf{F_N}$ and **d** is $\theta = 90°$, and $\cos 90° = 0$, the work done by $\mathbf{F_N}$ is zero.
c) The gravitational force is also perpendicular to the floor, and to **d**. Because the angle between $\mathbf{F_{grav}}$ and **d** is $\theta = 90°$, and $\cos 90° = 0$, the work done by $\mathbf{F_{grav}}$ is zero too.
d) First, since $F_N = mg = (20 \text{ kg})(10 \text{ N/kg}) = 200$ N, we have $F_f = \mu_k F_N = (0.4)(200 \text{ N}) = 80$ N. However, the direction of the vector $\mathbf{F_f}$ is opposite to the direction of **d**, so the angle between $\mathbf{F_f}$ and **d** is $\theta = 180°$. Because $\cos 180° = -1$, the work done by the friction force is $(80 \text{ N})(6 \text{ m})(-1) = -480$ J.
e) To find the total work done on the crate, we just add up the work done by each of the forces that acts on the crate. In this case, then, we'd have

$$W_{total} = W_{\text{by F}} + W_{\text{by } F_N} + W_{\text{by } F_{grav}} + W_{\text{by } F_f} = (600 \text{ J}) + (0 \text{ J}) + (0 \text{ J}) + (-480 \text{ J}) = 120 \text{ J}$$

Here are a couple of things to notice about the example above:

1) Although work depends on two vectors for its definition (namely, **F** and **d**), work itself is *not* a vector. *Work is a scalar*. W may be positive, negative, or zero, but work has no direction.
2) In this example, there were four forces acting on the crate: the pushing force **F**, gravity, the normal force, and friction. Each force does its own amount of work, which is why each part had to specify for which force we wanted the work. Only in the last part, where the total work is desired, can we omit the specific force we're looking at (because we're considering them all).

Example 38-2: In the situation described in Example 38-1, what is the net force on the crate? How much work is done by $\mathbf{F}_{net}$?

Solution: The normal force cancels out the gravitational force, so the net force on the crate is just $\mathbf{F} + \mathbf{F}_f =$ (100 N) + (−80 N) = +20 N, where the + indicates that $\mathbf{F}_{net}$ points to the right. Now, since $\mathbf{F}_{net}$ is parallel to $\mathbf{d}$, the work done by $\mathbf{F}_{net}$ is just the product, $F_{net}d = (20\ N)(6\ m) = 120\ J$. Notice that this is the same as the total amount of work done on the crate, as we figured out in part (e) of Example 38-1. This wasn't a coincidence. The total work done (found by adding up the values of the work done by each force separately) is always equal to the work done by the net force.

Remember that work is a scalar and it can be positive, zero, or negative. Now here's how to know *when* W will be positive, zero, or negative. Because $W = Fd \cos \theta$, and F and d are magnitudes (which means they're positive), the sign of W depends entirely on the sign of $\cos \theta$.

The diagrams below show the three cases.

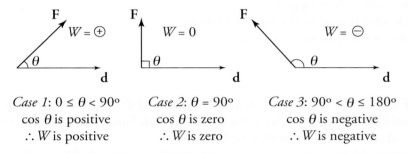

Case 1: $0 \leq \theta < 90°$
cos θ is positive
∴ W is positive

Case 2: $\theta = 90°$
cos θ is zero
∴ W is zero

Case 3: $90° < \theta \leq 180°$
cos θ is negative
∴ W is negative

In Case 1, the angle between $\mathbf{F}$ and $\mathbf{d}$ is less than 90° (an acute angle); since the cosine of such an angle is positive, the work done by this force will be positive.

In Case 2, the angle between $\mathbf{F}$ and $\mathbf{d}$ is 90°; since the cosine of 90° is zero, the work done by this force will be zero.

In Case 3, the angle between $\mathbf{F}$ and $\mathbf{d}$ is greater than 90° (an obtuse angle); since the cosine of such an angle is negative, the work done by this force will be negative.

Example 38-1 illustrated all three cases. The force that pushed the crate across the floor did positive work, gravity and the normal force did zero work, and sliding friction did negative work.

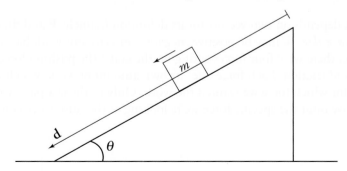

Example 38-3: In the situation pictured on the previous page, assume the mass of the block, *m*, is 20 kg and the coefficient of kinetic friction between the block and the ramp is 0.4. If *d* = 10 m and θ = 30°,

    a)   How much work is done by the normal force?
    b)   How much work is done by the force of friction?
    c)   How much work is done by gravity?
    d)   What is the total work done on the block?

Solution:

    a)   The normal force is perpendicular to the ramp, and to **d**. Since the angle between $\mathbf{F}_N$ and **d** is θ = 90°, and cos 90° = 0, the work done by $\mathbf{F}_N$ is zero. Forces acting perpendicular to the direction of travel always do zero work.

    b)   First, we know that since the block is on a ramp, we'll have $F_N = mg \cos θ$, where θ is the incline angle of the ramp. The magnitude of $\mathbf{F}_f$, the force of kinetic friction, is $\mu_k F_N$, so we get $F_f = (0.4)(20 \text{ kg})(10 \text{ N/kg}) \cos 30°$, which is approximately $(0.4)(200 \text{ N})(0.85) = 68$ N. Now, since the vectors $\mathbf{F}_f$ and **d** point in opposite directions (because **d** points down the ramp and $\mathbf{F}_f$ points up the ramp), the work done by $\mathbf{F}_f$ will be $-F_f d = -(68 \text{ N})(10 \text{ m}) = -680$ J.

    c)   There are two ways we can answer this part. One way is to remember that the force due to gravity acting parallel to the ramp is $mg \sin θ$, where θ is the incline angle. Since this component of the gravitational force is parallel to **d**, we can simply multiply $mg \sin θ$ by *d* to find the work done by gravity: $W = (mg \sin θ)(d) = (20 \text{ kg})(10 \text{ N/kg})(\sin 30°)(10 \text{ m}) = 1000$ J. Here's another way: the force $\mathbf{F}_{grav} = m\mathbf{g}$ points straight down, and the angle between $\mathbf{F}_{grav}$ and **d** is β, where β is the angle shown below. It's the complement of the incline angle θ; that is, β = 90° − θ.

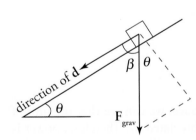

Since θ = 30°, we have β = 60°. Therefore, the work done by $\mathbf{F}_{grav}$ is $F_{grav} d \cos β = mgd \cos β = (20 \text{ kg})(10 \text{ N/kg})(10 \text{ m})(\cos 60°) = 1000$ J. You need to be very careful here; the formula for work reads, "$W = Fd \cos θ$," but the θ in this formula is *not* the same as the θ labeled in the figure. The angle in the formula for *W* is the angle between **F** and **d**, and this is not the same as the incline angle.

    d)   To find the total work done on the block, we just add up the work done by each of the forces that acts on the block. In this case, then, we'd have

$$W_{total} = W_{by\ F_N} + W_{by\ F_f} + W_{by\ F_{grav}} = (0 \text{ J}) + (-680 \text{ J}) + (1000 \text{ J}) = 320 \text{ J}$$

The formula $W = Fd \cos\theta$ can only be used if the force is constant during the motion. What if the force changes? In general, calculus is required, which is not needed for the MCAT. However, if a graph of force versus position is given (assuming $\theta = 0$), then the work done by that force is equal to the area *under the curve.*

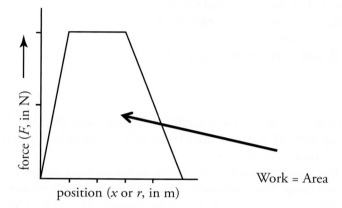

Work = Area

In Chapter 42, we will apply this to find the work required to compress or stretch a spring.

38.2 POWER

Power measures how fast work gets done. For example, if a force does 100 J of work in 20 seconds, then work is being done at a *rate* of

$$\frac{100 \text{ J}}{20 \text{ s}} = 5\frac{\text{J}}{\text{s}}$$

This is the power.

We use the letter P to denote power, and from the sample calculation above, we can see that the unit of power is the joule-per-second. This unit has its own name: the **watt**, abbreviated W. Therefore, power is measured in watts: $[P] = \text{J/s} = \text{W}$. (Don't confuse the abbreviation for the watt, W, with the usual variable used for work, W.)

The sample calculation above also shows us how we should define P in general:

Power

$$P = \frac{\text{work}}{\text{time}} = \frac{W}{t}$$

What if 100 J of work is done over a time interval of just 2 seconds? Then the power would be 50 W; it's easy to see that the faster work gets done, the greater the power.

A handy formula that you can also use to calculate P uses the fact that $v = d/t$:

$$P = \frac{W}{t} = \frac{Fd}{t} = F\frac{d}{t} = Fv \rightarrow P = Fv$$

(We're assuming here that $\mathbf{F}$ is parallel to $\mathbf{d}$, so that $W = Fd$, and that the object's speed, v, is constant.) To see how this formula would be used, let's answer this question: How much power must be provided to a toy rocket of mass 50 kg to keep it moving upward at a constant speed of 40 m/s? Ignoring air resistance, the engine thrust must provide an upward force that's equal to the weight of the rocket: $F = mg = (50 \text{ kg})$ $(10 \text{ N/kg}) = 500 \text{ N}$. Therefore, $P = Fv = (500 \text{ N})(40 \text{ m/s}) = 20{,}000 \text{ W} = 20 \text{ kW}$.

Example 38-4: A force of magnitude 40 N pushes on an object of mass 8 kg through a displacement of 5 m for 10 seconds. What's the power provided by this force?

Solution: Power is equal to work divided by time, so

$$P = \frac{W}{t} = \frac{Fd}{t} = \frac{(40 \text{ N})(5 \text{ m})}{10 \text{ s}} = 20 \text{ W}$$

Example 38-5: You're lifting bricks, each with a mass of 2 kg, from the floor up to a shelf that is 1.5 m high.

a) How much work do you perform lifting each brick?
b) If you can place 20 bricks on the shelf every minute, what is your power output?
c) If you continue this effort for an hour, how many Calories of work will you do (1 Cal = 4184 J)?

Solution:

a) The force you must provide to lift a brick is equal to the weight of the brick, which is $mg = (2 \text{ kg})(10 \text{ N/kg}) = 20 \text{ N}$. Since this force must act over a distance of 1.5 m to lift it up to the shelf, the work required is $W = Fd = (20 \text{ N})(1.5 \text{ m}) = 30 \text{ J}$.

b) If you can place 20 bricks on the shelf every 60 seconds, then on average you're lifting one brick every 3 seconds. If the work performed in 3 seconds is 30 J—as we found in part (a)—then your power output is

$$P = \frac{W}{t} = \frac{30 \text{ J}}{3 \text{ s}} = 10 \text{ W}$$

c) In an hour a power of 10 W amounts to $W = Pt = 10 \text{ J/s} \times 3600 \text{ s/hr} = 36{,}000 \text{ J}$. Unfortunately, that's only $36{,}000 \text{ J} \times 1/4184 \text{ Cal/J} \approx 9 \text{ Cal}$. However, our bodies are far from perfectly efficient, so we have to burn many more Calories than that to achieve that much work output. Moreover, there's a lot more to making a human body move than ideal work done against gravity in a frictionless process. After all, if you run for an hour on a horizontal treadmill, you have accomplished zero physical work, but obviously you will burn a lot of Calories!

Example 38-6: One month, your electric bill states that you used 500 kWh of electricity, at a cost of 8¢ per kWh. What is a kWh, and how much is your electric bill that month?

Solution: A kilowatt (kW) is a thousand watts; it's a unit of power. An hour (h) is a time interval. Therefore, a kilowatt-hour, kWh, obtained by multiplying power times time, Pt, has units of work. (1 kWh = (1000 W)(3600 s) = 3.6×10^6 J = 3.6 MJ.) The electric company performed 500 kWh of work pushing and pulling the electrons within the wires in your home to make electrical devices function, at a cost to you of (500 kWh)(8¢/kWh) = $40.

38.3 KINETIC ENERGY

An intuitive way to describe **energy** is that it's the ability to do work. Objects that move have this ability, since they can crash into something and thus exert a force over a distance. Therefore, objects that move have energy; specifically, we say they have **kinetic energy**, the energy due to motion.

To figure out how much kinetic energy a moving object has, imagine that an object of mass m is initially at rest (and thus has no kinetic energy). To get it moving, we have to exert a force **F** on it, over some distance d. (Let's assume, to keep things simple, that **F** points in the same direction as **d**.) How fast will the object be moving as a result? The acceleration is a constant $a = F/m$, so, using Big Five #5, we get

$$v^2 = v_0^2 + 2ad \;\rightarrow\; v^2 = 2ad \;\rightarrow\; v^2 = 2\frac{F}{m}d$$

Therefore, the final speed, v, will be $\sqrt{2Fd/m}$.

Now let's do a little algebra and rewrite the last equation above like this:

$$Fd = \frac{1}{2}mv^2$$

We recognize the product Fd as the work done by the force. So, we did work on the object to get it moving, and now because it's moving, it has kinetic energy. How much kinetic energy? This last equation tells us that we should consider the amount of kinetic energy to be $\frac{1}{2}mv^2$.

Kinetic Energy

$$KE = \frac{1}{2}mv^2$$

In words, this definition says that the kinetic energy of an object whose mass is m and whose speed is v is equal to one-half m times the square of the speed. Since $\frac{1}{2}mv^2$ is equal to the work Fd, we see right away that the unit of KE should also be the joule. In addition, like work, kinetic energy is a scalar.

Example 38-7: An object of mass 10 kg moves with a velocity of 4 m/s to the north. What is its kinetic energy? What would happen to the kinetic energy if the speed of the object doubled?

Solution: Kinetic energy is a scalar that cares only about the speed of an object; the direction of the object's velocity is irrelevant. So we find that

$$KE = \frac{1}{2}mv^2 = \frac{1}{2}(10 \text{ kg})(4 \text{ m/s})^2 = 80 \text{ J}$$

Because KE is proportional to v^2, if v were to increase by a factor of 2, then KE would increase by a factor of $2^2 = 4$.

The Work-Energy Theorem

The use of Big Five #5 on the previous page above (to motivate the definition $KE = \frac{1}{2}mv^2$) assumed that the initial speed of the object was zero. But what if the initial speed wasn't zero? Then we'd have

$$v^2 - v_0^2 = 2\frac{F}{m}d$$

$$v^2 = v_0^2 + 2ad \rightarrow v^2 - v_0^2 = 2ad \rightarrow \frac{1}{2}m(v^2 - v_0^2) = Fd$$

$$Fd = \frac{1}{2}mv^2 - \frac{1}{2}mv_0^2$$

$$W = KE_{\text{final}} - KE_{\text{initial}}$$

In other words, the total work done on the object is equal to the change in its kinetic energy. This fact is important enough that it's given a name:

Work-Energy Theorem

$$W_{\text{total}} = \Delta KE$$

This formula gives you another way to calculate work. You don't even need to know the force or the displacement! If you know the change in an object's kinetic energy, then you automatically know the total amount of work that was done on it.

Look back at the set of three diagrams showing when the work done by a force is positive, zero, or negative. In Case 1, the force is pulling in roughly the same direction as the object's displacement (more formally, the force **F** has a component that's in the same direction as **d**). We can think of such a force as "helping" the object move, and therefore causing its speed to increase. Is this consistent with the Work-Energy Theorem? Yes. This was the case of positive work being done, and according to the Work-Energy Theorem, positive work would automatically imply a positive change in kinetic energy. If the kinetic energy increases, then the speed increases.

In Case 3, the force is pulling in roughly the opposite direction from the object's displacement (more formally, the force **F** has a component that's in the opposite direction from **d**). We can think of such a force as "hindering" the object's motion, and therefore causing its speed to decrease. This is also consistent with the Work-Energy Theorem because Case 3 was the case of negative work being done, and according to the Work-Energy Theorem, negative work automatically implies a negative change in kinetic energy. If the kinetic energy decreases, then the speed decreases.

Example 38-8: An object of mass 10 kg is moving at a speed of 9 m/s. How much work must be done on this object in order to stop it?

Solution: We're asked to find W without being given **F** and **d**, so we use the Work-Energy Theorem. If we want to stop the object, we want to bring its final kinetic energy to zero. Therefore,

$$W = \Delta KE$$
$$= \tfrac{1}{2}mv^2 - \tfrac{1}{2}mv_0^2$$
$$= 0 - \tfrac{1}{2}mv_0^2$$
$$= -\tfrac{1}{2}(10 \text{ kg})(9 \text{ m/s})^2$$
$$\therefore W = -405 \text{ J}$$

The work that must be done on the object has to be negative, because only negative work causes a decrease in speed.

Example 38-9: An object of mass 3 kg is undergoing uniform circular motion. The object's speed is 4 m/s, and the radius of the path is 0.5 m.

a) What's the magnitude of the net force on the object?
b) How much work is done by the net force during each revolution of the object?

Solution:

a) The net force on an object undergoing uniform circular motion (UCM) is the centripetal force:

$$F_c = m\frac{v^2}{r} = (3 \text{ kg})\frac{(4 \text{ m/s})^2}{0.5 \text{ m}} = 96 \text{ N}$$

b) We can answer this part in two ways. The centripetal force points toward the center of the circular path, so it's always perpendicular to the object's velocity:

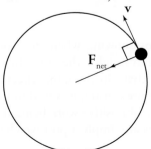

The work done by a force that's perpendicular to an object's motion is *zero* (remember: $\mathbf{F} \perp \mathbf{d}$ means $W = 0$.)

Another way is to use the Work-Energy Theorem. Since the object's speed is constant, its kinetic energy is constant too. No change in kinetic energy means no work is being done.

Example 38-10: A box of mass 4 kg is initially at rest on a frictionless horizontal surface. A horizontal force $\mathbf{F}$ of magnitude 32 N is exerted on the object and then removed. If the speed of the object is then 2 m/s, over what distance did $\mathbf{F}$ act?

Solution: By the Work-Energy Theorem, the work done by $\mathbf{F}$ was

$$W = \Delta KE = KE_f - KE_i = KE_f = \tfrac{1}{2}mv^2 = \tfrac{1}{2}(4 \text{ kg})(2 \text{ m/s})^2 = 8 \text{ J}$$

The question now is, "Given that $\mathbf{F}$ is parallel to $\mathbf{d}$ (so $W = Fd$), what's d?"

$$W = Fd \rightarrow d = \frac{W}{F} = \frac{8 \text{ J}}{32 \text{ N}} = 0.25 \text{ m}$$

Example 38-11: Consider the block described in Example 38-3. If the initial speed of the block was zero, what is the block's speed when it reaches the bottom of the ramp?

Solution: We figured out in part (d) of that example that the total work done on the block was 320 J. By the Work-Energy Theorem, we find that

$$W = \Delta KE = KE_f - KE_i = KE_f = \tfrac{1}{2}mv^2 \rightarrow v = \sqrt{\frac{2 \, W_{total}}{m}} = \sqrt{\frac{2(320 \text{ J})}{20 \text{ kg}}} = \sqrt{32 \text{ m}^2/\text{s}^2} \approx 5.6 \text{ m/s}$$

Example 38-12: Consider the crate described in Example 38-1.

a) If the initial speed of the crate was zero, what was the speed once the force $\mathbf{F}$ was removed after acting through the given displacement $\mathbf{d}$?
b) How far would the crate slide before coming to rest?

Solution:

a) We figured out in part (e) of that example that the total work done on the crate was 120 J. The Work-Energy Theorem then tells us that

$$W = \Delta KE = KE_f - KE_i = KE_f = \tfrac{1}{2}mv^2 \rightarrow v = \sqrt{\frac{2 \, W_{total}}{m}} = \sqrt{\frac{2(120 \text{ J})}{20 \text{ kg}}} = \sqrt{12 \text{ m}^2/\text{s}^2} \approx 3.5 \text{ m/s}$$

b)   Once the force **F** is removed, the only force acting on the crate that doesn't do zero work is friction. The work done by friction will be $-F_f d'$, where d' is the distance the crate will slide before coming to rest. By the Work-Energy Theorem, we have

$$W = \Delta KE = KE_f - KE_i = 0 - KE_i$$
$$-KE_i = -F_f d$$
$$F_f d = KE_i$$
$$d = \frac{KE_i}{F_f}$$

Since the crate had 120 J of kinetic energy right when the force **F** was removed, using the equation $F_f = \mu_k F_N = \mu_k mg$ gives us

$$d' = \frac{KE_i}{F_f} = \frac{KE_i}{\mu_k mg} = \frac{120\,\text{J}}{(0.4)(20\,\text{kg})(10\,\frac{\text{N}}{\text{kg}})} = 1.5\,\text{m}$$

38.4   POTENTIAL ENERGY

In the preceding section, we defined kinetic energy as the energy an object has due to its motion. **Potential energy** is the energy an object has by virtue of its *position*. There are different "kinds" of potential energy because there are different kinds of forces. For example, in our study of MCAT physics, we'll look at three types of potential energy: gravitational, electrical, and elastic. In this chapter, we'll study the first of these: *gravitational* potential energy.

Imagine a brick lying on the ground. Now, pick it up and place it on a shelf. You've just changed the position of the brick, and, since potential energy is the energy an object has by virtue of its position, you might expect that you've changed the brick's potential energy as well. You did. The brick's gravitational potential energy has been changed, because its position in a gravitational field has changed.

Now, let's be more specific. By *how much* did the brick's gravitational potential energy change? To find the answer, we need to look at the work done by the gravitational force (this is gravitational potential energy, after all). While the brick was being lifted, gravity did work on the brick. Let m be the mass of the brick and h be the height from the ground up to the shelf. The gravitational force on the brick is $\mathbf{F}_{grav} = m\mathbf{g}$, pointing downward; the displacement of the brick is h, upward.

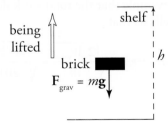

Because the force $\mathbf{F}_{grav}$ and the displacement $\mathbf{h}$ point in opposite directions, we know that the work done by $\mathbf{F}_{grav}$ will be the negative of F_{grav} times h: $W_{\text{by }\mathbf{F}_{grav}} = -F_{grav}h = -mgh$. The change in gravitational potential energy is defined to be the opposite of the work done by the gravitational force:

38.4

$$\Delta PE_{grav} = -W_{\text{by }F_{grav}}$$

In this case, then, we have $\Delta PE_{grav} = -(-mgh) = mgh$. If the brick had *fallen* from the shelf to the floor, so that its height *decreased* by h, then we would have had $W_{\text{by }F_{grav}} = F_{grav}h = mgh$ and $\Delta PE_{grav} = -mgh$.

The formulas on the previous page give the *change* in the gravitational potential energy of an object of mass m. If we designate the ground as our "$PE_{grav} = 0$" level, then we can say that the gravitational potential energy of an object at height h is equal to mgh.

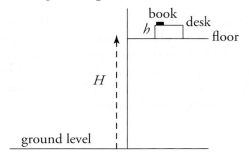

Potential energy is relative. Consider a book sitting on the desk in a second-floor office. Relative to the floor, the height of the book might be, say, half a meter. So, if the book has a mass of 1 kg, its gravitational potential energy is $mgh = (1\text{ kg})(10\text{ N/kg})(0.5\text{ m}) = 5\text{ J}$. But what if we were to measure the height of the book above the *ground*? Relative to the ground, the floor of the office might be at height $H = 5$ m, so the height of the book above the ground would be $H + h = 5.5$ m, and the book's gravitational potential energy is $mg(H + h) = (1\text{ kg})(10\text{ N/kg})(5.5\text{ m}) = 55\text{ J}$. Whenever we talk about "the" potential energy of an object, we must specify where we're choosing our "$PE = 0$" level.

The fact that potential energy is relative typically doesn't matter because only *changes* in potential energy are important and physically meaningful. Let's go back to our book on the office desk example. If the book falls off the desk to the floor, what is the change in its potential energy? To the person who calls the floor of the office their "$PE = 0$" level, the change in the book's potential energy will be

$$\Delta PE_{grav} = PE_{fi} - PE = 0 - mgh = -mgh = -(1\text{ kg})(10\tfrac{\text{N}}{\text{kg}})(0.5\text{ m}) = -5\text{ J}$$

Now, to the person who calls the ground their "$PE = 0$" level, the change in the book's potential energy will be the same:

$$\Delta PE_{grav} = PE_{fi} - PE = mgH - mg(H + h) = -mgh = -(1\text{ kg})(10\tfrac{\text{N}}{\text{kg}})(0.5\text{ m}) = -5\text{ J}$$

Both people will always agree on the *change* in an object's potential energy, even if they disagree about what the potential energy *is* at a certain height (because they choose different "*PE* = 0" levels). For this reason, it can be useful to memorize the gravitational potential energy equation as

$$\Delta PE_{grav} = mg\Delta h$$

Example 38-13: A brick that weighs 25 N is lifted from the ground to a shelf that's 2 m high. What is its change in gravitational potential energy?

Solution: Because mg = 25 N, we have $\Delta PE_{grav} = mg\Delta h = (25\ N)(2\ m) = 50\ J$. Notice that since the brick was lifted *up*, its change in gravitational potential energy is *positive*.

Example 38-14: A 1 N apple in a tree is at a height 4 m above the ground. The apple falls off its branch and lands on a branch that's only 1 m above the ground. What is the change in the apple's potential energy?

Solution: Because the apple *falls* a distance of Δh = 4 − 1 = 3 m, the change in its gravitational potential energy is $-mg\Delta h = -(1\ N)(3\ m) = -3\ J$. We could also have answered the question like this: First, we choose, say, the ground to be our "*PE* = 0" level. Then the initial potential energy of the apple is $PE_i = mgh_i = (1\ N)(4\ m) = 4\ J$, and the final potential energy of the apple is $PE_f = mgh_f = (1\ N)(1\ m) = 1\ J$. The change in the potential energy is, therefore, $\Delta PE = PE_f - PE_i = (1\ J) - (4\ J) = -3\ J$. Note that because the apple *falls*, the change in its gravitational potential energy must be *negative*.

Gravity is a Conservative Force

Suppose we want to move a brick from the floor up to a shelf. One way we could do it would be to simply lift the brick straight up. Another way would be to set up a ramp and then push the brick up the ramp to the shelf. Let's figure out how much work gravity does in each of these cases. We'll assume that the brick has a mass of 3 kg and that the shelf is 2 m high.

The first case is easy. The gravitational force on the brick is mg = (3 kg)(10 N/kg) = 30 N, directed straight downward. Since the displacement **h** of the brick is straight upward (that is, in the opposite direction from F_{grav}), we know that the work done by gravity is negative F_{grav} times h:

$$W_{by\ F_{grav}} = -F_{grav}h = -(30\ N)(2\ m) = -60\ J$$

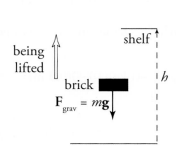

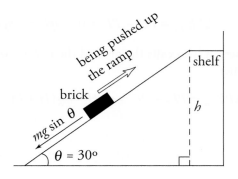

Now, let's look at the second case. Let's use a ramp whose incline angle θ is 30°. The gravitational force acting parallel to the ramp has magnitude $mg \sin \theta$, directed downward along the ramp. Because the displacement **d** is upward along the ramp (that is, in the opposite direction), we know the work done by gravity is negative, and equal to $-(mg \sin \theta)(d)$. Since the height of the shelf is $h = 2$ m, the length of the ramp (i.e., the hypotenuse of the right triangle) must be $d = h/(\sin \theta) = (2 \text{ m})/(\sin 30°) = 4$ m. Therefore, the work done by the gravitational force as the block is pushed up the ramp is

$$W_{\text{by } \mathbf{F}_{\text{grav}}} = -(mg \sin \theta)(d) = -(30 \text{ N})(\sin 30°)(4 \text{ m}) = -(15 \text{ J})(4 \text{ m}) = -60 \text{ J}$$

38.4

This is the same answer as we found before! Since the change in the gravitational potential energy is defined to be the opposite of the work done by the gravitational force, $\Delta PE_{\text{grav}} = -W_{\text{by } \mathbf{F}_{\text{grav}}}$, we can say that $\Delta PE_{\text{grav}} = -(-60 \text{ J}) = 60 \text{ J}$ in either case.

In the first case (lifting the brick straight upward), we exert a greater force over a smaller distance, while in the second case (moving the brick up a ramp), we exert a smaller force over a greater distance. However, the work done is the same in both cases.

These examples illustrate the following:

> *The work done by gravity*
>
> *depends only on the initial and final heights of the object,*
>
> *not on the path the object follows.*

Another way of saying this is to state that gravity is a **conservative** force. (In fact, it is the conservative nature of the gravitational force that allows us to define gravitational potential energy.)

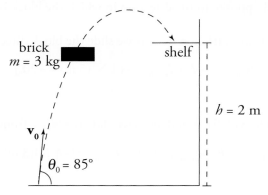

Example 38-15: In the situation pictured above, a brick is projected upward with an initial velocity $\mathbf{v}_0$ that makes an angle of 85° with the horizontal. The brick follows the path indicated and lands on the shelf. How much work did the gravitational force do on the brick?

Solution: The work done by gravity depends only on the initial and final positions of the object, not on the particular path the object takes. Since the initial height was $h_i = 0$ and the final height was $h_f = 2$ m, the change in the brick's gravitational potential energy is $\Delta PE_{\text{grav}} = mg\Delta h = (3 \text{ kg})(10 \text{ N/kg})(2 \text{ m}) = 60 \text{ J}$.

Therefore, the work done by the gravitational force is

$$W_{\text{by } \mathbf{F}_{\text{grav}}} = -\Delta PE_{\text{grav}} = -60 \text{ J}$$

just as we found before.

Friction Is NOT a Conservative Force

Gravity is a conservative force because the work done by gravity depends only on the initial and final positions of the object, not on the path taken. We'll now show that friction is *not* a conservative force; the work done by kinetic friction *does* depend on the path taken.

Consider a flat tabletop and mark two points on it, A and B. We're going to slide a block from Point A to Point B along two different paths; the work done will be different for the two paths, which will show that friction is not a conservative force. The figure below shows the two points, A and B, separated by a distance of 5 m. Another way to get from A to B is to move from A to C and then from C to B; I've chosen a point C that's 3 m from A and 4 m from B.

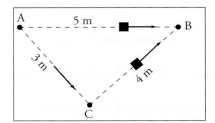

Assume the block has a mass of 1 kg; then its weight is $w = mg = (1 \text{ kg})(10 \text{ N/kg}) = 10 \text{ N}$, so the normal force on the block has magnitude 10 N also. If the coefficient of kinetic friction between the block and tabletop is 0.4, then, as the block slides, the magnitude of the force of kinetic friction is $F_f = \mu_k F_N = (0.4)(10 \text{ N}) = 4 \text{ N}$, always directed opposite to the direction in which the block is sliding.

Let's first figure out how much work friction does as we slide the block directly from A to B:

$$W_{\substack{\text{by } F_f \\ A \to B}} = -F_f \cdot d_{A \to B} = -(4 \text{ N})(5 \text{ m}) = -20 \text{ J}$$

Now let's figure out how much work friction does as we slide the block from A to B by way of C:

$$W_{\substack{\text{by } F_f \\ A \to C \to B}} = W_{\substack{\text{by } F_f \\ A \to C}} + W_{\substack{\text{by } F_f \\ C \to B}} = (-F_f \cdot d_{A \to C}) + (-F_f \cdot d_{C \to B}) = (-4 \text{ N})(3 \text{ m}) + (-4 \text{ N})(4 \text{ m}) = -28 \text{ J}$$

Even though we started at A and ended at B in both cases, we got a different amount of work done by friction for two different paths from A to B. Therefore, friction is *not* a conservative force. This means that there's no such thing as "frictional potential energy," because potential energy can be defined only for conservative forces.

38.5   TOTAL MECHANICAL ENERGY

Now that we've defined kinetic energy and potential energy, we can define an object's **total mechanical energy**, E. It's just the sum of the object's kinetic energy and potential energy:

Total Mechanical Energy

$$E = KE + PE$$

For example, consider an object of mass m sitting on a shelf that's at height h above the floor. Then, relative to the floor (where we'll set PE_{grav} equal to 0), the object's total mechanical energy is

$$E = KE + PE = 0 + mgh = mgh$$

Now, what if this same object falls off the shelf? What is its total mechanical energy when its height is, say, $h/2$? If v is the object's speed at this point, then the object's total mechanical energy is

$$E = KE + PE = \frac{1}{2}mv^2 + mg\frac{h}{2}$$

Using Big 5 #5, we can solve for the v in this equation:

$$v^2 = v_0^2 + 2ad = 0 + \left(2g\frac{h}{2}\right) = gh$$

Therefore,

$$E = \frac{1}{2}m(gh) + mg\frac{h}{2} = mgh$$

Notice that the object's total mechanical energy is the same at both points. This illustrates a very important concept: the **Conservation of Total Mechanical Energy**. If the only forces acting on an object during its motion are conservative (that means, for example, *no friction*), then the object's total mechanical energy will remain the same throughout the motion. Pick any two positions (or times) during the object's motion; for example, we could pick the initial position (initial time) and the final position (final time). Then

---

$$E_i = E_f$$

Writing E as $KE + PE$, we have

> **Conservation of Total Mechanical Energy
> (no outside forces)**
>
> $$KE_i + PE_i = KE_f + PE_f$$
>
> or
>
> $$\Delta KE + \Delta PE = 0$$

Example 38-16: An object of mass m is projected straight upward with an initial speed of v_0 at time $t = 0$. Use Conservation of Total Mechanical Energy to find its maximum height.

Solution: Noting that $v = 0$ at the maximum height h yields

$$\Delta KE = \tfrac{1}{2}\, mv_0^2$$

and $\Delta PE = mgh$

Therefore, by the second form of the Conservation of Total Mechanical Energy, we have

$$\Delta KE + \Delta PE = 0$$

$$\tfrac{1}{2}mv_0^2 = mgh$$

$$\therefore h = \frac{v_0^2}{2g}$$

This is the same answer we would find using the Big Five equations.

Another way to think about this problem is in terms of an energy *transformation*. At the moment the object was shot upward, it had only KE; at the top of its path, however, it has only PE. In other words, kinetic energy was transformed into gravitational potential energy:

$$KE \rightarrow PE \;\rightarrow\; \frac{1}{2}mv_0^2 = mgh \;\;\rightarrow\;\; \therefore h = \frac{v_0^2}{2g}$$

It can be very helpful to think of Conservation of Total Mechanical Energy in terms of energy transformations between KE and PE. (The MCAT likes to ask questions about such energy transformations.)

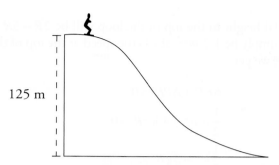

125 m

Example 38-17: A skier begins at rest at the top of a hill of height 125 m. If friction between her skis and the snow is negligible, what will be her speed at the bottom of the hill?

Solution: Let the bottom of the hill be $h = 0$, and call the top of the hill the skier's initial position and the bottom of the hill her final position. Then we have

$$KE_i + PE_i = KE_f + PE_f$$

$$0 + mgh = \tfrac{1}{2}mv^2 + 0$$

$$v = \sqrt{2gh}$$

$$= \sqrt{2(10 \text{ m/s}^2)(125 \text{ m})}$$

$$\therefore v = 50 \text{ m/s}$$

We could also think about this problem in terms of an energy transformation. At the top of the hill, the skier had only *PE*; at the bottom of the hill, she has only *KE*. In other words, gravitational potential energy was transformed into kinetic energy:

$$PE \rightarrow KE \rightarrow \quad mgh = \frac{1}{2}mv_0^2 \quad \rightarrow \quad \therefore v = \sqrt{2gh}$$

$h = 5R$

$v = ?$

R

Example 38-18: A roller-coaster car drops from rest down the track and enters a loop. If the radius of the loop is R, and the initial height of the car is $5R$ above the bottom of the loop, how fast is the car going at the top of the loop? Assume that $R = 15$ m and ignore friction.

Solution: Δh from the initial height to the top of the loop will be $2R - 5R = -3R$. Thus, $\Delta PE = -3mgR$. ΔKE starting from rest will simply be $1/2\ mv^2$, if v is the speed at the top of the loop. Using Conservation of Total Mechanical Energy, we get

$$\Delta KE + \Delta PE = 0$$

$$\frac{1}{2}mv^2 - 3mgR = 0$$

$$\frac{1}{2}v^2 = 3gR$$

$$v = \sqrt{6gR} = \sqrt{6\left(10\ \tfrac{m}{s^2}\right)\left(15\ m\right)}$$

$$\therefore v = 30\ \frac{m}{s}$$

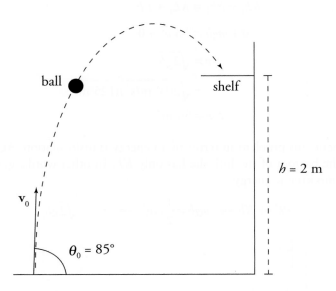

Example 38-19: In the situation pictured above, a ball is projected upward from the floor with an initial velocity $\mathbf{v}_0$ of magnitude 12 m/s that makes an angle of 85° with the horizontal. The ball follows the path indicated and lands on the shelf. How fast is the ball traveling as it hits the shelf? (Ignore air resistance.)

Solution: Let's call the floor our $h = 0$ level. At the object's initial position, we have $h_i = 0$ (so $PE_i = 0$). At the shelf (the final position), we have $h_f = 2$ m. The question is to find the speed of the ball, v, at this point. Using Conservation of Total Mechanical Energy, we get

$$KE_i + PE_i = KE_f + PE_f$$

$$\frac{1}{2}mv_0^2 + 0 = \frac{1}{2}mv^2 + mgh_f$$

$$\frac{1}{2}v_0^2 = \frac{1}{2}v^2 + gh_f$$

$$v = \sqrt{v_0^2 - 2gh_f}$$

$$= \sqrt{(12 \text{ m/s}^2)^2 - 2(10 \text{ m/s}^2)(2 \text{ m})}$$

$$\therefore v \approx 10 \frac{\text{m}}{\text{s}}$$

Notice that the direction of the initial velocity vector (given to be "at an angle of 85° with the horizontal") was irrelevant here. One of the most useful attributes of solving problems by Conservation of Total Mechanical Energy is that KE, PE, and E are all *scalars*. This makes it easier to solve questions because we don't have to worry about direction.

Using the Energy Method when There Is Friction

If friction acts during an object's motion, then total mechanical energy is no longer conserved. Consider this example: We give a block of mass 2 kg an initial speed of 6 m/s across a flat surface, where the coefficient of kinetic friction between the block and the surface is $\mu_k = 0.2$.

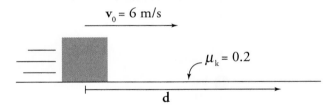

Kinetic friction will do work as the block slides. If d is the distance the block slides, then the work done by friction will be

$$W_{\text{by } F_f} = -F_f \cdot d = -\mu_k F_N d = -\mu_k mgd = -(0.4)(2 \text{ kg})(10 \tfrac{\text{N}}{\text{kg}})d = -(4 \text{ N})d$$

In particular, when $d = 9$ m, the work done by friction will be

$$W_{\text{by } F_f} = -(4 \text{ N})d = -(4 \text{ N})(9 \text{ m}) = -36 \text{ J}$$

Since the initial kinetic energy of the block was

$$KE_i = \frac{1}{2}mv_0^2 = \frac{1}{2}(2 \text{ kg})(6 \text{ m/s})^2 = 36 \text{ J}$$

then the Work-Energy Theorem tells us that the final kinetic energy of the block will be 0:

$$W = \Delta KE = KE_f - KE_i \rightarrow \quad KE_f = KE_i + W = \left(36\,\text{J}\right) + \left(-36\,\text{J}\right) = 0\,\text{J}$$

The block lost KE (and, therefore, E) as it moved because of friction. So, when friction acts, total mechanical energy is not a constant; in other words, it's not conserved.

Despite the fact that total mechanical energy is no longer conserved if friction acts, we can use a *modified* version of the Conservation of Total Mechanical Energy equation to handle questions with friction (or any force besides gravity). We can write this modified equation either in the form

$$E_i + W_{\text{by F}} = E_f$$

or as

> **Conservation of Total Mechanical Energy**
> **(with outside forces)**
> $$KE_i + PE_i + W_{\text{by F}} = KE_f + PE_f$$

Since $W_{\text{by } F_f}$ is negative, E_f will be less than E_i, just as we expect, since friction takes away mechanical energy.

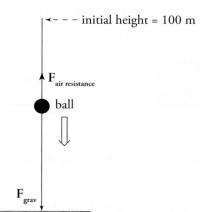

Example 38-20: A ball of mass 2 kg is dropped from a height of 100 m. As it falls, the ball feels an average force of air resistance of magnitude 4 N. What is the ball's speed as it strikes the ground?

Solution: Let's call the ground our $h = 0$ level. At the object's initial position, we have $h_i = 100$ m and $v_0 = 0$ (so $KE_i = 0$). As it hits the ground (the final position), we have $h_f = 0$ m (so $PE_f = 0$). The question is to find the speed of the ball, v, as it strikes the ground. Because the air resistance is given, and air resistance is friction exerted by the air on the moving object, we need to use the modified version of the energy equation, the one that includes the work done by friction.

Let's figure out the work done by the force of air resistance. Since the displacement of the ball is downward, the force of air resistance is upward; the opposite direction. This tells us that the work done by air resistance is negative, as we expect:

$$W_{\text{by } \mathbf{F}_f} = -F_f \cdot h = -(4\text{ N})(100\text{ m}) = -400\text{ J}$$

Therefore, using the modified equation for Conservation of Total Mechanical Energy, we find that

$$KE_i + PE_i + W_{\text{by } \mathbf{F}_f} = KE_f + PE_f$$

$$0 + mgh + (-400\text{ J}) = \frac{1}{2}mv^2 + 0$$

$$v = \sqrt{2gh - \frac{800\text{ J}}{m}}$$

$$= \sqrt{2(10\text{ m/s}^2)(100\text{ m}) - \frac{800\text{ J}}{2\text{ kg}}}$$

$$= \sqrt{1600\text{ m}^2/\text{s}^2}$$

Without air resistance, you can check that the ball's speed at impact would have been greater:

$$\sqrt{2000}\text{ m/s} \approx 45\text{ m/s}$$

38.6 SIMPLE MACHINES AND MECHANICAL ADVANTAGE

Simple machines are tools that allow us to accomplish a variety of tasks with less applied force. Some examples of common simple machines are inclined planes, pulleys, levers, screws, and wheel-and-axle systems. These machines generally have few or no moving parts. If the simple machine is used in the "ideal world" where there are only conservative forces (i.e., no loss of energy to friction, heat, etc.), the work done to complete the task using the machine is equal to the work that would be required to complete the task without the machine. The difference is that with less applied or effort force, a larger distance must be covered to satisfy the work requirements.

Let's consider the task of lifting a 3 kg brick up to a shelf that is 2 m above the ground.

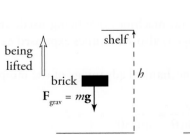
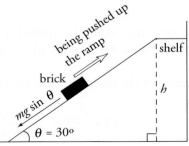

To move a mass straight upward, the applied force, $F_{app_{lift}}$, would need to be at least equal to the force of gravity acting on the mass. Thus, $F_{app_{lift}} \geq F_{grav} = mg = (3 \text{ kg})\left(10 \dfrac{\text{N}}{\text{kg}}\right) = 30 \text{ N}$. The minimum amount of work to lift the brick upward is

$$W_{lift} = F_{app_{lift}} \cdot d = mgh = 60 \text{ J}$$

Now, let's consider the inclined plane shown above. The plane allows us to push the brick up the ramp. If this is a frictionless ramp, the applied force on the ramp, $F_{app_{ramp}}$ would need to overcome the component of F_{grav} parallel to the plane. Thus,

$$F_{app_{ramp}} \geq mg \sin\theta = (3 \text{ kg})(10 \tfrac{\text{N}}{\text{kg}})(\sin 30°) = 15 \text{ N}$$

which will be less than $F_{app_{lift}} = mg$ (because the maximum value for $\sin\theta$ is 1). However, compared to lifting the box straight up through a distance h, the ramp requires you to push the brick over a longer distance, $d = \dfrac{h}{\sin\theta}$. Therefore, the work done to push the brick up the ramp is

$$W_{ramp} = F_{app_{ramp}} \cdot d = (mg \sin\theta) \cdot \left(\frac{h}{\sin\theta}\right) = mgh = 60 \text{ J}$$

The work required to move a brick to a height of h is the same, regardless of whether you lift it straight upward or push it up a ramp.

The fact that the inclined plane allows your effort force or applied force to be decreased in comparison to the straight lift is called **mechanical advantage**. Mechanical advantage can be quantified into a factor that describes precisely how much less force is required when using that particular simple machine. In other words, mechanical advantage tells us the factor by which the mechanism multiplies the input or effort force.

Mechanical Advantage

$$\text{mechanical advantage } (MA) = \frac{\text{resistance force}}{\text{effort force}} = \frac{F_{resistance}}{F_{effort}}$$

Resistance force is the force that would be applied if no machine were being used, and *effort force* is the force applied with the machine. Mechanical advantage is also sometimes expressed as F_{out} / F_{in}.

For the previous example of the inclined plane, the mechanical advantage of the ramp would be

$$MA = \frac{F_{resistance}}{F_{effort}} = \frac{mg}{mg \sin\theta} = \frac{1}{\sin 30°} = \frac{1}{\frac{1}{2}} = 2$$

Therefore, this specific inclined plane with an angle of $\theta = 30°$ has a mechanical advantage of 2, allowing it to "multiply" the input force $F_{app_{ramp}} = 15$ N by a factor of 2 to give the force that would have been required without the machine, $F_{app_{lift}} = 30$ N.

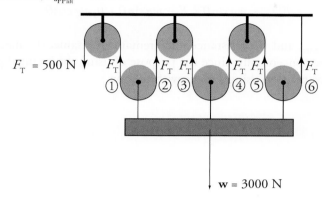

$F_T = 500$ N

F_T ① ② ③ ④ ⑤ ⑥

w = 3000 N

38.6

As another example, look back at Example 36-42 which shows a system consisting of 6 pulleys used to lift a plank. The plank weighs 3000 N, but we only have to exert a force of 500 N to lift it. The mechanical advantage is therefore equal to 3000 N/500 N = 6.

Efficiency

So far, we have described simple machines that are used in the ideal world. However, if the machine is used in the real world, we have to take into consideration the possibility of energy losses to the surroundings. In general, the actual mechanical advantage of a machine is less than its ideal mechanical advantage. The fact that the machine does not work as well in the real world leads us to the concept of **efficiency**. The efficiency of any machine measures the degree to which friction and other factors reduce the actual work output of the machine from its theoretical maximum. This can be calculated by examining the ratio of the useful energy output versus the supplied or input energy.

Efficiency

$$\text{Efficiency (\%)} = \frac{W_{output}}{\text{Energy}_{input}}$$

A machine that operates in the ideal world has an efficiency of 100% because it has no loss of energy to its surroundings. However, a machine with an efficiency of 50% has an output only one-half of its theoretical output. By calculating a machine's efficiency, we can determine what percentage of energy is being lost to heat, sound, light, etc.

How does an efficiency of less than 100% affect mechanical advantage? For the inclined plane example, the presence of friction would reduce the efficiency, since some of the work done to push the block up would be lost as heat. In terms of force, the minimum applied force (the effort force) would now have to be enough to balance the component of gravity down the inclined plane plus the force of kinetic friction.

$$F_{effort} = mg \sin\theta + F_f = mg \sin\theta + \mu_k mg \cos\theta$$

Since $MA = F_{resistance} / F_{effort}$, and the resistance force remains the same, the mechanical advantage will decrease. This makes sense conceptually, since the purpose of using the inclined plane is to reduce force. There will be less of an advantage to using a plane with friction.

38.6

Chapter 39
Thermodynamics

39.1 SYSTEMS, THERMAL PHYSICS, AND THERMODYNAMICS

As we've seen so far, work can be done on or by a physical system—a box on a ramp, a car's engine block hooked to several loops of rope attached to two pulleys, or a satellite launched into orbit are just a few examples—thereby increasing or decreasing the energy in that system. Broadly speaking, work is a *transfer of mechanical energy into or out of a system, from or to the environment.*

We ought to be careful here with our terms. In physics, as in chemistry and biology, you will hear a lot about *systems*. For our purposes, it is enough to define a system as the object or objects under examination and the ways they interact (which in physics typically means the forces among them). The *environment* is just the other objects and external forces outside the system. The environment may or may not be able to interact with the system. If the system is *closed*, then the environment cannot contribute matter to it; if it is *isolated*, the environment cannot contribute either matter or energy. If the system is *open*, then it is free to interact with the environment. This leads to a crucial point: systems obey conservation laws. Within the system, different forms of energy can *transform from one type to another but cannot spontaneously appear or cease to exist*. In other words, the only way the total energy in a system can change is if energy is *transferred* into or out of the system.

Consider a tennis ball in your hand. If you want to focus exclusively on the ball itself, you might call the ball "the system" and everything else "the environment." This is an open system; if you drop the ball, an external force in the environment (gravity) will do work on the ball, contributing to its increase in kinetic energy as it falls. Alternatively, you might want to look at the ball + the earth + gravity (the interaction between those two objects) as the system. In that case, when you drop the ball, one form of energy (gravitational potential energy) is transformed into another (kinetic energy).

But what about some other factors? For one thing, you could choose to throw the ball up in the air instead of just letting it idly drop to the ground. If we counted you as part of the environment, then we would say that the work you did on the ball in throwing it upward increased its kinetic energy: you transferred energy into the system. If we counted you as part of the system, we would have to explain the energy transformation in terms of the ATP turning to ADP and then AMP as your muscles contracted to allow you to throw the ball, and thus chemical potential energy was transformed into kinetic energy (for more on that, consult the biology section of this text). What about the air resistance the ball experiences as it falls through the air? As a frictional force, air resistance does what we have previously called "nonconservative" work on the ball, as it causes the ball to move more slowly (that is, to have less kinetic energy) than it would if there were no air. Is this a violation of what we have said so far about energy conservation or transferring to and from the environment?

It is not. The problem is that so far we have considered only a limited number of kinds of energy, and we have neglected an important mode of energy transfer. Consider the tennis ball a bit more closely. Even as it sits apparently still in your hand, on the molecular level there is a tremendous amount of random motion. This is another form of energy internal to the system, which we'll call *thermal energy* (or sometimes just *internal energy*, though as you know from chemistry, there are other forms of internal energy such as chemical or nuclear energies). **Temperature (T)** is the macroscopic measure of this thermal energy per molecule. As the tennis ball falls, the frictional effects of air resistance do negative work on the ball, slowing it down, but they also cause the temperature of the ball to increase, because all of those tiny collisions between the air molecules and the molecules in the ball increase the thermal energy of the ball's molecules (as well as that of the air molecules that interact with the ball directly). That is to say, the individual molecules of the surface of the ball are moving faster than before, but in random directions (in addition to all moving toward the ground while the ball is falling). If you were to catch and hold the now slightly warmer ball in your hand, over time it would cool back to the temperature of the surrounding air (or, more precisely, a temperature between that of the air and that of your hand). Its thermal energy would decrease, but it would be sitting perfectly still, so clearly it wasn't doing any work. It transferred energy to the environment by means of heat. **Heat (Q)** is the transfer of thermal energy between a system and its environment: $Q > 0$ when heat transfers *into* the system, $Q < 0$ when heat transfers *out* of the system. Please note this important distinction between *temperature* and *heat*, words that we use everyday in ways that can make them seem interchangeable. When we say *"it's hot* outside today," we're referring to the temperature, an indicator of the relatively high thermal energy per molecule of the local atmospheric system. When we then say "this weather *is making me hot* and sweaty," we're talking about heat, the transfer of the thermal energy from the atmosphere into our bodies. Note the difference in units as well: heat, as with energy, is measured in joules, whereas absolute temperature is measured in kelvins.

Another important difference between temperature and thermal energy contained within a system (and transferrable as heat) is that temperature is an *intensive* property, whereas thermal energy is an *extensive* one. That is to say, temperature (like density, for example) does not depend on the amount of a material present, but thermal energy (like mass) does. Imagine a block of stone at a temperature of 300 kelvins and containing 20,000 joules of thermal energy. If you split it in half, each half would still be 300 kelvins (not 150), but each would contain only 10,000 joules of thermal energy.

Thus, **thermodynamics** concerns how macroscopic systems transfer and transform energy. As such, it is perhaps the broadest subject you'll study in preparation for physics on the MCAT, taking into account not only everything we've looked at so far in this text, but also extending into all the other science topics on the exam.

39.2   THE ZEROTH LAW OF THERMODYNAMICS

Thermal physics depends upon the quantity *temperature* being well defined in such a way that, if we stick thermometers on two different objects and get the same reading, we know there is something fundamentally similar about those two objects. This is unlike, say, length: a 2 m long metal rod does not have anything fundamentally in common with a 2 m long wooden plank. The **Zeroth Law of Thermodynamics** provides this definition. It states that if one object is in thermal equilibrium with a second object, and that second object is in thermal equilibrium with a third object, then the first and third objects are in thermal equilibrium with each other. By *thermal equilibrium* we mean that, though the two bodies are in contact in such a way that heat is free to pass between them, no heat actually does so. Practically, what this means is that Objects 1 and 3 are the same temperature. Technically, this *defines* temperature as a fundamental property, or *state variable,* of a system. It tells us that if we measured the temperatures of two objects (like our metal rod and wooden plank) to be the same, we would know that when we put the two in contact with each other, no heat would be transferred between them (or, more technically, the same amount of heat would pass from each to the other).

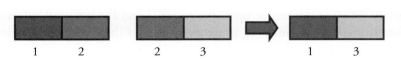

Objects 1 and 3 in thermal equilibrium, each at temperature T_0

The other *state variables* include pressure, volume, moles, and entropy. On the MCAT, as in your college coursework, discussion of these variables crosses over between physics and chemistry (and possibly other disciplines), and the connections among those discussions can be confusing. One unifying idea you should keep in mind in all applications is that these variables define a *state function* for a system, which means they are macroscopic properties that reflect the microscopic conditions of that system and predict the future behavior of the system. The specific relation between the microscopic average kinetic energy per atom of a monatomic ideal gas (wherein kinetic energy is the only form of energy) is given by the following equation, sometimes called the equipartition of energy equation for ideal gases (k_B is the Boltzmann constant and is equal to 1.38×10^{-23} J/K).

$$\frac{1}{2}mv^2_{avg} = \frac{3}{2}k_B T$$

Heat Transfer

In stating the Zeroth Law of Thermodynamics, we relied upon the idea that bodies can achieve thermal equilibrium by heat transfer, the movement of thermal energy from one point to another. There are three mechanisms by which this is achieved.

Conduction

An iron skillet is sitting on a hot stove, and you accidentally touch the handle. You notice right away that there's been a transfer of thermal energy to your hand. The process by which this happens is known as conduction. The highly agitated atoms in the handle of the hot skillet bump into the atoms of your hand, making them vibrate more rapidly, thus heating up your hand.

Example 39-1: The rate at which materials conduct heat varies widely. Metals conduct heat well, meaning that heat moves through them rapidly. Materials like fiberglass, which is often used to provide thermal insulation in buildings, conduct heat very poorly. The *conduction rate* is described by the equation

$$P_{cond} = \frac{\Delta Q}{\Delta t} = -kA\frac{\Delta T}{\Delta x} = kA\frac{T_i - T_f}{L}$$

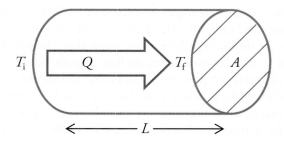

where k is a thermal conductivity constant dependent upon the material and the power P indicates the rate of thermal energy transfer. This energy is measured in joules as usual. (This is not an equation the

MCAT would expect you to have memorized.) Window glass typically has a thermal conductivity of $k = 1$ watt per meter per kelvin (recall that kelvins are a measure of absolute temperature with a scale equal to that of degrees Celsius). How many joules per second of heat are transferred out of a room at 25°C to an outside environment of at 0°C if there are two 2 × 1 meter single-paned windows in the room with a thickness of half a centimeter? Assume the walls are perfectly insulated.

Solution: Find the total area A by multiplying the dimensions of the windows and their total number: $A = 2 \times 2 \times 1 = 4$ m². Applying the given equation then yields

$$\frac{\Delta Q}{\Delta t} = kA\frac{T_i - T_f}{L} = (1)(4)\frac{25 - 0}{0.5 \times 10^{-2}} = 200 \times 10^2 = 2 \times 10^4 \text{ J/s}$$

This is quite a bit of power, which is why it is a good idea to use double-paned or otherwise insulated windows in climates where it gets cold outside!

Convection

As the air around a candle flame warms, it expands, becomes less dense than the surrounding cooler air, and thus rises due to buoyancy. (We'll study buoyancy in the next chapter.) As a result, heat is transferred away from the flame by the large-scale (from the atoms' point of view anyway) motion of a fluid (in this case, air). This is **convection**.

Example 39-2: During circulation, the relatively warm blood moves from the heart to the extremities, where it cools slightly before returning to the heart. What best describes this process?

  A) This is a free convection process, as warm blood rises to the head while relatively cold blood sinks to the feet.
  B) This is a free convection process, as the expansion of the warm blood in the heart pushes blood out to the extremities via the arteries, whereas cooler blood at the extremities condenses and sinks toward the heart via the veins.
  C) This is a forced convection process where the pumping action of the heart forces blood heated by the body's metabolic processes out to the extremities, which in turn forces the cooler blood back toward the heart (during which time it is heated).
  D) This is a forced convection process where the pumping action of the heart compresses and thereby heats the blood. Its motion to the extremities is a result of this pressurization.

Solution: The heart is a pump: you should know that blood's motion through the body is caused by the heart, not by some passive physical process. Choices A and B are eliminated for not making sense: don't ignore your biology knowledge when answering physics questions if it's pertinent! Along that line of thought, the heart is not a pressure cooker: the heat of our bodies is produced by metabolic processes, the conversion of chemical energy to other forms (such as kinetic energy and thermal energy due to friction in the contraction of muscles throughout the body, which is why you feel hotter when exercising vigorously). Choice D doesn't adequately explain this and is therefore eliminated. Choice C is correct: the movement of the warm fluid and displacement of the cooler fluid is convection, but it is *forced convection* due to the pumping action. The process by which a convection oven works is analogous: the forced movement of the fluid (air) in the oven due to a fan results in faster heat transfer than in a normal oven that relies on natural convection and conduction.

Radiation

Sunlight on your face warms your skin. Radiant energy from the Sun's fusion reactions is transferred across millions of kilometers of essentially empty space via electromagnetic waves. Absorption of the energy carried by these light waves defines heat transfer by **radiation**.

Thermal Expansion

Another response of materials to temperature difference is to change their physical dimensions, i.e., length and volume. Most materials expand as their temperature increases: this is why, for example, bridges have expansion slots, the metal grates you drive over every 10 meters or so. If the bridge got longer in response to an increase in temperature but had no room to expand, it would buckle and crack. The formula for linear thermal expansion is $\Delta L = \alpha L_0 \Delta T$, where ΔL is the change in length of the object, L_0 is its original length, and α is the coefficient of linear expansion of the material the object is made of. This is not typically an equation the MCAT expects you to have memorized.

39.3 THE FIRST LAW OF THERMODYNAMICS

Having defined two ways in which energy can transfer between the environment and a system (heat and work), as well as a way to measure the energy internal to the system (temperature), we are now ready to make a broader statement about conservation of energy than the ones we made in the preceding chapter. The First Law of Thermodynamics is just this statement: it says that *the total energy of the universe is constant*. Energy may be transformed from one form to another, but it cannot be created or destroyed.

The First Law of Thermodynamics can be expressed both tangibly and mathematically. To do this, consider the physical aspects of transferring energy into a system. Since energy cannot be created or destroyed, it must be in the form of heat (Q) or work (W). Thus, we have the following mathematical statement of the first law:

First Law of Thermodynamics

$$\Delta E = Q - W$$

Pay close attention to the sign conventions we're using. Q is considered positive when heat is moving into the system, negative when it is coming out of the system. W is considered positive when the work is *being done by the system on the environment*. W is considered negative when the work is *being done by the environment on the system*. Unfortunately, this convention for work is opposite what is typically used in chemistry books, so you may remember the formula as $\Delta E = Q + W$ (or with U in place of E and with lowercase letters). As long as you remember how the variables are being defined, when they are positive and negative, you shouldn't have any problems.

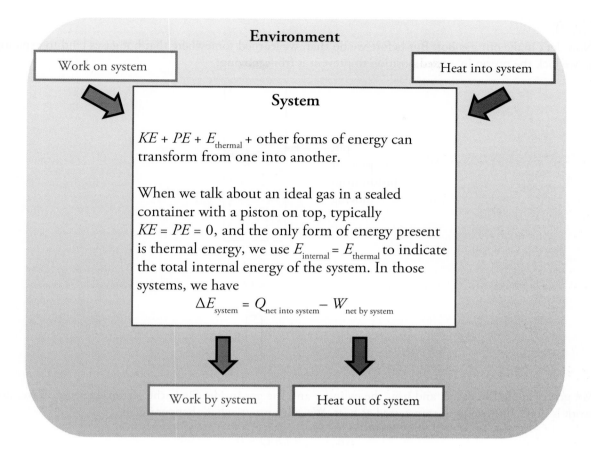

To analyze the first law equation, let's take a sample of ideal gas at room temperature and put it into a container to make a closed (but not isolated) system. Let's use a metal cylinder that's welded shut at one end and sealed on the other end with a piston.

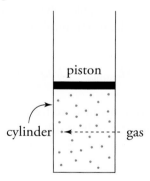

Starting with the energy component of the equation, we can consider the internal energy of the system (which for an ideal gas is simply the kinetic energy of all the molecules). The internal energy, $E_{internal}$, is proportional to the object's absolute temperature, T:

$$E_{internal} \propto T$$

Since this gas is at room temperature, we can say for sure that it has less $E_{internal}$ than a hot gas, and it has more $E_{internal}$ than a cold gas.

Heat

39.3

Now, let's make our gas hot. But before we do that, we learned somewhere that hot gases tend to expand, so we lock the piston in a fixed position to prevent it from moving:

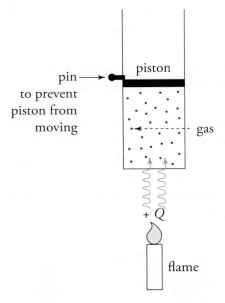

We gently apply the flame, and heat the cylinder and the gas inside. Since the piston does not move, no work is done, but energy is transferred as heat. We can sum up what's happening as

$$\Delta E_{internal} = Q, \ Q > 0$$

where we know that $E_{internal}$ has to increase because we feel that the gas and cylinder are getting hotter, and the additional energy is added to our system in the form of heat, Q.

If we let the hot gas and hot cylinder just sit on a table, what's going to happen over time? The hot cylinder and gas will cool down as they lose heat to the room, until they're at room temperature again. So, for this cooling down process, we'll have

$$\Delta E_{internal} = Q, \ Q < 0$$

where we know that $E_{internal}$ has to decrease because we feel that the gas and cylinder are cooling down, and energy is lost from our system in the form of heat, Q.

Work

Let's make the gas hot again. This time, let's remove the lock on the piston and allow it to move.

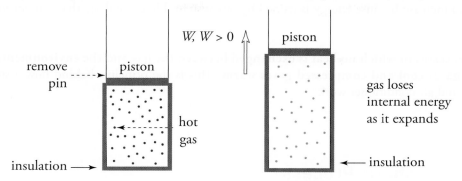

The hot gas pushes the piston up. Our gas is doing work, *W*, because it's applying a *force* and moving the piston a certain *distance*. As the piston moves, the volume of the gas increases since gases expand to fill their containers. Therefore, the ΔV in this example is positive. To quantify the work in a system, we not only need to know how much the volume of the system changes, but we also need to know how much pressure the gas exerts upward on the piston. Therefore, work can be defined as

$$W = P\Delta V$$

Due to an increase in volume, the work described in the case above has a positive value. A positive *W* is defined as work done *by* the system. When the weight on our piston moves up, it gains potential energy (the *h* in *mgh* is getting larger). Conservation of energy states that energy cannot be created or destroyed, but is simply moved around. Therefore, the energy gained by the weight must come from something else (the hot gas!). As long as the piston is well insulated, such that no heat (*Q*) can go in or out, we have

$$\Delta E_{internal} = -W, \ W > 0$$

where $E_{internal}$ of our gas has to decrease because energy is lost from our system in the form of doing work, *W*. Because the gas is losing energy as it expands and raises the piston, and we learned earlier that $\Delta E_{internal}$ is proportional to temperature, the *gas cools as it expands.*

Now, if after our gas has expanded and cooled as far as it's going to, we add more weight on the piston so that the piston and weights move down and compress the gas,

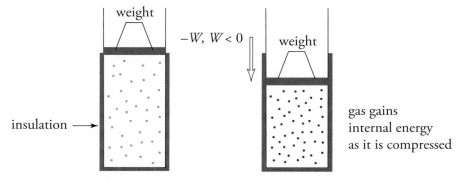

we have the situation for which

$$\Delta E_{internal} = -W, \ W < 0$$

Now, because ΔV is a negative value (because our gas has been compressed), this will lead to negative work being done *by the gas* (which is the same as *positive* work being done *on the gas*). In this situation, $E_{internal}$ has to increase because energy is gained by our system. Here, we'd see that our *gas warms as it is compressed*.

Thus, for processes in which no heat is exchanged between the gas and the environment, in general expanding gases cool and compressed gases warm. This is the principle behind how a steam engine, refrigerator, and air conditioner work.

Case 1: An Isobaric Process

An **isobaric** process is one that occurs at constant pressure. Consider heating our cylinder such that the volume of gas expands, pushing the piston upward, but the pressure remains constant because the weight of the piston is held constant. If we plot pressure versus volume for this process, the graph would look like this:

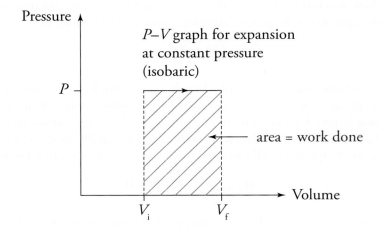

and the area under the curve would be equal to the work done by the gas on the piston. This means we can easily calculate W, without the use of calculus, since $W = P\Delta V$. **Note that this is positive because ΔV is positive; when the arrow goes backward in the graph indicating $\Delta V < 0$, the area should be considered negative.**

Case 2: An Isochoric Process

An **isochoric** process maintains a constant volume. Heating the gas with a locked piston would result in increasing pressure but no change in volume:

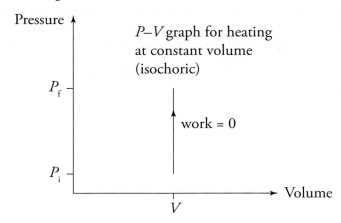

Therefore, no work is done. You can see this either by noticing that the area under the P-V graph is zero (since the graph is just a vertical line), or by realizing that if the volume didn't change, then the piston didn't move, and if there's no displacement of the piston, then there was no work done on the piston. Because $W = 0$, we know that $\Delta E = Q$.

Case 3: An Isothermal Process

When heat is allowed to pass freely between a system and its environment, an **isothermal** process can occur, where the temperature of the system remains constant. For example, for our gas to expand at constant temperature, the pressure must decrease (as governed by Boyle's Law).

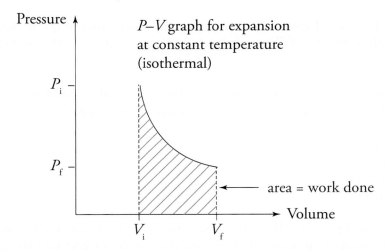

Again, the work done by the gas on the piston will be equal to the area under the curve. Since we know that E is directly proportional to T, we can say that in an isothermal process, $\Delta E = 0$ and $Q = W$.

Case 4: An Adiabatic Process

An **adiabatic** process occurs when no heat is transferred between the system and the environment, and all energy is transferred as work: The previous example with the insulated container is one instance. Another example is a rapidly expanding gas, which drops its pressure precipitously and simultaneously cools. This is the principle behind the release of compressed water vapor in a snow-making machine. The process happens so quickly that theoretically no heat is transferred; since $Q = 0$, we get $\Delta E_{internal} = -W$.

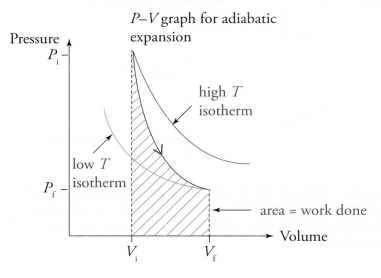

Example 39-3: For a perfectly insulated system, what are the values of $\Delta E_{internal}$ and Q if $W = +100$ J?

    A) $\Delta E_{internal} = -100$ J and $Q = 0$
    B) $\Delta E_{internal} = 0$ and $Q = -100$ J
    C) $\Delta E_{internal} = +100$ J and $Q = 0$
    D) $\Delta E_{internal} = 0$ and $Q = +100$ J

Solution: A perfectly insulated system allows no heat transfer (adiabatic), so $Q = 0$; this eliminates choices B and D. Now, by the First Law of Thermodynamics, $\Delta E_{internal} = Q - W = 0 - (+100 \text{ J}) = -100$ J, so the answer is choice A.

Example 39-4: Suppose you want to raise the temperature of an ideal gas while adding the lowest possible amount of heat and doing no work on the gas. Which process should you use?

    A) Isobaric
    B) Isochoric
    C) Isothermal
    D) Adiabatic

Solution: An isothermal process will not raise the temperature of the gas at all by definition, so choice C is eliminated. An adiabatic process will not allow the transfer of heat into the gas, so choice D is eliminated. If you add heat during an isochoric process, the change in internal energy of the gas (which is directly proportional to the change in temperature) will be $\Delta E = Q$, whereas during an isobaric process it will be $\Delta E = Q - P\Delta V$, because the gas will expand as it increases in temperature; rearranging gives $Q = \Delta E + P\Delta V$. Thus, the isochoric process will require less heat to increase E and therefore T by some arbitrary amount. The correct answer is choice B.

This example illustrates the difference between two ideal gas heating processes. This distinction is quantified by the difference between *molar specific heats*. An ideal gas at constant volume will increase in temperature according to $Q = nC_V\Delta T$, where n is the number of moles and C_V is called the constant volume molar specific heat. An ideal gas at constant pressure, on the other hand, will increase in temperature according to $Q = nC_P\Delta T$, where C_P is called the constant pressure molar specific heat. The units of molar specific heat are $[C] = [Q] / [n][T] = $ J/mol-K. The exact values of the molar specific heats depend upon the type of gas (monatomic, diatomic, polyatomic), and you are unlikely to need to know them. However, as you already know from the preceding example that a constant pressure process requires more heat for an equal change in temperature than a constant volume process, it is worth noting that, in general, $C_P = C_V + R$, where R is the gas constant.

Example 39-5: The P-V curve below represents a thermodynamic *cycle*, a series of reversible processes through which an ideal gas passes that return it to its initial state function. What area represents the net work done by the gas from steps 1 to 2 to 3 to 4 back to 1?

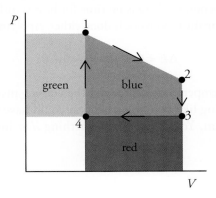

A) The blue trapezoid
B) The red rectangle
C) The blue trapezoid and the red rectangle
D) The blue trapezoid and both the red and green rectangles

Solution: The isochores 2→3 and 4→1 do no work, so we can ignore them. The process 1→2 does positive work $W_{1\rightarrow 2} = P\Delta V$, which is the sum of the blue and red areas. The process 3→4 does negative work, because the volume decreases (this would correspond to the piston moving down, compressing the gas), $W_{3\rightarrow 4} = P\Delta V$, which is the negative of the red area. Thus, the sum of the four processes yields (blue + red) + 0 + (−red) + 0 = blue. The correct answer is choice A.

This example illustrates a couple of important facts about **thermodynamic cycles**, sequences of processes that lead a gas back to its original state function. This means that $\Delta E = 0$ for the overall cycle, and thus $Q = W$. During a cycle, the system either converts heat to work (for a clockwise cycle, like the one shown) or work to heat (for a counterclockwise cycle). Thermodynamic cycles are important as models of ideal heat engines. Indeed, many of the breakthroughs in the science of thermodynamics were made by engineers attempting to understand how to make more efficient engines.

Example 39-6: An ideal gas is held under pressure in an isolated container behind a thin membrane separating it from vacuum, like an inflated balloon in a large evacuated room. The membrane is suddenly ruptured, like popping the balloon. What happens next?

A) Nothing: the membrane ruptures, but the gas is unaffected.
B) The pressure and temperature both decrease rapidly.
C) The temperature decreases rapidly, but the pressure stays constant.
D) The pressure decreases rapidly, but the temperature remains constant, since no heat is exchanged and no work is done.

Solution: If a gas is held under pressure and the source of the pressure is released, like suddenly removing the piston from the canister in the examples discussed previously, the pressure will spontaneously decrease to match that of the surroundings (this will be discussed in more detail in the next chapter on fluids). This eliminates choice A. The phenomenon described in this question is a special type of adiabatic process called a *free expansion:* it is nearly instantaneous, so there is no time for heat transfer, but because the membrane ruptures and there is nothing to push against, no work is done either. Applying the first law equation thus yields

$$\Delta E = Q - W = 0 - 0 = 0.$$

Therefore, there is no change in temperature either, and the correct answer is choice D. It might seem to you counterintuitive that something like popping a balloon could have such small apparent effect on the thermodynamic state of the system. You'd be right: something *does* increase, namely the *entropy* of the system.

39.4   THE SECOND LAW OF THERMODYNAMICS

As we have seen, the First Law of Thermodynamics is an expanded statement of conservation of energy, a principle we're familiar with from the realm of balls rolling down hills and blocks sliding across tables, as well as (now) gases being heated and expanding, doing work in the process. However, now that we have expanded our view of what counts as energy, it becomes apparent that many situations we would never expect to see do not in fact violate the principle of energy conservation. Imagine, for example, that you are looking at a wooden block resting on a normal horizontal table. All of the sudden, it begins sliding to the right. You'd be pretty surprised, and you'd probably start looking for the string (or the camera), because you would think that would violate the conservation of energy. However, suppose the block had a thermometer attached to it, and you noticed that as the block began to slide, its temperature began to lower. In that case, conservation of energy might not be violated: thermal energy was just transforming into kinetic energy. You would likely continue to object; it's one thing for a sliding block to slow down and stop due to friction, heating up in the process, but this doesn't typically work in reverse. Why *don't* things go backward? What directs the *arrow of time*? One answer is **entropy** and the **Second Law of Thermodynamics.**

Entropy is a measure of the *disorder* of a system. What does this mean? Imagine the Great Pyramid of Giza, built so carefully of stacked stones that it has stood for over 4500 years. Now imagine those same six billion kilograms of stone scattered around hundreds of square kilometers of desert. The pyramid is ordered, the scattered stone is disordered. A microscopic analogy would be a diamond crystal, with its extremely regular and predictable organization of carbon atoms, versus the carbon atoms in pencil shavings scattered on a desk. The carbon atoms in the pencil shavings have much greater entropy than those in the crystal.

Without stating any equations you won't need to know, we can say qualitatively that *predictability* is one measure of order. If I tell you the first five cards in a deck are the ace, 2, 3, 4, and 5 of spades, you will probably feel pretty comfortable guessing the next card will be the 6 of spades, a lot more comfortable than if I shuffled the deck and asked you to predict the sixth card (technically, this is a function of information entropy and not physical entropy, but the details aren't important). By analogy, the entropy will be lower whenever there's a higher likelihood that, given you know the locations and velocities of some particles, you can deduce the same of other particles. Under this criterion, solids, with their regular arrays of atoms, have greater order and therefore less entropy than liquids, which have in turn less entropy than gases. Entropy is another *state variable*, one whose value corresponds to the microscopic order of the particles making up the system, just as temperature corresponds to the microscopic kinetic energy of those particles. The MCAT doesn't care about the mathematical details of this correspondence, and you are really likely to see quantitative entropy problems only in chemistry or biochemistry, not in physics.

The Second Law of Thermodynamics states that the *entropy of an isolated system either stays the same or increases during any thermodynamic process*. If the system is closed, its entropy can decrease, but not without a corresponding greater increase in the entropy of the surrounding environment. Over a thermodynamic cycle, the rules are slightly different. If the entropy stays the same over a thermodynamic cycle, the cycle is said to be reversible, meaning that you could return from each state to the previous state by the same path in reverse (think of these paths as the curves on a P-V graph), and that on returning there would be no indication of any change.

This means also that it is impossible for a system to convert all of the input heat (disordered energy) into work (ordered energy) during a thermodynamic cycle: it must always output some heat as well. Similarly, it is impossible to move heat from a colder system to a hotter one without inputting some work (work which, we've just discovered, must itself involve some output of heat). If the entropy increases over a series of processes (thereby making it not a true cycle), this indicates the process is *irreversible*. In the real world, all macroscopic processes are irreversible due to friction and other "loss" effects. A wooden block sliding on a horizontal table comes to a stop due to friction. Energy is conserved, converted from kinetic to thermal, but entropy increases, which is why you will never see the block spontaneously accelerate backward from whence it came. Things really can't go back to just the way they were.

Example 39-7: A patient recovering from surgery is confined to a bed in a hospital room during the first couple of days of recovery: minimal movement is allowed. During that time, incisions begin to heal and organ function returns to normal. What best explains this?

    A) Entropy of the person decreases but the entropy of the surroundings increases more.
    B) Because the person does no work, she is an isolated system and thus her entropy increases.
    C) The person absorbs more heat from the environment than she emits, and therefore is able to increase her internal energy.
    D) There is no change to the entropy in the person because healing is a closed thermodynamic cycle.

Solution: Choice B is eliminated because humans are open systems that exchange matter and energy with their environments, not isolated (people eat, breathe, defecate, emit heat, etc. to stay alive). Choice C is not a good description of the physical situation: hospital rooms are not typically hotter than body temperature, and even if they were, the person would sweat to get rid of the excess thermal energy from the environment and more important from the chemical processes within the body (e.g., digestion). Also healing doesn't increase internal energy in any obvious way. Choice D is false because, again, a healing person is an open system and in any case, healing is not a closed cycle: your body isn't identical to its previous state regardless of having healed (aging, scar tissue, etc.). Choice A is correct because there are fewer ways to be healthy and functioning well than to be, say, cut up into bits (so the entropy of the person is likely lower), but the process of healing in that hospital room will increase the entropy of the surroundings due to the open-system interactions, the heating of the air around the body, etc.

Chapter 40
Fluids and Elasticity
of Solids

40.1 HYDROSTATICS: FLUIDS AT REST

In this section and the next, we'll discuss some of the fundamental concepts dealing with substances that can flow, which are known as **fluids**. *Both liquids and gases are fluids*, but there are distinctions between them. At the molecular level, a substance in the liquid phase is similar to one in the solid phase in that the molecules are close to, and interact with, one another. The molecules in a liquid are able to move around a little more freely than those in a solid, in which the molecules typically only vibrate around relatively fixed positions. By contrast, the molecules of a gas are not constrained and fly around in a chaotic swarm, with hardly any interaction. On a macroscopic level, there is another distinction between liquids and gases. If you pour a certain volume of a liquid into a container of a greater volume, the liquid will occupy its original volume, whatever the shape and size of the container. However, if you introduce a sample of gas into a container, the molecules will fly around and fill the *entire* container.

Density and Specific Gravity

The **density** of a substance is the amount of mass contained in a unit of volume. In SI units, density is expressed in kg/m^3, but you might also see on the MCAT g/cm^3.

$$\text{density} = \frac{\text{mass}}{\text{volume}}$$

$$\rho = \frac{m}{V}$$

There is one substance whose density you should memorize: the density of liquid water is taken to be 1000 kg/m^3 or 1 g/cm^3. (Another useful version of the same value: 1 kg/L, where L stands for a liter; a liter is 1000 cm^3.)

Sometimes the MCAT mentions **specific gravity**. This (poorly named) unitless number tells us how dense something is compared to water:

$$\text{specific gravity} = \frac{\text{density of substance}}{\text{density of water}}$$

$$\text{sp. gr.} = \frac{\rho}{\rho_{H_2O}}$$

For solids, density doesn't change much with surrounding pressure or temperature. For example, the density of marble is pretty close to 2700 kg/m^3 under most conditions. Liquids behave the same way: the density of water is pretty close to 1000 kg/m^3 under all conditions at which it's a liquid. However, the density of a gas changes markedly with pressure and temperature. (The Ideal Gas Law tells us that $PV = nRT$, so the density of a sample of an ideal gas is given by the equation $\rho_{gas} = m/V = mP/nRT$, which depends on P and T.)

Example 40-1: Turpentine has a specific gravity of 0.9. What is the density of this liquid?

Solution: By definition, we have

$$\rho_{turpentine} = (\text{sp. gr.}_{turpentine})(\rho_{H_2O}) = (0.9)(1000\,\tfrac{kg}{m^3}) = 900\,\tfrac{kg}{m^3}$$

Example 40-2: A 2 cm^3 sample of osmium, one of the densest substances on Earth, has a mass of 45 g. What's the specific gravity of this metal?

Solution: The density of osmium is

$$\rho = \frac{m}{V} = \frac{45\text{ g}}{2\text{ cm}^3} = 22.5\,\tfrac{g}{cm^3}$$

Since this is 22.5 times the density of water (which is 1 g/cm^3), the specific gravity of osmium is 22.5.

Force of Gravity for Fluids

When solving questions involving fluids, it is often handy to know how to find the force of gravity acting on the fluid itself or objects that are immersed in the fluid. In previous chapters, we have used $F_{grav} = mg$ without too much difficulty. However, with fluids, it is more difficult to remove a portion of fluid from a tank, place it on a scale, and find its mass. Using the relationship between mass, volume, and density, we can redefine the magnitude of F_{grav} for fluids questions:

$$\rho = \frac{m}{V} \;\rightarrow\; m = \rho V \;\rightarrow\; \therefore F_{grav} = mg = \rho V g$$

With this new formula $F_{grav} = \rho V g$, it is important to make sure that the density (ρ) and the volume (V) describe the properties of the correct object or fluid.

Pressure

If we place an object in a fluid, the fluid exerts a contact force on the object. If we look at how that force is *distributed* over any small area of the object's surface, we have the concept of **pressure**:

Pressure

$$P = \frac{\text{force}_\perp}{\text{area}} = \frac{F_\perp}{A}$$

The subscript ⊥ (which means "perpendicular") indicates that pressure is defined as the magnitude of the force acting *perpendicular* to the surface, divided by the area. Although the formula for pressure involves "force," pressure is actually a *scalar* quantity, because the perpendicular force is the same for all orientations of a surface exposed to a particular portion (or depth) of a static fluid. The unit of pressure is the N/m², which is called a **pascal** (abbreviated **Pa**). Because 1 N is a pretty small force and 1 m² is a pretty big area, 1 Pa is very small. Often, you'll see pressure expressed in kPa (or even in MPa). For example, at sea level, normal atmospheric pressure is about 100 kPa.

Let's imagine we have a tank of water with a lid on top. Suspended from the lid is a string attached to a thin metal sheet. The figures below show you two views of this.

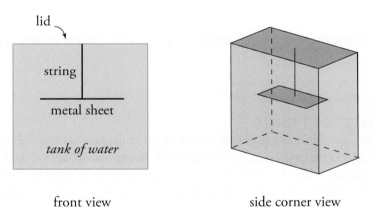

front view   side corner view

The weight of the water above the metal sheet produces a force that pushes down on the sheet. If we divide this force by the area of the sheet, w/A, we get the pressure, due to the water, on the sheet. The formula for calculating this pressure depends on the density of the fluid in the tank (ρ_{fluid}), the depth of the sheet (D), and the acceleration due to gravity (g).

$$P = \frac{w_{\text{fluid}}}{A} = \frac{m_{\text{fluid}}g}{A} = \frac{\rho_{\text{fluid}}V_{\text{fluid}}g}{A} = \frac{\rho_{\text{fluid}}ADg}{A} = \rho_{\text{fluid}}Dg$$

Hydrostatic Gauge Pressure

$$P_{gauge} = \rho_{fluid} gD$$

This formula gives the pressure due only to the fluid (in this case, the water) in the tank. This is called **hydrostatic gauge pressure**. It's called hydro*static*, because the fluid is at rest, and *gauge* pressure means that we don't take the pressure due to the atmosphere into account (the gauge reads zero before it is submerged in the water in the tank). If there were no lid on the water tank, then the water would be exposed to the atmosphere, and the *total* pressure at any point in the water would be equal to the atmospheric pressure pushing down on the surface *plus* the pressure due to the water (that is, the gauge pressure). So, below the surface, we'd have

$$P_{total} = P_{atm} + P_{gauge}$$

If the tank were closed to the atmosphere, but there were a layer of gas above the surface of the water, then the total pressure at a point below the surface would be the pressure of the gas pushing down at the surface plus the gauge pressure: $P_{total} = P_{gas} + P_{gauge}$. In general, we'll have

$$P_{total} = P_{at\ surface} + P_{gauge}$$

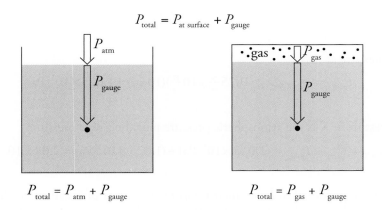

$$P_{total} = P_{atm} + P_{gauge} \qquad P_{total} = P_{gas} + P_{gauge}$$

in either case:

$$\boxed{P_{total} = P_{at\ surface} + P_{gauge}}$$

Notice that hydrostatic gauge pressure, $P_{gauge} = \rho_{fluid} gD$, is proportional to both the depth and the density of the fluid. *Total* pressure, however, is *not* proportional to either of these quantities if $P_{on\ surface}$ isn't zero.

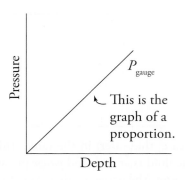

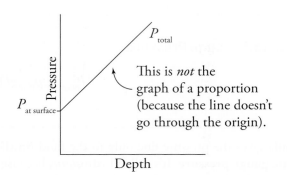

The lines in these graphs will be straight as long as the density of the liquid remains constant as the depth increases. Actually, ρ increases as the depth increases, but the effect is small enough that we generally consider liquids to be **incompressible**; that is, that the density of a liquid remains constant (so, in particular, the density doesn't increase with depth).

Example 40-3: The density of seawater is 1025 kg/m³. Consider a point X that's 10 m below the surface of the ocean.

   a)   What's the gauge pressure at X?
   b)   If the atmospheric pressure is 1.015×10^5 Pa, what is the total pressure at X?
   c)   Consider a point Y that's 50 m below the surface. How does the gauge pressure at Y compare to the gauge pressure at X? How does the total pressure at Y compare to the total pressure at X?

Solution:

   a)   The gauge pressure at X is

$$P_{\text{gauge}} = \rho_{\text{fluid}}gD = (1025\tfrac{\text{kg}}{\text{m}^3})(10\tfrac{\text{N}}{\text{kg}})(10 \text{ m}) = 1.025 \times 10^5 \text{ Pa}$$

   b)   The total pressure at X is the atmospheric pressure plus the gauge pressure:

$$P_{\text{total at X}} = P_{\text{atm}} + P_{\text{gauge}} = (1.015 \times 10^5 \text{ Pa}) + (1.025 \times 10^5 \text{ Pa}) = 2.04 \times 10^5 \text{ Pa}$$

   c)   Since P_{gauge} is proportional to D, an increase in D by a factor of 5 will mean the gauge pressure will also increase by a factor of 5. Therefore, the gauge pressure at Y will be $5\left(P_{\text{gauge at X}}\right) = 5.125 \quad 10^5$ Pa. The total pressure at Y is equal to the atmospheric pressure plus the gauge pressure at Y, so

$$P_{\text{total at Y}} = P_{\text{atm}} + P_{\text{gauge}} = (1.015 \times 10^5 \text{ Pa}) + (5.125 \times 10^5 \text{ Pa}) = 6.14 \times 10^5 \text{ Pa}$$

Notice that $P_{\text{total at Y}}$ is not 5 times $P_{\text{total at X}}$. *Total* pressure is *not* proportional to depth.

Example 40-4: A large storage tank fitted with a tight lid holds a liquid. The space between the surface of the liquid and the lid of the tank is filled with molecules of the stored liquid in the gaseous phase. At a depth of 40 m, the total pressure is 520 kPa, while at a depth of 50 m, the total pressure is 600 kPa. What's the pressure of the gas above the surface of the liquid?

Solution: Let P_{gas} be the pressure that the gas exerts on the surface of the liquid. Then we have

$$P_{\text{total at } D_1 = 40 \text{ m}} = P_{gas} + \rho_{fluid} g D_1 = P_{gas} + \rho_{fluid} g (40 \text{ m}) = 520 \text{ kPa}$$
$$P_{\text{total at } D_1 = 50 \text{ m}} = P_{gas} + \rho_{fluid} g D_2 = P_{gas} + \rho_{fluid} g (50 \text{ m}) = 600 \text{ kPa}$$

We have two equations and two unknowns (P_{gas} and ρ_{fluid}). If we subtract the first equation from the second, we get $\rho_{fluid} g (10 \text{ m}) = 80 \text{ kPa}$, which tells us that $\rho_{fluid} g = 8 \dfrac{\text{kP}}{\text{m}}$. Plugging this back into either one of the equations will give us P_{gas}. Choosing, say, the first one, we find that

$$P_{gas} + \left(8 \, \frac{\text{kPa}}{\text{m}} \right)(40 \text{ m}) = 520 \text{ kPa} \; \rightarrow \; P_{gas} = 200 \text{ kPa}$$

Example 40-5: A two identical tanks are filled with two fluids, A and B, such that the density of fluid B is three times the density of fluid A. What is the relationship between P_{gauge} at point 1 and P_{gauge} at point 2?

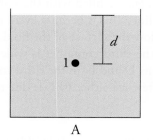
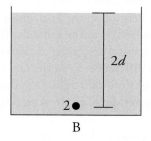

A

B

Solution: Isolate the variables necessary to set up the proportionality.

$$P_{gauge} = \rho_{fluid} g D \rightarrow P_{gauge} \propto \rho_{fluid} \text{ and } P_{gauge} \propto D$$

Gauge pressure is dependent on density and depth. Fluid B has three times the density and point 2 is located at double the depth beneath the surface, so the point 2 will have six times the gauge pressure.

Example 40-6: A two identical tanks are filled with two fluids, A and B, such that the density of fluid B is three times the density of fluid A (see previous example). What best characterizes the relationship between the total pressure P_1 at point 1 and total pressure P_2 at point 2?

- A) $P_1 = P_2$
- B) $6P_1 = P_2$
- C) $6P_1 < P_2$
- D) $6P_1 > P_2$

Solution: Pressure increases with depth and density, eliminating choice A. Total pressure must include the pressure at the surface of the tanks (likely atmospheric pressure), which as we've seen previously means that total pressure is not a direct proportion with respect to depth, or for that matter density in two different fluids (eliminating choice B). We know from the previous example that the gauge pressure at point 2 is six times the gauge pressure at point 1, which means that the total pressures are as follows:

$$P_1 = \rho_{\text{fluid 1}}gd + P_{\text{surface}} \text{ and } P_2 = 6\,\rho_{\text{fluid 1}}gd + P_{\text{surface}} < 6P_1$$

The correct answer is choice D.

Example 40-7: The containers shown below are all filled with the same liquid. At which point (A, B, C, D, E, or F) is the gauge pressure the lowest?

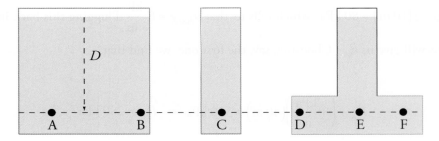

Solution: It's important to remember that the formula $P_{\text{gauge}} = \rho_{\text{fluid}}gD$ applies regardless of the shape of the container in which the fluid is held. If all the containers are filled with the same fluid, then the pressure is the *same* everywhere along the horizontal dashed line. This is because every point on this line (and within one of the containers) is at the same depth, D, below the surface of the fluid. The fact that the first container is wide, the second container is narrow, and the third container is wide at the base but has a narrow neck makes no difference. Even the fact that Points D and F (in the third container) aren't *directly* underneath a column of fluid of height D makes no difference either (this is due to Pascal's Law, which will be described in greater detail in a few pages).

Example 40-8: The following data are measured for total pressure as a function of depth in a given fluid. What would be the total pressure for a fluid with one half the density at a depth of 50 cm?

Depth	Total Pressure
10 cm	150 Pa
20 cm	200 Pa
30 cm	250 Pa
40 cm	300 Pa

Solution: Since the question asks for total pressure, we first should find the pressure at the surface. Note the linear relationship in the table: for each 10 cm interval, there is an increase of 50 Pa. This means that the surface pressure (D = 0 cm) is 100 Pa. Because gauge pressure is proportional to density, a fluid with half the density would will see an increase of 25 Pa for every 10 cm increase in depth, so at 50 cm it would have a total pressure of $P_{\text{total}} = P_{\text{gauge}} + P_{\text{surface}} = 125 \text{ Pa} + 100 \text{ Pa} = 225 \text{ Pa}$.

Buoyancy and Archimedes' Principle

Let's place a wooden block in our tank of water. Since the pressure on each side of the block depends on its average depth, we see that there's more pressure on the bottom of the block than there is on the top of it. Therefore, there's a greater force pushing up on the bottom of the block than there is pushing down on the top. The forces due to the pressure on the other four sides (left and right, front and back) cancel out, so the net fluid force on the block is upward. This net upward fluid force is called the **buoyant** force (or just **buoyancy** for short), which we'll denote by F_{Buoy} (or F_B).

We can calculate the magnitude of the buoyant force using Archimedes' principle:

Archimedes' Principle

The magnitude of the buoyant force
is equal to
the weight of the fluid displaced by the object.

When an object is partially or completely submerged in a fluid, the volume of the object that's submerged, which we call V_{sub}, is the volume of the fluid displaced.

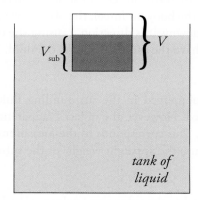

tank of liquid

By multiplying V_{sub} by the density of the fluid, we get the *mass* of the fluid displaced; then, multiplying this mass by g gives us the weight of the fluid displaced. So, here's Archimedes' principle as a mathematical equation:

Archimedes' Principle

$$F_{Buoy} = \rho_{fluid} V_{sub} g$$

When an object floats, its submerged volume is just enough to make the buoyant force it feels balance its weight. That is, for a floating object, we always have $w_{object} = F_{Buoy}$. If an object's density is ρ_{object} and its volume is V, its weight will be $\rho_{object}V_{object}g$. The buoyant force it feels is $\rho_{fluid}V_{sub}g$. Setting these equal to each other, we find that

---

Floating Object in Equilibrium on Surface

$$w_{object} = F_{Buoy}$$

$$\frac{V_{sub}}{V} = \frac{\rho_{object}}{\rho_{fluid}}$$

So, if $\rho_{object} < \rho_{fluid}$, then the object will float; and the fraction of its volume that's submerged is the same as the ratio of its density to the fluid's density. *This is a very helpful fact to know for the MCAT.* For example, if the object's density is 3/4 the density of the fluid, then 3/4 of the object will be submerged (and vice versa).

If an object is denser than the fluid, then the object will sink. In this case, even if the entire object is submerged (in an attempt to maximize the buoyant force), the object's weight is still greater than the buoyant force. This leaves a net force in the downwards direction, causing the object to sink by accelerating downwards. If an object just happens to have the same density as the fluid, it will be happy hovering (in static equilibrium) underneath the fluid.

For an object that is completely submerged in the surrounding fluid, the actual weight of the object ($w_{object} = \rho_{object}Vg$) remains unchanged. However, the object's "apparent" weight is less due to the buoyant force "buoying" the object upwards. This corresponds to the measurement of a scale placed at the bottom of a tank of liquid in order to measure the apparent weight of the submerged object, or the normal force acting on the object.

Since the volume of the object is equal to the submerged volume ($V = V_{sub}$), the buoyant force F_{Buoy} on the object is equal to $\rho_{fluid}Vg$. Therefore,

$$\frac{w_{object}}{F_{Buoy}} = \frac{\rho_{object}Vg}{\rho_{fluid}Vg} = \frac{\rho_{object}}{\rho_{fluid}}$$

If the fluid in which the object is submerged is water, the ratio of the object weight to the buoyant force is equal to the specific gravity of the object.

Example 40-9: Ethyl alcohol has a specific gravity of 0.8. If a cork of specific gravity 0.25 floats in a beaker of ethyl alcohol, what fraction of the cork's volume is submerged?

    A) 4/25
    B) 1/5
    C) 1/4
    D) 5/16

Solution: Because the cork has a lower density than the ethyl alcohol, we know that the cork will float. Furthermore, the fraction of the cork's volume that will be submerged is

$$\frac{V_{sub}}{V} = \frac{\rho_{object}}{\rho_{fluid}} = \frac{(0.25)\rho_{H_2O}}{(0.8)\rho_{H_2O}} = \frac{0.25}{0.8} = \frac{1/4}{4/5} = \frac{5}{16}$$

Therefore, the answer is choice D.

Example 40-10: The density of ice is 920 kg/m³, and the density of seawater is 1025 kg/m³. Approximately what percent of an iceberg floats above the surface of the ocean (in other words, how much is "the tip of the iceberg")?

A) 5%
B) 10%
C) 90%
D) 95%

Solution: Because the ice has a lower density than the seawater, we know that the iceberg will float. Furthermore, the fraction of the iceberg's volume that will be submerged is

$$\frac{V_{sub}}{V} = \frac{\rho_{object}}{\rho_{fluid}} = \frac{920\ \frac{kg}{m^3}}{1025\ \frac{kg}{m^3}} \approx \frac{900}{1000} = 90\%$$

However, the answer is not choice C. The question asked what percent of the iceberg floats *above* the surface. So, if 90% is submerged, then 10% is above the surface, and the answer is choice B. Watch for this kind of tricky wording; it is a common MCAT tactic.

Example 40-11: A ball floats in a vat of water with 4/5 of its volume submerged and feels a buoyant force of 15 N. It is placed in a separate container and feels a buoyant force of 9 N while being completely submerged. What is the density of the fluid in the second container?

Solution: We are given the values for F_{Buoy}, so we can set up a relationship between the two:

$$F_{Buoy\ 2} = 9\ N = \rho_{fluid\ 2}V_{submerged\ 2}g = \rho_{fluid\ 2}V_{object}g \rightarrow \rho_{fluid\ 2} = \frac{9\ N}{V_{object}g}$$

$$F_{Buoy\ 1} = 15\ N = \rho_{fluid\ 1}V_{submerged\ 1}g = \rho_{water}\left(0.8V_{object}\right)g = \left(800\ \frac{kg}{m^3}\right)V_{object}g \rightarrow V_{object}g = \frac{15\ N}{800\ \frac{kg}{m^3}}$$

$$\rho_{fluid\ 2} = \frac{9\ N}{V_{object}g} = \frac{9}{15}\left(800\ \frac{kg}{m^3}\right) = \frac{3}{5}\left(800\ \frac{kg}{m^3}\right) = 480\ \frac{kg}{m^3}$$

Example 40-12: A glass sphere of specific gravity 2.5 and volume 10^{-3} m^3 is completely submerged in a large container of water. What is the apparent weight of the sphere while immersed?

Solution: Because the buoyant force pushes up on the object, the object's *apparent weight*, $w_{apparent} = w - F_{Buoy}$, is less than its true weight, w. Because the sphere is completely submerged, we have $V_{sub} = V$, so the buoyant force on the sphere is

$$\begin{aligned} F_{Buoy} &= \rho_{fluid} V_{sub} g \\ &= \rho_{H_2O} V g \\ &= (1000 \tfrac{kg}{m^3})(10^{-3} \text{ m}^3)(10 \tfrac{N}{kg}) \\ &= 10 \text{ N} \end{aligned}$$

The true weight of the glass sphere is

$$\begin{aligned} w &= \rho_{glass} V g \\ &= (\text{sp. gr.}_{glass} \times \rho_{H_2O}) V g \\ &= (2.5 \times 1000 \tfrac{kg}{m^3})(10^{-3} \text{ m}^3)(10 \tfrac{N}{kg}) \\ &= 25 \text{ N} \end{aligned}$$

Therefore, the apparent weight of the sphere while immersed is

$$w_{apparent} = w - F_{Buoy} = 25 \text{ N} - 10 \text{ N} = 15 \text{ N}$$

Example 40-13: One way of measuring a person's body fat percentage is by comparing his weight in air to his weight while completely submerged in water. The principle is that fat is less dense than water (sp. gr. = 0.94), whereas bone and other tissues (average sp. gr. = 1.1) are more dense than water. If someone weighs 1050 N when weighed in air and 50 N when weighed fully submerged (with as little air in the lungs as possible), approximately what is his body fat percentage?

Solution: If the person has an apparent weight of 50 N when submerged, the buoyant force acting on him must be $w_{apparent} = w - F_B \rightarrow F_B = w - w_{apparent} = 1,050 \text{ N} - 50 \text{ N} = 1,000 \text{ N}$. According to Archimedes' principle, the ratio of the man's weight to the buoyant force while completely submerged yields the ratio of his density to that of the fluid (in this case, water).

$$\frac{w}{F_B} = \frac{\rho_{man}}{1,000 \text{ kg/m}^3} \rightarrow \frac{1,050 \text{ N}}{1,000 \text{ N}} = 1.05 = \frac{\rho_{man}}{1,000 \text{ kg/m}^3} \rightarrow \rho_{man} = 1,050 \text{ kg/m}^3$$

To achieve this density, the man must be some fraction of lean mass and the rest fat (note that we convert the given specific gravities of lean mass and fat to densities by multiplying by 1,000). Calling X the fraction of lean mass and omitting units for clarity:

$$1,100X + 940(1 - X) = 1,050 \rightarrow 1,100X - 940X = 160X = 110 \rightarrow X = \frac{110}{160} \approx \frac{2}{3}$$

Thus, the man is about 70% lean mass and is 30% body fat mass.

Example 40-14: A balloon that weighs 0.18 N is then filled with helium so that its volume becomes 0.03 m³. (Note: The density of helium is 0.2 kg/m³.)

a) What is the net force on the balloon if it's surrounded by air? (Note: The density of air is 1.2 kg/m³.)
b) What will be the initial upward acceleration of the balloon if it's released from rest?

Solution:

a) Remember that gases are fluids, so they also exert buoyant forces. If an object is immersed in a gas, the object experiences a buoyant force equal to the weight of the gas it displaces. In this case, the balloon is completely immersed in a "sea" of air (so $V_{sub} = V$), and Archimedes' principle tells us that the buoyant force on the balloon due to the surrounding air is

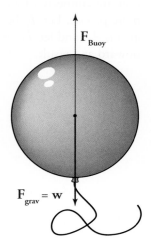

$$F_{Buoy} = \rho_{fluid} V_{sub} g$$
$$= \rho_{air} V g$$
$$= (1.2 \tfrac{kg}{m^3})(0.03 \text{ m}^3)(10 \tfrac{N}{kg})$$
$$= 0.36 \text{ N}$$

The weight of the inflated balloon is equal to the weight of the balloon material (0.18 N) plus the weight of the helium:

$$w_{total} = w_{material} + w_{helium}$$
$$= w_{material} + \rho_{helium} V g$$
$$= 0.18 \text{ N} + (0.2 \tfrac{kg}{m^3})(0.03 \text{ m}^3)(10 \tfrac{N}{kg})$$
$$= 0.18 \text{ N} + 0.06 \text{ N}$$
$$= 0.24 \text{ N}$$

Because $F_{Buoy} > w_{total}$, the net force on the balloon is upward and has magnitude
$$F_{net} = F_{Buoy} - w_{total} = (0.36 \text{ N}) - (0.24 \text{ N}) = 0.12 \text{ N}$$

b) Using Newton's Second Law, $a = F_{net} / m$, we find that

$$a = \frac{F_{net}}{m} = \frac{F_{net}}{\frac{w}{g}} = \frac{0.12 \text{ N}}{\left(\frac{0.24 \text{ N}}{10 \text{ m/s}^2}\right)} = \frac{(0.12 \text{ N}) \cdot (10 \text{ m/s}^2)}{0.24 \text{ N}} = \frac{10 \text{ m/s}^2}{2} = 5 \text{ m/s}^2$$

Pascal's Law

Pascal's Law is a statement about fluid pressure. It says that a confined fluid will transmit an externally applied pressure change to all parts of the fluid and the walls of the container without loss of magnitude. In less formal language, if you squeeze a container of fluid, the fluid will transmit your squeeze perfectly throughout the container. The most important application of Pascal's Law is to hydraulics.

Consider a simple hydraulic jack consisting of two pistons resting above two cylindrical vessels of fluid that are connected by a pipe. If you push down on one piston, the other one will rise. Let's make this more precise. Let F_1 be the magnitude of the force you exert down on one piston (whose cross-sectional area is A_1) and let F_2 be the magnitude of the force that the other piston (cross-sectional area A_2) exerts upward as a result.

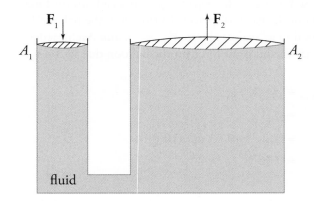

Pushing down on the left-hand piston with a force F_1 introduces a pressure increase of F_1 / A_1. Pascal's Law tells us that this pressure change is transmitted, without loss of magnitude, by the fluid to the other end. Since the pressure change at the other piston is F_1 / A_1, we have, by Pascal's Law,

$$\frac{F_1}{A_1} = \frac{F_2}{A_2}$$

Solving this equation for F_2, we get

$$F_2 = \frac{A_2}{A_1} F_1$$

So, if A_2 is greater than A_1 (as it is in the figure), then the ratio of the areas, A_2 / A_1, will be greater than 1, so F_2 will be greater than F_1; that is, *the output force, F_2, is greater than your input force, F_1*. This is why hydraulic jacks are useful; we end up lifting something very heavy (a car, for example) by exerting a much smaller force (one that would be insufficient to lift the car if it were just applied directly to the car).

This seems too good to be true; doesn't this violate some conservation law? No, since there's no such thing as a "Conservation of Force" law. However, there *is* a price to be paid for the magnification of the force. Let's say you push the left-hand piston down by a distance, d_1, and that the distance the right-hand piston moves upward is d_2. Assuming the fluid is incompressible, whatever fluid you push out of the left-hand cylinder must appear in the right-hand cylinder. Since volume is equal to cross-sectional area times distance, the volume of the fluid you push out of the left-hand cylinder is A_1d_1, and the extra volume of fluid that appears in the right-hand cylinder is A_2d_2.

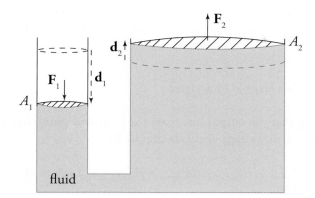

But these volumes have to be the same, so $A_1d_1 = A_2d_2$. Solving this equation for d_2, we get

$$d_2 = \frac{A_1}{A_2}d_1$$

If the area of the right-hand piston (A_2) is greater than the area of the left-hand piston (A_1), the ratio A_1 / A_2 will be *less* than 1, so d_2 will be less than d_1. In fact, the decrease in d is the same as the increase in F. For example, if A_2 is five times larger than A_1, then F_2 will be five times greater than F_1, but d_2 will only be *one-fifth* of d_1. We can now see that the product of F and d will be the same for both pistons:

$$F_2d_2 = \left(\frac{A_2}{A_1}F_1\right) \cdot \left(\frac{A_1}{A_2}d_1\right) = F_1d_1$$

Recall that the product of F and d is the amount of work done. What we have shown is that the work you do pushing the left-hand piston down is equal to the work done by the right-hand piston as it pushes upward. Just as when we discussed simple machines and mechanical advantage, we can't cheat when it comes to work. True, we can do the same job with less force, but we will always pay for that by having to exert that smaller force through a greater distance. This is the whole idea behind all simple machines, not just a hydraulic jack.

Example 40-15: A hydraulic lift is used to lift a car in a showroom on a circular platform with a 5 m diameter (connected to a central hydraulic cylinder pipe with a diameter of 40 cm) and negligible mass. If the hydraulic pump outputs a maximum pressure of 4×10^5 Pa, what is the maximum weight of the car that can be lifted?

Solution: Set up Pascal's Law, noting that the size of the platform is irrelevant: only the size of the hydraulic cylinder into which fluid is pumped to lift the platform matters. Also recall both that pressure is force / area and that diameter is twice the radius.

$$P_{pump} = \frac{F_{car}}{A_{cylinder}} = \frac{w_{car}}{\pi r^2} \rightarrow w_{car} = \pi r^2 P_{pump} \approx 3\left(20 \times 10^{-2}\ m\right)^2 \left(4 \times 10^5\ Pa\right) \approx 5 \times 10^4\ N$$

This is about twice as much as a large SUV weighs.

Example 40-16: Assuming that the output line from the hydraulic pump has an area of 10 square centimeters, what is the mechanical advantage of this hydraulic lift?

Solution: $MA = F_{resistance} / F_{effort} = F_{resistance} / (P_{pump} \times A_{pump\ output}) = 5 \times 10^4\ N / (4 \times 10^5\ Pa \times 10\ cm^2 \times 10^{-4}\ m^2/cm^2) = 1.2 \times 10^2 = 120$.

40.2 HYDRODYNAMICS: FLUIDS IN MOTION

Flow Rate and the Continuity Equation

Consider a pipe through which fluid is flowing. The **flow rate**, f, is the volume of fluid that passes a particular point per unit time, like how many liters of water per minute are coming out of a faucet. In SI units, flow rate is expressed in m^3/s. To find the flow rate, all we need to do is multiply the cross-sectional area of the pipe at any point, A, by the average speed of the flow, v, at that point:

Flow Rate

$$f = Av$$

Be careful not to confuse flow rate with flow speed; flow rate tells us how *much* fluid flows per unit time; flow speed tells us how *fast* the fluid moves. There's a difference between saying that a hose ejects 4 liters of water every second (that's flow rate) and saying that the water leaves the hose at a speed of 4 m/s (that's flow speed).

If a pipe is carrying a liquid, which we assume is **incompressible** (that is, its density remains constant), then the flow rate must be the same everywhere along the pipe. Choose any two points in a flow tube carrying a liquid, Point 1 and Point 2. If there aren't any sources or sinks between these points (i.e., no leaks and no additional liquid), then the liquid that flows by Point 1 must also flow by Point 2, and vice versa. In other words, $f_1 = f_2$, or, since $f = Av$, we get $A_1 v_1 = A_2 v_2$; this is called the:

> **Continuity Equation**
>
> $$A_1 v_1 = A_2 v_2$$

This tells us that when the tube narrows, the flow speed will increase; and if the tube widens, the flow speed will decrease. In fact, we can say that the flow speed is inversely proportional to the cross-sectional area (or to the square of the radius) of the pipe.

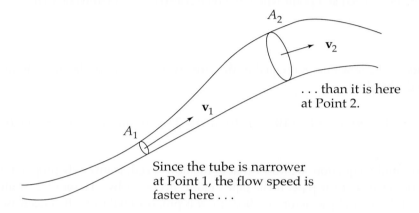

A_2

$\mathbf{v}_2$

... than it is here at Point 2.

$\mathbf{v}_1$

A_1

Since the tube is narrower at Point 1, the flow speed is faster here . . .

Example 40-17: In the pipe shown above, if $A_2 = 9A_1$, then which of the following will be true?

    A) $v_1 = 9v_2$
    B) $v_1 = 3v_2$
    C) $v_2 = 9v_1$
    D) $v_2 = 3v_1$

Solution: If the cross-sectional area at Point 2 is 9 times the cross-sectional area at Point 1, then the flow speed at Point 2 will be 1/9 the flow speed at Point 1. That is, $v_2 = v_1 / 9$, or, solving for v_1, we get $v_1 = 9v_2$ (choice A).

Example 40-18: Before using a hypodermic needle to inject medication into a patient, a nurse tests the needle by shooting a small amount of the liquid into the air. The barrel of the needle is 1 cm in diameter, and the tip is 1 mm in diameter. If the nurse pushes the piston with a speed of 2 cm/s, how fast does the liquid come out the tip?

    A)   4 cm/s
    B)   20 cm/s
    C)   40 cm/s
    D)   200 cm/s

40.2

Solution: Cross-sectional area is proportional to the square of the diameter of the flow tube. In this case, the diameter decreases by a factor of 10 (from 1 cm to 1 mm), so the cross-sectional area decreases by a factor of $10^2 = 100$. Now, according to the continuity equation, if A decreases by a factor of 100, then v increases by a factor of 100. Therefore, the speed of the liquid coming out of the tip is $100 \times (2 \text{ cm/s}) = 200 \text{ cm/s}$, choice D.

Example 40-19: A pipe of nonuniform diameter carries water. At one point in the pipe, the radius is 2 cm and the flow speed is 6 m/s.

   a)   What's the flow rate?

   b)   What's the flow speed at a point where the pipe constricts to a radius of 1 cm?

Solution:

   a)   At any point, the flow rate, f, is equal to the cross-sectional area of the pipe multiplied by the flow speed; therefore,

$$f = Av = \pi r^2 v = \pi (2 \times 10^{-2} \text{ m})^2 (6 \text{ m/s}) \approx 75 \times 10^{-4} \text{ m}^3/\text{s} = 7.5 \times 10^{-3} \text{ m}^3/\text{s}$$

   b)   By the continuity equation, we know that v, the flow speed, is inversely proportional to A, the cross-sectional area of the pipe. If the pipe's radius decreases by a factor of 2 (from 2 cm to 1 cm), A decreases by a factor of 4 because A is proportional to r^2. If A decreases by a factor of 4, then v will increase by a factor of 4. So, the flow speed at a point where the pipe's radius is 1 cm will be $4 \times (6 \text{ m/s}) = 24 \text{ m/s}$.

Bernoulli's Equation

The most important equation in fluid dynamics is Bernoulli's equation, but before we state it, it's important to know under what conditions it applies. Bernoulli's equation applies to **ideal fluid** flow. A fluid must satisfy the following four requirements in order to be considered an ideal fluid.

- *The fluid is incompressible.*
  This works very well for liquids; gases are quite compressible, but it turns out that we can use the Bernoulli equation for gases provided the pressure changes are small.
- *There is negligible viscosity.*
  Viscosity is the force of cohesion between molecules in a fluid; think of it as internal friction for fluids. For example, maple syrup is more viscous than water, and there's more resistance to a flow of maple syrup than to a flow of water. (While Bernoulli's equation gives good results when applied to a flow of water, it would not give good results if it were applied to a flow of maple syrup.)
- *The flow is laminar.*
  In a tube carrying a flowing fluid, a *streamline* is just what it sounds like: a "line" in the stream. If we were to inject a drop of dye into a clear glass pipe carrying, say, water, we'd see a streak of dye in the pipe, indicating a streamline. The entire flow is called streamline (as an adjective) or laminar if the individual streamlines don't cross. When the flow is laminar, the fluid flows *smoothly* through the tube.

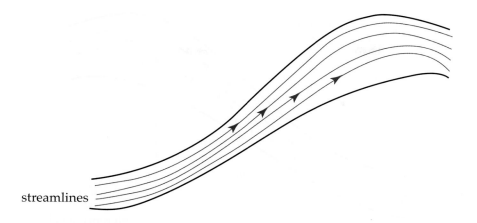

streamlines

The opposite of streamline flow is called **turbulent flow**. In this case, the flow is not smooth; it is chaotic (unpredictable). Turbulence is characterized by whirlpools and swirls (vortexes). At high enough speeds, all real fluids experience turbulent flow, and no simple equation can be applied to such a flow.

- *The flow rate is steady.*
  That is, the value of f is constant. If we're analyzing the water flowing through a garden hose connected to a faucet sticking out of the side of the house, turn the faucet handle to a particular setting and then leave it there. The flow rate through the hose must be steady while we're taking our measurements.

If these conditions hold—(1) the fluid is incompressible, (2) the flow is smooth (laminar), (3) there's no friction (viscosity), and (4) the flow rate is steady—then total mechanical energy will be conserved. *Bernoulli's equation is the statement of conservation of total mechanical energy for ideal fluid flow.* On the MCAT, you will often be told to consider a fluid to be ideal, allowing you to use Bernoulli's equation.

Bernoulli's Equation

$$P_1 + \tfrac{1}{2}\rho v_1^2 + \rho g y_1 = P_2 + \tfrac{1}{2}\rho v_2^2 + \rho g y_2$$

In this equation, ρ is the density of the flowing fluid, P_1 and P_2 give the pressures at any two points along a streamline within the flow, v_1 and v_2 give the flow speeds at these points, and y_1 and y_2 give the heights of these points above some chosen horizontal reference level.

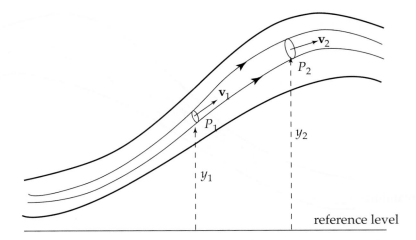

Although the equation may look complicated, notice that the two sides are the same, except all the subscripts on the left-hand side are 1s, while all the subscripts on the right-hand side are 2s. Also, each $\frac{1}{2}\rho v_1^2$ term looks very much like the kinetic energy (sometimes it's referred to as kinetic energy density), and each term ρgy looks very much like gravitational potential energy. So, just take the equation you already know for conservation of total mechanical energy, $KE_1 + PE_1 = KE_2 + PE_2$, change the ms to ρs, add P to both sides, and you've got Bernoulli's equation.

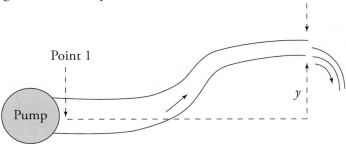

Example 40-20: In the figure above, a pump forces water at a constant flow rate through a pipe whose cross-sectional area, A, gradually decreases. At the exit point, A has decreased to 1/3 its value at the beginning of the pipe. If y = 60 cm and the flow speed of the water just after it leaves the pump (Point 1 in the figure) is 1 m/s, what is the gauge pressure at Point 1?

Solution: We'll apply Bernoulli's equation to Point 1 and the exit point, which we'll call Point 2. We'll choose the level of Point 1 as our horizontal reference level; this makes $y_1 = 0$. Now, because the cross-sectional area of the pipe decreases by a factor of 3 between Points 1 and 2, the flow speed must increase by a factor of 3; that is, $v_2 = 3v_1$. Since the pressure at Point 2 is P_{atm}, Bernoulli's equation becomes

$$P_1 + \tfrac{1}{2}\rho v_1^2 = P_{\text{atm}} + \tfrac{1}{2}\rho v_2^2 + \rho gy_2$$

This tells us that

$$P_1 - P_{atm} = \rho g y_2 + \tfrac{1}{2}\rho v_2^2 - \tfrac{1}{2}\rho v_1^2$$
$$= \rho g y_2 + \tfrac{1}{2}\rho(3v_1)^2 - \tfrac{1}{2}\rho v_1^2$$
$$= \rho(g y_2 + 4v_1^2)$$
$$= (1000\ \tfrac{\text{kg}}{\text{m}^3})[(10\ \text{m/s}^2)(0.6\ \text{m}) + 4(1\ \text{m/s})^2]$$

$$\therefore P_{\text{gauge at 1}} = 10^4\ \text{Pa}$$

Imagine that we punch a small hole in the side of a tank of liquid. We can use Bernoulli's equation to figure out the *efflux speed,* that is, how fast the liquid will flow out of the hole.

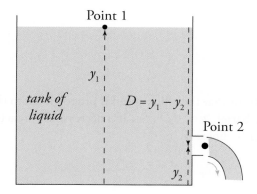

Let the bottom of the tank be our horizontal reference level, and choose Point 1 to be at the surface of the liquid and Point 2 to be at the hole where the water shoots out. First, the pressure at Point 1 is at atmospheric pressure; and the emerging stream at Point 2 is open to the air, so it's at atmospheric pressure too. Therefore, $P_1 = P_2$, and these terms cancel out of Bernoulli's equation. Next, since the area at Point 1 is so much greater than at Point 2, we can assume that v_1, the speed at which the water level in the tank drops, is much lower than v_2, the speed at which the water shoots out of the hole. (Remember that by the continuity equation, $A_1 v_1 = A_2 v_2$; since $A_1 \gg A_2$, we'll have $v_1 \ll v_2$.) Because $v_1 \ll v_2$, we can say that $v_1 \approx 0$ and ignore v_1 in this case. So, Bernoulli's equation becomes

$$\rho g y_1 = \tfrac{1}{2}\rho v_2^2 + \rho g y_2$$

Crossing out the ρ's, and rearranging, we get

$$\tfrac{1}{2}v_2^2 = g(y_1 - y_2)$$
$$= gD$$
$$v_2 = \sqrt{2gD}$$

That is, $v_{\text{efflux}} = \sqrt{2gD}$, where D is the distance from the surface of the liquid down to the hole. This is called **Torricelli's result.** This equation should look familiar; it's basically the same formula that tells us how fast an object is going after it has fallen a distance h from rest.

Example 40-21: The side of an above-ground pool is punctured, and water gushes out through the hole. If the total depth of the pool is 2.5 m, and the puncture is 1 m above ground level, what is the efflux speed of the water?

Solution: We apply Torricelli's result, $v = \sqrt{2gD}$, where D is the distance from the surface of the pool down to the hole. If the puncture is 1 m above ground level, then it's 2.5 – 1 = 1.5 m below the surface of the water (because the pool is 2.5 m deep). Therefore, the efflux speed will be

$$v = \sqrt{2gD} = \sqrt{2(10 \text{ m/s}^2)(1.5 \text{ m})} = \sqrt{30 \text{ m/s}^2} \approx 5.5 \text{ m/s}$$

Example 40-22: A hole is opened at the bottom of a full barrel of liquid. When the efflux speed has decreased to 1/2 the initial efflux speed, the barrel is:

    A) 1/4 full
    B) $1/\sqrt{2}$ full
    C) 1/2 full
    D) 3/4 full

Solution: Torricelli's result tells us that the efflux speed is proportional to the square root of the height to the surface of the liquid in the barrel: $v \propto \sqrt{D}$. So, if v decreases by a factor of 2, then D has decreased by a factor of 4, and the answer is choice A.

The Bernoulli or Venturi Effect

Consider the two points labeled in the pipe shown below:

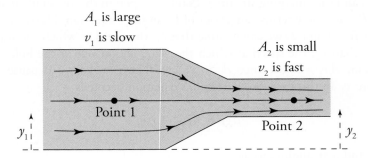

Since the heights y_1 and y_2 are equal in this case, the terms in Bernoulli's equation that involve the heights will cancel, leaving us with

$$P_1 + \tfrac{1}{2}\rho v_1^2 = P_2 + \tfrac{1}{2}\rho v_2^2$$

We already know from the continuity equation ($f = Av$) that the speed increases as the cross-sectional area of the pipe decreases. Since $A_2 < A_1$, we know that $v_2 > v_1$, and the equation above then tells us that $P_2 < P_1$. That is,

the pressure is lower where the flow speed is greater.

This is known as the **Bernoulli** or **Venturi effect**.

You may have seen a skydiver or motorcycle rider wearing a jacket that seems to puff out as they move rapidly through the air. The essentially stagnant air trapped inside the jacket is at a much higher pressure than the air whizzing by outside, and as a result, the jacket expands outward.

The drastic drop in air pressure that accompanies the high winds in a hurricane or tornado is another example. In fact, if high winds streak across the roof of a home whose windows are closed, the outside air pressure is reduced so much that the air pressure inside the house (where the air speed is essentially zero) can be great enough to blow the roof off.

Example 40-23: A pipe of constant cross-sectional area carries water at a constant flow rate from the hot-water tank in the basement of a house up to the second floor. Which of the following will be true?

    A) The speed at which the water arrives at the second floor must be lower than the speed at which it left the water tank.
    B) The speed at which the water arrives at the second floor must be greater than the speed at which it left the water tank.
    C) The water pressure at the second floor must be lower than the water pressure at the tank.
    D) The water pressure at the second floor must be greater than the water pressure at the tank.

Solution: Because the flow rate is constant and the cross-sectional area of the pipe is constant, the flow speed will be constant (this follows from the continuity equation, $f = Av = $ constant). This eliminates choices A and B. Now, if the flow speeds v_1 and v_2 are the same, Bernoulli's equation becomes

$$P_1 + \rho g y_1 = P_2 + \rho g y_2$$

Because $y_2 > y_1$, it must be true that $P_2 < P_1$ (choice C).

Example 40-24: In a healthy adult standing upright, blood pressure in the arms and legs should be roughly equal. Suppose the height difference between elbow and ankle is 1 m. If one assumes that blood is an ideal fluid flowing through smooth rigid pipes of equal diameter, what would be the pressure difference between the arm and leg (the density of blood is about 1,025 kg/m^3)?

Solution: According to Bernoulli's equation,

$$P_{arm} + \rho g y_{arm} + \tfrac{1}{2}\rho v^2_{arm} = P_{leg} + \rho g y_{leg} + \tfrac{1}{2}\rho v^2_{leg}$$

The question stem states that the diameter of the pipes (the arteries and veins) should be assumed constant, so according to the continuity equation, $v_{arm} = v_{leg}$. Thus, we have

$$\Delta P = P_{leg} - P_{arm} = \rho g y_{arm} - \rho g y_{leg} = \rho g(y_{arm} - y_{leg})(1{,}025 \text{ kg/m}^3)(10 \text{ m/s}^2)(1 \text{ m}) = 10{,}250 \text{ Pa}$$

For reference, this is about 80 torr, a huge pressure difference compared to typical healthy values of 120/80 torr. Clearly this result is suspicious. There are several reasons why one cannot validly apply Bernoulli's equation to blood flow, including that the heart is a pump (the flow is not under a constant pressure), the flexibility of the venous system, and the presence of valves in the circulatory system. However, one extremely important reason having to do with blood is its viscosity: blood is about 4 times more viscous than water (though the viscosity of blood varies depending upon several factors). This viscosity contributes to a resistance to flow, which leads to a pressure drop effect as blood gets further from the heart. One statement of **Poiseuille's Law** for viscous fluid flow gives this pressure drop per unit length as

$$\frac{\Delta P}{L} = \frac{8\eta f}{\pi r^4}$$

where η is the viscosity coefficient of the fluid, f is flow rate, and r is the radius of the pipe.

Example 40-25: Using Poiseuille's Law, we can determine the effects of vasoconstriction in limiting blood flow rate to tissues, as for example when arterioles constrict to minimize blood flow to the skin and thereby reduce radiative heat loss in cold weather. Suppose that a vein constricts to 80% of its original radius. Assuming the blood pressure remains constant in this portion of the circulatory system, what will be the approximate percentage of the new blood flow rate through the vein compared to its prior value?

    A) 80%
    B) 60%
    C) 40%
    D) 20%

Solution: We can assume that constricting the vessel does not affect its length or the viscosity of blood, and we are told the pressure does not change, so Poiseuille's Law yields:

$$\frac{\Delta P}{L} = \frac{8\eta Lf}{\pi r^4} \rightarrow f \propto r^4 = \left(8 \times 10^{-1}\right)^4 = 8^4 \times 10^{-4} \approx 6.5^2 \times 10^{-2} \approx 40 \times 10^{-2} = 40\%$$

The correct answer is choice C.

40.3 THE ELASTICITY OF SOLIDS

Support beams for a building are compressed slightly under the heavy load they support; thick steel cables may be stretched in the construction of a bridge; and the ends of a connecting rod in a structure can be pushed or pulled in opposite directions, causing the rod to bend. These are some examples of the type of problem we'll look at in this section: the relationship between the forces applied to a solid object and the resulting change in the object's shape.

Stress

We'll look at three ways forces can be applied to an object: **tension** (stretching) forces, **compression** (squeezing) forces, and **shear** (bending) forces:

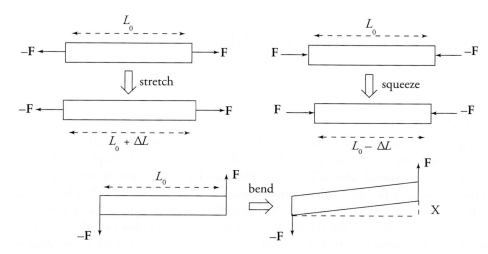

The magnitude of the force at either end, F, divided by the area over which it acts is called the **stress**:

Stress

$$\text{stress} = \frac{\text{force}}{\text{area}} = \frac{F}{A}$$

Stress is much like pressure, but they're not the same, because the force in the stress equation doesn't have to be perpendicular to the area over which it acts. For example, a shear force acts *parallel*, not perpendicular, to the areas at the ends. Nevertheless, we're still dividing a force by an area, so the unit of stress is the N/m^2, or pascal (Pa). It's *very important* to notice that stress is inversely proportional to the cross-sectional area, or, for an object with circular cross sections, inversely proportional to the *square* of the cross-sectional radius or diameter.

Strain

As a result of these forces, the object's shape will change. The ratio of the appropriate change in the length to the object's original length (see the figure above) is called the **strain**:

Strain

Tensile or Compressive	**Shear Strain**
$\text{strain} = \dfrac{\text{change in length}}{\text{original length}} = \dfrac{\Delta L}{L_0}$	$\text{strain} = \dfrac{\text{distance of shear}}{\text{original length}} = \dfrac{X}{L_0}$

The following mnemonic (though imprecise) may be helpful:

St__ress__ is p__ressure__. Str__ain__ is ch__ange__.

Hooke's Law

The idea is simple: *Stress causes strain.* As long as the stress isn't too large—so that we don't permanently deform the object once the stress is removed (that is, allowing the object to display some *elasticity*)—then *stress and strain are proportional.* This is known as **Hooke's Law**. For a tensile or compressive stress, the constant of proportionality is called **Young's modulus**; for a shear stress, it's called (what else?) the **shear modulus**. The modulus depends on the type of material the object is made of; generally, the stronger the intermolecular bonds, the greater the modulus. A material's modulus can also depend on the type of stress the material is subjected to. For example, for the kind of steel used in building construction, the shear modulus is less than half its Young's modulus; this tells us that structural steel is weaker when subjected to shear forces than to tension or compression forces (that is, it's easier to bend steel than it is to stretch or compress it). It's even possible to have a Young's modulus for tension and a different one for compression. For example, human bone has two Young's moduli: the value of the modulus for compact bone under a tensile stress is about twice the value of the modulus for a compressive stress. Bone is more resistant to tension than to compression.

Hooke's Law $\text{stress} = \text{modulus} \times \text{strain}$

Young's modulus is denoted by the letter Y or by E, while shear modulus is denoted by S or by G. Using E for Young's modulus (for tension and compression) and G for shear modulus, Hooke's Law yields the following easy-to-remember formulas for tension/compression and for shear:

Tension/Compression

$$\frac{F}{A} = E\frac{\Delta L}{L_0}$$

$$\therefore \Delta L = \frac{FL_0}{EA}$$

Shear

$$\frac{F}{A} = G\frac{X}{L_0}$$

$$\therefore X = \frac{FL_0}{AG}$$

We call these the *Flea* and *Flag* formulas.

Example 40-26: A piece of rubber, originally 18 cm long, is stretched to a length of 20 cm. What strain has it undergone?

Solution: The change in length is $\Delta L = 20 \text{ cm} - 18 \text{ cm} = 2 \text{ cm}$. Therefore, the strain is

$$\frac{\Delta L}{L_0} = \frac{2 \text{ cm}}{18 \text{ cm}} = \frac{1}{9}$$

Example 40-27: What are the units of Young's modulus and the shear modulus?

Solution: Hooke's Law says that stress = modulus × strain. Because strain has no units (we're dividing a length by a length), the units of the modulus must be the same as the units of stress: pascals.

Example 40-28: Two cylindrical rods with circular cross sections are identical except for the fact that Rod 2 has four times the diameter of Rod 1. If these two rods are subjected to identical compressive forces, how will the compression of Rod 2 compare to that of Rod 1?

Solution: First, the fact that Rod 2 has 4 times the diameter of Rod 1 means that Rod 2 has $4^2 = 16$ times the cross-sectional area. Therefore, if both rods experience identical compressive forces, the stress on Rod 2 will be 1/16 the stress on Rod 1 (because stress = force/area). Since the rods are made of the same material, their Young's moduli are the same, so, by Hooke's Law, the strain on Rod 2 will be 1/16 the strain on Rod 1. Finally, because the rods had the same original length, the change in length of Rod 2 will be 1/16 of the change in length of Rod 1.

Example 40-29: Two objects are subjected to identical tensile stresses. The object with the greater value of Young's modulus will undergo:

    A) a smaller change in length.
    B) a greater change in length.
    C) less strain.
    D) greater strain.

Solution: Hooke's Law says that stress = modulus × strain. If stress is a constant, then the strain is inversely proportional to the modulus. Therefore, the object with the greater value of Young's modulus will experience less strain (choice C). Notice that we can't say that choice A is correct, since we don't know the original lengths of the objects.

Example 40-30: Two metal beams have the same length and cross-sectional area, but Beam X has twice the shear modulus of Beam Y. If each beam is subjected to the same shear forces, which beam will bend more and by what factor?

    A) Beam X, by a factor of 2
    B) Beam X, by a factor of 4
    C) Beam Y, by a factor of 2
    D) Beam Y, by a factor of 4

Solution: If the beams have the same cross-sectional area and are subjected to the same shear forces, the shear stress on the beams will be the same (since stress = force/area). By Hooke's Law, then, the strain is inversely proportional to the modulus. If Beam X has twice the shear modulus, it will undergo 1/2 the strain. Since the beams had the same original length, Beam Y will bend more, by a factor of 2 (choice C).

Example 40-31: In a traumatic accident associated with large compressive forces, the tibia (the larger of the two bones of the lower leg) is more likely to fracture than the femur (the bone of the upper leg and the largest bone in the body). Which of the following best explains this?

    A) The tibia is shorter than the femur.
    B) The tibia has a lower Young's modulus than the femur.
    C) The tibia has a higher shear modulus than the femur.
    D) The tibia has a smaller radius than the femur.

Solution: The question stem mentions compressive force, so choice C can be eliminated because it has to do with shearing forces. Also, moduli are associated with material properties, so we could expect that bones would typically have the same moduli (eliminating choice B as well). There is no direct relationship suggested in the equation for Young's modulus and absolute length: fractional change in length characterizes strain (this eliminates choice A). The fact that the tibia has a smaller radius means that it also has a smaller cross-sectional area, meaning that for the same force, the tibia will experience a greater stress than will the femur. Choice D is correct.

Example 40-32: Hooke's Law for a spring says that the magnitude of the force required to stretch or compress the spring from its natural length is given by the simple formula $F = kx$, where k is a constant (which depends on the spring) and x is the amount by which the spring is stretched or compressed. Is this formula for Hooke's Law the same as the one given in this section?

40.3

Solution: Yes. Some of the letters may be different, but the idea is exactly the same: the force of tension or compression is proportional to the amount of stretch or compression. Let's take Hooke's Law as given in this section, express it in the form of the *Flea* formula, $\Delta L = FL_0\ /\ EA$, and rewrite it like this: $F = \left(EA\ /\ L_0\right) \cdot \Delta L$. Now, notice that this equation has exactly the same form as the equation $F = kx$:

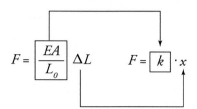

Chapter 41 Electrostatics, Electricity, and Magnetism

41.1 ELECTRIC CHARGE

An atom is composed of a central nucleus (which is itself composed of protons and neutrons) surrounded by a cloud of one or more electrons. The fact that an atom is held together as a single unit is due to the fact that protons and electrons have a special property: they carry **electric charge**, which gives rise to an attractive force between them.

Electric charge exists in two varieties, which are called **positive** and **negative**. By convention, we say that protons carry positive charge and electrons carry negative charge. (Neutrons are well-named: they're neutral, because they have no electric charge.) The charge of a proton is +e, where e is called the **elementary charge**, and the charge of an electron is −e. Notice that the proton and the electron carry exactly the same amount of charge; the only difference in their charges is that one is positive and the other is negative.

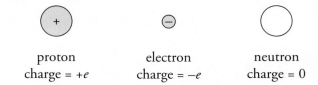

proton	electron	neutron
charge = +e	charge = −e	charge = 0

In SI units, electric charge is measured in **coulombs** (abbreviated **C**), and the value of the elementary charge, e, is 1.6×10^{-19} C.

Elementary Charge

$$e = 1.6 \times 10^{-19} \text{ C}$$

When an atom (or any other object) contains the same number of electrons as protons, its total charge is zero because the individual positive and negative charges add up and cancel. So, when the number of electrons (#e) equals the number of protons (#p), the object is *electrically neutral*. We say that an object is **charged** when there's an imbalance between the number of electrons and the number of protons. When an object has one or more extra electrons (#e > #p), the object is *negatively charged*, and when an object has a deficit of electrons (#e < #p), the object is *positively charged*. If a neutral atom has electrons removed or added, we say that it has been **ionized**, and the resulting electrically charged atom is called an **ion**. A positively charged ion is called a **cation**, and a negatively charged ion is called an **anion**. (An object can also become charged by gaining or losing protons, but these are usually locked up tight within the nuclei of the atoms. In virtually all cases, objects become charged by the transfer of *electrons*.)

Because an object can become charged only by losing or gaining electrons or protons, which can't be "sliced" into smaller pieces with fractional amounts of charge, the charge on an object can only be a whole number of ±e's; that is, charge is **quantized**. So, for any object, its charge is always equal to $n(\pm e)$, where n is a whole number. To remind us that charge is *q*uantized, electric charge is usually denoted by the letter q (or Q).

> ### Charge is Quantized
>
> $$q = n(\pm e)$$
>
> where $n = 0, 1, 2...$

It is interesting to note that this quantization of charge applies to all fundamental particles either found in nature or created in the laboratory (e.g., muons, pions, etc.).

In chemistry, it's common to talk about the charge of an atom in terms of whole numbers like +1 or –2, etc. For example, we say that the charge of the fluoride ion, F^-, is –1, and the charge of the calcium ion, Ca^{+2}, is +2. This is just a convenient way of saying that the charge of the fluoride ion is –1 elementary unit (in other words, $-1e$), and the charge of the calcium ion is +2 elementary units, $+2e$. When we want to find the electric force between ions, we will express their charges in the proper unit (coulombs), and say, for example, that the charge of the fluoride ion is $-1e = -1.6 \times 10^{-19}$ C and that the charge of the calcium ion is $+2e = +3.2 \times 10^{-19}$ C.

Finally, total electric charge is always conserved; that is, the total amount of charge before any process must always be equal to the total amount of charge afterward.[1]

Example 41-1: How much positive charge is contained in 1 mole of carbon atoms? How much negative charge? What is the total charge?

Solution: Every atom of carbon contains 6 protons, so the amount of positive charge in one carbon atom is $q_+ = +6e$. Therefore, if N_A denotes Avogadro's number, the total amount of positive charge in 1 mole of carbon atoms is

$$Q_+ = N_A \times q_+ = N_A \times (+6e) = (6.02 \times 10^{23}) \times (6)(+1.6 \times 10^{-19} \text{ C}) = +6 \times 10^5 \text{ C}$$

Because every neutral carbon atom also contains 6 electrons, the amount of negative charge in a carbon atom is $q_- = 6(-e) = -6e = -q_+$ so the total amount of negative charge in 1 mole of carbon atoms is $Q_- = N_A \times q_- = -Q_+ \approx -6 \times 10^5$ C. The total charge on the carbon atoms, $Q_+ + Q_-$, is zero.

---

[1] This does not mean that electric charge cannot be created or destroyed, which happens all the time. For example, in the reaction $e^- + e^+ \rightarrow \gamma + \gamma$, an electron ($e^-$) and its antiparticle (the positron, e^+, which is, in effect, a positively charged electron) meet and annihilate each other, producing energy in the form of two gamma-ray photons (γ), which carry no charge. Charge has been destroyed, but the total charge (zero, in this case) has been conserved. Conversely, charge can be created in the opposite process, when energy is converted to mass and charge (but always with zero total charge).

41.2 ELECTRIC FORCE AND COULOMB'S LAW

If two charged particles are a distance r apart,

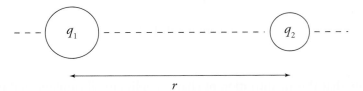

then the electric force between them, $\mathbf{F}_E$, is directed along the line joining them. The magnitude of this force is proportional to the charges (q_1 and q_2) and inversely proportional to r^2, as given by

---

Coulomb's Law

$$F_E = k \frac{|q_1 q_2|}{r^2}$$

The proportionality constant is k, and in general, its value depends on the material between the particles. However, in the usual case where the particles are separated by empty space (or by air, for all practical purposes), the proportionality constant is denoted by k_0 and called **Coulomb's constant**. This is a fundamental constant of nature (equal in magnitude, by definition, to 10^{-7} times the speed of light squared), and its value is $k_0 = 9 \times 10^9$ N·m²/C²:

Coulomb's Constant

$$k_0 = 9 \times 10^9 \, \tfrac{\text{N·m}^2}{\text{C}^2}$$

This is the value of k you should use unless you're specifically given another value (which would happen only if the charges were embedded in some insulating material that weakens the electric force).

The absolute value sign in the formula gives the magnitude of the force, whether repulsive or attractive. If direction (e.g., + or −) needs to be assigned, it should be done based on the fact that like charges (two positives or two negatives) repel each other, and opposite charges (one positive and one negative) attract. Note that the two electric forces in each of the following diagrams form an action–reaction pair.

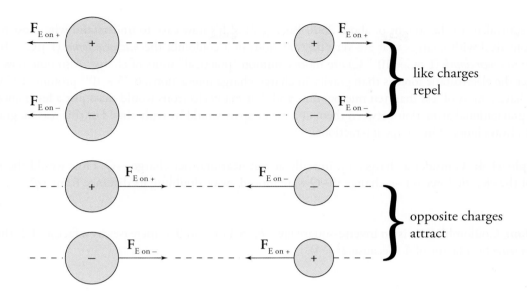

Example 41-2: Two charges, $q_1 = -2 \times 10^{-6}$ C and $q_2 = +5 \times 10^{-6}$ C, are separated by a distance of 10 cm. Describe the electric force between these particles.

Solution: Using Coulomb's Law, we find that

$$F_E = k_0 \frac{|q_1| q_2}{r^2} = (9 \times 10^9 \; \frac{\text{N·m}^2}{\text{C}^2}) \frac{(2 \times 10^{-6} \text{ C})(+5 \times 10^{-6} \text{ C})}{(10^{-1} \text{m})^2} = 9 \text{ N}$$

Since one charge is positive and one is negative, the force is attractive, and each charge feels a 9 N force toward the other.

Example 41-3: A coulomb is a *lot* of charge. To get some idea just how much, imagine that we had two objects, each with a charge of 1 C, separated by a distance of 1 m. What would be the electric force between them?

Solution: Using Coulomb's Law, we'd find that

$$F_E = k_0 \frac{q_1 q_2}{r^2} = (9 \times 10^9 \; \frac{\text{N·m}^2}{\text{C}^2}) \frac{(1 \text{ C})(1 \text{C})}{(1 \text{ m})^2} = 9 \times 10^9 \text{ N}$$

To write this answer in terms of a more familiar unit, let's use the fact that 1 pound (1 lb) is about 4.5 N, and 1 ton is 2000 lb:

$$F_E = (9 \times 10^9 \; \frac{\text{N·m}^2}{\text{C}^2}) \cdot \frac{1 \text{ lb}}{4.5 \text{ N}} \cdot \frac{1 \text{ ton}}{2000 \text{ lb}} = \text{one million tons}$$

That's equivalent to the weight of about 2500 Boeing 747s! It's now easy to understand why most real-life situations deal with charges that are very tiny fractions of a coulomb; the *microcoulomb* (1 μC = 10^{-6} C) and the *nanocoulomb* (1 nC = 10^{-9} C) are more common "practical" units of charge. Also note how much stronger the electrostatic force is than gravity in charge-charge interactions. 6.25×10^{18} protons (1 C worth) would have a mass of less than ten micrograms, and that many electrons would mass just a few nanograms, so the gravitational attraction between them at a meter apart would by truly tiny! For this reason, gravity is almost always ignored in charge interactions.

Example 41-4: Consider a charge, $+q$, initially at rest near another charge, $-Q$. How would the magnitude of the electric force on $+q$ change if $-Q$ were moved away, doubling its distance from $+q$?

Solution: Coulomb's Law is an inverse-square law, $F_E \propto 1/r^2$, so if r increases by a factor of 2, then F_E will *decrease* by a factor of 4 (because $2^2 = 4$).

The Principle of Superposition for Electric Forces

Coulomb's Law tells us how to calculate the force that one charge exerts on another one. What if two (or more) charges affect a third one? For example, what is the electric force on q_3 in the following figure?

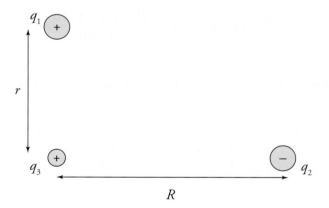

Here's the answer: if $\mathbf{F}_{1\text{-on-}3}$ is the force that q_1 *alone* exerts on q_3 (ignoring the presence of q_2) and if $\mathbf{F}_{2\text{-on-}3}$ is the force that q_2 *alone* exerts on q_3 (ignoring the presence of q_1), then the total force that q_3 feels is simply the vector sum $\mathbf{F}_{1\text{-on-}3} + \mathbf{F}_{2\text{-on-}3}$. The fact that we can calculate the effect of several charges by considering them individually and then just adding the resulting forces is known as the **principle of superposition**. (This important property will also be used when we study electric field vectors, electric potential, magnetic fields, and magnetic forces.)

The Principle of Superposition

The net electric force on a charge (q) due to a collection of other charges (Q's)

is equal to

the sum of the individual forces that each of the Q's alone exerts on q.

Example 41-5: In the preceding figure, assume that $q_1 = 2$ C, $q_2 = -8$ C, and $q_3 = 1$ nC. If $r = 1$ m and $R = 2$ m, which one of the following vectors best illustrates the direction of the net electric force on q_3?

A. ↖   C. ↘

B. ↗   D. ↙

Solution: The individual forces $\mathbf{F}_{1\text{-on-3}}$ and $\mathbf{F}_{2\text{-on-3}}$ are shown in the figure below. Adding these vectors gives $\mathbf{F}_{\text{on 3}}$, which points down to the right, so the answer is choice C.

q_1

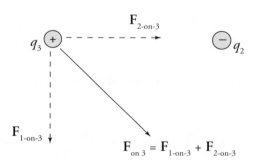

$$F_{1\text{-}on\text{-}3} = k_0 \frac{q_1 q_3}{r^2} = \left(9 \times 10^9 \, \frac{N \cdot m^2}{C^2}\right) \frac{(2 \text{ C})(1 \times 10^{-9} \text{ C})}{(1 \text{ m})^2} = 18 \text{ N}$$

(repulsive; away from q_1)

$$F_{2\text{-}on\text{-}3} = k_0 \frac{|q_2| q_3}{R^2} = \left(9 \times 10^9 \, \frac{N \cdot m^2}{C^2}\right) \frac{(8 \text{ C})(1 \times 10^{-9} \text{ C})}{(2 \text{ m})^2} = 18 \text{ N}$$

(attractive; toward q_2)

If the question had asked for the magnitude of the net electric force on q_3, then we'd use the Pythagorean Theorem to find the length of the vector $\mathbf{F}_{on\,3}$. The vector $\mathbf{F}_{on\,3}$ is the hypotenuse of the right triangle whose legs are $\mathbf{F}_{1\text{-on-}3}$ and $\mathbf{F}_{2\text{-on-}3}$, so the magnitude of $\mathbf{F}_{on\,3}$ is found like this:

$$(\mathbf{F}_{on\,3})^2 = (\mathbf{F}_{1\text{-on-}3})^2 + (\mathbf{F}_{2\text{-on-}3})^2$$
$$= 18^2 + 18^2$$
$$= (18^2)(2)$$
$$\therefore \mathbf{F}_{on\,3} = 18\sqrt{2} \approx 25\,\text{N}$$

$\mathbf{F}_{2\text{-on-}3}$

18 N

$\mathbf{F}_{on\,3} = 18\sqrt{2}\,N$

18 N $\Big\}$ $\mathbf{F}_{1\text{-on-}3}$

Example 41-6: In the figure below, assume that $q_1 = 1$ C, $q_2 = -1$ nC, and $q_3 = 8$ C. If q_4 is a negative charge, what must its value be in order for the net electric force on q_2 to be zero?

q_1 $\quad$ q_2 $\quad\quad\quad\quad\quad\quad$ q_3 $\quad\quad$ q_4

(+) - - - - - (−) - - - - - - - - - - - - - - - (+) - - - - - (−)

1 m $\quad\quad\quad$ 2 m $\quad\quad\quad$ 1 m

Solution: The individual forces $\mathbf{F}_{1\text{-on-}2}$, $\mathbf{F}_{3\text{-on-}2}$, and $\mathbf{F}_{4\text{-on-}2}$ are shown in the figure below. Notice that $\mathbf{F}_{1\text{-on-}2}$ and $\mathbf{F}_{4\text{-on-}2}$ point to the left, while $\mathbf{F}_{3\text{-on-}2}$ points to the right.

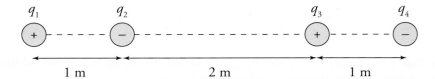

If we let $q_4 = -x$ C, then the magnitudes of the individual forces on q_2 are

$$F_{1\text{-on-}2} = k_0 \frac{|q_1||q_2|}{(r_{1-2})^2} = (9 \times 10^9 \,\tfrac{\text{N·m}^2}{\text{C}^2}) \frac{(1\,\text{C})(1\,\text{nC})}{(1\,\text{m})^2} = 9\,\text{N}$$

$$F_{3\text{-on-}2} = k_0 \frac{|q_2||q_3|}{(r_{2-3})^2} = (9 \times 10^9 \,\tfrac{\text{N·m}^2}{\text{C}^2}) \frac{(1\,\text{nC})(8\,\text{C})}{(2\,\text{m})^2} = 18\,\text{N}$$

$$F_{4\text{-on-}2} = k_0 \frac{|q_2||q_4|}{(r_{2-4})^2} = (9 \times 10^9 \,\tfrac{\text{N·m}^2}{\text{C}^2}) \frac{(1\,\text{nC})(x\,\text{C})}{(3\,\text{m})^2} = x\,\text{N}$$

In order for the net electric force on q_2 to be zero, the sum of the magnitudes of $\mathbf{F}_{1\text{-on-}2}$ and $\mathbf{F}_{4\text{-on-}2}$ must be equal to the magnitude of $\mathbf{F}_{3\text{-on-}2}$. That is, $9\,\text{N} + x\,\text{N} = 18\,\text{N}$, so $x = 9$. Therefore, $q_4 = -x$ C $= -9$ C.

41.3 ELECTRIC FIELDS

There are several advantages to regarding electrical interactions in a slightly different way from the simple "charge Q exerts a force on charge q," action-at-a-distance mode of thinking. In this more sophisticated interpretation, the very existence of a charge (or a more general distribution of charge) alters the space around it, creating what we call an **electric field** in its vicinity. If a second charge happens to be there or to roam by, it will feel the effect of the field created by the original charge. That is, we think of the electric force on a second charge q as exerted *by the field*, rather than directly by the original charge(s). (In an analogous way, the presence of mass creates a gravitational field filling the space around it, with which other masses then interact to experience a force of gravity.) Qualitatively, we can represent electrical interactions as follows:

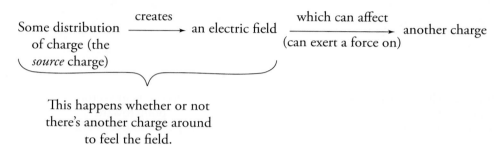

The charge(s) creating the electric field is/are called the **source charge(s)**; they're the source of the electric field. You may like to think of a source charge as a spider and its electric field as the spider's web. After a spider creates a web, when a small insect roams by, it is the web that ensnares the unfortunate bug, not the spider directly.

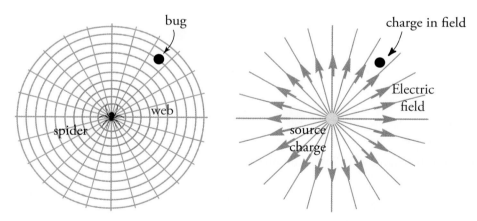

The figure on the right above illustrates one way to picture an electric field, but a few words of explanation are needed. First, an electric field is a **vector field**, which means that at each point in space surrounding the source charge, we associate a specific vector. The length of this vector will tell us the magnitude, or strength, of the field at that point, and the direction of the vector will tell us the direction of the resulting electric force that a *positive* test charge would feel if it were placed at that point. That's the convention: although the charge that finds itself in an electric field can of course be positive or negative, for purposes of *illustrating* the field, we always think of a *positive* test charge. Because of this convention, *electric field vectors always point away from positive source charges and toward negative ones*. Also, the closer we are to the source charge, the stronger the resulting electric force a test charge would feel (because Coulomb's Law is an *inverse*-square law). So, we expect the electric field vectors to be long at points close to the source charge and shorter at points farther away. The following figures illustrate the electric field due to a positive source charge and the electric field due to a negative source charge.

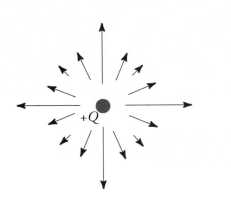

Electric field vectors
point away from
a positive source charge.

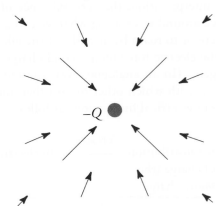

Electric field vectors
point toward
a negative source charge.

We can use Coulomb's Law to find a formula for the strength of the electric field due to a point charge. Remember that a source charge creates an electric field whether or not there's another charge in the field to feel it. It takes *two* charges to create an electric *force*, but it takes only *one* (the source charge) to create an electric *field*. So, let's imagine we have a single source charge, Q, and another charge, q, at a distance r from Q.

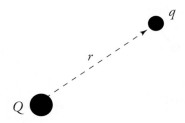

The force by Q, on the charge q, is, by Coulomb's Law,

$$F_{\text{by } Q} = k \frac{|Q||q|}{r^2}$$

Now we ask, "What if q weren't there? Do we still have something?" The answer is *yes*, we have the electric field created by the source charge, Q. "So, if q weren't there, what if we removed q from the formula for the force exerted on it by Q? Would we still have something?" The answer is *yes*, we'd have the formula for the electric field, **E**, created by the single source charge Q.

Electric Field

$$E_{\text{by } Q} = k\frac{|Q|}{r^2}$$

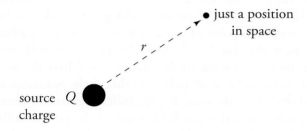

In the formula for the force by Q on q, the variable r represents the distance from Q to q. However, if q is not there, what does r mean now? Answer: It's simply the distance from Q to the point in space where we want to know the electric field vector.

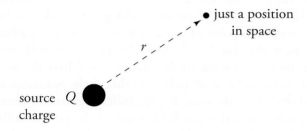

Example 41-7: Let $Q = +4$ nC be a charge that is fixed in position at the origin of an x-y coordinate system. What is the magnitude and direction of the electric field at the point (10 cm, 0)? At the point (–20 cm, 0)?

Solution: In the figure below, the point A is (10 cm, 0), which is 10 cm directly to the right of Q, and B is the point (–20 cm, 0), which is 20 cm directly to the left of Q.

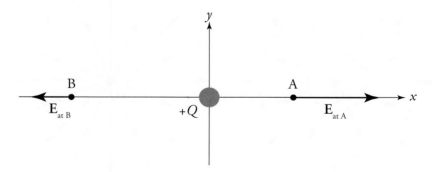

The electric field at point A is

$$E_{\text{at A}} = k_0\frac{Q}{(r_{\text{to A}})^2} = (9\times10^9\ \tfrac{\text{N·m}^2}{\text{C}^2})\frac{(4\times10^{-9}\ \text{C})}{(10^{-1}\ \text{m})^2} = 3600\ \tfrac{\text{N}}{\text{C}}$$

Since Q is positive, this means the electric field vector, $\mathbf{E}_{\text{at A}}$, points away from the source charge. Therefore, $\mathbf{E}_{\text{at A}}$ points in the positive x direction, which is usually written as the direction $\mathbf{i}$. So, if we wanted to write the complete electric field vector at point A, we'd write $\mathbf{E}_{\text{at A}} = (3600\ \text{N/C})\mathbf{i}$.

The electric field at point B is

$$E_{\text{at B}} = k_0 \frac{Q}{(r_{\text{to B}})^2} = (9 \times 10^9 \, \tfrac{\text{N·m}^2}{\text{C}^2}) \frac{(4 \times 10^{-9} \, \text{C})}{(2 \times 10^{-1} \, \text{m})^2} = 900 \tfrac{\text{N}}{\text{C}}$$

Once again, $\mathbf{E}_{\text{at B}}$ points away from the source charge. Therefore, $\mathbf{E}_{\text{at B}}$ points in the negative x direction, which is usually written as the direction $-\mathbf{i}$. So, if we wanted to write the complete electric field vector at point B, we'd write $\mathbf{E}_{\text{at B}} = (900 \text{ N/C})(-\mathbf{i})$ or $-(900 \text{ N/C})\mathbf{i}$.

Notice from the formula $E = k|Q|/r^2$ that the electric field obeys an inverse-square law, like the electric force. So the strength of an electric field from a single source charge decreases as we get farther from the source; in particular, $E \propto 1/r^2$. Also, for a given source charge Q, the electric field strength depends only on r, the distance from Q. So at every point on a circle (or more generally a sphere) of radius r centered on the source charge, the electric field strength is the same. In the electric field vector diagram below on the left, all the field vectors at the points on the smaller dashed circle have the same length, indicating that the electric field magnitude is the same at all points on this circle. Similarly, all the field vectors at the points on the larger dashed circle have the same length, indicating that the electric field magnitude is the same at all points on *this* circle. (Note that the field vectors at the points on the larger circle are shorter than those at the points on the smaller circle.) However, notice that the magnitude may be the same at every point on each circle (because they're all the same distance r from the source charge) but the directions of the electric field vectors are all different on each circle. Therefore, we're forced to say that the electric field isn't the same at every point a distance r from Q because the directions are all different.

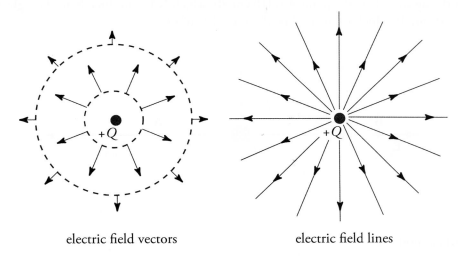

electric field vectors   electric field lines

The diagram on the left above and the two given earlier for the electric field produced by a positive source charge and by a negative source charge show the field represented by individual vectors. However, this is not the easiest way to draw an electric field.

Instead of drawing a bunch of separate vectors, we instead draw *lines* through them, like in the diagram on the right above. This drawing depicts the electric field using **field lines**. The direction of the field is indicated as usual; remember that, by convention, the electric field points away from positive source charges and toward negative ones and indicates the direction of the electric force that a positive test charge would feel if it were placed in the field.

Now that we've eliminated the separate vectors, it seems as though we've lost some information—namely, where the field is strong and where it's weak—because we got this information from the lengths of the individual vectors. (Where the vectors were long, the field was strong, and where the vectors were shorter, the field was weaker.) However, we can still get a general idea of where the field is strong and where it's weak by looking at the *density* of the field lines: where the field lines are cramped close together, the field is stronger; where the field lines are more spread out, the field is weaker.

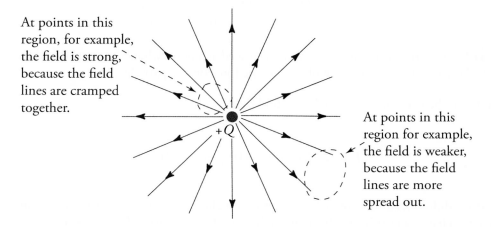

At points in this region, for example, the field is strong, because the field lines are cramped together.

At points in this region for example, the field is weaker, because the field lines are more spread out.

$+Q$

Now, let's imagine that we have a source charge Q creating an electric field, and another charge, q, roams in to the field. What force will q feel? We want to find an equation for the force on q due to the electric field. Recall the formulas above: $F_{on\,q} = k|Qq|/r^2$ and $E_{by\,Q} = k|Q|/r^2$. What would we need to do to E to get F? Just multiply it by q! That is, $F_{on\,q} = |q|E_{by\,q}$. It turns out that this very important formula works not just for the electric field created by a single source charge; it works for *any* electric field:

Electric Force and Field

$$\mathbf{F}_{on\,q} = q\mathbf{E}$$

Note that the absolute value symbol is useful when solving for the magnitude of force and electric field. The vector equation, $\mathbf{F}_E = q\mathbf{E}$, contains directional information and therefore does not need absolute values. Notice also from this formula that $E = F/|q|$, so the units of E are N/C, which you saw in Example 41-7. The equation $\mathbf{E} = \mathbf{F}/q$ also gives us the definition of the electric field: it's the force per unit charge.

Finally, before we get to some more examples, realize that we've had two important (boxed) formulas in this section on the electric field: $E = k|Q|/r^2$ and $\mathbf{F} = q\mathbf{E}$. In the first formula, Q is the charge that *makes* the field, while in the second formula, q is the charge that *feels* the field.

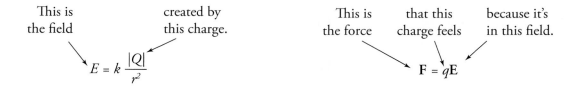

This is the field   created by this charge.   This is the force   that this charge feels   because it's in this field.

$E = k\dfrac{|Q|}{r^2}$ $\mathbf{F} = q\mathbf{E}$

41.3

Example 41-8: The magnitude of the electric field at a distance r from a source charge $+Q$ is equal to E. What will be the magnitude of the electric field at a distance $4r$ from a source charge $+2Q$?

Solution: The first sentence tells us that $kQ / r^2 = E$. Now, if we change Q to $2Q$ and r to $4r$, we find that E decreases by a factor of 8, because

$$E' = k\frac{Q'}{(r')^2} = k\frac{2Q}{(4r)^2} = \frac{2}{16} \cdot k\frac{Q}{r^2} = \frac{1}{8}E$$

Example 41-9: A particle with charge $q = 2\ \mu C$ is placed at a point where the electric field has magnitude 4×10^4 N/C. What will be the strength of the electric force on the particle?

Solution: From the equation $F_{on\ q} = qE$, we find that

$$F = (2 \times 10^{-6}\ C)(4 \times 10^{-4}\ \tfrac{N}{C}) = 8 \times 10^{-2}\ N$$

Notice that we didn't need to know what created the field. If E is given, and the question asks for the force that some charge q feels in this field, all we have to do is multiply, $F = qE$, and we're done.

Example 41-10: In the diagram on the left below, the electric field at Point A points in the positive y direction and has magnitude 5×10^6 N/C. (The source charge is not shown.) If a particle with charge $q = -3$ nC is placed at point A, what will be the electric force on the particle?

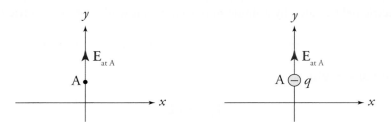

Solution: $\mathbf{E}_{at\ A}$ points in the positive y direction, sometimes, which for purposes of this question we will call "up," so $\mathbf{E}_{at\ A} = (5 \times 10^6\ \text{N/C})\mathbf{j}$. The equation $\mathbf{F}_{on\ q} = q\mathbf{E}$ then gives us

$$\mathbf{F} = (-3 \times 10^{-9})(5 \times 10^6\ \tfrac{N}{C})\mathbf{up} = (1.5 \times 10^{-2}\ N)(\mathbf{down})$$

That is, the force will have magnitude 1.5×10^{-2} N and point in the negative y direction. Notice that whenever q is negative, the force $F_{on\ q}$ will always point in the direction *opposite* to the electric field.

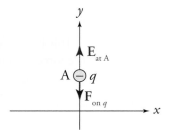

Example 41-11: A particle of mass m and charge q is placed at a point where the electric field is **E**. If the particle is released from rest, find its initial acceleration, **a**.

Solution: The acceleration of the particle is the force it feels divided by its mass: $\mathbf{a} = \mathbf{F}/m$. Because $\mathbf{F} = q\mathbf{E}$, we get

$$\mathbf{a} = \frac{\mathbf{F}}{m} = \frac{q\mathbf{E}}{m}$$

Notice that if q is negative, then **F** (and, consequently, **a**) will be directed *opposite* to the electric field **E**. Also, the question asked only for the *initial* acceleration, because once the particle starts moving, it will most likely move through locations where the electric field is different (in magnitude or direction or both), so the force on the particle will change; and if the force on the particle changes, so will the acceleration.

If a region contains a *uniform* electric field (that is, same magnitude and direction at all points within the region), then the electrostatic force and the particle's acceleration will likewise be uniform. The Big 5 kinematics equations can therefore be used to solve for final velocity, time, etc. In addition, the formula $W = Fd\cos\theta$ can also be used to calculate the work done by or against the electrostatic force to move a charge from one position to another. A large conducting plate that is charged (or a parallel plate capacitor, as detailed later in this chapter) creates an electric field that is approximately uniform.

Example 41-12: A uniform electric field of strength 4×10^6 N/C points to the left as shown in the figure on the next page. A particle with charge $q = -20$ nC and mass $m = 10$ g is initially placed at point B.

a)   If the particle is released from rest, toward which point will it move and how fast will it be traveling when it arrives?

b)   If the particle is again placed at point B and is now moved to point D, how much work is done "by the field"? (Note: In reality, forces do work, not fields; work done "by the field" is a commonly used expression.)

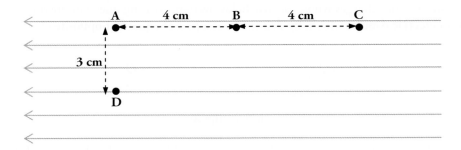

Solution:

a)   Negatively charged particles feel a force opposite the direction of the electric field, therefore, the particle will move to point C. To find the final speed, the acceleration must first be calculated using Newton's Second Law:

$$|q|E = ma$$

$$a = |q|E / m = (20 \times 10^{-9} \text{ C})(4 \times 10^6 \text{ N/C}) / (10 \times 10^{-3} \text{ kg}) = 8 \text{ m/s}^2$$

41.3

Using Big 5 #5,

$$v^2 = v_0^2 + 2ad = 0 + 2(8 \text{ m/s}^2)(0.04 \text{ m}) = 0.64 \text{ m}^2/\text{s}^2$$

v is therefore 0.8 m/s.

b) $W = Fd \cos\theta = |q|Ed \cos\theta$. Since $\theta > 90°$ the work done by the field is negative. $\triangle BAD$ is a 3-4-5 triangle, so $d = 5$ cm. More importantly, $\cos\theta = -4/5$. Therefore,

$$W = (20 \times 10^{-9} \text{ C})(4 \times 10^6 \text{ N/C})(0.05 \text{ m})(-4/5) = -3.2 \times 10^{-3} \text{ J}$$

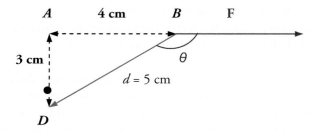

Notice that the work done by the field from point B to point D is the same as if the particle were moved from point B to point A. The field will only do work (whether positive or negative) if there is displacement in the direction of the electric field or opposite the field. This is similar to gravity, which only does work if there is displacement up or down. And as with gravity, the work done by the field is also path independent. This will be discussed in more depth later in the chapter.

The Principle of Superposition for Electric Fields

The pictures we've drawn so far have been of electric fields created by a single source charge. However, we can also have two or more charges whose electric fields overlap, creating one combined field. For example, let's consider an **electric dipole**, which, by definition, is a pair of equal but opposite charges:

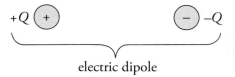

electric dipole

What if we regarded *both* of them as source charges; how would we find the electric field that they create together? By using the principle of superposition. If we wanted to find the electric field vector at, say, the point P in the diagram below,

P

we'd first find the electric field vector, $\mathbf{E}_+$, at P due to the +Q charge alone (ignoring the presence of the −Q charge) and then we'd find the electric field vector, $\mathbf{E}_-$, at P due to the −Q charge alone (ignoring the presence of the +Q charge). The net electric field vector at P will then be the vector sum, $\mathbf{E}_+ + \mathbf{E}_-$.

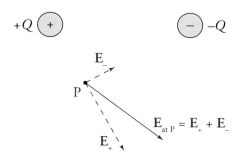

We can do this for as many points as we like and obtain a diagram of the electric field as a collection of vectors. The diagram in terms of electric field lines would look like this:

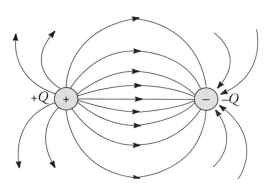

Notice that between the charges, where the field lines are dense, the field is strong; and as we move away from the charges, the field lines get more spread out, indicating that the field gets weaker.

Example 41-13: An electric dipole consists of two charges, +Q and −Q, where Q = 4 μC, separated by a distance of d = 20 cm. Find the electric field at the point midway between the charges.

Solution: The electric field at P due to the positive charge is $E_+ = k_0 Q / \left(\frac{1}{2}d\right)^2$, pointing away from +Q, and the electric field at P due to the negative charge is $E_- = k_0 Q / \left(\frac{1}{2}d\right)^2$, pointing toward −Q (which is in the same direction as $\mathbf{E}_+$).

$$+Q \,\bigoplus \qquad\qquad \mathrm{P} \cdot \overset{\mathbf{E}_+}{\underset{\mathbf{E}_-}{\longrightarrow}} \qquad \bigominus -Q$$

$$\overset{\longleftrightarrow}{\tfrac{1}{2}d} \qquad \overset{\longleftrightarrow}{\tfrac{1}{2}d}$$

By the principle of superposition, the net electric field at P is the sum: $\mathbf{E} = \mathbf{E}_+ + \mathbf{E}_-$. The magnitude of E_{atP} is E_{atP} is $E_+ + E_- = k_0 Q / \left(\frac{1}{2}d\right)^2 + k_0 Q / \left(\frac{1}{2}d\right)^2 = 2k_0 Q / \left(\frac{1}{2}d\right)^2$:

$$E = 2k_0 \frac{Q}{(\frac{1}{2}d)^2}$$
$$= 2(9 \times 10^9 \text{ } \tfrac{\text{N·m}^2}{\text{C}^2}) \frac{4 \times 10^{-6} \text{ C}}{(1 \times 10^{-1} \text{ m})^2}$$
$$= 7.2 \times 10^6 \text{ } \tfrac{\text{N}}{\text{C}}$$

The direction of $\mathbf{E}_{atP}$ is away from $+Q$ and toward $-Q$:

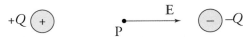

Example 41-14: A positive charge, $+q$, is placed at the point labeled P in the field of the dipole shown below. Describe the direction of the resulting electric force on the charge. Do the same for a negative charge, $-q$, placed at the point labeled N.

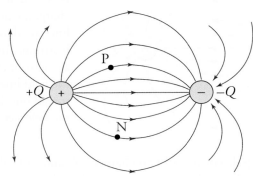

Solution: The electric field vector at any point is always *tangent* to the field line passing through that point and its direction is the same as that of the field line. Since $\mathbf{F} = q\mathbf{E}$, the force on a positive charge is in the same direction as $\mathbf{E}$ and the force on a negative charge is in the opposite direction from $\mathbf{E}$. The directions of $\mathbf{F}_{on\ q}$ and $\mathbf{F}_{on\ -q}$ are shown in the figure below.

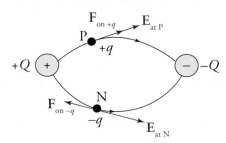

Conductors, Insulators, and Polarization

Most everyday materials can be classified into one of two major categories: *conductors* or *insulators* (also known as *dielectrics*). A material is a **conductor** if it contains charges that are free to roam throughout the material. Metals are the classic and most important conductors. In a metal, one or more valence electrons per atom are not strongly bound to any particular atom and are thus free to roam. If a metal is placed in an electric field, these free charges (called **conduction electrons**) will move in response to the field. Another example of a conductor would be a solution that contains lots of dissolved ions (such as saltwater).

Here's an interesting property of conductors: imagine that we place a whole bunch of electrons on a piece of metal. It's now negatively charged. Since electrons repel each other, they'll want to get as far away from each other as possible. As a result, all this excess charge moves (rapidly) to the surface. Any net charge on a conductor resides on its surface. Since there's no excess charge within the body of the conductor, there cannot be an electrostatic field inside a conductor. You can block out external electric fields simply by surrounding yourself with metal; the free charges in the metal will move to the surface to shield the interior and keep **E** = 0 inside.

By contrast, an **insulator** (**dielectric**) is a material that doesn't have free charges. Electrons are tightly bound to their atoms and thus are not free to roam throughout the material. Common insulators include rubber, glass, wood, paper, and plastic.

Now, let's study this situation: start with a neutral metal sphere and bring a charge (a positive charge) Q nearby without touching the original metal sphere. What will happen? The positive charge will attract free electrons in the metal, leaving the far side of the sphere positively charged. Since the negative charge is closer to Q than the positive charge, there'll be a net attraction between Q and the sphere. So, even though the sphere as a whole is electrically neutral, the separation of charge induced by the presence of Q will create a force of electrical attraction between them.

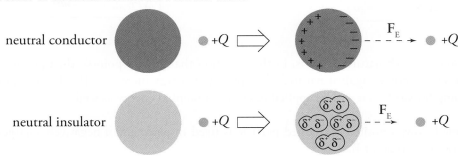

Now what if the sphere was made of glass (an insulator)? Although there aren't free electrons that can move to the near side of the sphere, the atoms that make up the sphere will become **polarized**. That is, their electrons will feel a tug toward Q, causing the atoms to develop a partial negative charge pointing toward Q (and a partial positive charge pointing away from Q). The effect isn't as dramatic as the mass movement of free electrons in the case of a metal sphere, but the polarization is still enough to cause an electrical attraction between the sphere and Q. For example, if you comb your hair, the comb will pick up extra electrons, making it negatively charged. If you place this electric field source near little bits of paper, the paper will become polarized and will then be attracted to the comb.[2]

---

[2] The same phenomenon, in which the presence of a charge tends to cause polarization in a nearby collection of charges, is responsible for a kind of intermolecular force: Dipole-induced dipole forces are caused by a shifting of the electron cloud of a neutral molecule toward positively charged ions or away from a negatively charged ion; in each case, the resulting force between the ion and the atom is attractive.

The **London dispersion force**, in which electrically neutral molecules temporarily induce polarization in each other, is a much weaker version of the same phenomenon—again, electron clouds shift a little bit to create dipoles.

41.4 ELECTRIC POTENTIAL AND POTENTIAL ENERGY

So far, we have viewed the electric field due to a source charge (or a more general charge distribution, such as a pair of charges or a plate) as a collection of vectors. This point of view allowed us to answer questions about other *vector* quantities, such as force and acceleration. The basic equations for finding these quantities were $\mathbf{F} = q\mathbf{E}$ and $\mathbf{a} = \mathbf{F}/m = q\mathbf{E}/m$.

What if we wanted to answer questions about *scalar* quantities, like energy, work, or speed? It turns out that the easiest way to answer these questions is to view the electric field in a different way, in terms of a scalar field. First, it is useful to review a few facts about gravitational potential energy. As you'll recall, if an object of mass m is dropped from rest from a height h and hits the ground, $W_{\text{by grav}} = +mgh$ while $\Delta PE_{\text{grav}} = -mgh$. Similarly, if the object is lifted from the ground to a height h, $W_{\text{by grav}} = -mgh$, $W_{\text{against grav}} = +mgh$ and $\Delta PE_{\text{grav}} = +mgh$.

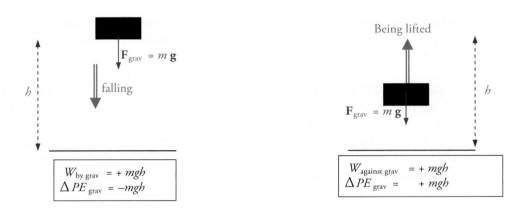

If an object moves "with nature" (that is, in the direction that gravity points), then potential energy decreases. If an object moves "against nature," then potential energy increases. This is an important fact to remember going forward, as it will be applied to electric potential energy as well.

In the example below, a positively charged particle is fixed in place and a negatively charged particle is moved from point A to point B.

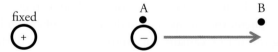

Without knowing the formula for electric potential energy, we can say that $\Delta PE_{\text{elec}} > 0$, since the particle is being moved "against nature."

Mathematically, we see that $W_{\text{by grav}} = -\Delta PE_{\text{grav}}$ and that $W_{\text{against grav}} = +\Delta PE_{\text{grav}}$. Similarly, we will be able to make an analogous statement about the relationship between the work done by or against the electric field and the change in electric potential energy. We will also be able to answer questions involving speed by using **Conservation of Mechanical Energy**.

41.4

To find the equation for electric potential energy, it is useful to first consider that charged particles not only create a vector field (that is, the electric field), they also create a scalar field.

This scalar field has a name: it's called **electric potential** (or just **potential** for short).

Let Q be a point source charge. At any point P that's a distance r from Q, we say that the electric potential at P is the scalar given by this formula:

Electric Potential

$$\phi = k\frac{Q}{r}$$

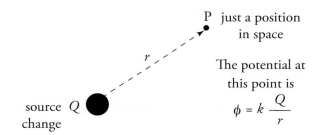

P just a position
in space

The potential at
this point is

$$\phi = k\frac{Q}{r}$$

source Q
change

Notice the differences between this formula and the one for the electric field. First, the potential is kQ divided by r, while the electric field is kQ divided by r^2. Second, the electric field has a specific direction at each point (because it's a vector quantity); the potential, on the other hand, is not a vector, so it has no direction. For this reason, no absolute value symbol is needed. The sign of the potential is important in determining the behavior of nearby charges if they are placed in the field. While the electric field has the same magnitude at every point a distance r from Q, the field has a different direction at every point on the circle (or, more generally, the sphere) of radius r centered on Q. Therefore, we're forced to say that the electric field isn't the same at every point a distance r from Q because the directions are all different. The potential, however, is easier because it has no direction: the potential *is* the same at every point that's a distance r from Q.

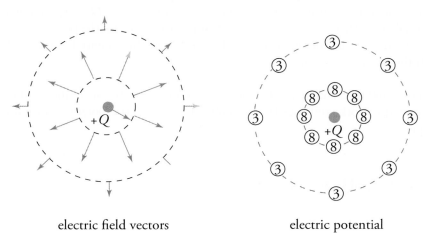

electric field vectors   electric potential

41.4

The dashed circles shown in the figure on the right above are called **equipotentials** ("equal potentials"), because the potential is the same at every point on them. For example, the potential is equal to 8 units everywhere on the inner dashed circle, and it is equal to 3 units everywhere on the outer dashed circle. As we move around on either dashed circle, the electric field changes (because the direction of **E** changes), but the potential doesn't change.

The formula given on the previous page for the potential, $\phi = kQ/r$, assumes that the potential decreases to 0 as we move far away from the source charges (that is, as $r \rightarrow \infty$); this is the standard, conventional assumption. With this formula, you can see that if Q is a positive charge, then the values of the potential due to this source charge are also positive (if Q is positive, then kQ/r is positive); on the other hand, the values of the potential due to a negative source charge are negative (if Q is negative, then kQ/r is negative). The sign of the potential (that is, whether it's positive or negative) is not an indication of a direction; remember, potential is a scalar, so it has no direction.

Before we get to some examples, it's important to mention that while there's no special name for the unit of electric field, there *is* a special name for the unit of electric potential:

$$[\phi] = [k]\frac{[Q]}{[r]} = (\tfrac{\text{N}\cdot\text{m}^2}{\text{C}^2})\frac{\text{C}}{\text{m}} = \frac{\text{N}\cdot\text{m}}{\text{C}} = \frac{\text{J}}{\text{C}}$$

A joule per coulomb (J/C) is called a **volt**, abbreviated V.

Example 41-15: In the figure below, the potential at Point A is 1,000 V. What's the potential at Point B?

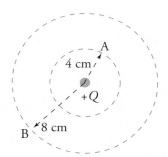

Solution: From the formula $\phi = k_0 Q / r$, we see that the potential is inversely proportional to r: Thus, $\phi \propto 1/r$. Because the distance from Q to B is twice the distance from Q to A, the potential at B should be half the potential at A. Therefore, $\phi_{at B} = 500\,\text{V}$. (Notice that because the potential at A is 1,000 V, the potential at *every* point on the inner circle is 1,000 V; and since the potential at B is 500 V, the potential at *every* point on the outer circle is 500 V.)

Now that we know how to calculate electric potential, how do we use it to answer questions about the scalar quantities energy, work, and speed? The applications of electric potential all follow from this one fundamental equation:

Change in Electrical Potential Energy

$$\Delta PE = q\Delta\phi = qV$$

That is, the change in potential energy of a charge q that moves between two points whose potential difference is $\Delta\phi$ is just given by the product, $q\Delta\phi$; it also can be expressed as qV, where V is defined in the change in potential and is known as the *voltage*. For example, let's say a charge $q = +0.03$ C moves from a point on the inner circle to a point on the outer circle in the figure accompanying the preceding example:

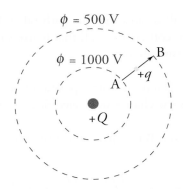

Then the change in the electrical potential energy of the charge q is

$$\Delta PE_{A \to B} = q\Delta\phi_{A \to B} = q(\phi_B - \phi_A) = (+0.03\,\text{C})(500\,\text{V} - 1000\,\text{V}) = -15\,\text{J}$$

We expected that the change in potential energy would be negative (that is, the potential energy would decrease), because the positive charge is moving farther from the positive source charge (that is, "with nature"). Because q moves in a way it naturally "wants" to move (since the positive charge q is naturally repelled by the positive charge Q), its potential energy should decrease.

If the charge q were instead pushed (by some outside force) from Point B to Point A (i.e., "against nature"), then its potential energy would increase:

$$\Delta PE_{B \to A} = q\Delta\phi_{B \to A} = q(\phi_A - \phi_B) = (+0.03\,\text{C})(1000\,\text{V} - 500\,\text{V}) = +15\,\text{J}$$

What if the charge q were moved from one point on the outer circle (Point B, say) to another point on the outer circle, B′?

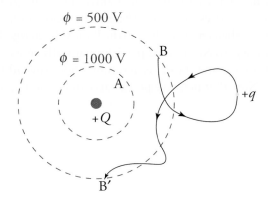

Its potential energy would not change. Because the potential is the same everywhere on the outer circle, the potential at B is the same as the potential at B′, so the potential *difference* between Points B and B′ is zero; and if $\Delta\phi = 0$, then $\Delta PE = 0$ as well. *A charge experiences no change in potential energy when its initial and final positions are at the same potential.*

The figure on the previous page also illustrates that the path taken by the charge is irrelevant. Like the gravitational force, the electric force is conservative; all that matters is where the charge began and where it ended; the specific path it takes doesn't matter.

Example 41-16: A charge $q = -8$ nC is moved from a position that's 10 cm from a charge $Q = +2$ μC to a position that's 20 cm away. What is the change in its electrical potential energy?

Solution: Let A be the initial point and B the final point; then the change in potential from Point A to Point B is

$$\Delta\phi = \phi_B - \phi_A = \frac{k_0 Q}{r_B} - \frac{k_0 Q}{r_A} = k_0 Q \left(\frac{1}{r_B} - \frac{1}{r_A} \right)$$
$$= (9 \times 10^9 \tfrac{\text{N} \cdot \text{m}^2}{\text{C}^2})(2 \times 10^{-6} \text{ C})\left(\tfrac{1}{0.2 \text{ m}} - \tfrac{1}{0.1 \text{ m}} \right)$$
$$= -9 \times 10^4 \text{ V}$$

Therefore, the change in potential energy of the charge q is

$$\Delta PE = q\Delta\phi = (-8 \times 10^{-9} \text{ C})(-9 \times 10^4 \text{ V}) = 7.2 \times 10^{-4} \text{ J}$$

We've seen that all charged particles naturally move to positions of lower potential energy. To accomplish this, notice in the preceding examples that *positively charged particles naturally tend toward lower potential and negatively charged particles tend toward higher potential.* To verify this mathematically, we have learned that $\Delta PE = q\Delta\phi$ or $\Delta\phi = \Delta PE / q$. Moving "naturally" means that ΔPE is negative. So if q is positive, then $\Delta\phi$ is $(-) / (+) = (-)$, which means that potential decreases. If q is negative, then $\Delta\phi$ is $(-) / (-) = (+)$, which means that potential increases.

A gravitational analogy may be useful. A positively charged particle can be thought of as any mass—it naturally "falls downward" when released from rest. Conversely, a negatively charged particle can be thought of as a helium balloon—it "rises upward." The electric field can be thought as **g**, which is a vector that points downward toward the center of the Earth. Positively charged particles therefore naturally move in the direction of **E** and negatively charged particles naturally move opposite **E**. Finally, potential can be thought of as height above ground. Positives naturally move toward lower potential and negatives move toward higher potential. Note that negative potentials can be thought of as "heights" below ground. The rules above still apply.

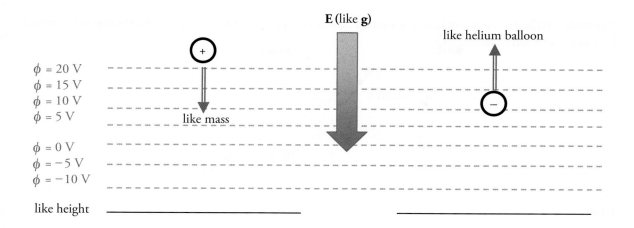

E (like g)

like helium balloon

$\phi = 20$ V

$\phi = 15$ V

$\phi = 10$ V

$\phi = 5$ V

like mass

$\phi = 0$ V

$\phi = -5$ V

$\phi = -10$ V

like height

Now that we've seen examples of how to calculate changes in potential energy in an electric field by using the concept of electric potential, how do we answer questions about work or kinetic energy? By using equations we already know from mechanics.

What if we want to find the work done by the electric field as a charge moves? If we move objects around in a *gravitational* field, we remember that the change in gravitational potential energy is equal to the opposite of the work done by the gravitational field. That is, $\Delta PE_{grav} = -W_{by\ gravity}$, which is the same as $W_{by\ gravity} = -\Delta PE_{grav}$. Applying this same idea to an electric field, we can say that the work done by the electric field is equal to $-\Delta PE_{elec}$:

Work Done by Electric Field

$$W_{by\ electric\ field} = -\Delta PE_{elec}$$

Now what about kinetic energy? Well, if there's no friction (which will be the case for charges moving around in empty space) or other forces doing work as a charge moves, then mechanical energy is conserved; that is, $KE + PE$ will remain constant. And if $KE + PE$ is constant, then $\Delta KE + \Delta PE = 0$.

So, as long as you remember the fundamental formula for potential energy changes in an electric field, $\Delta PE = q\Delta\phi$, you can answer questions about work or kinetic energy in an electric field by just using the formulas above.

41.4

Example 41-17: In the figure below, a particle whose charge q is +4 nC moves in the electric field created by a negative source charge, $-Q$.

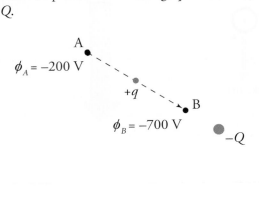

$\phi_A = -200$ V

A

+q

B

$\phi_B = -700$ V

$-Q$

Find:

a) the change in potential energy,
b) the work done by the electric field, and
c) the change in kinetic energy of the particle as it moves from position A to position B.
d) If the mass of the particle is 10^{-8} kg and it started from rest at Point A, what will be its speed as it passes through Point B?

Solution:

a) $\Delta PE = q\Delta\phi = q\left(\phi_B - \phi_A\right) = \left(4\times10^9\,\text{C}\right)\left[\left(-700\,\text{V}\right) - \left(-200\,\text{V}\right)\right] = -2\times10^{-6}\,\text{J}$

b) $W_{\text{by electric field}} = -\Delta PE_{\text{elec}} = -\left(-2\times10^{-6}\,\text{J}\right) = 2\times10^{-6}\,\text{J}$

c) $\Delta KE = \Delta PE_{\text{elec}} = -\left(-2\times10^{-6}\,\text{J}\right) = +2\times10^{-6}\,\text{J}$

d) If the particle started from rest at Point A, then $PE_{\text{at B}} = \Delta KE = +2\times10^{-6}$ J, so

$$\frac{1}{2}mv_B^2 = 2\times10^{-6}\,\text{J} \rightarrow v_B^2 = \frac{2(2\times10^{-6}\,\text{J})}{m} \rightarrow v_B = \sqrt{\frac{4\times10^{-6}\,\text{J}}{10^{-8}\,\text{kg}}} = \sqrt{400\,\text{m}^2/\text{s}^2} = 20\,\text{m/s}$$

Example 41-18: An electric field pulls an electron from one position to another such that the change in potential is +1 V. By how much does the electron's kinetic energy change?

Solution: The change in potential energy is

$$\Delta PE = q\Delta\phi = (-1.6\times10^{-19}\,\text{C})(+1\,\text{V}) = -1.6\times10^{-19}\,\text{J}$$

so the change in kinetic energy is the opposite of this, +1.6 × 10⁻¹⁹ C. This amount of energy is known as 1 **electron volt** (**eV**). In fact, the abbreviation for this unit makes the definition easy to remember: an electron (e⁻) moving through a potential difference of 1 V experiences a kinetic energy change of

$-q\Delta\phi = (e)(1\,\mathrm{V}) = 1.6\times10^{-19}\,\mathrm{J} = 1$ eV. While the joule is the SI unit for energy, it's too big to be convenient when discussing atomic-sized systems. The electron volt is commonly used instead.

Example 41-19: An electric field pushes a proton from one position to another such that the change in potential is –500 V. By how much does the kinetic energy of the proton increase, in electron volts?

Solution: The change in potential energy is

$$\Delta PE = q\Delta\phi = (+e)(-500\,\mathrm{V}) = -500\,\mathrm{eV}$$

so the change in kinetic energy, ΔKE, is $-\Delta PE = -(-500\text{ eV}) = +500$ eV.

The Principle of Superposition for Electric Potential

The formula $\phi = kQ/r$ tells us how to find the potential due to a single point source charge, Q. To find the potential in an electric field that's created by more than one charge, we use the principle of superposition. In fact, applying this principle is even easier here than for electric forces and fields because potential is a scalar. When we add up individual potentials, we're simply adding numbers; we're not adding vectors.

Let's illustrate with an example. In the figure below, the source charges Q_1 = +10 nC and Q_2 = –5 nC are fixed in the positions shown; the charges and the two points, A and B, form the vertices of a rectangle. What is the potential at Point A? At Point B?

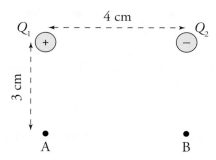

The potential at Point A due to Q_1 alone (ignoring the presence of Q_2) is

$$\phi_{A1} = k_0\frac{Q_1}{r_{A1}} = (9\times10^9\ \tfrac{\mathrm{N\cdot m^2}}{\mathrm{C^2}})\frac{+10\times10^{-9}\ \mathrm{C}}{3\times10^{-2}\ \mathrm{m}} = 3000\ \mathrm{V}$$

Since Point A is 5 cm from Q_2 (it's the hypotenuse of a 3-4-5 right triangle), the potential at Point A due to Q_2 alone (ignoring the presence of Q_1) is

$$\phi_{A2} = k_0\frac{Q_2}{r_{A2}} = (9\times10^9\ \tfrac{\mathrm{N\cdot m^2}}{\mathrm{C^2}})\frac{-5\times10^{-9}\ \mathrm{C}}{5\times10^{-2}\ \mathrm{m}} = -900\ \mathrm{V}$$

Therefore, the total electric potential at Point A, due to both source charges, is

$$\phi_A = \phi_{A1} + \phi_{A2} = (3000\,\text{V}) + (-900\,\text{V}) = 2100\,\text{V}$$

Similarly, the total electric potential at Point B is

$$\phi_B = \phi_{B1} + \phi_{B2} = k_0\frac{Q_1}{r_{B1}} + k_0\frac{Q_2}{r_{B2}}$$
$$= (9\times10^9\;\tfrac{\text{N·m}^2}{\text{C}^2})\frac{+10\times10^{-9}\;\text{C}}{5\times10^{-2}\;\text{m}} + (9\times10^9\;\tfrac{\text{N·m}^2}{\text{C}^2})\frac{-5\times10^{-9}\;\text{C}}{3\times10^{-2}\;\text{m}}$$
$$= (1800\,\text{V}) + (-1500\,\text{V})$$
$$= 300\,\text{V}$$

Example 41-20: A charge $q = 1$ nC is moved from position A to position B, along the path labeled *a* in the figure below. Find the work done by the electric field. How would your answer change if q had been moved from position A to position B, along the path labeled *b*?

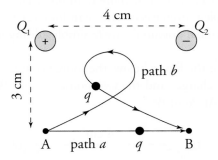

Solution: Path *a* begins at Point A, where $\phi_A = 2100\,\text{V}$, and ends at Point B, where $\phi_B = 300\,\text{V}$, so $\Delta\phi_{A\rightarrow B} = \phi_B - \phi_A = 300\,\text{V} - 2100\,\text{V} = -1800\,\text{V}$. Therefore, the change in potential energy of the charge q is

$$\Delta PE = q\Delta\phi = (1\times10^{-9}\;\text{C})(-1800\;\text{V}) = -1.8\times10^{-6}\,\text{J}$$

This means that the work done by the electric field, $W_{by\,E}$, is equal to $-\Delta PE = 1.8\times10^{-6}$ J. If q had followed path *b*, the change in potential energy and the work done by the electric field would have been the same as for path *a*. The shape or length of the path is irrelevant; all that matters is the initial point and the ending point, and both paths begin at Point A and end at Point B.

We can't use the formula "work = force × distance" here, because the force is not constant during the object's displacement. To calculate work in an electric field, we use electric potential and the formula $W_{by\,E} = -\Delta PE_{elec}$.

Example 41-21: An electric dipole consists of a pair of equal but opposite charges, $+Q$ and $-Q$, separated by a distance d. What is the electric potential at the point (call it P) that's midway between these source charges?

Solution: The potential at P due to the positive charge alone is $k(+Q)/\left(\frac{1}{2}d\right)$, and the potential at P due to the negative charge alone is $k(-Q)/\left(\frac{1}{2}d\right)$. Adding these, we get zero, which is the potential at P due to both charges. (Notice that although the potential at P is zero, the electric field at P is *not* zero. We can have the "opposite" situation as well; that is, it's possible to have a point where the electric field is zero, but the potential is not. For example, if we had two equal source charges of the *same* sign, say $+Q$ and $+Q$, separated by a distance d, then the potential at the point that's midway between them would not be zero [it would be $2k(+Q)/\left(\frac{1}{2}d\right)$] but the electric field there *would* be zero.)

Example 41-22: An electric dipole consists of a pair of equal but opposite charges, $+Q$ and $-Q$, separated by a distance d. The dashed curves in the figure below are equipotentials. (Notice that the equipotentials are always perpendicular to the electric field lines, wherever they intersect. This is true for *any* electrostatic field, not just for the field created by a dipole.)

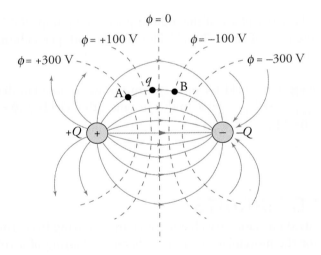

If a particle of mass $m = 1 \times 10^{-6}$ kg and charge $q = 5$ nC starts from rest at Point A and moves to Point B,

a) How much work is done by the electric field?
b) What is the speed of the particle when it reaches Point B?

Solution:

a) The work done by the electric field is equal to the opposite of the change in the particle's electrical potential energy $W_{\text{by E}} = -\Delta PE_{\text{elec}}$. Since the potential at Point A is $\phi_A = +300\,\text{V}$ (because A lies on the $\phi = +300\,\text{V}$ equipotential) and the potential at Point B is $\phi_B = -100\,\text{V}$ (because B lies on the $\phi = -100\,\text{V}$ equipotential), the change in potential from A to B is

$\phi_B - \phi_A = (-100\text{ V}) - (300\text{ V}) = -400\text{ V}$. Therefore,

$$W_{\text{by E}} = -\Delta PE_{\text{elec}} = -q\Delta\phi = -(5 \times 10^{-9}\text{ C})(-400\text{ V}) = 2 \times 10^{-6}\text{ J}$$

b) Since the total work done on the particle is equal to its change in kinetic energy (the Work-Energy Theorem), we have $\Delta KE = 2 \times 10^{-6}\text{ J}$. Because the particle started from rest at Point A, we have $KE_{\text{at B}} = \Delta KE_{\text{A} \to \text{B}} = 2 \times 10^{-6}\text{ J}$, so

$$\frac{1}{2}mv_B^2 = 2 \times 10^{-6}\text{ J} \rightarrow v_B = \sqrt{\frac{2(2 \times 10^{-6}\text{ J})}{1 \times 10^{-6}\text{ kg}}} = 2\tfrac{\text{m}}{\text{s}}$$

Example 41-23: During the active phase of the sodium-potassium pump, Na^+ ions are moved out of the cell against a potential difference of about 70 mV. How much work per sodium ion is done against the electric field during this process?

Solution: The work done against a field (or on a system, to use a more familiar phrasing for the same concept) is given by $W_{\text{against E}} = \Delta PE_{\text{elec}} = q\Delta\phi$. In this instance, that yields $q\Delta\phi = (1.6 \times 10^{-19}\text{ C})(7 \times 10^{-2}\text{ V}) \approx 11 \times 10^{-21}\text{ J} = 1.1 \times 10^{-20}\text{ J}$.

41.5 ELECTRIC CIRCUITS

So far we have mostly focused on stationary charges or charges moving freely through space. An **electric circuit** is a set pathway for the movement of electric charge, consisting of a voltage source, connecting wires, and other components.

Current

Current can be defined as the movement of charge, but for the purposes of analyzing an electric circuit, we need a more precise definition. For example, imagine picking up a metal paper clip and untwisting it to make it relatively straight. If we could look inside this piece of metal wire at the individual atoms, we would see a lattice with about one electron per atom free to roam freely, unbound to any particular atom. These free electrons are known as **conduction electrons**. The conduction electrons in a metal are zooming around throughout the lattice at very high speeds. However, we only have a current when there is a *net* movement of charge. Let's look at this a little more closely.

The figure below shows an imagined magnified view inside a metal wire. The conduction electrons move at an average speed on the order of a million meters per second ($v \sim 10^6$ m/s). If we chose any cross-sectional slice of the wire, we would see that these conduction electrons cross from left to right as often as they cross from right to left. So, while there is movement of charge, there's no *net* movement of charge; that is, there's no current.

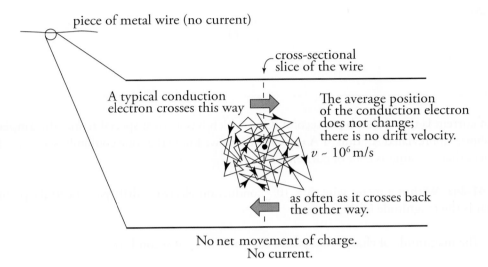

piece of metal wire (no current)

cross-sectional
slice of the wire

A typical conduction
electron crosses this way

The average position
of the conduction electron
does not change;
there is no drift velocity.

$v \sim 10^6$ m/s

as often as it crosses back
the other way.

No net movement of charge.
No current.

So how would this same piece of wire look if there *were* current in it? Superimposed on the conduction electrons' going-nowhere-fast zooming, we would see that there's a slight drift in one particular direction. This is known as the electrons' **drift velocity** (v_d). If we chose any cross-sectional slice of the wire, we'd see that these conduction electrons move across it from, say, left to right more often than they cross back. Thus, the average positions of the conduction electrons do change and there is a *net* movement of charge (in the case pictured below, negative charge to the right). This is **current**.

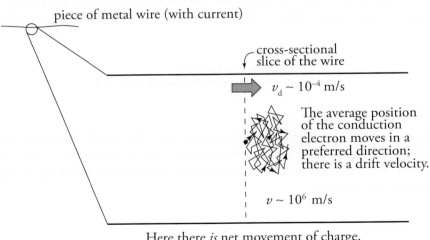

piece of metal wire (with current)

cross-sectional
slice of the wire

$v_d \sim 10^{-4}$ m/s

The average position
of the conduction
electron moves in a
preferred direction;
there is a drift velocity.

$v \sim 10^6$ m/s

Here there *is* net movement of charge.
This is current.

In the first figure, there was no drift velocity and, therefore, no preferred direction for the movement of charge and no current. In the figure above, however, there is a drift velocity, so there is a flow of charge: a current.

Now, how do we measure current? Since current is the flow of charge, it makes sense to measure current as the amount of charge that moves past a certain point per unit time. Current is denoted by the letter I, and it is equal to charge (Q) divided by time (t):

Current

$$I = \frac{Q}{t}$$

The unit of current is the coulomb per second (C/s), which has its own special name: the **ampère** (or just **amp**, for short), abbreviated **A**. Thus, 1 A = 1 C/s.[3] Since we know that one coulomb is a lot of charge, we would expect that one amp is a lot of current.

Example 41-24: Within a metal wire, 5×10^{17} conduction electrons drift past a certain point in 4 seconds. What is the magnitude of the current?

Solution: The magnitude of charge that passes the point in $t = 4$ seconds is

$$Q = ne = (5 \times 10^{17})(1.6 \times 10^{-19} \text{ C}) = 8 \times 10^{-2} \text{ C}$$

Therefore, the value of the current is

$$I = \frac{Q}{t} = \frac{8 \times 10^{-2} \text{ C}}{4 \text{ s}} = 0.02 \text{ A}$$

Example 41-25: A typical ion channel in a cellular membrane might allow the passage of 10^7 sodium ions to flow through in one second. What is the magnitude and direction of this ionic current?

Solution:

$$I = \frac{Q}{t} = \frac{(10^7)1.6 \times 10^{-19} \text{ C}}{1 \text{ s}} = 1.6 \times 10^{-12} \text{ A}$$

Because sodium ions are positive, the direction of current flow is the same as the one in which the charges are moving. (It is interesting to note that this current of ions into and out of the cell does not obey Ohm's Law—more on that one later on—generally, so predicting the current based upon voltage difference across the membrane is impossible.)

---

[3] Notice that current is defined in about the same way that we defined *flow rate*: amount of stuff per unit time. You can think of current as the flow rate of charge.

Voltage

Now that we know how to measure current, the next question is, *What causes it?* Look back at the picture of the wire in which there was a current. What would make an electron drift to the right? One answer is to say that there's an electric field inside the wire, and since negative charges move in the direction opposite to the electric field lines, electrons would be induced to drift to the right if the electric field pointed to the left:

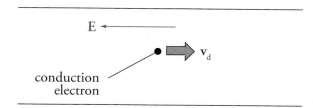

Another (equivalent) answer to the question, "What would make an electron drift to the right?" is that there's a potential difference (a voltage) between the ends of the wire. Because we know that negative charges naturally move toward regions of higher electric potential, electrons would be induced to drift to the right if the right end of the wire were maintained at a higher potential than the left end.

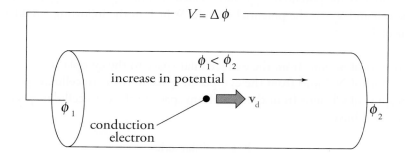

For our purposes in analyzing circuits, this second interpretation of the answer will be the one we use: that is, *it is a voltage that creates a current.* If there's no voltage (no potential difference), then the conduction electrons will just zoom around their original positions, going essentially nowhere; without a potential difference, they'd have no reason to do anything differently.

It is not uncommon to see the voltage that creates a current referred to as **electromotive force** (**emf**), since it is the cause that sets the charges into motion in a preferred direction. Notice, however, that calling it a "force" really isn't correct; it's a voltage.

Resistance

Now that we know what current is, how to measure it, and what causes it, the next question is, *How much do we get?* The answer is, *It depends.* If we took a paper-clip wire and touched its two ends to the terminals of a battery, we'd get a measurable current. Now imagine picking up a rubber band and cutting it so that it becomes essentially a straightened out "wire" of rubber. If we took this rubber wire and touched its two ends to the terminals of the same battery, we'd get essentially zero current. What's the difference? The metal wire and the rubber wire have very different **resistances**. Metals are conductors and rubber is an insulator. That is, metals have a very low intrinsic resistance, while insulators (like rubber) have a very high intrinsic resistance to the flow of charge. Since insulators have very few free electrons, there's going to be virtually no current, even with an applied voltage, which is why we got essentially zero current with our rubber wire.

Let V be the voltage applied to the ends of an object, and let I be the resulting current. By definition, the resistance of the object, R, is given by this equation:

Resistance

$$R = \frac{V}{I}$$

The unit of resistance is the volt per amp (V/A), which has its own special name: the **ohm**, abbreviated Ω (the Greek letter capital *omega*—get it? <u>ohm</u>ega). Thus, $1\ \Omega = 1$ V/A. Notice from the definition that for a given voltage, a large I means a small R, and a small I means a big R; that is, for a fixed voltage, resistance and current are inversely proportional.

Example 41-26: In neurons, the voltage difference between the cytoplasmic side and extracellular side is known as the resting membrane potential (V_m), and is calculated by $V_m = V_{in} - V_{out}$, where V_{in} is the electric potential inside the cell and V_{out} is the potential outside. Which of the following would act to increase the absolute magnitude of V_m?

A) Transport of K^+ ions from the extracellular space to the cytoplasm.
B) Transport of Na^+ ions from the cytoplasm space to the extracellular space.
C) Transport of Cl^- ions from the cytoplasm space to the extracellular space.
D) All of the above

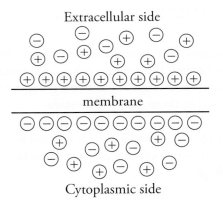

Extracellular side

membrane

Cytoplasmic side

Solution: First, note that the cytoplasmic potential is lower than the extracellular potential (this is something you should know from biology, but you can also tell that it must be so from the distribution of charges in the picture above). Thus $V_m < 0$. Since positive charges are associated with positive potential, V_m would become more negative due to increasing the negative charge inside the cell, increasing the positive charge outside of the cell, or both. Choice B is correct, as transport of Na^+ ions to the extracellular space would decrease V_{in} (make it more negative) and increase V_{out} (make it more positive), thus increasing $|V_m|$. Choices A and C are incorrect (and thus as is choice D) because they have the opposite effect, moving charges where they would tend to decrease the magnitude of the potential difference between the cytoplasm and the extracellular space. Note that choices A and C describe actions that would occur naturally if charges could redistribute to minimize electric potential energy. Such natural changes will never tend to increase the magnitude of overall potential difference.

Example 41-27: Glial cells, in contrast to neurons, have open channels that are permeable to potassium only, and the resulting resting potential (which is reached by the balance between the net concentration gradient and the net electrostatic force) is about 75 mV. A current of 1 nA is measured across the cell membrane. What is the internal resistance provided by the potassium channel?

Solution: Using the definition of resistance, we find that

$$R = \frac{V}{I} = \frac{75 \text{ mV}}{1 \text{ nA}} = \frac{7.5 \times 10^{-2} \text{ V}}{1 \times 10^{-9} \text{ A}} = 7.5 \times 10^{7} \ \Omega$$

There's another way to calculate the resistance, using a formula that does not depend on V or I. Instead, it expresses the resistance in terms of the material's *intrinsic* resistance, which is known as its **resistivity** (and denoted by ρ, not to be confused with the material's density):

Resistance and Resistivity

$$R = \rho \frac{L}{A}$$

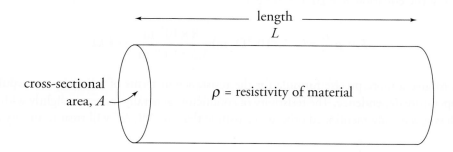

length
L

cross-sectional area, A

ρ = resistivity of material

Notice that resistance and resistivity are not the same thing. Each material has its own resistivity; its *intrinsic* resistance. However, the resistance R depends on how we shape the material. For example, if we had two aluminum wires, one that was long and thin and another that was short and thick, both would have the same resistivity (because they're both made of the same material, aluminum), but the wires would have different resistances. The long, thin wire would have the greater resistance because R is proportional to L and inversely proportional to A.

Example 41-28: Consider two copper wires. Wire #1 has three times the length and twice the diameter of Wire #2. If R_1 is the resistance of Wire #1 and R_2 is the resistance of Wire #2, then which of the following is true?

A) $R_2 = (2/3)R_1$
B) $R_2 = (4/3)R_1$
C) $R_2 = 6R_1$
D) $R_2 = 12R_1$

41.5

Solution: We're told that $L_1 = 3L_2$, and since $d_1 = 2d_2$, we know that $A_1 = 4A_2$ (because area is proportional to the *square* of the diameter). Since both wires have the same resistivity (because they're both made of the same material), we find that

$$\frac{R_2}{R_1} = \frac{\rho L_2 / A_2}{\rho L_1 / A_1} = \frac{L_2}{L_1} \cdot \frac{A_1}{A_2} = \frac{1}{3} \cdot 4 = \frac{4}{3} \;\rightarrow\; R_2 = \frac{4}{3}R_1$$

Thus, the answer is choice B.

Example 41-29: The wire used for lighting systems is usually No. 12 wire, in the American Wire Gauge (AWG) system. The diameter of No. 12 wire is just over 2 mm (which means a cross-sectional area of 3.3×10^{-6} m^2). What would be the resistance of half a mile (800 m) of No. 12 copper wire, given that the resistivity of copper is 1.7×10^{-8} Ω·m?

Solution: Using the equation $R = \rho L / A$, we get

$$R = \rho \frac{L}{A} = (1.7 \times 10^{-8} \, \Omega \cdot m) \frac{8 \times 10^2 \text{ m}}{3.3 \times 10^{-6} \text{ m}^2} \approx 4 \; \Omega$$

If we wanted to give a more precise formula for the resistance in terms of resistivity, we would have to include the temperature dependence. The resistivity of conductors generally increases slightly with temperature. However, unless specifically mentioned otherwise, assume that the MCAT will treat resistivity as a constant.

Ohm's Law

The definition of resistance, $R = V/I$, is usually written more simply as $V = IR$, and it is known as **Ohm's Law**.

> **Ohm's Law**
>
> $$V = IR$$

However, the actual statement of Ohm's Law isn't $V = IR$; rather, it's a statement about the behavior of certain conductors, and it isn't true for all materials. A material is said to obey Ohm's Law if its resistance, R, remains constant as the voltage is varied; another requirement is that the current must reverse direction if the polarity of the voltage is reversed.[4] On the MCAT, you can assume that materials are ohmic unless you are specifically told otherwise.

Resistors

A resistor is a component in an electric circuit that has a specific (and usually known) resistance. When we analyze a circuit, we generally ignore the resistance of the connecting metal wires and think of the resistance as being concentrated solely in the resistors placed in the circuit. We can do this because metal wires are such good conductors, i.e., their resistance is very low. Recall that in Example 41-28, we calculated that even half a mile of household wire has a resistance of only 4 Ω.

In the real world, a resistor is typically a little cylinder filled with an alloy (of carbon or of nickel and copper) and often encircled by colored bands to indicate the numerical value of its resistance, like this:

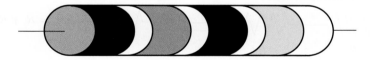

In circuit diagrams, however, a resistor is denoted by the following symbol:

Electric circuits on the MCAT may contain just one resistor, but it's more likely that they'll have two or more. There are two ways the MCAT will combine resistors: in series or in parallel. Two or more resistors are said to be in **series** if each follows the others along a single connection in a circuit. For example, these two resistors are in series, because R_2 directly follows R_1 along a single path.

---

[4] Some materials don't behave this way, and the relationship between voltage and current is more complex; on the MCAT, however, it's safe to assume that $V = IR$ applies unless you're told otherwise.

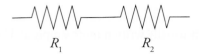

R_1 R_2

Resistors in Series

On the other hand, two or more resistors are said to be in **parallel** if they provide alternative routes from one point in a circuit to another. For example, the following two resistors are in parallel, because we get from Point P to Point Q in the circuit *either* by traveling through R_1 *or* by traveling through R_2; we don't go through both resistors like we would if they were in series.

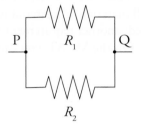

Resistors in Parallel

Typically, we analyze a circuit by first transforming it into a simpler one, one that contains just a single resistor. Therefore, we need a way to turn combinations of resistors (series combinations and parallel combinations) into a single, equivalent resistor; that is, one resistor that provides the same overall resistance as the combination. Here are the formulas:

resistors in series $\Rightarrow$ single equivalent resistor

$R_{eq} = R_1 + R_2$

R_1 R_2 R_{eq}

resistors in parallel $\Rightarrow$

$$\frac{1}{R_{eq}} = \frac{1}{R_1} + \frac{1}{R_2}$$

or

$$R_{eq} = \frac{R_1 R_2}{R_1 + R_2}$$

P R_1 Q R_{eq}

R_2

So, for resistors in series, we simply add the resistances. For example, if a 20 Ω resistor is in series with a 30 Ω resistor, this combination is equivalent to a single 50 Ω resistor, because 20 + 30 = 50. Notice that for a series combination, the equivalent resistance is always greater than the largest resistance in the combination; that's why the *R* is bigger in the figure above for the series combination.

41.5

For resistors in parallel, the formula is a little more complicated. If we have two resistors in parallel, we get the equivalent resistance by taking the product of the resistances (R_1R_2) and dividing this by their sum $(R_1 + R_2)$. For example, if a 3 Ω resistor is in parallel with a 6 Ω resistor, this combination is equivalent to a single 2 Ω resistor, because (3×6) divided by $(3 + 6)$ is equal to 2. For a parallel combination, the equivalent resistance is always less than the smallest resistance in the combination; that's why the R_{eq} is smaller in the figure above for the parallel combination.

The product over sum formula for parallel resistors only works for *two* resistors. If you have three or more resistors in parallel, they will probably have the same resistance, so using the reciprocal equation for $1/R_{eq}$ and adding the fractions will not be difficult.

For resistors in series, we just add the individual resistances, no matter how many we have in a row. For example, if we have the following four resistors in series: 10 Ω, 20 Ω, 30 Ω, and 40 Ω, then we can reduce this combination of four series resistors to a single equivalent resistance of 100 Ω, because $10 + 20 + 30 + 40 = 100$, but the equivalent resistance of two identical resistors in parallel is half the resistance of either resistor.

Example 41-30: What is the equivalent or total resistance of the following combination of resistors?

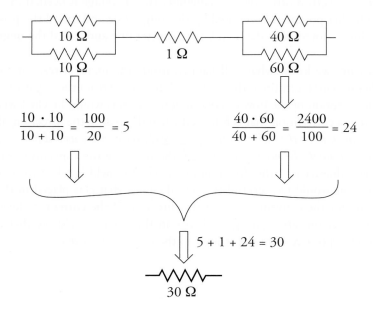

Solution: Here we have a mixture of parallel *and* series combinations. There's a parallel combination (the pair of 10 Ω resistors) that's in series with both a 1 Ω resistor and another parallel combination (the 40 Ω and 60 Ω resistors). To simplify this, we work in steps:

Therefore, the given combination of resistors is equivalent to a single 30 Ω resistor.

DC Circuits

Now that we know how to simplify series and parallel combinations of resistors, we're ready to analyze circuits. The simplest circuit consists of a voltage source (most commonly, it's a battery), a connecting wire between the terminals of the voltage source, and a resistor. As an example, imagine hooking up a light bulb to a typical flashlight battery; one wire connects the positive terminal of the battery to one of the leads on the light bulb, and another wire connects the other lead on the bulb to the negative terminal of the battery. This completes the circuit. The diagram on the right below shows the way this real-life circuit would be drawn schematically.

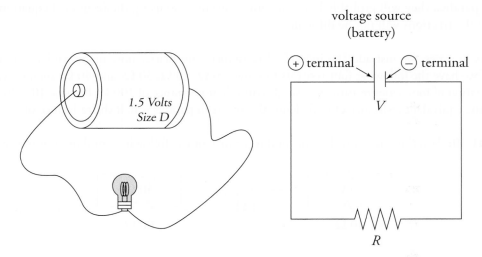

The pair of adjacent parallel lines denotes the voltage source. The job of the voltage source is to maintain a potential difference (a voltage) between its terminals; the value of this voltage is denoted by V or sometimes by ε, for emf (electromotive force). Remember that a voltage is needed to create a current. The terminal that's at the higher potential is denoted by the longer line and called the **positive terminal**; the terminal that's at the lower potential is denoted by the shorter line and called the **negative terminal**.

Once the circuit is set up, we know what will happen inside the metal wires: conduction electrons will drift toward the higher potential terminal; that is, they'll drift away from the negative terminal, toward the positive terminal. The direction of the flow of conduction electrons would be clockwise in the diagram as drawn. However, there is a convention that is followed when discussing the direction of the current. *The direction of the current is taken to be the direction that <u>positive</u> charge carriers would flow, even though the actual charge carriers that do flow might be negatively charged.* (Sounds like the convention for defining the direction of the electric field, doesn't it? "The direction of the electric field is taken to be the direction of the force that a positive charge would feel, even if the actual charge that gets placed in the field isn't positive." In fact, that's the reason for the convention about the direction of the current; to keep things consistent.) Even though we know electrons are drifting clockwise in this circuit, we'd say that the current, I, flows counterclockwise from the positive terminal around to the negative terminal.

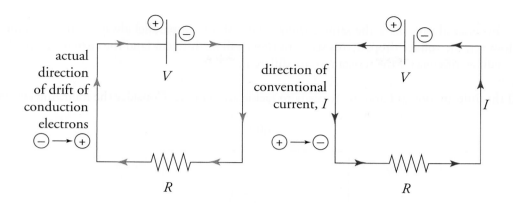

If we were asked for the value of the current in this circuit, this question would be easy to answer. We know V and R, and we want I. Using the equation $V = IR$, we'd say that

$$I = \frac{V}{R}$$

For example, if $V = 1.5$ V and $R = 150\ \Omega$, then $I = 0.01$ A. So, what made this problem so easy? The answer: there was only one resistor. This will usually be our goal: to simplify a circuit with multiple resistors into a circuit with just a single equivalent resistor. (We say usually because there are some question types that can be answered without changing the circuit into one with just a single resistor; we'll show you some examples of those too.)

In order to simplify a circuit with multiple resistors, we first need a way to turn resistors in series and resistors in parallel into a single equivalent resistor; this we already know how to do. However, there are two other important quantities in circuits besides R; namely, I and V. We also need to know what happens to these other quantities when we convert a series or parallel combination of resistors into a single resistor. The following figure contains this needed information:

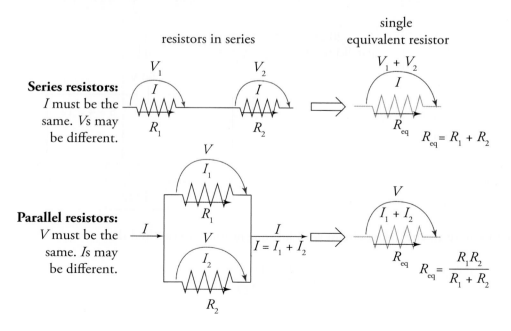

Resistors in series always share the same current, and resistors in parallel always share the same voltage drop. However, the voltage drops across series resistors will be different (and the currents through parallel resistors will be different) if the resistances are different.

With all this information at hand, we're ready to tackle an example. Consider the following circuit:

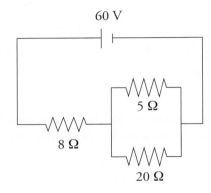

We'll find the current in the circuit, the current through each resistor, and the voltage across each resistor. The first stage of the solution involves simplifying this multiple-resistor circuit into a circuit with just a single equivalent resistor, like this:

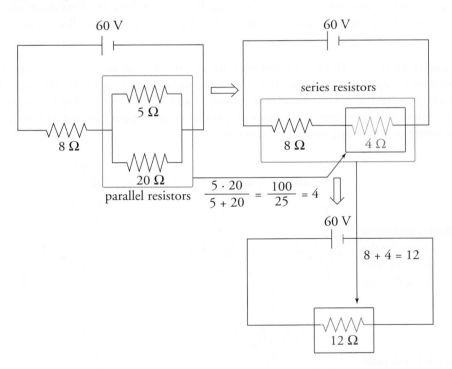

Now that we have an equivalent circuit with just one resistor, we can find the current:

$$I = \frac{V}{R} = \frac{60 \text{ V}}{12 \, \Omega} = 5 \text{ A}$$

If we want to find the currents through (and the voltages across) the individual resistors in the original circuit, we have to work backward. The key to working backward is to ask at each stage: "What am I going back to?" If the answer is, "a *series* combination," then the value you bring back is the *current*, because series resistors share the same current. If the answer is, "a *parallel* combination," then the value you bring back is the *voltage*, because parallel resistors share the same voltage.

going back to series combination → bring *I*

going back to parallel combination → bring *V*

Let me illustrate this working backward technique with our circuit above. You should read this figure starting at the bottom, then up, then to the left...in other words, in the *reverse* order from what we did before because now we're working backward:

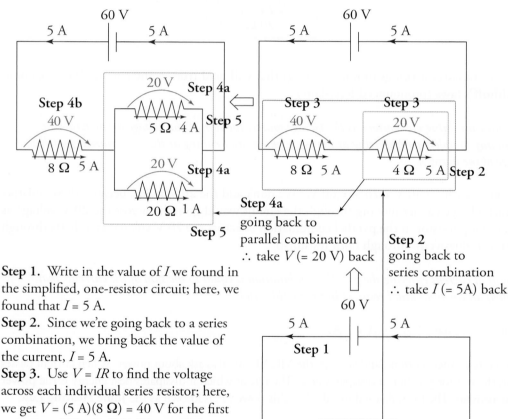

Step 1. Write in the value of *I* we found in the simplified, one-resistor circuit; here, we found that *I* = 5 A.

Step 2. Since we're going back to a series combination, we bring back the value of the current, *I* = 5 A.

Step 3. Use $V = IR$ to find the voltage across each individual series resistor; here, we get $V = (5\text{ A})(8\text{ }\Omega) = 40$ V for the first resistor and $V = (5\text{ A})(4\text{ }\Omega) = 20$ V for the second resistor.

Step 4a. Since we're going back to a parallel combination, we bring back the value of the voltage, *V* = 20 V.

Step 4b. Simply copy the information for the 8 Ω resistor, since that resistor doesn't change when we go back.

Step 5. Use $I = V/R$ to find the current across each individual parallel resistor; here, we get $I = (20\text{ V})/(5\text{ }\Omega) = 4$ A for the top resistor and $I = (20\text{ V})/(20\text{ }\Omega) = 1$ A for the bottom resistor.

Now that we have found all the information for the original circuit,

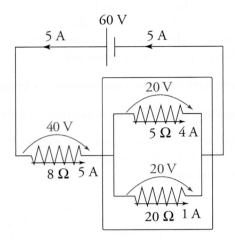

there are a couple of important things to notice, things that will hold true in any circuit. They are conse-quences of **Kirchhoff's laws** (pronounced Keer-koff).

- *For a circuit containing one battery as the voltage source, the sum of the voltage drops across the resistors in any complete path starting at the (+) terminal and ending at the (−) terminal matches the voltage of the battery.*

For our circuit above, we have 40 V + 20 V = 60 V. (We don't add the 20 V twice, because these resistors are in parallel; each charge carrier moving through the circuit would go *either* across the 20 V voltage as it drifts through the top resistor in the parallel combination *or* across the 20 V voltage as it drifts through the bottom resistor; it doesn't go through both resistors.)

- *The amount of current entering the parallel combination is equal to the sum of the currents that pass through all the individual resistors in the combination.*

For our circuit above, we have 5 A = 4 A + 1 A.

Besides asking about resistance, current, and voltage, the MCAT can also ask about power. When current passes through a resistor, the resistor gets hot: it dissipates heat. The rate at which it dissipates heat energy is the **power dissipated by the resistor**. The formula used to calculate this power, P, is known as the **Joule Heating Law**.

Power Dissipated by a Resistor: Joule Heating Law

$$P = I^2 R$$

So, for our circuit above, we find that

the power dissipated by the 8 Ω resistor is $I^2R = (5 \text{ A})^2(8 \text{ }\Omega)$ $\quad\quad$ = 200 W
the power dissipated by the 5 Ω resistor is $I^2R = (4 \text{ A})^2(5 \text{ }\Omega)$ $\quad\quad$ = $\quad$80 W
the power dissipated by the 20 Ω resistor is $I^2R = (1 \text{ A})^2(20 \text{ }\Omega)$ $\quad$ = $\quad$20 W
the total power dissipated by all resistors is the sum: $\quad\quad\quad\quad$ 300 W

The power *supplied* to the circuit by the voltage source (like a battery) is given by this formula: $P = IV$. So, for our circuit above, we find that

power supplied by the 60 V battery is $P = IV = (5 \text{ A})(60 \text{ V}) = 300$ W

Notice that these answers match:

power dissipated by all resistors = 300 W = power supplied by the battery

This is simply a consequence of Conservation of Energy, so it will be true in general:

- *The total power dissipated by the resistors is equal to the power supplied by the battery.*

Sometimes, a circuit may contain more than one battery, and in some of these cases, the battery with the lower voltage will be *absorbing* power from the battery with the higher voltage (that is, from the boss battery that supplies the power to the circuit). The power *absorbed* by a battery is also given by the formula $P = IV$, and the italicized statement above should then read:

- *The total power dissipated by the resistors and absorbed by other voltage sources (i.e., the total power used by the circuit) is equal to the power supplied to the circuit by the highest-voltage power source.*

One more note: the Joule Heating Law, $P = I^2R$, can be written as $P = I(IR) = IV$, so, in fact, we need just one formula for the power dissipated or supplied by *any* component in a circuit:

Power

$$P = IV$$

However, if you use the formula $P = IV$ to find the power dissipated by a resistor, *be careful* that you only use the V *for that resistor*, and not the V for the entire circuit. So, for our circuit above, we'd find that:

the power dissipated by the 8 Ω resistor is $\quad IV = (5 \text{ A})(40 \text{ V}) = 200$ W
the power dissipated by the 5 Ω resistor is $\quad IV = (4 \text{ A})(20 \text{ V}) = \quad$80 W
the power dissipated by the 20 Ω resistor is $\quad IV = (1 \text{ A})(20 \text{ V}) = \quad$20 W

giving us the same answers we found before when we used the formula $P = I^2R$.

Along with questions about power, there could also be questions about energy. Simply remember the definition: power = energy/time, so

$$\text{energy} = \text{power} \times \text{time}$$

For example, how much energy is dissipated in 5 seconds by the 5-ohm resistor in the circuit above? We calculated that the power dissipated by this resistor is $P = 80\ \text{W} = 80\ \text{J/s}$; so the energy dissipated in $t = 5$ seconds is $Pt = (80\ \text{J/s})(5\ \text{s}) = 400\ \text{J}$.

In some circuits (in practice, most of them), one or more of the resistors are actually doing something useful besides just heating up. However, the circuit diagrams and the calculations we do will be the same. For example, a motor will be shown as a resistor in an MCAT circuit; so will a light bulb (which is really just a resistor that happens to get so hot that some of the energy dissipated is emitted as light rather than heat). In either case, the calculations for these components are the same as treating each as a regular resistor. Notice that if you want to calculate the work that can be done by a motor, you'll wind up multiplying power by time.

Example 41-31: A portion of a circuit is shown below:

If the current through the 10-ohm resistor is 1 A, what is the current through the 20-ohm resistor?

    A) 0.25 A
    B) 0.5 A
    C) 1 A
    D) 2 A

Solution: Because these resistors are in series, they all share the same current. If the current in the first resistor is 1 A, then the current through each of the other resistors is also 1 A. The answer is choice C.

Example 41-32: A portion of a circuit is shown below:

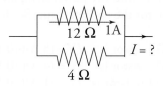

If the current through the 12-ohm resistor is 1 A, what is the value of the current I?

Solution: The voltage drop across the top resistor is $V = IR = (1 \text{ A})(12 \ \Omega) = 12$ V. Because the resistors are in parallel, the voltage drop across the bottom resistor must also be 12 V. Using $I = V/R$, we find that the current through the bottom resistor is $(12 \text{ V})/(4 \ \Omega) = 3$ A. Therefore, the total amount of current passing through the parallel combination is 1 A + 3 A = 4 A.

Example 41-33: A portion of a circuit is shown below:

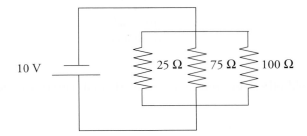

If the current entering the parallel combination is 12 A, how much current flows through the 120-ohm resistor?

Solution: Because the 60-ohm bottom resistor has half the resistance of the 120-ohm top resistor, twice as much current will flow through the bottom resistor as through the top one. So, if we let X stand for the current in the top resistor, then the current in the bottom resistor is $2X$. Because 12 A enters the parallel combination, we must have $X + 2X = 12$ A, so $X = 4$ A. Therefore, the current in the top resistor is 4 A (and the current in the bottom resistor is 8 A). Notice that the voltage drop across the top resistor is $V = IR = (4 \text{ A})(120 \ \Omega) = 480$ V, and the voltage drop across the bottom resistor is $V = IR = (8 \text{ A})(60 \ \Omega) = 480$ V. The fact that these voltages match (as they must for parallel resistors) verifies that our answer is correct.

Example 41-35: What is the current in the 100-ohm resistor shown below?

Solution: For this question, we don't need to begin by finding the single equivalent resistance of the given parallel combination, because we already know the voltage across the 100-ohm resistor. The parallel combination is attached directly to the terminals of the battery, so the voltage across each of the resistors must be 10 V. Because we know both V and R, we can find I in one step: $I = V/R = (10 \text{ V})/(100 \ \Omega) = 0.1$ A.

Example 41-34: A toaster oven is rated at 720 W. If it draws 6 A of current, what is its resistance?

Solution: Here, we're given P and I, and asked for R. Since $P = I^2R$, we find that

$$R = \frac{P}{I^2} = \frac{720 \text{ W}}{(6 \text{ A})^2} = 20 \ \Omega$$

Example 41-36: Current passes through an insulated resistor of resistance R, mass m, and specific heat c. The voltage across this resistor is V. If the resistor absorbs all the heat it generates, find an expression for the increase in temperature of the resistor after a time t. (All values are expressed in SI units.)

Solution: The amount of heat energy generated (and absorbed) by the resistor is $q = Pt$ (note that we're using lowercase q here, rather than the capital Q used in the thermodynamics chapter, because the formula we're going to use from chemistry is more familiar with that symbol), where $P = IV = (V/R)V = V^2/R$. Now, using the fundamental equation $q = mc\Delta T$ (from general chemistry), we have

$$\Delta T = \frac{q}{mc} = \frac{Pt}{mc} = \frac{\frac{V^2}{R}t}{mc} = \frac{V^2t}{Rmc}$$

All real batteries have **internal resistance**, which we denote by r. Let ε denote the emf of the battery; this is its ideal voltage (that is, the voltage between its terminals when there's no current). Once a current is established, the internal resistance causes the voltage between the terminals to be different from ε. If the battery is supplying current I to the circuit, then the **terminal voltage**, V, is less than ε and given by $V = \varepsilon - Ir$. (On the other hand, if the circuit is *supplying* current to the battery [charging it up] then the terminal voltage is greater than ε and given by the equation $V = \varepsilon + Ir$.) The internal resistance is actually *between* the terminals in a real battery, but in circuit diagrams, the internal resistance is drawn next to the battery, like this:

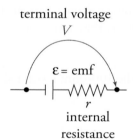

However, unless you are told otherwise, you may assume that all batteries are ideal and have no internal resistance.

41.5

Example 41-37: The battery shown in the circuit below has an emf of 100 V and an internal resistance of 5 Ω. What is its terminal voltage in this circuit? (*Note*: It's not uncommon to see a dashed box drawn around the battery and its internal resistance; this emphasizes that *r* is actually inside the battery.)

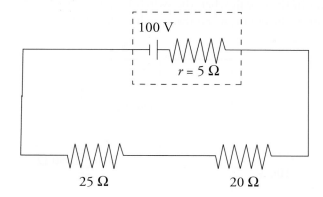

A) 80 V
B) 90 V
C) 100 V
D) 110 V

Solution: The three resistors in this circuit are in series, so the equivalent resistance for the circuit is 5 + 25 + 20 = 50 Ω. Because the emf is 100 V, the current in the circuit is

$$I = \varepsilon \, / \, R = (100 \text{ V})(50 \, \Omega) = 2 \text{ A}$$

The terminal voltage is therefore

$$V = \varepsilon - Ir = (100 \text{ V}) - (2 \text{ A})(5 \, \Omega) = 90 \text{ V}$$

The answer is choice B. (*Note*: You could eliminate choices C and D immediately; the terminal voltage must be *less* than the emf because the battery is supplying current to the circuit.)

Example 41-38: The diagram below shows a point X held at a potential of $\phi = 60$ V connected by a combination of resistors to a point (denoted by G) that is **grounded**. *The **ground** is considered to be at potential zero.* What is the current through the 100-ohm resistor?

Solution: The parallel resistors are equivalent to a single 20 Ω resistor, which is then in series with the 100 Ω resistor, giving an overall equivalent resistance of 20 + 100 = 120 Ω. Since the potential difference between points X and G is $V = \phi_X - \phi_G = 60 - 0 = 60$ V, the current in the circuit (and through the 100-ohm resistor) is

$$I = V \, / \, R = (60 \text{ V}) / (120 \, \Omega) = 0.5 \text{ A}$$

Example 41-39: The diagram below shows a battery with an emf of 100 V connected to a circuit equipped with a switch, S.

a) What is the current in the circuit when the switch is open?
b) What is the current in the circuit when the switch is closed?

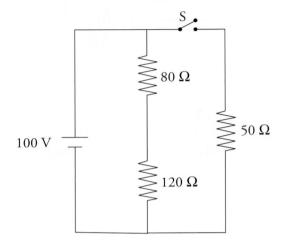

Solution:

a) With the switch open (as pictured above), the 50 Ω resistor is effectively taken out of the circuit; no current will flow in that branch. Current will flow only in the part of the circuit shown below:

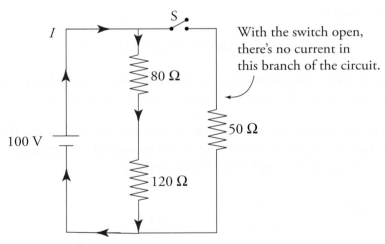

With the switch open, there's no current in this branch of the circuit.

The two resistors that *are* in the circuit when the switch is open are in series, so the total equivalent resistance is 80 + 120 = 200 Ω; thus, the current is

$$I = V / R = (100 \text{ V})/(200 \text{ Ω}) = 0.5 \text{ A}$$

b) With the switch closed, all the resistors are part of the circuit, and there will be current in all the branches. Let's find the equivalent resistance. The 80 Ω and 120 Ω resistors are in series, so they're equivalent to a single 80 + 120 = 200 Ω resistor, which is then in parallel with the 50 Ω resistor. This gives an overall equivalent resistance of 40 Ω because (200 × 50)/(200 + 50) is equal to 41. Therefore, the current supplied to the circuit in this case is $I = V/R_{eq} =$ (100 V)/(40 Ω) = 2.5 A.

Example 41-40: Three identical light bulbs are connected to a battery, as shown:

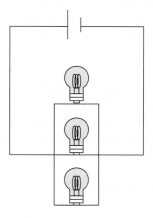

What will happen if the middle bulb burns out?

    A) The other two bulbs will go out.
    B) The light intensity of each of the other two bulbs will decrease, but they won't go out.
    C) The light intensity of each of the other two bulbs will increase.
    D) The light intensity of each of the other two bulbs will remain the same.

Solution: Let V be the voltage of the battery, and let R be the resistance of each light bulb. The current through each light bulb (that is, through each resistor) is $I = V/R$. If the middle bulb burns out, then the middle branch of the parallel combination is severed; however, current can still flow through the top and bottom bulbs, and the current through each will still be $I = V/R$. Because the intensity of the light is directly related to the power each one dissipates, the fact that the current doesn't change means that $P = I^2 R$ won't change, so the light intensity of the other two bulbs will remain the same. The answer is choice D. [What *will* change if the middle bulb burns out? Before the middle bulb burns out, the current through each of the three bulbs is $I = V/R$, so the battery must be providing a total current of $3I = 3V/R$. After the middle bulb burns out, the current through each of the other two bulbs is still $I = V/R$, so the battery need only provide a total current of $2I = 2V/R$. That is, the total current through the circuit will decrease (since, after all, there are only two bulbs to light, not three). In addition, the power supplied by the battery will also decrease, from $P = (3I)(V) = 3V^2/R$ to $P = (2I)(V) = 2V^2/R$, and the battery will last longer. Finally, notice that if the three bulbs were wired in *series* rather than in parallel, then if any one of the bulbs burned out, they'd all go out because the circuit would be broken.]

Measuring Circuit Values

To verify that a circuit is operating properly, or to troubleshoot one that is malfunctioning, we need to be able to measure the voltage and current in different parts of the circuit. **Voltmeters** are used to measure the potential difference between two points in a circuit, and **ammeters** are used to measure the current through a particular point in the circuit. At the core of each of these devices is a **galvanometer**.

A galvanometer on its own is an apparatus that sensitively measures current using the interaction between currents and magnetic fields (discussion of the particulars of this interaction is left to the final section of this chapter). Current enters the galvanometer and travels through a coil that is wound around the base of a needle. The coil is situated in an external magnetic field in such a way that whenever current runs through the coil, magnetic forces deflect the galvanometer needle. The degree of deflection indicates the amount of current running through the device.

To construct an ammeter, we need to have a small, known fraction of the current we are trying to measure running through the galvanometer (because the galvanometer is very sensitive, a large current will overload it). For instance, let's take a look at the circuit we discussed earlier in this section. Say that we want to measure the current flowing through each of the resistors. To do so, all we need to do is connect the ammeter in series with the resistor of interest.

To measure the current through the 8 Ω resistor:

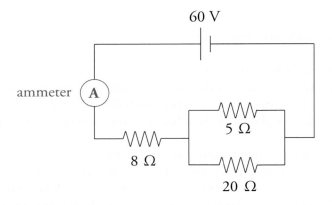

To measure the current through the 5 Ω resistor:

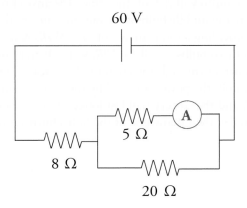

When we connect the ammeter to the circuit, we are adding an additional resistance to the circuit, known as the *internal resistance, r,* of the meter. In reality, this internal resistance is roughly equal to a small *shunt resistance, R_s,* connected in parallel with the ideal galvanometer (G) and its own much larger series resistance, R_g, used to ensure that only a small current actually passes through the galvanometer (the internal resistance of the galvanometer itself is approximated to be zero, a sound assumption given the large value of the R_g).

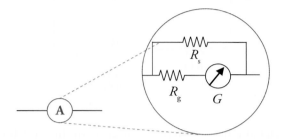

Since we don't want the ammeter to interfere with the circuit in the process of measuring it, we want our ammeter to have as low of an internal resistance as possible so that there is as little voltage dropped over this resistor as possible. The way to achieve this is for the shunt resistance to be very small, because the shunt resistance is very close to the total internal resistance of the ammeter:

$$r = \frac{R_s R_g}{R_s + R_g} = R_s \times \frac{R_g}{R_s + R_g} \xrightarrow{R_g \gg R_s} R_s \times 1 = R_s$$

Another way to think about this is that we want the equivalent resistance of the combination of the ammeter's internal resistance and the resistor of interest to be as close to the original resistance of the resistor as possible.

Example 41-41: A typical ammeter might have an internal resistance of $r = 0.1$ mΩ. If we are measuring the current through the 5 Ω resistor in the circuit above, what would be the equivalent resistance of the ammeter and resistor connected in series?

Solution: Just add the resistances: $R_{eq} = 5\ \Omega + 1 \times 10^{-4}\ \Omega \approx 5\ \Omega$.

Although a galvanometer is intrinsically a current-measuring device, it can also be used to measure voltage, since we know that current and voltage are proportional. To do this, we'll want to connect the voltmeter across the resistor of interest so that it can measure the potential difference from one side of the resistor to the other.

To measure the voltage across the 8 Ω resistor:

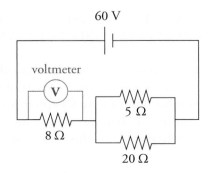

To measure the voltage across the 5 Ω resistor:

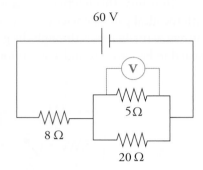

Just like an ammeter, a voltmeter also has an internal resistance. In this case, however, the internal resistance is connected in parallel to a resistor of interest. Again, we want to minimize any impact to the original circuit, so for the voltmeter we'll want the internal resistance to be as large as possible to minimize any current going through the voltmeter. A typical voltmeter might have an internal resistance of 10 MΩ. This is achieved by using a large resistance R_g in series with the galvanometer, as shown below. If we again assume the resistance of G is negligible, then $r = R_g$.

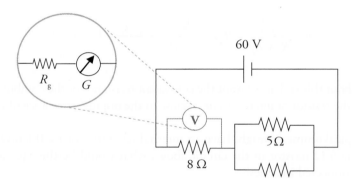

Example 41-42: When connecting a voltmeter to a circuit, we want the equivalent resistance of the combination to be as close to the original resistance as possible. In the circuit above, if $r = R_g = 10$ MΩ when measuring the voltage across the 8 Ω resistor, find

a) the equivalent resistance of the voltmeter and resistor, and
b) the measured voltage.

Solution:

a) The equivalent resistance is given by the product over sum rule for resistors in parallel:
    $R_{eq} = (10 \times 10^6 \ \Omega)(8 \ \Omega)/(10 \times 10^6 \ \Omega + 8 \ \Omega) \approx (10 \times 10^6 \ \Omega)(8 \ \Omega)/(10 \times 10^6 \ \Omega) = 8 \ \Omega$.

b) This is the same circuit we solved previously in the beginning of the subsection on DC circuits, when we found that the voltage across the 8 Ω resistor was 40 V. (This would be a good time to confirm you remember how to solve for currents and resistances across circuit elements by solving for this result again). Because we have just confirmed that the voltmeter does not appreciably affect the resistance across this circuit element, the measured value will be the same as the calculated value.

41.6 CAPACITORS

A pair of conductors that can hold equal but opposite charges is known as a **capacitor**. The conductors can be of any shape, but the most common capacitor consists of a pair of parallel metal plates; it's known as a **parallel-plate capacitor**:

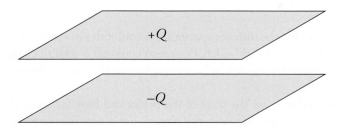

Notice that one plate carries a positive charge and the other plate carries an equal amount of negative charge. Therefore, the *net* charge on a capacitor is zero. However, whenever we talk about the charge on a capacitor, we always mean the magnitude of charge on either plate, which is $+Q$.

In circuit diagrams, a capacitor is denoted by either of these two symbols:

$$\left|\left|\quad \text{or} \quad \right|\right($$

The first question we'll answer is, "How do we create a charged capacitor?" Take an uncharged parallel-plate capacitor, and hook the plates to the terminals of a battery. Conduction electrons in the connecting wires will be repelled from the negative terminal and flow to one plate, while electrons from the other plate will be attracted toward the positive terminal of the battery. The current rises quickly at first, but it gradually dies out as the plates acquire charge. The plate that's connected to the positive terminal becomes positively charged, and the plate that's connected to the negative terminal becomes negatively charged. Since the positive plate has a higher potential than the negative plate, the potential difference between the plates opposes the potential difference of the battery. Charge will stop flowing when the potential difference between the plates matches the voltage of the battery because at that point the circuit will look like one that has two opposing voltage sources.

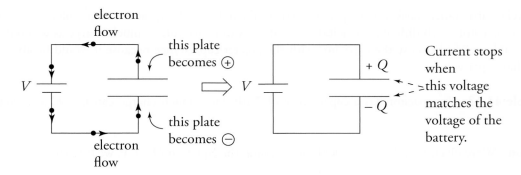

If V is the potential difference between the plates of a charged capacitor, and Q is the charge on the capacitor, then Q and V are proportional. The proportionality constant, C, is called the **capacitance**:

> ### Charge on a Capacitor
>
> $$Q = CV$$

41.6

From this equation we can see that the unit of capacitance is coulomb per volt (C/V), which has its own name: the **farad**, abbreviated F. Therefore, 1 C/V = 1 F. Because a coulomb is a lot of charge, we'd expect a farad to be a lot of capacitance. Most real-life capacitors have capacitances that are on the order of a few microfarads.

The capacitance is determined only by the sizes of the plates and how far apart they are (and, as we'll see a little later, whether there's anything between the plates). For a parallel-plate capacitor with empty space between the plates, C is given by the following equation:

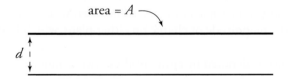

> ### Capacitance of a Parallel Plate Capacitor
>
> $$C = \varepsilon_0 \frac{A}{d}$$

where A is the area of each plate, d is their separation, and ε_0 is a fundamental constant of nature. (The constant ε_0 is known as the **permittivity of free space**; it's equal to $1/(4\pi k_0)$, where k_0 is Coulomb's constant, so the approximate numerical value of ε_0 is 8.85×10^{-12} F/m.)

The capacitance C depends only on A and d. Although $Q = CV$, the capacitance C does not depend on either Q or V; it only tells us how Q and V will be related. If you were given an uncharged capacitor, you could determine C without charging it up, by using the formula $C = \varepsilon_0 A/d$.

Intuitively, capacitance measures the plates' capacity for holding charge at a certain voltage. Let's say we had two capacitors with different capacitances, and we wanted to store as much charge as we could while keeping V low. We'd choose the capacitor with the greater capacitance because it would be able to hold more charge per volt.

Example 41-43: A capacitor has a capacitance of 2 nF. How much charge can it hold at a voltage of 150 V?

Solution: We're given C and V, and asked for Q. Using the equation $Q = CV$, we find that

$$Q = CV = (2 \times 10^{-9}\ \text{F})(150\ \text{V}) = 3 \times 10^{-7}\ \text{C}$$

(This means that the positive plate will have a charge of $+Q = 3 \times 10^{-7}$ C, and the negative plate will have a charge of $-Q = -3 \times 10^{-7}$ C.)

Example 41-44: A charged capacitor has charge Q, and the voltage between the plates is V. What will happen to C if Q is doubled?

Solution: Nothing. For a given capacitor, C is a constant. Because $Q = CV$, we see that Q is proportional to V. Doubling Q will not affect C; what *will* happen is that V will double.

Example 41-45: What will happen to the capacitance of a parallel-plate capacitor if the plates were moved closer together, halving the distance between them?

Solution: From the equation $C = \varepsilon_0 A/d$, we see that C is inversely proportional to d. Thus, if d is decreased by a factor of 2, then C will increase by a factor of 2.

Example 41-46: As ions diffuse across the cell membrane due to their respective concentration gradients, the movement of charge changes the electrical potential inside and outside of the cell. For example, when Na^+ moves into the cell as a current flow dictated by a battery (see figure below), the cytoplasm become more positive. R_{Na}, R_K, and R_{Cl} represent the effective resistances of the cell membrane to the flow of ions Na^+, K^+, and Cl^-, respectively; that is, the greater the resistance, the lower the permeability of the membrane to that ion. Increasing the permeability of the cell membrane to which of the following ions would act to increase the potential difference across the membrane (represented as the voltage across the capacitor C_m)?

    I. Na^+
   II. K^+
  III. Cl^-

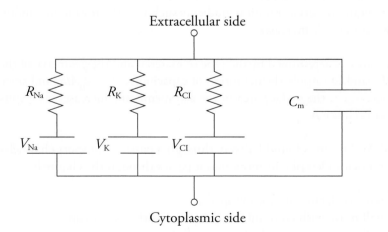

A) I only
B) II only
C) II and III only
D) I, II, and III

Solution: The cytoplasm is at a lower potential than the extracellular space, so items which would tend to make the cytoplasm more negative or the extracellular space more positive will increase the potential difference. Item I is false: Na^+ flowing into the cytoplasm causes an increase in its potential (making it less negative and the extracellular space less positive), thus reducing the potential difference. This eliminates choices A and D. Item III is true: Cl^- will flow to the cytoplasm (recall that negative charges flow opposite the current direction), increasing the potential difference. This eliminates choice B, so choice C is correct. Item II is indeed true: K^+ will flow to the extracellular space, increasing the potential difference.

Example 41-47: As shown in the schematic of the cell as circuit, the membrane acts as a capacitor between the extracellular and cytoplasmic sides of the cell. The specific membrane capacitance of a cell membrane is calculated as a capacitance per unit area of the membrane (usually in $\mu F/cm^2$). Given that the voltage across the cell membrane is measured as 70 mV, suppose that a square micrometer of membrane measures a total separation of charge of 0.63 fC (a femtocoulomb is 10^{-15} coulombs). What is the specific membrane capacitance C_m of this cell membrane?

Solution: We are given Q and V and asked for C / A, where A is the area of this patch of membrane. Apply the equation $Q = CV$ for the given patch area and then convert to the desired units.

$$C_m = \frac{Q}{V} = \frac{6.3 \times 10^{-16}\ C}{7 \times 10^{-2}\ V} = 9 \times 10^{-15}\ \frac{F}{\mu m^2} \times \frac{1\ \mu F}{10^{-6}\ F} \times \left(\frac{1\ \mu m}{10^{-4}\ cm} \right)^2 = 0.9\ \frac{\mu F}{cm^2}$$

Example 41-48: Which of the following changes to the cell would result in a net increase in the capacitance of the cell membrane?

    A) Increasing the size of the cell
    B) Reducing the resistance of the Na^+ voltage channel
    C) Increasing the resistance of the K^+ voltage channel
    D) Changing the concentration gradients such that the resting membrane potential between the cells increases

Solution: Capacitance is determined by the type of material and the geometry of the capacitor (this eliminates choices B, C, and D). Apply the definition of capacitance, $C = \varepsilon_0 A/d$, and since C is proportional to A, capacitance increases as the surface area of the cell membrane increases (as it must if the cell expands). The correct answer is choice A.

Example 41-49: An H^+ ion is found halfway through a passive transport channel and is not affected by a concentration gradient. Describe its motion as it passes through the channel:

    A) It will accelerate into the cytoplasm
    B) It will move with constant velocity towards the cytoplasm
    C) It will accelerate towards the extracellular space
    D) It will move with constant velocity towards the extracellular space

Solution: The particle is positively charged, so it will feel an electrostatic attraction towards the lower potential cytoplasm and a force from the charge distribution on either side of the cell membrane (effectively, it is between the plates of the capacitor C_m; choices C and D can be eliminated). Because the net force is not zero, the charge must accelerate (choice A is correct).

Now that we know the basic equation for capacitance ($Q = CV$) and how to calculate it ($C = \varepsilon_0 A/d$), the next question is, "What's a capacitor used for?" For MCAT purposes, a parallel-plate capacitor has two main uses:

1. to create a uniform electric field, and
2. to store electrical potential energy.

Let's go over each one.

When we studied electric fields, we noted that the electric field created by a plane of charge or capacitor was uniform, a constant independent of distance from the plane. The electric field, **E**, always points from the positive plate toward the negative plate.

Because **E** is so straightforward (it's the same everywhere between the plates), the equation for calculating it is equally straightforward. The strength of **E** depends on the voltage between the plates, V, and their separation distance, d. We call the equation Ed's formula:

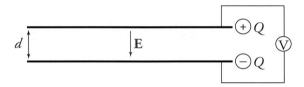

Ed's Formula

$$V = Ed$$

The equation $F = qE$ showed us that the units of E are N/C (because $E = F/q$). Ed's formula now tells us that the units of E are V/m (because $E = V/d$). You'll see both newtons-per-coulomb and volts-per-meter used as units for the electric field; it turns out that these units are exactly the same.

Example 41-50: The charge on a parallel-plate capacitor is 4×10^{-6} C. If the distance between the plates is 2 mm and the capacitance is 1 μF, what's the strength of the electric field between the plates?

Solution: Since $Q = CV$, we have $V = Q/C = (4 \times 10^{-6}$ C$)/(10^{-6}$ F$) = 4$ V. Now, using the equation $V = Ed$, we find that

$$E = \frac{V}{d} = \frac{4\text{ V}}{2 \times 10^{-3}\text{ m}} = 2000\,\tfrac{\text{V}}{\text{m}}$$

Example 41-51: A proton (whose mass is *m*) is placed on top of the positively charged plate of a parallel-plate capacitor, as shown below.

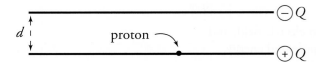

41.6

The charge on the capacitor is *Q*, and the capacitance is *C*. If the electric field in the region between the plates has magnitude *E*, which of the following expressions gives the time required for the proton to move up to the other plate?

A) $d\sqrt{\dfrac{eQ}{mC}}$

B) $d\sqrt{\dfrac{m}{eQC}}$

C) $d\sqrt{\dfrac{2eQ}{mC}}$

D) $d\sqrt{\dfrac{2mC}{eQ}}$

Solution: Once we find the acceleration of the proton, we can use Big Five #3, with $v_0 = 0$ (namely, $y = \frac{1}{2}at^2$) to find the time it will take for the proton to move the distance $y = d$. The acceleration of the proton is F/m, where $F = qE = eE$ is the force the proton feels; this gives $a = eE/m$. (We're ignoring the gravitational force on the proton because it is so much weaker than the electric force.) Now, since $E = V/d$ and $V = Q/C$, the expression for *a* becomes $a = eQ/mdC$. Substituting eQ/mdC for *a*, and *d* for *y*, Big Five #3 gives us

$$y = \frac{1}{2}at^2 \;\rightarrow\; d = \frac{1}{2}\cdot\frac{eQ}{mdC}t^2 \;\rightarrow\; t = d\sqrt{\frac{2mC}{eQ}}$$

The answer is choice D. Another way we could have attacked this question is to look at the answer choices and see if they make sense. If choice A were correct, then it would imply that a greater charge *Q* would *increase* the time required for the proton to move to the top plate. This doesn't make sense because a greater *Q* would create a greater force on the proton, giving it a greater acceleration, thus making it move faster, and causing *t* to decrease. We can also see that choice C can't be correct, for the same reason. Choice B could be eliminated because the units don't work out to be seconds, as shown below; therefore, the answer *had* to be choice D.

$$[d]\sqrt{\frac{[m]}{[e][Q][C]}} = \mathrm{m}\sqrt{\frac{\mathrm{kg}}{\mathrm{C}\cdot\mathrm{C}\cdot\frac{\mathrm{C}}{\mathrm{V}}}} = \mathrm{m}\sqrt{\frac{\mathrm{kg}}{\mathrm{C}\cdot\mathrm{C}\cdot\frac{\mathrm{C}}{\mathrm{J/C}}}} = \frac{\mathrm{m}}{\mathrm{C}^2}\sqrt{\mathrm{kg}\cdot\mathrm{J}} = \frac{\mathrm{m}}{\mathrm{C}^2}\sqrt{\mathrm{kg}\cdot\frac{\mathrm{kg}\cdot\mathrm{m}^2}{\mathrm{s}^2}} = \frac{\mathrm{kg}\cdot\mathrm{m}^2}{\mathrm{C}^2\cdot\mathrm{s}} \neq \mathrm{s}$$

Example 41-52: An electron is projected horizontally into the space between the plates of a parallel-plate capacitor, as shown below, where the electric field has a magnitude of 56 V/m. The initial velocity of the electron is horizontal and has a magnitude of $v_0 = 5 \times 10^6$ m/s.

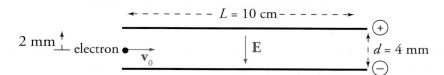

a) What is the force on the electron while it's in the region between the plates? (Neglect gravity.) What's the acceleration of the electron in this region? (Note: electron mass $\approx 9 \times 10^{-31}$ kg.)

b) How long would it take the electron to cover the horizontal distance L through the capacitor?

c) Describe the electron's trajectory through this region.

41.6

Solution:

a) Because the electric field **E** is constant between the plates, the force on the electron is also constant and given by $F = q\mathbf{E} = -e\mathbf{E}$; this force points upward, in the direction opposite to the electric field (because q is negative), toward the positively charged top plate. Substituting in the numerical values gives $F = eE = (1.6 \times 10^{-19} \text{ C}) \times (56 \text{ N/C}) = 9 \times 10^{-18}$ N. If the mass of the electron is m, then its acceleration, **a**, is F/m. Since $\mathbf{F} = -e\mathbf{E}$, we have $\mathbf{a} = -e\mathbf{E}/m$. Like **F**, the acceleration is uniform and vertical, pointing upward, toward the top plate. The magnitude of **a** is $a = F/m = (9 \times 10^{-18} \text{ J})/(9 \times 10^{-31} \text{ kg}) = 10^{13}$ m/s^2.

b) Because the acceleration of the electron is vertical, the electron's horizontal velocity will not change. Because v_{0x} is always equal to v_{0x}, the time require to traverse the 10 cm horizontal distance through the region between the plates is

$$x = v_x t \rightarrow t = \frac{x}{v_x} = \frac{x}{v_{0x}} = \frac{L}{v_{0x}} = \frac{10 \times 10^{-2} \text{ m}}{5 \times 10^6 \text{ m/s}} = 2 \times 10^{-8} \text{ s}$$

c) Because the acceleration is constant, we can use The Big Five to describe the motion of the electron. In fact, the motion of the electron between the plates is just like the motion of a projectile whose initial velocity is horizontal. The only difference is that while a projectile would curve downward in a half-parabola, the electron in the figure above will curve upward. Adapting Big Five #3 to vertical motion (in the y direction), we have $y = v_{0y} t + \frac{1}{2} a_y t^2$. Because $v_{0y} = 0$, this equation simplifies to $y = \frac{1}{2} a_y t^2$. Now, in the time t that the electron moves through the region between the plates (which we found in part b) its vertical displacement will be $y = \frac{1}{2}(10^{13} \text{ m/s}^2)(2 \times 10^{-8} \text{ s})^2 = 2 \times 10^{-3} \text{ m} = 2\text{mm}$. Therefore, the electron will just hit the right edge of the top plate.

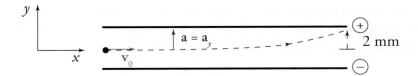

Now let's look at the second important use of a capacitor: as a storage device for electrical potential energy. We can think of the process of charging a capacitor as a transferal of electrons from one plate to the other. The plate that the electrons are taken from is left positively charged, and the plate the electrons are transferred to becomes negatively charged. Also, because we're simply transferring charge from one plate to the other, we are always assured at each moment that the plates carry equal but opposite charges.

During this charging process, an outside agent (the voltage source) must do work against the electric field that's created between the plates of the capacitor. Once we begin the process of transferring electrons from one plate to the other, it becomes increasingly difficult to transfer more. After all, it takes effort to remove more electrons from the plate that is left positively charged, *and* it takes effort to place them on the plate that is negatively charged. The fact that we have to fight against the system means we're storing potential energy.

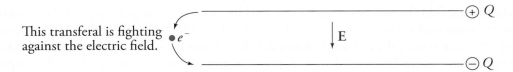

This transferal is fighting against the electric field.

To increase the charge on the capacitor, work is required to remove extra electrons from the positive plate and move them to the negative plate. This work against the electric field is stored as electrical potential energy.

Because it requires more work to transfer more charge, we'd expect that the amount of potential energy stored should depend on Q, the final charge on the capacitor; that is, as Q increases, so should the PE. We'd also expect that the amount of stored PE should depend on the voltage between the plates. After all, we defined potential difference, V, by the equation $\Delta PE = qV$, where q was the charge that moved between the points whose potential difference was V. Hence, the higher voltage V leads to an increase in stored potential energy. If the final charge on the capacitor is Q and the final resulting voltage is V, then PE is proportional to both Q and V. Here's how we can intuitively find the formula for PE in this case: we transferred a total amount of charge equal to Q, fighting against the voltage that prevailed at each stage. If the final voltage is V, then the average voltage during the charging process is $\frac{1}{2}V$. Since ΔPE is equal to charge times voltage, we get $\Delta PE = Q \cdot \left(\frac{1}{2}V\right) = \frac{1}{2}QV$. At the beginning of the charging process, when there was no charge on the capacitor, we had $PE_i = 0$, so $\Delta PE = PE_{fi} - PE = PE_{ff} - 0 = PE$. Therefore, we have $PE_f = \frac{1}{2}QV$:

Electrical PE Stored in a Capacitor

$$PE = \tfrac{1}{2}QV$$

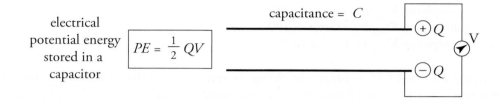

electrical potential energy stored in a capacitor

$$PE = \frac{1}{2}\,QV$$

capacitance $= C$

$+Q$

$-Q$

V

41.6

Using the fundamental equation $Q = CV$, we can rewrite this equation in terms of C and V, or in terms of Q and C:

$$PE = \frac{1}{2}QV = \frac{1}{2}CV^2 = \frac{Q^2}{2C}$$

If you lift a rock off the ground, you do work against the gravitational field of the Earth, and, as a result, you store gravitational potential energy. To recapture this stored energy, you let the rock fall back to the ground, transferring the gravitational potential energy into mechanical kinetic energy. Similarly, if you transfer electrons from one plate of a capacitor to the other, you do work against the electric field of the capacitor, and, as a result, you store electrical potential energy. To recapture this stored electrical energy, you let the electrons go back to their original plate, effectively **discharging** the capacitor. The movement of electrons can be used in a productive manner by providing a path for them and placing some electrical devices along the way. As a result, the electrons that return to the plate end up passing through, say, a light bulb, and the current causes the bulb to light. We've been able to tap into the energy stored in the capacitor to do useful work. When we connect the charged capacitor plates by a wire with some resistor(s) along it, the charge drains off rapidly at first, but the rate at which the charge leaves gradually decreases as time goes on. The same is true of the resulting current; it too starts off high and then gradually drops to zero as the capacitor discharges.

Discharging a Capacitor

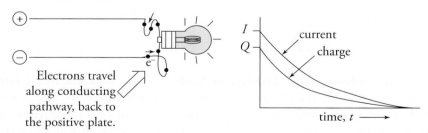

Electrons travel along conducting pathway, back to the positive plate.

I
Q

current

charge

time, t

Example 41-53: The Nernst equation (see Section 32.4) can be used to calculate the equilibrium potential for any ion X. At standard conditions, $RT/F = 25$ mV. The conversion factor from natural logs to base 10 logs is 2.3. Therefore, the Nernst equation can also be written as $E_{ion} = (58 \text{ mV}/z) \times \log ([X]_{out} / [X]_{in})$. Which of the following changes to K^+ concentrations would be needed to double the potential energy stored across a cell membrane characterized by C_m (see figure in Example 41-46)?

    A) multiplying K^+_{in} by a factor of 50
    B) multiplying K^+_{in} by a factor of 100
    C) multiplying K^+_{out} by a factor of 100
    D) multiplying K^+_{out} by a factor of 50

41.6

Solution: Apply $PE = 1/2\ CV^2$ to isolate the change in voltage across the membrane as the capacitance remains constant while K^+ moves from one side of the membrane to the other. $V \propto \sqrt{PE}$ so to double the PE, V would need to increase by a factor of $\sqrt{2} = 1.4$. This means that we need to obtain a log value between 10 and 100 (since $\log 10 = 1$ and $\log 100 = 2$). This eliminates choices B and C. Also, notice that the increase would have to occur outside the cell to increase the potential energy. Choice D is correct.

Example 41-54: A defibrillator contains a circuit whose primary components are a battery, a capacitor, and a switch. When the heart is undergoing ventricular fibrillation, the normally ordered electrical signals that organize the heart's pumping behavior are out of sync. The strong current delivered by the conducting paddles of the defibrillator can depolarize the entirety of the heart and potentially reset its orderly pumping triggered by the SA node. The defibrillator circuit first charges the capacitor with the battery. During the application and discharging of the circuit, a switch is closed to allow the capacitor to discharge through the paddles and the patient's tissue. Which of the following graphs best illustrates the voltage between the capacitor plates during this latter process?

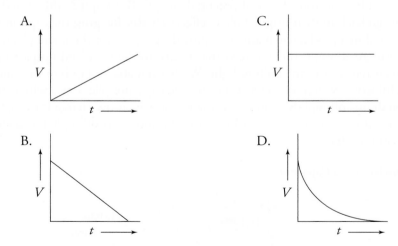

Solution: As the capacitor loses charge, Q decreases. Since $V = Q/C$, we know that V must decrease too. This eliminates choices A and C. The charge drains off rapidly at first, but the rate at which the charge leaves gradually decreases as time goes on; therefore, the decrease in Q (and therefore in V also) is not linear. Thus, the best graph is the one in choice D. (The defibrillator circuit will also feature an *inductor* or *solenoid*, described later in this chapter. This has the effect of slowing the discharge of the capacitor and prolonging the application of current sufficiently to completely depolarize the heart.)

Dielectrics

If the plates of a capacitor were touching at the start of the charging process, then we'd effectively have a single conductor, not a pair, and no transferal of electrons from one plate to the other could begin; it wouldn't work as a capacitor. And if the plates were ever allowed to touch during the charging process, the capacitor would discharge almost immediately, since the transferred electrons would have a direct route back to the positive plate. All the electrical potential energy that had been stored would be lost in an instant, without any useful work being done by the stored energy. So for a capacitor to be useful, we need to keep the plates from touching.

Let's consider ways to do that. One way would be to mount them on separate insulating handles, like this:

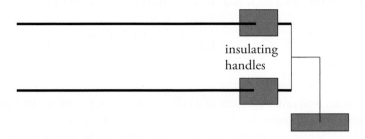

insulating
handles

That could work, but the way it's typically done is to sandwich a slab of insulating material between the plates. Such an insulator is known as a **dielectric**:

dielectric = slab of
insulating material
placed between
the plates of
a capacitor

Not only does a dielectric keep the plates from touching, but there's also a bonus: *The presence of a dielectric always increases the capacitance.* For the capacitor whose plates are mounted on insulating handles, with vacuum (or, for all practical purposes, air) between the plates, the capacitance is given by the equation we gave earlier: $C = \varepsilon_0 A/d$. However, if the capacitor is fitted with a dielectric, the capacitance is multiplied by a factor of K, where K is known as the **dielectric constant** of the insulating material. For example, wax paper is a dielectric, with a dielectric constant of about 3.5. If a parallel-plate capacitor were fitted with wax paper as a dielectric, the capacitance would be multiplied by 3.5. Other common dielectrics are teflon and certain plastics and ceramics.

Here's the formula for the capacitance of a parallel-plate capacitor with a dielectric:

> **Capacitance of a Parallel-Plate Capacitor with a Dielectric**
>
> $$C_{\substack{\text{with} \\ \text{dielectric}}} = K \cdot C_{\substack{\text{without} \\ \text{dielectric}}} = K \varepsilon_0 \frac{A}{d}$$

The value of K for vacuum is exactly 1, which makes sense since having empty space between the plates means there's *no* dielectric. The MCAT will assume that $K = 1$ for air as well because the actual value of K for air (~1.0005) is so close to 1. A capacitor with just air between its plates is known simply as an *air capacitor*. K is never less than 1, which is the reason dielectrics always increase capacitance.

Example 41-55: The area, A, of each plate of a parallel-plate capacitor satisfies the equation $\varepsilon_0 A = 10^{-10}$ F·m. If the plates are separated by a distance of 2 mm and this space is filled by a sheet of mica with a dielectric constant of 6, what is the capacitance of this capacitor?

Solution: The presence of the mica increases the capacitance by a factor of 6, so

$$C_{\substack{\text{with}\\\text{dielectric}}} = K \cdot C_{\substack{\text{without}\\\text{dielectric}}} = K\varepsilon_0 \frac{A}{d} = 6 \cdot \frac{10^{-10}\ \text{F}\cdot\text{m}}{2\times10^{-3}\text{m}} = 3\times10^{-7}\ \text{F}$$

Example 41-56: The inner and outer surfaces of a cell membrane act as plates in a parallel-plate capacitor. Consider a 1 μm^2 section of an axon: the dielectric constant of the membrane is 8 and the membrane is 6 nm thick. If the voltage across the membrane is 70 mV, what is the approximate magnitude of charge that resides on each side of this 1 μm^2 section? (*Note*: $\varepsilon_0 = 8.85 \times 10^{-12}$ C^2/N·m^2).

Solution: The capacitance is $C_{\text{with dielectric}} = K\varepsilon_0 A / d$, with $K = 8$, so

$$Q = CV = K\varepsilon_0 \frac{A}{d} \cdot V = (8)(8.85\times10^{-12}\ \tfrac{\text{C}^2}{N\cdot m^2}) \cdot \frac{1\ \mu\text{m}^2 \cdot \left(\frac{1\ \text{m}}{10^6\ \mu\text{m}}\right)^2}{6\times10^{-9}\ \text{m}} \cdot (70\times10^{-3}\ \text{V}) \approx 1\times10^{-15}\ \text{C}$$

Example 41-57: The capacitance of a certain air capacitor whose plates are separated by a distance of 1 mm is 4 pF. If the plates are moved apart to a distance of 2.2 mm to accommodate a slab of porcelain of thickness 2.2 mm that is then inserted between them, the capacitance becomes 12 pF. What is the dielectric constant of porcelain?

Solution: The capacitance without the porcelain is $C_{\text{without dielectric}} = \varepsilon_0 A / d_1$, and the capacitance with the porcelain is $C_{\text{with dielectric}} = K\varepsilon_0 A / d_2$. The ratio of these values is

$$\frac{C_{\text{with dielectric}}}{C_{\text{without dielectric}}} = \frac{K\varepsilon_0 A / d_2}{\varepsilon_0 A / d_1} = K\frac{d_2}{d_1} = K\frac{1\ \text{mm}}{2.2\ \text{mm}} = \frac{K}{2.2}$$

Now, because the capacitance increased by a factor of 3, we have

$$\frac{K}{2.2} = 3 \rightarrow \quad \therefore K = 6.6$$

The presence of a dielectric can affect other properties of a capacitor besides capacitance. However, the ways a dielectric affects the charge, voltage, and electric field depend on whether the capacitor is connected or disconnected from the battery that charged it.

Let's begin by looking at the case in which a capacitor without a dielectric is charged by a battery and then disconnected from it. What happens if we then insert a dielectric between the plates? First, since the capacitor is disconnected from the battery, the charge that exists on the plates is trapped and cannot change. Therefore, Q remains constant. Because the capacitance C increases, the equation $Q = CV$ tells us that the voltage will decrease; in fact, because Q stays constant and C increases by a factor of K, we see that V will decrease by a factor of K. Next, using the equation $V = Ed$, we see that because V decreases by a factor of K, so does E. Finally, using the equation $PE = \frac{1}{2}QV$, we conclude that since Q stays constant and V decreases by a factor of K, the stored electrical potential energy decreases by a factor of K.

We can look at this a little more closely: First, why does the electric field strength, E, decrease in this case? The dielectric is an insulator, so although the field between the plates won't move any free electrons through the material, it will polarize the molecules. That is, the electric field will create tiny dipole moments in the molecules of the insulator, with the negative (δ^-) ends closer to the positive plate and the positive (δ^+) ends closer to the negative plate. As a result, we'll have a layer of negative charge at the surface of the dielectric that's near the positive plate and a layer of positive charge at the surface of the dielectric that's near the negative plate. These layers of induced charge on the opposite surfaces of the dielectric are the source of a new electric field through the dielectric, $\mathbf{E}_{induced}$, a field that points in the opposite direction from the electric field created by the charged capacitor plates themselves (because electric fields always point from positive and toward negative source charges).

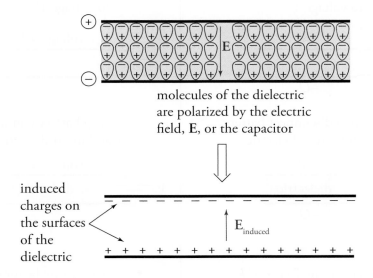

molecules of the dielectric
are polarized by the electric
field, **E**, or the capacitor

induced charges on the surfaces of the dielectric

$E_{induced}$

The total electric field between the plates is then the sum of the field created by the plates, $\mathbf{E}$, and the field created by the layers of induced charge on the surfaces of the dielectric, $\mathbf{E}_{induced}$. Because $\mathbf{E}_{induced}$ points in the direction *opposite* to $\mathbf{E}$, the *net* field strength is reduced to $E - E_{induced}$. This is the physical reason why the electric field magnitude is reduced in this case.

We also found that the potential energy would be reduced if we inserted a dielectric after disconnecting the capacitor from the charging battery. Where did this energy go? Most of it is stored as electrical potential energy inside those induced dipoles in the dielectric. (Unfortunately, that stored energy is hard to recapture in a useful way.) You would notice that as you began to place the dielectric between the plates, the electric field would actually pull it in; thus, some of the stored potential energy turns into kinetic energy of the dielectric as it was pulled into the space between the capacitor plates. Finally, there would be some heat production (the usual MCAT answer to "Where did the energy go?").

Now let's examine the case in which a capacitor without a dielectric is first charged up and then while it's still connected to its voltage source, we insert a dielectric between its plates. First, since the capacitor is still connected to the battery, the voltage between the plates must match the voltage of the battery. Therefore, V will not change.[5] Because the capacitance C increases, the equation $Q = CV$ tells us that the charge Q must increase; in fact, because V doesn't change and C increases by a factor of K, we see that Q will increase by a factor of K. Next, using the equation $V = Ed$, we see that because V doesn't change, neither will E. Finally, using the equation $PE = \frac{1}{2}QV$, we conclude that since V doesn't change and Q increases by a factor of K, the stored electrical potential energy increases by a factor of K. An important point to notice is that V doesn't change because the battery will transfer additional charge to the capacitor plates. This increase in Q offsets any momentary decrease in the electric field strength when the dielectric is inserted (because the molecules of the dielectric are polarized, as above) and brings the electric field strength back to its original value. Furthermore, as more charge is transferred to the plates, more electrical potential energy is stored.

The following figure summarizes the effects on the properties of a capacitor with the insertion of a dielectric in the two cases:

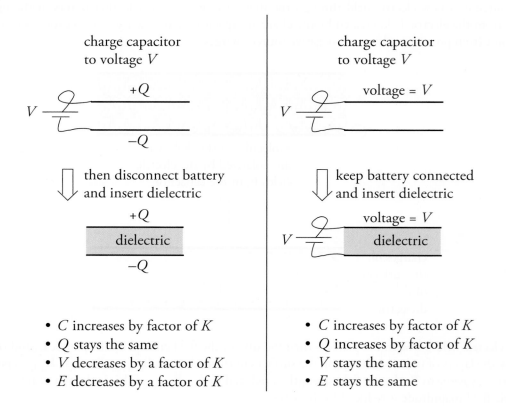

- C increases by factor of K
- Q stays the same
- V decreases by a factor of K
- E decreases by a factor of K

- C increases by factor of K
- Q increases by factor of K
- V stays the same
- E stays the same

---

[5] This analysis assumes that the circuit has no resistance, so the newly increased capacitance can be filled up instantaneously. In practice, voltage in the capacitor would drop at first but then rise quickly until it was again equal to the battery's voltage.

Example 41-58: A parallel-plate capacitor, with air between the plates, is charged to a voltage of $V = 1000$ V by a battery. The values of Q, E, and PE are also measured. The battery is then disconnected from the capacitor and a dielectric with dielectric constant $K = 4$ is inserted between the plates. The values of V, Q, E, and PE are measured again. Which of these values did *not* change?

    A) V
    B) Q
    C) E
    D) PE

Solution: Since the battery was disconnected from the capacitor after charging, the value of Q does not change: there's nowhere for charges to go and no source of new charges. The values of V, E, and PE will all decrease by a factor of K. The answer is choice B.

41.6

Example 41-59: Cell membranes have a dielectric number of about 9. If the internal potential of the cell is about 70 mV lower than the external potential, how much charge could accumulate on a square micrometer of phospholipid layer with a thickness of 8 nanometers ($\varepsilon_0 \approx 9 \times 10^{-12}$ F/m)?

Solution:

$$C = \frac{K\varepsilon_0 A}{d} = \frac{9(9 \times 10^{-12} \text{ F/m})(10^{-6} \text{ m})^2}{8 \times 10^{-9}} \approx 10^{-14} \text{ F}$$

Now the charge this cell membrane capacitor can hold at the given voltage is $Q = CV = (10^{-14}$ F$)$ $(70 \times 10^{-3}$ V$) = 7 \times 10^{-16}$ C. This may not seem like much, but considering that the charge of one sodium or potassium ion is 1.6×10^{-19} C, this amounts to about 4 thousand ions. This is NOT what actually happens to a living cell, mind you, because a living cell is not a passive participant in its local environment (and there are chemical considerations in addition to electrical ones).

Combinations of Capacitors

Like resistors, capacitors can also be placed in series and in parallel within a circuit. In this section, we'll see how to find the equivalent capacitance for each of these cases.

Capacitors in **parallel** all have the same voltage (like *resistors* in parallel), but the equivalent capacitance is the sum of the individual capacitances (like resistors in *series*):

equivalent capacitance
for capacitors in parallel
$$\boxed{C_{eq} = C_1 + C_2 + C_3 + \dots}$$

For example, in the figure below, the equivalent capacitance, C_{eq}, is 2 μF + 3 μF + 4 μF = 9 μF:

capacitors in parallel

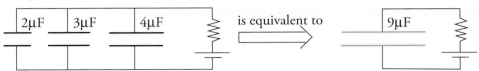

Capacitors in **series** all have the same charge (similar to *resistors* in series all having the same current), but the equivalent capacitance is found from the same formula that we used for resistors in *parallel*:

equivalent capacitance
for capacitors in series
$$\frac{1}{C_{eq}} = \frac{1}{C_1} + \frac{1}{C_2} + \frac{1}{C_3} + \dots$$

Equivalently, we could simplify the capacitors two at a time using the expression *product/sum*. For example, in the figure below, the equivalent capacitance, C_{eq}, is 2 μF, because 1/12 + 1/6 + 1/4 = 1/2. (We could also calculate it as (12 × 6)/(12 + 6) = 4 and (4 × 4)/(4 + 4) = 2.)

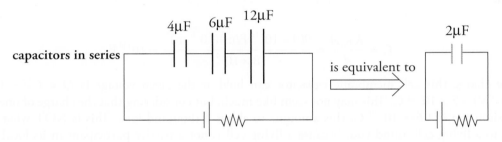

Example 41-60: Three uncharged capacitors are arranged in a circuit as shown.

After the switch S has been closed for a long time and electrostatic equilibrium is reached, how much charge is on the 6 μF capacitor?

Solution: The 3 μF and 6 μF capacitors are in series, so they're equivalent to a single 2 μF capacitor, because $(3 \times 6)/(3 + 6) = 2$. Therefore, the circuit shown above is equivalent to

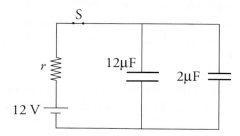

These two capacitors are in parallel, so both will have the same voltage: 12 V, since the plates of each are connected to the terminals of a 12 V battery. Now, using the equation $Q = CV$, we see that the charge on the 2 μF capacitor will be

$$Q = (2 \text{ μF})(12 \text{ V}) = 24 \text{ μC}$$

Since the 2 μF capacitor is equivalent to the series combination consisting of the 3 μF and 6 μF capacitors, the charge on each of these capacitors must be the same, 24 μC. (For extra practice, you may wish to verify the final voltages and charges on each of the three capacitors in the original circuit; the answers are shown below.)

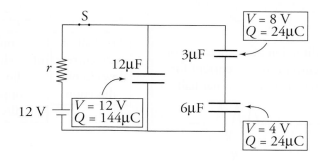

41.7 ALTERNATING CURRENT

In Section 41.5, we discussed circuits in which the current flowed in one direction only; such current is called **direct current** (DC). However, the electrical current that we use in our homes and offices every day is **alternating current** (AC), because the direction of the current changes: first one way, then the opposite way, then back again, and so on. The electrons that drift in the wires (and whose flow constitutes the current) are constantly forced to shuttle back and forth. While this may seem a little silly, producing an alternating voltage (and thus an alternating current) on a scale that supplies electricity to entire cities is far easier than producing a steady, direct voltage.

An AC generator creates a sinusoidally varying voltage. The voltage starts at, say, zero, and climbs to a peak value (called the amplitude), then falls back to zero; at this point, the polarity reverses, and the voltage again rises to its peak value then falls back to zero, and the cycle starts again. When we graph this time-varying voltage, we show the first half of the cycle as positive and the second half as negative; the negative voltage simply means that it points in the opposite direction from the voltage in the first half of the cycle. Thus, when the voltage is positive, the current flows in one direction. When the voltage is negative, the current flows in the opposite direction. In cases where the circuit contains only a source of alternating voltage and resistors, the current is in phase with the voltage, and we also consider Ohm's Law to hold: that is, the voltage and current are related by $v = iR_{eq}$, where R_{eq} is the equivalent resistance of the circuit.

Note: It's customary when discussing time-varying voltages and currents to use lower-case letters; v and i, rather than V and I. The capital letters then denote the *maximum* values of v and i.

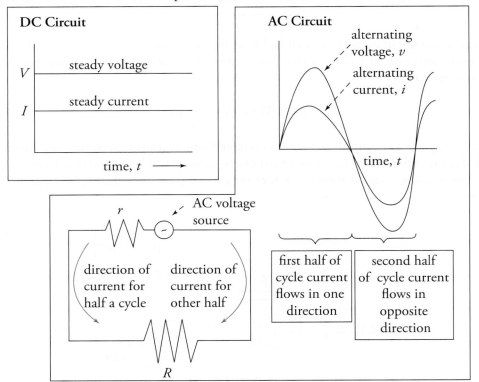

Notice that since v and i are constantly changing in an AC circuit, we can't talk about *the* voltage or *the* current. Instead, we talk about a kind of average voltage and average current. The particular average that is most useful is known as the **root-mean-square**, abbreviated **rms**. To form the rms of a quantity, we square it, average it over a cycle (that is, find the mean), then take the square root; it's the *root* of the *mean* of the *square* (hence root-mean-square). Fortunately, what all this boils down to is that the rms of a quantity is equal to its maximum divided by $\sqrt{2}$.

RMS Voltage and RMS Current

$$V_{rms} = \frac{v_{max}}{\sqrt{2}} = \frac{V}{\sqrt{2}} \quad \text{and} \quad I_{rms} = \frac{i_{max}}{\sqrt{2}} = \frac{I}{\sqrt{2}}$$

Recall that the power dissipated by a resistor in a DC circuit is given by the equation $P = I^2R$ and the power supplied by a voltage source is given by $P = IV$. For an AC circuit, we say that the average power dissipated by a resistor is $\bar{P} = I_{rms}^2 R$ and the average power supplied by the voltage source is $\bar{P} = I_{rms}V_{rms}$. This is why the rms average is one we use; it keeps the formulas the same as they were for DC circuits.

Example 41-61: Homes are typically supplied with 110 V rms.

a) What's the maximum voltage?
b) How much energy (in kWh) is used in 2 hours by a device whose resistance is 110 ohms?
c) How much would this cost if the electric company charges you 8¢ per kWh?

Solution:

a) Since 110 V is the rms voltage, we find the maximum voltage by multiplying V_{rms} by $\sqrt{2}$:

$$v_{max} = \sqrt{2} \cdot V_{rms} \approx (1.4)(110 \text{ V}) = 154 \text{ V}$$

41.8

b) Energy is power × time, so we can find the energy consumed by this device by multiplying the average power it consumes by the time. Since

$$\bar{P} = I_{rms}^2 R = \left(\frac{V_{rms}}{R}\right)^2 R = \frac{V_{rms}^2}{R} = \frac{(110 \text{ V})^2}{110 \text{ }\Omega} = 110 \text{ W}$$

we have

$$\text{energy} = \bar{P} \times t = (110 \text{ W})(2 \text{ h}) = 220 \text{ Wh} = 0.220 \text{ kWh}$$

c) To calculate how much this would cost, we multiply this by 8¢/kWh:

$$\text{cost} = 0.220 \text{ kWh} \times \frac{\$0.08}{\text{kWh}} = \$0.0175 = 1\tfrac{3}{4} \text{ cents}$$

41.8   MAGNETIC FIELDS AND FORCES

Electric fields are created by electric charges; **magnetic fields** are created by *moving* electric charges. If a charge is at rest, it produces an electric field in the surrounding space. If this charge were to move, it would create an additional force field, a magnetic field, in the surrounding space. Since charge in motion con- stitutes a current, we can also say that magnetic fields are produced by electric currents. A permanent bar magnet is a source of a magnetic field because of the multitude of microscopic currents due to motions of the orbiting electrons within the metal; therefore, even a bar magnet's magnetic field is ultimately due to charges in motion.

If we place a charge q in a given electric field, **E**, the force that the field will exert on this charge is given by the equation $\mathbf{F}_E = q\mathbf{E}$. We now need a similar formula to tell us the force that a magnetic field would exert on a charge q. First, a magnetic field can only exert a force on a charge that is *moving* through the field. A magnetic field is produced by moving charges and it exerts a force only on other moving charges. A magnetic field will exert no force on a charge that's at rest. The letter **B** is used to denote a magnetic field. The formula for the force that a magnetic field exerts on a charge q is as follows:

Magnetic Force

$$\mathbf{F}_\mathrm{B} = q(\mathbf{v} \times \mathbf{B})$$

---

where **v** is the velocity of the charge q. Notice that if **v** = 0 (that is, if the charge is at rest), then $\mathbf{F}_\mathrm{B}$ will also be 0.

The formula $\mathbf{F}_\mathrm{B} = q\left(\mathbf{v} \times \mathbf{B}\right)$ involves the *cross product* of **v** and **B**. You don't need to worry about calculating the vector components of the cross product; there is a much simpler way of finding $\mathbf{F}_\mathrm{B}$ that is more than adequate for the MCAT. First, the magnitude of $\mathbf{F}_\mathrm{B}$ is given by this equation:

Magnitude of Magnetic Force

$$F_\mathrm{B} = |q|\,vB\sin\theta$$

---

where θ is the angle between **v** and **B**. Notice that if **v** is parallel to **B**, then $\theta = 0$, and, since sin 0 = 0, we get $\mathbf{F}_\mathrm{B}$ = 0. So, a charge could be moving through a magnetic field and yet feel no force if its direction of motion is parallel to the magnetic field lines. The same will be true if **v** is anti-parallel to **B** (that is, if the direction of **v** is exactly opposite to the direction of **B**), since in this case, we have $\theta = 180°$ and sin 180° = 0, so again we get $\mathbf{F}_\mathrm{B}$ = 0. If **v** $\perp$ **B**, then $\theta = 90°$, and since sin 90° = 1, the magnitude of $\mathbf{F}_\mathrm{B}$ becomes simply $F_\mathrm{B} = |q|\,vB$. From this equation, we can find the SI unit for magnetic field strength:

$$[B] = \frac{[F_\mathrm{B}]}{[q][v]} = \frac{\mathrm{N}}{\mathrm{C} \cdot \mathrm{m/s}} = \frac{\mathrm{N}}{\frac{\mathrm{C}}{\mathrm{s}} \cdot \mathrm{m}} = \frac{\mathrm{N}}{\mathrm{A} \cdot \mathrm{m}}$$

One newton per amp-meter (1 N/A·m) is renamed one **tesla**, abbreviated **T**. That is, B is measured in teslas.

Now that we know how to find the magnitude of $\mathbf{F}_\mathrm{B}$, all we need is a way to find the direction. The direction of $\mathbf{F}_\mathrm{B}$ will depend on whether the charge q that moves through the field is positive or negative. Just like the force due to an electric field, the force due to a magnetic field also depends on the sign of the charge: If **B** exerts a force in a particular direction on a charge $+q$ moving with velocity **v**, then it would exert a force in the opposite direction on $-q$ moving with velocity **v**. In addition, magnetic forces have the following strange property: *The direction of $\mathbf{F}_\mathrm{B}$ is always perpendicular to both **v** and **B***. For example, if we had a magnetic field whose field lines pointed across this page (say, from left to right), and a positive charge q travels down the page, then the direction of the force $\mathbf{F}_\mathrm{B}$ that q feels would be out of the plane of the page. The direction of $\mathbf{F}_\mathrm{B}$ will always be perpendicular to the plane containing the vectors **v** and **B**, since we're now dealing with a situation in which we'll have vectors in *three* dimensions, we need a notation to indicate when a vector points into, or out of, the plane of the page. Here are the symbols:

means
out of
the plane of the page

means
into
the plane of the page

Now let's learn how to find the direction of the magnetic force, F_B, acting on a particle of charge q moving with velocity **v** through a magnetic field **B**. It involves the **right-hand rule**.[6] Here's how the rule works.

First, determine whether the charge moving through the magnetic field is positive or negative.

If q is *positive*, your *right*-hand rule will determine the direction you need.

If q is *negative*, your *right*-hand rule will determine the opposite direction of what you need, so remember to reverse the result!

When you use the right-hand rule, you will always follow these steps:

1. Orient your hand so that your thumb points in the direction of the velocity **v**.
2. Point your fingers in the direction of **B** (fingers = field).
3. The direction of F_B will then be perpendicular to your palm.

Think of your palm pushing with the force F_B; the direction it pushes is the direction of F_B.

Right-Hand Rule:

For determining the direction of
the magnetic force, F_B,
on a *positive* charge

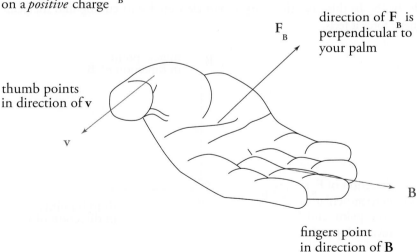

direction of F_B is
perpendicular to
your palm

F_B

thumb points
in direction of **v**

v

B

fingers point
in direction of **B**

---

[6] Another method which many people prefer is to use the left-hand rule for negative charges: everything else in the techniques described stays the same.

For example, let's say we have a positive charge q moving with velocity **v** to the right across the plane of this page through a magnetic field **B** directed toward the top of the page. How would you find the direction of the resulting magnetic force on this moving charge? Since q is positive, use your right hand, and lay it flat on this page with your palm facing up; notice that in this orientation, your thumb points to the right (as it should since your thumb always points in the direction of the particle's velocity, **v**) and your fingers point up toward the top of the page (as they should since your fingers always point in the direction of the magnetic field, **B**). The direction of $\mathbf{F}_B$ is perpendicular to your palm, pointing out of the plane of the page, and so we symbolize the direction of $\mathbf{F}_B$ by ⊙. In this case, the charged particle would start curling out of the plane of the page as a result of the magnetic force it feels.

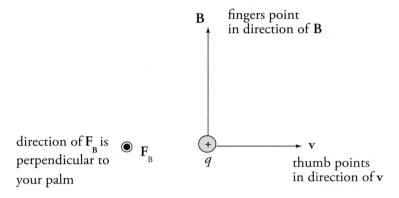

Now let's examine what would happen in the previous example if the charged particle had been *negative*. That is, we have a *negative* charge q moving with velocity **v** to the right across the plane of this page through a magnetic field **B** directed toward the top of the page. How would you find the direction of the resulting magnetic force on this moving charge? You would follow the exact same procedure *except you would reverse the final result*. The direction of $\mathbf{F}_B$ is perpendicular to your palm, but now pointing *into* the plane of the page, and so we symbolize the direction of $\mathbf{F}_B$ by ⊗. In this case, the charged particle would start curling into the plane of the page as a result of the magnetic force it feels.

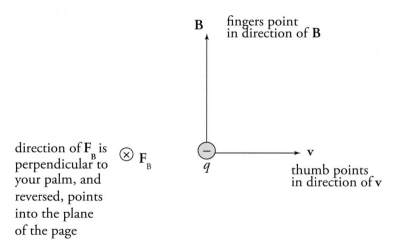

Practice the right-hand rule and verify each of the following:

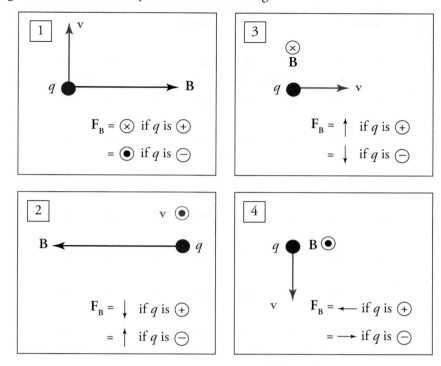

Because the magnetic force a charge feels is always perpendicular to the velocity of the charge, *magnetic forces do no work*. Recall that if a force **F** is perpendicular to the displacement **d** of an object, then this force **F** does zero work, because $W = Fd \cos \theta$ and $\theta = 90°$; since $\cos 90° = 0$, we get $W = 0$. Since magnetic forces never do work, they can never change the kinetic energy of a particle, meaning that *KE* is constant. (This follows from the Work-Energy Theorem, $W = \Delta KE$.) Since magnetic forces cannot change the kinetic energy of a particle, they can't change the speed of a particle. All magnetic forces can do is make charged particles change their direction; they can't make them speed up or slow down.

The formula given earlier for the magnitude of the magnetic force is $|q| vB \sin \theta$, where θ is the angle between **v** and **B**. On the MCAT, it's most common to have a constant magnetic field and $\mathbf{v} \perp \mathbf{B}$; in this case, $\theta = 90°$, and because $\sin 90° = 1$, the magnitude of $\mathbf{F_B}$ becomes $F_B = |q| vB$. Further, if $\mathbf{v} \perp \mathbf{B}$, the subsequent motion of the charged particle will be uniform circular motion, with the magnetic force providing the centripetal force. Recall that in uniform circular motion, the centripetal force is always perpendicular to the particle's velocity and the particle's speed is constant; all the particle does is continuously change direction as it moves in a circular path. This is consistent with what we said in the previous paragraph about magnetic forces: they don't change the speed of a particle, only its direction. The case of a charged particle executing uniform circular motion in a constant magnetic field is so important for the MCAT, that we'll do the following example in detail.

Example 41-62: A proton is injected with velocity **v** into a region of constant magnetic field **B** that points out of the plane of the page. The direction of **v** is to the right, in the plane of the page, as shown in the diagram below:

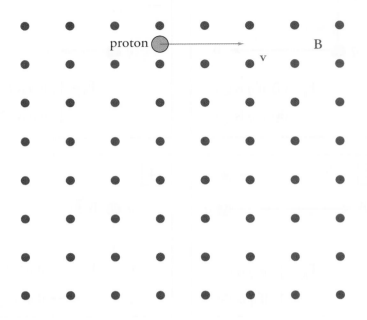

a) Describe the subsequent motion of the proton.
b) Find the radius of the circular trajectory it follows.

Solution:

a) Because the proton is a positive charge, we use the right-hand rule directly to find the direction of the magnetic force it feels. With **v** to the right and **B** out of the page, we find that **F**$_B$ points downward in the plane of the page:

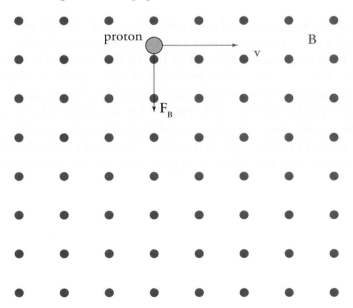

As a result, the proton will curve downward, and as it does, it is still continuously acted on by the magnetic force, but because the direction of **v** changes, so will the direction of $\mathbf{F}_B$. For example, when the proton is at the position shown in the following figure, the direction of $\mathbf{F}_B$ will be to the left:

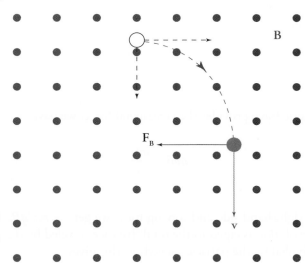

We can now see that the proton will continue to curve in a circular path, traveling clockwise:

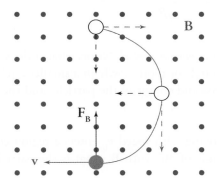
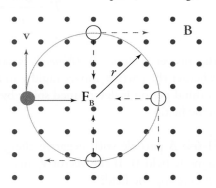

b) To find the radius of the circular path, we use the fact that the magnetic force provides the centripetal force to write

$$qvB = \frac{mv^2}{r}$$

where m is the mass of the proton. (We can drop the absolute value signs on the charge q because q is positive here.) Substituting $q = e$ (remember, it's a proton), then canceling one v from the right-hand side and solving for r, we get

$$r = \frac{mv}{eB}$$

Example 41-63: A particle with positive charge q and mass m moving with speed v undergoes uniform circular motion in a constant magnetic field **B**. If the radius of the particle's path is r, which of the following expressions gives the particle's orbit period (in other words, the time required for the particle to complete one revolution)?

A) $2\pi/qvB$
B) $2\pi m/qB$
C) $qvB/2\pi m$
D) $qB/2\pi m$

Solution: Since the magnetic force provides the centripetal force, we have

$$qvB = \frac{mv^2}{r}$$

Canceling one v from the right-hand side and solving for r, we get $r = mv/qB$. The time required for the particle to complete one revolution is equal to the total distance traveled by the particle in one revolution (the circumference, $2\pi r$) divided by the particle's speed, v. This gives

$$T = \frac{2\pi r}{v} = \frac{2\pi \times \dfrac{mv}{qB}}{v} = \frac{2\pi m}{qB}$$

Therefore, the answer is choice B. (*Note*: T is called the *cyclotron period*. Notice that it does *not* depend on r or v. Whether the particle moves rapidly in a large circle or more slowly in a smaller circle, it doesn't matter: the orbital period is determined solely by the mass and charge of the particle, and the magnitude of the magnetic field.)

Example 41-64: A particle with negative charge $-q$ moving with speed v_0 enters a region containing a uniform magnetic field **B**. If the vector $\mathbf{v}_0$ makes an angle of 30° with **B**, what is the particle's speed 8 seconds after entering the field?

A) $v_0/4$
B) v_0
C) $2v_0$
D) $4v_0$

Solution: Since magnetic forces do no work, the kinetic energy (and thus the speed) of the particle will be unchanged. The answer is choice B.

Example 41-65: A particle with charge q moves with velocity $\mathbf{v}$ through a region of space containing a uniform electric field, $\mathbf{E}$, *and* a uniform magnetic field, $\mathbf{B}$. Which of the following expressions gives the total electromagnetic force on the particle?

    A) $q(\mathbf{E} + \mathbf{B})$
    B) $q(\mathbf{v} \times \mathbf{E} + \mathbf{B})$
    C) $q\mathbf{v} \times (\mathbf{E} + \mathbf{B})$
    D) $q(\mathbf{E} + \mathbf{v} \times \mathbf{B})$

Solution: The electric force on the particle is $\mathbf{F}_E = q\mathbf{E}$, and the magnetic force is $\mathbf{F}_B = q(\mathbf{v} \times \mathbf{B})$. Therefore, the *total* electromagnetic force is

$$\mathbf{F}_E + \mathbf{F}_B = q\mathbf{E} + q(\mathbf{v} \times \mathbf{B}) = q(\mathbf{E} + \mathbf{v} \times \mathbf{B})$$

The answer is choice D.

Note: The total electromagnetic force is known as the **Lorentz force**.

41.8

Example 41-66: The figure below shows a charged parallel-plate capacitor with a uniform electric field, $\mathbf{E}$, in the space between its plates. A uniform magnetic field, $\mathbf{B}$, is also produced in the space between the capacitor plates by another device.

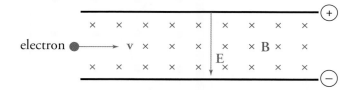

At what speed would an electron need to travel between the plates in order to pass through undeflected? (Ignore gravity.)

    A) E/B
    B) B/E
    C) EB
    D) EB^2

Solution: In between the plates, the direction of the electric force, $\mathbf{F}_E$, on the electron is upward. Using the right-hand rule and remembering to reverse the result because the particle is negatively charged, we find that the direction of the magnetic force, $\mathbf{F}_B$, is downward.

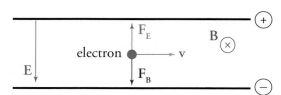

Therefore, these two forces point in opposite directions. They'll cancel (giving $\mathbf{F}_{net}$ = 0) and allow the particle to pass through undeflected if these forces have the same magnitude. The magnitude of the electric force is $F_E = |q|E = |-e|E = eE$, and the magnitude of the magnetic force is $F_B = |q|vB = |-e|vB = evB$. Therefore, we'll have $F_B = F_E$ when $evB = eE$. Solving this equation for v, we find that $v = E/B$, choice A.

Example 41-67: The figure below shows a simple mass spectrometer. It consists of a source of ions that are accelerated from rest through a potential difference V and then enter a region containing a uniform magnetic field $\mathbf{B}$ that points out of the plane of the page and is perpendicular to the initial velocity, $\mathbf{v}$, of the ion as it enters. Once an ion enters the magnetic field, it travels in a semicircular path until it strikes the detector, which records its arrival and the distance, d, from the opening.

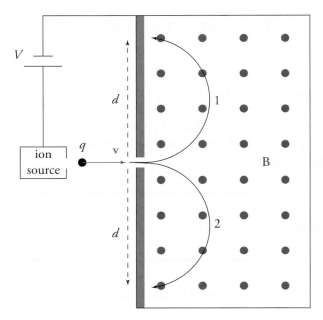

a)   An ion of charge $+q$ and mass m will enter the magnetic field with what speed? Write v in terms of q, m, and V.
b)   Which semicircular path would a cation follow: 1 or 2?
c)   If you were using this device in a lab to analyze a sample containing various isotopes of an element, how would you find the mass of a cation striking the detector if all you knew were q, V, B, and d?

Solution:

a)   The ion loses electrical potential energy in the amount qV, and as a result, gains kinetic energy, $\frac{1}{2}mv^2$. Therefore, $\frac{1}{2}mv^2 = qV$, so $v = \sqrt{2qV/m}$.

b) The right-hand rule (for a positive charge) tells us that if **v** points to the right and **B** points out of the plane of the page, then **F**$_B$ points downward:

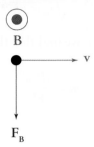

Since **F**$_B$ points downward when the particle is at the opening, a cation would follow path 2, because **F**$_B$ provides the centripetal force and thus points toward the center of the path. The following diagram illustrates this:

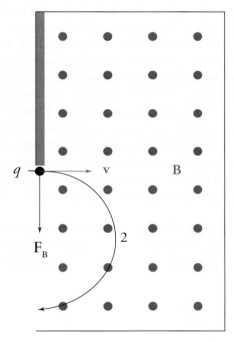

c) Since the magnetic force provides the centripetal force, we have

$$qvB = \frac{mv^2}{r}$$

Canceling one v from the right-hand side and solving for m (the mass of the cation) gives

$$m = \frac{qBr}{v}$$

From the diagram, we see that $r = \frac{1}{2}d$, and from part (a), $v = \sqrt{2qV/m}$, so we get

$$m = \frac{qB \cdot \frac{1}{2}d}{\sqrt{2qV/m}}$$

Squaring both sides and solving for m, we find that the mass of the cation is

$$m = \frac{qB^2d^2}{8V}$$

Sources of Magnetic Fields

Now that we know how a given magnetic field affects a charged particle, we'll look at how the magnetic field was created in the first place. Recall that charges *in motion* produce a magnetic field. A current is charge in motion, so electric currents produce magnetic fields. Let's take the simplest possible case: an electric current moving in a straight line. The magnetic field lines created by the current wrap around the current, forming closed loops. To find the direction of these magnetic field loops, we use the right-hand rule because by convention we consider a current I to be the direction that positive charges would move.[7] Imagine grabbing the wire in your right hand in such a way that your thumb points in the direction of the velocity of the charges (that is, in the direction of I). The way that your fingers wrap around the wire gives the direction of the magnetic field. Verify the directions of the **B**-field loops for the wires shown below; remember, magnetic field lines are actually circles that wrap around the wire. (That's the end of the right-hand rule in this situation. We are not trying to figure out the direction of the magnetic force that a given magnetic field exerts on a charged particle; we're now finding the magnetic field. Your thumb and fingers mean the same thing now as they did before: your thumb points in the direction of the motion of the relevant charge (the charge making the field), and your fingers point in the direction of the magnetic field, **tt**).

current-carrying wire perpendicular to page with current coming *out* of the plane of the page

current-carrying wire perpendicular to page with current going *into* the plane of the page

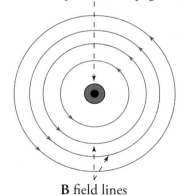

B field lines

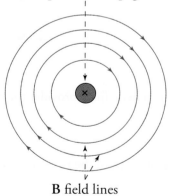

B field lines

---

[7] Though it's uncommon on the MCAT, it's possible you'll be asked about the field produced by a single moving charge, not a current. If the charge is positive, you simply use the method given here; if the charge is negative, you could use the left-hand rule, or use the right-hand rule and then reverse the direction of the answer; in other words, the field lines created by a negative charge circle in the opposite direction from those created by a positive charge.

In these next two diagrams, the **B**-field circles look like ellipses because of perspective; here the current-carrying wires lie in the plane of the page, and the **B**-field circles are perpendicular to the page, going into (or out of) the page above the wire and out of (or into) the page below the wire.

With the current pointing to the left, the B field lines go into the page above the wire . . .

With the current pointing to the right, the B field lines come out of the page above the wire . . .

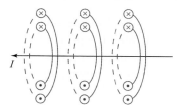

and come out of the page below the wire.

and go into the page below the wire.

The magnitude of the magnetic field created by a straight wire carrying a current I is proportional to I and inversely proportional to the distance r from the wire:

$$B \propto \frac{I}{r}$$

Hence, the magnetic field will be stronger if the current is increased or if we are positioned closer to the wire.

Circular wire loops that carry current also create magnetic fields. In the figure below, notice that the field lines are nearly vertical near the center of the circular wire loop that lies along the central axis. At the center of the loop, the magnitude of **B** is proportional to the current, I, and inversely proportional to the radius of the wire loop ($B \propto I/r_{loop}$). If the current in the wire loop had been traveling in the opposite direction (that is, clockwise), then each of the arrows on the **B**-field lines would point in the opposite direction.

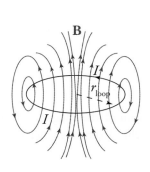

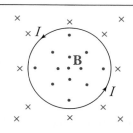

counterclockwise current:
B field points out of page inside the loop and points into the page outside the loop

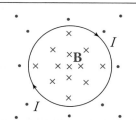

clockwise current:
B field points into page inside the loop and points out of the page outside the loop

Imagine taking a long wire and wrapping it tightly around a cylinder, like a paper-towel tube. The result will look like a spring; we can also consider it to be like a lot of circular loops close together. Such a helical coil of wire is called a **solenoid**. The magnetic field it produces inside the cylinder is parallel to the central axis and achieves its maximum magnitude *on* the central axis, getting weaker as we move away from the center, closer to the coils:

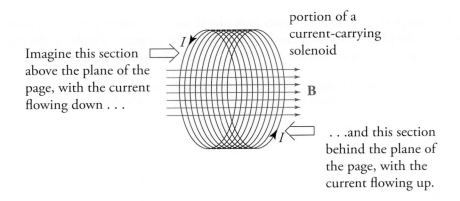

Imagine this section above the plane of the page, with the current flowing down . . .

I

portion of a current-carrying solenoid

B

. . .and this section behind the plane of the page, with the current flowing up.

I

If the solenoid has many windings and if the length is much greater than its diameter, then the magnetic field in the interior is nearly uniform and is proportional to the current (I) and to the number of turns per unit length (N/L): $B \propto I(N/L)$. Hence, the magnetic field will be stronger if the current is increased or if the solenoid wire loops are tightly packed.

Example 41-68: The figure below shows a long straight wire carrying a current, I. An electron is projected above the wire and initially parallel to it.

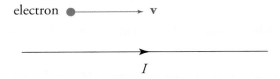

electron • ——————→ **v**

——————————→

I

Which of the following best illustrates the direction of the magnetic force on the electron at the position shown?

A. ↓   C. ⊗

B. ⊙   D. ↑

Solution: Since the current in the wire points to the right, the direction of the magnetic field **B** above the wire is out of the plane of the page. Using the left-hand rule (since the electron is a negative charge),

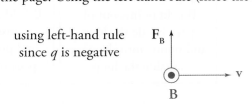

using left-hand rule since q is negative

$\mathbf{F}_B$ ↑

⊙ ——→ **v**

B

we find that the direction of the magnetic force $\mathbf{F}_B$ is upward, away from the wire, so choice D is correct.

41.8

Example 41-69: The figure below shows two long, straight wires carrying current. The top wire carries a current $I_1 = I$ to the left, while the bottom wire carries a current $I_2 = 2I$ to the right.

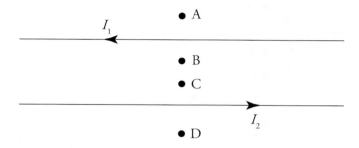

Points A and B are equidistant from the top wire, and Points C and D are equidistant from the bottom wire. Furthermore, the distance between Points B and C is the same as the distance between B and the top wire, which is also the same as the distance between C and the bottom wire. Of these four points, where is the total magnetic field the weakest?

Solution: First, we notice that the magnetic field created by the top wire, $\mathbf{B}_1$, encircles the wire, with the magnetic field circles centered on the top wire and pointing into the plane of the page above the wire and out of the page below it. Similarly, the magnetic field created by the bottom wire, $\mathbf{B}_2$, also encircles the wire, with the magnetic field circles centered on the bottom wire and pointing out of the plane of the page above the wire and into the page below it:

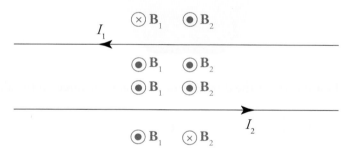

So, we can immediately rule out choices B and C; between the wires, the individual magnetic fields point in the same direction, so their magnitudes add, giving a strong field in this region. However, above the top wire and below the bottom wire, the individual magnetic fields point in opposite directions, so their magnitudes subtract; therefore, of the choices given, the field is weakest at either Point A or Point D. Because $I_2 = 2I$, Point D is closer to the higher-current wire, so to calculate the net $\mathbf{B}$ field at Point D, we'd subtract a small quantity (the contribution from the weaker-current, which is also farther away) from a large quantity (the contribution from the close higher-current). By contrast, to calculate the net $\mathbf{B}$ field at Point A, the quantity we'd subtract is larger than the one we subtracted to find the field at Point D and the positive term here is smaller than the positive term in the calculation of the field at Point D. Therefore, we expect the field at Point A to be weaker than at Point D. If this intuitive argument is unconvincing, let's do some math to back it up:

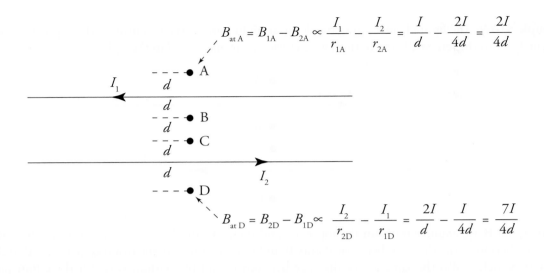

$$B_{at\,A} = B_{1A} - B_{2A} \propto \frac{I_1}{r_{1A}} - \frac{I_2}{r_{2A}} = \frac{I}{d} - \frac{2I}{4d} = \frac{2I}{4d}$$

$$B_{at\,D} = B_{2D} - B_{1D} \propto \frac{I_2}{r_{2D}} - \frac{I_1}{r_{1D}} = \frac{2I}{d} - \frac{I}{4d} = \frac{7I}{4d}$$

Example 41-70: The figure below shows a portion of a long narrow solenoid carrying a current, *I*. An alpha particle (α) is projected with velocity **v** down the central axis of the solenoid, as shown:

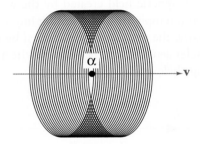

Which of the following best illustrates the direction of the magnetic force on the alpha particle?

A. ↓

C. ↑

B.

D. None of the above

Solution: At the position of the alpha particle, the magnetic field **B** created by the current-carrying solenoid is directed along the central axis; that is, either in the same direction as **v** or in the opposite direction from **v**, depending on the direction of the current in the wire loops. In either case, though, the magnetic force will be zero. (Remember that if **v** is parallel [or anti-parallel] to **B**, then $F_B = 0$.) The answer is choice D.

Magnets

A permanent bar magnet creates a magnetic field that closely resembles the magnetic field produced by a circular loop of current-carrying wire:

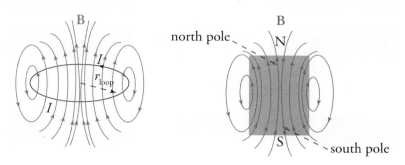

By convention, the magnetic field lines emanate from the end of the magnet designated the **north pole** (**N**) and then curl around and re-enter the magnet at the end designated the **south pole** (**S**). The magnetic field created by a permanent bar magnet is due to the electrons; they have an intrinsic spin (remember the spin quantum number, m_s, from general chemistry) and they orbit their nuclei; therefore, they are charges in motion, the ultimate source of all magnetic fields. If a piece of iron is placed in an external magnetic field (for example, the one created by a current-carrying solenoid) the individual magnetic dipole moments of the electrons will be forced to more or less line up. Because iron is *ferromagnetic*, these now-aligned magnetic dipole moments tend to retain this configuration, thus permanently magnetizing the bar and causing it to produce its own magnetic field.

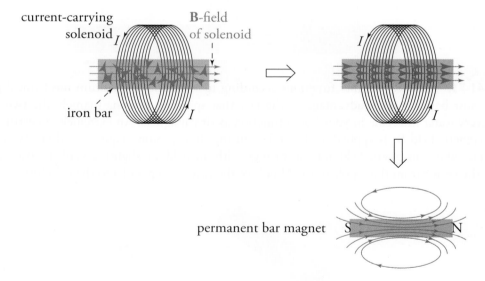

As with electric charges, like magnetic poles repel each other, while opposite magnetic poles attract each other:

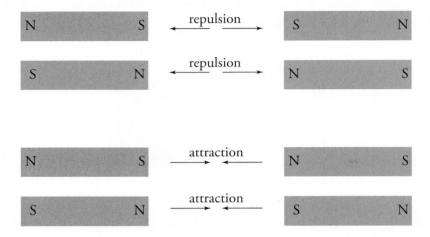

However, while you can have a positive electric charge all by itself, you can't have a single magnetic pole all by itself: the existence of a lone magnetic pole has never been confirmed. That is, there are no magnetic *monopoles*; magnetic poles always exist *in pairs*. If you cut a bar magnet into two pieces, you wouldn't get a piece with just an N and another piece with just an S; you'd get two separate and complete magnets, each with a N–S pair:

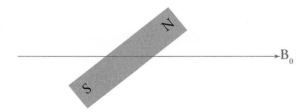

Example 41-71: An MRI scanner functions according to some subtle quantum mechanical principles, but at its most basic, it takes advantage of the fact that spinning protons (namely the two hydrogen nuclei in every water molecule in your body) function as tiny magnets. An extremely powerful, constant external magnetic field $\mathbf{B}_0$ is applied to the body, causing these proton magnets to align. Why? When a magnet is placed in a magnetic field, it tends to align with the field (or, slightly less likely, exactly opposite it), so that the vector from the S pole to the N pole of the magnet is parallel to the field lines.

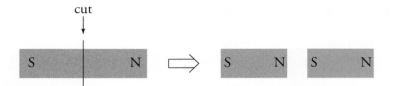

Given that the uniform magnetic field $\mathbf{B}_0$ in the figure above exerts the same magnitude of force on the N pole as it does on the S pole and the magnetic force on a pole is along the field line, what can you say about the net force and net torque on the magnet?

Solution: Because the $\mathbf{B}_0$ field will exert a force $\mathbf{F}_B$ on the N pole and a force of $-\mathbf{F}_B$ on the S pole, the net force on the magnet will be zero ($\mathbf{F}_B + -\mathbf{F}_B = 0$). However, the net torque will not be zero, since the magnetic force produces a clockwise torque on each pole, tending to align the magnet parallel to the field line.

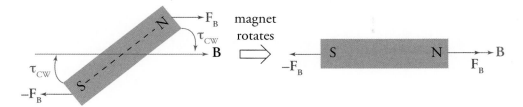

Example 41-72: Two bar magnets are fixed in position, and a proton is projected with velocity **v** into the region between adjacent opposite poles, as shown below:

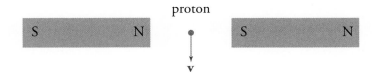

Which of the following best illustrates the direction of the magnetic force on the proton at the position shown?

A. ⟵   C. ⊗

B. ⊙   D. ⟶

Solution: On the outside of the magnet(s), **B** points from the N pole to the S pole.

Using the right-hand rule (for a positive charge) where **B** points to the right and **v** is downward, then $\mathbf{F}_B$ points out of the plane of the page:

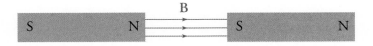

Therefore, the answer is choice B.

Chapter 42
Oscillations, Waves, and Sound

42.1   OSCILLATIONS

Any motion that regularly repeats is referred to as **periodic** or **harmonic motion**. Common examples include an object undergoing uniform circular motion, a mass oscillating on a spring and a pendulum. This type of motion can be characterized by its **period** or **frequency**.

Period

The time it takes an object to move through one full cycle of motion is called the period. For an object undergoing uniform circular motion, the period is the time it takes to make one revolution. For a mass on a spring or a pendulum, it is the time it takes to make a round trip (i.e., the final position and velocity must be the same as the initial values). The period is denoted by T and is measured in seconds.

Example 42-1: The bob on a pendulum moves from point A to point B in 0.5 seconds. What is the period of oscillation?

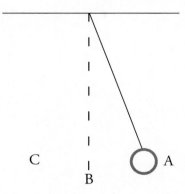

Solution: A to B represents one-quarter of a period. A full period is the time it takes for the bob to move from A to B to C to B and back to A. So $T = 4(0.5 \text{ s}) = 2 \text{ s}$.

Frequency

Rather than timing one cycle to find the period, we can instead count the number of cycles that occur in one second. This is known as the frequency, denoted by f. The units of f are cycles per second, or **hertz** (Hz).

Now the first thing we notice is that period and frequency are reciprocals. After all, the period is the number of seconds per cycle, and the frequency is the number of cycles per second. So, we have these fundamental relationships:

> **Period and Frequency**
>
> $$f = \frac{1}{T} \quad \text{and} \quad T = \frac{1}{f}$$

Every type of oscillation has a period and a frequency, but there is a special class of oscillations in which these quantities have a unique property. This ideal type of oscillatory motion is referred to as **simple harmonic motion** (often abbreviated SHM). A mass oscillating on a spring exhibits SHM.

The spring in the series of diagrams below is fixed at its left end and has a block attached to its right end. When the spring is neither stretched nor compressed (i.e., when it's at its natural length, as shown in Diagram 1 below) we say the spring is at its **equilibrium position**. In general, the point at which the net force on the block is zero, which in this case is when the spring is at its natural length, is called the equilibrium position, and we label it $x = 0$.

Now, imagine that we stretch the spring (Diagram 1 to Diagram 2) and let go. Once released, the spring pulls back to the left, going through its equilibrium position and then to the point of maximum compression. From here, the spring pushes back to the right, passing again through its equilibrium position, and returning to the point of maximum extension. If friction is negligible, this back-and-forth motion will continue indefinitely, and the time it takes for the block to go through one period, for example, from Diagram 2 to Diagram 6, is a constant.

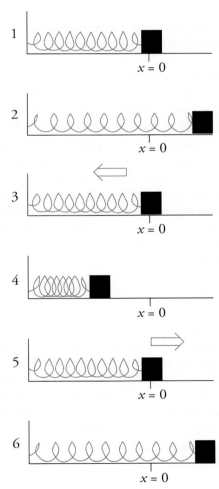

The Dynamics of SHM

Force

Let's first describe the motion of the block attached to the spring from the point of view of the force it feels. The spring exerts a force on the block that's proportional to its displacement. If we call the equilibrium position $x = 0$, then the force exerted by the spring is given by

---

Hooke's Law

$$\mathbf{F} = -k\mathbf{x}$$

The proportionality constant, k, called the **spring constant**, tells us how strong the spring is; the greater the value of k, the stiffer (and stronger) the spring.

As we can see from Hooke's Law, the units of k are newton/meter. Since a meter is a large distance to stretch or compression a spring, the values for k are often large.

What is the role of the minus sign in Hooke's Law? Look back at the diagrams on the previous page. Since we're calling the equilibrium position $x = 0$, when the block is to the right of equilibrium, its position, x, is positive. At this point, the stretched spring wants to pull back to the left; because the direction of the force of the spring is to the left, we indicate this direction by calling it negative. Similarly, when the block is to the left of equilibrium, its position, x, is negative. At this point, the compressed spring wants to push back to the right; because the direction of the force of the spring is to the right, we indicate this direction by calling it positive. We see that the direction of the spring force is always directed opposite to its displacement from equilibrium, and for this reason, the minus sign is needed in Hooke's Law. Furthermore, because the spring is always trying to restore the block to equilibrium, we say that spring provides the **restoring force**; it's this force that maintains the oscillations. The fact that the restoring force exerted by the spring obeys Hooke's Law (i.e., the force is directly proportional to the distance from equilibrium) is the reason why the block undergoes simple harmonic motion.

Energy

Unfortunately, knowing an equation for the force doesn't allow us to solve directly for other things, such as the speed of the block at some later time or the work done by or against the spring: the force changes as the block moves, so acceleration is not uniform. However, there is a way to figure out these quantities by using energy. When we pull on the spring to get the oscillations started, we're exerting a force over a distance; that is, we're doing work. Because we're doing work against the spring, the spring stores potential energy, called **elastic potential energy**. If we once again call the equilibrium position of the spring $x = 0$, then the potential energy of a stretched or compressed spring is given by this equation:

Elastic Potential Energy

$$PE_{\text{elastic}} = \tfrac{1}{2}kx^2$$

It follows that $W_{by\ spring} = -\Delta PE_{elastic}$ and $W_{against\ spring} = \Delta PE_{elastic}$.

We can also use conservation of energy to find the speed of a oscillating mass on a spring at any given position. When we release the block from rest, the spring is stretched and the block isn't moving, so all the energy is in the form of elastic potential energy. This potential energy turns into kinetic energy, until at $x = 0$ (equilibrium), all the energy has been converted to kinetic energy. As the block rushes past equilibrium, this kinetic energy gradually turns back into elastic potential energy until the point where the spring is at maximum compression and it's all transformed back to potential energy. The compressed spring then pushes outward, converting its potential energy back to kinetic; the block rushes through equilibrium again, and kinetic energy is transformed back to potential energy, until it reaches its starting point at maximum extension. At this instant, we're back to our full reserve of elastic potential energy (and no kinetic energy), and the process is ready to repeat.

As a result, we can look at the motion of the block from the point of view of the back-and-forth transfer between elastic potential energy and kinetic energy.

The maximum displacement of the block from equilibrium is called the **amplitude**, denoted by A. This positive number tells us how far to the left and right of equilibrium the block will travel. So, in the series of diagrams above, the block's position at maximum extension is $x = +A$, and its position at maximum compression is $x = -A$.

We can summarize the dynamics of the oscillations in this table:

	at $x = -A$	at $x = 0$	at $x = +A$
magnitude of restoring force	max	0	max
magnitude of acceleration	max	0	max
$PE_{elastic}$ of spring	max	0	max
KE of block	0	max	0
speed (v) of block	0	max	0

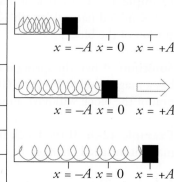

Because we're ignoring any frictional forces during the oscillations of the block, total mechanical energy will be conserved. That is, the sum of the block's kinetic energy, $\frac{1}{2}mv^2$, and the spring's potential energy, $\frac{1}{2}kx^2$, will be a constant. We can use this fact to figure out the maximum speed of the block. At the instant the block is passing through equilibrium, all the potential energy of the spring has been transformed into kinetic energy of the block. If the amplitude of the oscillations is A, then the maximum elastic potential energy, $\frac{1}{2}kA^2$ (the value of $\frac{1}{2}kx^2$ when $x = \pm A$), is completely converted to maximum kinetic energy at $x = 0$. This gives us

$$PE_{\text{elastic, max}} \rightarrow KE_{\text{max}}$$

$$\tfrac{1}{2}kA^2 = \tfrac{1}{2}mv^2$$

$$\therefore v_{\text{max}} = A\sqrt{\frac{k}{m}}$$

Example 42-2: A block of mass 200 g is oscillating on the end of a horizontal spring of spring constant 100 N/m and natural length 12 cm. When the spring is stretched to a length of 14 cm, what is the acceleration of the block?

Solution: When the spring is stretched by 2 cm, Hooke's Law tells us that the force exerted by the spring has a magnitude of $F = kx = (100\text{ N/m})(0.02\text{ m}) = 2$ N. Therefore, by Newton's Second Law, the acceleration of the block will have a magnitude of $a = F/m = (2\text{ N})/(0.2\text{ kg}) = 10$ m/s^2.

Example 42-3: If the block in Example 42-2 were replaced with a block of mass 800 g, how would its maximum speed change?

Solution: The equation derived above, $v_{\text{max}} = A\sqrt{k/m}$, tells us that v_{max} is inversely proportional to the square root of the mass of the oscillator. Therefore, if m increases by a factor of 4, v_{max} will decrease by a factor of 2.

The Kinematics of SHM

Earlier it was mentioned that a mass oscillating on a spring exhibits ideal oscillatory motion, which is called simple harmonic motion, and that this motion is the result of Hooke's Law (i.e., the restoring force is directly proportional to the distance from equilibrium). But what makes this motion different than non-ideal oscillations? It turns out (using calculus) that the frequency and period only depend on the spring constant, k, and the mass of the block, m.

$$f = \frac{1}{2\pi}\sqrt{\frac{k}{m}} \quad \text{and} \quad T = 2\pi\sqrt{\frac{m}{k}}$$

Notice that neither f *nor* T *depends on* A, *the amplitude.* This is why we call the motion of the block on the spring *simple* harmonic motion. This is not an obvious statement. If a mass on a spring is pulled back 1 cm or pulled back 10 cm (assuming the spring is still within its elastic limit), the time it takes to complete one cycle is exactly the same. As an example of an oscillating system that does not exhibit simple harmonic motion, imagine a ball bouncing. Removing air resistance and assuming that the bounces are completely elastic, the ball will continue to bounce to the same height from which it was released. However, dropping the ball from 1 cm will take less time to fall and rise than dropping it from 10 cm (which can be proven with the Big 5 equations).

It's possible for a system to oscillate because of a restoring force that is not directly proportional to the displacement. If this were the case, the frequency and period would depend on the amplitude; we'd still call the motion *harmonic*, which just means back-and-forth, but we wouldn't call it *simple* harmonic.

Pendulums

Besides the spring-block simple harmonic oscillator, there's another oscillator that the MCAT will expect you to know about: the simple pendulum. If the connecting rod or string between the suspension point and the object at the end of a pendulum has negligible mass (so that all the mass is in the object at the end of the rod or string), and if there is no friction at the suspension point during oscillation, we say the pendulum is a **simple pendulum**.

The displacement of the mass is not taken as a distance from equilibrium (as in the spring-block case), but rather as the angle it makes with the vertical. The vertical (shown as a dashed line in the figure below) is the equilibrium position, $\theta = 0$. The restoring force here is gravity; specifically, it's equal to $mg \sin \theta$, which is the component of the object's weight in the direction toward equilibrium.

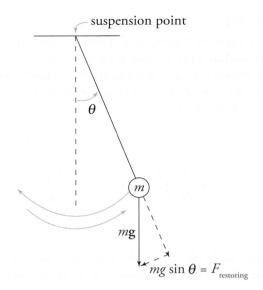

Strictly speaking, a pendulum does not undergo simple harmonic motion because the restoring force is not proportional to the displacement ($mg \sin \theta$ is not exactly proportional to θ). However, if the angle is small, then $\sin \theta \approx \theta$ (in radians), so the restoring force can be approximated as $mg\theta$, which is proportional to θ.[1] In this case, we can treat the motion as simple harmonic, and the frequency and period are given by the following equations:

$$f = \frac{1}{2\pi}\sqrt{\frac{g}{l}} \text{ and } T = 2\pi\sqrt{\frac{l}{g}}$$

where l is the length of the pendulum and g is the acceleration due to gravity. Observe that in the case of simple harmonic motion of a simple pendulum, the mass of the swinging object does not affect the frequency or period of oscillation.

Example 42-4: The bob (mass = m) of a simple pendulum is raised to a height h above its lowest point and released. Find an expression for the maximum speed of the pendulum.

Solution: When the bob is at height h above its lowest point, it has gravitational potential energy equal to mgh (relative to its lowest point). As it passes through the equilibrium position, all this potential energy is converted to kinetic energy. Therefore, $mgh = \frac{1}{2}mv_{max}^2$, and we get $v_{max} = \sqrt{2gh}$. This is the speed of the bob as it passes through equilibrium, which is where it attains its maximum speed.

---

[1] The conversion between degrees and radians is as follows: 180 degrees = π radians. If the angle is given in degrees, the restoring force is approximately $mg\,\theta(\pi/180°)$, which is still proportional to θ.

42.2 WAVES

A **mechanical wave** is a series of disturbances (oscillations) within a medium that transfers energy from one place to another. The medium itself is not transported, just the energy. Examples included a vibrating string or sound. Mechanical waves cannot exist without a medium. In the next chapter, we will discuss **electromagnetic waves**, which do not need a medium. This is because the electric and magnetic fields oscillate rather than physical matter.

Transverse Waves

Perhaps the simplest example of wave is one we can create by wiggling one end of a long rope:

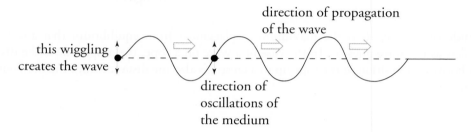

This wave uses the rope as the medium, traveling from one end to the other. Notice that the wave is moving horizontally, but the rope itself is moving up and down. That's why this is called a **transverse** wave: the wave travels (propagates) in a direction that's *perpendicular* to the direction in which the medium is vibrating.

Frequency and Period

The most fundamental characteristic of a wave is its frequency. If we pick a spot on the rope and count how many times it moves up and down (the number of round trips it makes) in one second, we've just measured the **frequency**, f, which we express in hertz (cycles per second).

The **period** of a wave, T, is the reciprocal of the frequency, and it is the amount of time it takes any spot on the rope to complete one cycle (in this case, one up-and-down round trip).

These definitions for frequency and period are same as for a mass on a spring or a pendulum. Each particle of rope oscillates up and down with simple harmonic motion. However, we can also think of the frequency and period of a wave in a different way. Instead of focusing on the oscillations, we can observe "pulses" moving the right. Frequency can be thought as the number of pulses that pass a given point per unit time, while period is the time it takes between pulses.

Wavelength and Amplitude

The figure below identifies the **crests (peaks)** and **troughs** of the wave. The distance from one crest to the next (the length of one cycle of the wave) is called the **wavelength**, denoted by λ, the Greek letter lambda. We can also measure the wavelength by measuring the distance from one trough to the next, or, in fact, between any two consecutive corresponding points along the wave.

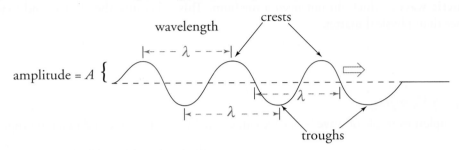

The **amplitude** of a wave, A, is the maximum displacement from equilibrium that any point in the medium makes as the wave goes by. In the case of a wave on a rope, the amplitude is the distance from the original horizontal position of the rope up to a crest; it's also the distance from the horizontal position down to a trough.

Wave Speed

To figure out how fast the wave travels, we just notice that the wave travels a distance of λ in time T; that is, λ is the length of one wave cycle, and T, the period, is the time required for one wave cycle to go by. Since distance = rate × time, we get $\lambda = vT$. Solving this for v gives us $\lambda(1/T) = v$ and since $f = 1/T$, the equation becomes $v = \lambda f$. *This is the most important equation for waves and one of the most important equations for the MCAT.*

Wave Equation

$$v = \lambda f$$

Two Big Rules for Waves

Notice that the second equation for the wave speed shows that v does not depend on f (or λ). While this may seem to contradict the first equation, $v = \lambda f$, it really doesn't. The speed of the wave depends on the characteristics of the rope; how tense it is, and what it's made of. We can wiggle the end at any frequency we want, and the speed of the wave we create will be a constant. However, because $\lambda f = v$ must always be true, a higher f will mean a shorter λ (and a lower f will mean a longer λ). Thus, changing f doesn't change v: it changes λ. This brings up our first Big Rule for waves:

Big Rule 1: The speed of a wave is determined by the type of wave and the characteristics of the medium, *not* by the frequency.

For a transverse wave on a rope, there's another equation we can use to figure out the wave speed:

$$v = \sqrt{\frac{\text{tension}}{\text{linear density}}}$$

The linear density of a rope is its mass per unit length.

Notice that two different types of wave can move with different speeds through the same medium; for example, sound and light move through air with very different speeds. There are exceptions to Big Rule 1, but the only one the MCAT will expect you to know about is *dispersion*, which is discussed in Chapter 43, on Optics. Any other exception would be discussed in the passage; otherwise, you can assume the rule applies.

Our second Big Rule for waves concerns what happens when a wave passes from one medium into another. Because wave speed is determined by the characteristics of the medium, a change in the medium implies a change in wave speed, but the frequency won't change.

> **Big Rule 2: When a wave passes into another medium, its speed changes, but its frequency does *not*.**

The reasoning behind this makes sense if you focus on a wave as a series of pulses. Frequency is the number of pulses that pass by per unit time. It stands to reason that, if a certain number of pulses per second arrives at the boundary between two different media, then the same number of pulses per second must leave, passing into the new medium. In other words, rate in = rate out. This is similar to the Equation of Continuity in fluids and the rule for electric current passing through resistors in series.

Because f is constant, Big Rule 2 tells us that the wavelength is proportional to wave speed.

Notice that Big Rule 1 applies to different waves in one medium, while Big Rule 2 applies to a single wave in different media. Memorize these rules. The MCAT loves waves.

Example 42-5: A transverse wave of frequency 4 Hz travels at a speed of 6 m/s along a rope. What would be the speed of a 12 Hz wave along this same rope?

Solution: Big Rule 1 for waves says that the speed of a wave is determined by the type of wave and the characteristics of the medium, not by the frequency. If all we do is change the frequency, the wave speed will not change: the wave speed will still be 6 m/s. (What *will* change? The wavelength. Because $\lambda = v/f$, a change in f with no change in v will change λ.)

Example 42-6: Which one of the following statements is true concerning the amplitude of a wave?

A) Amplitude increases with increasing frequency.
B) Amplitude increases with increasing wavelength.
C) Amplitude increases with increasing wave speed.
D) None of the above

Solution: The amplitude is determined by how much energy we put into the wave to get it started. If we wiggle the rope up and down through a large distance (a large amplitude), this takes more energy on our part, and as a result, the wave carries more energy. However, the amplitude doesn't depend on f, λ, or v. The answer is choice D.

Example 42-7: An electrocardiogram responds to changes in the electric potential of the heart from a number of different angles and distances, and it represents a different pair combinations of these signals (voltages) as deflections of several needles under which runs graph paper moving horizontally at a constant speed. Suppose a patient has a resting heart rate of 60 beats per minute and the tape runs through the machine at 4 cm/s. What is the wavelength over which the pattern should repeat?

Solution: 60 beats/min = 1 beat/s, or a period of 1 s and frequency of 1 Hz. The wave speed, v, is simply the speed at which the tape runs under the needle: v = 4 cm/s. Thus, $\lambda = v/f$ = 4 cm/s / 1 Hz = 4 cm.

Example 42-8: What happens when the wave shown below passes from the thick, heavy rope into the thinner, lighter rope?

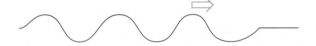

Solution: According to Big Rule 2 for waves, when a wave passes into another medium, its speed changes, but its frequency does not. How does the speed change? Because the rope is lighter (i.e., it has a lower linear density), the equation for wave speed on a string (given above) tells us that v will *increase*. So, if v increases but f doesn't change, then λ will also increase because $\lambda = v/f$.

42.3   SOUND WAVES

Sound waves don't travel in the same way that waves on a rope do. The waves we've looked at so far are transverse waves: the direction in which the particles of the conducting medium oscillate is perpendicular to the direction in which the wave travels. If, however, the direction in which the particles of the conducting medium oscillate is *parallel* to the direction in which the wave travels, we call the wave **longitudinal**. Sound waves (also known as compression waves) are longitudinal waves in gas, liquid, or solid; when a compression wave's frequency is between 20 Hz and 20 kHz, humans can perceive it as what we commonly call sound.

Let's take a closer look at sound waves. As a stereo speaker, vocal fold, or tuning fork vibrates, it creates regions of high pressure (**compressions**) that alternate with regions of low pressure (**rarefactions**). These pressure waves are transmitted through the air (or some other medium) and can eventually reach our ears and brain, which translate the vibrations into sound.

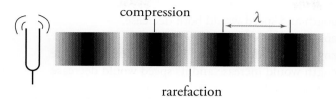

Like other waves, a longitudinal compression wave has a wavelength, a speed, a frequency, a period, and an amplitude. The equation $v = \lambda f$ holds, as do the two Big Rules for waves.

Sound can travel in any medium: gas, liquid, or solid. Its speed depends on two things: the medium's resistance to compression (quantified by its *bulk modulus B*) and its density, according to the equation $v_{sound} = \sqrt{\dfrac{B}{\rho}}$.

On the MCAT, knowing the relationship is good enough—you won't have to calculate the speed of sound in a given medium. However, you should know that in general, *sound travels slowest through gases, faster through liquids, and fastest through solids.* The speed of sound in air is about 340 m/s (that's about 760 miles per hour), but it varies slightly with temperature, pressure, and humidity.

Example 42-9: A sound wave of frequency 440 Hz (this note is *concert A*, or the A above middle C) travels at a speed of 344 m/s through the air in a concert hall. How fast would a note one octave higher, 880 Hz, travel through the same concert hall?

    A) 172 m/s
    B) 344 m/s
    C) 516 m/s
    D) 688 m/s

Solution: Altering the frequency will not affect the wave speed. Remember Big Rule 1 for waves. Therefore, the answer is choice B.

Example 42-10: A siren produces sound waves in the air. If the frequency of the waves is gradually decreasing, which of the following changes to the waves is most likely also occurring?

    A) The wavelength is increasing.
    B) The wave speed is decreasing.
    C) The amplitude is decreasing.
    D) The period is decreasing.

Solution: Because the wave speed is set by the medium (the air, in this case), the wave speed is a constant. Since $v = \lambda f$, this means that λ and f are inversely proportional. So, if f is decreasing, then λ must be increasing, choice A.

Example 42-11: A typical medical ultrasound scan uses frequencies in the MHz range. What would happen to an ultrasound signal as it passed from air into body tissues?

A) Its wavelength and speed would both decrease.
B) Its wavelength and speed would both increase.
C) Its wavelength would decrease and its speed would increase.
D) Its wavelength would increase and its speed would decrease.

Solution: When a wave passes into a new medium, its frequency does not change (the specific frequency range is irrelevant). Therefore, when traveling through the body, the frequency of the sound wave will be the same as it was in the air. However, we know that sound waves generally travel faster through liquids and solids than they do through gases, so we'd expect the wave speed through the body to be faster. Because the equation $v = \lambda f$ is always true, the same f at a faster v means a greater wavelength. Therefore, the answer is choice B. (Note that almost all of the ultrasound wave would reflect off the skin if it were incident on it from air: this is why a gel is first applied to the skin before the emitter/detector is placed on the skin, so that no air interrupts the signal.)

42.4 INTERFERENCE OF WAVES AND BEATS

When two or more waves are superimposed on each other, they will combine to form a single resultant wave. This is called **interference**. The amplitude of the resultant wave will depend on the amplitudes of the combining waves *and* on how these waves travel relative to each other.

If crest meets crest, and trough meets trough, we say that the waves are **in phase** with each other. Their amplitudes will *add*, and we say the waves interfere **constructively**. However, if the crest of one wave coincides with the *trough* of the other (and vice versa), we say that the waves are exactly **out of phase** with each other. In this case, their amplitudes *subtract*, and we say that the waves interfere **destructively**.

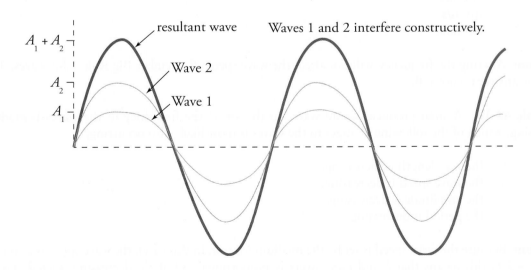

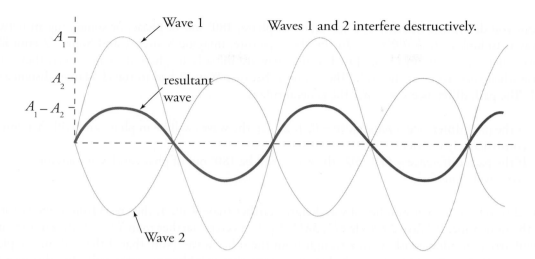

Wave 1

Waves 1 and 2 interfere destructively.

A_1

A_2

resultant wave

$A_1 - A_2$

Wave 2

A passage might also say that waves that are directly opposite each other in amplitude are *180 degrees out of phase*, or *π radians out of phase*; it is common to refer to a whole cycle or wave as being 360 degrees or 2π radians, as if it were a circle. If the waves aren't exactly in phase (0°, 360°, or 2π radians) or exactly out of phase (180° or π radians), the amplitude of the resultant wave will be somewhere between the difference and the sum of the amplitudes of the interfering waves.

The preceding pictures of waves that are in phase and out of phase can also be thought of as graphs representing the displacement at a fixed location as a function of time. As an example, imagine a cork floating in calm water. Source 1 creates a wave, which travels through the water, causing the cork to bob up and down. A graph of the cork's motion as a function of time would be sinusoidal (that is, it looks like Wave 1 in the picture except that the distance from maximum to maximum is the period rather than the wavelength).

Similarly, if Source 2 were acting alone, Wave 2 would cause the cork to bob up and down. The graph of this motion as a function of time would look similar to the picture of Wave 2. If Wave 1 and Wave 2 both arrive at the cork, they will interfere. If the waves are in phase when they arrive at the cork (that is, crests arrive at the same time, troughs arrive at the same time, etc.), or if they are 180° out of phase when they arrive at the cork (that is, the crest of one wave arrives simultaneously with the trough of the other), the graph of the cork's motion as a function of time would look like the resultant waves in the picture. Note that if the waves have different frequencies (and wavelengths), then the graph of the cork's motion will not look like a sine or cosine, but will be more complicated. An example of this is **beats**, which are discussed below.

Be careful on the MCAT. If you see a picture of a sine or cosine, make sure you can determine whether it is an actual wave (pictured at a fixed time), or a graph of one particle's motion as a function of time.

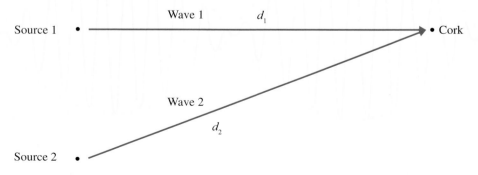

Source 1 • Wave 1 d_1 • Cork

Wave 2

d_2

Source 2 •

How can you determine whether two waves are in phase, 180° out of phase, or something in between? One way is to look at *path difference*. In the above picture, imagine Source 1 and Source 2 emit identical waves that are exactly in phase. Just because they are initially in phase does not mean they will be in phase when they arrive at the cork. The reason is because Wave 2 had to travel a larger distance than Wave 1. The path difference = $d_2 - d_1$. The general rule is

- If the path difference = $n\lambda$ and, ($n = 0, 1, 2, \ldots$), the waves will be in phase and will therefore constructively interfere.
- If the path difference = $(n + \frac{1}{2})\lambda$, the waves will be 180° out of phase and will therefore destructively interfere.

If Wave 2 travels an integer number of wavelengths farther than Wave 1, the crests from each will still arrive at the same time. If Wave 2 travels $\lambda/2$, $3\lambda/2$, $5\lambda/2$, et cetera, farther than Wave 1, the crest from one wave will arrive simultaneously with a trough from the other wave. Note that if the cork in the picture experiences constructive interference, it does not mean that neighboring corks will. The distance from the sources to the other corks would be different. An example of this is Young's Double-Slit experiment, where the two sources are small holes in a screen emitting light that is in phase. On the opposite wall is a screen that features alternating bright and dark fringes. Bright fringes are the result of constructive interference, and dark fringes are the result of destructive interference. They alternate, since the path difference changes as you move up or down the screen.

Beats

If two sound waves with slightly different frequencies (the difference is less than about 10 Hz) combine, the product is a pulsating, wobbling resultant wave. This produces the phenomenon known as **beats**. Because the frequencies don't match, sometimes the waves are in phase and sometimes they're out of phase. When they're in phase, their amplitudes add; when they're out of phase, their amplitudes subtract. The combined waveform reaches its maximum amplitude when the waves interfere constructively and its minimum amplitude when they interfere destructively, and these points alternate. Maximum amplitude sounds loud and minimum amplitude sounds soft, so we hear loud, soft, loud, soft, et cetera. The resulting equally spaced moments of constructive interference (the loud moments) are the beats.

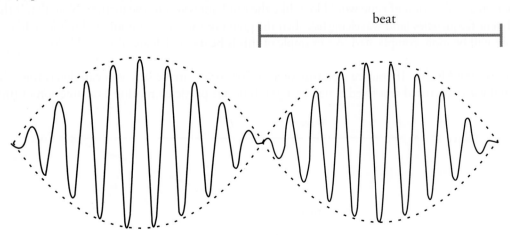

The frequency at which the beats are heard (the **beat frequency**) is equal to the difference between the frequencies of the two original sound waves. Therefore, if one of these waves has frequency f_1 and the other has frequency f_2, then $f_{beat} = |f_1 - f_2|$.

Beat Frequency

$$f_{beat} = |f_1 - f_2|$$

Example 42-12: A piano tuner strikes a tuning fork at the same time he strikes a piano key with a note of similar pitch. If he hears 3 beats per second, and the tuning fork produces a standard 440 Hz tone, then what must be the frequency produced by the struck piano string?

  A) 437 Hz
  B) 443 Hz
  C) 437 Hz or 443 Hz
  D) 434 Hz or 446 Hz

Solution: If f_{beat} = 3 Hz, then the frequencies of the tuning fork and piano string are "off" by 3 Hz. The frequency produced by the piano string might be 3 Hz lower or 3 Hz higher than the tuning fork; without more information, we don't know which one. If the tuning fork produces a tone of frequency 440 Hz, the piano string produces a frequency of either 440 − 3 = 437 Hz or 440 + 3 = 443 Hz. Choice C is the answer.

42.5   STANDING WAVES ON STRINGS, SOUND WAVES IN PIPES

Let's say that we have a long rope with one end in our fingers and the other end attached to a wall. We wiggle the rope up and down at a certain frequency, f, and create waves of frequency f that travel down the length of the rope. When they hit the wall, they'll be reflected. We now have two waves on the same rope (the wave we continue to generate plus the reflected wave) with the same frequency and amplitude but traveling in opposite directions. These waves will interfere. If the frequency is just right, the resulting wave seems to stand still; the rope continues to vibrate up and down, but the resultant wave no longer travels. The combination of these traveling waves produces a **standing wave**, with the horizontal positions of the crests and troughs remaining fixed.

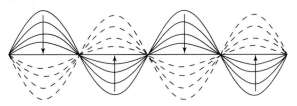

Notice that each point along the rope has its own amplitude. Some points don't vibrate up and down at all; these points are called **nodes** (points of <u>no</u> displacement). Halfway between any two consecutive nodes are points where the amplitude is maximized; these positions are called **antinodes**. Every other point has an amplitude that's smaller than the amplitude at the antinode positions.

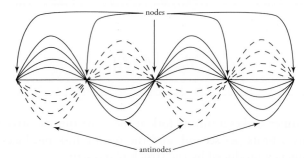

To figure out the conditions under which a standing wave will be formed, we'll look at the three simplest standing waves. In the figure at the top of the next page, we have a rope of length L. The first picture shows the simplest standing wave that can form if we have nodes at the two ends; the second and third pictures show the next simplest standing waves that the rope could support.

The distance between any two consecutive nodes is always one-half of the wavelength. The first picture shows us that one of these half-wavelengths is equal to L; in the second picture, two half-wavelengths are equal to L; and in the third picture, three half-wavelengths are equal to L.

Notice the pattern that emerges relating the length of the rope and the wavelength of the standing wave.

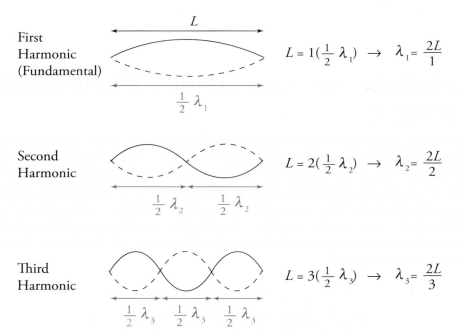

First Harmonic (Fundamental)

$$L = 1\left(\frac{1}{2}\lambda_1\right) \rightarrow \lambda_1 = \frac{2L}{1}$$

Second Harmonic

$$L = 2\left(\frac{1}{2}\lambda_2\right) \rightarrow \lambda_2 = \frac{2L}{2}$$

Third Harmonic

$$L = 3\left(\frac{1}{2}\lambda_3\right) \rightarrow \lambda_3 = \frac{2L}{3}$$

The only standing waves that can be supported are those for which the length of the rope is equal to a whole number of half-wavelengths, so the wavelength must be twice the length of the rope divided by a whole number:

Standing-Wave Wavelengths for Two Fixed Ends

$$\lambda_n = \frac{2L}{n} \quad \text{where} \quad n = 1, 2, 3\ldots$$

The number n is called the **harmonic number**. The first harmonic is usually called the **fundamental** because once we know the **fundamental wavelength**, λ_1, we automatically know all the other harmonic wavelengths, because we can write λ_n in terms of λ_1, like this: $\lambda_n = \lambda_1/n$.

Because the equation $v = \lambda f$ must always be true, and only certain wavelengths are allowed for a standing wave, then only certain frequencies will give standing waves. To find the harmonic frequencies, we just write $\lambda_n f_n = v$ and solve for f_n:

Standing-Wave Frequencies for Two Fixed Ends

$$f_n = \frac{n}{2L} v \quad \text{where} \quad n = 1, 2, 3\ldots$$

In the same way that the fundamental wavelength can be used to figure out all the other harmonic wavelengths, the fundamental frequency can be used to figure out all the other harmonic frequencies: $f_n = nf_1$. Memorizing this equation is helpful for the MCAT.

It is possible to create standing waves with only one fixed end (node) and one non-fixed end (antinode), but the appropriate formulas to find frequency and wavelength for this situation are discussed in Chapter 43. Regardless of the type of standing wave, the formula to find the appropriate harmonic from the fundamental frequency still holds ($f_n = nf_1$).

Example 42-13: If a rope of length 6 m supports a standing wave with exactly four nodes (which includes the ends of the rope), what is the wavelength of the standing wave?

Solution: Draw the standing wave. It should look just like the third harmonic drawn on the previous page. Therefore, the wavelength is $\lambda_3 = 2L/3 = 2(6 \text{ m})/3 = 4 \text{ m}$.

Example 42-14: The speed of a transverse traveling wave along a certain 4-meter-long rope is 24 m/s. Which of the following frequencies could cause a standing wave to form on this rope, assuming both ends of the rope are fixed?

- A) 32 Hz
- B) 33 Hz
- C) 34 Hz
- D) 35 Hz

Solution: The fundamental frequency for this rope is $f_1 = (1/2L)v = 3$ Hz. All harmonic frequencies are whole-number multiples of the fundamental, so any frequency that could cause a standing wave to form on the rope must be a multiple of 3 Hz. Of the choices given, only choice B, 33 Hz, is a multiple of 3 Hz.

Example 42-15: For a particular rope, it's found that the fundamental frequency is 6 Hz. What's the third-harmonic frequency?

Solution: From the equation $f_n = nf_1$, we get $f_3 = 3f_1 = 3(6$ Hz$) = 18$ Hz.

Example 42-16: The second-harmonic wavelength for a rope fixed at both ends is 0.5 m. How fast do transverse waves travel along this rope if the fundamental frequency is 4 Hz?

Solution: Using the equation $\lambda_n = \lambda_1/n$, we get $\lambda_2 = \lambda_1/2$. This means that $\lambda_1 = 2\lambda_2 = 2(0.5$ m$) = 1$ m. Now, multiplying any harmonic wavelength by its corresponding harmonic frequency will give us the wave speed. In particular, we have $v = \lambda_1 f_1$, so $v = (1$ m$)(4$ Hz$) = 4$ m/s.

Just as we can have standing waves on a rope caused by the interference of two oppositely directed transverse waves with equal amplitudes, standing sound waves in a pipe can be caused by the interference of two oppositely-directed longitudinal waves of equal amplitude.

The analysis of these standing waves is similar to that of a string attached at each end. In that case, the ends correspond to nodes (because there is no motion). Since the distance between nodes is some whole number of half-wavelengths, this gave us formulas for the different frequencies and wavelengths that the standing waves can have. In the case of pipes, we also need to know what corresponds to each end. The ends of a pipe can either be open to the atmosphere or closed.

It turns out that the open end of a pipe (technically, just beyond it) corresponds to an antinode. To be more specific, these are often referred to as displacement antinodes (maximum displacement). They are also called pressure nodes (constant pressure). The closed end of a pipe corresponds to a displacement node (no motion) or a pressure antinode (maximum pressure fluctuations). The pressure varies most where there is no motion and the motion varies most where there is constant pressure.

Pipes are often classified as *open pipes* (open on each end) or *closed pipes* (open on one end and closed on the other).

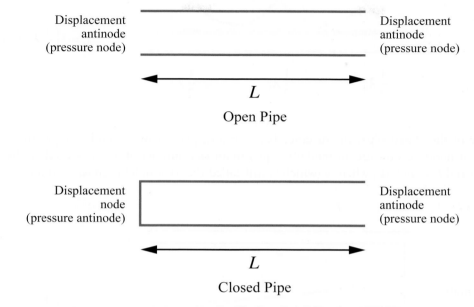

Displacement antinode (pressure node)

Displacement antinode (pressure node)

L

Open Pipe

Displacement node (pressure antinode)

Displacement antinode (pressure node)

L

Closed Pipe

In the case of the open pipe, the distance between displacement antinodes (or pressure nodes) is equal to a whole number of half-wavelengths. The formulas for wavelength and frequency are therefore the same as for the string attached at each end: $\lambda_n = 2L\,/\,n$ and $f_n = nv\,/\,2L$, where the harmonic number, n, is any positive whole number, and v now refers to the speed of sound in air.

To visualize the harmonic modes, it is convenient to represent the standing waves as transverse.

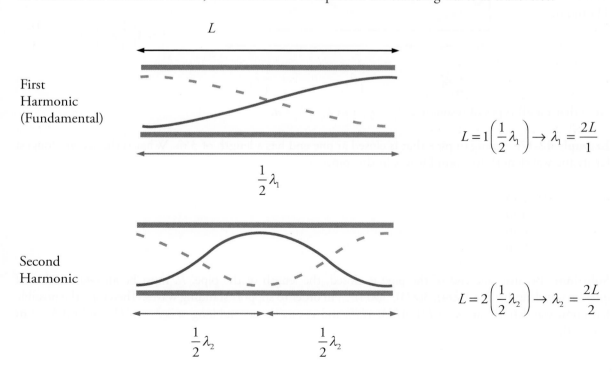

L

First Harmonic (Fundamental)

$\dfrac{1}{2}\lambda_1$

$$L = 1\left(\frac{1}{2}\lambda_1\right) \rightarrow \lambda_1 = \frac{2L}{1}$$

Second Harmonic

$\dfrac{1}{2}\lambda_2$

$\dfrac{1}{2}\lambda_2$

$$L = 2\left(\frac{1}{2}\lambda_2\right) \rightarrow \lambda_2 = \frac{2L}{2}$$

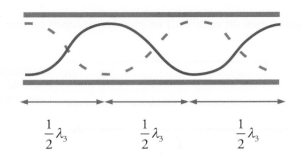

Third Harmonic

$$L = 3\left(\frac{1}{2}\lambda_3\right) \rightarrow \lambda_3 = \frac{2L}{3}$$

$$\frac{1}{2}\lambda_3 \qquad \frac{1}{2}\lambda_3 \qquad \frac{1}{2}\lambda_3$$

In the case of the closed pipe, the distance between a displacement antinode (or pressure node) and a displacement node (or pressure antinode) is equal to an *odd* number of *quarter*-wavelengths. As a result, $\lambda_n = 4L / n$ and $f_n = nv / 4L$, where n (which is still called the harmonic) is an *odd* number.

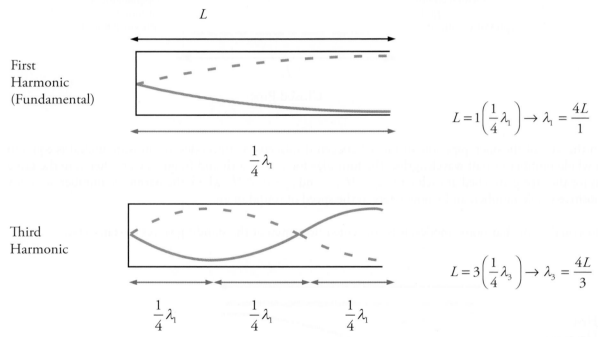

L

First Harmonic (Fundamental)

$$L = 1\left(\frac{1}{4}\lambda_1\right) \rightarrow \lambda_1 = \frac{4L}{1}$$

$$\frac{1}{4}\lambda_1$$

Third Harmonic

$$L = 3\left(\frac{1}{4}\lambda_3\right) \rightarrow \lambda_3 = \frac{4L}{3}$$

$$\frac{1}{4}\lambda_1 \qquad \frac{1}{4}\lambda_1 \qquad \frac{1}{4}\lambda_1$$

Note that for all types of resonance, $f_n = nf_1$ and $\lambda_n = \lambda_1 / n$.

Example 42-17: An organ pipe that is closed at one end has a length of 3 m. What is the second-longest harmonic wavelength for sound waves in this pipe?

    A) 3 m
    B) 4 m
    C) 6 m
    D) 9 m

Solution: Because one end of the pipe is closed, the length of the pipe, L, must be an *odd* number of *quarter*-wavelengths: $L = 1(\lambda/4)$, $3(\lambda/4)$, $5(\lambda/4)\ldots$, in order to support standing waves. Therefore, the possible harmonic wavelengths are $\lambda = 4L/1$, $4L/3$, $4L/5$, and so on. The second longest is $\lambda = 4L/3 = 4(3 \text{ m})/3 = 4$ m, choice B.

Example 42-18: An organ pipe that is open at both ends has a length of 3 m. What is the second-longest harmonic wavelength for sound waves in this pipe?

    A) 3 m
    B) 4 m
    C) 6 m
    D) 9 m

Solution: Because both ends of the pipe are open, the length of the pipe, L, must be a whole number of half-wavelengths: $L = 1(\lambda/2), 2(\lambda/2), 3(\lambda/2)\ldots$, in order to support standing waves. Therefore, the possible harmonic wavelengths are $\lambda = 2L/1, 2L/2, 2L/3$, and so on. The second longest is $\lambda = 2L/2 = L = 3$ m, choice A.

42.6 INTENSITY AND INTENSITY LEVEL

Intensity and intensity level are closely related quantities. The **intensity** of a sound wave (or, indeed, any wave) is the energy it transmits per second (the power) per unit area. It is measured in W/m^2. For a point source (that is, one that creates waves that travel uniformly in all directions), the area in the equation is the surface area of a sphere, which equals $4\pi r^2$. Each wavefront in the figure below can be thought of as a bundle of energy that is expanding in size, much like a balloon being blown up. The farther a detector is from the source, the larger the bundle of energy will be, and therefore the detector will receive a smaller fraction of it.

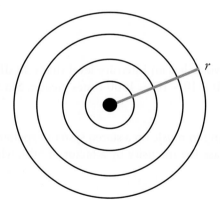

Mathematically, the important fact to remember is that, for a point source, intensity varies inversely as the square of the distance r from that source: $I \propto 1/r^2$. If the detector of a wave doubles his distance from the source, the power produced by the wave will spread out over an area that is $2^2 = 4$ times larger, causing the detector to receive ¼ as much. Intensity is also proportional to the square of the amplitude of a wave.

Since the intensity that we can hear spans an impressively large range (about twelve orders of magnitude!), we use logarithms to make the numbers easier to handle. The **threshold of hearing**, which is roughly the lowest intensity the human ear can perceive as sound at the common middle frequencies, is equal to 10^{-12} W/m^2; this intensity is denoted by I_0. The **intensity level** (or **sound level**) of a sound wave whose intensity is I is equal to the base-10 logarithm of the ratio I/I_0. The unit of intensity level is the **bel**, abbreviated **B**. Usually, we multiply this by 10 to get the intensity level, β, in **decibels** (dB):

Intensity Level in Decibels

$$\beta = 10 \log_{10} \frac{I}{I_0}$$

The most important relationship to get from this equation can be summarized as follows:

> Every time we *multiply* I by 10, we *add* 10 to β.
>
> Every time we *divide* I by 10, we *subtract* 10 from β.

For example, if the intensity is multiplied by 10,000, which is $10 \times 10 \times 10 \times 10$, the intensity level in decibels is increased by adding $10 + 10 + 10 + 10 = 40$. If we divide by the intensity by, say, $100,000 = 10^5$, then the decibel level decreases by 50.

Example 42-19: At a distance of 1 m, the intensity level of a soft whisper is about 30 dB, while a normal speaking voice is about 60 dB. How many times greater is the power delivered per unit area by a normal-speaking voice than by a whisper?[2]

- A) 2.5
- B) 30
- C) 1000
- D) 3000

Solution: The normal speaking voice has an intensity level that's 30 dB greater than the whisper. Therefore, the intensity must be $10 \times 10 \times 10 = 10^3 = 1000$ times greater. Since power delivered per unit area *is* intensity, the answer is choice C.

Example 42-20: A person listening to music on a stereo system experiences a sound level of 70 dB. If the volume dial is turned up to increase the intensity by a factor of 500, what sound level would this person hear now?

- A) 97 dB
- B) 105 dB
- C) 115 dB
- D) 120 dB

Solution: If the intensity had increased by a factor of 100, which is 10×10, the sound level would have increased by $10 + 10 = 20$ dB. If the intensity had increased by a factor of 1000, which is $10 \times 10 \times 10$, the sound level would have increased by $10 + 10 + 10 = 30$ dB. The fact that the intensity increased by a factor

---

[2] Our perception of loudness is completely different from both intensity and intensity level. Roughly speaking, a difference in intensity level of 10 dB (and therefore a factor of 10 in intensity) corresponds to a perceived loudness difference of a factor of 2.

of 500, which is between 100 and 1000, means that the sound level increased by between 20 dB and 30 dB. If the original sound level was 70 dB, then the new sound level must be between 70 + 20 = 90 dB and 70 + 30 = 100 dB. Only choice A falls in this range.

Example 42-21: Suppose one moves 10 times further away from a loud siren of constant power. What is the resultant decrease in sound level?

    A) 10 dB
    B) 20 dB
    C) 40 dB
    D) 100 dB

Solution: Increasing distance by a factor of 10 decreases intensity by a factor of 100, which is 10 × 10. Therefore, sound level will be reduced by 10 + 10 = 20 dB, choice B.

42.7

42.7   THE DOPPLER EFFECT

Suppose a train that is loudly sounding its horn is approaching a passenger waiting on a platform. As the train is approaching, the person hears the pitch at a higher frequency than does the engineer on the train. As the train is moving away, the person on the platform hears a lower frequency than does the engineer. These differences in frequency are the result of the **Doppler effect**, which arises whenever a source of waves is moving relative to the detector. The result is that the perceived or *detected* frequency will be different from the frequency of the sound that was emitted from the *source*.

Normally when a sound is emitted from a source, the rate of the compressions (or frequency, f) is detected as the wave travels at speed v towards the detector. The most important fact to remember is that if the source and detector are moving *closer* together (no matter which is moving), the detected frequency with be *higher* than the emitted frequency. Similarly, if the source and detector are moving *farther apart,* the detected frequency will be *lower* than the emitted frequency.

> **Doppler Effect**
>
> approaching ⟷ higher detected frequency
>
> receding ⟷ lower detected frequency

For sound, if the detector moves toward the source or if the source moves toward the detector, the detected frequency will be higher than the emitted frequency. But the reasons are different.

If a detector moves toward (or away from) a stationary source, the relative speed of sound changes. As an example, if a sound wave is moving toward the detector at 340 m/s and the detector moves toward the source at 20 m/s, the wave will appear to be moving at 360 m/s in the detector's frame of reference.

Similarly, if the detector is moving away from the source at 20 m/s, the wave will appear to moving at 320 m/s. The wavelength (i.e., the spacing between wavefronts) will not change. According to the wave equation, $v = \lambda f$, an increase (or decrease) in perceived wave speed with a constant wavelength will cause an increase (or decrease) in perceived frequency.

If the source moves, the waves themselves become distorted. Say a source emits a pulse that spreads out in all directions. The wavefront is a sphere, though in 2 dimensions it looks like a circle. If the source moves to the right the next pulse it emits would again look like a circle, but whose center is to the right of the previous pulse's center. The wavefronts bunch up on the right and spread out on the left. The wavelength has therefore changed. If the detector is at rest, then the speed of the wave hasn't changed. According to the wave equation, $v = \lambda f$, an increase (or decrease) in wavelength with a constant wave speed will result in a decrease (or increase) in frequency.

42.7

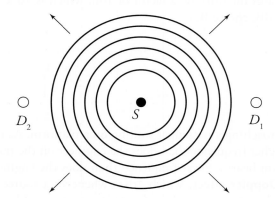

No relative motion between the source (S) and detectors (D_1 and D_2)

Each wave compression emitted by S arrives at the same speed when perceived by D_1 and D_2. The perceived frequency is the same.

No Doppler shifts.

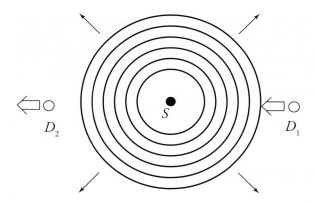

Here, there *is* relative motion between the source (S) and detectors (D_1 and D_2).

D_1 is approaching S, so each compression of the wave emitted from S requires less time to reach D_1. The perceived wave speed at D_1 is faster, and thus the frequency at D_1 is higher.

D_2 is receding from S, so each compression of the wave requires more time to reach D_2. The perceived wave speed at D_2 is slower, and thus the perceived frequency is lower.

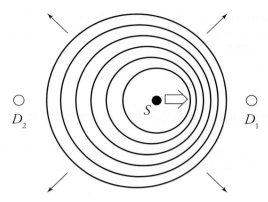

Here, there *is* relative motion between the source (*S*) and detectors (*D*₁ and *D*₂).

S is approaching D_1, so the compressions of the wave emitted from *S* are closer together. The perceived wavelength at D_1 is shorter, and thus the frequency at D_1 is higher.

S is receding from D_2, so the compressions of the wave emitted from *S* are farther apart. The perceived wavelength at D_2 is longer, and thus the frequency at D_2 is lower.

42.7

To predict exactly what the perceived frequency will be, we need an equation. Despite the fact that there are lots of individual cases to consider (whether the source and/or the detector are stationary or in motion), we can summarize everything in a single equation:

Doppler Effect

$$f_D = f_S \frac{v \pm v_D}{v \mp v_S}$$

In this equation:

> f_D = the frequency heard by the detector
> f_S = the frequency emitted by the source
> v_D = the speed at which the detector is moving
> v_S = the speed at which the source is moving
> v = the speed of the wave

What we need to do to make this one equation fit all the possible cases is use the conceptual relationships given in the box on the previous page to decide whether to use the + or − in the numerator and whether to use + or − in the denominator.

Notice that we have written ± in the numerator and ∓ in the denominator; one way to memorize the sign conventions for this equation is by the mnemonic "top sign is toward." When the motion of the detector is toward the source, you use the top of ±, or the "+" sign, in the numerator. When the motion of the source is toward the detector, you use the top of ∓, or the "−" sign, in the denominator.

For example, suppose the source is stationary and the detector is moving toward it. Because $v_S = 0$, there's no decision to make in the denominator. Since the detector is moving <u>toward</u> the source, we choose the <u>top</u> sign, +, in the numerator.

$$f_D = f_S \frac{v + v_D}{v}$$

If the detector is moving away from the stationary source, we would choose the − in the numerator.

Now, suppose the detector is stationary and the source is moving <u>toward</u> it. Since $v_D = 0$, there's no decision to make in the numerator. In the denominator, we choose the <u>top</u> sign, − .

$$f_D = f_S \frac{v}{v - v_S}$$

If the source is moving away from the stationary detector, we choose the + sign in the denominator.

If both the source and the detector are moving, we have two decisions to make (one in the numerator and one in the denominator). The key is to make the two decisions separately, using the same rule. For example, let's say you're the detector, driving in your car following a police car whose siren is wailing. In this case, both the source (the police car) and the detector (you) are moving. To decide what to do in the numerator, ask yourself, *what's the detector doing?* It's moving <u>toward</u> the source, so we choose the <u>top</u> sign, + in the numerator. Now, *what's the source doing?* It's moving away from the detector, so we choose the bottom sign, +, in the denominator.

$$f_D = f_S \frac{v + v_D}{v + v_S}$$

If your speed is greater than that of the police car, you're gaining on it, so the relative motion is motion *toward*. We'd expect f_D to be greater than f_S. If $v_D > v_S$, then the fraction multiplying f_S is bigger than 1, so f_D will indeed be greater than f_S. On the other hand, if your speed is less than that of the police car, it's pulling away from you, so the relative motion is motion *away*. In this case, we'd expect f_D to be lower than f_S. Further, if $v_D < v_S$, then the fraction multiplying f_S is less than 1, so f_D will indeed be lower than f_S. Finally, it's important to notice what happens if your speed is the same as the police car's speed. If $v_D = v_S$, then the fraction multiplying f_S is equal to 1, so $f_D = f_S$. Therefore, even though you're both moving, there's no Doppler shift because there's no *relative* motion between you.

The Doppler effect also applies to electromagnetic waves, such as visible light. The same qualitative relationships continue to hold: motion *toward* results in a frequency shift upward, while motion *away* results in a frequency shift downward. An astronomer observing a star moving away from the earth observes the light emitted as being shifted downward in frequency, toward the red end of the visible spectrum (in fact, this is known as the **redshift**). Furthermore, by measuring the shift, the astronomer can calculate how fast the star is moving away from us.[3]

---

[3] For light waves, the equation that is used to calculate the magnitude of the Doppler effect is different. This is because of a postulate of special relativity: the speed of light is the same in all frames of reference. The detector, therefore, cannot perceive the speed of light to be faster or slower than 3×10^8 m/s. Another way of saying this is that we can always treat the detector as being at rest while the source may move.

Example 42-22: A speaker emitting a sound with a constant frequency approaches a detector. Which of the following wave characteristics will have a greater value at the detector than at the source?

   I. Frequency
  II. Wavelength
 III. Speed

Solution: Since the source is approaching the detector, the detected frequency will be higher than the emitted frequency. The wavelength will be shorter, and the wave speed will be the same. Therefore, only characteristic I will have a greater value at the detector than at the source.

Example 42-23: Your grandfather pushes the "star" key on his flip phone with giant buttons, generating a tone with a frequency of about 1080 Hz. However, the button gets stuck and the tone is continuous. Exasperated, he tosses drop the broken phone off a bridge. What is the frequency of the tone he hears at the instant the phone's speed is 20 m/s (speed of sound in air = 340 m/s)?

Solution: Since your grandfather (the detector) is stationary, $v_D = 0$. Now, because the source of the sound (the broken phone) is moving away from him, we use the plus sign on v_S in the denominator of the Doppler effect equation to find that

$$f_D = f_S \frac{v}{v + v_S} = (1080 \text{ Hz}) \cdot \frac{340 \text{ m/s}}{340 \text{ m/s} + 20 \text{ m/s}} = (1080 \text{ Hz}) \cdot \frac{340}{360} = (3 \text{ Hz}) \cdot 340 = 1020 \text{ Hz}$$

Note that, because the phone is *accelerating* away from him, the magnitude of v_S is increasing as the phone falls, and thus the frequency he detects is *decreasing* as a function of time.

Example 42-24: As a high-speed chase begins, a police car travels at a speed of 40 m/s directly toward the suspect's getaway car, which is traveling at a speed of 70 m/s, trying to outrun the pursuing police. The frequency that the suspect hears will be what percentage of the frequency of the police car's siren? (speed of sound = 340 m/s)

Solution: Use the Doppler effect equation, choosing the signs carefully. The suspect in the getaway car is the detector (so v_D = 70 m/s), moving *away* from the source. The source is the police car (v_S = 40 m/s), moving *toward* the detector. Therefore,

$$f_D = f_S \frac{v \pm v_D}{v \mp v_S} = f_S \frac{340 \text{ m/s} - 70 \text{ m/s}}{340 \text{ m/s} - 40 \text{ m/s}} = f_S \frac{270}{300} = f_S \frac{90}{100} = (90\%) f_S$$

In order to find the correct value of f_D, it was necessary to plug in the values for v_D and v_S, and to change the top and the bottom of the equation separately; we couldn't just use the relative velocity of 30 m/s. However, if all the problem had asked for was the qualitative effect (i.e., whether the detected frequency was higher or lower than that of the source), then we could have worked out that the frequency was lower simply by noticing that the detector was getting farther away from the source.

42.7

Example 42-25: A technician is using his ultrasound scanner to detect a fetal heartbeat. The scanner emits short pulses of frequency 5 MHz, which then bounce off the beating heart and return to the scanner (functioning as a detector). The detector compares the final received frequency, f_2, with the original emitted frequency, f_1, and converts the difference in frequency into the speed and direction of the heart's motion. The difference in frequency, $\Delta f = f_2 - f_1$, is equal to $\pm 2vf_1/v_{sound}$, where v is the speed of the heart and $v_{sound} = 1500$ m/s is the speed of the ultrasound pulses. If $\Delta f = -100$ Hz, then the observed heart is:

- A. expanding at 1.5 cm/s.
- B. contracting at 1.5 cm/s.
- C. expanding at 7.5 cm/s.
- D. contracting at 7.5 cm/s.

42.7

Solution: First, the fact that Δf is negative means that f_2 is lower than f_1, and if the final detected frequency is *lower* than the frequency emitted by the source, then the heart surface must be moving *away from* the source (i.e., contracting). This eliminates choices A and C. Now, to figure out the value of the heart's speed, v, we just use the given formula:

$$\Delta f = -\frac{2vf_1}{v_{sound}} \rightarrow v = -\frac{v_{sound}\Delta f}{2f_1} = -\frac{(1,500 \text{ m/s})(-100 \text{ Hz})}{1 \times 10^7 \text{ Hz}} = 1.5 \times 10^{-2} \text{ m/s}$$

This is equal to 1.5 cm/s, and choice B is correct.

Chapter 43
Light, Optics, and
Quantum Physics

43.1 ELECTROMAGNETIC WAVES

We've seen that if we oscillate one end of a long rope, we generate a wave that travels down the rope and whose frequency is the frequency with which we oscillate.

You can think of an electromagnetic wave in a similar way: an oscillating electric charge generates an **electromagnetic (EM)** wave, which is composed of oscillating electric and magnetic fields. These fields oscillate with the same frequency at which the electric charge that created the wave oscillated. The fields oscillate in phase with each other, perpendicular to each other and to the direction of propagation. For this reason, electromagnetic waves are transverse waves. The direction in which the wave's electric field oscillates is called the direction of **polarization** of the wave.

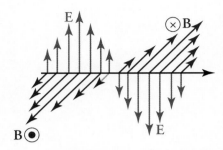

Most EM waves have electric fields oscillating in all perpendicular directions to propagation equally and are thus *unpolarized*.

Unlike waves on a rope or sound waves, electromagnetic waves do not require a material medium to propagate; they can travel through empty space (vacuum). When an EM wave travels through vacuum, its speed is a constant. It is one of the fundamental constants of nature and a value you should memorize for the MCAT:

Speed of Light in Vacuum

$$c = 3 \times 10^8 \, \text{m/s}$$

All electromagnetic waves, regardless of frequency, travel through vacuum at this speed. The most important equation for waves, $v = \lambda f$, is also true for electromagnetic waves. For EM waves traveling through vacuum, $v = c$, so the equation becomes $c = \lambda f$.

The frequencies for electromagnetic waves span a huge range, and different ranges have been given specific names. This assignment of names to specific regions based on frequency (or wavelength) is known as the **electromagnetic spectrum** and is shown here.

Notice that visible light occupies only a small part of the electromagnetic spectrum. When waves from all over the visible spectrum are mixed together, the resulting light is perceived as white. You should memorize the order of the colors of the visible spectrum from lowest frequency (longest wavelength) to highest frequency (shortest wavelength): ROYGBV (Roy-Gee-Biv), which stands for red, orange, yellow, green, blue, and violet. In terms of wavelengths, violet light has a wavelength (in vacuum) of about 400 nm and red light has a wavelength of about 700 nm; the other colors are in between.

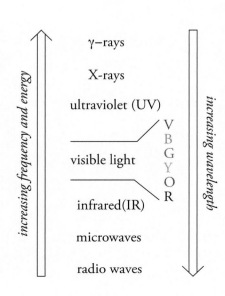

43.2 REFLECTION AND REFRACTION

When a beam of light strikes the boundary between two transparent media, some of the light will be reflected from the surface. In the figure below, some of the sunlight will be reflected off the water in the tank.

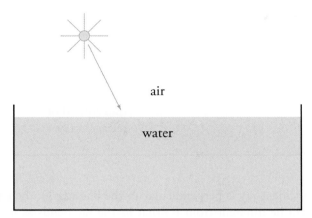

When a ray of light passing through one medium is reflected from the surface of another, the angle at which it bounces off the new medium is equal to the angle at which it strikes. In other words, *the angle of reflection is equal to the angle of incidence*. This fact is known as the **Law of Reflection**. Notice that, by definition, the angles of incidence and reflection are measured with reference to a line that's perpendicular to the plane of interface between the two media; that is, the angle of incidence and the angle of reflection are the angles that the incident and reflected rays make with *the normal*, not with the surface.

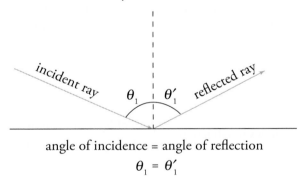

angle of incidence = angle of reflection

$$\theta_1 = \theta_1'$$

Example 43-1: In the figure above, assume that a ray of sunlight strikes the water, making an angle of 60° with the surface. What is the angle of reflection?

  A) 15°
  B) 30°
  C) 60°
  D) 90°

Solution: Be careful. If the incident ray makes an angle of 60° with the surface, then it makes an angle of 30° with the normal. Therefore, the angle of incidence is 30°. By the law of reflection, the angle of reflection is 30° also. Choice B is the answer.

In the figure below, not all of the sunlight that encounters the surface of the water is reflected; some is transmitted into the water. Unless the angle of incidence is 0°, the light will be *bent* as it enters the water. The bending is called **refraction**. The **angle of refraction** is the angle that the **transmitted** (or **refracted**) ray makes with the line that's perpendicular to the plane of interface between the two media.

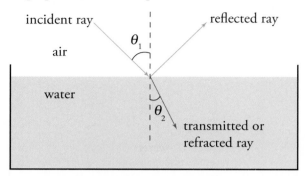

If $\theta_1 = 0°$ (that is, if the incident ray is perpendicular to the boundary), then $\theta_2 = 0°$. However, if θ_1 is any other angle, then θ_2 will be different from θ_1; that is, the ray bends as it's transmitted. In order to figure out the angle of refraction, we first need to discuss a medium's index of refraction.

Index of Refraction

Light travels at speed $c = 3 \times 10^8$ m/s when traveling in a vacuum. However, when light travels through a material medium such as water or glass, its transmission speed is less than c. Every medium, in fact, has an **index of refraction** that tells us how much slower light travels through that medium than through empty space.

Index of Refraction

$$\text{index of refraction} = \frac{\text{speed of light in vacuum}}{\text{speed of light in medium}}$$

$$n = \frac{c}{v}$$

The index of refraction of vacuum is, by definition, exactly equal to 1. Because the index for air is very close to 1, we simply use $n = 1$ for air as well. (The MCAT will use this approximation unless otherwise specified.) Notice that n has no units, it's never less than 1, and the greater the value of n for a medium, the slower light travels through that medium. For most materials, the value of n is between 1 and 2.5. Glass has an index of refraction of about 1.5 (but varies depending on the type of glass), while diamond has a particularly high value of n, about 2.4. Values of n above 2.5 are rare.

Example 43-2: Light travels through water at an approximate speed of 2.25×10^8 m/s. What is the refractive index of water?

  A) 0.75
  B) 1.33
  C) 1.50
  D) 2.25

Solution: First, eliminate choice A: the index of refraction is never less than 1. Now, by definition,

$$n = \frac{c}{v} = \frac{3 \times 10^8 \text{ m/s}}{2.25 \times 10^8 \text{ m/s}} = \frac{3}{2.25} = \frac{3}{2\frac{1}{4}} = \frac{3}{\frac{9}{4}} = 3 \cdot \tfrac{4}{9} = \tfrac{4}{3} \approx 1.33$$

Therefore, the answer is choice B.

Now that we know about the index of refraction, we can state the rule that's used to figure out the angle of refraction. It's called the Law of Refraction, or Snell's Law:

> ### Law of Refraction (Snell's Law)
>
> $$n_1 \sin\theta_1 = n_2 \sin\theta_2$$

In this equation, n_1 is the refractive index of the medium through which the incident ray is traveling, and n_2 is the refractive index of the medium through which the transmitted (or refracted) ray is traveling.

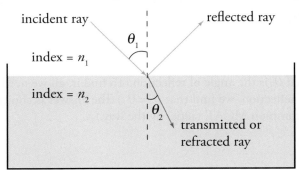

It follows from Snell's Law that if $n_2 > n_1$, then $\theta_2 < \theta_1$. That is, if the transmitting medium has a higher index of refraction than the incident medium, then the ray will bend *toward* the normal. Similarly, if $n_2 < n_1$, then $\theta_2 > \theta_1$. That is, if the transmitting medium has a lower index of refraction than the incident medium, then the ray will bend *away from* the normal. You should memorize both of these facts.

Example 43-3: A ray of light traveling through air is incident on a piece of glass whose refractive index is 1.5. If the sine of the angle of incidence is 0.6, what's the sine of the angle of refraction?

Solution: Using the law of refraction, we find that

$$n_1 \sin\theta_1 = n_2 \sin\theta_2 \rightarrow \quad (1)(0.6) = (1.5)(\sin\theta_2) \quad \rightarrow \quad \sin\theta_2 = \frac{0.6}{1.5} = \frac{\frac{3}{5}}{\frac{3}{2}} = \frac{2}{5} = 0.4$$

Notice that $\sin\theta_2$ is less than $\sin\theta_1$; this immediately tells us that $\theta_2 < \theta_1$. The light is traveling from air ($n_1 = 1$) into glass, whose refractive index is higher. If the transmitting medium (the second one) has a higher index of refraction than the incident medium (the first one), then θ_2 *will* be less than θ_1; that is, the ray will bend toward the normal.

Example 43-4: Consider the diagram below, showing an incident ray, reflected ray, and transmitted ray:

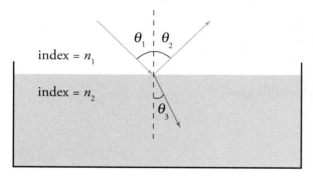

What information is needed to find θ_2?

        A) n_1, n_2, and θ_1
        B) n_1, n_2, and θ_3
        C) n_1 only
        D) θ_1 only

Solution: The angle labeled θ_2 is the angle of reflection. To find it, all we need to know is the angle of incidence, θ_1. (By the law of reflection, we find that $\theta_2 = \theta_1$.) The answer is choice D. (This unconventional labeling of the angles is a common MCAT tactic, by the way.)

Total Internal Reflection

When a light ray traveling in a medium of high refractive index approaches a medium of lower refractive index (for example, a light ray traveling in water towards the interface with the air), it may or may not escape into the second medium. If the ray's angle of incidence exceeds a certain **critical angle**, the light ray will undergo **total internal reflection**: all of the incident ray's energy will be reflected back into its original medium; there will be no refracted ray.

Critical Angle for Total Internal Reflection

$$\sin \theta_{crit} = \frac{n_2}{n_1}$$

In this equation, n_1 is the refractive index of the medium through which the incident ray is traveling, and n_2 is the refractive index of the medium on the other side of the boundary. The angle θ_{crit} is the critical angle. What this means is that if the angle of incidence, θ_1, is greater than θ_{crit}, then total internal reflection will occur.[1] However, if θ_1 is less than θ_{crit}, then total internal reflection will not occur. (If θ_1 just happens to equal θ_{crit}, then the refracted beam skims along the boundary with $\theta_2 = 90°$.)

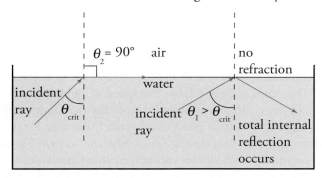

Notice that there can be a critical angle for total internal reflection *only if n_1 is greater than n_2*. For example, a beam of light incident in the air and striking the surface of the water can never experience total internal reflection because $n_1 < n_2$. In other words, there'll be some reflection and some refraction, as usual. In this case, some of the light's intensity will always be transmitted into the water.

Example 43-5: A beam of light is incident on the boundary between air and a piece of glass whose index of refraction is $\sqrt{2}$. When would total internal reflection (TIR, for short) of this beam occur?

Solution: First, in order to have TIR, the beam would have to start in the glass, trying to exit into the air. (If the beam were traveling in the air and incident on the glass, then TIR could not occur.) Furthermore, the angle of incidence would have to be greater than the critical angle, which we calculate as follows:

$$\sin \theta_{crit} = \frac{n_2}{n_1} = \frac{1}{\sqrt{2}} = \frac{\sqrt{2}}{2} \rightarrow \theta_{crit} = 45°$$

---

[1]   If you forget the formula for the critical angle, there's another way to know that total internal reflection occurs: if you plug numbers into the law of refraction and find that $\sin \theta > 1$ (which is impossible), that tells you there is no angle of refraction, so there must be total internal reflection.

Example 43-6: Fiber optics technology makes use of total internal reflection: a core of flexible glass tubing surrounded by a different cladding material have light pulses sent down the core at angles greater than the crucial angle between the core and cladding, so that the light bounces back and forth inside the core tube down the length of the cable, emerging on the other side. An *endoscope* bundles many such fiber optic tubes. Some of the tubes are used to transmit light into the body, others to transmit the reflected light out of the body to the eyepiece. All of the following are plausible concerns in medical imaging using light EXCEPT:

    I.   Blurring of X-ray images due to refraction and diffraction
   II.   Burning of tissue due to endoscopic light intensity
 III.   Doppler shift of light frequencies due to movement of the endoscope

    A) I and II only
    B) II only
    C) III only
    D) II and III only

Solution: This is a Roman numeral question, so the best strategy is to begin with the item that appears precisely twice (item III). That item is clearly false: the speed of light waves is so much faster than the speed at which a doctor could physically move an endoscope that the Doppler effect would be completely negligible. This eliminates choices C and D. Next check item I. Because X-rays are a form of light, they do indeed refract and diffract when passing through the body, and so item I is true, eliminating choice B. Choice A is correct. Item II is indeed true: significant light intensity is maintained in an endoscope due to total internal reflection over a very small core area, so presumably if a bright enough light is sent through the tubes responsible for illuminating tissue, that light could burn said tissue if exposure occurred over too long a time due to negligence (this has in fact been recorded in medical journals).

43.3   WAVE EFFECTS

Diffraction

Simply put, waves, whether they're water waves, sound waves, EM waves, etc., don't always travel in a single direction when they encounter an obstruction. This redistribution of the wave's intensity is known as **diffraction**. Water waves bend around a rock sticking up out of the water, for example. The obstruction can even be a hole. For example, water or light incident on a hole in a barrier will pass through and *spread out* beyond the barrier. These effects are observed when the size of the object or opening is comparable to the wavelength of the waves.

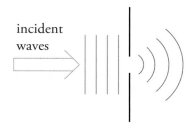

Polarization

Normally, the electric-field components of the waves in a beam of light vibrate in *all* planes. **Polarized** light is light whose direction of polarization has been restricted somehow. For example, all the waves in a beam of **plane-polarized** light have their electric-field components vibrating in a single plane.

It is possible to transform unpolarized light into polarized light by several methods. One method is the use of a *polarizing filter.* The filter has a polarization axis, so that when unpolarized light strikes the filter, only the portion of the waves vibrating in that direction pass through while the portion of the waves vibrating perpendicular to the axis is absorbed. The light that emerges is now polarized in in direction of the axis and has half the intensity of the original unpolarized light.

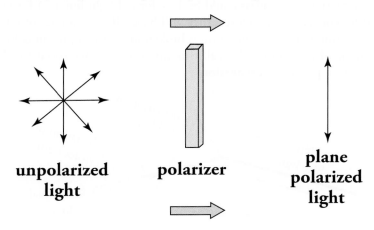

unpolarized light   **polarizer**   **plane polarized light**

If polarized light passes through a second polarizer, the amount of light that passes through or is absorbed depends on the angle between the direction of polarization of the incident light and the axis of the polarizer. As an example, if vertically polarized light is incident upon a horizontally polarizing filter, none of the light will pass through.

If two light waves of equal amplitude vibrate perpendicular to each other and have a 90° phase difference (the "crest" of one wave interferes with the "0" of the other), the light is *circularly polarized.*

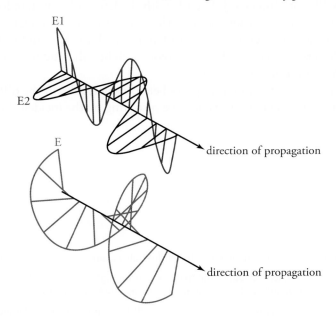

As a result, the electric field appears to be rotating.

Dispersion

When light moves from one medium to another, some wavelengths are bent more than others. The reason for this is that electromagnetic waves of different frequencies travel at slightly different speeds when traveling through a material medium like glass or water. Although Big Rule 1 for waves states that the speed of a wave is determined by the medium, not by the wave's frequency, light waves traveling through a material medium are an exception to this rule.[2] (In fact, they're the only exception that's at all likely to appear on the MCAT.) When light travels through a material (not vacuum), different frequencies will have different speeds. Thus, when we say that the index of refraction for a piece of glass is 1.5, what is really true is that the index varies slightly as the color of the light varies. For example, the index of refraction of the glass could be 1.47 for red light but 1.54 for violet light.[3] Because different colors have different refractive indexes, they will have different angles of refraction. This is why when white light passes through a prism, the beam is broken into its component colors. Each color leaves the prism at its own angle of refraction.[4] We call this variation in wave speed for different frequencies (and the effects this variation produces) **dispersion**.

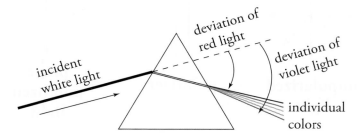

Example 43-7: *Circular dichroism spectroscopy* is a technique used to measure secondary structure in proteins and polypeptides. In this technique, differential absorbances of light occur due to the different handedness and spacing of different structures (such as alpha helix and beta sheet). Which property of light is most helpful in this technique and why?

A) Plane polarization, because the vertical and horizontal orientations of the electric field oscillations interact differently with the left- and right-handed structures.

B) Circular polarization, because the clockwise and counterclockwise rotations of the electric field vectors interact differently with the left- and right-handed structures.

C) Dispersion, because different colors of light will bend by different amounts in passing through different structures.

D) Diffraction, because the spaces between molecules in the different protein foldings will cause different amounts of wave spreading by the incident light.

---

[2] This isn't the case when electromagnetic waves travel through vacuum, where *all* frequencies travel at the same speed, *c*.

[3] In general, as in this example, the higher the frequency of the light, the lower the speed. However, there are complicated exceptions to this rule of thumb, and there's no need to memorize it or learn about the exceptions for the MCAT.

[4] The greater the index of refraction, the more the light will be bent on entering the medium from air or vacuum, so high-frequency violet light will generally bend more than red light.

Solution: The biggest clues in the question stem are the word "circular" and the reference to the handedness of the secondary structures, as both mirror the description of the rotation of circularly polarized light (choice B is correct). Otherwise there aren't good justifications for the other answer choices. It's not clear why unidirectional oscillations of the electric field would particularly interact with curving structures in proteins, so choice A can be eliminated. Dispersion happens in *any* translucent material due to the frequency dependence of index of refraction, so choice C doesn't make sense. Choice D sounds tempting, and indeed X-ray diffraction is used as a technique for observing protein's crystal structure. However, there is not enough information in the question stem to support this particular type of spectroscopy being based upon diffraction (this could be a case where you need to remind yourself to rely on the information on the screen more than your prior knowledge if you recalled that X-ray diffraction studies of proteins were a method).

Example 43-8: What wave phenomena (or wave effects) are observed in sound waves as well as light waves?

Solution: Sound waves reflect and refract, the latter because sound changes speed when it goes from one medium to another. Diffraction occurs when waves encounter obstacles or pass through holes that are on the order of the size of the wavelength. This phenomenon applies equally well to sound and light waves (and other waves as well). Dispersion, the differential changing of direction of waves of different frequencies due to those frequencies traveling at different speeds in a new medium, actually does happen with sound waves (acoustic dispersion) as well as light. The one wave effect that definitely does NOT apply to sound is polarization. Because sound is a longitudinal wave, the medium through which the wave passes only oscillates in one direction (parallel to the propagation). Polarization requires eliminating some directions of oscillation in favor of others, which can only happen for a transverse wave, which has infinitely many possible directions of oscillation of the medium (or of the electromagnetic field) perpendicular to the direction of propagation.

43.4 MIRRORS

A **mirror** is a surface, usually made of glass or metal, that forms an image of an object by *reflecting* light.

Plane Mirrors

A **plane** mirror is an ordinary flat mirror. If you put an object in front of a plane mirror, the image will appear to be behind the mirror. The image will be the same size as the object and will appear to be as far behind the mirror's surface as the object is in front of it. The image will also appear upright; it won't be inverted.

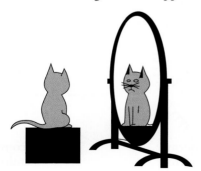

Curved Mirrors

We all have experience with plane mirrors, but a **curved** mirror presents us with images that are less familiar. The purpose of this section is to find a systematic way to describe the images formed by curved mirrors.

There are essentially two types of curved mirrors: concave and convex. The shiny (reflecting) surface of a **concave** mirror appears like the entrance to a cave from the point of view of the object. The reflecting surface of a **convex** mirror bends away from the object. As a simple demonstration of the difference, imagine holding a polished spoon. If you look into the spoon, you're looking at a concave surface; if you turn it around and look at the back of the spoon, you're looking at a convex surface.

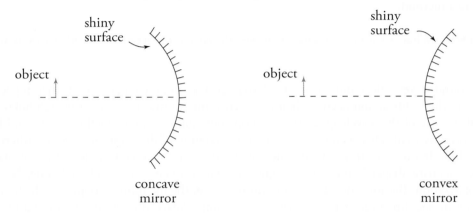

The curved mirrors we'll consider could be termed **spherical** mirrors, because near the center of the mirror, the surface is spherical (that is, part of a sphere).

When light parallel to the central **axis** of a concave mirror strikes the surface, it's reflected through a point called the **focus** (or **focal point**), denoted by F. This point is halfway to the **center of curvature**, C, of the mirror, which is the center of the sphere that the mirror is cut from. The distance between the center of curvature and the mirror is called the **radius of curvature**, *r*. (The radius of curvature is also sometimes denoted by *RC*.) Because the focal point is halfway between the mirror and C, the distance from the mirror to the focal point, the all-important **focal length**, *f*, is half the radius of curvature: $f = \frac{1}{2}r$.

When light parallel to the central axis of a *convex* mirror strikes the surface, it's reflected directly *away from* the imaginary **focal point** behind the mirror.

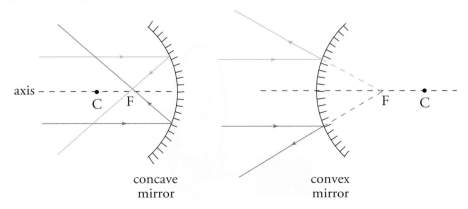

We see an image in a mirror at the point where the rays reflected off the mirror intersect *or* at the point from where the reflected rays seem to intersect (and therefore emanate from) behind the mirror. When a very distant object is placed in front of a mirror, the light rays that strike the mirror are approximately parallel, like the rays shown above. This illustrates the significance of the focal point. *The image of a distant object will appear at the focal point, for all curved mirrors.* This turns out to be true for thin lenses as well. But what if the object is not distant?

The following figures illustrate the process of image formation by curved mirrors:

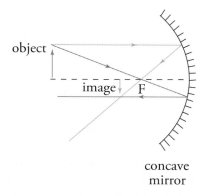

concave
mirror

The ray diagram for the concave mirror shows two incident rays reflecting off the mirror. One ray, parallel to the axis, is reflected through the focal point. Another ray, which goes through the focal point, is reflected parallel to the axis. The intersection point of these reflected rays determines the location of the image.

Note that the light rays still cross after reflecting off the mirror, but the image is located behind the focal point. If the object is moved closer to the mirror (i.e., inside the focal point), the reflected rays no longer cross and the image forms behind the mirror.

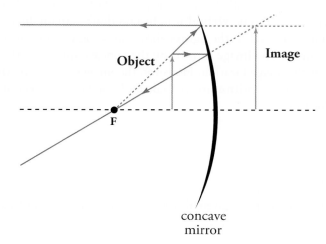

concave
mirror

One ray, parallel to the axis, is again reflected through the focal point. Another ray, which is directed as if it came from the focal point, is reflected parallel to the axis.

The ray diagram for the convex mirror also shows two incident rays reflecting off the mirror. One ray, parallel to the axis, is reflected directly away from the focal point. Another ray, which hits the center of the mirror (the point where its axis of symmetry intersects the mirror surface), is reflected at the same angle below the axis. Following these reflected rays back behind the mirror, their intersection point determines the location of the image.

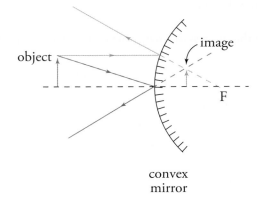

convex
mirror

Ray diagrams (like the ones drawn in the figures above) can be used to determine the approximate location of the image, but they usually can't give precise answers to all the questions we may be asked about the image formed by a mirror. What we want is a systematic way to get precise answers to these four questions:

1. Where is the image?
2. Is the image real or is it virtual?
3. Is the image upright or is it inverted?
4. How tall is the image (compared to the object)?

Before we discuss how to answer these questions, let's first define the terms *real* and *virtual*. An image is said to be **real** if light rays actually focus at the position of the image. A real image can be projected onto a surface. An image is said to be **virtual** if light rays don't actually focus at the apparent location of the image. For example, look back at the figures above, showing the formation of images by a concave mirror and by a convex mirror. The image formed by the concave mirror in the first diagram is real: light rays actually intersect at the image location. However, the images formed by the concave mirror in the second diagram and by the convex mirror are virtual: no light rays intersect at its location; they just seem to come from that location.

The Mirror Equation

To answer the first two questions given above, we use the mirror (and lens) equation:

***

Mirror (and Lens) Equation

$$\frac{1}{o} + \frac{1}{i} = \frac{1}{f}$$

***

Here, *o* stands for the object's distance from the mirror, and it is always positive. The value of *f* represents the focal length of the mirror. The value of *i* that satisfies this equation gives us the image's distance from the mirror. Both *f* and *i* are positive if they are on the same side as the human observer in relation to the mirror or lens. In the case of a mirror, the human observer is on the same side as the object. In the case of a lens, the human observer is on the opposite side of the object. Using the mirror (and lens) equation, we can find the location of the image, answering the first question.

The second question is also answered using the mirror equation. If we get a *positive* value for *i*, that tells us that the image is in front of the mirror and it's *real*; a *negative* value for *i* means the image is behind the mirror and is *virtual*. For example, let's say that *o* = 2 cm and *f* = 6 cm. Substituting these values into the mirror equation, we find that *i* = −3 cm. Therefore, the image is 3 cm behind the mirror and it's virtual. Note that you can use any unit for the measurement of distance, as long as it is the same unit for *o*, *i*, and *f*.

The Magnification Equation

To answer the last two questions, we then use the magnification equation:

Magnification Equation

$$m = -\frac{i}{o}$$

The value of *m* is the **magnification factor**; multiplying the height of the object by *m* gives us the height of the image. The sign of *m* tells us whether the image is upright or inverted. If *m* is *positive*, the image is *upright*; if *m* is *negative*, the image is *inverted*. To illustrate this, let's continue our example above, with *o* = 2 cm and *f* = 6 cm. We found that *i* = −3 cm. Therefore, the magnification factor is *m* = −(−3 cm)/(2 cm) = +1.5. This tells us that the height of the image is 1.5 times the height of the object, and (because *m* is positive) the image is upright.

The object distance, *o*, is always positive. If *i* is positive, then *m* is negative; if *i* is negative, then *m* is positive. In other words,

Real images are inverted, and virtual images are upright.

Now, the only thing that's left to do is to find the way to tell the mirror equation whether we have a concave mirror or a convex mirror. The rule is simple: when using the mirror equation, we write the focal length of a *concave* mirror as a *positive* number, and we write the focal length of a *convex* mirror as a *negative* number. Here's a summary of mirrors:

Mirrors

Concave mirror
f is positive

Convex mirror
f is negative

$$\frac{1}{o} + \frac{1}{i} = \frac{1}{f}$$

i positive $\longrightarrow$ real image (in front of mirror)

i negative $\longrightarrow$ virtual image (behind mirror)

$$m = -\frac{i}{o}$$

m positive $\longrightarrow$ image upright

m negative $\longrightarrow$ image inverted

- Concave mirrors can create real and virtual images.
- Convex mirrors can only create virtual images.

Example 43-9: Describe the image formed in a plane mirror.

- A) Real and upright
- B) Real and inverted
- C) Virtual and upright
- D) Virtual and inverted

Solution: First, eliminate choices A and D; *real* always goes with *inverted*, and *virtual* always goes with *upright*. We know from common experience that the image formed in a flat mirror is upright, so the answer must be choice C.

Example 43-10: If an object is placed very far from a concave mirror, where will the image be formed?

- A) Halfway between the focal point and the mirror
- B) At the focal point
- C) At the center of curvature
- D) At infinity

Solution: Use the mirror equation. "The object is placed very far from a mirror" means that we take $o = \infty$, so $1/o = 0$. The mirror equation then says $1/i = 1/f$, so $i = f$. That is, the image is formed at the focal point of the mirror, choice B.

Example 43-11: An object is placed 40 cm in front of a concave mirror with a radius of curvature of 60 cm. Locate and describe the image.

Solution: Because $f = \frac{1}{2}r$, we know that $f = 30$ cm. The mirror equation now gives

$$\frac{1}{40 \text{ cm}} + \frac{1}{i} = \frac{1}{30 \text{ cm}} \rightarrow \frac{1}{i} = \frac{1}{30} - \frac{1}{40} = \frac{4-3}{120} = \frac{1}{120} \rightarrow \therefore i = 120 \text{ cm}$$

(Be careful: The MCAT often gives the radius of curvature, r. What you want is f, the focal length, which is half of r.) Since i is positive, we know the image is real; also, it's located 120 cm from the mirror on the same side of the mirror as the object. (*Virtual* images are located *behind* the mirror.) Since $m = -i/o = -(120 \text{ cm})/(40 \text{ cm}) = -3$, we know that the image is 3 times the height of the object and inverted.

Example 43-12: An object is placed 40 cm in front of a convex mirror with a radius of curvature of -60 cm. Locate and describe the image.

Solution: Because $f = \frac{1}{2}r$, we know that $f = -30$ cm. The mirror equation now gives

$$\frac{1}{40 \text{ cm}} + \frac{1}{i} = \frac{1}{-30 \text{ cm}} \rightarrow \frac{1}{i} = \frac{1}{-30} - \frac{1}{40} = \frac{-4-3}{120} = \frac{-7}{120} \rightarrow \therefore i = -\frac{120}{7} \text{ cm}$$

Since i is negative, we know the image is virtual; also, it's located $120/7 \approx 17$ cm from the mirror on the opposite side of the mirror from the object. Since $m = -i/o = -(-\frac{120}{7} \text{ cm})/(40 \text{ m}) = +3/7$, we know that the image is 3/7 times the height of the object and upright. Comparing this example to the preceding one, notice how critical the sign of f was. It changed everything about the image.

Example 43-13: A convex mirror forms an upright image 12 cm behind the mirror when an object of height 15 cm is placed 20 cm in front of it. What is the height of the image?

Solution: To find the height of the image, we need the magnification. We're given that $o = 20$ cm and $i = -12$ cm. (We know that i is negative because not only do convex mirrors only form virtual images [a good fact to remember, by the way], but the question also says that the image is formed "behind the mirror." Images formed behind the mirror are virtual.) Therefore, $m = -i/o = -(-12 \text{ cm})/(20 \text{ cm}) = 3/5$. Multiplying the height of the object by the magnification gives the height of the image. Therefore, the height of the image is $(3/5)(15 \text{ cm}) = 9$ cm.

43.5 LENSES

A **lens** is a thin piece of clear glass or plastic that forms an image of an object by *refracting* light. The purpose of this section is to find a systematic way to describe the images formed by lenses.

There are essentially two types of lenses: converging and diverging. **Converging** lenses are thicker in the middle than they are at the ends, and they refract light rays that are parallel to the axis *toward* the focal point on the other side of the lens. **Diverging** lenses are thinner in the middle than they are at the ends, and they refract light rays that are parallel to the axis *away from* the "imaginary" focal point that's in front of the lens.

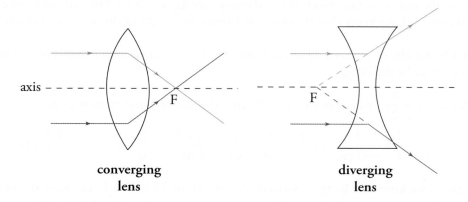

converging
lens

diverging
lens

We want to be able to answer the same four questions for lenses as we did for mirrors. Fortunately, *virtually everything we did for mirrors carries over unchanged to lenses.* For example, the mirror equation is also the lens equation, and the magnification equation is also the same. The conventions for positive and negative *i* and *m* are also the same for lenses as they are for mirrors.

We distinguish between the two types of lenses in the same way we distinguished between the two types of mirrors. When using the lens equation, we write the focal length of a *converging* lens as a *positive* number, and we write the focal length of a *diverging* lens as a *negative* number.

Here's an important note. The MCAT uses the terms *concave* and *convex* to refer to different mirrors and lenses. The diagrams above show us that the surfaces of a converging lens are convex, and the surfaces of a diverging lens are concave. Thus, a concave lens is the same as a diverging lens, and a convex lens is the same as a converging lens. Now for a warning: for a concave *mirror, f* is positive; for a convex *mirror, f* is negative. When these terms are applied to lenses, things necessarily switch: for a concave *lens, f* is negative; for a convex *lens, f* is positive. *Be careful* when you see the words *concave* or *convex*. Whether these terms describe a mirror or a lens will make a critically important difference in whether you write the focal length as a positive or as a negative number.

Besides the fact the lenses form images by refracting light (rather than by reflecting light, as is the case for mirrors), there's really only one difference: For lenses, *real* images are formed on the *opposite* side of the lens from the object, while *virtual* images are formed on the *same* side of the lens as the object.

Here's a summary of lenses:

Lenses

Converging lens
(convex lens)
f is positive

Diverging lens
(concave lens)
f is negative

$$\frac{1}{o} + \frac{1}{i} = \frac{1}{f}$$

i positive $\Rightarrow$ real image (other side of lens)
i negative $\Rightarrow$ virtual image (same side of lens as object)

$$m = -\frac{i}{o}$$

m positive $\Rightarrow$ image upright
m negative $\Rightarrow$ image inverted

- Converging (convex) lenses can create real and virtual images.
- Diverging (concave) lenses can create only virtual images.

Example 43-14: An object is placed 10 cm in front of a diverging lens with a focal length of −40 cm, then the image will be located:

    A) 5 cm in front of the lens.
    B) 5 cm behind the lens.
    C) 8 cm in front of the lens.
    D) 8 cm behind the lens.

Solution: We use the lens equation to find i:

$$\frac{1}{10\text{ cm}} = \frac{1}{i} = \frac{1}{-40\text{ cm}} \rightarrow \frac{1}{i} = \frac{1}{40} - \frac{1}{10} = \frac{-1-4}{40} = \frac{-5}{40} = -\frac{1}{8} \rightarrow \therefore i = -8\text{ cm}$$

This eliminates choices A and B. Because i is negative, the image is virtual, and for lenses, virtual images are formed on the same side of the lens as the object. Therefore, the answer is choice C.

Example 43-15: An object of height 10 cm is held 50 cm in front of a convex lens with a focal length of magnitude 40 cm. Describe the image.

Solution: The fact that the lens is convex means that it's a converging lens with a *positive* focal length; therefore, $f = +40$ cm. The lens equation now gives us i:

$$\frac{1}{50\text{ cm}} = \frac{1}{i} = \frac{1}{40\text{ cm}} \rightarrow \frac{1}{i} = \frac{1}{40} - \frac{1}{50} = \frac{5-4}{200} = \frac{1}{200} \rightarrow \therefore i = 200\text{ cm}$$

Because i is positive, we know the image is real; also, it's located 200 cm from the lens on the *opposite* side of the lens from the object. Because $m = -i/o = -(200\text{ cm})/(50\text{ cm}) = -4$, we know that the image is 4 times the height of the object and inverted.

Lens Power

A lens with a short focal length refracts light more (i.e., through larger angles) than a lens with a longer focal length. We say that the lens of short focal length has a greater *power* than a lens with a longer focal length.

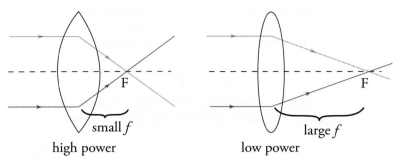

small *f*

high power

large *f*

low power

The **power** of a lens is defined to be the reciprocal of *f*, the focal length. When *f* is expressed in *meters*, the unit of lens power is called the **diopter** (abbreviated **D**).

Lens Power

$$P = \frac{1}{f} \text{, where } f \text{ is in meters}$$

For example, to find the power of a lens whose focal length is 40 cm, we first write *f* in meters: *f* = 0.4 m. Since 0.4 = 2/5, the reciprocal of 0.4 is 5/2 = 2.5. Therefore, the power of this lens is 2.5 diopters. Since the focal length of a converging lens is positive, the power of a converging lens is positive. Similarly, since the focal length of a diverging lens is negative, the power of a diverging lens is negative.

If two (or more) lenses are placed side by side, the power of the lens combination is equal to the sum of the powers of the individual lenses. In the case of two lenses, $P = P_1 + P_2$. For example, if we place a converging lens with a power of 3 D right next to a converging lens with a power of 1 D, then the power of the lens combination will be 4 D.

Example 43-16: A lens has a focal length of –20 cm. Is the lens converging or diverging? What is the power of this lens?

Solution: The fact that the lens has a negative focal length means that it's a diverging (or concave) lens. Rewriting *f* in meters, we have $f = -\frac{1}{5}$ m. Therefore, the power of this lens is

$$P = \frac{1}{f} = \frac{1}{-\frac{1}{5} \text{ m}} = -5 \text{ D}$$

Example 43-17: The human eye is typically about 1.7 cm from cornea to retina. Which of the following best describes the optics of the typical eye when viewing a distance object?

    A) The lensing system of the eye has a power of about +60 D, and it forms a real image on the retina.

    B) The lensing system of the eye has a power of +60 D, and it forms a virtual image on the retina.

    C) The lensing system of the eye has a power of −60 D, and it forms a real image on the retina.

    D) The lensing system of the eye has a power of −60 D, and it forms a virtual image on the retina.

Solution: Note that for a distant object, $o \to \infty$, so $i = f$. Since a real image must fall on the retina, which is essentially the projection screen at the back of the eye (eliminating choices B and D), the image distance is +1.7 cm, and so is the focal length (this eliminates choice C). 1/(0.017 m) is about 60 D.

43.6   PHOTONS AND QUANTIZATION

We've seen that electromagnetic waves, including visible light, exhibit many of the same wave phenomena as do mechanical waves like sound or waves on a string. However, when electromagnetic radiation interacts with matter (absorption and emission), we find that it carries energy, and that the energy is quantized. That is, the energy associated with EM radiation is absorbed or emitted by matter in packets; individual bundles. Each such bundle of energy is called a **photon**, and the energy of a photon is directly proportional to the frequency:

Photon Energy

$$E = hf = h\frac{c}{\lambda}$$

The constant of proportionality, h, is called **Planck's constant**. In SI units, its value is about 6.6×10^{-34} J·s.

The fact that electromagnetic radiation carries energy in packets (photons), which we can think of as a particles of light, gives rise to the idea of **wave-particle duality** for electromagnetic radiation: EM radiation travels like a wave but interacts with matter like a particle. One peculiarity of this duality is that, for waves, energy is proportional to the square of amplitude (recall the intensity relation from the previous chapter), whereas for particles (photons), energy is proportional to frequency. Earlier we noted that these two properties were independent of one another. Thus, the wave and particle models for light differ significantly in their predictions, and yet each is sometimes true.

Example 43-18: Which one of the following statements is true regarding red photons and blue photons traveling through vacuum?

A) Red light travels faster than blue light and carries more energy.
B) Blue light travels faster than red light and carries more energy.
C) Red light travels at the same speed as blue light and carries more energy.
D) Blue light travels at the same speed as red light and carries more energy.

Solution: All electromagnetic waves, regardless of frequency, travel through vacuum at the same speed, c. This eliminates choices A and B. Now, because blue light has a higher frequency than red light (remember ROYGBV, which lists the colors in order of increasing frequency), photons of blue light have higher energy than photons of red light. Therefore, the answer is choice D.

The discovery of this wave-particle duality of light was one of the first important results of the new **quantum physics** around the turn of the twentieth century. The word "quantum" refers to a specific amount of something measurable, like mass, charge, wavelength, momentum, energy, and the like. Quantum physics, then, is the physics associated with discrete values and changes in the values of such quantities; that is, their **quantization**. We've already encountered an example of this phenomenon with charge: only charges that are integer multiples of the elementary charge $e = 1.6 \times 10^{-19}$ coulombs will ever be observed, because you can't have half a proton or two thirds of an electron. Thus, charge is **quantized**.

Quantum physics is a complex and fascinating field that describes myriad strange phenomena and underlies many of our most important technological advances, such as computers, MRIs, and lasers. For MCAT purposes, you will need to understand the basic quantum model of the atom and the Pauli exclusion principle, the quantization of EM energy and the photoelectric effect, and the Heisenberg uncertainty principle.

43.7   THE BOHR MODEL OF THE ATOM

When a diffuse elemental gas is energized by heating or passing a current through it, the gas glows with a particular hue. If that light is passed through a prism, then dispersion will cause the light to separate into its component colors, corresponding to frequencies and wavelengths. This pattern of distinct bright lines of color is called the element's **emission spectrum**.

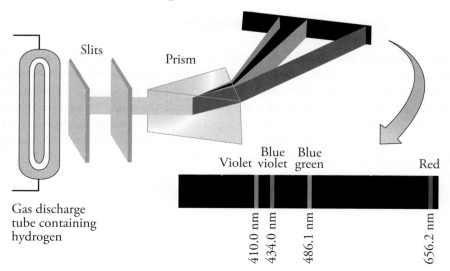

Recall that the energy of a photon is given by

$$E_{photon} = hf = hc \,/\, \lambda$$

where h is Planck's constant, 6.63×10^{-34} joule-seconds. Thus, one can use the measured wavelengths of light to determine the energies of the atomic transitions that produced the light. The assumption is that the particular frequencies of photons emitted by the atoms in the gas correspond to the energy losses of the atoms as their electrons transition from higher to lower energy states. Because only these characteristic frequencies are observed for a given element under normal conditions, this indicates that only certain electron transitions can occur.

Example 43-19: The wavelength of the red Hα spectral line characteristic of the visible hydrogen spectrum is 656 nm. How much energy does a hydrogen atom lose when it emits an Hα photon? Use $h = 6.63 \times 10^{-34}$ J·s.

Solution: Use the equation for the energy of a photon in terms of wavelength:

$$E_{photon} = \frac{hc}{\lambda} = \frac{\left(6.63 \times 10^{-34} \text{ J·s}\right)\left(3 \times 10^{8} \text{ m/s}\right)}{656 \times 10^{-9} \text{ m}} \approx 3 \times 10^{-19} \text{ J}$$

The energy of the emitted photon corresponds exactly to the energy lost by the hydrogen atom.

Danish physicist Niels Bohr explained these discrete and characteristic emission spectra by modifying the classical Rutherford atomic model, which depicted the atom as a planetary system, with a tiny but massive central positive charge orbited by distant electrons. The Rutherford model explained many experimental results, but it failed to account for the discrete emission spectra. Bohr concluded that electrons orbiting s nucleus are restricted to certain specific radii and energy levels. The radii, often referred to as shells, are labeled with the letter n, where $n = 1, 2, 3, \dots.$

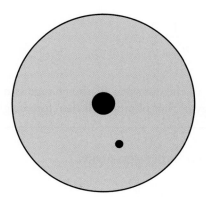

Rutherford Model
Electrons assume arbitrary orbits

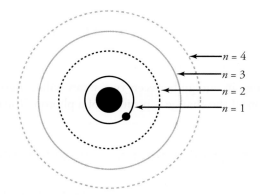

Bohr Model
Electrons assume quantized orbits

The Bohr model assumes that atoms have electron orbitals with quantized energy levels and that a transition between levels requires the absorption or emission of a photon:

Energy of a Photon Emitted or Absorbed under the Bohr Model

$$E_{\text{photon}} = |\Delta E_{\text{atom}}|$$

The energy of the atomic energy levels is expressed in terms of electron-volts (eV), that is, the product of the elementary charge e with volts V. Because the elementary charge is equal to 1.6×10^{-19} C, converting from joules to eV requires dividing by this number. This yields

---

Energy Level of a Hydrogen Atom

$$E_n = -13.6 \text{ eV} / n^2$$

where n = 1, 2, 3

Be sure you understand why this energy is negative. Electrons orbiting a nucleus are energetically bound to it and must absorb more energy to move further from that nucleus or to escape (thereby ionizing the atom). Thus, the energy of the orbital has to become increasingly positive as n increases, up to zero as n approaches infinity (which means ionization has occurred).

Bohr's model thus explains the emission spectra of hydrogen and, by extension, the other elements: any single change in n entails a discrete change in energy according to

$$\Delta E = -13.6 \text{ eV} \left(\frac{1}{n_{\text{final}}^2} - \frac{1}{n_{\text{initial}}^2} \right)$$

This change in energy between two states will correspond to the emission (if the change is negative) or absorption (if the change is positive) of a photon. The energy of that photon will therefore be given by

---

The Energy of a Photon Emitted or Absorbed by a Hydrogen Atom

$$hf = |\Delta E| = \left| 13.6 \text{ eV} \left(\frac{1}{n_{\text{final}}^2} - \frac{1}{n_{\text{initial}}^2} \right) \right|$$

Example 43-20: What is the frequency of a photon that, when absorbed, will ionize a hydrogen atom that begins in the $n = 2$ state? Planck's constant is $h = 4.14 \times 10^{-15}$ eV·s.

Solution: When an atom is ionized, its final state is $n \to \infty$, so applying the preceding equation yields

$$hf = \left| 13.6 \text{ eV} \left(0 - \frac{1}{2^2} \right) \right| = 3.4 \text{ eV}$$

$$f = \frac{3.4 \text{ eV}}{4.14 \times 10^{-15} \text{ eV·s}} \approx 8 \times 10^{14} \text{ Hz}$$

43.8   THE PAULI EXCLUSION PRINCIPLE

A few years after Bohr refined his model, Wolfgang Pauli devised an explanation for the fact that the elements exhibited patterns of chemical behavior related to the number of electrons. For example, atoms with even numbers of electrons are in general more chemically stable than those with odd numbers. Pauli determined that these groupings of elements and their behaviors could be explained that so long as only one electron was allowed to occupy a particular *quantum state*, defined not only by the principal quantum number n but three additional quantum numbers. For MCAT purposes, understanding the **Pauli exclusion principle** usually means recognizing that each atomic orbital can hold only two electrons of opposite *spin*, a quantum number that defines the intrinsic angular momentum of the electron. However, the Pauli exclusion principle applies to protons and neutrons as well, and asserts more broadly that there is a limit to how many such particles can be confined in a small space.

43.8

43.9   THE PHOTOELECTRIC EFFECT

In the late nineteenth century, long before Bohr's quantum atomic model, it was noticed that a spark would jump between two charged plates when a strong light was shone on the negative plate, and the spark would diminish or disappear altogether when a filter was used to block the ultraviolet component of the light. Because the light is giving rise to an electric current, the effect is called the **photoelectric effect**. Below is a picture of the apparatus used to measure this effect.

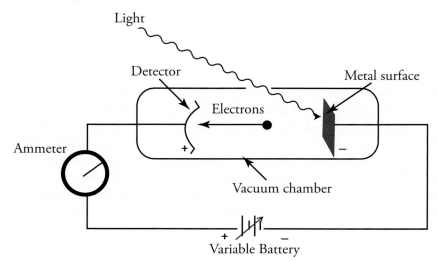

The ammeter will register a current only when *photoelectrons* (that is, electrons ejected by the incident light) pass from the metal surface to the detector. Note that the voltage of the battery can be varied and that its polarity can be reversed.

According to the classical theory of light as a wave, the energy absorbed by the metal surface depends only upon the amplitude of the light wave, that is, the light's brightness. The energy delivered by this continuous wave increases with time; the longer a light of a given intensity shines on a surface, the more energy will be absorbed. The binding energy of the metal for its surface electrons (the ones most likely to be ejected) is called the metal's **work function**, ϕ.

Based upon the wave theory of light, electrons would be ejected if the light had a large enough intensity to overcome the work function or if the light shone on the metal for a long enough period of time. Surprisingly, these expectations were contradicted by experimental results. Though increasing the intensity of the light did yield more current when there was a current to begin with, light below a certain frequency would not generate any current, regardless of intensity. Similarly, an increase in time of exposure to light below a certain frequency had no effect.

In 1905, Einstein published the paper that explained these findings (the paper for which he later won the Nobel Prize). Einstein's explanation of the photoelectric effect developed the photon model of light previously mentioned. There are three important points in this model that explain the experimental results better than does the wave model of light.

- Electromagnetic radiation (that is, light) of a certain frequency is made up of discrete bundles of energy (now called "photons"), each with energy $E = hf$.
- Photons of light are absorbed or emitted as single instantaneous interactions (as opposed to the mechanism provided by the wave model for gradually absorbing or emitting energy).
- When a photon strikes the surface of a metal, it interacts with a single electron, imparting all of its energy in the form of increased kinetic energy for the electron. If this energy is greater than the work function of the metal, the electron will be ejected from the metal with kinetic energy given by the following expression (note the subscript indicating that this is the maximum kinetic energy for an ejected electron: many electrons ejected will be deeper in the metal and thus will lose more energy in the process of ejection).

Kinetic Energy of a Photoelectron

$$KE_{max} = hf - \phi$$

Example 43-21: Almost all modern medical imaging (that doesn't rely on actual film) relies on a simple principle: translating electromagnetic or ionizing radiation signals from the imaging device into electrical signals, which can then be translated into an image on a screen. In the operation of a positron emission tomography (*PET*) scan, for example, a radioactive tracer is injected into a patient. The tracer undergoes β+ decay, and the positrons annihilate electrons in their vicinity in a matter-antimatter interaction that releases gamma radiation. The gamma radiation is then picked up by a so-called gamma camera composed of an array of scintillating crystals (which absorbs the gamma photon and reemits a photon of lower energy) and *photomultiplier tubes* (which absorb these secondary photons). The principle of operation of the photomultiplier tubes is the photoelectric effect: incident photons are converted to photoelectrons, which are absorbed and amplified as a cascading electric current measured and recorded by a computer. These flashes of current are eventually composed into an image.

Suppose the photomultiplier tubes in a gamma camera use cesium to absorb the incident photons. Cesium has a work function of 2.1 eV. What is the maximum wavelength of incident light that would eject a photoelectron from cesium?

Solution: First, recognize that the *maximum* wavelength of light will correspond to the *minimum* frequency and therefore energy. The minimum kinetic energy an electron could have when ejected would be 0, meaning the electron just barely overcame the work function of the metal. Applying the equation for the kinetic energy of the ejected photoelectron yields

$$0 = hf_{min} - \phi = \left(4.1 \times 10^{-15} \text{ eV}\right) f_{min} - 2.1 \text{ eV}$$

$$f_{min} = \frac{2.1}{4.1 \times 10^{-15}} \approx 5 \times 10^{14} \text{ Hz}$$

Now convert this minimum frequency into a maximum wavelength:

$$c = f\lambda \rightarrow \lambda_{max} = \frac{c}{f_{min}} = \frac{3 \times 10^8}{5 \times 10^{14}} = 6 \times 10^{-7} \text{ m}$$

43.9

Example 43-22: Suppose a photoelectric experiment is conducted and the applied voltage is varied over a range of values to generate a graph of current versus voltage similar to that shown above. If the intensity of the light is increased but all other aspects of the experiment are kept the same, which of the following aspects of the generated graph would change?

   I.   The slope of the line from V_{stop} to $V = 0$
  II.   The location of V_{stop}
 III.   The maximum value of the current

   A.   I only
   B.   II only
   C.   I and III only
   D.   I, II, and III

Solution: The stopping voltage depends upon the maximum kinetic energy of the photoelectrons, which in turn depends upon the *frequency* of the incident light and the work function of the metal target. Therefore, changing the *intensity* of the incident light will not alter the stopping voltage, so Item II is false, eliminating choices B and D. Increasing the intensity will, however, increase the number of photons striking the target, and therefore will increase the number of photoelectrons and therefore the maximum current, meaning Item III is true, eliminating choice A. Choice C is correct, and Item I is true because if the stopping voltage stays the same but the maximum current increases, the slope of the line from V_{stop} up to the now higher *y*-intercept must be greater.

43.10 THE HEISENBERG UNCERTAINTY PRINCIPLE

In 1927, Werner Heisenberg was working with Niels Bohr in Copenhagen to further develop the new quantum physics. While Bohr was away skiing, Heisenberg recognized a surprising but critical consequence of wave-particle duality: uncertainty. To measure the position of a particle extremely accurately, one had to shine a very short wavelength light on it, because the wavelength itself is a limitation on the determination of position. A short wavelength corresponds to a high frequency and high energy, and when a high energy photon interacts with a particle like an electron, it imparts some of its energy and momentum to the particle. (The relation between energy and momentum is given by $E = p^2/2m$, which you should confirm to yourself using the classical formulas for kinetic energy and momentum. The latter formula you do not need to know, but it is $p = mv$.) This means the momentum of the particle changes, which introduces an uncertainty into the measure of the momentum. Conversely, a longer wavelength, lower energy light beam would allow one to measure the momentum of the particle it interacted with to greater precision, but the long wavelength means a greater uncertainty in the position of the particle. Using capital deltas to represent the uncertainty in a quantity, Heisenberg's uncertainty relation can be written as

The Heisenberg Uncertainty Relation

$$\Delta x \Delta p \geq h/2\pi$$

where x represents to the position of the particle (or object more generally) and h is Planck's constant.

Example 43-23: Determine the uncertainty of the momentum of an electron in the $n = 1$ state.

Solution: The diameter of the hydrogen atom in the ground state is known to be about 10^{-10} m. An electron in the $n = 1$ state therefore could be found anywhere within that diameter, meaning $\Delta x = 10^{-10}$ m. The uncertainty of its momentum is therefore given by

$$\Delta x \Delta p \geq \frac{h}{2\pi} \rightarrow \Delta p \geq \frac{6.63 \times 10^{-34}}{2\pi \times 10^{-10}} \approx 10^{-24} \text{ kg} \cdot \text{m/s}$$

Though the math is slightly beyond the level of the MCAT, it is straightforward to show using the relation $E = p^2/2m$ that, given this uncertainty in momentum, were the electron to be confined to a smaller radius, the uncertainty in its energy would necessarily be greater than 13.6 eV, the energy of the hydrogen ground state. In other words, a lower state than the ground state would, according to the Heisenberg uncertainty principle, have to have a *higher* energy. This is a contradiction, proving that the ground state in the Bohr model of hydrogen indeed must be the lowest energy state.

Part 8

MCAT
Critical Analysis and Reasoning Skills

Chapter 44
Introduction to MCAT
Critical Analysis
and Reasoning Skills

GOALS

1) To understand the structure and scoring of the Critical Analysis and Reasoning Skills Section
2) To learn the fundamentals of Critical Analysis and Reasoning Skills strategies

You are well on your way to significantly raising your MCAT score and getting into your top-choice medical school. We understand that the Critical Analysis and Reasoning Skills (CARS) section presents many challenges to the typical MCAT student. We want our students to have every available tool, so we have devoted ourselves to developing the most rigorous CARS materials possible, based on intensive study of the MCAT itself and of the best strategies that lead to success on this test.

44.1   THE CRITICAL ANALYSIS AND REASONING SKILLS (CARS) SECTION

Structure

- CARS is the second section of the test.
- It consists of nine passages, which typically average 500–700 words each.
- Each passage is followed by 5–7 questions (with four answer choices per question), for a total of 53 questions.
- You will have 90 minutes to complete the section. You can do the questions and passages in any order that you choose within the 90-minute limit.
- You will be able to scroll up and down within the passage text. The questions are displayed one at a time on the right, with the passage (and any highlighting you have done in the passage text) always displayed on the left. Click on the Next and Previous buttons on the bottom of the screen to go back and forth between the questions and passages within the section. Clicking Next from the last question for a passage takes you to the next passage and the first question for that passage. Once the 90 minutes are up, however, you cannot go back to any of the CARS passages or questions.

Pacing

You do not necessarily need to complete all nine passages to get a competitive score. Many people will maximize their score by randomly guessing on at least one passage and focusing on getting a high percentage of the rest of the questions correct. Also, keep in mind that there is no guessing penalty. Never leave a question blank; always select a random guess for questions that you choose not to complete. You have a 25 percent chance of getting those questions right.

Content

The passages may be on any subject in the humanities and social sciences. Passage topics may include philosophy, ethics, archeology, economics, history, political science, literature and literary theory, psychology, sociology, anthropology, cultural studies, geography, population health, and art history and theory. This range of topics may seem overwhelming. However, unlike the other multiple-choice sections of the test, CARS does not test your outside knowledge of the subject. In fact, using your own factual knowledge or opinions can lead you to pick incorrect answers; the questions require you to use only the information provided in the passage. Clearly, you can't prepare for or approach this section of the test in the same way as physics or chemistry!

44.2   DEVELOPING YOUR CRITICAL REASONING SKILLS

The Critical Analysis and Reasoning Skills section can be intimidating for many people taking the MCAT. You have been studying hard for many years, packing your brain with lots of science knowledge and refining your memorization skills. But now, as you confront the CARS section, all those facts and mnemonics are useless, and you have to employ an entirely different approach. Even if you have taken a lot of humanities and social science courses and have been speaking and reading English for many years, you might find the CARS section to be challenging at first. This is because you need to adapt to the specific nature and requirements of this section of the MCAT.

There are many false beliefs regarding the CARS section, one of which is that your score depends on luck. That is, if you happen to get "good" passages, all is well, but if you don't, you are in trouble. However (and thankfully!), this is entirely untrue. There are ways that you can improve your CARS score regardless of the passages you happen to get on your test. BUT...to achieve this improvement, many if not most of you will need to fundamentally change how you read the passages and go about answering the questions. You will need to develop new skills that have little to do with memorization and everything to do with reading efficiently and thinking critically. The good news is that these are skills that everyone can develop and improve through practice and careful self-evaluation. These core skills fall into three basic categories.

Working the Passage

- **Reading the passage efficiently:** identifying the most important points made by the author while moving quickly through the details
- **Following the logical structure of the author's argument:** identifying such things as key shifts in direction, comparisons and contrasts, conclusions, and author's tone
- **Synthesizing the Bottom Line of the entire passage:** identifying the author's Main Idea and Attitude

Attacking the Questions

- **Correctly identifying and translating the questions:** knowing what each question is asking you to do in order to choose the correct answer
- **Using the passage (and only the passage) as a resource:** quickly locating the relevant passage information for each question
- **Answering in your own words:** predicting what the correct answer will do before considering the answer choices
- **Using Process of Elimination (POE):** eliminating down to the "least wrong" choice rather than just picking an answer that "sounds good"

General Test Strategy

- **Time management:** getting what you need from the passage without getting bogged down in irrelevant facts or spending too much time on one question
- **Pacing and accuracy:** not going so fast that you miss a high percentage of the questions that you complete, or so slow that you overthink the questions or do not get to enough questions to reach your target score
- **Stress management:** thinking clearly and working efficiently under stressful conditions

44.3   FUNDAMENTALS: THE SIX STEPS

Based on these core skills, here are the six steps to follow when working the CARS section.

■ STEP 1: RANK AND ORDER THE PASSAGES

Ranking

The passages are not necessarily, or even usually, presented in order of difficulty. There is no reason to waste time on the hardest passage or passages, only to skip or rush through an easy passage at the end of the section. So your first step, as you reach each new passage, is to decide if it is a Now (or easier) passage, a Later (or harder) passage, or a Killer passage (one that you will do last of all if you are doing all nine or simply randomly guess on if you are completing eight or fewer). To assign a rank, skim a few sentences of the passage and see if you can easily paraphrase them. If you can, it's most likely an easier passage to understand. If not, it is likely to be a harder passage that you should either come back to later during your 90 minutes or just randomly guess on.

Ordering

If a passage is a Now passage, go ahead and work it through, completing all of the questions. If it is a Later or Killer passage, click though each question, marking it and filling in a random guess, and move on to ranking the next passage. Also note the passage number on your noteboard. Once you have completed the Now passages in the section, go back through the section and complete the Later passages, and make sure that you have filled in your random guesses on any Killer passages that you will not be completing. (See Sections 47.3 and 47.8 of this book for more information on Ranking and Ordering.)

■ STEP 2: PREVIEW THE QUESTIONS

Knowing what topics show up in the questions will help you work the passage more quickly and effectively. Before working the passage, read through the question stems from first to last (not the answer choices), identifying and highlighting any words or phrases that indicate important passage content. Do not worry at this stage about understanding the question or identifying the question type. (See Section 44.6 of this book for more information on Previewing the Questions.)

STEP 3: WORK THE PASSAGE

Stay on the screen for the last question and work the passage from here (your highlighting will stay and appear in the passage text regardless of which question for that passage you are working on). As you read through the passage, use the highlighting function (sparingly) to annotate the most important references in the text. This includes things like: question topics, topic sentences, shifts in direction or continuations, the author's tone, different points of view, and conclusions. As you move through the passage, articulate the Main Point of each chunk of information (usually, each paragraph). Use your noteboard, especially on difficult passages, to jot down these main points. As you read, think about how these chunks relate to each other; that is, track the logical structure of the author's argument in the passage. (See Chapter 45 of this book for more information on Active Reading and Annotation.)

STEP 4: BOTTOM LINE

After you have read the entire passage, sum up the Bottom Line: the Main Idea and tone of the entire passage. For particularly difficult passages, write this down on your noteboard to make sure that you have a reasonably clear idea of the point and purpose of the passage as a whole. (See Chapter 45 for more information on finding the Bottom Line.)

STEP 5: ATTACK THE QUESTIONS

Here is an example of how the question will be formatted on the screen.

1. The author probably intends the final paragraph to:

    A) introduce a new perspective on the central theme.
    B) summarize the principle components of the argument presented throughout the passage.
    C) qualify the reasoning of the paragraph directly before.
    D) describe an application of the position introduced in the first paragraph.

Work through the questions backwards, so that you don't need to click back to the first question for that passage. As you work each question, follow these steps:

- Read the question word for word and identify the question type.
- Translate the question task into your own words, thinking about what the question is asking you to do with or to the passage.
- When the question stem provides a specific reference to the passage, go back to the passage before reading the answer choices and find the relevant information (reading at least five lines above and below the reference).
- Paraphrase the passage information. Then, with the question type firmly in mind, think about what the correct answer will need to do.
- As you go through the choices, use POE actively. Look for reasons to strike out incorrect choices, and select the "least wrong" of the four. (See Chapters 45 and 46 for more information on identifying and answering different question types.)
- If you hit a particularly difficult question, skip over it for the moment and complete the other easier questions. Then click forward through the questions toward the next passage, completing any questions you initially skipped.

44.4

■ **STEP 6: INSPECT THE SECTION**

At or before the 5-minute mark (ideally, before you begin your last passage), double-check to make sure that you haven't left anything incomplete. You can use the Review function at this stage. Do NOT re-think questions you have already completed. Your goal in this step is simply to make sure that you have selected an answer for each question.

44.4 GUIDELINES FOR USING YOUR STUDY MATERIALS

Focus on Accuracy

Whenever you're acquiring a new skill, you need to learn to do it well before learning to do it quickly. Many students feel that speed is their number one concern. This often leads them to rush through the initial "learning to do it well" phase. Unfortunately, this is entirely counterproductive and will ultimately keep you from scoring as well as you possibly can.

As you begin working practice passages, do the passages untimed; focus on following the techniques and on improving your accuracy. Once you become comfortable with these techniques, set a timer to count *up* as you do each passage (or, note your start and end times with a watch). Record how long it takes you to do a passage, but don't attempt to complete the passage within a set time limit. Wait until you have settled into a consistent and methodical approach before you start to do lots of strictly timed passages and practice tests.

Even after you have been studying for some time and have taken many practice tests, it is still useful to do some untimed passages, focusing on avoiding the types of mistakes you tend to make. Then bring that same focus into the next set of timed passages you complete or the next practice test that you take.

Build Endurance

At first, work on only a few passages at a time, developing the skills you've learned. Allowing yourself this time to practice slowly but accurately gives you a strong foundation for accurate timed practice. Always do passages at least two at a time to practice ranking and ordering them. After a couple of weeks, try to do a number of practice passages at once, and don't take any breaks between the passages. Also, at this stage, don't check your answers after every one or two passages. You need to get used to working through each new passage without the reassurance or feedback from knowing how you did on the previous passage. Build up your endurance over time so that you can eventually maintain your concentration at its peak over the course of an entire 90-minute section. Set aside a daily time for CARS work and stick to your schedule. Keep in mind the particular strategies you should be focusing on depending on where you are in this book and in your preparation process.

Control Your Environment

Give your full attention to the passages when you practice. That is, don't do homework while watching TV or conversing with friends. However, when you take the actual MCAT you'll be in a room full of people who are muttering to themselves, sniffling and coughing, typing loudly, standing up and sitting down at different times, and generally behaving in a distracting or annoying manner (unintentionally, we hope!). Therefore, practice working in less-than-ideal conditions. Go to a reasonably quiet coffeehouse, a room in the library where there are people moving around (but not talking loudly), or some other location with low-level distractions. Learn how to tune out what is going on around you and to keep your focus on the passages in front of you. (Note: Basic foam earplugs in a factory sealed package are allowed on the MCAT. You will also be provided with noise-reduction headphones in the testing center.)

Evaluate Your Work

Constant self-evaluation is the key to continued improvement. Don't just answer the questions and tally your score at the end. Use the materials to teach yourself how to improve. What kinds of questions do you consistently miss? What kinds of passages slow you down? What kinds of answer traps do you tend to fall for? What caused you to pick the wrong answer to each question that you missed?

However, don't just think about the questions you got wrong—also analyze how you arrived at the credited response when your answers are correct. Did you avoid a common trap? Are there question types on which you are particularly strong? Did you successfully apply one of our techniques?

Use the charts and the Self-Evaluation Survey provided at the end of this chapter to identify patterns in the mistakes you are making. Only by identifying your mistakes can you learn to correct them. The next section provides you with guidance on how to use those resources.

44.5   SELF-EVALUATION

Every student has different strengths and weaknesses on the MCAT CARS section. To improve on your weaknesses, you must first recognize them. From now on, keep a log of every passage that you do (sample logs are provided later on in this section).

The time you spend reviewing your work is just as important as the time spent doing the passages. After you do a passage, go through each question and answer choice. Pay particular attention to those questions that you got wrong. In order to increase your score, you'll need to assess and change the way that you think. Often we continue to take the same steps or read in the same way, even when we've seen that this way is not successful. You may not even realize that you're making the same mistake over and over again until you see it logged into your chart several times. Look for patterns in your mistakes and successes; based on those patterns, define ways in which you need to change how you read and think in order to raise your score.

There are three resources provided at the end of this chapter to help you with the self-evaluation process.

I. Individual Passage Log

Fill out this log for every passage that you do from this book or other resources, and for every question within the passage that you miss. Also fill out the log for every question that you got right but were unsure of the correct answer when you picked it (for example, you were down to two choices and then guessed).

At the end of the next four chapters there are two Individual Passage Logs to use on the practice passages for those chapters. To use the Individual Passage Logs on other practice materials (such as online practice passages), make clean copies of the logs or follow the same structure on notebook paper or in a Excel spreadsheet.

II. Test Assessment Log

Fill out this log for each full CARS test section that you do. Complete it as soon as you can after the test; once a few hours have passed, it will be difficult to remember why you made the choices that you did. As with the Individual Passage Log, either make multiple clean copies of the log for future use or follow the same structure on notebook paper or in a spreadsheet.

Following the blank version of that log you will find a filled-out sample log. It doesn't correspond to any particular test; it is provided to give you an idea of how you should be filling out your own logs.

III. Self-Evaluation Survey

Complete the Self-Evaluation survey for every full CARS test section that you do. It consists of a series of questions to help you to analyze your overall performance on the section and on each question within it. It is generally best to fill out the Test Assessment Log first, while the questions are still fresh in your mind, and then use the Survey to sum up your analysis and set goals for future tests.

I. Individual Passage Log

Key for Passage Log

Passage # and Time spent on passage   Indicate the location of the passage and how long it took you to complete it (when you are doing timed passages).

Q # and Q type   For each question you miss in a passage, indicate the number and the type of question. Refer to the list of question types in Chapter 46.

Attractors   For the first 15 individual logs that you fill out, list what was wrong with every wrong answer, including the ones that you did not pick. After that, you can list only the wrong answers that you chose or seriously considered choosing.

Refer to the Attractors described and listed in Chapters 44, 46, and 47.

What did you do wrong?   Describe the error that led you down the path to the wrong answer, and how you will avoid making that same mistake in the future. Below is a (non-exhaustive) list of common mistakes. Choose one or more items from this list (there may be more than one misstep involved in picking a wrong answer), or, if none fits, describe the error in your own words. If time after time you cannot figure out why you chose the wrong answer, it is very likely that you are working too quickly and/ or too carelessly. Did you

- misread the question?
- fail to go back to the passage?
- fail to read all four of the answer choices?
- fail to read the entire answer choice?
- over-interpret the passage or the answer choice?
- forget the "EXCEPT/LEAST/NOT" in the question?
- pick an answer choice that was
    …out of scope or not the issue?
    …too extreme or absolute?
    …from the wrong part of the passage?
    …half right, half wrong?
    …strengthening when it should have been weakening (or vice versa)?
    …too narrow on a general question?

Using the Individual Passage Log, take the time to assess how your current thought processes led you to a tempting but wrong answer choice, and how a different way of thinking on the question would have been more successful. The log will help you to see how the test is constructed, and most importantly, how you are responding to it. **You can't change the test, but you can change your responses to it.** This process will allow you to work through the MCAT CARS section more quickly and with greater accuracy.

Individual Passage Log

Passage # _____ Time spent on passage _____

Q#	Q type	Attractors	What did you do wrong?

Revised Strategy _____

Passage # _____ Time spent on passage _____

Q#	Q type	Attractors	What did you do wrong?

Revised Strategy _____

II. Test Assessment Log

Use this worksheet to record and monitor your performance on full nine-passage sections, and to continue the self-evaluation process. In particular, use it to see if you are spending the time you need on the easier passages in order to get most of those questions right. Keep track of how much time you spent (roughly) on the Now passages and on the Later passages. If you find that you are spending the bulk of your 90 minutes on the harder passages with a low level of accuracy, you need to reapportion your time. Also evaluate your ranking; are you choosing the right passages?

44.5

Now Passages

Now Passage #	Q # and Type (for questions you got wrong)	Attractors (for wrong answers you picked or seriously considered)	What did you do wrong?

Approximate time spent on Now passages _____

Total Now passages attempted _____

Total # of Q's on Now passages attempted _____

Total # of Now Q's correct _____

% correct of Now Q's attempted _____

Later Passages

44.5

Later Passage #	Q # and Type (for questions you got wrong)	Attractors (for wrong answers you picked or seriously considered)	What did you do wrong?

Approximate time spent on Later passages _____

Total Later passages attempted _____

Total # of Q's on Later passages attempted _____

Total # of Later Q's correct _____

% correct of Later Q's attempted _____

Final Analysis

Total # of passages attempted (including partially completed) _____

Total # of questions attempted _____

Total # of correct answers: _____

Total % correct of attempted questions: _____

Revised Strategy

Pacing	
Passage choice/ranking	
Working the Passage	
Attacking the Questions	

Sample Completed Test Assessment Log—Now Passages

44.5

Now Passage #	Q # and Type (for questions you got wrong)	Attractors (for wrong answers you picked or seriously considered)	What did you do wrong?
1	None		Spent a bit too much time—was *overly* cautious
3	Q12: Main Point	Q12 D: too narrow	Q12: got it down to two and guessed—didn't compare choices or reread the question stem
4	Q23: Inference	Q23 A: out of scope	Q23: Got it right but took too much time—should have gone back to the passage before POE (almost talked myself into an answer that was clearly wrong once I went back to passage)
7	Q39: Weaken Q41: New Information Q42: Inference	Q39 B: opposite Q41 C: opposite Q42 C: reversal	All three: shouldn't have done this passage at all—it was a killer. Didn't understand the passage at all (very abstract and confusing), and got the author's argument all turned around.
9	None!		Nothing!

Approximate time spent on Now passages **a little less than an hour**

Total Now passages attempted **5**

Total # of Q's on Now passages attempted **28**

Total # of Now Q's correct **23**

% correct of Now Q's attempted **82%**

Sample Completed Test Assessment Log—Later Passages

Later Passage #	Q # and Type (for questions you got wrong)	Attractors (for wrong answers you picked or seriously considered)	What did you do wrong?
2	Q7: Analogy Q10: New Information/ Weaken	Q7 A: half right, half wrong Q10 D: opposite	Q7: didn't read the whole choice (or the rest of the answer choices) carefully—made up my mind too fast Q10: lost track of question type—picked what would be strengthened, not weakened
5	Q26: Retrieval	Q26 B: words out of context	Q26: didn't read carefully enough when went back to passage. Easy question.
6	Q33: Evaluate Q35: Analogy Q37: Inference	Q33 A: half right, half wrong Q35 D: out of scope Q37 C: too extreme	Q33: didn't make sure that the description matched Q35: panicked and didn't think about the logic/theme of the relevant part of the passage Q37: saw the strong language but picked it anyway because was rushed
8	Q43: Inference Q44: Weaken Q46: Structure Q47: Retrieval	Q43 B: too extreme Q44 C: opposite Q46 D: right answer, wrong question Q47 A: words out of context	Q43: didn't pay enough attention to strength of language Q44: forgot the question type and picked something supported by the passage (as if was answering Inference question) Q46: forgot the question type and picked answer that was supported by passage but not the purpose of the reference Q47: picked answer because sounded like what I remembered from the passage—in reality, was never mentioned Overall: was rushing because running out of time

Approximate time spent on Later passages __**35 minutes**__

Total Later passages attempted ____**4**____

Total # of Q's on Later passages attempted ____**25**____

Total # of Later Q's correct ____**15**____

% correct of Later Q's attempted ____**60%**____

44.5

Final Analysis

Total # of passages attempted (including partially completed)   **9**

Total # of questions attempted   **53**

Total # of correct answers: **38/53**

Total % correct of attempted questions: **72%**

Revised Strategy

Pacing	Slow down—only do 8 passages.
Passage choice/ranking	Skip over more Later/Killer passages in first pass. Take difficulty of abstract passage texts seriously—skip or do Later.
Working the Passage	Pay more attention to author's opinion and contrasting points of view (so that I don't mix them up later). Write down the main points and Bottom Line on harder passages.
Attacking the Questions	Read the question carefully and reread it when down to two. Go back to the passage more, and read more carefully when I do. Read THE WHOLE answer choice word for word and paraphrase it. Compare choices to each other when down to two. Pay more attention to strength of language and tone.

III. CARS Self-Evaluation Survey

This section consists of a series of questions intended to help you evaluate your performance on each practice test.

Before answering the questions in this section, you should review your score report, go back over the questions that you missed, and fill out your Self-Evaluation Passage Logs or Test Assessment Logs. You may wish to look through the questions in this survey first and then review your exam using the score report. Finally, come back and select your answers for the survey and read the feedback corresponding to your responses.

Do this one exam at a time—that is, answer these survey questions after each exam you take. Don't answer them for multiple exams in a group. The survey is extensive; you may even wish to break up your evaluation of a single exam into two or more chunks of time. Note that it is important to answer the survey questions, especially those regarding the reasons why you missed particular questions, as soon as possible after taking the exam, when your reasoning is fresh in your mind. Therefore, answer the questions in Part III within a day of taking the practice test. However, you can fill in your responses for Parts I and II a day or two later.

There is space under each question to list the answer choice or choices (for some of the survey questions, you may be selecting more than one choice). Compare your responses for each practice test to look for trends.

After completing the survey for each test that you take, write down at least three things that you will focus on during your next practice test, or during your next set of practice passages. Space is provided at the end of the survey for you to write down these goals.

PART I: OVERALL ACCURACY AND PACING

1. Approximately what percentage of the 53 questions did you get correct?

Test 1 _____

Test 2 _____

Test 3 _____

Test 4 _____

Test 5 _____

44.5

A. 85–100%

Your accuracy is excellent. Define the strategies that led to your correct answers and apply them to the practice MCATs that you take in the future. If you missed any questions, carefully diagnose the reasons why, so that you can achieve an even higher level of accuracy in the future.

B. 70–84%

Your accuracy is reasonably good. Make a list of at least three reasons why you missed the questions that were incorrect, and focus on not making those same kinds of mistakes on the practice passages and MCATs that you take in the future. Also define some of the strategies that led to correct answers, and apply those to future practice tests as well.

C. 55–69%

You need to work on improving your accuracy, especially if you are on the low end of this range. Make a list of at least three reasons why you missed the questions that were incorrect, and focus on not making those same kinds of mistakes on the practice MCATs you take in the future. Also compare the questions you got wrong to the questions that you got right in order to diagnose the strategies that were and were not working for you.

D. 40–54%

Your accuracy is relatively low. In the prep you do in the near future, focus on getting a higher percentage of the questions that you complete correct, even if that means slowing down for now and not completing all of the questions. Make a list of at least three reasons why you missed the questions that you got incorrect, and focus on not making those same kinds of mistakes on the practice MCATs you take in the future. Also compare the questions you got wrong to the questions that you got right in order to diagnose the strategies that were and were not working for you.

E. Less than 40%

Your accuracy is low. You will need to significantly increase your percentage correct in order to get a competitive score. That will likely involve slowing down and randomly guessing on at least one passage in the section. Make a list of at least three reasons why you missed the questions that were incorrect, and focus on not making those same kinds of mistakes on the practice MCATs you take in the future.

2. Is your accuracy:

Test 1 _____

Test 2 _____

Test 3 _____

Test 4 _____

Test 5 _____

A. highest in the beginning of the section and falling off toward the end?

Work on building up your endurance by studying for longer and longer periods of time. Taking as many mock MCATs as you can will also help you keep your concentration at a high level throughout a test. You may also have been lingering too long on the questions in the beginning, and then rushing the questions at the end.

Also, many test takers will maximize their score by randomly guessing on a certain percentage of the questions in a CARS section. If you had to rush through many of the questions and if you got many of those questions wrong, this is an indication that at this point in your preparation process you should not be trying to work through all of the passages or questions.

B. highest in the middle of the section?

It is likely that it took you some time to warm up in the beginning, and then you tired out (or got impatient or rushed) at the end. Try warming up a bit by working through a passage before you take your next test. Take little 5–10 second breaks every 10–15 minutes during a test, so that you can maintain your energy and focus at the end of the section.

C. highest at the end of the section?

It is likely that you gradually warmed up as you went through the test. The good news is that endurance was not a problem for you. To achieve a high level of accuracy from beginning to end, try warming up by working through a passage before you take your next practice test.

D. about the same all the way through the section?

Good work, if your accuracy was relatively good. On the MCAT, your goal is to hit the ground running, and to keep your focus and energy high through the entire test.

3. **For the questions that you missed, on average, what was your level of confidence as you answered those questions?**

Test 1 _____

Test 2 _____

Test 3 _____

Test 4 _____

Test 5 _____

A. Fairly high

If you commonly felt very confident while picking answers that were in fact incorrect, and if you answered those questions relatively quickly, you may have been answering based on memory rather than by using the passage actively. If this is the case, in the future go back to the passage, find the relevant information, and base your answer closely on the passage text. Alternatively, you may have misread the question stem and/or answer choices, or selected a response before reading through all four choices. Look back at the questions you missed to determine if this was the case. In the future, make a conscious effort to slow down when you read the question stem and answer choices, and read all four choices before selecting your response.

However, if you spent a great deal of time on the questions before picking the wrong answer, and if you read through the answer choices multiple times or spent a lot of time debating between two choices, you may have been overthinking the question and talking yourself into a wrong answer. In the future, limit yourself to two careful passes through the answer choices, select an answer (based on the passage information and question task), and then move on.

B. Moderate

It is normal to have a moderate level of confidence on most of the questions that you miss. If you missed quite a few questions (more than 16), however, your confidence and accuracy will increase if you read the question, the answer choices, and the relevant passage text more carefully, and if you base your answers more closely on the information in the passage. Use the feedback for your responses to the survey, especially questions 8–10, to diagnose specific reasons for your mistakes.

C. Fairly low

If you only missed a few questions, it is normal to have a low level of confidence on those questions; they were likely among the hardest questions in the test. However, if you missed many questions (more than 15), it is likely that you were not using the passage information actively enough. If you read the question stem and answer choices more carefully and go back to the passage text more consistently to find the relevant information, your level of confidence and your accuracy (and potentially your speed as well) will increase.

4. **For the questions that you got correct, what was your average level of confidence while answering the question?**

    Test 1 _____

    Test 2 _____

    Test 3 _____

    Test 4 _____

    Test 5 _____

A. Fairly high

If you completed the section in the time allowed, and if you had excellent accuracy (that is, missed 8 or fewer), a high level of confidence is a sign that your approach to the questions was solid. However, if you had trouble completing the section (that is, did not get to one or more passages and/or had to rush at the end and missed many of those final questions), you may have been overcautious. If your experience fits this scenario, don't double or triple check your answers. Once you have eliminated three of the choices and have a reasonable answer left, select that choice and move on.

B. Moderate

If your accuracy was fairly good (that is, you missed 12 or fewer), a moderate level of confidence on the questions that you got correct is normal. However, if your accuracy was significantly lower than this, it can improve through a combination of reading the passage text more carefully (at least the part that is relevant to the question), thinking through the question task more carefully, and paying attention to every word in each answer choice. Use the feedback for your responses to this survey, especially questions 8–10, to diagnose specific reasons for your mistakes.

C. Fairly low

If your accuracy was fairly good (you missed 12 or fewer questions and you completed the section), having a low level of confidence is not necessarily a bad thing. You do not need to understand every idea or detail in the passage in order to get most questions correct. If your accuracy was significantly lower, however, it most likely means that in general you may not be reading the questions carefully enough, using the passage actively enough, or reading and analyzing the answer choices closely enough. Focus on reading the question stem and answer choices word for word, and on finding specific information in the passage to support your response.

PART II: GENERAL TESTING STRATEGIES

44.5

5. **Did you read the question stems (not the choices) before you read the passage text?**

    Test 1 _____

    Test 2 _____

    Test 3 _____

    Test 4 _____

    Test 5 _____

A. Yes

This is an effective approach for most test takers. When you preview the questions, don't worry at that stage about the question type. Rather, look for words in the question that relate to passage content to help you focus in on the key parts of the passage as you read it the first time through.

B. No

On the MCAT, previewing the questions (just the stem, not the choices) can be a very useful technique. If you haven't tried it, or if you have only tried it a few times and then abandoned the technique, it is worth practicing to see if it will pay off for you. On your next set of practice passages or practice test, try quickly reading through the question stems before reading the passage. Don't worry about the question type at that stage. Instead, pick out and highlight the words and phrases that relate to the content of the passage. This will allow you to focus on the most important parts of the passage, and to highlight words in those sections to help you go back efficiently to find the necessary information as you answer the questions.

However, if you have in fact practiced it for a month or more, and have implemented it on several tests without seeing a payoff in accuracy and/or speed, then not previewing the questions is a reasonable choice for you.

6. **Did you use your noteboard as you took the test?**

   Test 1 _____

   Test 2 _____

   Test 3 _____

   Test 4 _____

   Test 5 _____

44.5

A. No

Using the noteboard (provided by the test center on the real MCAT) is a very useful strategy. Writing down a few words to express the main point of each paragraph or big chunk of information, as well as the main point or Bottom Line of the whole passage, can help you to understand and keep track of the key parts of the author's argument, especially on the harder passages. It can also be quite helpful to keep track of your Process of Elimination on Roman numeral and EXCEPT/LEAST/NOT questions. If you are not used to using the noteboard, make sure to practice with it on several practice passages and then on at least two practice tests. Once you practice it, you will most likely find that it improves both your accuracy and your speed.

B. Yes

If you are using the noteboard already, the next step is to think about how you can use it even more effectively than you are now. In particular, make sure that it is well organized and that you are writing clearly. If you are writing quite a bit, work on paring it down (for example, limiting yourself to 4–5 words to express the main point of a paragraph or of the passage as a whole). Also, you may not need to write down the main point of every paragraph for every passage. If the passage is easy to follow and understand, you might define some or all of the main points as a mental step without writing them all down. If you are making notes on the passage but never on the questions, try using it (sparingly) to write down brief notes to help you clarify and organize your thought process on difficult questions.

PART III: ATTACKING THE QUESTIONS AND POE

44.5

7. **When you went back over the questions that you missed, which of the following reactions did you often have? Select all that apply and read the feedback for those responses.**

Test 1 _____

Test 2 _____

Test 3 _____

Test 4 _____

Test 5 _____

A. "The correct answer looks obvious in retrospect, and I don't know why I didn't pick it."

If the correct answer looks obvious in retrospect and/or if you don't remember why you made the choices that you did during the test, this is often due to going too fast and choosing based on intuition rather than on test-appropriate reasoning. Don't just pick the first answer that "sounds good." Instead, base your answer closely on the question task and the passage text.

B. "I see why the right answer could be right, but I still think the answer I picked is right too."

In MCAT CARS, many wrong answers are written to sound very good, but they have something, sometimes something fairly subtle, in them that makes them worse than the credited response. The correct answer is the "least wrong" answer. That is, it may not be perfect, but the other three are even worse. Furthermore, the correct answer must be based on the passage, not on outside knowledge or your own opinion. Go back to the questions that you missed, compare the right answers to your wrong answers, and identify the differences between them that make the credited response the best of the four choices.

C. "I see why the right answer is right and the wrong answer is wrong, but I think that I would still pick the wrong answer in the future."

A big part of maximizing your CARS score is learning the logic of the test itself. Each time you break down the logic of a question that you missed, you prepare yourself to get similar questions right in the future. Always review questions that you missed, not only to see why the right answer was right, but to diagnose what caused you to disregard it. Your ultimate goal is to get points; if you understand the logic of the test, you can begin to answer more strategically, and avoid picking wrong answers in the future.

D. "I still don't get it."

Make sure to read the explanations for these questions especially carefully. Then go back through the question step by step. Paraphrase what the question is really asking, identify and paraphrase the relevant information in the passage text, and go through the choices one more time, comparing them to each other and identifying differences between them. Even if this process takes some time, on most questions you will come to see the logic of the test, and questions will make more and more sense to you in the future.

8. **For which of the following question types did you miss two or more questions? Select all that apply and read the corresponding feedback below each response.**

Test 1 _____

Test 2 _____

Test 3 _____

Test 4 _____

Test 5 _____

A. Inference and Retrieval questions

The key to getting these questions right is sticking as closely as possible to the information in the passage. Compare your wrong answers to the credited responses and identify how the right answers are better supported by the text. In the future, whenever possible, answer in your own words (based only on the passage text) before you evaluate the answer choices.

B. Main Point, Primary Purpose, and Tone/Attitude questions

The answers to these general question types must include, explicitly or implicitly, the whole passage, not just a part of it. Commonly, wrong answers for these types will be too narrow, too strong, or have a word or phrase within them that is inconsistent with the passage. Identify the Bottom Line of the passage (including the author's tone) before you go through the answer choices. Make sure to track the author's tone or attitude throughout the passage and highlight the relevant words. When you are down to two answers, look for differences in tone and scope.

C. Structure and Evaluate questions

To get these questions right, you need to identify the logical structure of the relevant part of the passage. You must see how different statements in the passage relate to each other, which includes separating the author's claims or conclusions from the support for those claims. Often, wrong answers are true based on the passage, but they do not answer the question being asked. When attacking these questions, generate an answer in your own words, based not just on content but also on the logical structure of the passage, before you go through the answer choices.

D. New Information questions

These questions require you to summarize the theme of the new information in the question stem, and then apply it to the relevant information in the passage text. When you get these questions wrong, identify whether or not you correctly understood the point of the new information. If you did, see if you might have lost track of the relevant issue in the passage, and/or picked an answer that took the wrong direction (e.g., it was inconsistent with the passage, but the question asked how the author would respond). In the future, first identify the theme of the new information, then describe its relationship to the passage, including whether the question requires an answer consistent or inconsistent with the passage. Keep track of this direction as you evaluate each answer choice.

9. **For which of the following question types or formats did you miss two or more questions? Select all that apply and read the corresponding feedback below each response.**

Test 1 _____

Test 2 _____

Test 3 _____

Test 4 _____

Test 5 _____

A. Strengthen and Weaken questions

These questions require you to accept the new information in the answer choices as true, and to find the correct answer that goes in the right direction. The answer must be strong enough to have a significant impact on the relevant part of the author's argument. Look at your wrong answers and identify if they were too weak to "most strengthen" or "most undermine" the passage, if they went in the opposite direction (for example, strengthened instead of weakened), or if they were not directly relevant to the passage. In the future, define what the correct answer needs to do before evaluating the answer choices. You may benefit from jotting this on your noteboard, especially on Weaken questions.

B. Analogy questions

These questions ask you to find an answer with the same logic as the relevant part of the passage. In most cases, the correct answer will not be about the same subject matter as the passage. Look at your wrong answers to see if they match the content/topic but not the passage logic, or if they are part right/part wrong (one piece matches, another does not). In the future, describe the logic of the relevant part of the passage in generic terms before looking at the answer choices (e.g., if the passage states "increased food production led to a population explosion," you could write "an increase in A led to a large increase in B").

C. Roman numeral questions

These questions provide you with three statements, and ask you to select the answer choice that includes all the statements that correctly answer the question and none that do not. Look at your wrong answers: Did you include too many (you were not strict enough) or too few (you eliminated statements that were not quite as good as those most obviously correct, but that were still good enough)? In the future, use your noteboard to keep track of your evaluation of each statement as you go. Also, if you are sure that a statement is correct, eliminate answer choices that do not include it, and compare the remaining choices. If you are sure a statement is incorrect, eliminate choices that do include it and compare what remains.

D. EXCEPT/LEAST/NOT questions

These questions ask you to select the "worst" answer. For example, when a question asks "All of the following can be inferred EXCEPT," the three wrong answers will be supported by the passage, and the correct answer will not. Look at the questions you missed to see if you lost track of the EXCEPT, LEAST, or NOT. In the future, use your noteboard to keep track of why you are eliminating each choice as you go.

10. For which of the following reasons did you miss one or more questions? Select all that apply and read the suggestions below each selection.

Test 1 _____

Test 2 _____

Test 3 _____

Test 4 _____

Test 5 _____

44.5

A. "I misunderstood the question."

Read the question stem word for word and put it into your own words before you read the answer choices.

B. "I misunderstood the passage."

If you read the passage text very quickly, slow down a bit and pay more attention to (at least!) the most important statements. When you go back to the passage while answering the question, read the relevant part carefully and paraphrase it. If you spent quite a bit of time reading the passage, however, you may have overthought it. Stick to what is explicitly stated, and don't spend time speculating about what the author might have meant.

C. "I answered from memory, and my memory was inaccurate."

Go back to the passage and read the relevant part carefully when answering the questions.

D. "I based my answer on the wrong part of the passage."

Make sure to keep track of the precise issue raised in the question stem, and to identify all the parts of the passage that may be relevant to it. Previewing the questions before you work the passage will help you to do this most effectively and efficiently.

E. "I misunderstood or misread one or more of the answer choices."

Read each answer choice word for word the first time through. Paraphrase complicated choices to make sure that you understand what they are saying.

F. "I talked myself into the wrong answer."

The correct answer should not take a lot of effort to justify. Stick to the question task, the passage, and the exact wording of the answer choice. Use Process of Elimination aggressively; look for reasons to strike out choices.

G. "I got it down to two and then picked the wrong one."

This happens because there is often at least one wrong answer that is written to be very attractive. When down to two choices, reread the question, compare the two choices to each other, and, if needed, go back to the passage again. Remember to pick the "least wrong" answer, not just the answer that "sounds best."

44.5

11. **On average, how often did you read all or part of the passage before answering a question?**

Test 1 _____

Test 2 _____

Test 3 _____

Test 4 _____

Test 5 _____

A. Once

This is fine if you had a high level of accuracy. If you had a low level of accuracy, use the passage more actively (as if you are taking an open book test).

B. Twice

This is usually appropriate. Most of the time you will read the passage as a whole once, and then go back at least once to the relevant section or sections as you answer each question.

C. Three times

This can be appropriate for harder questions. However, make sure that you are reading the relevant section thoroughly enough and pausing to paraphrase it. Often reading the appropriate part of the passage more completely and thoughtfully earlier on (during the process of answering the question) will eliminate the need to go back to it again and again. Also focus more on answering the question in your own words in order to increase your efficiency and speed.

D. Four or more times

You may be reading and rereading bits and pieces of the passage out of context, which then requires you to go back and forth between the answer choices and the passage too often. Focus on reading and paraphrasing the entire relevant chunk, and on answering in your own words so that you can increase your efficiency and speed.

Also ask yourself if you are overworking the questions, rethinking them or rereading parts of the passage over and over, even when you have a solid basis for picking an answer and moving on. If so, give yourself a limit on the number of times you can go back to the passage (for example, twice). Once you have hit that limit, select an answer and go on to the next question.

12. **On average, how many times did you read through the set of answer choices before making a final selection?**

   Test 1 _____

   Test 2 _____

   Test 3 _____

   Test 4 _____

   Test 5 _____

A. Once

This is appropriate if you had a high level of accuracy (you missed 8 or fewer questions). If your accuracy was significantly lower, take two passes through the choices, at least on the more difficult questions. Eliminate the one or two most clearly wrong answers the first time through, and then compare the remaining choices before making a final selection.

B. Twice

This is usually appropriate. In most cases, you will eliminate one or two choices the first time through, and then compare the remaining answers in order to make a final decision.

C. Three times

This can be necessary on the more difficult questions. However, if you are going through the choices three times on most questions, you can increase your efficiency (and accuracy) by answering in your own words first whenever possible, and by reading the choices word for word (and paraphrasing complicated statements) the first time through.

D. Four or more times

If you are often reading through the choices four or more times, you need to work on attacking the questions more efficiently. Make it a goal to eliminate at least one or two choices on your first read through, based on the question task and the relevant passage information. Whenever possible, answer the question in your own words first so that you have more information in hand up front. When you are down to two choices, compare them to each other, reread the question, and go back to the passage rather than just rereading the choices over and over. Keep your focus on what is wrong with each choice, and on selecting the "least wrong" answer.

Goals for Test 2:

1)

2)

3)

44.5

Goals for Test 3:

1)

2)

3)

Goals for Test 4:

1)

2)

3)

Goals for Test 5:

1)

2)

3)

Goals for Real MCAT:

1)

2)

3)

Chapter 45
CARS: Active Reading

GOALS

1) To develop new—and more effective—active reading habits
2) To read for logical structure and get to the Bottom Line
3) To use annotation in order to be able to retrieve information quickly and accurately

45.1 BASIC APPROACH: THE SIX STEPS

First, here is a review of the six basic steps to approaching the CARS section that we discussed in Chapter 44. In the rest of this chapter, we will focus on steps two, three, and four.

■ STEP 1: RANK AND ORDER THE PASSAGES

Decide whether to do the passage Now, Later, or Never, based on the difficulty level of the passage text.

■ STEP 2: PREVIEW THE QUESTIONS

Read through the question stems from first to last (not the answer choices) before you read the passage. Look for and highlight words and phrases that indicate important passage content. Do not worry at this stage about identifying the question type.

■ STEP 3: WORK THE PASSAGE

As you read through the passage (staying on the screen that includes the last question of the set for that passage), use the highlighting function (sparingly) to annotate the most important references in the passage, especially words that indicate the logical structure of the author's argument and references that appeared in your preview of the questions. Notice topic sentences that help you to identify conclusions made by the author. Articulate the Main Point of each chunk of information (usually, each paragraph). Use your noteboard, especially on difficult passages, to jot down these main points. As you read, think about how these chunks relate to each other, and identify the structure of the passage.

■ STEP 4: BOTTOM LINE

After you have read the passage, sum up the Bottom Line: the Main Point and tone of the entire passage.

■ STEP 5: ATTACK THE QUESTIONS

Start with the last question in the set for that passage. Read the question word for word, identifying the question type and translating the question task into your own words. Go back to the passage before reading the answer choices and find the relevant information (reading at least five lines above and below the reference). Think about what the correct answer will need to do, and generate an answer to the question in your own words. Use Process of Elimination (POE) actively. Select the "least wrong" answer.

If a question looks especially difficult, skip over it the first time through, and answer it after the easier questions as you click forward through the questions towards the next passage.

■ STEP 6: INSPECT THE SECTION

At or before the 5-minute mark (ideally, before you begin your last passage), double-check to make sure that you haven't left anything blank. You can use the Review function at this stage. Do NOT rethink questions you have already completed.

45.2   ACTIVE READING: READING FOR STRUCTURE AND THE BOTTOM LINE

What is the Bottom Line?

When you read a CARS passage for the first time, you must read it in a very different way than you would read most other texts. For example, when you are studying for a bio exam in a class, you are trying to understand and memorize every fact and detail in the course material. If you read a CARS passage in that way, however, you will not only waste a great deal of precious time, but you will also overlook the things that are really important: the main points being made by the author, and how they fit together to communicate the core idea or Bottom Line of the entire passage. In this chapter, we will first discuss what you are reading FOR the first time through a passage: the logical structure and core ideas of the passage. Then we will lay out HOW you should be working the passage by using your highlighter and noteboard to map out those basic aspects of the passage.

As you've no doubt noticed, MCAT CARS passages are often dense, convoluted, and full of details that you ultimately don't need to know in order to answer the questions. Such passages are impossible to read as closely as you would read a text for school, especially given the time constraint. On the MCAT, your goal is not to develop a deep understanding of every aspect of the passage; your goal is to find the information you need to answer the questions, and to pay as little attention as possible to everything else.

Therefore, do not attempt to understand or memorize every detail. This is time-consuming and counterproductive. Instead, visualize the passage as comprised of several large chunks of information. Each chunk, which may span part or all of a paragraph, has a Main Point and serves a particular function within the passage as a whole.

As you read, separate the central point of each paragraph from the evidence used to support that point. Translate the Main Point of each paragraph into your own words. What is the author trying to prove? Pay close attention to words that indicate the author's opinion or attitude. Jot down a few words or a short sentence indicating the Main Point of the chunk and/or paragraph on your noteboard. Link this theme with the Main Points of the previous paragraphs. Imagine that you are reading a mystery novel, following a twisty plot line and adding up the major clues to the story as you go.

After you have read and identified the Main Point of the last paragraph, define the main idea and tone of the passage as a whole: this is the Bottom Line of the entire passage.

How to Get the Bottom Line

In order to read the passages effectively (that is, quickly and with a reasonable degree of comprehension), you must become an *active reader*. Don't read passively; imagine yourself attacking and taking control over each passage. Think of the passage as an argument that you are breaking down into its most basic parts.

Here are the basic principles for active reading.

1) Preview the questions for content (not for question type). Predict what issues will be especially important in the passage you are about to read.
2) Note the author's tone and purpose. What side is the author on? Why is he or she writing this passage?
3) Notice pivotal words and other transitions: use them to identify the "chunks" of an argument and how those chunks relate to each other.
4) Highlight the words that indicate the logical structure of the passage—that is, how the parts of the passage relate to each other. Also highlight topics that appeared in the questions.
5) Translate the Main Point of each paragraph or chunk of information into your own words. Link it to what you've already read and predict what is to come next.
6) Articulate the Bottom Line of the whole passage to yourself before answering the questions.

Reading For Structure

The structure of a passage can be identified on three levels.

- **Level 1:** The structure of individual sentences. Look for how the parts of the sentence work together, and how the words used by the author indicate the meaning of that sentence. Don't get caught up in parsing out the structure of every line of every paragraph. But, when sentences contain **indicator words** like *however, although, therefore, on one hand, for example*, etc., it is important to use those words to figure out the meaning of that sentence.

  For example, pivotal words such as *however* or *but* signal a shift in meaning or subject. When you identify a pivotal word in the sentence, ask, "What is it shifting from, and what is it shifting to? How do the two parts of a sentence (or the pair of sentences, if the indicator words come at the beginning of a sentence) relate to each other, and what does this tell me about the author's argument?" Or, if you see the word *therefore*, your immediate question should be, "What is the conclusion or claim being made and where is the evidence supporting that claim?" (especially important for answering Reasoning questions). The words *for example* should raise the question, "what larger claim is being supported by this example, and how does it connect to the author's argument in the passage as a whole?"

  By paying attention to indicator words, you can identify the sentences that will play a particularly important role in constructing the author's argument, and skim over the sentences that are less important at this stage.

- **Level 2:** The structure of a paragraph or chunk of information. If you ask these questions about individual sentences, it naturally leads you to the structure and intent of the entire paragraph. Did it introduce an opposing point of view? Did it provide specific evidence and support for a conclusion drawn earlier? Does it introduce another stage of development, or continue to develop a description of a particular phase?

Separate the paragraph into **claims** and **evidence**. The claims being made are important in understanding the main point of the paragraph, whereas the details of the evidence supporting those claims are usually important only when answering the questions.

Look for **topic sentences.** Often (but not always) the author uses the first or last sentence of the paragraph to sum up the theme or main point of the paragraph as a whole.

- **Level 3:** The structure of the passage as a whole. The relationship between the individual paragraphs creates or constructs the logical structure of the author's argument. This leads you naturally into an understanding of the Bottom Line (logic of the passage). Having this map of the passage in mind also helps you to quickly locate the information you need as you are answering the questions.

Some common passage structures are:

- compare and contrast
- cause and effect
- thesis with evidence
- rebuttal
- narration or description
- analysis of different aspects of an issue or idea
- old and new theory
- chronology

45.3 THE MAPS OF A PASSAGE

There are four basic components to any passage that, when clearly identified and articulated, give you a firm grounding in the overall structure and argument of the text and build a foundation for the process of answering the questions.

These components are the **MAPS** or

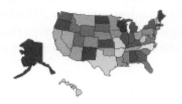
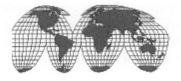

Main Point

Attitude

Purpose

Support

1) The **MAIN POINT** of each paragraph encapsulates the core of *what* the author is trying to communicate. It includes the main idea of each paragraph or chunk of information, and defines and delimits the scope of the passage. The **MAIN POINT** of the passage is the Bottom Line.
2) The **ATTITUDE** expresses *who* the author is through the tone of the passage. Is the author presenting himself or herself as a critic? An advocate? A neutral observer?
3) The **PURPOSE** is the intent of each chunk of the passage and of the passage as a whole. *Why* did the author write it? Was it to compare and contrast two theories? To propose a new theory? To trace the evolution of an idea? To describe a process?
4) The **SUPPORT** is the evidence the author uses to support his or her claims. *How* does the author construct the passage?

Think about a real map. It is constructed in a particular way with a particular purpose: to guide you to your destination. When you use a map, you don't need to pay attention to every street or highway or reference; you only need to find the streets and the connections between those streets which are relevant to your particular goal at that particular time. Memorizing the entire map is not only unnecessary, it's impossible. If you look at the entire picture without separating out the important from the unimportant sections, you will be lost—it's just too much information!

By breaking a passage down into MAPS, you define both Logic and Location. The Logic gives you the Bottom Line, which is crucial for all questions. Location "labels" the different parts of the passage, enabling you to use your map to find the specific information you need as you are answering each question.

So, let's look at our four MAPS components in more detail in connection to passage structure. To follow the process you actually go through as you work a passage, we will reverse the components to SPAM, starting at the lowest level and working up to the Main Point.

Support

How does the passage use evidence to support the author's larger claims?

All passages, even neutral explanatory passages, are made up of big claims and specific evidence supporting those claims. As we discussed above, your main goal the first time through a passage should be to identify the author's main points and overall purpose; the evidence or support should be skimmed or read more quickly so that you don't get bogged down in the details. So, you need to be able to identify the support used by the author in order to 1) decide to skim through it in your first read-through, as it is less important to the logic of the passage, and 2) relocate it, if and when it becomes relevant to the questions. Also, many CARS questions require you to enumerate or to characterize evidence presented in a passage. While you should not dwell on the support during your first reading of the passage, you should ask yourself, "What larger point is being supported here?

So, how do you recognize the support?

There are many ways to support a Main Point. The following are the most common:

1) **Examples:** The author illustrates the Main Point with an example from the real world or with a hypothetical example meant to reflect the real world. Examples are often introduced with standard words or phrases that help you to identify them: *in this case, in illustration, for example.*

2) **Generalizations:** To make a point about Christmas, for example, an author might generalize about something larger—like holidays in general. Or the author might make a point about Christmas by discussing Christmas trees. In other words, a generalization supports a main idea by giving an example of something larger—or something smaller—than the subject.

3) **Steps/stages:** Many passages describe the development of an idea, a historical time line, or an evolutionary process. Generally, each paragraph will describe one of those stages. Or, a passage may describe how one thing preceded another in order to support a larger claim about cause and effect.

4) **Comparisons/contrasts:** An effective way to explain something is to compare it to, or contrast it with, something else. Through differences and similarities, the specific characteristics of an idea can be highlighted. A specific type of comparison is an *analogy*, where one situation is described in order to communicate something about another, supposedly similar situation.

5) **Statistics:** Statistics can be any type of numerical information—percentages, ratios, probabilities, populations, prices, etc. It is especially important to avoid getting bogged down in these details. You will be able to find them again later, if you need to.

6) **Studies:** The author cites studies, research, or polling data to support a conclusion.

7) **Definitions:** The author defines key terms in order to communicate something about the context or issues within which those terms are used.

8) **Quotes or citation of others:** The passage includes either direct quotes or citation of other works. It is important to ask yourself if the author is agreeing or disagreeing with these other writers or speakers.

9) **General opinion:** The author describes a past or present common belief. Authors often do this in order to introduce a different or alternative idea. Always define if the common belief is consistent or inconsistent with the author's point of view.

10) **Anecdotes:** The author tells a story, often from his or her personal experience.

Purpose

Why was the passage written?

Purpose is closely related to structure, and it can be broken down to three levels in a similar way.

1) **W**hat is the purpose of the support provided by the author? What larger claim is being supported? Answering this question will lead you to the next level.

2) **W**hat is the purpose of the paragraph? What role does it play within the logical structure of the passage? How do the different paragraphs connect to each other? Answering this question leads you to the final level.

3) **W**hat is the purpose of the passage as a whole? Why did the author write it? What overall claim or point is being made?

The purpose of the passage as a whole is very closely tied to the author's attitude. The intent of neutral passages is to describe or explain something. In a purely descriptive passage, it is likely that each paragraph will deal with a different characteristic of the thing being described.

An explanatory passage often includes both generalizations as well as specific examples as illustrations of those generalizations. Identify transition words to ascertain when the author is moving from one point to another (*additionally, also, furthermore*, etc.) or from a generalization to a specific case or illustration (*for example*).

On the other hand, evaluative, critical, or persuasive passages often present one idea or position, a contrasting idea or position, and the author's opinion, which may involve choosing one of those sides over the other or presenting a separate alternative altogether. A common purpose is to contrast old with new theories, or to present and evaluate a debate or controversy.

Keep in mind the strength of the tone and the language. For example, the author may be rejecting the validity of a claim, or may simply be raising questions about or problems with that claim. Keep track of pivotal words (*however, but, yet, conversely, although*, etc.) that indicate when the author is shifting in the discussion from one side to the other, or introducing a qualification. (Pivotal words, however, are not limited to opinionated passages, just as transitional words do not appear exclusively in neutral passages.) Difficult passages may have several such shifts.

Attitude

Who wrote the passage? What is the author's tone?

When asking yourself "who wrote the passage," don't take the question literally, and don't speculate about what kind of person the author might be in real life. Rather, connect this to the purpose of the passage and to how the author presents him or herself through the passage text. An author may position herself as a neutral observer, simply describing or explaining without expressing an opinion. The author may even describe a debate or conflicting points of view without directly entering into that debate.

In other passages, the author is more present—speculating, evaluating, criticizing, praising, or advocating. To define the attitude of the author, look for words that indicate the tone of the passage (for example, *unfortunately, shamefully, at last, thankfully*, etc.), or statements that embody the voice or opinion of the author. If the author does have an opinion, evaluate how strongly negative or positive it is. Look out for qualifying language (for example, *might, could, in some cases, while it is sometimes true that*, etc.) that authors often use to moderate their tone.

Occasionally, a question will directly ask for the attitude or tone of the author. However, attitude can play a role in any question type. It is particularly central to Main Point or Primary Purpose questions, to any question that asks how the author would respond to new information, and to Strengthen and Weaken questions.

Main Point

What is the passage trying to prove?

Articulating the Main Point or Main Idea (that is, the Bottom Line of the passage) is one of the most important steps you can take to maximize both your accuracy and your speed in working through the questions. A question may directly ask for the main point or central thesis. However, even if there is no such question, the main point can be used on a variety of question types to quickly eliminate answer choices that are out of scope or not the issue of the passage. The main point may be summarized in the first or last paragraph of the passage, but this is not always the case. In many passages, parts of the main point are scattered throughout, and it can be defined only by synthesizing or piecing together the main idea of each chunk of information.

Students often fall into one of two traps when attempting to identify the main point. On the one hand, they might state it too broadly, as a vague category or idea that includes—but goes beyond—the passage. On the other hand, they may define it too narrowly, focusing on only one among several of the points made by the author.

45.4 MAPS EXERCISE

To break down and explore each of these components in more detail in the context of tracking the structure of the passage, let's visit a sample MCAT CARS passage, which is reproduced on the following pages.

Preview the questions and work the passage. For each example provided, ask yourself why the author uses that example. Identify wording that indicates the author's tone. For each paragraph, identify how that paragraph relates to the rest of the passage. Articulate the Bottom Line of the passage.

Then answer the questions, specifically looking for how your understanding of MAPS and passage structure applies. Finally, read through the explanation that follows.

<u>Note</u>: On the computer-based test, each question will be displayed on a separate page.

Passage 1 (Questions 1–7)

From Romania to Germany, from Tallinn to Belgrade, a major historical process—the death of communism—is taking place. The German Democratic Republic does not exist anymore as a separate state. And the former GDR will serve as the first measure of the price a post-Communist society has to pay for entering the normal European orbit. In Yugoslavia we will see whether the federation can survive without communism, and whether the nations of Yugoslavia will want to exist as a federation. (On a larger scale, we will witness the same process in the Soviet Union.)

One thing seems common to all these countries: dictatorship has been defeated and freedom has won, yet the victory of freedom has not yet meant the triumph of democracy. Democracy is something more than freedom. Democracy is freedom institutionalized, freedom submitted to the limits of the law, freedom functioning as an object of compromise between the major political forces on the scene.

We have freedom, but we still have not achieved the democratic order. That is why this freedom is so fragile. In the years of democratic opposition to communism, we supposed that the easiest thing would be to introduce changes in the economy. In fact, we thought that the march from a planned economy to a market economy would take place within the framework of the *nomenklatura* system, and that the market within the Communist state would explode the totalitarian structures. Only then would the time come to build the institutions of a civil society; and only at the end, with the completion of the market economy and the civil society, would the time of great political transformations finally arrive.

The opposite happened. First came the big political change, the great shock, which either broke the monopoly and the principle itself of Communist Party rule or simply pushed the Communists out of power. Then came the creation of civil society, whose institutions were created in great pain, and which had trouble negotiating the empty space of freedom. And only then, as the third moment of change, the final task was undertaken: that of transforming the totalitarian economy into a normal economy where different forms of ownership and different economic actors will live one next to the other.

Today we are in a typical moment of transition. No one can say where we are headed. The people of the democratic opposition have the feeling that we won. We taste the sweetness of our victory the same way the Communists, only yesterday our prison guards, taste the bitterness of their defeat. And yet, even as we are conscious of our victory, we feel that we are, in a strange way, losing. In Bulgaria the Communists have won the parliamentary elections and will govern the country, without losing their social legitimacy. In Romania the National Salvation Front, largely dominated by people from the old Communist *nomenklatura,* has won. In other countries democratic institutions seem shaky, and the political horizon is cloudy. The masquerade goes on: dozens of groups and parties are created, each announces similar slogans, each accuses its adversaries of all possible sins, and each declares itself representative of the national interest. Personal disputes are more important than disputes over values. Arguments over labels are fiercer than arguments over ideas.

1. Which of the following best describes the author's main point?

A) Democracy is a superior political system to Communism.
B) The fall of Communism in Eastern Europe has occurred more rapidly than most of the democratic opposition expected.
C) Political change is difficult, particularly when economic systems are in transition.
D) Post-Communist countries, while gaining in freedom, have not yet established stable democratic political institutions.

2. The author describes a set of previously shared expectations about the emergence of a democratic order. The first significant change was expected to be:

A) the destruction of totalitarian political power in favor of growing civil institutions.
B) an economic transition expanding private ownership.
C) a decrease in the power of the Communist Party.
D) an explosive market collapse provoked by the failures of Communist economic policies.

3. Which of the following is true, according to the passage, regarding the relationship of democracy to freedom?

A) Freedom is a necessary component of democracy, but does not necessarily spur the development of democracy.
B) When a country experiences increases in freedom, it is likely that democracy will also increase.
C) In the absence of democracy, freedom is harder to achieve and to sustain.
D) Both freedom and democracy can and do exist separately from one another.

4. Which of the following best describes the author's attitude towards the political, economic, and social changes described in the passage?

A) Approval of the new governments in specific countries, such as Bulgaria and Romania, but disapproval of other countries where governments are more shaky
B) Pessimism that the reversed order of changes in the transition away from Communism signals an inevitable instability in the fledgling democracies
C) A celebration of the overthrow of totalitarianism, alongside concern about whether the progress is sustainable
D) Optimism that market forces will continue to push governments towards an emerging democratic order

5. In the phrase, "the price a post-Communist society has to pay" (paragraph 1), the word "price" most nearly refers to which of the following?

A) The death of some citizens
B) A loss of political autonomy
C) Economic penalties and hardships
D) A reduction in freedom

6. Which of the following does the author cite as contributing to a sense in post-Communist countries that the democratic movement may be losing?

   I. Too little emphasis on democratic ideals by those running for political office
  II. Certain economic and political transformations occurring in a different order than was expected
 III. The continued political power held by former Communist party elites

A) I only
B) II only
C) I and III only
D). I, II, and III

7. It can be inferred from the passage that the author would be most favorable to which of the following hypothetical events in one of the countries described in the passage?

A) The assassination of a totalitarian leader by a freedom party activist
B) The emergence of several new, small political parties, each promising improved economic conditions
C) A fair parliamentary election in which a Communist-leaning party retains a majority but loses seats to a more democratic party
D) A nation's government suspending all elections so that it can focus fully on reducing unemployment and building up infrastructure

Answers to MAPS Exercise

1) **D**
2) **B**
3) **A**
4) **C**
5) **B**
6) **C**
7) **C**

Support

This passage supports its main thesis by contrasting what *actually* happens with the expectation that formerly communist nations would evolve into democracies, and then it cites specific cases in the first and last paragraphs to illustrate the point. Your paragraph-by-paragraph outline might look like this.

1) Examples of the death of communism
2) Generalization and contrast nature of freedom and democracy
3) Expected progression
4) Real progression
5) Examples of incomplete transition

Knowing where and how the author supports his claims is particularly important in answering questions 2, 5, and 6.

Purpose

In this passage, the purpose is to analyze how and why sociopolitical transformation in the formerly communist nations did not follow the expected path, and to express regret that this has left their evolution into democracies incomplete.

Take a look at questions 3, 5, and 7, and consider the role played by the Purpose of the author in each of the credited responses.

Attitude

The author is clearly present in this passage. Note the repeated use of the word "we"; the author presents as a participant (paragraph 3) as well as an informed expert (paragraph 1), not as a disinterested outsider. Note also the tone and language of the passage. Democracy is something to be "achieved," from which we can infer that it is a desirable thing. The author speaks of the "sweetness of our victory," telling us that freedom in this sense, while limited, is greatly appreciated. Yet at the same time the author feels that "we are, in a strange way, losing." This indicates the author's discontent with the incomplete nature of the transformation.

Now take a look at question 4, which directly asks for the author's attitude. Choices A and D are too positive (the author is critical of the two countries mentioned in choice A, and the suggestion in choice D that market forces will produce political change is contradicted by the author's analysis). Choice B is too negative. The word "inevitable" is too extreme and it is not clear that the reversal of the steps is the source of the author's concern. Only choice C reflects the mixture of appreciation and regret that defines the author's attitude in this passage.

Main Point

In this passage, the author argues that many formerly communist nations have overthrown totalitarian regimes and achieved political freedom. However, because the transformation of the economy and civil society of these countries is as yet incomplete, true democracy does not exist. A student without a firm grasp on the driving theme and scope of the argument might incorrectly identify the main point as, "One can have freedom without democracy," which is too broad. A student who gets too caught up in one part of the passage might say the Main Point is that, "In Bulgaria and Romania, members of the old communist order still hold positions of power." A student who gets it just right, however, might say that the Main Point is something like this: "Many countries have overthrown communism and are now free, but they have not yet achieved democracy."

Now take a look in particular at questions 1, 3, 4, and 7. Notice how useful it is to have a clear statement of the Main Point as a tool to eliminate traps and choose the correct answer.

45.5   PASSAGE ANNOTATION AND MAPPING

Now that we have broken down what you are reading for during your first time through a passage, let's get into the mechanics of working a passage. That is, what you should be doing with your pencil and the highlighter in order to keep your focus on the logic and structure of the passage, and to set up the process of answering the questions as accurately and efficiently as possible.

Why Annotate?

Annotation is a crucial part of active reading. Like any successful traveler, you need a *map* to help you navigate the passage. Intelligent annotation can help you to create this map. A smart annotation system is neither too sparse nor too elaborate.

In the course of your undergraduate studies, you may have become accustomed to highlighting large chunks of text. However, this approach is not going to help you on the MCAT. If you highlight everything that "looks important" in the passage, in the end, all you will have is some big blocks of yellow text. This won't help you to understand the logic of the argument as you read, and you will have to reread huge chunks of text to find the relevant information as you answer the questions.

You must have a specific strategy for annotating or mapping the text of the passage. While you do not need to write down all aspects of the four parts of MAPS that we discussed above, your physical mapping of the passage is based on the logical structure of the passage that you identified through reading for MAPS. Mapping is an active process that keeps you engaged with the text. It forces you to decide which points are most crucial to the author's argument, and how those points relate to each other to create the Bottom Line. It also marks the breaks between logically important chunks of the passage, which helps you locate information necessary for answering the questions.

Mapping

There are two tools you have to map the passage: *making notes on your noteboard* and *highlighting the passage*.

Making Notes

Use your noteboard to jot down the Main Point of each paragraph and the Bottom Line of the passage. Do this for every passage now; eventually, you may only need to write it down for the harder passages. Do NOT, however, use your noteboard to list every fact mentioned in each paragraph; your goal is to identify the core idea of that chunk, not to write down a detailed outline of it. Also, if there is a time line in the passage, write it down so that you can use it as you answer the questions. You can also use your noteboard to write down translations of difficult questions and answer choices.

What to Highlight

Question Topics   When you see words or phrases that you recognize from your preview, highlight them. However, don't jump out of the passage to answer the question at this point (you don't know yet what else the author might have to say about that subject!). By highlighting them, you make it easy to come back and find them when you do answer the question.

Transitions: Pivotal words   Pivotal words are especially important, so let's discuss them in more detail.

MCAT CARS passages rarely contain a single point reiterated over and over again. Rather, a chain of reasoning is more likely to change direction one or more times. These turns in the overall direction of a passage are often marked by **pivotal words**. Here are some common pivotal words and phrases.

but	although	however
yet	despite	nevertheless
nonetheless	except	admittedly
in spite of the fact that	in contrast	even though

These words indicate *change* or *contrast*. Pivotal words signal that the author is about to shift the course of the argument by:

- placing a condition on the argument
- introducing an antithetical point
- shifting from a simple to a more complex level of argument
- making a concession to an opposing viewpoint

Think of pivotal words as signposts that appear at crucial turns or refinements in the argument. Highlight them as you work through the passage. Marking pivotal words serves at least two functions.

- First, it increases the visibility of the parts of the passage that are likely to contain key ideas.
- Second, stopping to highlight a pivotal word lets you know that you need to determine *why* a transition is occurring at that point. In other words, the most valuable aspect of marking pivotal words— indeed, of annotating in general—is that it alerts you to the parts of the passage to which you need to pay the most attention, and it helps you track the logic of the author's argument.

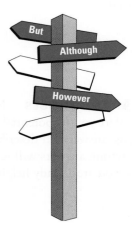

45.5

Transitions: Continuations
These words indicate that the author is further developing or explaining the point he or she has just made. Noticing and highlighting them will help you to distinguish different parts of the author's argument from each other. Here are words commonly used to indicate continuations.

furthermore
additionally
also
moreover

Conclusions
Authors use these words to sum up their Main Points. Finding and highlighting these words will help you to do the same. Here are some common conclusion indicators.

therefore	thus
so	consequently
clearly	hence
for this reason	

Opinion Indicators
One of the most important aspects of the Bottom Line is the author's tone. To accurately identify the author's point of view, look for and highlight phrases that express opinion, and words like

finally
fortunately
thankfully
unfortunately
sadly

Emphasis Words
Authors use words like these to catch your attention, because what follows is especially important. Here are some examples of emphasis words.

most important
primarily
chiefly
key
crucial

Comparisons And Contrasts
Not only are these words important to the logical structure of the passage, they also alert you to potential traps in the questions. When the passage describes two things as different, a wrong answer will describe them as similar, and vice versa. When the author discusses a change over time, wrong answers will reverse the chronology. By locating and highlighting comparison/contrast indicators, you are already helping yourself get the questions right. Here are some examples.

similarly	like
analogy	unlike
in contrast	later
the difference between	before/after

All of the categories of words discussed above indicate that something important to the Bottom Line is being discussed by the author; that is, major claims that deserve some attention on your first reading of the passage. These last three categories, however, tend to indicate details or support for those major claims. Highlight these markers to indicate location of the support, but read through what follows them in the text more quickly. You can follow your highlighting back to the relevant part of the passage if you need to as you are answering the questions.

Examples   These words tell you that what follows is an example or illustration of a larger, more important point. Highlight them so that you can find these details if they become important to the questions. These markers are especially useful for answering questions that ask you if, or how well, the author's claims are supported. What you should be *thinking* about now as you read, however, is the conclusion being supported by the example. This is what will give you the Main Point of the chunk and eventually the Bottom Line of the passage. Here are some common example indicators.

> for example
> because
> since
> in this case
> in illustration

List Markers   When the author provides a string of claims or examples, it can be difficult to pull out the relevant item from that list when you are answering the questions. Highlight just the markers, not the entire list. But, just as with example indicators, define what this list is illustrating as you read: What is it a list of? List markers might be

> first
> second   There are three factors
> thirdly

Names   Highlight names now so that you don't have to reread large chunks of text to find them when they show up in the question stems and answer choices.

45.6   CARS EXERCISES: ACTIVE READING

Exercise 1: Working the Passage

Previewing the Questions

Read through the five questions below. Identify and highlight the words and phrases that indicate the issues in the passage that will be relevant to answering these questions. Don't try to identify the question type at this stage; focus only on clues to passage content. After you preview the questions and answer the question that follows, you will move on and read the passage attached to them.

1. According to the author, which of the following constitutes a fundamental human characteristic?

2. Which of the following, based on information in the passage, would most strengthen the author's claim in paragraph 6 that the work of economists is necessary to the advancement of civilization?

3. The author claims that human beings find it difficult to survive. What explanation is offered in support of this conclusion?

4. According to the passage, why do economists have such significant influence over society?

5. It can be inferred from the passage that economists are relatively unknown because:

Summing it up: What will this passage be about? _____

_____

_____

The questions you have just previewed are about the passage (presented paragraph by paragraph) on the following pages. As you work through those paragraphs, keep in mind what you learned from these questions.

Defining the Main Points and the Bottom Line

What we have here is an entire passage. These paragraphs have already been highlighted for you, as an illustration of what you should be (and shouldn't be) highlighting. As you read, think about *why* those words have been highlighted, and what those highlighted words tell you about the important parts of the author's argument.

For each paragraph, define the Main Point of that chunk. Write down the Main Point in the space provided before you move on to the next paragraph. Don't make a list of all the information included. Focus on the claims being made, not the evidence supporting those claims. At the end, articulate the Bottom Line of this passage.

45.6

The very fact that man has had to depend on his fellow man has made the problem of survival extraordinarily difficult. Man is not an ant, conveniently equipped with an inborn pattern of social instincts. On the contrary, he is preeminently the creature of his will-o'-the-wisp whims, his unpredictable impulses, and his selfishness. Man is torn between a basic need for gregariousness—to coexist peaceably with his neighbors—and a pronounced tendency toward greediness. Often, his tendency to guard his own interest is at odds with his need to survive in a community. And it is to this clash and conflict that the first great economists addressed themselves.

Main Point: _____

_____

_____

One would think that in a world torn by economic problems, a world in which we constantly worry about economic affairs and talk of economic issues, the great economists would have an important place in history and be as familiar to us as the great philosophers or statesmen. Yet they seem to be only shadowy figures of the past. In the 1760s an educated traveler in England would probably have heard of Adam Smith, a professor at the University of Glasgow, but today a great many educated people do not know that this gentleman was the father of economics.

Main Point: _____

_____

_____

No economist has ever been either a national hero or a national villain. Yet what economists have done has been more decisive for history than many acts of statesmen who basked in brighter glory. Often their deeds have been more profoundly disturbing than the shuttling of armies back and forth across frontiers, more powerful for good and bad than the edicts of kings and legislatures. Since economists have shaped and swayed men's minds they have necessarily shaped and swayed the world.

Main Point: _____

_____

_____

Few economists ever lifted a finger in action. They worked, in the main, as scholars: quietly, inconspicuously, and without much regard for what the world had to say about them.

Main Point: _____

_____

_____

Economists are not well known because most people do not understand the significance of economics and believe it to be a rather uninteresting academic pursuit. But a man who thinks that economics is only a matter for professors forgets that this is the science that has sent men to their battle stations. A man who has looked into an economics textbook and concluded that economics is boring is like a man who has read a primer on logistics and decided that the study of warfare must be dull.

Main Point: _____

_____

_____

To be sure, not all the economists were titans. Adam Smith was a stunningly interesting character. But thousands of his followers wrote texts, some of them monuments of dullness, and explored minutiae with all the zeal of medieval scholars. Nonetheless, economists are the worldly philosophers, and their work is essential to the growth and continuation of advanced civilizations. Economists have sought to embrace in a scheme of philosophy the most worldly of man's activities: his drive for wealth. It is not, perhaps, the most elegant kind of philosophy, but there is no more intriguing or important.[1]

45.6

Main Point: _____

_____

_____

Bottom Line of the passage as a whole: _____

_____

_____

---

[1] Material used in this particular passage has been adapted from the following source: R. L. Heilbroner, *The Worldly Philosophers.* © 1999 by Simon & Schuster Inc.

Answers for Exercise 1: Working the Passage

Previewing the Questions
Summing it up: What will this passage be about?

This passage will be about human nature and survival, economists and their relationship to society, and why economists are not well known.

Defining the Main Points and the Bottom Line:

NOTE: Your own notes may be briefer; these are written out in more complete terms than you may need for your own understanding.

1) Man's independence conflicts with his need to be part of a group for survival.
2) Economists surprisingly fade into the background of history.
3) Economists have great influence over history.
4) Economists are scholarly, removed from the world.
5) People don't "get" economics, and so don't know economists.
6) Economists are vital to civilization.

Bottom Line of the passage as a whole: Although they fade into history, economists are crucial to the advancement of society.

Exercise 2: Annotation and Active Reading—Putting It All Together

Read and annotate the following passage. As you read, stop and write down the Main Point of each paragraph on your noteboard. When you have read the whole passage, write down the Bottom Line. Then turn the page and read through the sample annotations and explanation of the passage. The sample passage also indicates what sections of the passage you should skim or move through more quickly.

Passage for Annotation Exercise 2

There are two major systems of criminal procedure in the modern world—the adversarial and the inquisitorial. The former is associated with common law tradition and the latter with civil law tradition. Both systems were historically preceded by the system of private vengeance in which the victim of a crime fashioned his own remedy and administered it privately, either personally or through an agent. The vengeance system was a system of self-help, the essence of which was captured in the slogan "an eye for an eye, a tooth for a tooth." The modern adversarial system is only one historical step removed from the private vengeance system and still retains some of its characteristic features. Thus, for example, even though the right to institute criminal action has now been extended to all members of society, and even though the police department has taken over the pretrial investigative functions on behalf of the prosecution, the adversarial system still leaves the defendant to conduct his own pretrial investigation. The trial is still viewed as a duel between two adversaries, refereed by a judge who, at the beginning of the trial, has no knowledge of the investigative background of the case. In the final analysis, the adversarial system of criminal procedure symbolizes and regularizes punitive combat.

By contrast, the inquisitorial system begins historically where the adversarial system stopped its development. It is two historical steps removed from the system of private vengeance. Therefore, from the standpoint of legal anthropology, it is historically superior to the adversarial system. Under the inquisitorial system, the public investigator has the duty to investigate not just on behalf of the prosecutor but also on behalf of the defendant. Additionally, the public prosecutor has the duty to present to the court not only evidence that may lead to the conviction of the defendant but also evidence that may lead to his exoneration. This system mandates that both parties permit full pretrial discovery of the evidence in their possession. Finally, in an effort to make the trial less like a duel between two adversaries, the inquisitorial system mandates that the judge take an active part in the conduct of the trial, with a role that is both directive and protective.

Fact-finding is at the heart of the inquisitorial system. This system operates on the philosophical premise that in a criminal case the crucial factor is not the legal rule but the facts of the case and that the goal of the entire procedure is to experimentally recreate for the court the commission of the alleged crime.

Material used in this particular passage has been adapted from the following source:

M. A. Glendon, *Comparative Legal Traditions in a Nutshell.* © 1982 by West Publishing Company.

Sample Annotation (Annotation Exercise 2)

There are two major systems of criminal procedure in the modern world—the adversarial and the inquisitorial. The former is associated with common law tradition and the latter with civil law tradition. Both systems were historically preceded by the system of private vengeance in which the victim of a crime fashioned his own remedy and administered it privately, either personally or through an agent. The vengeance system was a system of self-help, the essence of which was captured in the slogan "an eye for an eye, a tooth for a tooth." The modern adversarial system is only one historical step removed from the private vengeance system and still retains some of its characteristic features. Thus, for example, even though the right to institute criminal action has now been extended to all members of society, and even though the police department has taken over the pretrial investigative functions on behalf of the prosecution, the adversarial system still leaves the defendant to conduct his own pretrial investigation. The trial is still viewed as a duel between two adversaries, refereed by a judge who, at the beginning of the trial, has no knowledge of the investigative background of the case. In the final analysis, the adversarial system of criminal procedure symbolizes and regularizes punitive combat.

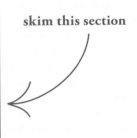

skim this section

By contrast, the inquisitorial system begins historically where the adversarial system stopped its development. It is two historical steps removed from the system of private vengeance. Therefore, from the standpoint of legal anthropology, it is historically superior to the adversarial system. Under the inquisitorial system, the public investigator has the duty to investigate not just on behalf of the prosecutor but also on behalf of the defendant. Additionally, the public prosecutor has the duty to present to the court not only evidence that may lead to the conviction of the defendant but also evidence that may lead to his exoneration. This system mandates that both parties permit full pretrial discovery of the evidence in their possession. Finally, in an effort to make the trial less like a duel between two adversaries, the inquisitorial system mandates that the judge take an active part in the conduct of the trial, with a role that is both directive and protective.

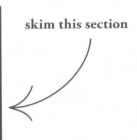

skim this section

Fact-finding is at the heart of the inquisitorial system. This system operates on the philosophical premise that in a criminal case the crucial factor is not the legal rule but the facts of the case and that the goal of the entire procedure is to experimentally recreate for the court the commission of the alleged crime.

Explanation of the Passage

This passage presents a clear argument, using detailed descriptions to support it. The trick to understanding this argument is to keep track of the three kinds of legal systems: the adversarial, the inquisitorial, and the system of private vengeance, and the differences among them.

Notice that there are three major chunks of information here. They roughly correspond to the three legal systems, but they do not correspond to the three paragraphs; paragraph 1 contains two chunks: a description of the system of private vengeance and of the adversarial system. Paragraphs 2 and 3 work together as one chunk to describe the features of the modern inquisitorial system. Your annotation and summation of the Main Points in the passage should focus on the contrast drawn by the author between the three different systems. Good annotation and "chunking" will help you to get to the Bottom Line of a passage and to find the details necessary to answer the questions.

Your understanding of the Bottom Line of the passage should be something like: "The adversarial system of criminal law is similar to the traditional system of private vengeance and is therefore less developed than the modern inquisitorial system."

On the following page is an example of what your noteboard might look like. You will notice that these notes are very brief. Remember that you may be expressing the main points and Bottom Line with just a few words; only you—no one else—needs to be able to understand your notes.

45.6

45.6

P1: *Private vengeance: self-help

*Adversarial came next: similar features

P2: *Inquisitorial more developed: public actors greater role*

P3: *Inquisitorial: goal of discovering facts*

BL: *Inquisitorial more developed than adversarial*

—less like private vengeance

45.7   HABITS OF EFFECTIVE READERS

Here are some suggestions for learning to read not only faster but more efficiently, the first time through the passage.

- **Focus on big ideas and skim the details.** Don't get bogged down in long descriptions. Practice using the clues provided in the author's wording to distinguish the major claims from the (potentially irrelevant) details.
- **Hit the right pace.** If you read too fast, you won't get anything out of the passage, and will end up rereading the entire passage as you answer the questions. If you go too slowly, however, you will lose focus and/or overthink what you are reading.
- **Don't try to memorize.** Remember, this is essentially an open book test. You will be going back to the passage for the facts you need for the questions.
- **Practice reading in chunks of words.** Rather than "sounding out" each word in your mind as if you were reading out loud, think about seeing the words in groups of two or three to get a sense of what is being said. When you are answering the questions, however, always read word-for-word.
- **Push your eyes forward toward the end of the sentence.** Keep your momentum; don't linger on or ponder every word.
- **Visualize as you read.** When you hit an important point in the passage, create an image in your mind that captures the author's meaning.
- **Sit back and relax!** If you have your nose up against the screen, it is harder to think about the "big picture." You will get tired and stiff, and it will be harder to keep focused.

45.8   DOS AND DON'TS FOR ACTIVE READING

Do

- highlight key words and phrases
- link and predict major themes
- take notes on your noteboard
- keep it simple
- translate the main idea of each paragraph into your own words
- summarize the main point and tone of the whole passage before attacking the questions

Don't

- focus on the details
- read parts of the passage text over and over (instead, move on!)
- memorize
- copy words or phrases on to your noteboard without knowing what they mean

WANT MORE PRACTICE?

Go online to your Student Tools to access 4 full-length practice exams or buy a copy of *MCAT Workout, 2nd Edition* for tons of practice passages and drills.

Chapter 46
CARS Question Types and Strategies

GOALS

1) To learn the types of questions that are likely to be asked and strategies for attacking them
2) To refine the use of Process of Elimination (POE)

46.1   ATTACKING THE QUESTIONS

In order to continue to improve your CARS skills, you will need to refine your approach to the questions. In this chapter, we will discuss the five basic steps you should take in answering any question and the specific tactics appropriate to each question type.

Five Steps For Answering Questions

1) Read the question word for word and identify the question type.
2) Translate the question into your own words: identify what the question task is asking you to do with the information in the passage.
3) Identify any key words that refer to specific parts of the passage. If key words are provided, *go back to the passage* to locate that information.
4) Answer in your own words: articulate what the correct answer will need to do based on the question type and the information in the passage.
5) Use Process of Elimination (POE), and choose the *least wrong* answer choice.

Let's look at each step in more detail.

1) **Read the question word for word; identify the question type.**
   WHY?
   - If you misread or misinterpret the question now, you may never catch your mistake. Now is not the time to skim, or to get only a vague impression of what the question is asking.
   - No matter how good your annotation and mapping of the passage, if you're headed to the wrong destination, those signposts do you no good. You could have an excellent map of the United States, but if you're supposed to get to Boston, and you think your destination is Biloxi, you are in big trouble. Know your destination!
   - The MCAT writers are highly skilled at predicting likely misinterpretations and at giving you wrong answers with which you could be perfectly happy. If you've ever completed a passage, pleased with how quickly and smoothly it went, only to realize upon checking your answers that you got many questions wrong, you may be reading the questions too carelessly.
   - Different kinds of questions ask for different kinds of information. Most importantly, General questions require general answers and can usually be answered with your own statement of the Bottom Line. Specific answer choices can be very narrow and always require going back to the passage. Reasoning and Application questions will usually also require you to go back to the passage, but they also ask you to either describe the logic or structure of the author's argument, or to apply new information to it. Identifying the question type is important because that will guide the rest of the process.

HOW?

- Read the question as if you have never seen it before. Focus on each word rather than taking it in as a chunk.
- Think of the question as assigning you a task: What mission do you need to accomplish in answering the question? Do you need to find information that matches the passage? Describe the author's argument in the passage (in part or the whole)? Strengthen or weaken the author's argument? Apply new information from the question stem?

2) **Translate the question into your own words; identify what the question task is asking you to do.**
   WHY?

- You may have noticed by now that questions are not always phrased in an easily comprehensible way. The test-writers do this on purpose to see if you can understand difficult, complex writing and ideas.

HOW?

- When you come across a long, complex, and convoluted question, take it out of MCAT-speak and put it into your own words. You may find it useful to jot down a few words on your noteboard.
- The benefits of translation are two-fold. First, it helps you to clarify exactly what the question is asking. Second, it will enable you to remember exactly what you're looking for when you go back to the passage.

For example, a question for a passage on Abstract Expressionism may ask,

1. Which of the following would most undermine the author's argument that the generally accepted critical appraisal underestimates the influence of Jackson Pollock on the development of Abstract Expressionism?

When you cut away the extraneous stuff and clarify the convoluted wording, all this question is asking is,

1. Which answer choice gives evidence that Pollock did not have such a significant influence on Abstract Expressionism?

3) **Identify any key words that refer to specific parts of the passage. If key words are provided, go back to the passage to locate that information.**
   WHY?

- Going back to the passage to answer questions with specific lead words is fundamental. You simply don't have time to memorize the details. Relying on your ability to recall facts under time pressure will only get you into trouble.
- If you don't check your answers against the text, you are likely to pick a choice that contains words from the passage taken out of context, or one that is true in the real world, but not supported by the passage.

- Going back to the passage before you read the answer choices will not only increase your accuracy, but will also increase your overall speed. If you already have a solid grounding in the passage, you will more quickly recognize the correct choice, and you are much less likely to get stuck between two answers.

HOW?

- A key word or phrase is something in the question that appears only a few times in the passage, and it guides you toward the relevant sections in the passage that you'll need to reread.
- Looking again at the sample question above, the phrase "Abstract Expressionism" would not make a good key phrase if the whole passage is about Abstract Expressionism; it's likely to appear many times throughout the passage. The name Jackson Pollock, however, is likely to lead you right to the relevant sections for that particular question.
- Once you've identified the key words, *scan* the passage (using your annotations) until you locate those words, and then read a few sentences above and below until you find what you need. "Five lines above and five lines below" is a good guide. However, you should start reading where the relevant information begins, and keep reading until the passage moves on to another issue.
- Pay attention to the logical structure of the author's argument. For example, if the sixth line below begins with a word like *yet* or *additionally*, you need to keep reading. Pivotal and transitional words indicate that the author may be qualifying what he or she has just said, or adding an additional point that you need to take into account.
- Some Specific (such as, "With which of the following statements would the author be most likely to agree?") and Application questions do not give you lead words as clues. For these questions, eliminate the choices that are inconsistent with the Bottom Line (or, for a Weaken question, that are consistent with the passage), and then go back to the passage to check each of the remaining possibilities.
- For General questions, you can usually use your own articulation of the Bottom Line. You may, however, still need to go back to the passage when you are down to two choices.

4) **Answer in your own words; articulate what the correct answer will need to do, based on the question type and the information in the passage.**
   WHY?

- Think of the answer choices as a minefield, full of potentially fatal missteps and pitfalls. Before you enter that minefield, you want to have a detailed map of what a strong answer choice will accomplish.
- The wording of the credited response may be quite different from what you expect, but with your own answer as a guide, you will recognize it while avoiding the traps.

   HOW?

- Once you've located the relevant information—and not before—articulate your own answer to the question. For particularly difficult questions, you may wish to jot this down on your noteboard.
- This does not mean, however, that you should try to predict the exact wording of the credited response. Instead, come up with a guide to what the correct answer needs to *do* (such as, in the sample question above, to show that Jackson Pollock had little or no influence).

5) **Use Process of Elimination (POE) to choose the *least wrong* answer choice.**
   WHY?
   - POE is the best friend of every strategic test taker. Very often on the MCAT, there is no perfectly correct answer among the given choices, only better and worse choices. On particularly difficult passages, the credited response can even be a pretty bad answer. However, it will be *less bad* than the other three.
   - There are a number of standard ways in which the MCAT writers make loser choices look like winners. The answer that at first glance "looks good" may in fact be a trap. See the rest of this chapter and Chapter 47 for more information on types of wrong answers.

   HOW?
   - Use your own understanding of the question task and of what the correct choice needs to do in order to eliminate the most clearly wrong answers. This will usually take you down to two choices.
   - Reread the question and compare the choices you have left to each other. Identify what is wrong, if anything, with each choice. The winner is the choice that has the *least wrong* with it. You may not like that winner very much, but you score a point, which is all that matters in this game.
   - When you are down to two choices, actively look for the types of Attractors that commonly appear for that question type.

46.2 QUESTION TYPES AND FORMATS

There are 10 basic questions types that you will encounter in an MCAT CARS section. These ten types fall into four categories.

Specific
1) Retrieval
2) Inference

General
3) Main Idea/Primary Purpose
4) Tone/Attitude

Reasoning
5) Structure
6) Evaluate

Application
7) Strengthen
8) Weaken
9) New Information
10) Analogy

Specific questions ask you for the answer that is best supported by a particular part of the author's argument. General questions ask you what is true of the passage as a whole. Reasoning questions ask you to describe some aspect of the logical structure of the author's argument. Finally, Application questions require you to apply new information (provided either in the question stem or in the answer choices) to the passage.

Occasionally, there can be a variation within a category. For example, a Tone/Attitude question could refer to a particular part of the passage rather than the passage as a whole, and so qualify as a Specific question. Or, a Structure question could ask for the overall organization of the passage, which would make it a General Reasoning question.

These 10 types can appear in one of three formats.

1) **Standard:** The question task is direct.
2) **EXCEPT/LEAST/NOT:** The question asks you to find the exception.
   That is, the choice that does NOT address, or that LEAST addresses, the question task (e.g., the statement that is *not* supported by the passage). The three wrong answers will in fact address the task (e.g., *will be* supported by the passage).
3) **Roman numeral:** The question offers you three items. The correct answer will include all of the items that do appropriately address the question task and none that do not.

A firm knowledge of all of these types and of the common trap answers that appear in each is necessary for dealing with the questions quickly and accurately. Before you take the MCAT, you will be able to easily identify each question and know immediately what strategy you will need to employ.

As you move through the set of questions for a passage, use your understanding of question types to attack the questions in the order that works best for you. If you hit a particularly difficult question, skip over it for the moment, and continue answering the easier questions on that passage. Then click back through the set of questions one more time, answering the harder questions. Here is the most efficient approach:

1) Preview the questions from first to last.
2) Work the passage from the screen containing the last question for that passage (remember—your highlighting will not disappear).
3) Then work backwards through the questions, answering the easier ones and skipping harder ones as you go.
4) Finally, click forward through the set of questions, answering the ones you left blank the first time through.
5) Click "Next" from the last question to move on to the next passage.

In the next part of this chapter, we will go through each question type in the Standard format, as well as the EXCEPT/LEAST/NOT and Roman numeral formats. After a discussion of the basic approach to the type, you will find a sample question and a description of how to apply the Five Steps to that question. The sample questions are attached to the passage on criminal procedure that you annotated for an Active Reading Exercise in the previous chapter. The passage is reproduced here; first rework the passage so that it is fresh in your mind.

46.3   QUESTION TYPES: SAMPLE PASSAGE AND QUESTIONS

There are two major systems of criminal procedure in the modern world—the adversarial and the inquisitorial. The former is associated with common law tradition and the latter with civil law tradition. Both systems were historically preceded by the system of private vengeance in which the victim of a crime fashioned his own remedy and administered it privately, either personally or through an agent. The vengeance system was a system of self-help, the essence of which was captured in the slogan "an eye for an eye, a tooth for a tooth." The modern adversarial system is only one historical step removed from the private vengeance system and still retains some of its characteristic features. Thus, for example, even though the right to institute criminal action has now been extended to all members of society, and even though the police department has taken over the pretrial investigative functions on behalf of the prosecution, the adversarial system still leaves the defendant to conduct his own pretrial investigation. The trial is still viewed as a duel between two adversaries, refereed by a judge who, at the beginning of the trial, has no knowledge of the investigative background of the case. In the final analysis, the adversarial system of criminal procedure symbolizes and regularizes punitive combat.

By contrast, the inquisitorial system begins historically where the adversarial system stopped its development. It is two historical steps removed from the system of private vengeance. Therefore, from the standpoint of legal anthropology, it is historically superior to the adversarial system. Under the inquisitorial system, the public investigator has the duty to investigate not just on behalf of the prosecutor but also on behalf of the defendant. Additionally, the public prosecutor has the duty to present to the court not only evidence that may lead to the conviction of the defendant but also evidence that may lead to his exoneration. This system mandates that both parties permit full pretrial discovery of the evidence in their possession. Finally, in an effort to make the trial less like a duel between two adversaries, the inquisitorial system mandates that the judge take an active part in the conduct of the trial, with a role that is both directive and protective.

Fact-finding is at the heart of the inquisitorial system. This system operates on the philosophical premise that in a criminal case the crucial factor is not the legal rule but the facts of the case and that the goal of the entire procedure is to experimentally recreate for the court the commission of the alleged crime.

Material used in this particular passage has been adapted from the following source:

M. A. Glendon, *Comparative Legal Traditions in a Nutshell.* © 1982 by West Publishing Company.

46.3

Type 1: Specific—Retrieval Questions

Retrieval questions test your ability to locate information in the passage. They may also involve simple paraphrasing and summarizing, but they do not require any substantial analysis or interpretation. They will include some reference to a detail in the passage (a person's name, a theory, a time period, etc.).

Retrieval questions may be phrased in the following ways:

- "According to the passage, the three components of Brown's theory are…"
- "The passage states that Brown's theory is rejected by…"
- "Which of the following statements is *not* mentioned as a characteristic of Brown's theory?" (EXCEPT/LEAST/NOT format)

Sample Question 1:

1. According to the author, one trait of the adversarial system that resembles private vengeance is:

   A) that it stands just one step removed from physical combat.
   B) that the defendant is expected to engage in a pretrial investigation distinct from the police inquiry.
   C). that the judge functions as a referee, with both directive and protective powers.
   D) that the police conduct a pretrial investigation on behalf of the prosecution.

1) **Read the question word for word and identify the question type.**
   The words "according to the passage" tell you that this is a Retrieval question.

2) **Translate the question into your own words: identify what the question task is asking you to do with the information in the passage.**
   Retrieval questions tend to be fairly straightforward. Here, the question is asking you to locate information in the passage about the inquisitorial system, and to find an answer choice that is best supported by that information.

3) **Identify any key words that refer to specific parts of the passage. If key words are provided, go back to the passage to locate that information.**
   "Adversarial system" appears throughout the passage. However, "private vengeance" is only in the middle of paragraph 1. That is where you will find information to answer the question.

4) **Answer in your own words: articulate what the correct answer will need to do, based on the question type and the information in the passage.**
   The correct answer will come from the examples that follow the phrase "and still retains some of its characteristic features." Similarities include that the adversarial system still leaves the defendant to conduct his own investigation, and that the trial is still viewed as a duel.

5) **Use Process of Elimination (POE) to choose the *least wrong* answer choice.**
   As we indicated earlier, each question usually has at least one trap or Attractor answer, that is, a choice that "sounds good" but in fact has some significant flaw. (See Chapter 47 for further discussion of Attractors.)
   Because Retrieval questions tend to be relatively easy, the MCAT writers often try to distract you from the credited response by pairing it with an answer choice that sounds very similar to

the passage but *is not* directly supported by it. These Attractors often copy words and phrases directly from the passage text, but they don't capture the meaning of those words in the passage. The test writers may also give you an answer choice that *is* directly supported by the text, but that is not an appropriate answer to that particular question. They may also change or reverse a relationship (for example, the passage says A leads to B, and the wrong answer says that B leads to A).

The only way to spot and avoid these traps is to go back to the passage and reread the relevant sections.

Let's take a look at each answer choice for our sample question.

A: No. This choice takes words from the passage out of context, but it doesn't directly address the question asked. Violence and combat are referenced in the passage as possible aspects of a private vengeance system and so are NOT "one step removed" from private vengeance.

B: **Yes. The passages states that the adversarial system "still leaves the defendant to conduct his own pretrial investigation," a continuation of the "self-help" nature of the private vengeance system. This choice is directly supported by the relevant part of the passage.**

C: No. This answer choices combines descriptions of the judge's role from each system. In the last sentence of the second paragraph, the judge's role in the inquisitorial system is described as "both directive and protective."

D: No. This choice is tricky because it does reference information from the correct paragraph and section. But the sentence states that "even though" the police have taken over pretrial functions, the similarities with private vengeance remain. So the police role represents a difference between the adversarial system and private vengeance, not a similarity.

Type 2: Specific—Inference Questions

Inference questions are the most common question type in the CARS section. They require you to choose the answer that is best supported by the passage. They may ask you what can be inferred or concluded, what the author would agree with, what is implied or suggested by the author, what the author assumes to be true, or what the author means by a particular word or phrase.

There is no such thing as being "too close" to the passage to qualify as a correct answer to an Inference question. An answer that directly paraphrases the passage may in fact be the credited response. On the other hand, the correct answer may seem debatable (that is, you could argue that it isn't literally deducible from the passage information), but it will still be better supported by the passage text than the other three choices.

46.3

To approach an Inference question, find the relevant section or sections of the passage. Check each answer choice against that information, choosing the one that has the most support. The credited response may seem like a stretch (for example, something that you think is not particularly "reasonable" to conclude), but it will be the best supported of the four. Be flexible; the correct answer may be something that you would never have come up with on your own, but there will be some solid evidence for it in the passage.

There are a variety of ways in which Inference questions can be phrased. Some of the most common phrasings are:

- "It can inferred from the passage that…"
- "An assumption underlying the author's discussion of Brown's theory is that…"
- "The author implies that Brown's theory is most closely linked to…"
- "Implicit in the passage is the contention that Brown's theory is…"
- "By *only dimly perceived*, the author most likely means:"
- "The author suggests that…"
- "Based on information in the passage, it can be most reasonably concluded that…"
- "With which of the following statements would the author be most likely to agree?"
- "Which of the following statements is best supported by the passage?"

Sample Question 2:

2. The passage implies that, in comparison with the adversarial system, the inquisitorial system incorporates more of which of the following?

A) Information available to the judge and defense attorney
B) Just outcomes for defendants
C) A resemblance to punitive combat
D) A difficult role for the judge in the proceedings

1) **Read the question word for word and identify the question type.**
   The words "The passage implies that" identify this as an Inference question.
2) **Translate the question into your own words: identify what the question task is asking you to do with the information in the passage.**
   This question is asking you what increases in the shift to the inquisitorial system.
3) **Identify any key words that refer to specific parts of the passage. If key words are provided, *go back to the passage* to locate that information.**
   This is where many students falter, thinking that they don't need to go back to the passage because the question is asking us to infer something (or, in this case, what is suggested). The correct answer still must be closely based on the passage text, not on your own ideas or deductions.

The words "inquisitorial" and "adversarial" appear in multiple places. However, the words "in contrast" at the beginning of paragraph 2 indicate that this is the beginning of the author's discussion of the differences between the two systems. Your annotation should alert you to the fact that there are a variety of differences listed in this paragraph. Don't reread the whole paragraph at this point, but you will need to check the answer choices against it.

4) **Answer in your own words: articulate what the correct answer will need to do, based on the question type and the information in the passage.**
   The credited response will need to describe something there is more of in the inquisitorial system than there is in the adversarial system.

5) **Use Process of Elimination (POE) to choose the *least wrong* answer choice.**
   A wide variety of Attractors appear in Inference answer choices. One of the most common is a statement that puts information from the passage into overly absolutist or extreme language. For example, the passage may say that something *often* occurs, while the trap answer will say that same thing *always* occurs.

   Do not, however, eliminate a choice for an Inference question only because it is narrower or more moderate than the scope or wording of the passage.

   Be careful to eliminate answer choices that are out of scope; that is, answer choices which refer to issues that could be tangentially related but that are never discussed in the passage. Just like for Retrieval questions, look out for Attractors that take words out of context, or that are supported by the passage but not relevant to the question.

Let's take a look at each answer choice for our sample question.

A: **Yes. Paragraph 2 states that the inquisitorial system "mandates that both parties permit full pretrial discovery of the evidence in their possession." This contrasts with the statement in the first paragraph that the judge in the adversarial system "at the beginning of the trial, has no knowledge of the investigative background of the case." From this you can conclude that both judge and defense attorney have greater access to prosecutorial evidence in the inquisitorial system.**

B: No. This answer choice involves too much outside knowledge or speculation. There is no reference to just or fair outcomes in the text.

C: No. This answer choice is reversed. It is the adversarial system that is more similar to combat.

D: No. Although the author does talk about the change in the role played by judges between the two systems, the author says nothing to indicate that the role becomes more difficult. This sort of attractor may sound reasonable, but is too much of a stretch beyond what can be supported with passage information.

Type 3: General—Main Idea/Primary Purpose Questions

These questions require you to summarize claims and implications made throughout the passage in order to formulate a general statement of the central point or primary activity of the passage. Think of the passage as an argument. The Main Idea is the overall claim, supported by specific evidence in the various paragraphs, which the author wants to convince you to accept as true. The Primary Purpose is then very closely related; it will express what the author *does* in order to convey the Main Idea.

Good active reading is the key to these questions; don't wait until you encounter a Main Idea question to think about the Main Point or Bottom Line of the passage. Synthesize the major themes as you read the passage. Distill these themes into a summary of the content and tone of the author's argument or presentation. Don't ignore the author's attitude as expressed in the passage. An answer may have the correct content and scope, but if the tone or attitude doesn't match the passage, the choice is incorrect.

Main Idea questions are often phrased in the following ways:

- "The main idea of the passage is that…"
- "The central thesis of this passage is…"

Primary Purpose questions are often phrased as follows:

- "The author's primary purpose is to explain that…"

Sample Question 3:

3. The primary purpose of the passage is to:

A) enumerate reasons why the inquisitorial system of justice is superior to the adversarial system.
B) argue that both the inquisitorial and adversarial systems of justice should be understood as extensions of an older practice of private vengeance.
C) survey the development and evolution of modern criminal justice procedure.
D) analyze and contrast two different systems of criminal justice.

1) **Read the question word for word and identify the question type.**
   General questions are generally very easy to identify. Here, the words "primary purpose" tip you off.

2) **Translate the question into your own words: identify what the question task is asking you to do with the information in the passage.**
   The question is asking you to summarize the author's overall goal in writing this passage. A good translation of this question would be: "Why did the author describe the two modern criminal procedure systems, as well as the pre-modern system of private vengeance?"

3) **Identify any key words that refer to specific parts of the passage. If key words are provided, *go back to the passage* to locate that information.**

46.3

On Main Idea and Primary Purpose questions, you will not usually need to go back to the passage before reading the choices. Use your original articulation of the Bottom Line to take a first pass or cut through the choices. You may, however, need to go back to the passage when you are down to two or three choices.

4) **Answer in your own words: articulate what the correct answer will need to do, based on the question type and the information in the passage.**

For this type, the correct answer needs to include (explicitly or implicitly) all of the major themes of the passage, without going beyond the scope of the author's argument. Your own answer to this question would be something like: "The author describes the pre-modern system of private vengeance in order to set up contrast between the adversarial and inquisitorial systems; the adversarial system is closer to the system of private vengeance, and the inquisitorial system is more highly evolved."

5) **Use Process of Elimination (POE) to choose the *least wrong* answer choice.**

Common Attractors for Main Idea and Primary Purpose questions will understate or overstate the author's point. Choices that summarize the main idea of a paragraph or two but which leave out other major themes are too narrow. Vague or overly inclusive choices that go beyond the scope of the passage are too broad. Take the "Goldilocks approach": eliminate what is too big or too small, and find the one that is the best fit.

For Primary Purpose questions, focus in part on the verb in each answer choice, and eliminate the ones that are inappropriate; that is, too opinionated, too neutral, or that go in the opposite direction from the passage.

Eliminate choices that are too extreme. Is the author really *proving* or *disproving* a claim, or just *supporting* or *challenging* that claim? Eliminate any verb that expresses an opinion (*criticizing, propounding,* etc.) on a neutral passage (*explaining, describing,* etc.), and vice versa. Be very careful to read and evaluate all parts of each answer choice. An answer choice may begin beautifully, but change halfway through to bring in something inconsistent with or irrelevant to the author's argument. If any part of the choice is wrong, the whole thing is wrong.

Let's take a look at the choices for this question.

- A: No. The verb "enumerate" does not correctly describe the passage. The author does state that the inquisitorial system is "historically superior," but this is the context of explaining how it is further removed from private vengeance and focused on fact-finding.
- B: No. This answer choice is too narrow. In addition to linking these systems of justice to the earlier private vengeance system, the author contrasts the two systems.
- C: No. This choice is too broad. The passage does not provide a general survey of criminal justice procedure. It only discusses and contrasts two systems.
- **D: Yes. While this choice does not explicitly mention the system of private vengeance, it doesn't need to; the author discusses the pre-modern system of private vengeance in order to argue that the inquisitorial system is historically superior to the adversarial system (because the adversarial system is closer to the system of private vengeance).**

Type 4: General—Tone/Attitude Questions

Tone and Attitude questions ask you to evaluate whether or not the author expresses an opinion regarding the material in the passage, and if so, to judge how strongly positive or negative that opinion is. Or, the question may ask you who or what the author is most likely to be. Pure Tone or Attitude questions are somewhat rare (however, Main Idea and Primary Purpose questions always involve assessing the tone of the passage).

Just as for Main Idea and Primary Purpose questions, you must identify the tone of the author through active reading before you begin any of the questions.

When pure Tone/Attitude questions do appear, they are usually general questions, as in the following:

- "In this passage, the author's tone is one of…"
- "The author's attitude can best be described as…"
- "The passage makes it clear that the author is…"

However, Tone/Attitude questions may also appear in Specific form, asking about the author's attitude towards a particular part of the passage (in which case they are Specific Tone/Attitude question), as in:

- "The author's attitude toward Brown's claim can best be described as…"
- "What is the tone of the author's response to Brown's critics?"
- "The author's attitude towards the controversy surrounding Brown's theory can best be characterized as exhibiting…"

Sample Question 4:

4. In the context of the passage discussion of differences between the adversarial and inquisitorial systems, the author's attitude towards the adversarial system appears to be one of:

A) explicit condemnation.
B) mild disapproval.
C) tempered admiration.
D) puzzled exasperation.

1) **Read the question word for word and identify the question type.**
   The word "attitude" is a pretty clear indication of a tone question. Given that the question asks about the author's attitude toward the adversarial system in the context of the contrast between the two systems (i.e., what the passage as a whole is about), this is a General Tone/Attitude question.
2) **Translate the question into your own words: identify what the question task is asking you to do with the information in the passage.**
   This question is asking you what the author's feelings are toward the adversarial system.
3) **Identify any key words that refer to specific parts of the passage. If key words are provided, *go back to the passage* to locate that information.**
   As with most General questions, you already have an answer, based on the passage, in mind. Therefore, you may not need to go back to the passage before you begin evaluating the answer choices. However, you may well need to refer back to the passage during POE.

4) **Answer in your own words: articulate what the correct answer will need to do, based on the question type and the information in the passage.**

The correct answer must be somewhat negative in tone. Although the author is not forcefully condemning the adversarial system, the author does describe it as less evolved and similar to private vengeance. The organization of the passage and the claim that the inquisitorial system is "historically superior" does suggest that it is preferable for a justice system to focus on facts rather than vengeance.

5) **Use Process of Elimination (POE) to choose the *least wrong* answer choice.**

Common Attractors on Attitude and Tone questions are choices that take the author's opinion to extremes. If the passage expresses qualified or moderate admiration, for example, an Attractor may incorrectly describe the author as "enthusiastic." If the author expresses both positive and negative thoughts about a subject, incorrect answer choices may leave out the positive or ignore the negative. Also, positive and negative comments don't cancel each other out to create a neutral tone. If the passage is neutral, any choice that expresses an opinion one way or the other is incorrect.

Beware of choices that express strange attitudes rarely seen in MCAT passages. For example, if you see a choice like "obtuse ambiguity," you should be highly suspicious of it.

Let's apply POE to our sample question:

A: No. This choice is too strong—and too negative. The author does not denounce or explicitly reject the adversarial system.

B: Yes. Although much of the passage is descriptive, the author does suggest that certain characteristics of the adversarial system are somewhat primitive from a modern judicial perspective. Based on the passage information, this is the least wrong choice.

C: No. This choice is too positive. The author does not admire the adversarial system.

D: No. "Exasperation" (irritation or annoyance) would be a strange attitude for an author, and there is nothing to indicate the author is puzzled.

Type 5: Reasoning—Structure Questions

Structure questions ask you to describe how the author makes his or her argument. They differ from other questions in that they address the passage's construction or logical structure along with its content. This is what puts them into the category of Reasoning Questions, even though they almost always relate to one specific area of the passage. Structure questions may ask you for the purpose of a particular reference within the passage. That reference could be to an example, a conclusion, a contrasting point of view, etc. For example, the question stem may cite evidence from the passage and ask you to find the answer that describes the claim or larger point being supported by that evidence. This version of a Structure question often includes the wording "in order to," as in: "The author states X in order to…."

Alternatively, a Structure question might cite a claim from the passage and ask you how, or if, that claim is supported by the author. Similarly, the question may ask what kinds of support are not used in the passage, or what claims are not supported in a particular way; for example: "Which of the following statements is NOT supported by an example or explanation?"

To answer these questions, it is crucial to identify the Main Point of the paragraph or chunk of information in which a reference cited in the question appears, and to separate the claims made by the author from the evidence (if any is given) supporting those claims. Look for words—like *for example* or *for instance*—that indicate that what comes next is the support or evidence, and conclusion words—like *therefore*, *thus*, *so*, or *hence*—that indicate that what comes next is the claim being supported.

It is also possible for Structure questions to appear in General form, asking you to describe the organization of the passage as a whole. When answering a General Structure question, separate the choices into pieces and check for pieces that are out of order, that have an inappropriate tone, or that describe things that never happened in the passage.

Specific Structure questions may be worded as follows:

- "The author probably mentions the controversy surrounding Brown's ideas in order to…"
- "The three experiments carried out by Brown are cited in the passage as evidence that…"
- "The author describes Brown's unique methodology in order to make the point that…"

or

- "Which of the following items of information presented in the passage provides the most support for the author's claim that Brown's methodology is unique?"
- "The author's claim that Brown's methodology is unique is supported by…"
- "Which of the following claims made by the author regarding Brown's methodology is NOT supported by example or reference to authority?"

General structure questions can be phrased as

- "Which of the following best describes the overall organization of the passage?"
- "Which of the following statements best describes the logical progression of the author's argument?"

Sample Question 5:

5. The author quotes the phrase "an eye for an eye and a tooth for a tooth" in order to:

A) give a historical foundation for why self-help is an important aspect of the legal tradition.

B) criticize the violence inherent in pre-modern systems of justice.

C) characterize an aspect of the private vengeance system that has parallels in the modern adversarial system.

D) set up an implicit contrast with the more humane punishments associated with the inquisitorial system.

1) **Read the question word for word and identify the question type.**
The words "in order to" tell you that this is a Structure question.

2) **Translate the question into your own words: identify what the question task is asking you to do with the information in the passage.**
The question is asking you to describe why the author used this phrase at this point in the passage.

3) **Identify any key words that refer to specific parts of the passage. If key words are provided, *go back to the passage* to locate that information.**
The quote "An eye for an eye…" appears in paragraph 1. The author argues that it "captures the essence" of the private vengeance system, in which "the victim of a crime fashioned his own remedy and administered it privately…."

4) **Answer in your own words: articulate what the correct answer will need to do, based on the question type and the information in the passage.**
The correct answer must connect the quote to the system of private vengeance, and describe it as elucidating the notion of self-help characteristic of that system.

5) **Use Process of Elimination (POE) to choose the *least wrong* answer choice.**
For Structure questions, beware of Attractors that describe claims that are made in the passage but that are not relevant to or directly supported by the reference given in the question. Also beware of half right, half wrong choices. All parts of the correct answer choice must check out.

The correct choice must be consistent with the Main Point and tone of the relevant chunk of passage, as well as with the Bottom Line of the passage as a whole.

Let's evaluate the answer choices for our sample questions.

A: No. Although the quote does expand on the notion of "self-help," the context is not an argument about the importance of self-help, but rather a comparison of private vengeance and the adversarial system.

B: No. The tone of this choice is too extreme and too negative for the passage. While the quote does suggest that violence was part of private vengeance system, the tone here is descriptive.

C: Yes. The quote appears in a sentence describing private vengeance as "a system of self-help." Later in the paragraph, the author describes self-help aspects of the adversarial system, since the defendant is personally responsible for his own defense and since the trial takes on characteristics of a duel.

D: No. This answer choice is out of scope. The author gives no indication that this phrase is linked to anything in the description of the inquisitorial system. No punishments in the inquisitorial system are discussed.

Type 6: Reasoning—Evaluate Questions

Evaluate questions are similar to Structure questions in that you need to identify the logical structure of the author's argument. Evaluate questions, however, go a step farther by asking *how well* an author supports his or her claims. That is, the question asks you to evaluate whether or not the author does a good job justifying his or her conclusions.

The answers for these questions often come in two parts. One part will be some version of "strongly" or "weakly" supported. The other part will be the explanation or justification for that evaluation (for example, that it is weakly supported *because* no examples are given, or, strongly supported *because* relevant examples are provided). When choosing an answer, make sure to check that both parts of the choice are supported by the text; that is, both the judgment itself (strongly or weakly) and the justification for that judgment.

Alternatively, an Evaluate question may ask you whether or not the author's logic is valid or internally consistent. The answers to this form of the question may not include the words "strongly" or "weakly," but they will still judge the strength of the author's argument.

These questions may be phrased as follows:

- "The author asserts that Brown's theoretical model is 'dangerously incomplete.' The support offered for this conclusion is…"
- "Is Brown's analysis of the implications of Herrera's theoretical model well supported?"
- "The author's assertion that Brown's model is incomplete is…"

Sample Question 6:

6. How well supported is the author's assertion that the adversarial system is only one-step removed from private vengeance?

A) Strongly supported by the contrast between the adversarial and inquisitorial systems of justice
B) Strongly supported, since the author elaborates on certain overlapping traits of the two systems
C) Strongly supported by a quotation from a respected source
D) Weakly supported, since no other connection between the adversarial system and private vengeance is discussed

1) **Read the question word for word and identify the question type.**

The question asks *how well* supported the author's claim is, which makes it an Evaluate question. Notice that it doesn't just ask *what* the author's claim is (this would be a Retrieval or Inference question).

2) **Translate the question into your own words: identify what the question task is asking you to do with the information in the passage.**

The question is asking to what extent the author chooses to and succeeds in providing relevant evidence for the claim that the adversarial system is closely related to a system of private vengeance.

3) **Identify any key words that refer to specific parts of the passage. If key words are provided, *go back to the passage* to locate that information.**

This question sends you back to paragraph 1. The claim cited in the question comes in the middle of the paragraph. Immediately after the claim, the author discusses particular similarities (as well as some differences) between private vengeance and the adversarial system.

4) **Answer in your own words: articulate what the correct answer will need to do, based on the question type and the information in the passage.**

Read through the examples supporting the claim: The defendant must conduct "his own pretrial investigation," and "the trial is still viewed as a duel between two adversaries." This leads the author to the conclusion that the adversarial system "symbolizes and regularizes punitive combat;" punitive combat characterizes private vengeance. Because the author gives relevant examples, and draws reasonably well-supported conclusions based on those examples, you can say that the claim is strongly supported.

5) **Use Process of Elimination (POE) to choose the *least wrong* answer choice.**

Answer choices are incorrect if they either mischaracterize the strength of the argument or misrepresent the type of evidence in the passage or the way the evidence connects to this claim. Make sure the answer choice looks at the author's explicit argument and evidence for the claim; do not create speculative connections in the text.

Let's go through the answer choices for our sample question:

A: No. While the author does contrast the adversarial and inquisitorial systems, the question is about the author's claim about a different relationship: that between the adversarial system and the system of private justice. The difference between the first two does not support the author's claim about the similarity between the latter two.

B: **Yes. The fact that the defendant must carry out his own pretrial investigation, and that the trial is still seen as a duel, show that the adversarial system retains aspects of private vengeance, even if they are in a somewhat more symbolic or institutionalized form. By showing these similarities, the author provides direct, relevant evidence for the claim that the adversarial system is only one-step removed from private vengeance.**

C: No. While the author does include the "eye for an eye" quotation, this quotation illustrates the nature of private vengeance. It does not provide evidence about the adversarial system.

D: No. Direct, relevant evidence is in fact given (note the phrase "for example" in the passage, directly following the claim cited in the question).

Type 7: Application—Strengthen Questions

A Strengthen question asks you to find the answer that most supports the passage (as opposed to Structure and Evaluate questions, which ask how, if, or how well the author has supported his or her own argument). That is, the correct answer will make the author's argument more convincing than it already was.

Notice that Strengthen questions often use the phrase, "which of the following, if true…." Take those words *if true*—whether implied or explicitly stated—seriously. Do not try to find the answer choices *in* the passage. Take each statement as if it were true and find the one that does what it needs to do *to* the relevant part of the passage. These questions are quite different from Specific, General, and Reasoning questions in that they give you new information in the answer choices; the correct answer will change (for the better), not just describe or reflect, the passage. These questions are also distinct from other question types (except for Weaken questions) in that it is impossible for an answer to be "too extreme" to be correct. You want the answer that goes the farthest in the correct direction.

Strengthen questions may be phrased as follows:

- "Which of the following, if valid, would provide the best support for the author's conclusion in the last paragraph?"
- "Which of the following, if true, would most strengthen the author's claims?"

Strengthen EXCEPT/LEAST/NOT

Strengthen questions can also appear in the EXCEPT/LEAST/NOT format. EXCEPT/LEAST/NOT Strengthen questions have a bit of a twist, compared to most other questions in this format; the correct answer may do the opposite (in this case, Weaken), but they may also just do nothing (have no effect or be irrelevant), or not go as far in the strengthening direction as the three wrong answers (that is, barely strengthen the passage, but less so than the other choices). It is especially crucial to compare choices to each other and pick the one that is the farthest away from strengthening as possible.

The correct answer is the one that goes the farthest to the left along this spectrum.

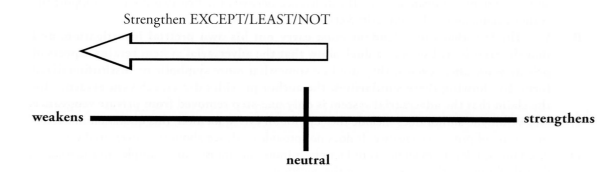

Sample Question 7:

7. Which of the following, if true about typical inquisitorial justice practices, would provide the strongest support for the claim that the inquisitorial system is based on establishing facts?

A) Neither the prosecution nor the defense is allowed to let witnesses testify if they know the witness will make false statements to the court.

B) Prosecutors often describe in detail for the jury the way in which they claim the crime was committed and may even recreate this version in the courtroom.

C) The judge's role is less like a referee and more focused on ensuring that the law is appropriately carried out for each case.

D) The police conduct thorough investigations before the trial to unearth evidence about who committed the crime.

1) **Read the question word for word and identify the question type.**
   The words "provide the strongest support" tell you that this is a Strengthen question.

2) **Translate the question into your own words: identify what the question task is asking you to do with the information in the passage.**
   You will need to take each choice as true, rather than looking for support for the right answer in the passage. The question is asking you to find new evidence (not currently in the passage) that makes the author's claim that the inquisitorial system is based on fact-finding more credible.

3) **Identify any key words that refer to specific parts of the passage. If key words are provided, *go back to the passage* to locate that information.**
   The author claims that the inquisitorial system is based on fact-finding at the beginning of paragraph 3. Read above and below to clarify the claim and see what evidence is already present. The author elaborates that it is establishing the facts of the case (and not just legal rules) that is of central importance in this system.

4) **Answer in your own words: articulate what the correct answer will need to do, based on the question type and the information in the passage.**
   The correct answer will provide new evidence that the inquisitorial system does indeed prioritize establishing the facts of the case over other concerns.

5) **Use Process of Elimination (POE) to choose the *least wrong* answer choice.**
   When using POE on Strengthen questions, eliminate choices that are irrelevant to the cited part or issue in the passage (that is, that are out of scope). Remember, however, that the correct answer will bring in new information—"irrelevant" is not the same thing as "never mentioned."

Do *not* eliminate choices on the basis of absolute or extreme wording. It is impossible on these questions (in contrast to Specific, General, and Reasoning questions) for an answer to be wrong solely on the basis of being too strong. The more it strengthens the passage, the better. In fact, choices on this question type may be wrong because they don't go far enough to have a significant impact on the author's argument. Also, make sure to look out for wrong answers that weaken instead of strengthen by suggesting that the inquisitorial system is not based on fact-finding.

Let's use POE on our sample question.

A: **Yes. This new information about trial rules in the inquisitorial system strengthens the claim that the truth of the facts is a high priority. False testimony would detract from that value and so is disallowed.**

B: No. This choice does not go far enough to strengthen the claim that the truth of the facts of the case is a priority. Notice that only the prosecutor, not the defense, is mentioned, and it is "the way in which *they claim* the crime was committed [emphasis added] that is presented.

C: No. This choice entails the judge's role in enforcing laws, not in establishing the facts of the case.

D: No. While this answer choice does suggest a focus on facts, it does not go far enough to strengthen the claim about the inquisitorial system. This occurs before there even is a court case. Also, the description of the police pre-trial investigation is equally compatible with the account of the adversarial system in the first paragraph.

Type 8: Application—Weaken Questions

A Weaken question requires you to find the answer choice that most undermines or calls into question the claim or claims made by the author.

Notice that just like Strengthen questions, Weaken questions often use the phrase, "which of the following, if true…." Take those words *if true*—whether implied or explicitly stated—seriously. Do not try to find the answer choices *in* the passage. Take each statement as if it were true and find the one that is most *inconsistent* with the relevant part of the passage. These questions are quite different from Specific, General, and Reasoning questions in that they give you new information in the answer choices; the correct answer will change the passage by making the author's argument less convincing than it originally was. These questions are also distinct from other question types (except for Strengthen questions) in that it is impossible for an answer to be "too extreme" to be correct. You want the answer that goes the farthest in the correct direction.

Weaken questions are often phrased as follows:

- "Which of the following, if valid, would most *weaken* the author's point?"
- "Which of the following, if true, would most *undermine* the author's claims?"
- "Which of the following results, if proven to be valid, would most call into question the author's conclusion regarding Brown's methodology?"

You might also see a variation on Weaken questions that cites a statement from the passage and asks you to decide which *answer choice* would be most weakened by that statement. For example,

- "The claims made by Brown, if true, would cast the most *doubt* on which of the following statements?"

Regardless of the wording, you are doing the same thing in answering any Weaken question in the Standard format: finding the answer choice that is *most inconsistent* with the cited part of the passage.

Weaken EXCEPT/LEAST/NOT

As with Strengthen questions, Weaken questions can appear in the EXCEPT/LEAST/NOT format, as in, "Which of the following would LEAST weaken the claims made by the author?" EXCEPT/LEAST/NOT Weaken questions have the same twist as Strengthen questions in this format; the correct answer may do the opposite (Strengthen), but they may also just do nothing (have no effect or be irrelevant), or not go as far in weakening as the three wrong answers (i.e., weaken a little bit but less than the other choices). It is especially crucial to compare choices to each other and pick the one furthest along the spectrum we discussed for Strengthen EXCEPT/LEAST/NOT questions, but in this case in the opposite direction.

The correct answer is the one that goes the farthest to the right along this spectrum.

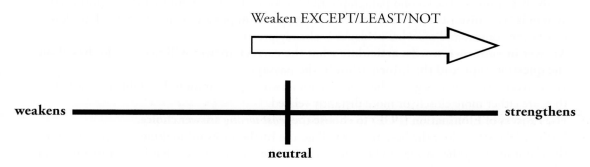

Sample Question 8:

8. The author's claim that the inquisitorial system is two historical steps removed from the system of private vengeance would be most *undermined* if which of the following were established?

A) There is a great temptation for both prosecutors and defense lawyers to try to conceal evidence that they don't want the opposing counsel to know about.

B) The modern inquisitorial system still contains certain forms of symbolic combat.

C) It is the state, not the injured party, who is responsible for determining the appropriate punishment for a convicted defendant.

D) Recently discovered documents indicate that certain adversarial components of the common law tradition were preceded by and evolved from practices more focused on truth-finding than on combat.

46.3

1) **Read the question word for word and identify the question type.**
   The words "most undermined" identify this as a Weaken question. The question is asking you to undermine the author's central argument.

2) **Translate the question into your own words: identify what the question task is asking you to do with the information in the passage.**
   You will need to take each choice as true, rather than looking for support for the right answer in the passage. You will still need to go back to the passage, however, to pin down the credited response. You need the response that most undermines the claim that the inquisitorial system is two steps removed from private vengeance.

3) **Identify any key words that refer to specific parts of the passage. If key words are provided, *go back to the passage* to locate that information.**
   At the beginning of the second paragraph, the author makes the claim that the inquisitorial system is "two historical steps removed from the system of private vengeance." Look back to clarify the context and see what evidence is already present.

4) **Answer in your own words: articulate what the correct answer will need to do, based on the question type and the information in the passage.**
   The correct answer will suggest that there is not a two-step separation. It might suggest that they are either more closely or more distantly related.

5) **Use Process of Elimination (POE) to choose the *least wrong* answer choice.**
   For a Weaken question, the best answer will go the furthest toward making it impossible for the claim made in the passage to be true. Look for the answer choice that is most inconsistent with the relevant part of the passage.

   When using POE on Weaken questions, eliminate choices that are irrelevant to the cited part or issue in the passage (that is, that are out of scope). Remember, however, that the correct answer will bring in new information: "irrelevant" is not the same thing as "never mentioned."

   Do *not* eliminate choices on the basis of absolute or extreme wording. It is impossible on these questions (in contrast to all other question types except for Strengthen questions) for an answer to be wrong solely on the basis of being too strong. The more it weakens the passage, the better.

   In fact, choices on this question type may be wrong because they don't go far enough to have a significant impact on the author's argument.

   Finally, look out for Attractors that strengthen instead of weaken.

Let's use POE on our sample question.

A: No. This information is consistent with the description of the inquisitorial system. That lawyers are tempted does not undermine the claim that the system values truth more than vengeance.

B: No. This does not go far enough to weaken the claim. Although it may contain "certain forms of symbolic of combat," it is still is further removed from vengeance than the adversarial system.

C: No. This choice strengthens the claim, providing additional evidence of separation from private vengeance.

D: Yes. This new evidence challenges the author's description of the timeline by which the inquisitorial system evolved from the adversarial system. If aspects of the inquisitorial system preceded the adversarial system, the author's argument about two-step removal is weakened. That is, it might be even further removed from the system of private vengeance than the author claims. Thus, choice D is the best answer.

Type 9: Application—New Information Questions

All New Information questions have one thing in common: they provide new facts or scenarios in the question stem that are never mentioned in the passage. That said, the question may require you to do a variety of things with that new information. New Information questions break down into two general types.

Type 1: New Information/Inference questions

These questions give you new facts that are in the same general issue area of the passage and then ask what, according to the passage, is likely to be true. In essence, you're inserting the new facts into the existing passage, and then drawing an inference from both the new and the old information. Before you read the answer choices, answer the question in your own words, based on the information already in the passage and on the new facts in the question stem.

For example, the question might ask

- "If China experienced an unusually rainy winter, what would also be true, based on the passage?"
- "According to the passage, what would likely happen if China experienced an unusually rainy winter?"
- "What would the author recommend as the best way to predict whether China is likely to experience an unusually rainy winter next year?"
- "If a meteorologist were to claim that China's climate can be studied in isolation, how would the author respond?"

Type 2: New Information/Strengthen/Weaken questions

These questions provide you with new facts in the question stem (as opposed to pure Strengthen or Weaken questions that give the new information only in the answer choices). They then ask you to evaluate what effect those new facts would have on the author's argument as a whole, or on one specific claim made or described in the passage.

Use the passage much like you do Strengthen, Weaken, and Structure questions. Identify the issue of the question, and go back to the passage to find the relevant sections. Pay close attention to the logical structure of the author's argument. Define what the correct answer needs to do based on the passage, the information in the question stem, and the direction (strengthen or weaken) the correct choice must take.

46.3

This type of New Information question may be phrased as follows:

- "Suppose it was shown to be true that when winters in China are unusually rainy, summers in Latin America are unusually dry. What effect would this have on the author's argument as it is described in the passage?"
- "Which of the following claims made in the passage would be most strengthened by data showing that industrialization has affected global weather patterns?"
- "Recent studies have shown that the jet stream has shifted 10 degrees in latitude over the past five years. This fact tends to *undermine* the author's claim that…"
- "El Niño has been proven to be a recurring and invariant pattern. This fact tends to support the author's claims in paragraph 2 because…"

The following sample question falls into the *Type 1* category.

Sample Question 9:

9. Suppose that within an inquisitorial system, a prosecutor is misdirecting a trial by introducing inaccurate scientific data. The judge would be expected to:

A) intervene only if the defense team objects.
B) admonish the prosecution and have the inaccurate information expunged.
C) ignore the issue, as the judge's responsibility regards points of law rather than points of fact.
D) wait to see whether or not the testimony influences the jurors' decisions.

1) **Read the question word for word and identify the question type.**
   The word "suppose" is our first indication that this is a New Information question. What follows is a scenario that does not already appear in the passage. The question asks you what the author of the passage would advise, making this a *Type 1* question.

2) **Translate the question into your own words: identify what the question task is asking you to do with the information in the passage.**
   The question is asking you to find an answer choice that is consistent both with the passage and with the new situation in the question stem; in this new scenario, the judge discovers that the prosecution is breaking the rules.

3) **Identify any key words that refer to specific parts of the passage. If key words are provided, *go back to the passage* to locate that information.**
   The role of the judge in the inquisitorial system is described at the end of paragraph 2. The judge must "take an active part in the conduct of the trial, with a role that is both directive and protective."

4) **Answer in your own words: articulate what the correct answer will need to do, based on the question type and the information in the passage.**
   Based on the passage, the judge in this situation must take action to protect the defense from the unfair tactics used by the prosecution, and must direct the trial in a way consistent with the system's rules.

5) **Use Process of Elimination (POE) to choose the *least wrong* answer choice.**
A common Attractor for any New Information question is an answer choice that focuses on the wrong part of the passage. Also beware of answer choices that are inconsistent with the passage (for all but the Weaken version of this question type), or that deal with irrelevant issues. This means choices that do not connect to the passage, or that are not relevant to the theme of the new information in the question.

For *Type 1* questions, beware of extreme language. The correct answer can't go too far beyond the scope and tone of the passage.

For *Type 2* questions, beware of choices that go in the opposite direction (e.g., that strengthen instead of weaken, or vice versa).

Let's go through POE on our sample question.

A: No. This is inconsistent with the claim that the judge must take an active role in the proceedings in service of the goal of finding the truth.

B: Yes. This is consistent with the judge's active role and the importance of fact-finding to the court. It correctly responds to the new information and the appropriate passage material.

C: No. This contradicts the passage description of an inquisitorial system in which the court is committed to fact-finding.

D: No. As in choice A, this is inconsistent with the author's claim that judges in the inquisitorial system must play an active role.

Type 10: Application—Analogy Questions

These questions ask you to take something described in the passage, abstract or generalize it, and then apply it to an entirely new situation. They differ from New Information questions in that the new information is in the answer choices, not in the question stem. They differ from Strengthen questions in that the new information in the correct choice will not make the original argument stronger than it already was. It will be similar to it in logic, but is likely to be on a different issue or subject matter.

These questions can be tricky, as all the answers at first glance may seem to have nothing to do with the passage. However, you are matching the logic or purpose of the author's argument, not the informational content of the passage. Therefore, the correct answer can match the logic of the passage (or relevant part of the passage) while still bringing in entirely new content.

Take, for example, a passage in which the author argues the following: "Weather is the result of a global interactive system. Therefore, to understand and predict the weather in a particular region, you must analyze how the climates of all regions interact with each other, and not limit your focus to the weather patterns in that region alone."

46.3

The question might ask

- "Which of the following approaches to educational reform would most likely be advocated by a school board member following the same logic as the author of the passage?"

To answer this question, you must *first* generalize the author's own claims to create an abstracted model that could be applied to other situations. For example, you might say, "Large interactive systems cannot be understood by looking at the parts in isolation from the whole; you must understand how those parts relate to and affect each other," or, more simply, "the whole is more than the sum of its parts."

Now, take this generalized version into the answer choices, and look for a choice that has the same theme. The school board member might place the school system within the context of larger socioeconomic forces that also affect educational performance. Or, she might argue that the school itself is a large interactive system, and that you can't improve education by addressing only one piece of the puzzle (standardized testing, for example). As you can see, a wide variety of answer choices are possible. Don't waste time coming up with specific scenarios; generalize the passage's argument as much as possible, and then match each answer choice against that abstracted model.

Remember that the correct answer must depend solely on the content of the passage, not on outside information or your own opinion!

Sample Question 10:

10. As portrayed in the passage, the historical relationship between the adversarial and inquisitorial systems would be most similar to the relationship between:

A) two competing political parties with different ideals of justice.
B) one style of painting that loses adherents while another style becomes more appreciated and widespread.
C) an old martial arts form closely related to military training exercises and a later form in the same tradition focused more on physical health.
D) the original form of a language and a later dialect that develops from it.

1) **Read the question word for word and identify the question type.**
   The phrase "most similar to" tells you that this is an Analogy question.
2) **Translate the question into your own words: identify what the question task is asking you to do with the information in the passage.**
   The question is asking you to describe and match the logic of the historical relationship between the two justice systems.
3) **Identify any key words that refer to specific parts of the passage. If key words are provided, *go back to the passage* to locate that information.**
   Look back to the passage to clarify what needs to be matched. The historical relationship is described in the second paragraph. The inquisitorial system begins where the adversarial ends and is further removed from private vengeance.

4) **Answer in your own words: articulate what the correct answer will need to do, based on the question type and the information in the passage.**
   You need an answer that matches a historical relationship where one thing evolves from another, moving further away from an original source.

5) **Use Process of Elimination (POE) to choose the *least wrong* answer choice.**
   Keep in mind that all of the answer choices may be on different topics (i.e., not on criminal procedure). The correct choice will be the one that is most similar in logic to the author's portrayal of this historical relationship between the two systems. Be careful to eliminate choices that describe a different logical relationship.

   When you are down to two, eliminate the choice that has any relevant difference when compared to the relationship described in the passage, and pick the choice that has the most similarities. If one of the two remaining choices has one similarity, but the other remaining choice is similar in two ways, the latter choice will be the credited response.

Let's use POE on our sample answer choices.

A: No. Although this answer choice describes a contrast, there is no historical relationship of one evolving from the other.

B: No. Again, this choice does not indicate that one style evolved from the other. Also the passage does not indicate that the adversarial system has become less common.

C: Yes. This choice describes a relationship in which a later form evolves from an earlier one and moves further away from the original source. It is the least wrong of the answer choices.

D: No. This choice is tempting as it does include one form evolving from another. Notice, however, that in the choice, the first language is the original form. This does not match the logic of the passage, since the adversarial system derives from private vengeance and is not an original form.

Now that we have looked at the 10 question types in the Standard format, let's look at examples of the other two formats: EXCEPT/LEAST/NOT and Roman numeral questions.

EXCEPT/LEAST/NOT Questions

This question type can appear in combination with most of the question tasks described above. Because of its potentially confusing structure (looking for the worst instead of the best), students often misread or misapply the question. In fact, the correct answer to this question type can be the wacky or totally irrelevant answer choice that you are used to eliminating first.

To avoid making a mistake, use your noteboard. Write down the passage number (if you haven't already) and the number of the question. Next to the question number jot down a translation of the question, including what kind of choices you will be eliminating. Do this before looking at the answer choices. For example, for a Weaken EXCEPT question, write down

"eliminate what weakens, pick what strengthens or has no effect."

46.3

Also jot down the four letters. As you evaluate each answer choice, write Y (in this case, for *yes*, it does weaken the passage) or N (for *no*, it does not significantly weaken the passage) next to the choice. Cross it off on your noteboard as you strike it out on the screen. At the end, you should have three Ys and one N. Pick the one that is not like the others!

Sample Question 11:

11. All of the following statements are supported by the passage EXCEPT that:

A) the judge's role is more active under the inquisitorial system.

B) in an adversarial system, a prosecutor is unlikely to share evidence with the defendant.

C) the inquisitorial system is more widely practiced in the modern world than is the adversarial system.

D) the vengeance system might well involve a family member of a murder victim seeking to arrange the killing of the suspected murderer.

1) **Read the question word for word and identify the question type.**
   EXCEPT/LEAST/NOT questions are quite easy to recognize. Here, the key word is "EXCEPT." This is an Inference question ("supported by the passage") in EXCEPT/LEAST/NOT format.

2) **Translate the question into your own words: identify what the question task is asking you to do with the information in the passage.**
   This question is asking you to eliminate the choices that are supported by the passage (that is, statements that the author of the passage would accept as true), and to pick the one that is most inconsistent with the author's argument.

3) **Identify any key words that refer to specific parts of the passage. If key words are provided, *go back to the passage* to locate that information.**
   In this question, there is no specific reference to the passage. You will need, however, to go back to the passage as you work through the answer choices. If the question had given you a specific reference (e.g., to "the police department"), you would go back to the passage and read above and below that reference before moving on to the next step.

4) **Answer in your own words: articulate what the correct answer will need to do, based on the question type and the information in the passage.**
   The correct choice will contradict the passage in some way. The incorrect answers will be consistent with the passage information as well as consistent with the author's tone and purpose.

5) **Use Process of Elimination (POE) to choose the *least wrong* answer choice.**
   As you might predict, the most common Attractor is the opposite: a choice that would be the correct answer to a Standard Format question. Approach EXCEPT/LEAST/NOT questions carefully and methodically to avoid falling into this (very annoying) trap.
   Keep in mind that your reasons for eliminating choices on a Standard question (e.g., language that is too extreme, or a statement that mixes up two different things in the passage) now become your reasons for keeping and perhaps selecting an answer.

Let's take a look at our answer choices.

A: No. This choice is directly supported by the end of paragraph 2.

B: No. This choice is supported by the author's contrast between the two forms of justice. Full pretrial discovery and the prosecutor's obligation to potentially exonerate the defendant are presented as traits of the inquisitorial system not shared by the adversarial system.

C: Yes. This answer choice is out of scope. There is no information provided about how widely practiced either form is. So for an EXCEPT question, this is the credited response.

D: No. This choice is consistent with the portrayal of the vengeance system and the "eye for an eye" quotation.

Roman Numeral Questions

Like EXCEPT/LEAST/NOT questions, Roman numeral questions can appear in combination with a variety of question tasks.

To approach these questions, evaluate numeral I (unless it appears in all four choices, in which case it must be true). If it is not an appropriate answer to the question, strike it out, as well as all of the choices that include it. If it *is* appropriate, eliminate the choices that do *not* include it. (If you are not sure about a numeral, leave it and look at the next numeral before eliminating any more answer choices.) Compare the choices you have left with each other. If numeral II or III appears in all of them, read it but don't overthink it. Unless there is something terribly wrong with it, it must also be true based on the combinations you have.

Sample Question 12:

12. Identify which of the following are, according to the passage, obligations of a prosecutor in the inquisitorial system.

    I.   To give to the defense team evidence harmful to her or his own case

    II.   To assist in establishing and recreating the facts of the crime committed

    III.   To elicit testimony from the defendant concerning the facts of the case

    A) II only
    B) III only
    C) I and II only
    D) I and III only

1) **Read the question word for word and identify the question type.**

   This is a Retrieval question ("According to the passage") in Roman numeral format.

2) **Translate the question into your own words: identify what the question task is asking you to do with the information in the passage.**

   The question is asking which of the three statements accurately represent things that are required of a prosecutor within the inquisitorial system.

3) **Identify any key words that refer to specific parts of the passage. If key words are provided, *go back to the passage* to locate that information.**

   The inquisitorial system is described in paragraphs 2 and 3. Prosecutor's duties are specifically mentioned in the context of pretrial discovery, in the second half of paragraph 2 (after the word "additionally," and before the word "finally").

4) **Answer in your own words: articulate what the correct answer will need to do, based on the question type and the information in the passage.**

   Prosecutors in the inquisitorial system must permit full disclosure of all evidence they have uncovered, even if that evidence would help the defense. They must also comply with all of the other rules of the inquisitorial system.

5) **Use Process of Elimination (POE) to choose the *least wrong* answer choice.**

   In some ways, you are approaching the choices just as you would for a Standard question (in our Sample, a Retrieval task). For each numeral, ask yourself if this statement accomplishes the question task (here, if it describes a prosecutor's duty in the inquisitorial system).

   However, you can also often use the combinations in the answer choices to your advantage. You should start with a numeral that appears in exactly two answer choices to maximize the chance that you will be able to eliminate wrong answers immediately. However only eliminate choices based on a single Roman numeral if you are sure that it either is or is not supported. So, for example, if numeral I appears in two answer choices and you are sure it is supported, then you can eliminate the two answers that don't include it.

   If you tend to miss Roman numeral questions, diagnose the most common reasons for your mistakes. If you tend to pick incomplete answers that are missing one or two numerals, you may be reading the numerals too quickly, picking only the ones that are the most obvious, and missing the more subtly supported statements. If you tend to pick choices that include too many, you may not be going back to the passage enough to check your answers carefully against the text.

Let's go through POE on our sample question item by item.

   I: **True. This statement is supported by the author's discussion of pretrial discovery in paragraph 2. Therefore, you can eliminate choices A and B, because neither includes Roman numeral I. You are now down to choices C and D. The difference between them is that choice C includes II but not III, and choice D includes III but not II. It is now a battle between II and III—only one of them can be correct!**

   II: **True. This is also supported by the author's description goal of the overall trial procedure and the prosecutor's role as part of that system. Note that you essentially have the correct answer at this stage, as there is no answer that includes all three numerals.**

   III: False. This is out of scope. Although the prosecutor must turn over relevant evidence, there is no indication of a duty to have the defendant testify.

   So, your credited response is **choice C: I and II only.**

46.4 EXERCISE: IDENTIFYING QUESTION TYPES

Here are 10 sample questions. Read each question carefully, and identify the question type and format. Also think about what this question type is asking you to do.

1. The author references Adam Smith in order to:

2. If it is shown that embrace of Unitarianism occurred only at Harvard and one other New England school, the author would most likely conclude that:

3. The passage suggests which of the following to be true of weaving practices prior to the Industrial Revolution.

4. According to passage information, Beethoven's earliest works:

5. Which of the following claims, if true, would most *undermine* the author's contention that graphic novels have achieved a new prominence in the 21st century?

6. Which of the following is most similar to the experimental methodology described by the author in the fourth paragraph?

7. By "duty" the author most likely means:

8. All of the following strengthen the author's claim that the ADA has not assisted those with mental disabilities EXCEPT:

9. How well supported is the author's claim that rhetoric denying a difference between human and animal suffering undermines the animal rights movement?

10. Which of the following claims is NOT supported by the author's argument in the passage?

Answers for CARS Exercise 1: Identifying Question Types

1. **Structure:** What role does this reference play in the author's argument?
2. **New Information *Type 1*:** What would the author say is true about Unitarianism, based both on the new information and on the existing information in the passage?
3. **Inference:** Which statement about weaving before the Industrial Revolution is best supported by information in the passage?
4. **Retrieval:** Which statement about Beethoven's earliest works is best supported by information in the passage?
5. **Weaken:** Which answer choice goes furthest to suggest that graphic novels did not gain new prominence?
6. **Analogy:** Which choice most describes the same kind of methodology or process as that described in paragraph 4?
7. **Inference:** Which definition of duty best fits with the author's use of that word in the passage?
8. **Strengthen EXCEPT:** Which choice either weakens that claim (by indicating that the ADA has helped those with mental disabilities) or has no effect on that claim? *Eliminate* the choices that confirm the ADA has not helped them.
9. **Evaluate:** Is the author's criticism of rhetoric equating human and animal suffering supported by evidence? If so, how much and what type: is it directly relevant to the claim and of sufficient strength to make the claim believable?
10. **Inference/NOT:** Look for the answer that is least supported by the passage. *Eliminate* the choices that are most supported by the information presented in the passage.

46.4

Individual Passage Log

Passage # _____

Q#	Q type	Attractors	What did you do wrong?

Revised Strategy _____

Passage # _____

Q#	Q type	Attractors	What did you do wrong?

Revised Strategy _____

Chapter 47
CARS: The Process of Elimination (POE) and Attractors

GOALS

1) To learn the principles and steps of working through questions using the Process of Elimination (POE)
2) To recognize patterns in Attractors

47.1 THE PROCESS OF ELIMINATION

As we discussed in the last chapter, there are five basic steps you must take in answering any CARS question.

1) **Read the question word for word and identify the question type.**
2) **Translate the question into your own words: identify what the question task is asking you to do with the information in the passage.**
3) **Identify any key words that refer to specific parts of the passage. If key words are provided, *go back to the passage* to locate that information.**
4) **Answer in your own words: articulate what the correct answer will need to do based on the question type and the information in the passage.**
5) **Use Process of Elimination (POE), and choose the *least wrong* answer choice.**

In this chapter, we'll focus in more detail on Step 5, Process of Elimination, or **POE**.

It is more effective to attack the question by eliminating the three wrong answer choices than by searching for the perfect choice. The MCAT writers are highly skilled at hiding the credited response in obscure and convoluted language, and at creating wrong answer choices that at first glance look good, but have a subtle yet fatal flaw. Your mission is to avoid the traps on your way to the correct choice.

Here are the basic steps of POE. In most cases, you will need to take two "cuts" through the choices as you narrow them down.

First Cut

Read Every Word of Every Choice Carefully.

This is not the time to skim! Once you have misinterpreted or skipped over something, it is very difficult to recognize your mistake.

Eliminate Choices Using the Bottom Line of the Passage.

Remind yourself of the Main Point and tone of the passage and read through each answer choice, eliminating any that violate, or directly contradict, the author's argument (unless it's a Weaken or EXCEPT/LEAST/NOT question). Understanding the passage's Bottom Line will also allow you to quickly eliminate choices that, although they may not contradict the author's points, are not relevant to the passage and thus are out of scope.

Eliminate Choices Inconsistent with Your Own Answer (When Possible, Given the Question Type).

Use your own answer to the question (which should be based closely on the passage and on the question task) as a guideline for eliminating answer choices. Do not, however, eliminate a choice just because it's not a perfect match. Be flexible.

As you gain experience predicting the answer, trust yourself more and more. Don't let an inconsistent answer make you second guess yourself. Your prediction is your life raft: don't abandon it on a whim! On the other hand, if none of the choices are consistent with your prediction, don't force a round peg into a square hole and talk yourself into one that "kind of sounds like" what you were looking for. Carefully re-read the question and go back into the passage to see what you might have missed the first time.

Second Cut

Reread the Question Stem.

Remind yourself (or improve your understanding) of the question type and issue.

Compare the Remaining Choices to Each Other.

Notice strength of language, scope, content references, and any other relevant differences between them.

Go Back to the Passage Again to Pin It Down (When Necessary).

Keep the differences between the choices in mind to help you find where you need to go.

Choose the Least Wrong Answer Choice.

When making your final choice, it's important to keep two things in mind.

1) **Be highly suspicious of absolute or extreme statements.**
   EXCEPT on Strengthen or Weaken questions, correct MCAT answer choices will rarely make an extreme claim. Do not use this test carelessly, however. Simple declarative statements (such as, *The inquisitorial system is historically superior to the adversarial system*) are not necessarily extreme. Look for words that may indicate absolute statements such as *any, all, none, never, always, totally, must, only, exactly, impossible,* etc. Also look out for statements that make extreme claims even without using any of these words.

Notice the wishy-washy or equivocal wording in the previous statement; these words *may*, not *must*, indicate statements that are too extreme for the passage. Whether or not a particular word or statement is extreme depends on how it is used within the context of the answer choice.

2) **If part of an answer choice is wrong, then it's all wrong.**

Pay attention to every word: one incorrect word or phrase will make the entire answer choice wrong. This is one reason why searching for the correct choice—instead of the three wrong choices—may lead you to an incorrect choice. Don't talk yourself into an answer just because you really like one thing about it; something really good about part of an answer can't outweigh a definitively bad part of that same answer. A wrong answer may have something attractive about it, but the credited response won't have anything incorrect in it (or will at least be the best supported of the four).

Any word can make an answer choice wrong. If the answer choice implies that something is true *all* of the time, and the passage suggests that it is true *some* (but *not all*) of the time, then the answer choice cannot be supported by the passage. Pay special attention to words of negation (such as *no, not, none, never*).

47.2   ATTRACTORS

Usually, if you understand the Bottom Line of the passage, it is easy to eliminate two of the four answer choices. But students commonly express this lament: "I always get it down to two choices, and then I pick the wrong one!" That's because the test is designed to make you do this.

For each question, there is usually at least one **Attractor**: an answer choice designed to tempt you into choosing it. It will have something attractive about it, such as words from the passage or concepts similar to those discussed by the author. If you're in too much of a hurry, looking only for the "right" answer, you'll fall for an Attractor much of the time. Remember, the test-writers know how students think and what kind of logical mistakes they tend to make. Take the control away from them by predicting and avoiding the traps.

Typical Attractors

If you look for them, you'll see some patterns appear in the answer choices. The MCAT utilizes a core group of Attractors to tempt those who rush or who do not understand basic ideas presented in the passage. Here are the most common Attractors, grouped into categories. Learn them, look for them, and, thus, defend yourself against them.

Decoys

These choices are written to sound just like the passage. However, they include something that doesn't match up, either with the passage text or the question task.

- **Words out of context**

  This Attractor uses vocabulary right from the passage. It "sounds good," but the meaning of the words is changed. That is, the answer choice uses the right words but carries the wrong meaning. This is a trap in particular for people who are not going back to the passage, or who are not rereading the relevant parts of the passage carefully enough.

- **Half-right/half-wrong**

  These are "bait-and-switch" answers. Part or most of the choice is exactly what you are looking for, but another part is not supported by the passage (e.g., too extreme or out of scope). This is a trap set for people who make up their minds before they read the entire choice, or who try to "rehabilitate" an answer because part of it sounds so good. Remember that one word is enough to make a choice wrong.

- **Opposite/Negations**

  These choices take a sentence or idea directly from the passage, but add or remove a crucial "not" or "un." The statement therefore sounds just like the passage, but in fact directly contradicts it.

- **Reversals**

  This answer choice extracts a relationship from the passage but then reverses it to go in the opposite direction. It may flip a sequence of cause and effect, or confuse the order of events in a chronology.

- **Garbled language**

  This choice gives you some familiar words, but is difficult or impossible to understand. The test-writers are hoping that you will pick it thinking that because it is confusing it must be correct. However, another version of this trap is to put the correct choice into confusing language, with the hope that you will immediately eliminate it because it doesn't "sound good." So, when you see garbled language, don't automatically pick it, but don't automatically eliminate it either. And don't spend five minutes trying to decipher it. Use POE aggressively: there may be a better choice, or it may be the only one left after you have eliminated the other three.

- **Right answer/wrong question**

  The statements in these Attractors, unlike in the other members of this category, are in fact directly supported by the passage. However, they aren't relevant to the question being asked. When you are down to two choices, always reread the question stem in order to avoid this trap.

- **Wrong point of view**

  This is a variation on the right answer/wrong question Attractor. If there is more than one point of view described in the passage, a wrong answer might describe a point of view different from the one referred to in the question stem.

Extremes

These choices go too far in one direction or the other.

- **Absolutes**

  This type of wrong answer uses language that is much stronger than the language in the passage. It may include extreme words such as *none, always, never, only,* etc. Keep in mind, however, that a strongly worded passage may support a strongly worded choice. Also remember that a choice doesn't have to include one of the standard extreme words to be making a claim that is too extreme or absolute in its meaning.

- **Superlatives**

  These wrong answers include words like *first, last, best, most, worst, least* (or anything else ending in *-est*), or *primary*. For instance, it may describe a theory as the *first* or the *best* theory, but the author simply says that it's an important theory.

- **Judgments and recommendations**

  The choice passes judgment on whether something is good or bad, but that thing is described by the author in a neutral tone. Or, the answer choice states that a proposal should be implemented or rejected, when that policy or action is merely described in the passage, or the choice may describe a moderate point of view in overly extreme terms. Finally, a wrong answer may tempt you to intuit the author's state of mind or personal beliefs in a way that is not supported by the passage text.

- **Not strong enough**

  This Attractor is specific to Strengthen and Weaken questions. Rather than being too extreme, it is too wishy-washy to significantly affect the author's argument in the passage. Always compare choices to each other; for this question type, you want the choice that goes farthest in the right direction.

Out of Scope

These answer choices introduce facts, issues, or claims that are never addressed in the passage, or, they do not match the scope of the question task.

- **Not the issue**

  This answer choice brings in ideas or facts that are not discussed in the passage. You will usually eliminate these in your first cut.

- **Outside knowledge**

  The wrong answer makes a statement that is true based on your own knowledge, but isn't directly supported by the text of the passage. Remember that the CARS section tests your ability to read actively and analyze the passage; it does not test your general knowledge.

- **Crystal ball**

  The wrong answer predicts the future (but the passage doesn't) or goes beyond the timeframe of the passage.

- **No such comparison**

  This incorrect choice will take something that is mentioned in the passage and compare it to something that is not. Or, it may take two things that are mentioned by the author and compare them in a way that is not supported by the passage (often by stating that one option is better than the other).

- **Too narrow/too broad**

  The "too narrow" Attractor is typical on General questions: it mentions or contains only part of the author's argument. Keep in mind, however, that correct answers to Specific questions (including Inference questions) can be quite narrow. Wrong answers that are too broad have the opposite problem: they overgeneralize or go beyond the author's argument. They may describe a general category into which the topic of the passage would fit. On General questions, use the "Goldilocks Approach": eliminate any answer choices that are too narrow or too broad, and choose the one that is the best fit.

47.3   POE DOS AND DON'TS

Do

- read and identify the question carefully—predict the traps
- read each answer choice word for word the first time, and consider all parts of every choice
- read all four answer choices carefully and with an open mind before deciding
- be suspicious—look for traps
- notice extreme or absolute wording and compare it to the passage text
- eliminate using the Bottom Line
- eliminate using your own answer
- compare the choices to each other
- go back to the passage often

Don't

- skim the answer choices
- pick the first choice that "sounds good"
- ignore information in a choice, or add something to it, in order to make it fit. (That is, don't force a square peg into a round hole.)
- eliminate choices on Strengthen or Weaken questions because of strong wording
- eliminate choices on Inference questions because of moderate wording
- pick choice D without reading it carefully just because you've eliminated choices A, B, and C
- answer based on memory

47.4   THE SIX STEPS IN ACTION: MODEL PASSAGE

This exercise is intended to give you a picture of what an "ideal" process of attacking a passage looks like. One of your online CARS passages is reproduced on the next two pages.

- First, work through the passage on your own.
- Next, compare your progress through the passage to the model that follows in the book, which takes you from Previewing the Questions all the way through POE.
- The highlighting and noteboard in the sample passage provide a picture of what actual good highlighting and passage notes would look like and why. Keep in mind, however, that it isn't important to have matched them exactly—use the model to see if you caught and highlighted the most important things in the passage text and if you correctly understood the key parts of the author's argument. The questions that follow the highlighted passage are annotated to illustrate the thought process involved in translating the question, using the passage to generate an answer, and doing good POE.

Passage 2 (Questions 1–6)

It is strange that a novelist as superbly imaginative as John Fowles should be content to write within the canons of conventional textbook realism. Of the four stories in *The Ebony Tower*, three are simple, linear structures—situation, complication, resolution—the incidents rationally linked through the probable interactions of credible characteristics, the action and theme neatly illustrating each other. The fourth story is somewhat more open-ended and covert: a picnic in the country that ends in a disappearance and, by implication, a suicide. One has to draw the connections for oneself and see the sudden gathering storm at the end as an epiphany. But this is a technique that Joyce was practicing in *Dubliners* at the turn of the century, and it is still being practiced, from week to week, in the pages of *The New Yorker* and elsewhere.

Yet each of these stories [by Fowles] is anything but obvious or thin. However conventionally they begin and proceed, there comes a point when their issues dramatically engage and take on complexity and power—it's as though one had picked up a simple, familiar object, casually examined it, and suddenly found it shaking in one's hands. By the same token, Fowles' seemingly typecast characters—a lascivious old artist meets his decorous young critic, a timid literary scholar is ripped off by an aggressive hippie—have a way of slipping out of their mold, surprising us first as individuals and then as the strange faces that our most intense experiences tend to take on.

The popular writer turns life into clichés, the artist of realism turns clichés back into life. But why start with clichés in the first place and why tie yourself down to the restrictions and reductions of a plot? Why all this outmoded literary law and order? It's as though a brilliant playwright came upon the scene, a master of illusion, who insists upon practicing the three unities.

One may believe Fowles enjoys being so clever and also the rewards it has brought him as a writer of highly intelligent books that manage to be very popular. But judging from *The Aristos*, his "intellectual self-portrait," Fowles has more ambitious goals in view: in his quiet, detached way, just as much as Mailer does in his very different way, Fowles wants to create a revolution in the consciousness of his time. Still, if this is so, surely he must suspect that his fiction is going about it in the wrong way. Tidy narrative structures, well-rounded characters, consistent point of view, lucid prose, accurate descriptions of times and places—aren't these the techniques at our late state of modernism, that confirm the most retrograde bourgeois tastes,

that are valuable only so that they can then be superseded or, better yet, destroyed by the writer's innovations? Learn the rules so that you know what you're doing when you break them—so the young writer is told. Learn the craft so that you can then practice the art: craft being what all writers are supposed to be able to do, art being what only the individual writer can do because true art is the creation of new *forms* of consciousness, which only the individualist can achieve. Right?

Wrong. Partly wrong in theory and increasingly wrong in practice. New consciousness does not necessarily require new forms in literature any more than it does in any other field of writing. When Shakespeare wrote the "Dark Lady" sonnets, he was doing something original in love poetry, and hence for love itself, though he left the sonnet form undisturbed. And while it is true that new literary forms can provoke new consciousness, it tends more often to work the other way around. In any case, modernism, which has tended to identify individuality with formal innovation exclusively, has left the writers who still subscribe to it increasing high and dry: i.e., rarefied and empty. Or as Fowles himself put it in *The Aristos*: "There is a desperate search for the unique style, and only too often the search is conducted at the expense of content. This accounts for the enormous proliferation in styles and techniques…and for that only too characteristic coupling of exoticism, of presentation, and banality of a theme." If you don't think he is right, pick an anthology of current experimental fiction or poetry and see how much genuine new consciousness you find and how much of the same surreal solipsism, forlorn, or abrasive. Talk about conventionality.

Material used in this particular passage has been adapted from the following source:
T. Solotaroff, *A Few Good Voices in My Head: Occasional Pieces on Writing, Editing, and Reading My Contemporaries* © 1987 by Reed Business Information.

1. The author's example of Shakespeare is used to:

A) describe how Shakespeare changed the sonnet form.
B) illustrate how new forms of literature are required to bring new consciousness.
C) support the claim that writers should not necessarily learn the rules with the goal of eventually breaking them.
D) provide an example of a modernist work.

2. The author states that Joyce and other authors use plotlines similar to Fowles' fourth story in *The Ebony Tower* in order to suggest that:

A) Fowles' prose is more conventional than it seems.
B) Fowles' usage of open-ended and covert plotlines contributes to his ambition to create a revolution in consciousness.
C) the impact of Fowles' work comes more from its content than from formal innovation.
D) Fowles' work is just as good as Joyce's *Dubliners*.

3. Which of these characters or plots from novels would exemplify the author's description in paragraph 2 of Fowles' work?

    I. A private investigator falls for his client. He later discovers that she is his long-lost daughter.
    II. A suburban mother watches as her daughter is slowly dying of a mysterious illness. In the final chapter of the novel, it is revealed that the mother has been poisoning her daughter all along.
    III. The son of a small-town pastor leads the church choir to winning a national singing competition.

A) I only
B) II only
C) I and II
D) I, II, and III

4. Some literary theorists claim that the impact of a literary work is defined not by the intent of the author, but rather by the interaction between reader and text, and that different readers may have very different and at times contradictory reactions to and interpretations of the same text. If valid, what impact would this theory have on Fowles' goal of creating a revolution in consciousness?

A) It would suggest that Fowles could not succeed in his goal because for a revolution to occur there must be agreement on what new views should replace the old way of thinking.
B) It would suggest that Fowles succeeded in his goal because the popularity of his work ensured that it had impact on the thinking of a significant number of people.
C) It would suggest that Fowles misunderstood the complexity involved in creating a revolution in consciousness through literature.
D) It would suggest that achieving Fowles' goal of creating a revolution in consciousness depends on factors that go beyond using conventional forms to express original ideas.

5. What is "conventional textbook realism" as it is defined in the passage?

A) A novel with a simple story structure and believable outcome
B) Stories that are based on real-life events
C) A story based on use of stereotypical characters
D) Stories that begin conventionally and then reveal unexpected levels of complexity

6. Which of the following statements, if true, would most *undermine* the author's argument?

A) Rules are not valuable only when they are destroyed by a writer's innovative techniques.
B) Mailer's writing is often described as aggressive.
C) Literature that contributes to a transformation in consciousness is often only recognized as such many decades after it is written.
D) Fowles intended for *The Aristos* to be partially autobiographical.

Ranking the Passage

Abstract passage content = Later/Killer passage

Previewing the Question Stems

Below are the question stems only. The key words to note in the Preview stage are highlighted. Remember, you are only looking for references to passage content at this point in the process.

1. The author's example of Shakespeare is used to:

2. The author states that Joyce and other authors use plotlines similar to Fowles' fourth story in *The Ebony Tower* in order to suggest that:

3. Which of these characters or plots from novels would exemplify the author's description in paragraph 2 of Fowles' work?

4. Some literary theorists claim that the impact of a literary work is defined not by the intent of the author, but rather by the interaction between reader and text, and that different readers may have very different and at times contradictory reactions to and interpretations of the same text. If valid, what impact would this theory have on Fowles' goal of creating a revolution in consciousness?

Note: When a question is this long, you may want to skip it in the Preview stage.

5. What is "conventional textbook realism" as it is defined in the passage?

6. Which of the following statements, if true, would most *undermine* the author's argument?

Note: There is no reference to specific passage content here—skip it in the Preview stage.

47.4

TONE · LIST INDICATORS—CONTRAST

QUESTION TOPICS

PIVOTAL WORD

TONE

PIVOTAL WORDS— CONTRAST

PIVOTAL WORD/ LEADING QUESTION

SUGGESTED PIVOT

ACTUAL PIVOT

COMPARISON/ CONTRAST

QUESTION TOPIC

SUGGESTED PIVOT/ LEADING QUESTION

COMPARISON

AUTHOR'S/ FOWLES' POSITION

QUESTION TOPIC

PIVOTAL WORDS/ CONTRAST

TONE

It is strange that a novelist as superbly imaginative as John Fowles should be content to write within the canons of conventional textbook realism. Of the four stories in *The Ebony Tower*, three are simple, linear structures—situation, complication, resolution—the incidents rationally linked through the probable interactions of credible characteristics, the action and theme neatly illustrating each other. The fourth story is somewhat more open-ended and covert: a picnic in the country that ends in a disappearance and, by implication, a suicide. One has to draw the connections for oneself and see the sudden gathering storm at the end as an epiphany. But this is a technique that Joyce was practicing in *Dubliners* at the turn of the century, and it is still being practiced, from week to week, in the pages of *The New Yorker* and elsewhere.

Yet each of these stories [by Fowles] is anything but obvious or thin. However conventionally they begin and proceed, there comes a point when their issues dramatically engage and take on complexity and power—it's as though one had picked up a simple, familiar object, casually examined it, and suddenly found it shaking in one's hands. By the same token, Fowles' seemingly typecast characters—a lascivious old artist meets his decorous young critic, a timid literary scholar is ripped off by an aggressive hippie—have a way of slipping out of their mold, surprising us first as individuals and then as the strange faces that our most intense experiences tend to take on.

The popular writer turns life into clichés, the artist of realism turns clichés back into life. But why start with clichés in the first place and why tie yourself down to the restrictions and reductions of a plot? Why all this outmoded literary law and order? It's as though a brilliant playwright came upon the scene, a master of illusion, who insists upon practicing the three unities.

One may believe Fowles enjoys being so clever and also the rewards it has brought him as a writer of highly intelligent books that manage to be very popular. But judging from *The Aristos*, his "intellectual self-portrait," Fowles has more ambitious goals in view: in his quiet, detached way, just as much as Mailer does in his very different way, Fowles wants to create a revolution in the consciousness of his time. Still, if this is so, surely he must suspect that his fiction is going about it in the wrong way. Tidy narrative structures, well-rounded characters, consistent point of view, lucid prose, accurate descriptions of times and places—aren't these the techniques at our late state of modernism, that confirm the most retrograde bourgeois tastes, that are valuable only so that they can then be superseded or, better yet, destroyed by the writer's innovations? Learn the rules so that you know what you're doing when you break them—so the young writer is told. Learn the craft so that you can then practice the art: craft being what all writers are supposed to be able to do, art being what only the individual writer can do because true art is the creation of new forms of consciousness, which only the individualist can achieve. Right?

Wrong. Partly wrong in theory and increasingly wrong in practice. New consciousness does not necessarily require new forms in literature any more than it does in any other field of writing. When Shakespeare wrote the "Dark Lady" sonnets, he was doing something original in love poetry, and hence for love itself, though he left the sonnet form undisturbed. And while it is true that new literary forms can provoke new consciousness, it tends more often to work the other way around. In any case, modernism, which has tended to identify individuality with formal innovation exclusively, has left the writers who still subscribe to it increasing high and dry: i.e., rarefied and empty. Or as Fowles himself put it in *The Aristos*: "There is a desperate search for the unique style, and only too often the search is conducted at the expense of content. This accounts for the enormous proliferation in styles and techniques… and for that only too characteristic coupling of exoticism, of presentation, and banality of a theme." If you don't think he is right, pick an anthology of current experimental fiction or poetry and see how much genuine new consciousness you find and how much of the same surreal solipsism, forlorn, or abrasive. Talk about conventionality.

Material used in this particular passage has been adapted from the following source:
T. Solotaroff, *A Few Good Voices in My Head: Occasional Pieces on Writing, Editing, and Reading My Contemporaries* © 1987 by Reed Business Information.

Model Noteboard Notes

This is what your noteboard for this passage might look like:

Passage [#] Q 1–6

¶ 1)   Fowles—conventional techniques
¶ 2)   But surprising complexity
¶ 3)   So why use conventions?
¶ 4)   Misguided approach?
¶ 5)   No—new form ≠ new consciousness

BL: Fowles' conventional form for new consciousness (author supports)

Attacking the Questions

The questions below are annotated to represent the thought process you would go through in answering the questions, not to represent the actual appearance of the screen. Remember, on the test, you can only strike out or select entire answer choices; partial strikeouts are not possible. The explanations to the right of each choice model a first cut through the answers: what you may have eliminated and why, and what you might have left in. The "Down to Two" explanations to the left describe the reasoning that you would use to eliminate down to the correct answer in your second cut.

47.4

1. The author's example of Shakespeare is used to:

A. describe how Shakespeare ~~changed~~ the sonnet form. **Opposite—he didn't**

B. illustrate how new forms of literature ~~are required~~ to bring new consciousness. **(Left it in)**

C. support the claim that writers should not necessarily learn the rules with the goal of eventually breaking them. **(Left it in)**

D. provide an example of a modernist work. **Words out of context—example makes larger point about literature, not just about modernism**

> **Question Type:** Structure
> **Translation:** Why does the author discuss Shakespeare?
> **Back to the Passage:** Last paragraph—Shakespeare did something original but used existing sonnet form
> **Answer:** To show that position described at end of previous paragraph is wrong

> **Down to Two—Compare:**
> Choices B and C are opposites of each other. Choice C fits the Bottom Line, although it is tricky—have to see relationship between paragraphs 4 and 5, and that paragraph 5 is denying validity of the position described at end of paragraph 4 ("Right? Wrong.").

2. The author states that Joyce and other authors use plotlines similar to Fowles' fourth story in *The Ebony Tower* in order to suggest that:

A. Fowles' prose is more conventional ~~than it seems.~~ **(Left it in)**

B. Fowles' usage of open-ended and covert plotlines contributes to his ambition to create a revolution in consciousness. **Contradicts point of the paragraph and Bottom Line—it wasn't his plotlines that did this**

C. the impact of Fowles' work comes more from its content than from formal innovation. **(Left it in)**

D. Fowles' work is ~~just as good as~~ Joyce's *Dubliners*. **Not the issue/No such comparison on quality**

> **Question Type:** Structure
> **Translation:** Why does the author state that other authors use similar plotlines?
> **Back to the Passage:** First paragraph—part of discussion of Fowles' use of conventional textbook realism (later says that issues within them are complex)
> **Answer:** To provide evidence that Fowles did not use innovative techniques to achieve his effect

> **Down to Two—Compare:**
> Both have idea of conventional form, but choice A suggests that it seemed unconventional, while passage argues the opposite. Seeing the validity of choice C requires connecting paragraph 1 to the Bottom Line.

3. Which of these characters or plots from novels would exemplify the author's description in paragraph 2 of Fowles' work?

I. A private investigator falls for his client. He later discovers that she is his long-lost daughter. **Twist/unexpected: yes**

II. A suburban mother watches as her daughter is slowly dying of a mysterious illness. In the final chapter of the novel, it is revealed that the mother has been poisoning her daughter all along. **Twist/unexpected: yes**

III. The son of a small-town pastor leads the church choir to winning a national singing competition. **Totally expected: No**

A. I only
B. II only
C. I and II
D. I, II, and III

Eliminate anything with III. I and II are so similar that you can't include one without the other.

Question Type: Analogy
Translation: Which is most similar to Fowles' work as it's described in second paragraph?
Back to the Passage: Begins conventionally, but complex and powerful
Answer: Begins in familiar way, then surprises us with more complexity (maybe character that does something unexpected)

47.4

4. Some literary theorists claim that the impact of a literary work is defined not by the intent of the author, but rather by the interaction between reader and text, and that different readers may have very different and at times contradictory reactions to and interpretations of the same text. If valid, what impact would this theory have on Fowles' goal of creating a revolution in consciousness?

A. It would suggest that Fowles could not succeed in his goal because for a revolution to occur there must be agreement on what new views should replace the old way of thinking. **Too extreme/Out of scope**

B. It would suggest that Fowles succeeded in his goal because the popularity of his work ensured that it had impact on the thinking of a significant number of people. **Too extreme/Out of scope**

C. It would suggest that Fowles misunderstood the complexity involved in creating a revolution in consciousness through literature. **(Left it in)**

D. It would suggest that achieving Fowles' goal of creating a revolution in consciousness depends on factors that go beyond using conventional forms to express original ideas. **(Left it in)**

Question Type: New Information (Strengthen/Weaken)
Translation: If it's true that effect of work depends on various reader interpretations, not just author, how would this affect Fowles' goal?
Back to the Passage: Fowles' goal most directly discussed in paragraph 4. Passage never discusses role of readers' interpretations.
Answer: Would have to take this additional factor into account.

Down to Two—Compare:
Choice C indicates that Fowles was unaware of this, but we don't know that. Choice D only indicates that there are additional factors. Choice D is more moderate, and within the scope of the passage and question stem information.

5. What is "conventional textbook realism" as it is defined in the passage?

(A) A novel with a simple story structure and believable outcome (**Left it in**)

~~B.~~ Stories that are based on ~~real-life events~~
Out of scope/Outside "knowledge"

~~C.~~ A story based on use of ~~stereotypical characters~~
Fowles' characters only *seem* typecast or stereotypical

~~D.~~ Stories that begin conventionally and then ~~reveal unexpected levels of complexity~~ (**Left it in**)

Question Type: Inference

Translation: What is "conventional textbook realism," as described in passage?

Back to the Passage: Paragraph 1—simple, linear structure, credible, not innovative

Answer: What the passage said

Down to Two—Compare:

Both choices A and D describe Fowles' work, which uses conventional realism. But only choice A is given as part of the description of realism more generally, while choice D is specific to Fowles' work. Choice A is a close paraphrase of the passage description.

6. Which of the following statements, if true, would most *undermine* the author's argument?

~~A.~~ Rules are ~~not~~ valuable only when they are destroyed by a writer's innovative techniques. (**Left it in**)

~~B.~~ Mailer's writing is often described as aggressive.
No effect on passage (paragraph 4—author already says Mailer different)

(C) Literature that contributes to a transformation in consciousness is often only recognized as such many decades after it is written. (**Left it in**)

~~D.~~ Fowles intended for *The Aristos* to be partially autobiographical. **Strengthens/Consistent with "intellectual self-portrait" (paragraph 4)**

Question Type: Weaken

Translation: What would be most inconsistent with author's claims in the passage?

Back to the Passage: Bottom Line—Fowles' conventional form for new consciousness (author supports)

Answer: Either that innovative form does/might lead to new consciousness, or that conventional form does not

Down to Two—Compare:

Choice A has tricky wording and connects to tricky relationship between last two paragraphs. But when translated, it's consistent with author's real position in last paragraph: it strengthens, not weakens. Connection of choice C to passage is less obvious, but it's inconsistent with argument in last paragraph: it suggests that "current experimental fiction or poetry" might eventually lead to a new consciousness.

Individual Passage Log

Passage # _____

Q#	Q type	Attractors	What did you do wrong?

Revised Strategy _____

Passage # _____

Q#	Q type	Attractors	What did you do wrong?

Revised Strategy _____

Chapter 48
CARS Section-Wide Strategy

GOALS

1) To better understand the organization of the MCAT CARS section
2) To learn to assess the difficulty levels of passages
3) To improve your strategy for attacking the section as a whole

48.1 FOCUS ON PACING

Now that you have the basic strategies for attacking a passage down, it is time to refine your approach, not only to individual passages, but to the section as a whole. This means making good choices about how and where you spend your time. By this point, you should begin timing yourself on your practice passages. If your reasonable goal is to complete eight passages with high accuracy and randomly guess on one passage, as a rule of thumb, it should take you about 11 minutes per passage. If your reasonable goal is to complete all 9 (which is only reasonable if you are already scoring well), that entails taking about 10 minutes per passage. Keep in mind that this is only an approximation. A passage with seven questions will take you a bit longer than a passage of equal difficulty with only five questions, and a more difficult passage will legitimately take you a little longer to complete than an easier passage.

Here are some specific guidelines to help you to decide on an appropriate pacing plan for your target score.

Pacing Guidelines

The sections on the following pages describe the appropriate pacing for various CARS target score levels. Use your CARS score on your most recent practice test to determine which targets are most appropriate. If you are not hitting the accuracy goals for your current target level, you should not be trying to speed up or answer more questions. Once you are consistently hitting those targets, you may be ready to attempt the next level.

Current Score Level: Below Average

Target Score: Average

Pacing and Accuracy Goals: 7–8 Passage Pace
In this score range, it is critical that you identify easier (Now) passages and perform with high accuracy. Do not waste time on Killer passages, or spend too much time on Later passages. Plan to skip over at least three or four passages on your first pass through the section.

Now Passages (4):
You should spend 11–12 minutes on each of these passages. The reading should take 4–5 minutes and each question should take on average 1–1.5 minutes. Work carefully and use POE in order to avoid errors.

Accuracy Goal:
0–1 mistakes per passage

Later Passages (3):
You should spend 13–14 minutes on each of these passages. The reading should take 5–6 minutes and each question should take on average 1–2 minutes. If you are taking a very long time on a question or just don't understand it, guess on that question and move on.

Accuracy Goal:
0–2 mistakes per passage

Killer Passages (2):
You should mostly be guessing on these passages. If after finishing the other passages, you have a few minutes left, pick another passage and read just the first and last sentences of the text. Then look for Specific questions with paragraph references or lead words. Use aggressive POE. Don't spend too much time on any one question. Make sure you have guessed on every question before time runs out.

Accuracy Goal:
At least 1 correct answer

Current Score Level: Average
Target Score: Average-High

Pacing and Accuracy Goals: 8–9 Passage Pace
In this score range, it is critical that you not become distracted by the hard or Killer passages early in the test. Plan to skip at least two or three passages on your first pass through the test. Make sure you start with a Now passage and at your target pace.

Now Passages (5):
You should spend 10–11 minutes on each of these passages. The reading should take 3–4 minutes and each question should on average take 1–1.5 minutes. Work carefully and use POE in order to avoid errors.

Accuracy Goal:
0–1 mistakes per passage with ideally at least two perfect passages

Later Passages (3):
You should spend 11–12 minutes on each of these passages. The reading should take 4–5 minutes and each question should on average take 1–1.5 minutes. If a question is taking a very long time, or you don't understand it at all, use aggressive POE, pick an answer, and move on. You may also choose to randomly guess on several of the hardest questions in some of the passages that you complete.

Accuracy Goal:
0–2 mistakes per passage

Killer Passages (1):
You should be mostly guessing on one passage. If you start working on a passage early in the test and realize it is a killer, immediately move on to easier passages. If you have time after completing the Now and Later passages, go to the remaining passage and read just the first and last sentence of each paragraph. Then look for Specific questions (or, if there are no Specific questions, Structure questions) with paragraph references and/or lead words from the passage. Use aggressive POE. Don't spend too much time on any single question. Make sure you have guessed on every question before time runs out.

Accuracy Goal:
At least 1 correct answer

Current Score Level: Average-High
Target Score: High

Pacing and Accuracy Goals: 9 Passage Pace
You should only be attempting a 9-passage pace if you have consistently achieved the accuracy goals of previous levels. At this pace, plan to skip at least one or two passages on your first pass through the test. Make sure you start with a passage that is not too difficult and to hit a good pace at the beginning.

Now Passages (6–7):
You should spend 8–9 minutes on each of these passages. The reading should take 2.5–3.5 minutes and each question should on average take 1 minute or less. Work carefully and use POE in order to avoid errors.

Accuracy Goal:
0–1 mistakes per passage with at least three perfect passages

Later Passages (1–2):
You should spend 10–11 minutes on each of these passages. The reading should take 3.5–4.5 minutes and each question should on average take 1 minute or less. If a question is likely to take longer than 1.5 minutes or is confusing, skip it and look at it again before moving on to the next passage. You may also choose to "cherry-pick," that is, randomly guess on 2–3 of the hardest questions in these passages. If you employ this strategy, you will need to get almost every other question correct in order to achieve the target score.

Accuracy Goal:
0–1 mistakes per passage, with at least two perfect passages

Killer Passages (1):
Your approach to your last passage will depend on how much time you have left. To get a score at the top of the scale, you have to attack every passage and get almost all of the questions correct. However, you don't necessarily have to attempt every single question. You should not spend more time than usual reading the passage; instead, keep your focus on main points and tone. Use aggressive POE and don't spend too much time on any single question. However, don't rush through all the questions if you are running out of time. Make a good attempt at most of them, and if needed, guess on one or two particularly difficult questions within the set. Make sure you have answered every question before time runs out.

Accuracy Goal:
At least 3 correct answers

Diagnosing Pacing Problems

If you are not hitting the right pace to achieve your target score, you must

1) diagnose what is wrong with your current pace, and
2) adjust accordingly.

So, let's first look at four basic pacing issues.

1) **Going too fast**
   There are three signs that your score will improve if you slow down and do fewer questions.
   - You are finishing nine passages but consistently missing two or more questions on every passage, or if you often miss more than half of the questions for a passage (that is, you do well on some passages but crash and burn on others).
   - You realize that you often miss easy questions. This means that when you go over a test, many or most of the questions that you got wrong look obvious in retrospect. You can't imagine why you didn't pick the credited response, and you can't really remember why you liked that wrong answer so much.
   - You are completing all nine passages and not getting a significantly above-average score.

2) **Going too slow**
   If one or more of the following describes you, increasing your speed and efficiency will improve your score:
   - You consistently get all or almost all of the questions that you do correct, but you are doing eight or fewer passages.
   - You spend a disproportionately high amount of time on a few passages or a few questions.
   - You spend 6 or more minutes reading the passage text the first time through.
   - You find yourself over-thinking the passage and/or the questions, spending a lot of time talking yourself into wrong answers.

3) **Getting bogged down in a Killer passage**
   Let's imagine two hypothetical students and compare their different approaches to the Killer passage:
   - **What the first student, untrained in strategy, does with the Killer passage:**
     She slows down, gets lost and distracted while reading, and spends too much time going back and rereading long sections of the passage. She gets caught up in deciphering fancy vocabulary words.
     When she moves into the questions, she goes even slower; she has spent so much time reading the passage that she feels that she has to get all of the questions right to justify it. At some point, the student realizes anxiously that too much time has passed and she guesses on the last two or three questions of the passage before moving on, stressed out and perspiring. She then speeds through the other easier passages, trying to make up for lost time, making foolish errors and throwing away easy points.
   - **What the second, trained student does with the Killer passage:**
     Skips it (or does it last of all)
     By randomly filling in all of the answer choices on the Killer Passage, the second student frees up at least 10–15 minutes that may well have been wasted on getting questions wrong. And if she does complete it, she does it last so that it doesn't negatively affect how she does on the easier passages.

4) **Getting bogged down on a Killer question**

Even Now and Later passages can have a question that is extremely hard for you. You can't allow yourself to get sucked into that one question, if doing so means you are losing the opportunity to answer two or more easier questions down the road.

48.2 REFINING YOUR PACING

Once you have decided if you need to slow down or speed up, the next question is HOW?

Slowing Down

This is not as obvious as it seems. Don't spend the time that you save by doing fewer questions or passages on excessive rereading. Also, don't sit and ponder difficult parts of the passage at great length, or come up with elaborate justifications for why a variety of answer choices might be correct. It is still important to be tightly focused and efficient, even when slowing down your pace.

Instead, invest the extra time in the following:

- translating the question and clearly identifying the question type and task,
- reading the answer choices more carefully: that is, word for word,
- comparing choices to each other and specifically looking out for common traps,
- and—most importantly—in going back to the passage to find the relevant information and defining what the correct answer needs to do.

Speeding Up

There are four common ways in which students get bogged down and lose time. To pick up your pace, focus on avoiding these traps.

1) **Reading the passage too carefully the first time through**

If you are reading every word, and highlighting the passage heavily, then you're reading the passage like a college course book rather than a CARS passage. You may feel safer going into the questions having consistently spent 6 or more minutes with the passage, but the test doesn't allow you the time to do so. Cut to the chase the first time through, and save the more careful rereading for answering the questions. (Review Chapter 44.)

2) **Not reading and translating the question carefully**

If you go back into the passage without a clear idea of what you're looking for, you are likely to get lost and waste precious time backtracking to reread the question, or getting stuck in the answer choices because nothing fits what you first thought the question was asking. Spend a few more seconds translating the question, and the correct answers will come a lot more quickly. (Review Chapter 45.)

3) **Not aggressively using POE**

You can waste a huge amount of time looking for a perfect answer instead of the "least wrong" answer. Trying to make a watertight case for the credited response when it is one of those "not great, but the best of what I've got" answers will not only suck up a lot of time and energy, it will also often cause you to talk yourself out of the correct choice. Maintain a critical focus through the entire POE process. (Review Chapter 47.)

4) **Overcommitting to one question or one passage**

- Learn to recognize quickly whether you understand a test question or not. Are you rereading it over and over? Are you bouncing repeatedly (three or more times) from passage to question and back again? If so, these are clear signs that this question is not working for you (that is, it's very difficult). Many people become stubborn about seeing a question through; they think that because they have devoted some time already to the question, they can't abandon that question because doing so means they have wasted time. But spending even more time on a question that is particularly difficult means nothing more than wasting more time. You can't change the past, but you don't have to continue in an effort that is unlikely to yield a point.

- If you doubt this logic, consider the following analogy. If you have dated someone for six months and realize that the person is a jerk, do you say, "Well, I don't want to have wasted the past six months, so I better get married to the jerk?" No! You move on, chalk up the episode to experience, and look for someone easier to get along with. Bringing it back to the world of the MCAT, in this situation use POE, take your best shot, and move on.

- However, don't go to the opposite extreme. If you are getting it down to two and then guessing on a majority of questions, your accuracy will significantly suffer and your score will go down, not up.

- Don't spend a high percentage of your resources on a single passage. More difficult passages should take a bit more time, but you need to keep moving. Remember that in many cases, hard passages have been edited in such a way that some things are never fully explained or clarified; you could read it ten times over and still not really "get it." Luckily, in most cases you don't need to understand every aspect of the passage to get most of the questions right.

Try the pacing exercise on the next page if your accuracy is good but you need to increase your speed.

Avoiding Killer Passages

Use your previous experience to refine your ranking technique. Each time you rank a passage as Now, and it turns out to be a Later or Killer, go back and re-evaluate the passage and the questions to see what made it harder than you expected, and how you could have recognized it earlier.

Conversely, every time you misidentify an easy passage as a difficult passage, do the same. Look in particular for passages with unfamiliar subject matter that you ranked as Later or Killer that were relatively easy once you got into them.

It is dangerous to rank passages on the basis of familiarity; it is really the difficulty of the language and of the question types that makes for a hard passage.

Exercise 1: Speeding Up Your Pacing

Do this exercise if you have excellent accuracy on the passages that you actually complete, but can only complete a limited number of passages under timed conditions. You may wish to spread this exercise out over a few days or weeks.

Do a nine-passage section (or look at your most recent practice test), and note the average time spent per passage here._____

Now do four more passages back to back (or, an entire nine-passage test section), but give yourself one less minute per passage. Use the suggestions in this chapter to diagnose areas where you may be wasting time, and to work through those areas more efficiently. If you complete those passages with good accuracy, reduce your time per passage by another 30–60 seconds and do another set of passages.

Continue this process until your accuracy begins to suffer. Note the average time spent per passage here._____

Carefully diagnose the reasons for your mistakes, and continue to work at that pace until your accuracy improves to your previous level.

Continue this exercise until you hit the appropriate pace for you.

Exercise 2: 5-Minute Drill

If you have about 5 minutes left when you've finished a passage, do not begin to carefully read the next Later or Killer passage in your ranking. If you do, you will run out of time with few or no questions answered. Instead, quickly read the first and last line of each paragraph. If it's a two-sentence paragraph, just read the first line. Next, click through the questions and pick out the easier Specific questions (such as Retrieval, and Inference questions with lead words and/or paragraph references) and do those first, going back to the passage to hunt down and read the relevant sections. You have a good chance of getting those easier questions right, even with little time remaining.

If you have time left after doing these Specific questions, take a shot at any Main Idea or Primary Purpose questions, using what you have now learned about the major themes of the passage. Be sure to rely heavily on POE, thinking actively about identifying and avoiding common Attractors. Even if you only have a minute left, you can probably at least eliminate one or two answer choices on one General question, or even a Reasoning or Application question.

So, imagine that the 5-minute warning has come up on the screen, just as you have completed a passage. Your goal now is to get what you can out of the seven questions for the passage on the next pages in the few minutes you have left.

Passage 3 (Questions 1–7)

Formal and informal reactions to crime are distinguished by whether they are administered by representatives of the state. Government officials administer formal reactions, such as penal sanctions. Informal reactions are sanctions imposed by non-state functionaries, usually ordinary citizens. These sanctions include all the detrimental consequences that convicted offenders experience that are not formally specified by law or pronounced by a judge in the disposition. To lose one's job or be ridiculed by others are examples of informal sanctions. Since equality before the law is such a symbolically important part of the criminal justice system, many investigators have examined the legal and extralegal determinants of formal sanctions. For example, the effects of offense and offender characteristics on variations in criminal sentences have been investigated extensively. By contrast, informal reactions to crime have received minimal analytic attention. This failure to explore the determinants of informal sanctions distorts understanding of the links between social structure and social control.

Position in the stratification hierarchy is one of the factors that determine susceptibility to law. Those in low positions are more susceptible to law in that, among other things, their crimes are more harshly sanctioned. The same is true for non-governmental forms of social control. Just as inequality in wealth and power influences decision-making in courtrooms, it also affects how offenders are treated in workplaces and in the community. Criminal conviction has been shown to reduce the employment opportunities of working-class defendants. Case studies of powerful corporate executives who have committed egregious offenses find that they often continue to hold respected positions in both the economic and social worlds. These studies suggest that the "stigmatizing effects" of criminal conviction are not damaging for some white-collar offenders.

Less powerful white-collar offenders may be more stigmatized by criminal conviction than business executives. For example, professionals and public-sector workers convicted of white-collar crimes lose occupational status more often than business executives convicted of similar offenses. The consequences of legal stigma may be influenced more by the offender's class position than by his or her criminal conduct.

The extent of social condemnation presumably varies directly with the seriousness of offense and severity of the criminal sentences received. In theory, those who commit minor offenses provoke little censure from the community-at-large and receive lenient treatment in the legal system. Those who commit more serious offenses do not fare as well: they may receive both stronger social condemnation and harsher punishment. Since judges supposedly deem informal sanctions, such as loss of status, sufficient punishment for white-collar offenders, they may impose less severe sentences on those who experience those sanctions. Consequently, formal and informal reactions to white-collar crime may not be consistent.

Material used in this particular passage has been adapted from the following source:

M. L. Benson, "The Influence of Class Position on the Formal and Informal Sanctioning of White-Collar Offenders," *Sociological Quarterly.* © 1989.

1. It can be inferred from the passage that the courts would treat social isolation of an accused business executive as:

A) an expected consequence of public accusations but not relevant to the judicial process.
B) a more potent form of punishment than even a prison sentence.
C) a situation that, since not truly measurable, cannot be considered punitive.
D) a legitimate form of punishment that is often considered before a sentence is determined.

2. According to the passage, which of the following is a ramification of the failure to examine the determining factors of informal sanctions?

A) A misunderstanding of the relationship between the structure of society and sanctions that are used to control criminal behavior
B) A reduction of employment opportunities for working-class defendants
C) An inability to establish effective punitive measures using formal sanctions on criminal behavior
D) The ability of numerous business executives convicted of criminal offenses to maintain respectable positions

3. Which one of the following best describes the author's reaction to the two forms of sanctions discussed in the passage?

A). Frustration that class position is a factor in the severity of both formal and informal sanctions
B) Concern about the injustices frequently occurring because governmental and non-governmental sanctions against offenders are both solely determined by the hierarchy of class position
C) Advocating further study of non-governmental sanctions to address inconsistent treatment of criminal offenders
D) Favoring formal sanctions as the fairest method of punishing criminal offenders

4. The phrase "'stigmatizing effects' of criminal conviction" (paragraph 2) refers to which one of the following?

A) The severity of formal sanctions imposed upon working-class defendants after criminal convictions
B) The less severe formal sanctions received by white-collar criminals after criminal convictions
C) The informal sanctions a defendant receives as a result of being convicted of a crime
D) The inequality of treatment before the law of working-class and white collar offenders

5. Which of the following questions about the two forms of sanctions could not be answered by using the information provided in the passage?

A) What is the difference between formal and informal sanctions?
B) Why have formal sanctions received extensive analytic treatment?
C) Why have informal sanctions not received thorough investigation?
D) Why are formal and informal sanctions of white-collar crimes sometimes inconsistent?

6. Which of the following sentences would best serve as a completion to the passage?

A) As the justice system progresses, the determinants of informal sanctions should receive more investigation.
B) Accordingly, judges should not consider informal sanctions when imposing sentences on criminal offenders, regardless of their position on the social hierarchy.
C) If this trend continues, it will remain impossible for criminal defendants to receive fair sentences until more attention is paid to the study of informal sanctions.
D) It is clear that the seriousness of the offense alone should determine the formal sanctions imposed upon criminal conviction.

7. Which of the following best expresses the main idea of the passage?

A) The extent to which a person is stigmatized by criminal conviction depends in large part on their social status or class.
B) To understand how individual behavior is influenced by society, we must learn more about the effect of social stigma on criminal offenders.
C) Informal sanctions have an even greater effect than formal sanctions on those accused or convicted of crimes and so must be studied in more depth.
D) The workings of law and society cannot be studied in isolation from each other; the two are inherently intertwined in our institutions and cultural beliefs.

Answers to 5-Minute Drill

1) **D**
2) **A**
3) **C**
4) **C**
5) **C**
6) **A**
7) **B**

Exercise 3: Test Assessment Log

This Log should look familiar; there is a copy of it in Chapter 44. If you haven't been using it to evaluate your practice tests, now is the time to start.

In particular, use it to evaluate your pacing. Are you spending the time you need on the easier passages in order to get most of those questions right? Keep track of how much time you spent (roughly) on the Now passages and on the Later passages. If you find that you are spending the bulk of your 90 minutes on the harder passages with a low level of accuracy, you need to reapportion your time. Also evaluate your ranking: Are you choosing the right passages?

Now Passages

Now Passage #	Q # and Type (for questions you got wrong)	Attractors (for wrong answers you picked or seriously considered)	What did you do wrong?

Approximate time spent on Now passages _____

Total Now passages attempted _____

Total # of Q's on Now passages attempted _____

Total # of Now Q's correct _____

% correct of Now Q's attempted _____

48.2

Later Passages

Later Passage #	Q # and Type (for questions you got wrong)	Attractors (for wrong answers you picked or seriously considered)	What did you do wrong?

Approximate time spent on Later passages _____

Total Later passages attempted _____

Total # of Q's on Later passages attempted _____

Total # of Later Q's correct _____

% correct of Later Q's attempted _____

Final Analysis

Total # of passages attempted (including partially completed) _____

Total # of questions attempted _____

Total # of correct answers _____

Total % correct of attempted questions _____

Revised Strategy

Pacing	
Passage choice/ranking	
Working the Passage	
Attacking the Questions	

48.3   RANKING AND ORDERING

Why Rank the Passages?

As we have discussed, to maximize your efficiency and accuracy within each passage, you must take control of the material and not let the material control you. In the same way, you'll maximize your score by taking control of the section *as a whole*, working through the passages in a way that helps you get the easy questions and not waste time on the most difficult questions.

The first part of this section outlines what you need to know about how the MCAT CARS section is organized in terms of level of difficulty, and how you can assess any nine passages to design your best plan of attack.

How Are the MCAT CARS Passages Organized?

The MCAT does not follow a strict pattern in how they organize the nine passages; they are presented more or less randomly. Needless to say, the AAMC will not disclose specific information concerning how the passages are chosen, how many are at an easy, medium, or difficult level, etc. Moreover, each administration is different, and every time the test is administered there are multiple forms of the test. So, where does that leave us?

Let's begin with what we know. During the many years that we have been developing these materials, we have discovered some patterns. A lot of experience has led us to the following conclusions about the structure of the CARS section.

Passage Organization

Although one might think that the nine passages would be arranged in order of level of difficulty (that is, easy passages first, medium next, and difficult last), this is generally *not* the case. What would be the point of putting all the difficult passages at the end in a section that students sometimes don't finish? In fact, the passages are in a seemingly random order; often, the last passage in the section is an easy or medium passage that you want to be sure to complete, and the hardest passage is in the middle of the section.

Most CARS sections will have at least one passage that merits the rank of Killer, meaning it's so difficult that spending even 30 or 40 minutes wouldn't allow you to answer all—or even most of—the questions correctly. Killer passages are not worth your valuable time—guess on the questions or, at least, do them last.

Therefore, it's up to you to strategically reorganize your nine passages in order to address them most effectively.

Passage Division

Division of the nine passages generally breaks down into:

- 2–4 easy passages
- 3–5 medium passages
- 1–2 difficult passages

Unless your reasonable goal is to score at the very top of the scale, you probably should be randomly guessing on at least one passage; that is, the one or two most difficult passages in the section. And if your reasonable goal is to score in the 98th or 99th percentile, you may still do best by guessing on a few of the most difficult questions you encounter.

48.4   ASSESSING DIFFICULTY LEVEL: NOW, LATER, AND KILLER

Your first objective when beginning the section is to assess the relative difficulty of the passages. A passage should be ranked Now if it seems relatively straightforward. The passages that appear to be more challenging should be ranked as Later. The most difficult passage or passages (the ones on which you may be randomly guessing) get a rank of Killer.

Although it's tempting to associate topic or subject matter with difficulty level, remember that—unlike the science sections—the CARS section of the MCAT does not test outside knowledge. Everything you need to correctly answer the questions is in the passage. In fact, bringing in outside knowledge can actually hurt your score.

Students will often want to skip easier passages simply because they're about, say, poetry or opera (or any other topic that tends to be unfamiliar). However, what really makes a passage difficult is the way it's written (and in some cases the types of questions that are asked about it). Just because a topic is boring or foreign to you doesn't mean the passage is written in an inaccessible way, and even though a topic may be interesting or familiar, the passage can be written in a dense, convoluted way.

The Passage Text

What Should You Look For?

The following criteria should be used to evaluate the difficulty of the passage text itself.

1) **Level of concreteness or abstraction:** Passages that are highly theoretical and that discuss abstract concepts will be much harder to follow than passages that are concrete and descriptive. Would you rather read a passage about the "philosophic contemplation of the Not-Self" or one on the "doubling of the cost of living in the last ten years"? And again, subject matter is not the key to difficulty. For example, an art passage that is essentially a painter's biography may be very concrete and factual, and therefore quite easy to comprehend.

2) **Language level:** While the CARS section cannot expect you to know technical language specific to a particular discipline (without defining the terms in context), difficult passages will often include esoteric language that no one really uses in everyday conversation. If the author uses many such words as *lugubrious*, *phlegmatic*, *synesthesia*, or *flagitious* in the first few sentences, she's probably not going to start using "plain English" in the next few. Lots of unfamiliar vocabulary will make the passage more difficult to understand, regardless of the topic.

3) **Sentence structure:** Extremely long, convoluted sentences are harder to read, especially under a time constraint. Short, direct sentences will be easier to follow.

How to Evaluate the Passage Text

Skim the first few sentences of the first or second paragraph. Try to paraphrase what you have just read. If your reaction is essentially "huh???," and all you can do is repeat the exact wording of the passage because the meaning of those words is so unclear, this indicates a more difficult passage. If, on the other hand, you can easily put the meaning of those lines into your own words, the passage is likely to be fairly straightforward.

Think of it this way: If in 15 seconds, you could explain to your six-year-old sister what those two sentences are saying, then the passage will probably make sense to you too.

Do NOT rank a passage solely on the basis of its length. The few moments it may take you to read five or six extra lines will not significantly affect your performance, but choosing a short yet difficult passage over a longer but easier passage certainly will.

The Questions

Adapting to Difficulty Level

Given that the questions are displayed one at a time, on separate screens, for most test takers it is too cumbersome and time-consuming to click through and look at each question, evaluate the difficulty level of the set, and then incorporate that into a ranking decision. Therefore, most of your ranking decisions should be based on the apparent difficulty of the passage text.

However, once you have decided to do a passage and are previewing the questions, if you notice a high percentage of very difficult question types (in particular, Application and Structure-Evaluate questions) or unusually lengthy question stems and/or answer choices, you may decide at that point to skip over that passage (marking and guessing on the questions and making a clear noteboard note) and move on to the next. Do not, however, employ this strategy more than once or twice at the most during a CARS section. Otherwise, you will spend too much time previewing questions without answering them, and your efficiency and pacing will suffer.

48.5   ORDERING THE SECTION

Now that you have the criteria with which to rank your passages, let's discuss the overall ordering of the section.

The Two-Pass System

1) For the first passage, write down the passage number and question range on your noteboard (e.g., "Passage 1 Q 1–7").

2) Read the first two or three sentences of the passage and try to paraphrase. If it's a Now passage, do it now. If it's a Later or Killer passage, write "SKIPPED" under the passage heading on your noteboard, Mark and randomly guess on each question, and move on to ranking the next passage. Go through the entire section in the same way: writing the passage heading on your noteboard, completing the Now passages, and noting, marking, and guessing on the Later or Killer passages. This is your first pass.

3) Once you've completed all the Now passages, take a second pass through the section and do all the Later passages. You can use the Review function, if necessary, to find the passages you have marked and guessed on.

At or before the 5-minute mark (ideally before you begin your last passage), inspect the section to make sure that you haven't left any questions blank.

If you have a few extra minutes left over for a Killer passage, quickly read the first and last line of each paragraph. Identify the easiest questions (especially Retrieval questions and Inference questions with paragraph references and/or lead words), and do as many as you can by going to the relevant sections of the passage text. Again, be careful to leave time to fill in random guesses for the questions you cannot complete.

48.6   CARS EXERCISES: RANKING

Exercise 1: Evaluating the Passage Text

Each of the following paragraphs represents the first two sentences of a CARS passage. Using the criteria described earlier, decide if these are likely to be Now, Later, or Killer passages. You can find answers at the end of the exercise.

Passage I

With Chicago School economic theory at its apex, the emphasis on rational choice as the paradigm for interpreting human behavior throughout the social sciences seemed to offer a new scientific foundation to a variety of disciplines. A more rigorous sociology/psychology of human behavior, however, suggests that a unilateral focus on rationality (a surprisingly slippery concept) may misrepresent human motivations as often as explain them.

Passage II

Found in some form in nearly all cultures, weaving has a rich history. Straddling the divide between craft and art form, the tradition of weaving intersects with industrialization, imperialism, and today, the digital revolution.

Passage III

The modern animal rights movement remains apparently oblivious to the way in which its terminology reflects a narrow class identity and social elitism. The irony here is that a language of animal rights rooted instead in more traditional and religious language would likely achieve the ends of the movement much more effectively.

Passage IV

The graphic novel as literary genre is now well-established enough to no longer shock even the most traditional scholars. From **Watchmen** to **Persepolis** to even **Fun Home**, we have seen how graphic novels can achieve literature status.

Passage V

Its embrace of science constitutes only one of several ways in which 18th Century Unitarianism continues to surprise modern students of history or religion who stumble upon it. This distinctively American movement (the hubris of planning to recreate Christianity without a Christ!) for a while influenced, if not actually dominated, New England intellectual life.

Passage VI

To translate poetry seems impossible. If a poem, by its nature, plays on the delicate interaction between meaning and sound, how can that perfect symbiosis possibly be reassembled in a new language, in which not only the vocabulary but the actual phonemes are utterly different?

Passage VII

When it was ratified in 1990 the Americans with Disabilities Act (ADA) promised, by reducing discrimination, to improve the lives of Americans with all types of disabilities. Ramps, interpreters, dogs, and, most importantly, legal protection against employment discrimination would remove the barriers separating those with disabilities from full social participation.

Passage VIII

Although critics for more than a decade now have bemoaned (or sometimes applauded) the effect of social media on mental health, surprisingly little quantitative analysis is available. Instead the literature relies on historical correlations impossible to untangle from confounding variables.

Passage IX

Was Beethoven ever subtle? It has become a trope within musical criticism to categorize Beethoven as one of those composers whose grand emotionality dominates his musical oeuvre.

Passage X

If Buber exemplifies the individualist wing of Jewish existentialist philosophy, Franz Rosenzweig must be credited with re-articulating how a more traditional Jewish conception of duty might co-exist with this radical self. The genius of Jewish existentialism is to stand against the inevitable secularization of rationalism, but the question of whether halakhah can be preserved from an existentialist starting point threatens the project at its roots.

48.6

Explanations for Exercise 1: Evaluating the Passage Text

1. **Killer:** This paragraph addresses abstract themes, such as rationality and motivation. The vocabulary level is also high: "paradigm," "unilateral."

2. **Now:** This passage seems straightforward and factual.

3. **Later:** The topic is addressed in an academic and abstract fashion. Concepts such as the terminology of class identity and social elitism may be difficult to paraphrase.

4. **Now:** This passage seems straightforward, and it seems to have a clear viewpoint.

5. **Later:** A passage about "intellectual life" is likely to be fairly abstract.

6. **Later/Killer:** The topic is highly abstract. The author is raising a question and the answer may be difficult to explain.

7. **Now:** The topic of the passage (the ADA) seems fairly concrete and the language is not difficult.

8. **Now:** The topic of the passage is clearly stated and, although the vocabulary is a bit difficult, the ideas would not be difficult to paraphrase.

9. **Now/Later:** Some of the more difficult language (for example, "trope," and "oeuvre") suggests the reading may be somewhat difficult. The topic, though, is clear.

10. **Killer:** This paragraph has an extremely abstract topic as well as multiple points of view and some unfamiliar vocabulary.

48.6

Exercise 2: Evaluating the Questions

In most cases, your passage ranking will be based only on the passage text. However, to be able to adapt your ranking, if needed, to an unusually difficult set of questions during the preview stage, you need to be able to recognize what tends to make questions easier or harder. Classify each of the following CARS questions as Easy or Hard. You can find answers at the end of the exercise.

1. It can be inferred from the passage that the most significant influence on economic decision-making is:

2. Which of the following would most strengthen the standard interpretation of American secularization while challenging the author's criticism of that interpretation?

3. Which of the following would most *undermine* the author's claim that the digital revolution is transforming the practice of weaving?

4. Suppose it was demonstrated that social media has a less significant effect on mental health than previously thought. What impact would this have on the author's claims in the second paragraph?

5. According to the passage, what is the aspect of Beethoven's composition style most overlooked by critics?

6. The phrase "literary purpose" (paragraph 2) refers to:

7. The author's attitude towards the Americans with Disabilities Act can best be describes as:

8. In describing Buber's contribution to Jewish philosophy, the author states that Buber did all of the following EXCEPT:

9. Which of the following would be most parallel to the transformation in the discourse of animal rights that the author of the passage recommends?

10. The author claims that translating poetry is more difficult than translating any other literary form. How well supported is this claim?

Explanations for Exercise 2: Evaluating the Questions

1. **Easy:** Inference questions with specific references to the passage often have straightforward answers. In this case, you would probably just need to find where these records are discussed in the passage.

2. **Hard:** This is a Strengthen question that involves two perspectives—you need to keep both in mind and strengthen the first while weakening the second.

3. **Hard:** A Weaken question requires taking new information provided in the answer choices and using reasoning to apply it to the passage.

4. **Hard:** The word "suppose" indicates that this question is going to require evaluating new information in the question stem and then taking multiple steps to answer the question. Also, the question stem is quite lengthy.

5. **Easy:** This is a Retrieval question, so the answer can be found in the passage text.

6. **Easy:** This question tells you where to go to find the information you need. As long as you remember to read above and below, it should not be difficult to answer.

7. **Easy:** The author's attitude can usually be determined with little difficulty.

8. **Easy:** The wording "The author states" tells you that this is a Retrieval question. The fact that it is an "EXCEPT" question shouldn't make it significantly more difficult, as long as you keep track of the question format, and of why you are eliminating each choice.

9. **Hard:** The phrase "most parallel" indicates that this is an Analogy question, which involves a higher level of reasoning and abstraction than do most question types.

10. **Easy:** This is an Evaluate question. Discovering whether or not there is evidence for the claim may be straightforward. However, the need to evaluate the strength or relevance of any such evidence is more challenging.

48.6

Exercise 3: Evaluate Your Ranking

Ranking is a skill, like any other, that needs to be learned, practiced, and refined over time. If you ever rank an easy passage as Later (or Killer), or a difficult passage as Now, review the passage to see what made it easy or difficult and how you could have evaluated it better the first time through.

Compare the ranking you gave each passage to your eventual performance (taking into account both your accuracy and your efficiency/pacing) on that passage. Determine the order of attack that would have worked best for you.

- Were there any Killer passages that you should have skipped and guessed on? How could you have known it was a Killer before you wasted any time on it?
- Did you fail to get to any easy passages lurking at the end of the section?
- How will you change your approach on the next MCAT Practice Test you take?

48.6

Individual Passage Log

Passage # _____ **Time spent on passage** _____

Q#	Q type	Attractors	What did you do wrong?	

Revised Strategy _____

Passage # _____ **Time spent on passage** _____

Q#	Q type	Attractors	What did you do wrong?	

Revised Strategy

48.7   MAXIMIZING YOUR SCORE

Now is the time to ask yourself a serious question: are you diligently and consistently implementing and refining a strategic approach to the test? Or are you just doing passage after passage and taking test after test in the belief that simple repetition will continue to improve your score? If it's the latter, you must ask yourself WHY you are making the mistakes that you are and HOW you can change to improve your performance.

The Big Picture

Imagine two students. The first (say, the one who isn't using these materials) approaches the CARS section as she would any test in college. The second, a student using this book, uses the strategies she has learned. How will these students use their time on the test?

First Student, With No Specialized Test Strategy

- **On Easier Passages:** Overconfident and complacent, this student rushes through the easier passages, relying on her memory and failing to check her answer choices back to the passage text. She chooses the first answer that sounds good, and she is perfectly happy with her choices, not realizing that she has fallen into all of the test writers' traps.
- **On Harder Passages:** This student, doing the passages in the order given by the test writers, hits a difficult passage in the middle of the section. Frustrated and confused, she slows down, reading everything three times, trying to understand exactly what the author is saying. She spends five minutes on a question, believing that she can't move on until she is sure of the correct answer. She becomes more and more anxious about the time, which makes it even harder to focus on the passage. This student tries to use sheer effort where strategy would be more effective.

Second Student, With MCAT-Appropriate Strategies

- **On Easier Passages:** Knowing that the majority of her correct answers will come from the easier passages, this student works through them with steadiness and focus. She clearly articulates the Bottom Line of the passage before answering the questions. She answers the questions in her own words before attacking the answer choices, and she checks each choice back to the passage.
- **On Harder Passages:** This student knows that not all passages will be completely comprehensible, and she has an appropriate strategy for the harder passages. She uses POE to the fullest, remembering that she is looking for the "least wrong" choice, not an ideal answer. She asks questions of the answer choices (such as, *Is the language too extreme to be an inference? Is this choice too narrow for a Main Idea question?*) based on her knowledge of question types and common Attractors. This student gains points based on her intelligent, test-appropriate strategy.

Narrowing It Down

Let's revisit our first student. When asked why she misses questions, she responds, "I don't know. I always get it down to two choices, and then I pick the wrong one."

The second student, having done an extensive evaluation of her own performance to date, might respond, "On Inference questions, I tend to forget to look for absolute language, and I pick choices that are too extreme. Sometimes I get too impatient to define the Bottom Line, and then I pick Main Point answer choices that are too narrow. I also sometimes have too much confidence in my own memory, don't go back to the passage, and then miss easy Retrieval questions by choosing answer choices from the wrong part of the passage." The second, self-aware student knows exactly what she needs to work on over the next few weeks, and she has a clear path to continued improvement. The first student will most likely continue to make the same mistakes over and over again. Remember, those who don't know and understand their own history are doomed to repeat it.

If you are identifying a bit too much with our first student, now is the time to ask yourself the following questions:

1) **Are you having trouble articulating the Bottom Line?**
   Is it difficult to locate the relevant parts of the passage when you are working the questions?
   The Diagnosis
   Both of these issues go back to articulating the main point of each paragraph or chunk and synthesizing those themes as you read. If you don't identify the author's main points as you read, separating out the claims from the evidence, it is almost impossible to distill it down at the end to a core argument. And, if you aren't identifying the location of these different themes, the passage runs together in your mind as an undifferentiated block of information, and you will have trouble remembering and locating where different topics appeared.

   The Cure
   Review Chapter 45 on Active Reading.
   Break the argument into chunks and define the Main Points as you read; don't wait to think about it until after you have finished reading the passage. If you haven't been using your noteboard much (or at all), make yourself write down the Main Points as you go. Articulate how each new chunk logically relates to what you have already read. Preview the questions for content, so that you have some context within which to translate what you are reading, and so you are alerted to some of the important issues in the passage.

2) **Do you tend to miss certain question types?**
   The Diagnosis
   Use your passage and practice test logs to identify which types give you the most trouble. Is it an overall category (e.g., Specific questions)? Is it a few particular question types or formats?

   The Cure
   Review Chapter 46 on Question Types.
   Identifying these patterns is the first step towards figuring out the exact causes of your mistakes. Here are some common problem areas and solutions.
   - Main Point/Primary Purpose: Pay attention to tone, and break down the passage by defining its logical structure. Avoid choices that are too narrow.
   - Specific questions: Keep track of the specific reference in the question stem, and go back to the passage *before* you take the first cut through the answer choices.

- Structure: Pay attention to words in the passage that distinguish claims (*therefore, thus, in conclusion*) from evidence (*for example, in illustration, in these three cases*).
- New Information: Treat the new information in the question stem like a paragraph of the passage: What is the main point of this chunk, and how does it relate to the logic of the author's argument? Use your noteboard to translate complicated questions.
- Strengthen and Weaken: Clearly define what the correct answer needs to do: What is the relevant issue, and must the correct answer be consistent or inconsistent with the passage? With what part of the passage? Keep close track of direction.
- EXCEPT/LEAST/NOT: Define not only what the right answer needs to do but what kind of choices you will be eliminating. Use your noteboard to keep track of POE.

3) **Do you tend to fall for certain types of Attractors?**
The Diagnosis
Use your logs and look for patterns!

The Cure
Review Chapter 47 on POE.
Each time you do a new passage or test section, pick out ahead of time two types of Attractors you will be on the lookout for. Define a specific tactic for recognizing and avoiding these traps, such as the following:

- Extreme wording: Look out for words like *only, most, all, must, never,* etc. Also, evaluate the strength of the statements in each choice; an answer choice can be too extreme even if it doesn't use these particular words.
- Partially correct: Force yourself to read the entire choice word for word. Actively look for that one word that can make it incorrect. Suspend all judgment on the validity of the choice until you have read every word.
- Right answer/wrong question: Always go back to the passage, with the specific reference in the question clearly in mind. Reread the question before you take your second cut through the choices.

48.7

48.8   VARIATIONS ON A THEME: REFINING YOUR STRATEGY

Through your preparation you are learning a standard approach to the CARS section that has been tested and refined over decades, based in part on the experience and input of hundreds of thousands of students. However, different people process information somewhat differently. Once you have mastered the approach, you may benefit from experimenting with variations on those techniques in order to make them work optimally for you.

Unfortunately, there are no secret "tricks" to the CARS section. Making score improvements in this section requires a lot of practice, hard work, and vigilant review. It is easy to get into a rut, doing the same thing over and over without thinking about how to further improve your line of attack. This section is intended to spark, or add fuel to, that thought process.

Pacing and Accuracy

As we discussed in the previous sections, the way for many students to maximize their score is to attempt eight of the nine passages, randomly guessing on the hardest passage in the section. However, if your reasonable goal (based on your performance to date) is to score significantly above average, you will most likely need to attempt some or all of a ninth passage. And, if you are currently completing six or seven passages, unless you have close to perfect accuracy, you will need to pick up the pace in order to achieve an average or bit above average score. The question is then, how can you speed up without a significant loss of accuracy?

Ironically, you might find that going a bit faster not only gets you through more questions, but it also improves your accuracy. This may be the case if you tend to overthink the passage or the questions, making the passage more confusing than it needs to be, or talking yourself out of correct answers.

On the other hand, if you are missing a large number of questions because you did not read carefully enough, or did not think enough about the meaning of what you read, then slowing down (especially if you are doing all nine passages) may pay off. No one really wants to randomly guess on questions (everyone would prefer to do all of the questions and get them all right); however, many students have found that once they do slow down, focusing more on accuracy and less on speed, they not only have the time to do what needs to be done, but they also think more clearly and efficiently.

Below are suggestions and variations on the standard approach that may improve your speed, your accuracy, or both. Always try new approaches on multiple passages and tests to gather enough data to see if they are really working for you. Also, test one new approach at a time, rather than trying to do a massive overhaul.

Ranking and Ordering: The Three-Pass System

Most test takers do best with the Two-Pass system of ordering the passages; that is, doing the Now passages the first time through as you find them, then coming back for a second pass to do the Later passages. However, if you find that you struggle with separating out the Nows from the Laters from the Killers, AND that you are often making bad choices in the passages you attempt to the extent that it hurts your score, it is worth trying the Three-Pass system.

1) First Pass: Rank all nine passages Now, Later, or Killer
2) Second Pass: Do the Now passages
3) Third pass: Do the Later passages and check the Review screen for incompletes

The Three-Pass system may take a bit more total time than the Two-Pass System. However, if you are consistently making bad ranking decisions and wasting time struggling with difficult passages, comparing all nine passages before beginning your Now passages may pay off.

Working the Passage

1) **Push the Pace**

   a) It is comforting to read the whole passage word for word, translating and understanding every point and nuance within the author's argument. However, most questions don't require a deep understanding of the passage. And, many parts of the passage never become relevant to the questions. Try pushing yourself through the passage faster on your first reading, accepting the fact that there will be some sections that you do not fully understand. If you know what was discussed, even if you don't really get the author's meaning, you can always find it again if you need it.

   b) If your reading speed is very slow and you have problems with reading comprehension, one technique to try is to read just the first and last sentence of each paragraph the first time through the passage. You may also want to try this approach if you commonly get bogged down in the passage text, losing too much time and/or comprehension.

   CAUTION: This generally only works well on easier passages. This is also quite risky, as there may well be important information in the middle of the paragraph (and neither the first nor the last sentence of the paragraph is guaranteed to be a topic sentence). However, some people find that it gets them through the passage fast enough (with at least a basic comprehension of the Bottom Line and understanding of the location of different parts of the author's argument) that they can spend their time more productively on the questions. They may also get to more questions this way, and their overall percentage correct increases. This is definitely a strategy that you want to test on a wide range of passages and on multiple practice tests before you settle on it, but for a few people, it does pay off. Make sure that you evaluate your accuracy, not just the number of questions you are able to attempt. If you come out behind score-wise and in terms of overall percentage correct (taking guessing into account), this is not the strategy for you.

2) **Separate Claims From Evidence**

   One way to push the pace is to vary your reading speed, paying attention to the major claims (often the main point of the paragraph or chunk) and skimming through (that is, reading faster, not word for word) the evidence supporting those claims. Look for topic sentences (if they exist) to help you make these decisions. Use "MAPS" (see Chapter 45) to help out as well. If you see data, studies, examples, descriptions, explanations, anecdotes, etc., they are highly likely to be evidence in support of a larger claim. As long as you know where they are and what they are supporting, the details are of little importance the first time through the passage.

48.8

For example, here is a sample paragraph (with highlighting).

> Sedentarization is also having a perverse effect on the roles and position of women. For example, in their traditional nomadic state, with men away on caravans or other business, the domestic domain, including the tending of goat herds, education of children, etc., was the preserve of women. The transition from tent to village is being associated with a marked diminution of the domestic responsibilities and authority of women.

The first sentence of the paragraph sets out the main claim being made by the author. The rest of the paragraph supports that claim. If you understand that the paragraph is about the negative effects of sedentarization on women, you don't really need the rest of the details unless they appear in the questions.

3) **Write Less**

You should be writing down the main point of each paragraph (or chunk) and the Bottom Line of the passage on your noteboard for the first several weeks of your preparation. You are training yourself to read differently, and writing it all down at that stage is crucial. However, once defining those aspects of the passage comes more easily to you, and you are more and more accurate in your understanding, you can cut down the amount that you are writing to a couple of words per paragraph and for the Bottom Line. You may even find that it becomes a tool you can use on the harder passages or more confusing paragraphs only, while the rest of the time you do it as a mental step (while still highlighting within the text). This can be especially useful if you find that you usually have a good understanding of the chunks and how they relate to each other (i.e., the logical structure of the passage), but you struggle and get bogged down when putting it into your own words.

This is one area in which there is significant variation between students. Some people who consistently get high scores are writing brief notes for every paragraph and passage because it contributes both to their speed and to their accuracy, while others in the same scoring range use writing more selectively. Find what level of writing works best for you.

4) **Visualize**

a) Visualizing as you read engages a different part of your brain. When you hit an important part of the passage (especially when you go back to the passage as you answer the questions) and it isn't really making sense, create a visual image in your head. Imagine people waving signs and blocking the streets while the city stagnates around them, or elitist historians thumbing their noses at the common people, or humanists admiring Greek statues while turning a group of robed scholars away from a church, or an adult artist frowning in concentration as she paints while a carefree child spontaneously creates artwork next to her. By the way, the difficulty in visualizing an abstract argument, compared to a concrete and descriptive one, is one thing that tends to make abstract passages Laters or Killers.

b) Another way of using visualization is to create a picture in your mind of the structure of the passage. When you hit a pivotal word, imagine a detour sign. At a continuation, think of a bridge. When the author expresses an opinion, picture a smiley or frowny face. Of course, these are all things that you should also be highlighting. You may even choose to write down some quick symbols on your noteboard, such as a "+" or "−"

for positive and negative tone, or a Δ (delta) for a significant shift or change. One reason students often find it harder to process a passage on the computer screen than on paper is that it is easier to have a visual map of a whole page than of a scrolled passage. If you put some effort into creating visual map markers as you read, it takes little time and can really pay off when you use them to efficiently find information in the passage as you answer the questions.

5) **To Preview or Not to Preview**

Previewing the questions is one way of moving faster through the passage; knowing the question topics ahead of time helps you to prioritize. However, if you are spending an appropriate amount of time previewing (20–30 seconds) and still not retaining enough information to make it useful, there are a few things to try.

a) First, make sure you are focusing on and highlighting the lead words that indicate passage content, not the question type (question types, while crucial to define as you are answering the questions, are irrelevant at this stage). Picture the lead words as little bursts of information. Focus on each burst as a distinct chunk, rather than skimming through every word of the question with equal attention. Engage your visual memory and your pattern recognition skills. You don't need to fully understand the words at this stage; you just need to fix them in your memory so that you can recognize them in the passage. And, if the question is long and complicated, or if it looks like a New Information question (which usually start with the words "Suppose" or "If"), skip over it during the preview.

b) Second, if you still can't retain the information, try jotting down a word or two for each content-containing question on your noteboard. While this will take a bit of time, if you are getting bogged down in the passage, or if you are spending an inordinate amount of time hunting for information as you work the questions, it can pay off in the long run.

c) Third, if no matter what you do, you can't make the preview work for you, then don't do it. That is, if you have practiced it for at least a month, and used it on at least three practice tests and at least 25 practice passages, and it is still not paying off, then those 20–30 seconds are better spent on answering the questions.

Attacking the Questions

1) **Simplify**

Even difficult questions can be amazingly straightforward when you look at them with clear eyes and a calm brain. If you are struggling with a question, stop and remind yourself that you may be overcomplicating it. Imagine a triangle connecting the question stem, the relevant part of the passage, and the correct answer. When you are stuck, ask yourself: "What was the question asking, what did the author say about it, and what answer is most closely connected to both of those things?" Staying with the geometrical theme, also ask yourself if you have left the world of the "MCAT CARS box." Are you bringing in outside knowledge? Are you speculating about what the author might think, rather than basing your answer on what the author explicitly said? Are you debating an imperfect answer, rather than asking, "Is it the least wrong of the four?" Sometimes when you just relax, use your brain, and relocate yourself within the passage and the question task, things look a lot clearer.

48.8

2) **Use Aggressive POE**

If you are going back to the passage multiple times to prove the right answer right, or cycling through the choices multiple times, remember that eliminating the other three choices is a perfectly legitimate way to get the right answer. Use the Bottom Line, tone, the main point of the relevant chunk or chunks, the strength of the language in the passage and in the answer choices, and when possible your own answer (based on the passage) to weed out what you can. If you are left with one choice still standing, a choice you can't find anything wrong with, pick it and move on, even if you aren't thrilled with it.

3) **Triage**

Some questions are not worth saving. Unless your reasonable goal is to get a perfect score, you are going to miss some questions. It can be useful to think of this as a strategy, not a failure. That is, your strategy is to allow yourself to miss some questions in order to maximize your score, rather than to try to get every single question right. If you are the kind of person who can't move on until you are 100% sure you have a question right, push yourself to take your best shot and move on (once you have been through the appropriate procedure). If you have carefully reread the question, compared the remaining choices, gone back to the passage again, looked for Attractors, and you are still stuck between two choices, pick one and move on. Even if three more minutes on that one question would produce a correct answer, it isn't worth sacrificing the two or three other questions you could have answered correctly in those three minutes.

4) **Cherry Pick**

Cherry picking is a somewhat extreme form of triage. Generally, you want to work through every question attached to a passage. Otherwise, you are wasting some of your investment of time in reading and working the passage. However, if you ALWAYS (or almost always) get the hardest question on a passage wrong, whatever you do, then take an educated guess on that question once you recognize it. If you ALWAYS (or almost always) get a particular type of Reasoning or Application question, or the longest questions, wrong, then try guessing on that type when you find it. Compare your performance on several tests, some doing eight passages working all of the questions and others doing nine passages using cherry picking; follow the strategy that has the best outcome.

5) **Tone Questions**

If you tend to get Tone/Attitude questions wrong, or if you miss other question types because you missed or mistook the tone of the passage, this often goes back to how you are working the passage, and to whether or not you are looking for and highlighting tone indicators as you read. However, this can also be due to how you are doing POE on questions where tone is particularly relevant. Make sure to identify the "attitude words" in each choice. For example, imagine that you have four answer choices that begin as follows:

    A) To defend…
    B) To recommend…
    C) To show…
    D) To contradict…

Make sure that you are focusing particular attention on those tone words. While you should always read all four choices carefully and fully, if you are stuck on the question and you know that the passage was entirely neutral, choice C is your best shot.

6) **Order the Questions Within a Passage**

If you are always doing every question in order, regardless of question difficulty, consider taking a consistent "two-pass" approach within the set of questions for a passage. As described in the Ranking and Ordering section, first preview the questions for a passage from first to last. Then, while on the last question, work the passage. Next, work backwards through the set for that passage, skipping over the harder questions and completing the easier ones. Finally, click forward through the set, completing the harder questions (and making sure that you are not leaving any blank).

Dealing With (or Not Dealing With) Killer Passages

Identify a set of difficult passages from your practice materials. Do at least five of them, giving yourself five minutes per passage, and at least five other passages at ten minutes per passage. Compare the results.

1) If you do about the same with five or ten minutes, and your accuracy is low (that is, if you miss a majority of the questions), and if you are completing nine passages during a test without approaching your target score, that is a clear sign that you should slow down to seven and a half or eight passages. That is, your payoff on that last hard passage is very low, and you would be better off spending much or all of that time on improving your accuracy on the other passages.

2) If you do about the same on both sets and your accuracy is high (you miss on average one or zero questions per passage) and you are normally completing eight or fewer passages in a test, these are signs that you may well be able to speed up without losing accuracy.

3) If you do significantly better on a Killer passage when you have ten minutes as opposed to five minutes (getting all or almost all of the questions right in ten minutes) and you have a high level of accuracy overall, you may well want to try cherry picking or aggressive triage in order to get to all nine passages.

4) If you do better on hard passages when you spend five minutes than when you spend ten minutes, and you are doing eight or fewer passages, that is a very clear sign that you should try speeding up. You may well be overthinking the passages and the questions, especially the more difficult ones, and the faster pace may be forcing you to simplify and stick to the information in front of you.

Final Words

Take control of the test by taking ownership over your own method and strategy. If you have prepared not only by learning and practicing our techniques, but also by undergoing a rigorous process of self-analysis and self-correction, all you need to do in order to do well on the day of the MCAT is show up, relax, and use your brain!!

PASSAGE PERMISSIONS INFORMATION

Index

Symbols

ΔG and Temperature	659
(+) RNA Viruses	244
1,3-diaxial interaction	780
¹H Nuclear Magnetic Resonance (NMR) Spectroscopy	66
5'UTR	209
(first) ionization energy	625
(–) RNA Viruses	244
α-tubulin	288
α,β-unsaturated carbonyl compound	825
β–particle	607
β-pleated sheet	120
β-tubulin	288

A

a band	437
abbreviated line structures	750
abiotic synthesis	328
ABO blood group	383
Abraham Maslow	542
absolute configuration	784
absolute poverty	517
absolute refractory period	336
absolute threshold	360
acceleration	869, 873
accessory organs	422
acetal formation	816
acetals and hemiacetals	815
acetylcholinesterase	441
achieved statuses	529
achiral	782
acid anhydrides	832
acid-base equivalence point	727
acid-base titration	726
acid derivative reactivity	834
acid-dissociation constant	712, 841
acid halides	832
acid hydrolases	270
acidic amino acids	113
acid-ionization constant	712
acidity	423, 626, 764
acidity and enolization	810
acini	421
acinus	421
acquisition	553
acrosomal process	470
acrosome	460, 470
acrosome reaction	470
actin	290, 437
action potentials	330
action–reaction pair	885
activated complex	686
activation energy (E_a)	108, 686
activator proteins	230
active site	127
active site model	127
active transport	282
actor-observer bias	523

actualizing tendency	538
acyl carrier protein (ACP)	173
adaptation	352
addiction	577
adenine	180
adenohypophysis	365
ADH	414
adiabatic process	956
adipocytes	388, 450
adrenal gland	351
adrenaline	351
adrenal medulla	351
adrenergic tone	379
adsorption	240
adult stem cells	96
advertising bias	42
aerobic conditions	143
afferent arteriole	413
afferent neurons	339
affinity chromatography	56, 95
affinity tag	57
age	513
age cohorts	513
ageism	513
age-specific birth rates	509
aggregate	525
aggression	533
Albert Bandura	559
albumin	381
aldehydes and ketones	809
aldol condensation	823
aldosterone	414
alertness and sleep	574
algorithm	572
alimentary canal	418
alkyl amines	818
allantois	473
alleles	298
allosteric regulation	129
allosteric sites	129
allotropes	661
all-trans form	358
alpha	606
alpha waves	574
alpha (α) decay	607
altering expression	93
alternating current (AC)	1061
alternative splicing	213
altruistic behavior	533
alveolar capillaries	396
alveolar duct	391
alveoli	391
alveolus	391
Alzheimer's Disease	545
amalgamation	521
ambiguity	196
amides	833
amines	818
amino acid acceptor site	215

amino acid activation	217, 218
amino-acid derivatives	362
amino acid reactivity	841
amino acids	112, 836
amino acid sequence	120
aminoacyl-tRNA synthetase enzymes	218
ammeters	1042
ammonium group	843
amnion	473
amoeboid movement	290
amp	1022
ampère	1022
amphiarthroses	453
amphipathic	162, 858
amphoteric	117, 715, 841
amplitude	1087, 1092
ampullae	355
amu	593
amygdala	580
anabolic reactions	418
anabolism	110
anaerobes	253
anaerobic conditions	143
anaerobic respiration	254
analogous structures	326, 461
anal sphincter	427
anaphase	292
anaphase I	302
androgens	456, 462
anergic	406
angiotensin-converting enzyme (ACE)	416
angiotensin I	416
angiotensin II	414, 416
angiotensinogen	416
angle of refraction	1116
angstrom	591
anhydride linkage	178
anion	606, 992
annealing	184
Anne Treisman's Attenuation Model	569
anode	733
anomeric carbon	852
anomers	852
anomie	521
anterior chamber	356
anterior pituitary	364
anterograde amnesia	545, 564
antibodies (Ab)	402
anticodon	215
anti conformation	778
antidiuretic hormone	414
antigen (Ag)	403
antigen-presenting cells (APCs)	405
antinodes	1100
antiparallel orientation	183
antiparallel β-pleated sheet)	121
antiports	281
anus	427
aortic semilunar valves	373
apical surface	291, 419
apoptosis	295
appearance	532
appendicular components	449
appendix	406, 427
aqueous humor	356
aqueous solution	701
archea	247
archenteron	473
Archimedes' Principle	969
arousal	457, 465, 541
Arrhenius equation	691
arteries	370
arterioles	370
arthritis	453
articular cartilage	453
artificial chromosomes	82
artificial selection	325
aryl amines	818
ascending limb	415
ascribed statuses	529
asexuality	515
assimilation	521
associative learning	552
aster	288
asymmetric center	782
atherosclerosis	286
atomic mass unit	593
atomic number	604
atomic radius	625
atomic structure	611
atomic weight	605
atoms	604
ATP synthase	147
atria	372
atrioventricular (AV) node	378
atrioventricular valve (AV valve)	373
attachment	240
attended channel	568
attention	568, 570
attitude	546
attraction	532
attribution	522
attributional biases	522
attribution theory	522
attrition	486
auditory canal	353
auditory cortex	355
auditory hair cell	351
auditory tube	353
Aufbau principle	616
auricle	353
autoimmune reaction	406
autoimmunity	406
autonomic division	340
autonomic nervous system	420
autonomic PNS anatomy	348
autophagy	270
autosomal dominant	318

autosomal recessive	318
autotrophs	252
auxotroph	253
availability heuristic	573
avascular	453
AV bundle (bundle of His)	378
average velocity	868
Avogadro's Law	673
Avogadro's number	593
avoidance	557
axial components	449
axial hydrogens	779
axis	1124
axons	330

B

backbone	117, 847
back stage	532
bacteria	247
bacterial lawn	252
bacterial life cycle	254
bacterial shape	249
bacterial transformation	81
bacteriophage	237
bacteriophage life cycles	240
Baddeley's model of working memory	571
balanced	596
balancing equations	597
barbiturates	576
basal body	289
basal ganglia	545
basal nuclei	344
basal structure	250
base-dissociation constant	713
base-ionization constant	713
basement membrane	419
base plate	238
base units	590, 864
basic amino acids	113
basilar membrane	354
basolateral surface	291, 419
b cells	403, 406
beat frequency	1099
beats	1097, 1098
behavioral neuroscience	583
behaviorist perspective	538
bel	1105
belief bias	573
belief perseverance	573
beliefs	507
Benedict's test	856
Bernoulli effect	983
Bernoulli's Equatio	978
beta	606
beta (β) decay	607
B.F. Skinner	554
B.F. Skinner's behaviorist model	581
bicarbonate	387
bicuspid valve	373

bile	388, 426
bile acids	426
bile salts	429
bilirubin	381
bimolecular	805
binary fission	254
bindin	460, 470
binomial classification	326
bipolar	330
bipolar cells	356
birth	478
bisexual	514
bivalent	301
blastocyst	471
blastopore	473
blastula	473
blastulation	471
blind spot	357
blood pressure	380
blood typing	383
blotting	76
blue-green algae	247
Bohr effect	386
Bohr model of the atom	612, 1134
boiling-point elevation	276
bolus	420, 423
bond dissociation energy (BDE)	632
bond length and bond dissociation energy	632
bone marrow	406, 451
bone marrow stem cells	381
bone structure	450
Bowman's capsule	413
Boyle's Law	672
brain lesions	583
brainstem	343
Broadbent Filter model of selective attention	568
Broca's aphasia	582
Broca's area	582
bronchi	390
bronchioles	390
bronchoconstriction	400
Brønsted-Lowry acids and bases	710
brush border	424
brush border enzymes	426
budding	239
buffer	381, 723
buffering domain	727
buffering region	727
buffer solutions	723
bulbourethral glands	456
buoyancy	969
buoyant force	969
bureaucracy	530
bystander effect	526

C

calcitriol	454
calculation of ΔHrxn	652
calmodulin	446

calorie	650
calorimetry	649
calyces	410
calyx	410
canaliculi	452
Cannon-Bard Theory	579
capacitance	1045
capacitated	470
capacitor	1045
cap-dependent translation	223
capillaries	370
cap-independent translation	223
capitalism	505
capsid	238
capsid head	238
capsule	250, 411
carbanions	760
carbocations	760
carbohydrates	431, 849
carbon dioxide	387
carbonic acid	387
carbonic anhydrase	387, 417
carbonium ions	760
carboxylic acid derivatives	828
carboxylic acids	827
carboxypeptidase	428
cardiac conduction system	375
cardiac cycle	373
cardiac muscle	375, 436
cardiac output (CO)	374
cardiac sphincter	423
Carl Rogers	538
carrier	403
carrier proteins	280, 281
carrying capacity	255, 509
cartilage	453
case fatality rate	510
case studies	494
caspases	295
caste system	517
catabolic reactions	418
catabolism	110
catalase	270
catalyst	108, 687
catalytic receptors	286
category	525
cathode	733
cation	606, 992
cecum	427
cell adhesion	290
cell diagram	734
cell junctions	290
cell-surface receptors	272
cell theory	247
cellular expression	93
center of curvature	1124
central canal	452
central chemoreceptors	399
Central Dogma	195
central executive	571
central nervous system (CNS)	342
central route	548
centrioles	288
centripetal	903
centripetal force	903
centromere	188, 262
cerebellum	343
cerebral cortex	343
cerebral hemispheres	343
cerebrospinal fluid (CSF)	342
cerebrum	343
cervix	464
chair form	778
channel proteins	272, 280
chaperones	231
charge on a capacitor	1046
charismatic authority	505
Charles Cooley	519
Charles's Law	672
chemical kinetics	108
chemically equivalent hydrogens	66
chemical shift	68
chemical synapses	336
chemoautotrophs	252
chemoheterotrophs	109, 252
chemoreceptors	351
chemotaxis	384
chemotrophs	252
chief cells	423
chiral	782
chiral centers	782
chirality	782
cholecystokinin (CCK)	424, 428
cholesterol	271
chondrocytes	450, 453
chorion	469, 471
choroid	355
chromatin	186
chromatin remodeling	224
chromatography	50
chromosome	186, 262
chromosome amplification	205
C—H Stretches	65
chunking	562
chylomicron remnants	430
chylomicrons	169, 388, 430, 432
chyme	424
chymotrypsin	428
chymotrypsinogen	428
cilia	289, 354
ciliary muscle	356
circular layer	419
circulatory system	370
citrate	145
citric acid cycle	145
civil unrest	516
class	326
classical conditioning	552

class system	517
clathrin	286
cleavage	471
cleavage furrow	293
clitoris	463
clockwise	913
clonal selection	404
closed complex	212
CNS anatomical organization	342
coacervate	328
cochlea	353
cocktail party effect	568
coding RNA	189, 209
codominance	309
codon	195
coefficient of kinetic friction	894
coefficient of static friction	895
coenzyme	128
coercive organizations	530
cofactors	128
cognition	570
cognitive development	571
cognitive dissonance theory	548
cognitive routes	548
cohabitation	503
cohort studies	513
collagen	450
collagenase	428
collecting duct	410, 411, 414, 415
colligative properties	276
colon	408, 427
colonic bacteria	427
colonization	511
colony	252
columnar	391
column (flash) chromatography	52
combinations of capacitors	1059
combined gas law	673
common bile duct	426
common ion	706
common-ion effect	706
common names	849
competitive inhibition	133
competitive inhibitors	133
complementary DNA	82
components of blood	381
compression forces	985
compressions	1094
compressive strain	986
Computerized Tomography (CT) scans	584
concave mirror	1124
concentration	596
concentration and dilution	409, 414
concentration cell	738
concentration measurements	274
concrete operational stage	572
conditioned reinforcers	555
conditioned response (CR)	553
conditioned stimulus (CS)	553
conduction	948
conduction electrons	1009, 1020
conduction zone	389, 390
conductor	1009
cones	356
confederates	528
confirmation bias	572
conflict theory	499
conformational isomers	775
conformity	528
confounding factors	46
confounding variables	485
conjugate acid	711
conjugate base	711
conjugated system	761
conjugation	254, 256
conjugation bridge	251, 256
conjugation mapping	257
connective tissue	450
consciousness	574
consciousness-altering drugs	576
consensus	522
conservation	572
conservation of mechanical energy	1010
conservation of total mechanical energy	935, 940
conservative force	933
consistency	522
constant region	402
constitutional isomerism	775
constitutional isomers	775
constitutive activity	129
constructively	1096
construct validity	46
continuity equation	977
contractility	376
control group	485
controlled tasks	570
convection	949
converging lenses	1130
conversion factor	865
convex mirror	1124
cooperatively	132, 385
coordinate covalent bond	634
copy number variation	194
core enzyme	212
cornea	355
corona radiata	466, 470
corpora cavernosa	457
corpus callosum	343
corpus luteum	466
corpus spongiosum	457
correlation	44
correlational studies	493
cortex	351, 410
cortical reaction	471
cortisol	365
coulombs	992
Coulomb's Constant	994
Coulomb's Law	994

counterclockwise	913
countercurrent multiplier	416
covalent	600
covalent bond	633
covalent modification	129, 232
cranial nerves	347
creatine phosphate	442
crests	1092
cristae	146, 264
critical angle	1118
critical period	582
critical point	667
cross	304
cross bridge	438
cross bridge formation	438
crossed aldol condensation	824
crossing over	301
crude birth rate (CBR)	509
crude death rate (CDR)	509
cubic centimeter	669
cued recall	563
cultural assimilation	521
cultural capital	517
cultural differences	503
cultural diffusion	508
cultural lag	508
cultural transmission	508
cultural universals	507
culture	507
culture shock	508
current	1020
curved mirror	1124
cuspids	422
cyanohydrin formation	818
cyclic AMP (cAMP)	286
cytochromes	147
cytokinesis	292
cytosine	180
cytoskeleton	288

D

Dalton's law of partial pressures	678
daughter	606
daughter DNA	196
DCC coupling	847
DC Circuits	1030
DCT	414
debriefing	492
decay	564
decay constant	609
decibels	1105
decision making	572
dedifferentiation	477
defecation	427
degenerate	196
degree of unsaturation	758
deindividuation	526
delta waves	575

dementia	545
demographic structure	512
demographic transition (DT)	512
denaturation	120, 184
dendrites	330
dense connective tissue	450
density	591, 962
deoxynucleoside triphosphates	180
deoxyribose sugar	179
dependent variable	41, 483
depolarization	331
depressants	576
depth of processing	562
descending limb of the loop of Henle	415
descriptive statistics	34
desmosomes	290, 291
destructively	1096
detergents	859
determined	476
deterministic	538
developing	50
dextrorotatory	789
diamagnetic atoms	618
diaphragm	394
diaphysis	450
diarthroses	453
diastereomers	790
diastole	373
diastolic pressure	380
dielectric constant	1055
dielectrics	1055
diencephalon	343
difference threshold	361
differentiation	475
diffraction	1120
diffusion	278
digestive tract	418
dihydrotestosterone	460
dimension	864
diopter	1132
diploid germ cells	458
dipole-dipole forces	641
dipole-induced dipole force	641
dipole moment	633
direct current (DC)	1061
directional selection	325
direct reversal	206
disaccharide	138, 849
disclosure	492
discrimination	524, 553
dishabituation	552
dispersion	1122
displacement	866
dispositional attribution	522
dissociation curve	386
dissolution	701
distal convoluted tubule (DCT)	413
distal nephron	414
distillations	58

distinctiveness	522
disulfide bond	119
disulfide bridges	117
diuresis	414
divergent selection	325
diverging lenses	1130
divided attention	569
divorce	503
DNA Fingerprinting	88
DNA gyrase	186
DNA Methylation	224
DNA polymerase	198, 200
DNA Repair	206
DNA replication	196
DNA sequencing and Genomics	85
DNA Structure	180
dNTP	180
domain	247, 326
domain Archaea	258
dominant	299
dominant groups	512
dopamine	337
Doppler effect	1107, 1109
dorsal root ganglion	348
double blind	485
double bonds	629
double bond stretches	63
double-strand break repair	207
double-stranded DNA viruses	245
doubling time	253
downward mobility	517
dramaturgical approach	500
dramaturgical perspective	532
drift velocity	1021
drive	540
Drive Reduction Theory	541
drives / negative feedback systems	540
dual coding hypothesis	562
ductus deferens	456
duodenal enzymes	426
duodenal hormones	427
duodenum	424
dynamic equilibrium	498, 702
dynamics	883
dynamics of SHM	1086
dynein	289
dyssomnias	575

E

early adults	513
early brain development	560
early gene	240
Eastern Blotting	78
echoic memory	562
eclipsed conformation	775
economic interdependence	516
ectoderm	473, 474
Ed's Formula	1049
educational	503

effector caspases	295
effectors	339
efferent arteriole	413
efferent neurons	339
efficiency	943
effusion	679
egg activation	471
ego	536
Einstein's equations for mass-energy equivalence	611
ejaculation	457
ejaculatory duct	456
elaboration likelihood model	548
elastic cartilage	453
elasticity of solids	985
elastic potential energy	1086
elastin	450
elease factor	221
electrical synapses	336
electric charge	992
electric circuit	1020
electric dipole	1006
electric field	999, 1101
electric force and field	1003
electric potential	1011
electrode	733
Electroencephalography (EEG)	585
electrolysis	739
electrolytes	275, 381, 701
electrolytic cell	739
electromagnetic (EM) wave	1114
electromagnetic receptors	352
electromagnetic spectrum	1114
electromagnetic waves	1091
electromotive force (emf)	1023
electron	604
electron affinity	626
eectron capture	607
electron configurations	616
electron configurations of ions	621
electron-donating	760
electronegativity	626
electronegativity effects	765
electron spin	615
electron transport chain	141, 147
electron volt (eV)	1016
electron-withdrawing	760
electrophile	634, 772
electrophilicity	772
electrophoresis	74
elementary charge	992
elongation	212, 221
embryo	471, 475
embryogenesis	471
embryonic disk	473
embryonic stem cells (ESCs)	96
emigration	511
Émile Durkheim	498
emission	457
emission spectrum	611, 1134

emotion	577
emotion and cognition in prejudice	524
emotion and memory	580
empirical formula	592
enamine formation	820
enantiomeric stereoisomers	837
enantiomers	788
encoding	561
endergonic	106
endochondral ossification	454
endocrine	421
endocrine gland	361
endocrine pancreas	428
endocrine system	361
endocytosis	285
endoderm	473
endolymph	354
endometrium	464
endonuclease	78
endoplasmic reticulum (ER)	265
endosome	285
endospore formation	256
endospores	256
endosymbiotic theory	265
endothelial cells	370
endothermic	106
endothermic reaction	651
end plate potential (EPP)	441
energy	926, 1086
energy shell	614
energy subshell	615
enolate ion	810
enteric nervous system	420
enterogastrone	427
enterokinase	426, 428
enteropeptidase	426
enthalpy	106, 651
entropy	106, 657, 664, 958
environmental injustice	517
environment-gene interaction	475
enzymatic hydrolysis	418
enzyme kinetics	131
enzyme-linked immuno-sorbent assay (ELISA)	71
epididymis	456
epiglottis	390, 423
epimeric carbon	795
epimers	795
epinephrine	351
epiphyseal line	454
epiphyseal plate	454
epiphysis	450
episodic buffer	571
episodic memory	563
epistasis	309
epithelium	290
epitope	403
equatorial hydrogens	779
equilibrium	107, 694, 917
equilibrium constant	694
equilibrium position	1085
equilibrium potential	335
equipotentials	1012
erectile tissue	457
erection	457
Erik Erikson	537
erythrocytes	381, 382
erythropoietin	382
escape	557
esophagus	423
esterification reaction	829
esters	832
estradiol	166
estrogens	462
ethnicity	514
ethnographic studies	493
eticular formation	574
euchromatin	187, 262
eukaryotes	247
eukaryotic cilia	289
eukaryotic plasmids	82
eukaryotic replication	201
eukaryotic transcription	212
eukaryotic translation	222
eustachian tube	353
evaporative water loss	389
evolution	323
evolutionary comparisons	92
excision	241
excision repair	206, 207
excitatory	337
excitatory postsynaptic potentials (EPSPs)	338
excited state	59, 612
excretion	408
excretory system	408
executive functions	580
exergonic	106
exocrine	421
exocrine glands	361
exocrine pancreas	428
exocytosis	285
exome and targeted sequencing	90
exothermic	106
exothermic reaction	651
experimental design	482
expiration	393
expiratory reserve volume (ERV)	395
expressive functions	525
extended family	503
external locus of control	519
external migration	511
external sphincter	410
external validity	46, 490
exteroceptors	351
extinction	553
extrachromosomal genetic elements	249
extractions	48
extraneous variables	485

F

F1 generation	304
facilitated diffusion	280
facultative anaerobes	253
false consensus	523
false memories	565
family	326, 502, 619
farad	1046
faraday	735
Faraday's Law of Electrolysis	742
fascicles	436
fast block to polyspermy	471
fast sodium channels	375, 444
fats	432
fat-soluble	434
fat-soluble vitamins	168
fatty acids	160
fatty acid structure	857
fatty acid synthase	173
feature detection theory	360
feedback inhibition	130, 364
female reproductive system	463
female sexual act	465
feminist theory	501
fermentation	143
fertility and mortality	509
fertilization	470
fetus	475
F (fertility) factor	256
fibrin	384
fibrinogen	381, 384
fibroblast	450
fibrous cartilage	453
field lines	1002
filament	250
filtrate	409
filtration	409, 413
fimbriae	251, 464
First Law of Thermodynamics	648, 950
fischer projection	836
fitness	323
Five-Factor Model	539
fixation	572
fixed-interval schedule	556
fixed-ratio schedule	556
flagella	250, 289
flagellum	289
flavoprotein	140
flow cytometry	91
flow rate	976
fluid mosaic model	273
fluids	962
fluorescence in situ hybridization	90
focal length	1124
focal point	1124
focus	1124
folkways	520
follicle	465

follicle stimulating hormone (FSH)	460
follicular phase	467
food desert	506
force	883
forced expiration	394
force diagram	900
forebrain	342
formal charge	629
formal norms	520
formal operational stage	572
formed elements	381
formula weight	593
fovea centralis	357
fractional distillation	58
frameshift mutations	204
frank-starling mechanism	374
free energy (Gibbs free energy)	106
Free Fall	878
free recall	563
freezing-point depression	277
frequency	1084, 1091
frequency of recombination	315
frequency summation	442
friction	894
frontal lobes	344
front stage	532
frustration-aggression principle	533
fulcrum	911
functional fixedness	572
functional groups	748
functional imaging	584
functionalism	498
functional magnetic resonance imaging (fMRI)	585
functional residual capacity (FRC)	396
functional syncytium	375, 420, 444
fundamental	1101
fundamental attribution error	522
fundamentalists	504
Fundamentals of Acid/Base Chemistry	841
fundamental wavelength	1101
furanoses	851
futile cycling	153

G

Gabriel-Malonic Ester Synthesis	840
gallbladder	426, 428, 429
gallstone	429
galvanic cells	733
galvanometer	1042
gametogenesis	458
gamma	606
gamma-aminobutyric acid (GABA)	337
gamma (γ) decay	607
ganglia	342
ganglion cells	356
gap junctions	290
gas	664, 669
gas chromatography	57

gas exchange 396
gas laws 672
gastric 423
gastric glands 421
gastrin 424
gastrointestinal (GI) tract 418
gastrula 473
gastrulation 473
gauche conformation 778
Gay-Lussac's Law 672
g cells 424
gel electrophoresis 845
gender 513
gender expression 514
gender roles 514
gene 298
gene expression 209
gene pool 321
general fertility rate 509
generalization 553
generalized other 520
generations 513
gene repressor proteins 230
genes 194
genetic code 194
genetic mutation 203
genetics 298
genome 186, 262
genomic imprinting 225
genomics 87
genotype 299
gentrification 512
genus 326
geometric isomers 799
George Herbert Mead 519
George Ritzer 531
germ cells 458
germination 256
ghrelin 430
GI Accessory Organs 428
Gibbs free energy 659
GI Epithelium 419
GI lumen 418
GI motility 419
GI Secretions 421
GI Smooth Muscle 419
GI tract 422
glial cells 335
global inequality 517
globalization 516
global stratification 517
glomerular basement membrane 413
glomerular filtration rate (gfr) 416
glomerulus 413
glucagon 154, 428
glucocorticoids 351
gluconeogenesis 151
glutamate 358
glyceraldehyde 837

glycerol phosphate shuttle 150
glycocalyx 250
glycogen metabolism 155
glycogenolysis 155
glycolipids 271
glycolysis 140, 141
glycosidic linkage 138, 854
goblet cells 391, 421
golgi apparatus 269
golgi tendon organs 352
gonadotropin releasing hormone (GnRH) 462
government and economy 505
G-protein-linked receptor 286
Graafian follicle 466
Graham's Law of Effusion 679
Gram-negative 249
Gram-positive 249
Gram staining 249
granulosa cells 465
gravitational acceleration 878
greater vestibular glands 465
Grignard reagents 813
ground 1039
grounded 1039
ground state 59, 612
ground substance 450
group 525, 619
group polarization 527
group pressure 528
groupthink 527
growth media 252
guanine 180
gustation 353
gustatory receptors 351
gut 418

H

habit 552
habituation 552
hair cells 354
half-life 609
hallucinogens 576
halo effect 523
haploid gametes 458
hapten 403
Hardy-Weinberg equilibrium 322
Hardy-Weinberg Law 321
harmonic motion 1084
harmonic number 1101
Harry Harlow 560
hCG 469
health and medicine 505
healthy user bias 42
heart 370, 372
heart rate (HR) 374
heat 947, 952
heat capacity 649
heating curve 666
heat of formation 652

heat of fusion	656
heat of reaction	651
heat of transition	656
heat of vaporization	656
heats of phase changes	656
heat transfer	948
heavy chains	402
Heisenberg uncertainty relation	1140
hematocrit	381
hematopoiesis	449
heme	385
hemiacetal	852
hemodynamics	379
hemoglobin	382, 385
hemolytic disease of the newborn	383
hemophilia	385
hemostasis	384
Henderson–Hasselbalch	842
Henry's Law	397
hepatic portal system	429
hepatic portal vein	387, 425, 429
heritability	493
hertz	1084
Hess's Law	653
heteroatoms	70
heterochromatin	187, 262
heterogeneous nuclear RNA	189, 210
heterolytic bond cleavage	632
heteronormative beliefs	515
heterosexual	514
heterotrophs	252
heterozygote	299
heuristics	572
hexokinase	142
Hfr (high frequency of recombination) cell	256
high culture	507
high-energy phosphate bond	178
high performance liquid chromatography (HPLC)	54
hindbrain	342
hippocampus	580
histamine	424
histones	186
holoenzyme	212
homeostasis	363, 409
homologous chromosomes	298
homologous pairs	292
homologous recombination	207
homologous structures	326
homology-dependent repair pathways	206
homolytic bond cleavage	632
homosexual	514
homozygote	299
homunculus	346
hook	250
Hooke's Law	986, 1086
hormonal changes during pregnancy	469
hormone	361
hormone inhibin	460
hormone receptor	361
hormone types	361
human chorionic gonadotropin	469
human development	560
humanistic perspective	538
humanistic theory	538
humoral immunity	402
Hund's Rule	616
hyaline cartilage	453
hybridization	184, 637, 759
hybridization effect	69
hybrid orbitals	637
hydration	701
hydrogen bonding	643, 827
hydrolase	240
hydrophilic substances	160, 857
hydrophobic effect	122
hydrophobic/hydrophilic interactions	122
hydrophobic interaction	161, 858
hydrophobicity	160, 857
hydrophobic (nonpolar) amino acids	114
hydrostatic gauge pressure	965
hydrostatics	962
hydroxyapatite	451
hyperosmotic	278
hyperpolarized	336
hypertonic solution	278
hyperventilation	389
hypoosmotic	278
hypophysis	364
hypothalamic-pituitary portal system	364
hypothalamus	364, 580
hypoventilation	389
hypoxia	370
H zone	437

I

I bands	437
iconic memory	562
id	536
ideal fluid flow	978
Ideal Gas Law	671
identity formation	518
ileocecal valve	427
ileum	424
imine formation	819
immigration	511
immigration controls	515
immigration status	515
immune system	402
immunoglobulins (Ig)	381, 402
immunohistochemistry	91
implantation	472
implanted	469
implants	472
implicit memory	563
important stretching frequencies	63
impression management	531
incentives	541
incentive theory	541

incidence rate	510
incisors	422
incline angle	897
inclined plane	897
inclusive fitness	533
incomplete dominance	308
incompressible	966, 976
incongruence	538
incus	353
independent variable	41, 483
index of refraction	1116
indicator	725
induced	476
induced fit model	127
inducible enzymes	226
inductive effect	760, 768
industrialization	511
inertia	883
infantile amnesia	563
infant mortality rate	510
Inferential statistics	41
inferior vena cava	372
influence of individuals	519
informal norms	520
information-processing models	570
infrared (IR) spectroscopy	63
in-group	525
inguinal canal	456
inhibitory	338
inhibitory interneuron	340
inhibitory postsynaptic potentials (IPSPs	338
initiation	212, 221
Initiator caspases	295
inner cell mass	471
inner ear	353
inner membrane	146
in phase	1096
insecurely attached	561
in situ hybridization	91
insomnia	575
inspiration	393
inspiratory capacity (IC)	396
inspiratory reserve volume (IRV)	395
instinct	540
institutional discrimination	524
instrumental conditioning	554
instrumental functions	525
insulator (dielectric)	1009
insulin	154, 428
integral membrane proteins	267, 272
integration	68
integrative function	339
intensity	1105
intensity level	1105
intercalated disks	375, 444
intercellular clefts	387
intercostal muscles	394
interference	564, 1096
intergenerational mobility	517

intergenic regions	194
interleukins	405
intermediate filaments	288
intermediates	684
intermembrane space	146
intermolecular forces	641
internal locus of control	519
internal migration	511
internal resistance	1038
internal sphincter	410
internal validity	46, 491
internodal tract	378
interoceptors	351
inter-rater reliability	46
interstitial cells	456
intestinal villus	425
intragenerational mobility	517
intrinsic factor	427
invagination	473
Inverse-Square Law	890
ion-dipole forces	641
ion-electron	732
ion exchange chromatography	52
ionic	600
ionic bond	634
ionic radius	625
ionic solid	645
ionizability factor	275, 701
ionization energy	625
ionized	992
ion product	705
ions	606
iris	356
Iron Law of Oligarchy	531
irritant receptors	400
ischemia	370
islets of Langerhans	421, 428
isobaric process	954
isochoric process	955
isoelectric point	843
isoelectronic	621
isomerism	775
isoosmotic	278
isothermal process	955
isotopes	605
Ivan Pavlov	552

J

James-Lange Theory	578
Jean Piaget	571
jejunum	424
joint	453
joint capsule receptors	352
joule	920
Joule Heating Law	1034
justification of effort	547
just world phenomenon	523
juveniles	513
juxtaglomerular apparatus (JGA)	416

juxtaglomerular (JG) cells	416

K

Karl Marx	499
karyon	212
karyotyping	90
K-complex	574
keratin	291
keto-enol tautomerism	812
ketogenesis	171
ketone bodies	171
kidneys	409
kinase	129
kinematics	866
kinematics of shm	1089
kinetic concerns	281
kinetic control	825
kinetic energy	926
kinetic energy of a photoelectron	1138
kinetic friction	894
kinetic-molecular theory	669
kinetochore fibers	288
kinetochores	188
kingdom	248, 326
kin selection	325
Kirchhoff's laws	1034
Kitty Genovese	526
Krebs cycle	145

L

labia majora	463
labia minora	463
labioscrotal swellings	463
labor contractions	478
lac operon	226
lactase	139, 855
lactation	478
lacteals	388, 425, 433
lactose intolerant	139, 855
lactose malabsorbers	139, 855
lacunae	452
lagging strands	200
lag phase	255
lamellae	452
language	581
language acquisition	581
large intestine	408, 427
larynx	390
late adults	513
late gene	240
latent functions	498
lattice structure	645
launch angle	880
Law of Conservation of Mass	596
Law of Independent Assortment	304
Law of Refraction (Snell's Law)	1117
Law of Segregation	304
leading strands	200

leak channels	331
learned helplessness	519
leaving groups	773
Le Châtelier's principle	697
left bundle branches	378
lens	356, 1130
lens power	1132
leptin	430
lesbian and gay relationships	503
leukocytes	381
lever arm	914
levorotatory	789
Lewis acid	634, 772
Lewis base	634, 771
Lewis Dot Structures	628
Lewis dot symbol	628
life expectancy	510
ligaments	453
ligand	286
ligand-gated	280
ligand-gated ion channels	286
light chains	402
limbic system	344
limiting reagent	599
lingual lipase	423
linkage	312
lipases	162
lipemia	388, 433
lipid bilayer	163, 271, 859
lipid bilayer membranes	271, 859
lipids	857
lipoprotein lipase	433
lipoproteins	381
liposomes	328
liquid	664
liquid-liquid extraction	48
liter	669
liver	408, 428
local autoregulation	381
localization signals	267
locus	262, 298
locus of control	519
log phase	255
London dispersion forces	641
longitudinal layer	419
longitudinal method	493
Long-term memory	562
longitudinal muscle	420
longitudinal wave	1094
looking-glass self	519
loop of Henle	415
loose connective tissues	450
Lorentz force	1071
loss of heterozygosity	206
loudness	355
lower esophageal sphincter	423
lowering blood glucose	429
lubrication	457
Ludwig Gumplowicz	499

lumen	263
lung elasticity	393
luteal phase	467
Luteinizing hormone (LH)	460
lymph	401
lymphatic system	401
lymph nodes	401, 406
lymphokines	405
lysogen	241
lysogenic cycle	240, 241
lysosome	270
lysozyme	240, 402, 423
lytic cycle	240

M

macrophages	270, 384
macula	357
macula densa	416
magnetic fields	1063
magnetic force	1064
magnetic resonance imaging (MRI)	584
magnetoencephalography (MEG)	585
magnets	1079
magnification equation	1127
magnification factor	1127
magnitude of magnetic force	1064
major histocompatibility complex (mhc)	405
male reproductive system	456
male sexual act	457
malleus	353
maltase	139, 855
malthusian catastrophe	512
malthusianism	512
manifest functions	498
Margaret Harlow	560
Mary Ainsworth	561
Maslow's Hierarchy of Needs	542
mass	883, 889
mass defect	610
mass number	604
mass spectrometry	60
master status	529
mastication	422
material culture	507
maternal experience	477
maternal inheritance	458
matter	596
maturation	560
Max Weber	499, 530
mean	35
mechanical advantage	942
mechanical wave	1091
mechanism of hearing	354
mechanoreceptors	351
media	252
median	36
medium	252
medulla	343, 351, 410
medullary pyramids	410

megakaryocytes	384
meiosis	300
meiosis I	300
meiosis II	300
meiotic division	458
melting	184
membrane-bound organelles	247
membrane structure	271
memory	561
memory cells	403
memory construction and source monitoring	565
memory dysfunctions	564
memory storage	562
Mendelian Genetics	304
meninges	348
menopause	469
menstrual cycle	467
menstruation	467
mental set	572
mere exposure effect	532
mere presence	526
meritocracy	517
meso compounds	796
mesoderm	473
mesophiles	251
message characteristics	548
messenger RNA	189, 209
mesylates and tosylates	814
metallic solid	645
metaphase	292
metaphase I	301
metaphase plate	293
method of loci	562
metric units	590
MHC I	405
MHC II	405
micelle	161, 429, 858
microfilaments	288, 290
microRNA	190
microscopic	451
microspheres	328
microtubule	288
microtubule organizing center (MTOC)	288
microvilli	419, 424
midbrain	342
middle adults	513
middle ear	353
migration	323, 511
milk let-down	478
mindguarding	527
mineralocorticoids	351
miniature EPP (MEPP)	441
Minorities	512
mirror	1123
Mirror (and Lens) Equation	1126
misinformation effect	565
mismatch repair pathway	207
missense mutation	204
mitochondria	264

mitochondrial traits 318
mitosis 292
mitotic spindle 288
mitral valve 373
mixed-type inhibition 133, 135
mks system 864
mnemonic 562
mobile gas phase 57
mobile liquid phase 50
mode 37
modeling 558
molarity (*M*) 274, 590, 596
molar solubility 702, 704
mole 593
molecular formula 591
molecular geometry 636
molecular polarity 640
molecular solid 645
molecular weight (MW) 593
molecule 591
mole fraction 275, 596
monocistronic 209
monosaccharide 138, 849
monosomy 303
monosynaptic reflex arc 339
monotrichous 250
mood-dependent memory 564
morbidity 510
mores 520
mortality 510
morula 471
motile 250
motility 424
motivation 540
motor end plate 440
motor function 339
motor neurons 339
motor unit recruitment 441
mouth 422
mRNA Surveillance 231
mucociliary escalator 289, 389, 391
mucus membrane 421
Müllerian ducts 460
Müllerian inhibiting factor (MIF) 460
multiculturalism 521
multinucleate syncytia 436
multipolar 330
multipotent 476
multisubunit complex 124
muscle fibers 436, 443
muscle spindle 352
muscle stretch reflex 339
muscle tissue 436
mutarotation 852
mutation 323
myelin 334
myenteric plexus 420
myofibers 436
myofibrils 436

myoglobin 442
myometrium 464
myosin 437
myosin binding site 438
myosin light-chain kinase (MLCK) 446

N

n + 1 RULE 67
Na+/K+ ATPase 331
NADH dehydrogenase 147
naked viruses 239
narcolepsy 575
nasal cavit 390
nasopharynx 353
natural selection 323
meeds 541
negative charge 992
negative correlation 44
negative feedback 130, 364, 540
negative punishment 557
negative reinforcement 555
negative terminal 1030
neo-Malthusianism 512
nephron 411
nernst equation 335
networks 530
network solid 645
neural crest cells 474
neural folds 474
neural networks 560
neural plate 474
neuritic plaques 545
neuroendocrine cells 365
neurofibrillary tangles 545
neurohypophysis 365
neuroimaging techniques 584
neuromuscular junction (NMJ) 440
neuron 330
neurotransmitters 346
neurulation 474
neutralization reaction 721
neutral stimulus 553
neutrons 604
neutrophils 384
newton 885
Newton's Law of Gravitation 889, 890
Newton's laws 883
Newton's Second Law 884
Newton's Third Law 885
night terrors 576
Noam Chomsky 582
noble gases 617
nociceptors 351
nodes 1100
nodes of Ranvier 334
nomadism 511
nomenclature basics 748
nomenclature of alcohols 755

nomenclature of alkanes 752
nomenclature of haloalkanes 753
nonassociative learning 552
non-coding RNA 189, 210
noncompetitive inhibition 133
noncompetitive inhibitors 133
nondisjunction 303
nonelectrolytes 275, 701
non-experimental studies 492
nonhomologous end joining 208
non-material culture 507
nonpolar bond 633
non-random mating 323
nonsense codons 196
nonsense mutation 204
nonverbal communication 532
norepinephrine 337
normal boiling point 667
normal distribution 38
normal force 893
normal melting point 667
normative behavior 520
normative organizations 530
norms 507, 520
Northern Blotting 76
north pole (N) 1079
nose 390
nuclear binding energy 610
nuclear envelope 261, 263
nuclear family 503
nuclear localization sequence 263
nuclear matrix 262
nuclear pores 263
nuclear scaffold 262
nuclear shielding 624
nuclease 78, 428
nuclei 342
nucleic acids 180
nucleolus 262
nucleons 604
nucleophiles 771
nucleophilic substitutions 804
nucleoside 180
nucleosomes 186
nucleotides 179, 180
nucleus 261, 604
nucleus accumbens 577
null hypothesis 487
nutrition 252

O

object permanence 572
obligate aerobes 253
obligate anaerobes 253
obligate intracellular parasite 236
observational learning 538, 558
occipital lobes 344
octet 617
ohm 1024

Ohm's Law 1027
O—H Stretch 64
Okazaki fragments 200
olfaction 353
olfactory bulbs 353
olfactory receptors 351
oligosaccharide 849
oncogenes 294
oncotic pressure 381, 388
oogenesis 465
oogonia 300, 465
open complex 197, 212
open reading frame 209
operant conditioning 554
operational definition 484
opiates 576
opsin 358
optical activity 789
optic disk 357
optic nerve 356
optimism bias 523
orbital 615
orbital orientation 615
order 326
order of acidity 768
organelle 261
organizations 530
organ of corti 354
organogenesis 475
organometallic reagents 813
orgasm 457, 465
origin of life 328
origin of replication 197
oscillations 1084
osmosis 278
osmotic pressure 279
ossicles 353
osteoblasts 454
osteoclasts 454
osteocyte 450, 452, 454
osteon 452
outer ear 353
outer membrane 146
out-group 525
out of phase 1096
outsourcing 516
oval window 353
ovarian cycle 467
overconfidence 573
overpopulation 509
ovulated 465
ovulation 465
ovulatory phase 467
ovum 470
oxaloacetate 145
oxidant 732
oxidation 109, 732
oxidation number 600, 732
oxidation-reduction 732

oxidation-reduction reactions	732
oxidation state	600, 732
oxidative catabolism	110
oxidative decarboxylation	144
oxidative phosphorylation	141, 147, 148
oxidizing agent	732
oxygen	385
oxygen Utilization	253
oxytocin	478

P

pacemaker of the heart	376
pacinian corpuscles	351
pancreas	428
pancreatic acinar cells	421
pancreatic amylase	428
pancreatic duct	426
pancreatic lipase	428
pancreatic proteases	428
pansexual	515
papilla	410
papillae	410
paradoxical sleep	575
parallel-plate capacitor	1045
parallel processing	360
parallel β-pleated sheet	121
paramagnetic atoms	618
parasite	258
parasitic bacteria	258
parasomnias	576
parasympathetic	340
parent	606
parental DNA	196
parietal lobes	344
parietal pleura	393
Parkinson's Disease	545
partial pressure	678
parturition	478
pascal	670, 964
Pascal's Law	974
passive transport	279
Pauli exclusion principle	616, 1137
peaks	1092
Pearson correlation	493
peer pressure	528
pendulums	1089
penetrance	309
pentose phosphate pathway	156
pepsin	423
pepsinogen	423
peptide bond	117, 846
peptide hormones	362
peptides	362
peptide YY	430
peptidoglycan	249
peptidyl transferase	221
percentile	40
percent saturation (% sat.)	386

perception	570
perforating canals	452
perfusion	370
perilymph	354
period	619, 1084, 1091
periodic motion	1084
Periodic Table	619
periodic trends	624
peripheral chemoreceptors	399
peripheral membrane proteins	272
peripheral nervous system (PNS)	342
peripheral resistance	379
peripheral route	548
periplasmic space	249
peristalsis	420
peritrichous	250
peritubular capillaries	413
permittivity of free space	1046
peroxisomes	270
personal identity	518
personality	536
personality trait	539
person-situation controversy	539
persuasion	548
Petri dish	252
Peyer's patches	425
phagocytic vesicle	270
phagocytosis	270, 286
pharynx	390, 423
phase	599, 664
phase diagram	667
phase transition diagram	666
phase transitions	664
pH Calculations	719
phenomenological studies	494
phenotype	299
phonological loop	571
phosphatases	129
phosphodiester bonds	182
phosphoenolpyruvate carboxykinase (PEPCK)	152
phosphofructokinase (PFK)	142, 153
phospholipids	163, 271, 859
phosphorylases	129
photoautotrophs	109, 252
photoelectric effect	1137
photoheterotrophs	252
photon	1133
photon energy	1133
photoreceptors	352, 358
photosynthesis	109
phototrophs	252
phylum	326
physical attractiveness stereotype	523
physical changes	664
physical dependence	577
physiological arousal	577
physiological endpoint	363
physiological pH	842
pili	251

pinna	353	porin proteins	146
pinocytosis	286	porins	281
pitch	355	portal systems	371
pivot point	911, 912	positive charge	992
pi (π) Bonds	639	positive correlation	44
placebo effect	485	Positive punishment	557
placenta	469, 472	Positive reinforcement	555
placental villi	472	positive terminal	1030
Planck's constant	611, 1133	positive transfer	564
plane mirror	1123	positron	607
plane-polarized light	1121	positron emission	607
plaque	252	positron emission tomography (PET)	585
plasma	381	posterior chamber	356
plasma cells	403	posterior pituitary	365
plasma membrane	270	postganglionic neuron	348
plasmid	78, 80, 249	post-implantation development	473
plateau phase	377	post-replication repair	206
platelet plug	384	post-replication repair	207
plating	252	post-translational modification	231
pleasure principle	536	postzygotic	325
pleiotropism	309	potassium leak channels	283
pleura	393	potential energy	930
pleural pressure	393	power	924, 1035
pleural space	393	power dissipated by the resistor	1034
pluralism	521	power stroke	438
pluripotent	475	precapillary sphincters	379
PNS Anatomical Organization	347	precipitation	702
Poiseuille's Law	984	prefrontal cortex	580, 583
polar amino acids	114	preganglionic neuron	348
polar body	465	pregnancy	477
polar bond	633	prejudice	524
polar fibers	288	preoperational stage	572
polarity	273, 633	pre-screening bias	42
polarizability	771	pressure	669, 670, 964
polarization	1114, 1121	prevalence rate	510
polarized	331	prezygotic	325
polar stationary phase	50	pribnow box	212
polyatomic ions	592	primacy effect	561
polygenism	309	primary active transport	282
polymerase chain reaction (PCR)	83	primary bronchi	390
polymers	139	primary germ layers	473
polymorphisms	88	primary groups	525
polynucleotides	182	primary immune response	404
polyprotic	715	primary reinforcers	555
polyribosome	248	primase	198
polysaccharide	139, 849	priming	563
polysomnography (PSG)	574	primordial follicle	466
polyspermy	471	principle of aggregation	547
pons	343	Principle of Superposition for Electric Fields	1006
popular culture	507	Principle of Superposition for Electric Potential	1017
population	509	prions	245
population agin	513	proactive interference	564
population equilibrium	509	problem solving	572
population genetics	321	procarboxypeptidase	428
population-lag effect	509	procedural memory	563
population momentum	509	procollagenase	428
population projections	509	productive cycle	243
population studies	509	products	596
pore	281	proenzymes	232

projectile motion 879
projection bias 523
prokaryotes 247
prokaryotic replication 201
prokaryotic transcription 212
prokaryotic translation 220
prolactin 478
proliferative phase 467
proline 116
proofreading function 201
prophage 241
prophase 292
prophase I 301
proprioception 352
proprioceptors 352
prostaglandins 168
prostate 456
protease 118
protein domains 92
protein folding 231
protein interactions 92
proteinoids 328
protein quantification 94
proteins 432, 846
proteolysis 118
proteolytic cleavage 118, 129
proteolytic enzyme 118
proteomics 94
protobionts 328
proton 387, 604
proton gradient 148
protooncogenes 294
protoplast 249
provirus 243
proximal convoluted tubule (PCT) 413
Proximity 532
psychoanalytic perspective 536
psychoanalytic theory 536
psychological dependence 577
psychological disorder 543
psychologically fixated 537
psychrophiles 251
PTH (parathyroid hormone), calcitonin 454
public declaration 547
pulley 899
pull factors 511
pulmonary capillaries 396
pulmonary circulation 371, 396
pulmonary edema 396
pulmonary valves 373
Pulmonary Ventilation 393, 395
pulse 374
punishment 557
Punnett square 305
pure-breeding strain 304
purine base 179
purines 180
purkinje fibers 378
push factors 511

p-value 42, 488
pyloric sphincter 424
pyranoses 851
pyrimidine base 179
pyrimidines 180
pyrophosphate 178
pyruvate carboxylase 152
pyruvate dehydrogenase complex 140, 144
pyruvic acid 140

Q
qualitative 484
quantitative 484
quantitative polymerase chain reaction (qPCR) 85
quantization 1134
quantized 992, 1134
quantum physics 1134

R
race 514
racemic mixture 789
racemization 812
racism 514
radiation 950
radioactive 606
radioactive decay 606
radioimmunoassay (RIA) 73
radius of curvature 1124
radius vector 912
raising blood glucose 429
random Drift 323
randomized block technique 486
random sample 42
range 37, 882
rapid behavior acquisition 555
rapid extinction 555
rapid eye movement 574
rarefactions 1094
rate constant 690
rate-determining step 685
rate law 689
rate of population change 509
rational choice 501
rational choice theory 501
rationalization 531
rational-legal authority 505
reactants 596
reaction coordinate diagram 686
reaction coupling 125
reaction intermediates 760
reaction mechanism 684
reaction quotient 696
reaction rate 686
reaction rate (V, for velocity) 131
reality principle 536
recall 563
recency effect 561
receptor-mediated endocytosis 286

receptors	286
recessive	299
reciprocal control	153
reciprocal determinism	559
reciprocal inhibition	340
recognition	563
recombinant DNA	78
recombinant protein	78
recombination	301
rectum	427
red marrow	451
redox	732
red oxidative	443
redox pair	110
redox titrations	738
red slow twitch	443
reducing agent	732
reducing environment	328
reducing sugars	856
reductant	732
reduction	109, 732
reduction of carboxylic acids	827
reference group	525
reflex	339
refracted	355, 1116
refraction	1116
refractory period	336
refugees	511
regulation of ventilation rate	399
rehearsal	562
reinforcement	555
reinforcement schedule	555
relative poverty	517
relative refractory period	336
relaxed	385
relearning	563
releasing and inhibiting factors	364
releasing and inhibiting hormones	364
reliability	46
reliable	487
religion	504
religiosity	504
remodeling	454
REM sleep	575
renal artery	410
renal cortex	415
renal medulla	415
renal pelvis	410
renal tubule	409, 411
renal vein	410
renin	416
replacement fertility rate	509
replicating telomeres	202
replication	210
replication forks	199
repolarization	331, 332
repolarized	333
representativeness heuristic	573
reproductive isolation	325

residential segregation	517
residual volume (RV)	396
residue	117, 847
resistance	379, 1023, 1024
resistivity	1025
resistors	1027
resistors in parallel	1028
resistors in series	1028
resolution	458, 465, 793
resonance effects	765
resonance hybrid	631, 761
resonance stabilization	761
resonance structures	630
resource model of attention	569
respiration	389
respiratory alkalosis	389
respiratory bronchiole	390, 391
respiratory control center	399
respiratory epithelium	391
respiratory membrane	398
respiratory zone	391, 389
resting membrane potential	283, 331
restoring force	1086
restriction endonucleases	78
restriction fragment length polymorphism (RFLP)	88
retention interval	564
retina	356
retinal	358
retrieval	563
retrieval cues	563
retroactive interference	564
retro-aldol reaction and dehydration	825
retrograde amnesia	564
retroviruses	244
reverse culture shock	508
reverse migration	511
reverse transcriptase-polymerase chain reaction	84
reverse transcription	244
reversibility	661
revolutions	508
Rh blood group	383
ribose	209
ribose sugar	179
ribosomal RNA	190, 210
ribosome	195, 219
ribosome binding site	221
ribozymes	190, 210
right bundle branches	378
right-handed double helix	185
right-hand rule	1065
rigor mortis	442
ring strain	774
rites of passage	513
RNA-dependent RNA polymerase	244
RNA Interference	231
RNA Translocation	231
rod	250, 356
role conflict	530
role exit	530

role-playing	547
roles	529
role strain	530
root-mean-square	1062
rotational equilibrium	917
rough ER	265
round window	353
rule of addition	308
rule of multiplication	308
running	50
rural flight	511

S

saccule	353, 355
saliva	422
salivary amylase (ptyalin)	422
salivary glands	428
salt	722
saltatory conduction	334
salt bridge	733
sample size	41, 488
sampling bias	42
sanctions	520
Sapir-Whorf hypothesis	582
saponification	162
sarcolemma	436
sarcomeres	437
sarcoplasmic reticulum (SR)	441
saturated fatty acids	857
saturated solution	702
Schachter-Singer Theory	579
schema	565
schwann cells	334
sclera	355
secondary active transport	282, 283
secondary group	525
secondary immune response	404
secondary reinforcers	555
secondary sexual characteristics	462
second ionization energy	625
Second Law of Thermodynamics	657, 958
second messenger	286
second trimester	477
secretin	427
secretion	409, 414
secretory phase	467
securely attached	561
selective attention	568
selective permeability	280
selective priming	569
selective reabsorption	409, 413
self-actualization	538
self-concept	518, 538
self-consciousness	518
self-efficacy	519
self-esteem	519
self-fulfilling prophecy	524
self-handicapping	531

self-identity	518
self-presentation	531
self-reference effect	518
self-schemas	518
self-selection bias	42
self-serving bias	523
semantic memory	563
semen	456
semicircular canals	353, 355
seminal vesicles	456
seminiferous tubules	456
semipermeable membrane	278
senescence	296
sensitization	552
sensorimotor stage	572
sensory function	339
sensory memory	562
serial position effect	561
series	1027
serotonin	337
serum	381
settlers	511
sex	513
sex chromosomes	310
sex-linked traits	311, 318
sex pilus	251
sexual orientation	514
sexual selection	325
shear forces	985
shear modulus	986
shear strain	986
sheath	238
shielding	624
shielding effect	624
shine-dalgarno sequence	221
short tandem repeat (STR)	88
short-term memory	562
sick role	506
side chain	112, 836
sigma factor (σ)	212
sigma (σ) Bonds	638
Sigmund Freud	537
signal recognition particle (SRP)	266
signal sequence	266
signal transduction	286
significant difference	487
silent mutation	204
similarity	533
simple diffusion	280
simple distillation	58
simple harmonic motion	1085
simple pendulum	1089
simple sugar	849
single bond	629
single circular chromosome	186
single nucleotide polymorphisms	194
single-strand binding proteins (SSBPs)	197
single-stranded	209
sinoatrial (SA) node	376, 378

sister chromatids	292
situational attribution	522
size exclusion chromatography	55
skeletal muscle	340, 436
skin	402, 408
sleep apnea	575
sleep disorders	575
sleep spindles	574
sliding friction	894
slow block to polyspermy	471
slow calcium channel	375
slow channels	444
small interfering RNA	190
small Intestine	424
small nuclear RNA	190
smooth ER	265
smooth muscle	419, 436, 445
SN2 Mechanism	804
soaps	858
social behavior	532
social behaviorism	519
social capital	517
social change	508
social cognition	523
social cognitive perspective	538
Social Cognitive Theory	559
social construct	500
social constructionism	500
social cues	539
social development and attachment	560
social dysfunction	498
social exchange theories	501
social exchange theory	501
social facilitation	526
social facilitation effect	526
social factors	559
social facts	498
social geography	511
social identity	518
social institutions	502
social interactions	531
socialism	505
socialization	520
social learning	558
social loafing	526
social mobility	517
social network	530
social perception	523
social reproduction	517
social roles	529
social stratification	517
social structures	529
social support	533
society	498
sociobiology	507
sociocultural evolution	508
socioeconomic status (SES)	517
sociology	498
sodium leak channels	376
solenoid	1075
solid	645, 664
Solomon Asch	528
solubility	702
solubility computations	704
solubility product constant	703
solution	701
solutions and solubility	701
solvation	701
solvation shell	161, 858
solvent	701
soma	330
somatic division	340
somatic PNS anatomy	348
somatostatin	428
somnambulism	576
sound level	1105
sound waves	1094
source characteristics	548
source charge(s)	999
source monitoring	565
sources of magnetic fields	1074
source traits	539
Southern Blotting	76
south pole (S)	1079
spatial summation	338
species	325, 326
specific gravity	962
specific heat	649
specific real area	42
specific rotation	789
spectroscopy	59
speed	868
speed of light	1114
spermatogenesis	456, 458
spermatogonia	300
spermatozoa	458
spherical mirrors	1124
sphincter of Oddi	426
sphincters	424
sphingolipids	166
spicules	452
spike potentials	446
spinal cord	342
spinal nerves	347
spin-spin splitting phenomenon	67
spirometer	395
spirometric graph	395
spirometry	395
spleen	406
spliceosome	213
splicing	213
splitting	67
spontaneous recovery	553
spring constant	1086
S (synthesis) phase	196
stabilizing selection	325
stage 1 sleep	574
stage 2 sleep	574

stage 3 sleep	575
stages of sleep	574
staggered conformation	775
standard conditions	652
standard deviation	38
standard heat of formation	652
standard molar volume	673
Standard Temperature and Pressure (STP)	670
standing wave	1099
Stanley Milgram	528
stapes	353
state	539, 664
State capitalism	505
States	539
states of Consciousness	574
static equilibrium	917
static friction	894
stationary liquid phase	57
stationary phase	255
statistical power	41
statistics	34
status	529
stem cells	96
stereocenter	782
stereogenic center	782
stereoisomerism	781
stereoisomers	781
stereotypes	523
stereotype threat	524
steroid hormones	362
steroids	165
sticky ends	78
stigma	527
stigma and deviance	527
stimulants	576
stimulus duration	352
stimulus intensity	352
stimulus location	352
stimulus modality	352
stoichiometric coefficients	596
stomach	423
stop codons	196
storage	570
strain	986
stranger anxiety	560
stratification and inequality	517
Strecker Synthesis	839
stress	581, 985
striated muscle	419
stroke volume (SV)	374
strong acid	712
strong electrolytes	275, 701
strong nuclear force	606
structural formulas	758
structural imaging	584
structure of the ear	353
subculture	521
submucosal plexus	420
sub-replacement fertility	509

substantia nigra	545
substrates	127
subunit	124
suburbanization	511
suburbs	511
subviral particles	245
sulfur-containing amino acids	115
summation	338
supercoils	186
superego	536
superior vena cava	372
surface tension	392
surface traits	539
surfactant	392
sustentacular cells	456
symbiotic bacteria	258
symbolic culture	507
symbolic interactionism	499, 519
sympathetic	340
symports	281
synapse	336
synapsis	301
synaptic cleft	330
synaptic knobs	330
synaptic transmission	330, 336
synarthroses	453
syn conformation	778
syngamy	458
synonyms	196
synovial capsule	453
synovial fluid	453
systemic arterial pressure	380
systemic circulation	371
systole	373
systolic pressure	380

T

taboo	520
Talcott Parsons	506
tandem repeats	194
target characteristics	548
targeting signals	267
taste-aversion	554
taste buds	353
taste hairs	353
taste pore	353
tautomers	812
taxonomy	247, 326
T cell clone	406
T cell receptor	405
T cells	405
tectorial membrane	354
telecommunications	516
telencephalon	343
telomerase	203
telomeres	188, 202, 262
telophase	292
telophase I	302

temperature	251, 669, 946	torque	911
template-driven polymerization	210	Torricelli's result	981
temporal lobes	344	total fertility rate	509
temporal summation	338	total internal reflection	1118
tendons	436, 453	total lung capacity (TLC)	396
tense	385	total mechanical energy	935
tensile strain	986	totipotent	475
tension/compression	987	trabeculae	452
tension forces	985	trachea	390, 423
terminal bronchioles	390	traditional authority	505
terminal voltage	1038	trait perspective	539
termination	212, 221	traits	539
terpenes	164	trait versus state controversy	539
terrorism	516	trajectory	879
tesla	1064	transcription	194, 210
testcross	304	transcription bubble	212
testosterone	166, 460	transduction	242, 256
test-retest reliability	46	transesterification	830
tetrad	301	transfer RNA	190, 210
The Big Five	873	transformation	256
thecal cells	466	transfusion reaction	383
the digestive system	418	transgender	514
the gastrointestinal tract	422	transition shock	508
T helpers	405	transition state	686
theories of population change	512	translation	195
theory of mind	583	translational equilibrium	917
thermal expansion	950	translocation	205, 221
thermodynamic cycles	957	transmembrane domains	267, 272
thermodynamics	106, 107, 648, 947	transmembrane transport	274
thermophiles	251	transmissible spongiform encephalopathies	246
thermoreceptors	352	transmitted	1116
theta mechanism	201	transport of gases	385
theta replication	201	transposons	194
theta waves	574	transverse tubules	441
the trp operon	229	transverse waves	1091
thick filaments	437	triacylglycerols (TG)	161, 859
thin filaments	437	trial and error	572
thin-layer chromatography (TLC)	50	tricarboxylic acid cycle (TCA cycle)	145
Third Law of Thermodynamics	658	tricuspid valve	373
third trimester	477	triglyceride	161, 859
Thomas Robert Malthus	512	triple bonds	629
thoracic duct	401	triple bond stretch	64
three components of emotion	577	triple point	667
threshold of hearing	1105	trisomy	303
threshold potential	331	tRNA loading	217
thrombin	384	troph	252
thrombus	385	trophoblast	471
thymine	180	tropic hormones	363
thymus	405, 406	tropomyosin	439
thyroid hormone	365	troponin	439
tidal volume (TV)	395	troponin-tropomyosin complex	439
tight junctions	290, 419	troughs	1092
T killers	405	trp operon	226
tocopherols	168	trypsin	428
tolerance	406	trypsinogen	426, 428
tolerant anaerobes	253	t-test	42
tonicity	278	T-tubules	375, 441
tonsils	406	tumor suppressor genes	294
topoisomerases	197	turbulent flow	979

twin studies	493
twitch	441
tympanic membrane	353
Type II Fast Twitch Fibers	443
Type I Slow Twitch Fibers	443
types of learning	552

U

ubiquinone	147
ultraviolet/visible (UV/Vis) spectroscopy	61
unattended channel	568
uncompetitive inhibition	133
uncompetitive inhibitor	134
unconditioned reinforcers	555
unconditioned response (UR)	553
unconditioned stimulus (US)	553
uniform circular motion	902
uniformly accelerated motion	873
unimolecular	807
uniports	281
UNITS and dimensions	864
universal emotions	578
universal recipients	383
unsaturated fatty acids	857
upper esophageal sphincter	423
upward mobility	517
uracil	209
urban blight	512
urban decline	511
urban growth	511
urbanization	511
urban renewal	511
urban sprawl	511
urea	381
ureter	410
urethra	456
urethral opening	463
urinary bladder	410
urinary system	410
uterine cycle	467
uterine tubes	464
uterus	464
utilitarian organizations	530
utricle	353, 355

V

vaccination	404
vagal tone	378
vagina	464
vagus nerve	347, 378
valence	620
valence shell electron-pair repulsion (VSEPR) theory	635
validity	46
values	507
valves	373
van der Waals equation	675
van der Waals forces	122
van't Hoff equation	279

van't Hoff factor	275, 701
vapor pressure	276, 644
vapor-pressure depression	276
variable (antigen binding) region	402
variable-interval schedule	556
variable-ratio schedule	556
variables	41
vasa recta	416
vasopressin	414
vector field	999
veins	370
velocity	867
venous return	374
ventilation	389
ventricles	372
venturi effect	983
venules	370
verbal communication	532
vicarious	538
vicarious learning	558
Villi	424
villus	424
viral genomes	243
viroids	246
viruses	236
visceral pleura	393
visual cortex	360
visuospatial sketchpad	571
vital capacity (VC)	396
vitamin K	427
vitamins	434
vitreous chamber	356
vitreous humor	356
vocal cords	390
volatile	644
volt	1012
voltage	1023
voltage-gated	280
voltage-gated sodium channels	331
voltmeters	1042
volume	669
Vsepr Theory	635

W

water-soluble	434
Watson-Crick Model	183
watt	924
wave effects	1120
wave equation	1092
wavelength	1092
wavenumber	63
wave-particle duality	1133
waves	1091
wave speed	1092
waxes	167
weak acid	712
weak electrolytes	275, 701
Weber's Law	361

weight 889
welfare capitalism 505
Wernicke's aphasia 582
Wernicke's area 582
western blotting 77
Wobble Hypothesis 216
wolffian ducts 460
work 920, 953
Work-Energy Theorem 927
work function 1138
working memory 571

X

X chromosomes 310
X-linked dominant 319

Y

Y chromosomes 310
yellow marrow 451
Yerkes-Dodson Law 578
yolk sac 473

Z

Zeroth Law of Thermodynamics 648, 947
Z lines 437
zona pellucida 466, 470
zwitterion 843
zygote 458, 470
zymogen 232, 423, 428

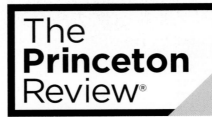
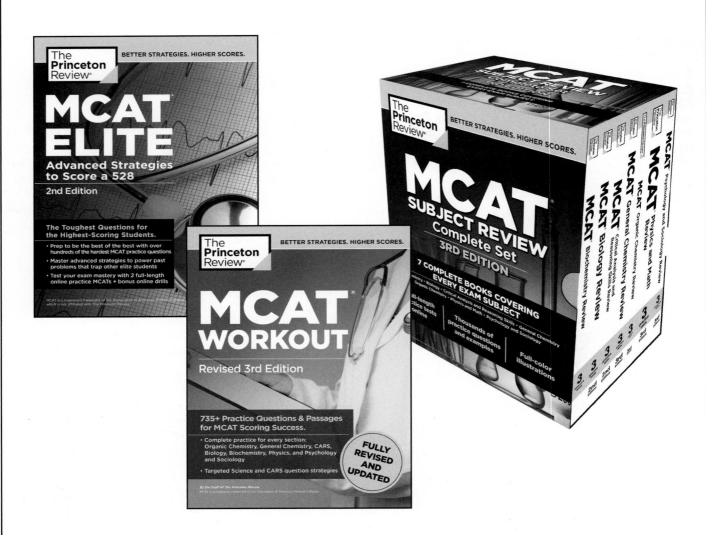

BIOLOGY AND BIOCHEMISTRY

THE CELL

The plasma membrane

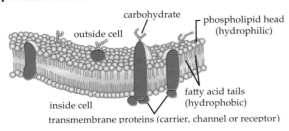

outside cell

carbohydrate

phospholipid head (hydrophilic)

fatty acid tails (hydrophobic)

inside cell

transmembrane proteins (carrier, channel or receptor)

ORGANELLES

- **Ribosome:** protein synthesis via translation
- **Nucleus:** houses the genome in chromosomes
- **Mitochondria:** cell respiration and energy production
- **Rough ER and Golgi:** protein trafficking and modification
- **Lysosome:** autophagy and degradation

ENZYMES AND CELLULAR METABOLISM

REGULATION

- **Reversible inhibition:** competitive inhibitors bind to active site; noncompetitive inhibitors to an allosteric site; uncompetitive inhibitors to the enzyme substrate complex

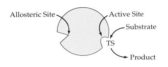

Allosteric Site

Active Site

Substrate

TS

Product

METABOLISM

Glycolysis occurs in the cell cytoplasm; produces 2 net ATP, 2 pyruvate, and 2 NADH.

Fermentation occurs in anaerobic conditions. Pyruvate is converted into lactic acid (in muscle) or ethanol (in yeast).

Respiration occurs in aerobic conditions.

- **Pyruvate decarboxylation:** Pyruvate converted to Acetyl-CoA in the mitochondrial matrix.
- **Citric acid cycle:** Acetyl-CoA enters, reduced electron carriers (NADH, $FADH_2$) and CO_2 exit.
- **Electron transport chain:** $NADH/FADH_2$ oxidized, electrons passed from carrier to carrier, proton gradient generated across inner mitochondrial membrane
- **Oxidative phosphorylation:** Proton gradient provides energy for ATP synthase to phosphorylate ADP into ATP.

Glycogenesis/Glycogenolysis occurs in the liver and skeletal muscle and is a means of storing/releasing glucose.

Gluconeogenesis occurs in the liver when dietary glucose is unavailable and glycogen stores are depleted; conversion of non-carbohydrate precursors into glucose.

The **pentose phosphate pathway** creates ribose-5 phosphate (precursor to nucleotide synthesis) and NADPH (reducing energy for other anabolic pathways).

Fatty acid oxidation a repeated series of four reactions that liberate an acetyl-CoA in addition to generating $FADH_2$ and NADH.

Fatty acid synthesis is a repeated series of reactions that adds two carbons at a time until a 16-carbon fatty acid is produced. It requires NADPH.

MOLECULAR GENETICS

Nucleic acid

- Basic unit: nucleotide (sugar, nitrogenous base, phosphate)
- Sugar in DNA is deoxyribose; sugar in RNA is ribose.
- 2 types of bases: double-ringed purines (adenine, guanine) and single-ringed pyrimidines (cytosine, thymine, uracil)
- DNA double helix; antiparallel strands joined by hydrogen bonding between base pairs (A=T, G ≡ C)
- RNA is usually single-stranded: A pairs with U, not T

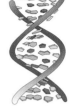

DNA Replication

- Key enzymes are helicase (unwinds the DNA), primase (lays down RNA primer), and DNA polymerases (synthesize DNA).

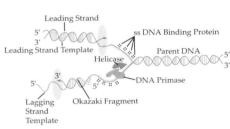

Leading Strand

5′
3′

Leading Strand Template

ss DNA Binding Protein

Parent DNA

5′
3′

Helicase

DNA Primase

5′
3′

Lagging Strand Template

Okazaki Fragment

MUTATIONS

Point: One nucleotide is substituted by another; they are silent if the amino acid sequence doesn't change.

Frameshift: Insertions or deletions shift reading frame; generally serious mutations because many amino acids are affected.

Transcript Regulation in Prokaryotes

Operon: An operator and promoter control transcription of one or more genes.

- Operator: binding site of repressor protein
- Promoter: binding site of RNA polymerase
- Generates polycistronic transcripts that are translated by polyribosomes
- Inducible systems need an inducer for transcription to occur; common in catabolic processes
- Repressive systems need a corepressor to inhibit transcription; common in biosynthetic pathways

EUKARYOTIC PROTEIN SYNTHESIS

- **Transcription:** RNA polymerase synthesizes hnRNA using DNA, "antisense strand" as a template.
- **Post-transcriptional processing:** Introns are cut out of hnRNA, exons spliced to form mRNA; mRNA is 5' and 3' capped and exported out of the nucleus.
- **Translation** occurs on ribosomes in the cytoplasm.

Post-translational modifications: made before the polypeptide becomes a functional protein, include disulfide bridge formation, glycosylation, phosphorylation, and clipping

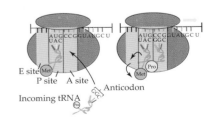

E site

P site   A site

Anticodon

Incoming tRNA

MICROBIOLOGY

Viruses
- Acellular structures of double or single-stranded DNA or RNA in a protein capsid
- Lytic cycle: virus kills the host
- Lysogenic cycle: virus enters host genome
- Retroviruses are RNA viruses that create DNA versions of themselves to insert in a host-cell genome.

Bacteria
- Single-celled prokaryotes
- Single circular DNA genome
- Gram + have thick cell walls, Gram—have thin cell walls and an outer membrane
- Reproduce by binary fission

Prions: abnormal protein that can induce structural changes in the normal version of the protein; responsible for spongiform encephalopathies

CLASSICAL GENETICS

Law of independent assortment: Alleles of unlinked genes assort independently in meiosis.
- If both parents are *Rr*, the alleles separate to give a genotypic ratio of 1:2:1 (RR:Rr:rr) and a phenotypic ratio of 3:1 (dom:rec).
- For two traits: *AbBb* parents will produce *AB*, *Ab*, *aB*, and *ab* gametes.
- The phenotypic ratio for an AaBb × AaBb cross is 9:3:3:1.

Statistical calculations
- The probability of A and B occurring together is the product of their individual probabilities (Prob A × Prob B).
- The probability of A or B occurring (assuming they are mutually exclusive) is the sum of their individual probabilities (Prob A + Prob B).

NERVOUS SYSTEM:

The **neuron** is the basic cell.
The signal generated by a neuron is called an **action potential**.
The **CNS** is the brain and the spinal cord.
The **PNS** can be divided into the somatic (voluntary) and autonomic (involuntary) divisions.
- The somatic system controls the skeletal muscles.
- The autonomic system can be divided into the parasympathetic (rest and digest) division and the sympathetic (fight or flight) division.

CIRCULATION

The **heart**: The pathway of blood through the heart is: body → RA → tricuspid valve → RV → pulmonary seminlunary valve → pulmonary artery → lungs → pulmonary veins →LA → bicuspid valve → LV → aortic semilunar valve → aorta → body.

Arteries carry blood away from the heart and **veins** carry blood toward the heart. **Capillaries** are the sites of exchange between blood and tissue.

Blood pressure is directly proportional to cardiac output and peripheral resistance.

RESPIRATORY SYSTEM

The **respiratory system** functions in gas exchange and pH regulation.

The **conduction zone** is for ventilation only and includes the nose, nasal cavity, pharynx, larynx, trachea, right and left primary bronchi, bronchioles, and terminal bronchioles.

The **respiratory zone** is for respiration (gas exchange) and includes the respiratory bronchioles, the alveolar ducts, and the alveoli.

Ventilation rate is controlled by pH. A high pH reduces ventilation rate and a low pH increases ventilation rate.

RENAL SYSTEM

The **kidneys** produce urine, regulate blood pressure, regulate ion and water balance, regulate pH, activate vitamin D, and secrete erythropoietin.

The functional unit of the kidney is the **nephron**. It uses filtration, reabsorption, and secretion to produce urine.

IMMUNE SYSTEM

The body distinguishes between "self" and "nonself."

HUMORAL IMMUNITY (SPECIFIC DEFENSE)

B lymphocytes

Memory cells
Remember antigen, speed up secondary response

Plasma cells
Make and release antibodies (IgG, IgA, IgM, IgD, IgE), which induce antigen phagocytosis

CELL-MEDIATED IMMUNITY

T lymphocytes

Cytotoxic T cells destroy cells directly.

Suppressor cells regulate B cells and T cells to decrease anti-antigen activity.

Helper T cells activate B cells and T cells and macrophages by secreting lymphokines.

Memory cells

Nonspecific immune response includes skin, passages lined with cilia, macrophages, acidic stomach and vagina, inflammatory response, and interferons (proteins that help prevent the spread of a virus).

Autoimmunity is when the immune system attacks and destroys normal body proteins.

ENDOCRINE SYSTEM

Direct hormones directly stimulate organs; tropic hormones stimulate other glands. Mechanisms of hormone action: **Peptides (P)** act via binding a receptor on the PM and inducing second messengers. **Steroids (S)** diffuse across the plasma membrane and act via hormone/receptor binding to DNA.

<table>
<tr><td></td><td>Anterior Pituitary</td><td>Action</td></tr>
<tr><td rowspan="11">Peptides</td><td>Follicle-stimulating (FSH)</td><td>Follicle maturation, spermatogenesis</td></tr>
<tr><td>Luteinizing (LH)</td><td>Ovulation, testosterone synthesis</td></tr>
<tr><td>Adrenocorticotropic (ACTH)</td><td>Stimulates adrenal cortex</td></tr>
<tr><td>Thyroid-stimulating (TSH)</td><td>Stimulates thyroid gland</td></tr>
<tr><td>Prolactin</td><td>Milk production</td></tr>
<tr><td>Growth hormone</td><td>Whole body growth, increase metabolism</td></tr>
<tr><td>Posterior Pituitary</td><td>Action</td></tr>
<tr><td>Oxytocin</td><td>Uterine contractions, milk ejection</td></tr>
<tr><td>Antidiuretic (ADH, vasopressin)</td><td>Increase water retention</td></tr>
<tr><td>Thyroid Gland</td><td></td></tr>
<tr><td>Thyroid hormones (T4, T3)</td><td>Increase metabolism</td></tr>
<tr><td></td><td>Calcitonin</td><td>Decrease blood calcium</td></tr>
<tr><td></td><td>Parathyroid Glands</td><td></td></tr>
<tr><td></td><td>Parathyroid hormone (PTH)</td><td>Increase blood calcium</td></tr>
<tr><td></td><td>Adrenal medulla</td><td></td></tr>
<tr><td></td><td>Epinephrine</td><td>Increases "fight or flight" response</td></tr>
<tr><td></td><td>Pancreas</td><td></td></tr>
<tr><td></td><td>Insulin</td><td>Reduces blood sugar</td></tr>
<tr><td></td><td>Glucagon</td><td>Increases blood sugar</td></tr>
<tr><td rowspan="8">Steroids</td><td>Adrenal Cortex</td><td></td></tr>
<tr><td>Cortisol</td><td>"stress hormone" controls blood sugar, regulates metabolism, memory formation</td></tr>
<tr><td>Aldosterone</td><td>Increase renal sodium reabsorption</td></tr>
<tr><td>Testes</td><td></td></tr>
<tr><td>Testosterone</td><td>Male secondary sex characteristics</td></tr>
<tr><td>Ovaries/Placenta</td><td></td></tr>
<tr><td>Estrogen</td><td>Female secondary sex characteristics, endometrial growth</td></tr>
<tr><td>Progesterone</td><td>Endometrial maintenance</td></tr>
</table>

DIGESTION

Alimentary Canal:
- mouth: grind food, begin starch digestion
- esophagus: tube to stomach
- stomach: storage tank, acid hydrolysis, limited digestion/absorption
- sm. intestine: most digestion/absorption
- lg. intestine: water reabsorption, store feces

Accessory Organs:
- liver: make bile
- gallbladder: store/ concentrate bile
- pancreas: secrete digestive enzymes and bicarbonate

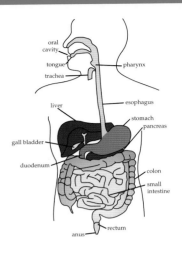

REPRODUCTION

Cell division

- G_1: cell growth and metabolism
- S: DNA replication
- G_2: same as G_1
- M: the cell divides in two

SEXUAL REPRODUCTION

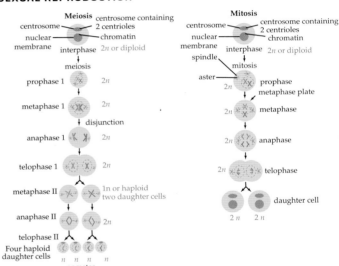

In humans
- Spermatogenesis in males (making sperm in the seminiferous tubules of the testes) and oogenesis (making ova in the ovaries) in females are examples of meiosis.

FOUR STAGES OF EARLY DEVELOPMENT
Cleavage: mitotic divisions of the zygote to form the morula
Implantation: blastocyst (trophoblast and inner cell mass) implants into the uterus wall
Gastrulation: ectoderm, endoderm, and mesoderm form
Neurulation: develop a nervous system and all other body organs

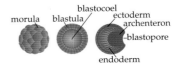

MUSCULAR SYSTEM

Sarcomere
- Contractile unit of the skeletal muscle
- Contains thin actin and thick myosin filaments

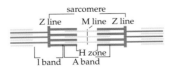

SKELETAL MUSCLE CONTRACTION
- ACh release from a neuron leads to action potential
- Ca^{2+} in the sarcoplasm increases
- Actin released from troponin/tropomyosin regulation
- Myosin and actin interact and cause muscle contraction
- Sarcomeres, H zone, and I band shorten

PSYCHOLOGY AND SOCIOLOGY

SOCIETY

Society: the group of people who share a culture and live/interact with each other within a definable area

Socialization: the process through which people learn to be proficient and functional members of society

Norms are society's rules and expectations for the behavior of its members. They are enforced by **sanctions**.

- **Formal Norms** (for example, laws) are generally written down, clearly defined, and accompanied by strict penalties for those who violate them.
- **Informal Norms** (for example, how to behave at a funeral) are generally understood by all but are less clearly defined, and carry no specific punishments for those who violate them.

Mores are norms that are highly important for the benefit of society and so are often strictly enforced.

Folkways are norms that are less important but shape everyday behavior (for example, styles of dress).

Taboos are norms that are so strong that their violation is considered forbidden and oftentimes punishable through formal or informal methods. Taboo behaviors result in disgust toward the violator.

Non-normative behavior challenges shared values and institutions, threatening social structure and cohesion. These behaviors are seen as abnormal and thus discouraged.

Deviance describes actions that violate dominant social norms, either formal or informal.

Assimilation occurs when an individual forsakes aspects of his or her own cultural tradition to adopt those of a different culture.

Amalgamation occurs when majority and minority groups combine to form a new group.

THEORETICAL APPROACHES TO SOCIOLOGY

Functionalism is a view that conceptualizes society as a living organism with many different parts and organs, each of which has a distinct purpose.

Conflict Theory views society as a competition for limited resources, which results in inequality.

Symbolic interactionism starts at the micro (close-up) level and sees society as the buildup of every-day typical interactions; this theory focuses on communication, the exchange of information through language and symbols.

Social constructionism argues that people actively shape their reality through social interactions; it is therefore something that is constructed, not inherent.

Feminist Theory is concerned with the differing social experiences of men and women, including how social structures contribute to gender differences (macro-level) and the effects of gender differences on individual interactions (micro-level).

Rational-Choice and Social-Exchange Theory both suggest that human behavior is driven by a desire to maximize benefit and minimize loss.

Social loafing: tendency for people to exert less effort in a group than if they were individually accountable

Group polarization: phenomenon in which the average view of a member of a group is accentuated after like-minded group members confer

Groupthink: phenomenon in which group members value harmony and agreement over a careful consideration of the problem/issue and therefore come to a faulty consensus decision

Conformity: behavior in accordance with what others are doing

Obedience: action in accordance with the explicit instructions of an authority figure

SOCIAL BEHAVIOR

Impression management: conscious or unconscious attempt to manage one's own image by influencing the perceptions of others

Dramaturgical perspective: within symbolic interactionism, a theory that posits that we imagine ourselves playing certain roles when interacting with others, like actors on a stage

The **mere exposure effect** suggests that people prefer things that they have been repeatedly exposed to.

Inclusive fitness suggests that altruism among organisms who share genes increases the chances those genes will be passed on to subsequent generations.

SOCIAL STRUCTURES

Status: a broad term that refers to all socially defined positions within a society; **ascribed statuses** are assigned to a person by society regardless of the person's own efforts, while **achieved statuses** are due largely to the individual's efforts

Social roles: expectations for people of a given social status

Role conflict: conflict in society's expectations for *multiple statuses* held by the same person

Role strain: phenomenon in which a single status results in conflicting expectations

Role exit: phenomenon in which disengaging from a role that has become closely tied to one's self-identity to take on another

Social stratification: the subdivision of society by status according to wealth, education, power, or some other status marker

Caste system: a closed stratification in which people can do nothing to change the category they are born into.

Class system: a type of stratification that considers both social variables and individual initiative; classes are open, meaning that people can strive to reach a higher class (or fall to a lower one)

Social mobility: the ability to move up or down in social class

Socioeconomic status (SES) can be defined in terms of power (influence over others), property (possessions and income) and prestige (reputation in society).

Social reproduction refers to the structures and activities in place in a society that serve to transmit and reinforce social inequality from one generation to the next.

Cultural capital: the non-financial social assets that promote upward social mobility (e.g., education, credentials)

Social capital: social networks that promote upward social mobility

SOCIAL INTERACTIONS

Attribution Theory is rooted in social psychology and attempts to explain how individuals view behavior, both our own behavior and the behavior of others; this can lead to many biases.

Prejudice: thoughts, feelings, and attitudes about another group that are not based on actual experience

Discrimination: bias actions, usually negatively, toward a group

Group: a collection of people (two or more) who regularly interact and identify with each other, sharing similar norms, values, and expectations

Primary groups: (for example, families) groups that play a more important role in an individual's life; these groups are usually smaller, more intimate, and longer-term. Primary groups serve expressive functions by meeting emotional needs.

Secondary groups: (for example, classmates, coworkers) groups that are usually larger and more impersonal, and may interact for specific reasons for shorter periods of time

Reference groups are those which one compares themselves to

Social network: a web of social relationships, including directly links and indirect connections

Organization: large, less personal collections of individuals that come together to pursue specific goals; tend to be complex and hierarchically structured

Utilitarian organizations: organization in which members are paid or otherwise compensated for their efforts

Normative organizations: type of organization that members join because of shared moral goals

Coercive organizations: type of organization that members are forced to join

Bureaucracy: an organization designed to specifically accomplish work tasks. Bureaucracies include division of labor, management, structure, and are designed to be very efficient.

McDonaldization: social phenomenon in which a culture or geographic area adopts characteristics and values of a fast-food restaurant

Iron Law of Oligarchy: tendency of all social structures to develop systemic inequality and other characteristics of oligarchy as they evolve over time

Social facilitation: tendency of people to perform simple, well-learned tasks better in front of other people, and more complex tasks more poorly

Deindividuation: tendency that when situations are highly arousing and individuals feel a low sense of responsibility, people are more likely to lose their sense of restraint and their individual identity in exchange for a mob mentality

Bystander Effect: phenomenon in social psychology that a person is less likely to provide help when there are other bystanders

IDENTITY

Personal identity: one's own sense of personal attributes

Social identity: social definitions of who you are

Self-esteem: an individual's overall evaluation of their self-worth

Charles Cooley posited the idea of the looking glass self

George Herbert Mead developed the theory of symbolic interactionism

PERSONALITY

Sigmund Freud developed the psychoanalytic theory of personality, which asserts that our personalities are made up of patterns of thoughts, feelings, and behaviors, and are shaped by our unconscious thoughts, feelings, and memories.

Erik Erikson extended Freud's theory of developmental stages by emphasizing social and interpersonal factors and by including stages through adulthood, to supplement Freud's focus on early childhood.

Carl Rogers developed the humanistic theory of personality development.

Behaviorist perspective: based on the theory of operant conditioning, the deterministic view of personality that personality is shaped completely by positive and negative reinforcements and punishments

Social cognitive perspective: the belief that our personalities are shaped through conditioning and observational learning

Trait perspective: the belief that our personalities are defined by specific traits; source traits underlie our personality and behavior

THEORIES EXPLAINING BEHAVIOR

Drive-Reduction Theory: theory of motivation that organisms act to reduce physiological drives

Maslow's hierarchy of needs suggests that physiological needs must first be met before higher level needs.

ATTITUDES

Attitudes better predict behavior when

- social influences are reduced
- general, rather than specific, patterns of behavior are observed
- specific, rather than general, attitudes are considered
- self-reflection occurs

Behavior influences attitudes when

- role-playing occurs
- we publicly declare our intentions
- we are trying to justify our efforts

Cognitive dissonance theory explains that we feel tension ("dissonance") whenever we hold two thoughts or beliefs ("cognitions") that are incompatible, or when attitudes and behaviors don't match.

PSYCHOLOGICAL DISORDERS

See Chapter 22, Table 2

LANGUAGE

Behaviorist Model: The theory of language acquisition that states that infants are trained to acquire language through operant conditioning.

Noam Chomsky proposed that we all possess an innate ability to learn language through exposure to language before the critical period.

Broca's area: brain region responsible for speech or language production

Wernicke's area: brain region responsible for language comprehension (verbal and written)

LEARNING

Nonassociative Learning: learning that results from exposure to a repeated stimulus, including habituation, dishabituation, sensitization, and desensitization

Associative Learning: learning in which an association is formed, which includes classical conditioning (one stimulus is paired with another, Pavlov) and operant conditioning (reinforcement or punishment changes the likelihood of a behavior occurring again, Skinner)

MEMORY

Encoding: the process of transferring sensory information into memory

Serial position effect: the phenomenon that we are more likely to remember the first and last items in a list, also known as the **primacy effect** and the **recency effect**, respectively

Processes that aid in memory include mnemonics, chunking, and the self-reference effect.

The types of memory: sensory memory (iconic and echoic memory), short-term memory, and long-term memory

RETRIEVAL, FORGETTING, AND ERRORS

Retrieval: the process of locating information in memory; types of retrieval include

- **Free recall:** retrieval without any cues or hints
- **Cued recall:** retrieval with a cue or hint
- **Recognition:** identification of information from a set
- **Priming:** prior activation of certain memory nodes subconsciously affects an individual's response to a stimulus

Anterograde amnesia: an inability to encode new memories

Retrograde amnesia: an inability to recall previously encoded information

Proactive interference: phenomenon in which previously learned information interferes with information learned later

Retroactive interference: phenomenon in which newly learned information interferes with previous information

BEHAVIOR

The **elaboration likelihood model** attempts to explain how people will be influenced or persuaded.

Harry and Margaret Harlow conducted important studies on monkeys to learn about the effects of isolation and social deprivation on development (which was later applied to humans).

Mary Ainsworth conducted experiments on infant attachment and found that parenting style has an impact on whether an infant is securely or insecurely attached.

ATTENTION

Selective Attention: the process by which one input is attended to and the rest are tuned out

The **"cocktail party effect"** occurs when we immediately detect words of importance (such as our name) originating from unattended stimuli.

Divided Attention: occurs when and if we are able to perform multiple tasks simultaneously

COGNITION

WORKING MEMORY

Baddeley's Model of Working Memory (See Chapter 24, Figure 3)

PIAGET'S STAGES OF COGNITIVE DEVELOPMENT

Stage	Age	Hallmarks
Sensorimotor Stage	0–1.5/2	Infants experience world through senses/movement; object permanence marks transition to 2nd stage
Preoperational Stage	1.5/2–7	Children learn that symbols represent things, but they still lack logical reasoning; children are egocentric
Concrete Operational Stage	7–12	Children think logically about concrete events, learn mathematical concepts, obtain principle of conservation
Formal Operational Stage:	12–adulthood	Ability to think about abstract concepts, gain skills such as logical thought, deductive reasoning, and systematic planning

PROBLEM-SOLVING TERMS TO KNOW

Trial and error: a problem-solving technique that involves employing repeated, varied attempts until a problem is solved

Algorithm: a problem-solving technique that involves employing a step-by-step procedure to solve a problem

Heuristics: a problem-solving technique that involves employing mental shortcuts to solve a problem

Insight: experienced as a sudden flash of inspiration to help us solve a problem

Confirmation bias: the tendency to only seek information that confirms what we believe, and ignore information that refutes our beliefs

Fixation: a type of limitation on problem-solving in which an individual is unable to see the problem from a fresh perspective

Mental set: a type of limitation on problem-solving in which an individual fixates on solutions that worked in the past though they may not apply to the current problem

Functional fixedness: the tendency to perceive the functions of objects as fixed and unchanging

Belief bias: the tendency to judge arguments based on what we believe about their conclusions rather than on whether they use sound logic

Belief perseverance: the tendency to cling to beliefs despite the presence of contrary evidence

Overconfidence: the tendency of most people to overestimate the accuracy of our knowledge and judgments

CONSCIOUSNESS

Consciousness: an awareness that we have of our internal states, the environment, and ourselves

Alertness and arousal: the ability to remain attentive to what is going on; controlled by the reticular formation (or reticular activating system, RAS)

Sleep Stage	EEG	EMG	EOG
Stage 1	Theta waves (waves of low to moderate intensity and intermediate frequency)	moderate activity	Slow rolling eye movements
Stage 2	Theta waves interspersed with K-complexes and sleep spindles	moderate activity	No eye movement
Stage 3	Slow wave sleep, characterized by delta waves (high amplitude, low frequency waves)	moderate activity	No eye movement
REM	Beta waves, most similar to those seen during wakefulness, dreaming occurs in this stage	Little to no activity	Quick bursts of eye movement

Dyssomnias: abnormalities in the amount, quality, or timing of sleep

Parasomnias: abnormal behaviors that occur during sleep

Consciousness altering drugs alter actions at the neuronal synapses, enhancing, dampening, or mimicking the activity of the brain's natural neurotransmitters.

EMOTION

Universal emotions are expressed by all normal humans, regardless of culture, including: happiness, sadness, fear, surprise, anger, and disgust.

The **limbic system** in the brain is primarily responsible for the experience of emotion. See Chapter 24, Figure 7 for the three major theories of emotion.

GENERAL CHEMISTRY

MOLE RELATIONSHIPS

A **mole** is a unit of amount, equal to Avogadro's number of things, or 6.02×10^{23}

$$\text{Moles} = \frac{\text{mass}}{\text{molar mass}}$$

Percent composition by mass: $= \dfrac{\text{Mass of element}}{\text{Mass of compound}} \times 100\ (\%)$

Mole fraction: $\dfrac{\text{\# of mol of compound}}{\text{total \# of moles in system}}$†

Molarity: $\dfrac{\text{\# of mol of solute}}{\text{liter of solution}}$†

NUCLEAR AND ATOMIC STRUCTURE

$$^{\text{mass number (protons + neutrons) } A}_{\text{atomic number (\# of protons) } Z}\!X$$

Molar mass: the mass in grams of one mole (mol) of a given element or compound; expressed in terms of g/mol

Isotopes: atoms with the same number of protons but different numbers of neutrons

The Bohr atom: Electrons reside in discrete energy levels around the nucleus. Electrons can absorb energy and move to higher levels of energy or lose energy as photons and settle to lower energy states: $E_{\text{photon}} = hf = hc/(\lambda)$.

Principal quantum number (n): The larger the integer value of n, the higher the energy level and radius of the electron's orbit. The maximum number of electrons in energy level n is $2n^2$.

ELECTRON CONFIGURATION

Electrons are filled in order, from top to bottom, left to right, along the periodic table. The shell in which electrons fall is dictated by their row. The subshell is dictated by their block. For s and p electrons, $n = $ # of row, for d electrons, $n = $ row # − 1, and for f electrons $n = $ row # − 2.

Hund's rule: within a given subshell, half-fill orbitals with electrons before pairing; maximize parallel spins

Valence electrons: electrons of an atom that are in its outer energy shell or that are available for bonding

Unstable nuclei decay, becoming new stable nuclei through the emission of a number of different particles (α, β, γ, etc.). In any nuclear chemistry reaction, the total mass and total atomic number in the reactants must equal the total mass and atomic number of the products.

Summary of Radioactive Decay		
N−2, Z−2	Alpha Decay	$^{A}_{Z}X \xrightarrow{\ \alpha\ } {}^{A-4}_{Z-2}Y + {}^{4}_{2}\alpha$
N−1, Z+1	Beta⁻Decay	$^{A}_{Z}X \xrightarrow{\ \beta^{-}\ } {}^{A}_{Z+1}Y + {}^{0}_{-1}\beta^{-}$
N+1, Z−1	Positron Emission	$^{A}_{Z}X \xrightarrow{\ \beta^{+}\ } {}^{A}_{Z-1}Y + {}^{0}_{+1}\beta^{+}$
N+1, Z−1	Electron Capture	$^{A}_{Z}X + {}^{0}_{-1}e^{-} \xrightarrow{\ EC\ } {}^{A}_{Z-1}Y$
N & Z remain the same	Gamma Decay	Decreases energy of an excited nucleus $^{A}_{Z}X^{*} \xrightarrow{\ \gamma\ } {}^{A}_{Z}X + \gamma$

Half-life: the amount of time it takes a sample of radioactive material to decay to half its original mass

$$M_t = \frac{M_0}{2^{T/t_{1/2}}}$$

Where M_t = final amount of isotope, M_0 = initial amount of isotope T = total decay time, $t_{1/2}$ = half-life

BONDING AND INTERMOLECULAR FORCES

Formal charge $=$ Valence electrons $-\dfrac{1}{2}N_{bonding} - N_{nonbonding}$

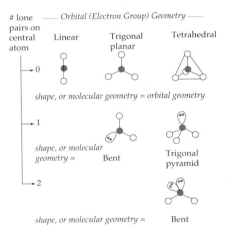

lone pairs on central atom — Orbital (Electron Group) Geometry —

Linear, Trigonal planar, Tetrahedral

0 — *shape, or molecular geometry = orbital geometry*

1 — *shape, or molecular geometry =* Bent, Trigonal pyramid

2 — *shape, or molecular geometry =* Bent

Hydrogen bonding: The partial positive charge of a H atom bonded to an F, O, or N atom interacts with the partial negative charge located on the electronegative atoms (F, O, N) of nearby molecules.

Dipole-dipole interactions: Polar molecules orient themselves such that the positive region of one molecule is close to the negative region of another molecule.

Dispersion forces: The bonding electrons in covalent bonds may appear to be equally shared between two atoms, but at any point in time they will be located randomly throughout the orbital. This permits unequal sharing of electrons, causing rapid polarization and counter-polarization of the electron clouds of neighboring molecules, inducing the formation of more dipoles.

Strength of IMFs: ion-ion > ion-dipole > hydrogen bonds > dipole-dipole > dipole-induced dipole > London dispersion (instantaneous dipole-induced dipole)

Bond order	Single	Double	Triple
Bond type	Sigma	Sigma / pi	Sigma / 2 pi
Hybridization	sp^3	sp^2	sp
Angles	109.5º	120º	180º
Example	C-C	C=C	C≡C

PERIODIC TRENDS

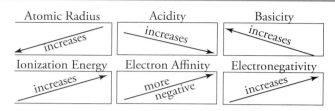

electronegativity of some common atoms:

$$F > O > (N \approx Cl) > Br > (I \approx S \approx C) > H$$

THERMODYNAMICS AND THERMOCHEMISTRY

First Law of Thermodynamics: $E_{universe}$ is constant. $\Delta E = Q - W$

Second Law of Thermodynamics: In any thermodynamic process that moves from one equilibrium to another, the entropy of the universe will either increase or remain unchanged.

Third Law of Thermodynamics: $S = 0$ for pure crystal at $T/0$ K; standard conditions (25°C or 298 K, and 1 atm) used when measuring standard enthalpy, entropy, Gibbs free energy, and voltage

Specific heat (c): the amount of energy required to raise 1 g of a substance by 1°Celsius

$q = mc\Delta T$, where q is the heat absorbed or released in a given process, m is the mass, c is the specific heat, and ΔT is the change in temperature

$q > 0$ means heat is gained,

$q < 0$ means heat is lost [units: joules or calories]

Enthalpy (H) is used to express heat changes at constant pressure. $\Delta H < 0$, exothermic, $\Delta H > 0$, endothermic. Enthalpy is a state function, and independent of path.

Standard heat of formation ($\Delta H°_f$): the enthalpy change that would occur if one mole of a compound were formed directly from its elements in their standard states

Standard heat of reaction ($\Delta H°_{rxn}$): the hypothetical enthalpy change that would occur if the reaction were carried out under standard conditions

$$\Delta H°_{rxn} = (\text{sum of } \Delta H°_f \text{ of products}) - (\text{sum of } \Delta H°_f \text{ of reactants})$$

Heat of phase change: the quantity of heat required to change the phase of 1 mol of a substance

Hess's Law states that enthalpies of reactions are additive.

The reverse of any reaction has an enthalpy of the same magnitude as that of the forward reaction, but its sign is opposite.

Bond dissociation energy: an average of the energy required to break a particular type of bond in one mole of gaseous molecules

Entropy (S): the measure of the disorder, or randomness, of a system

$$\Delta S \text{ universe} = \Delta S \text{ system} + \Delta S \text{ surroundings}$$

Gibbs free energy (G) combines the two factors that affect the spontaneity of a reaction—changes in enthalpy, ΔH, and changes in entropy, ΔS.

$$\Delta G = \Delta H - T\Delta S$$

If $\Delta G < 0$, then rxn is spontaneous.

If $\Delta G > 0$, then rxn is not spontaneous.

If $\Delta G = 0$, the system is in a state of equilibrium; thus $\Delta H = T\Delta S$.

ΔH	ΔS	Outcome
−	+	Spontaneous at all temps
+	−	Nonspontaneous at all temps
+	+	Spontaneous only at high temps
−	−	Spontaneous only at low temps

$$\Delta G° = -RT\ln K_c$$

GASES

1 atm = 760 mm Hg = 760 torr   °C + 273 = K

STP (0°C or 273 K, and 1 atm) used for gas law calculations

Boyle's Law: $PV = k$ or $P_1 V_1 = P_2 V_2$

Charles's Law: $\dfrac{V}{T} = k$ or $\dfrac{V_1}{T_1} = \dfrac{V_2}{T_2}$

Avogadro's Law: $\dfrac{n_1}{V_1} = \dfrac{n_2}{V_2}$

Combined Gas Law: $P_1 V_1 / T_1 = P_2 V_2 / T_2$

Ideal Gas Law: $PV = nRT$

van der Waals: $\left(P + \dfrac{an^2}{V^2}\right)(V - nb) = nRT$

Dalton's Law of Partial Pressures: $P_{tot} = \sum p_i$

Graham's Law of Effusion: $\dfrac{\text{rate of effusion of gas 2}}{\text{rate of effusion of gas 1}} = \sqrt{\dfrac{m_1}{m_2}}$

KINETICS

The following factors affect reaction rates: reactant concentrations, temperature, surface area, catalysts.

Catalysts increase reaction rate without being consumed by lowering the E_a.

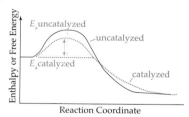

Experimental determination of rate law: The values of k, x, and y in the rate law equation (rate $= k [A]^x [B]^y$) must be determined experimentally for a given reaction at a given temperature. The rate is usually measured as a function of the initial concentrations of the reactants, A and B.

Rate determining step (RDS): The slowest step in a reaction mechanism, used to write the rate law if given a reaction mechanism. The coefficients of reactants in the RDS become the order of reaction with respect to their concentrations. For example, if the RDS is $A + 2B \rightarrow C$, then rate $= k[A][B]^2$.

Average rate of reaction:

$$-\frac{1}{\text{coeff}} \frac{\Delta[\text{reactant}]}{\text{time}} \quad \text{or} \quad +\frac{1}{\text{coeff}} \frac{\Delta[\text{product}]}{\text{time}}$$

Arrhenius equation: $k = Ae^{-E_a/RT}$

EQUILIBRIUM

Law of mass action

$$a\,A + b\,B \rightleftharpoons c\,C + d\,D$$

$$K_c = \frac{[C]^c [D]^d}{[A]^a [B]^b}$$

K_c is the equilibrium constant (c stands for concentration).

K_p is used when reactants and products are gases and partial pressures replace molar concentrations in the K expression.

Q is the reaction quotient, obtained from using nonequilibrium concentrations in the K ratio.

Properties of the Equilibrium Constant

- Pure solids/liquids don't appear in expression.
- K_{eq} is constant at a given temperature.
- If $K_{eq} \gg 1$, equilibrium reaction mixture will have more products than reactants.
- If $K_{eq} \ll 1$, equilibrium reaction mixture will have more reactants than products.
- If K_{eq} is close to 1, an equilibrium mixture will contain approximately equal amounts of reactants and products.

Le Châtelier's Principle: When a stress is imposed on a reaction at equilibrium, the reaction will respond to relieve the stress and re-establish equilibrium. Stresses must change the Q of the reaction. These stresses include: changing the concentration of any reactant or product in the K expression, changing the volume of the container (for gaseous systems only), or changing the temperature of the reaction.

$Q < K$, reaction shifts towards products

$Q = K$, reaction is at equilibrium

$Q > K$, reaction shifts toward reactants

ACIDS AND BASES

Brønsted definition: acid = proton donor; base = proton acceptor

Lewis definition: acid = e^- pair acceptor; base = e^- pair donor

Neutralization: Acids and bases neutralize each other, forming a salt and (often, but not always) water.

$$a \times [A] \times V_A = b \times [B] \times V_B$$

where a = # of H^+ in the acid; b = # of OH^- in the base

$$H_2O(l) \rightleftharpoons H^+(aq) + OH^-(aq) \qquad K_w = [H^+][OH^-] = 10^{-14} \text{ at } 25°C$$

$$pH = -\log[H^+] \qquad pOH = -\log[OH^-] \qquad pH + pOH = 14 \text{ at } 25°C$$

$$K_a = \frac{[H_3O^+][A^-]}{[HA]} \qquad pK_a = -\log K_a \qquad K_a K_b = K_w$$
$$\text{(for a conjugate pair)}$$

$$K_b = \frac{[BH^+][OH^-]}{[B]} \qquad pK_b = -\log K_b$$

Henderson-Hasselbalch equation: used to calculate the pH or pOH of a buffer solution

$$pH = pK_a + \log \frac{[A^-]}{[HA]} \qquad pOH = pK_b + \log \frac{[BH^+]}{[B]}$$

Titration

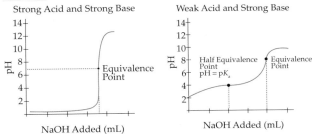

Strong Acid and Strong Base / Weak Acid and Strong Base

Titration is a procedure used to determine the molarity of an acid or base by reacting a known volume of solution of an unknown concentration with a known volume of a solution of a known concentration.

REDOX REACTIONS AND ELECTROCHEMISTRY

Rules for determining oxidation state (OS):[1]

1) OS of pure element = 0
2) sum of OS's = 0 in neutral molecule, or charge on ion
3) Group 1 metals: $OS = +1$
   Group 2 metals: $OS = +2$
4) OS of F = -1
5) OS of H = $+1$
6) OS of O = -2
7) OS of halogens = -1; of O family = -2

Rule higher in list takes precedence if rules contradict.

Oxidation: loss of electrons; **Reduction:** gain of electrons

Oxidizing agent: causes another atom to undergo oxidation, and is itself reduced

Reducing agent: causes another atom to be reduced, and is itself oxidized

Galvanic cell: Electrons flow spontaneously from the anode to the cathode: $E_{cell}° > 0$.

Electrolytic cell: Electron flow must be forced by an external power source from the anode to the cathode; the reaction is nonspontaneous. The sum of the oxidation potential at the anode and the reduction potential at the cathode is negative: $E_{cell}° < 0$.

Faraday's Law of Electrolysis:

The amount of chemical charge is proportional to the amount of electricity that flows through the cell.

$$\Delta G = -nFE_{cell} \qquad F = \text{faraday} = 96,500 \text{ C/mol } e^-$$

Nernst equation: $E = E° - \dfrac{0.06}{n} \log Q$

PHASES AND PHASE CHANGES

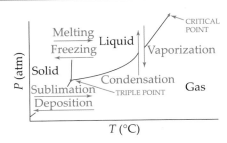

These rules work 99 percent of the time.

ORGANIC CHEMISTRY

NOMENCLATURE

- Find the longest carbon chain containing the most oxidized functional group.
- Number the carbon chain so that the principle functional group gets the lowest number (1).
- Proceed to number the chain so that the lowest set of numbers is obtained for the substituents.
- Name the substituents and assign each a number.

#'s of Cs	IUPAC base name	#'s of Cs	IUPAC base name
1	meth-	6	hex-
2	eth-	7	hept-
3	prop-	8	oct-
4	but-	9	non-
5	pent-	10	dec-

List substituents in alphabetical order, place commas between numbers and dashes between numbers and words.

Functional Group	Suffix	Functional Group	Suffix
Carboxyl	-oic acid	Ketone	-one
Ester	-oate	Thiol	-thiol
Acyl halide	-oyl halide	Alcohol	-ol
Amide	-amide	Amine	-amine
Nitrile	-nitrile	Imine	-imine
Aldehyde	-al	Ether	-ether
Alkene	-ene	Alkyne	-yne

Nitrogen Containing Compounds

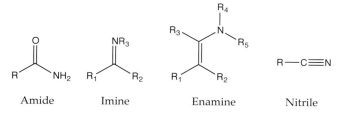

| Amide | Imine | Enamine | Nitrile |

R/S CONFIGURATION AND E/Z NOTATION

For chiral centers, assign priority to each substituent:
- Give highest priority to group with highest atomic number, then atomic weight.
- Go to first point of difference on chains.
- Count multiple bonds as higher priority.
- With #4 group in back of molecule, a clockwise trace of groups $1 \rightarrow 2 \rightarrow 3$ is R; a counterclockwise trace is S.
- For alkenes, if highest priority groups are on the same side of bond = Z; if on opposite = E.

ISOMERIC RELATIONSHIPS

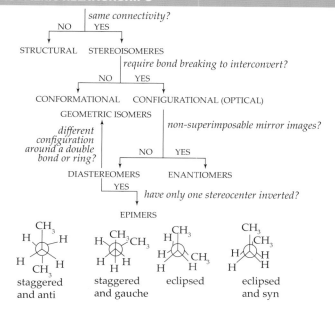

STABILIZATION/REACTIVITY

Induction: electron deficient groups like carbocations are more stable when substituted by electron-donating alkyl groups.

$$\oplus CH_3 < H_3C-\overset{H}{\underset{\oplus}{\overset{|}{C}}}-H < H_3C-\overset{H}{\underset{\oplus}{\overset{|}{C}}}-CH_3 < H_3C-\overset{CH_3}{\underset{\oplus}{\overset{|}{C}}}-CH_3$$

Electron rich groups (carbanions) are more stable when less substituted, or when adjacent to electron withdrawing groups.

$$\ominus CH_3 > H_3C-\overset{H}{\underset{\ominus}{\overset{|}{C}}}-H > H_3C-\overset{H}{\underset{\ominus}{\overset{|}{C}}}-CH_3 > H_3C-\overset{CH_3}{\underset{\ominus}{\overset{|}{C}}}-CH_3 \left(\text{and } CF_3\overset{\ominus}{CH_2} > CH_3\overset{\ominus}{CH_2} \right)$$

Resonance: Compounds can be stabilized through delocalization of π electrons and charge if the charge is adjacent to the π bond. More resonance structures generally leads to more stability.

Leaving groups (weak bases best) $I^- > Br^- > Cl^-$

Nucleophilicity and basicity

$$CH_3^- > NH_2^- > RO^- \approx HO^- > RCO_2^- > ROH \approx H_2O$$

Nucleophicity $I^- > Br^- > Cl^-$

Oxidation of Alcohols

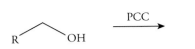

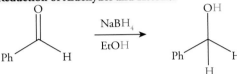

Hydride Reduction of Aldehydes and Ketones

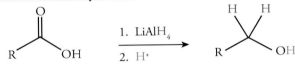

Reduction of Carboxylic Acids

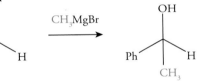

Grignard Reaction

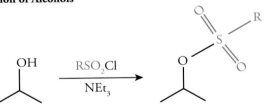

Protection of Alcohols

Acetal Formation

Cyanohydrin Formation

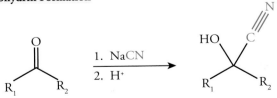

Imine Formation

Enamine Formation

Aldol Condensation

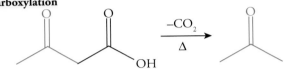

Decarboxylation

Acid halide can only be synthesized from acid directly.

$$RCOOH + SOCl_2 \longrightarrow$$

Esterification

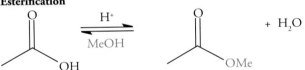

Saponification

$$+ MeOH$$

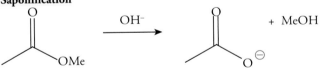

Unimolecular Substitution (S$_N$1)

racemic mixture

Bimolecular Substitution (S$_N$2)

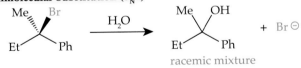

Strecker Synthesis of Amino Acids

AMINO ACIDS, PEPTIDES, AND PROTEINS

Amino acids have four components: amine group, carboxyl group, hydrogen, and R group. They are **amphoteric** (can act as acids or bases).

amino acid   zwitterion

Isoelectric point: the pH at which an amino acid will be in its zwitterionic (overall neutral) form

- For a polar or nonpolar amino acid: pI = ½(pK_a COOH + pK_a NH_3^+)
- If pH > pI, AA is –. If pH < pI, AA is +. If pH = pI, AA is neutral.

Amino Acid Classification	Names	3-letter (1-letter) abbreviations
Acidic	Aspartic acid, Glutamic acid	Asp (D), Glu (E)
Basic	Lysine, Arginine, Histidine	Lys (K), Arg (R), His (H)
Polar	Serine, Cysteine, Tyrosine, Threonine, Asparagine, Glutamine	Ser (S), Cys (C), Tyr (Y), Thr (T), Asn (N), Gln (Q)
Non-polar	Glycine, Alanine, Valine, Leucine, Isoleucine, Phenylalanine, Tryptophan, Methionine, Proline	Gly (G), Ala (A), Val (V), Leu (L), Ile (I), Phe (F), Trp (W), Met (M), Pro (P)

PROTEIN STRUCTURE

Primary: sequence of amino acids; determined by peptide bonds
Secondary: α-helix, β-pleated sheet; backbone H bonds
Tertiary: folding to lowest energy conformation; interactions of R groups (S–S bonds, ionic bonds, van der Waals, H bonds)
Quaternary: association of multiple peptides; H bonds, R groups, disulfide bonds

SUGARS

(D) Sugar   (L) Sugar
OH on Right   OH on Left

α- anomer   β- anomer

OH group down   OH group up

LAB TECHNIQUES

Extraction: separates based on solubility. Compounds with 5 Cs or more with only one polar functional group are more soluble in the organic layer. Compounds with fewer than 5 Cs are more soluble in water.
- RNH_2 extracted with HCl only
- RCOOH extracted with $NaHCO_3$ or NaOH
- PhOH extracted with NaOH only

TLC separates based on polarity.
High polarity = low R_f values   Low polarity = high R_f values
R_f = distance compound travels/distance solvent travels
HPLC separates based on polarity. Reverse-phase HPLC is conventional form (nonpolar components elute first).
GC separates small amounts of material based on boiling point.
High bp comes off column late; Low bp comes off column early.
Size-exclusion: Larger molecules travel around polymer beads and elute first; smaller molecules travel through pores in polymer beads and elute last.
Ion-exchange: cation exchange elutes cations last; anion exchange elutes anions last. Species of the appropriate charge are slowed by electrostatic attractions to polymeric beads in the column.
Distillation separates large amounts of material based on boiling point. Simple: solvents with very different bps; fractional: solvents with similar bps
Electrophoresis separates amino acids or peptides based on their charge at a specific buffered pH
- + charged molecules are attracted to the – end of the gel
- – charged molecules are attracted to the + end of the gel
- zwitterions (neutral species) do not move

Spectroscopy:
IR

Functional group	Wave number
C=O	1720 cm^{-1}
C=C	1650 cm^{-1}
O–H	3200–3600 cm^{-1}
C≡C, C≡N	2100–2260 cm^{-1}

^{1}H NMR—spectrum tells four things about structure.
1. # of nonequivalent Hs = # signals
2. # of nonequivalent neighboring Hs = splitting pattern (follows $n + 1$ rule where n = # neighboring Hs)
3. # of Hs in each signal = integration
4. chemical environment of Hs = chemical shift

PHYSICS

KINEMATICS

Displacement (d): the vector change in position that goes in a straight-line path from the initial position to the final; it is independent of the path taken (SI unit: m)

Distance: the length of the particular path

Average velocity: $\mathbf{v} = \dfrac{\mathbf{d}}{\Delta t}$ (SI units: m/s)

Average speed: $\dfrac{distance}{\Delta t}$

Acceleration: the vector rate of change of an object's velocity; if acceleration is constant (uniform): $\mathbf{a} = \dfrac{\Delta \mathbf{v}}{\Delta t}$ (SI units: m/s²)

Linear motion

$d = vt = \left(\dfrac{v_0 + v}{2}\right)t$

$v = v_0 + at$

$d = v_0 t + \dfrac{1}{2}at^2$

$v^2 = v_0^2 + 2ad$

- To choose an equation, list the given variables and the one you want. The remaining, missing variable tells you which equation to use.
- To find max height, remember that the vertical velocity of the projectile is 0 at the highest point of the path.

Projectile motion

- vertical component of velocity: $v\sin\theta$
- acceleration $= a_y = -g$
- horizontal component of velocity: $v\cos\theta = v_x$ (constant)
- $(d_x = v_x t)$ $R = v_x t$

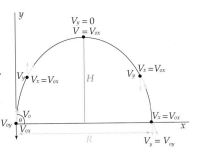

WORK, ENERGY, AND MOMENTUM

Work: For a constant force $\mathbf{F}$ acting on an object that moves through a displacement $\mathbf{d}$, the work is $W = Fd\cos\theta$, where θ is the angle between $\mathbf{F}$ and $\mathbf{d}$. (For a force perpendicular to the displacement, $W = 0$.) [SI unit: joule (J) $= N{\cdot}m$]

Power: The rate at which work is performed, found by using

$$P = \dfrac{W}{t} \text{ (SI unit: watt = J/s) or } P = Fv\cos\theta$$

Kinetic energy is the energy associated with moving objects. It is found by using $KE = \dfrac{1}{2}mv^2$ (SI unit: J).

Potential energy is the energy associated with a body's position, well defined only as a change between initial and final positions. The change in gravitational potential energy of an object is expressed as $\Delta PE = mg\Delta h$ (SI unit: J).

Work-Energy Theorem: Relates the work performed by all forces acting on a body in a particular time interval to the change in kinetic energy during that time. The expression is $W_{TOTAL} = \Delta KE$.

Conservation of Energy: When there are not any nonconservative forces (such as friction) acting on a system, the total mechanical energy remains constant: $\Delta E = \Delta KE + \Delta PE = 0$.

Momentum is a vector quantity. It's given by $\mathbf{p} = m\mathbf{v}$ (SI unit: kg·m/s).

Impulse is a vector quantity. It's given by $\mathbf{J} = \Delta\mathbf{p} = \mathbf{F}_{ave}\Delta t$.

Conservation of momentum: When there are no net external forces acting on a system of objects (e.g., during a collision), total momentum is conserved: $\mathbf{p}_{TOTAL\,before} = \mathbf{p}_{TOTAL\,after}$.

Elastic collision is a collision where KE is conserved.

Inelastic collision is a collision where KE is not conserved.

Perfectly inelastic collision is a collision where the objects stick and move together.

NEWTON'S LAWS

Newton's First Law (law of inertia): A body in a state of constant velocity motion or at rest will remain in that state unless acted upon by a net force.

Newton's Second Law: When a net force is applied to a body of mass m, the body will be accelerated in the same direction as the force applied to the mass. This is expressed by the formula $\mathbf{F}_{net} = m\mathbf{a}$ (SI unit: newton (N) = kg·m/s²).

Newton's Third Law: If body A exerts a force on body B, then B will exert a force back onto A that is equal in magnitude, but opposite in direction. This can be expressed as $\mathbf{F}_{b\,on\,a} = -\mathbf{F}_{a\,on\,b}$.

Newton's Law of Gravitation: All masses experience an attractive force to other masses. The magnitude of this force is represented by $F_g = \dfrac{Gm_1m_2}{r^2}$.

FRICTIONAL FORCES

Static friction (f_s) is the force that must be overcome to set an object in motion. If the applied force is less than the maximum frictional force, f_s max $= \mu_s F_N$, then $f_s = F_{applied}$.

Kinetic friction (f_k) opposes the motion of objects moving relative to each other. It has the formula $f_k = \mu_k N$.

UNIFORM CIRCULAR MOTION:

F_c is the force needed to keep an object moving in a circular motion. It is equal to the net force acting on an object toward its center of revolution.

$a_c = \dfrac{v^2}{r}$

$F_c = \dfrac{mv^2}{r}$

CENTER OF MASS AND TORQUE

Center of mass: the location where a system of objects would balance:

$x_{cm} = \dfrac{m_1 x_1 + m_2 x_2 + \ldots}{m_1 + m_2 + \ldots}$

Torque: For a force acting on an object at a distance r from its pivot point, $\tau = rF\sin\theta$, where θ is the angle between $\mathbf{F}$ and $\mathbf{r}$. [SI units: newton-meter $(N-m)$]

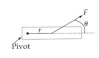

THERMODYNAMICS

Heat Q: $Q > 0$ for heat transferred into a system; $Q < 0$ for heat transferred out of a system (SI units: joules)

The internal energy of a system is proportional to its temperature:

$$E \propto T \text{ (SI units: kelvins = K)}$$

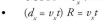

The First Law of Thermodynamics states that the internal energy of a system is equal to the heat input into the system minus the work done by the system, which is expressed as $\Delta E = Q - W$.

The work done by an ideal gas is expressed as: $W = P\Delta V$.

The four thermodynamics processes for an ideal gas are

- Isochoric: V = constant
- Isobaric: P = constant
- Isothermal: T = constant
- Adiabatic: $Q = 0$

FLUIDS

Density $\rho = \dfrac{m}{V}$, where V is volume [SI units: kg/m³]

Pressure: a scalar quantity defined as force per unit area:

$$P = \frac{F}{A} \quad \text{[SI Units: pascal (Pa) = N/m²]}$$

- **Standard atmospheric pressure:** $P_{atm} \spadesuit 10^5 \, \text{Pa}$
- **Gauge pressure:** $P_{gauge} = \rho g d$
- **Absolute pressure:** In a static fluid due to gravity, a depth d below the surface is given by:

$$P = P_0 + \rho g d, \text{ where } P_0 \text{ is the pressure at the surface.}$$

Buoyant force: the upward force exerted by a fluid on an object totally or partially submerged, equal to the weight of the displaced fluid:

$$F_b = \rho_{fluid} V_{submerged} g$$

Flow rate: $f = Av$ [SI unit: m³/s]

Continuity equation: $A_1 v_1 = A_2 v_2$

Bernoulli's equation: $P + \dfrac{1}{2}\rho v^2 + \rho g h$ = constant

ELECTROSTATICS

Coulomb's Law

$$F = \frac{k q_1 q_2}{r^2}$$

[SI units: newtons]

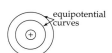

Opposite charges attract;
like charges repel.

Electric field

$$E = \frac{F}{q} = \frac{kq}{r^2}$$

[SI units: N/C or V/m]

field lines

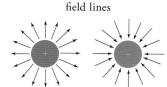

- A positive point charge will move in the same direction as the electric field vector; a negative charge will move in the opposite direction.

Electric potential (φ)

$$\varphi = \frac{PE}{q} = \frac{kq}{r} \quad \text{[SI unit: volts (V) = J/C]}$$

equipotential curves

Electric potential energy (PE)

The electric potential energy stored by two point charges:

$$PE = \frac{k q_1 q_2}{r}$$

Work done by the electrostatic force = $-\Delta PE = -q\Delta\varphi$
Work done against the electrostatic force = $+\Delta PE = +q\Delta\varphi$

DC AND AC CIRCUITS

DIRECT CURRENT

Current: the flow of electric charge. Current is given by:

$$I = \frac{\Delta q}{\Delta t} \quad \text{[SI units: amp (A) = C/s]}$$

(The direction of current is the direction positive charge would flow, or from high to low potential.)

Ohm's Law and resistance

$V = IR$ (can be applied to entire circuit or individual resistors)

Resistance: opposition to the flow of charge; $R = \dfrac{\rho L}{A}$ (Resistance increases with increasing temperatures with most conductors.)

[SI Units: ohm (Ω) = V/A]

CIRCUIT LAWS

Kirchhoff's laws:

1. Elements in series have the same current.
2. Elements in parallel have the same voltage.

Alternating current

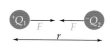

$$V_{rms} = \frac{V_{max}}{\sqrt{2}}$$

$$I_{rms} = \frac{V_{max}}{\sqrt{2}}$$

$$P_{avg} = I_{rms} V_{rms}$$

Series circuits

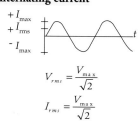

$$R_{eq} = R_1 + R_2 + R_3 + \ldots$$
$$I = I_1 = I_2 = I_3 = \ldots$$
$$V = V_1 + V_2 + V_3 + \ldots$$

Parallel circuits

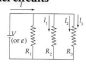

$1/R_{eq} = 1/R_1 + 1/R_2 + 1/R_3$
For two resistors:

$$R_{eq} = \frac{R_1 R_2}{R_1 + R_2}$$

$I = I_1 + I_2 + I_3 + \ldots$
$V = V_1 = V_2 = V_3 = \ldots$

Power dissipated by resistors

$$P = IV = \frac{V^2}{R} = I^2 R$$

(Can be applied to entire circuit or individual resistors)

CAPACITORS

Capacitance is the ability to store charge per unit voltage. It is given by:

$C = \dfrac{Q}{V}$. [SI unit: farad(F) = C/V]

Capacitors in parallel add:
$C_{eq} = C_1 + C_2 + C_3$

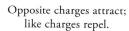

Energy stored by capacitors: $P_E = \dfrac{1}{2}QV = \dfrac{1}{2}CV^2 = \dfrac{1}{2}Q^2 / $

Electric field between the capacitor plates: $V = Ed$

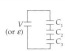

Adding a dielectric always increases the capacitance:

$$C = \kappa \frac{\varepsilon_0 A}{d}$$

Capacitors in series add as reciprocals:

$$\frac{1}{C_{eq}} = \frac{1}{C_1} + \frac{1}{C_2} + \frac{1}{C_3} \cdots$$

MAGNETISM

Right-hand rule for direction of B field produced by current-carrying wires

- Right thumb points in the direction of current flow.
- Wrap your fingers around the wire as if you were grabbing it with your palm.
- The direction that the fingers curl is the direction of the magnetic field.

[SI Units = tesla (T) = N·s/m·C]

Force on a moving charge

A charge moving in a magnetic field experiences a force.

$F_B = qvB\sin\theta$ where θ is the angle between **v** and **B**

The magnetic force is zero when charges move parallel or antiparallel to the magnetic field.

Right-hand rule for finding direction of force

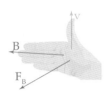

Note that the right-hand rule gives the direction of magnetic force on a positive charge. The direction of force on a negative charge is simply the opposite direction of the force on a positive charge (or you may use a left-hand rule).

PERIODIC MOTION

Period: T is the time it takes to complete one cycle.

Frequency: $f = \frac{1}{T}$ [SI unit: hertz (Hz)=1/s]

Simple harmonic motion is periodic motion where the period (and frequency) are independent of amplitude.

Mass spring: $F_s = -kx,\ PE = \frac{1}{2}kx^2,\ f = \frac{1}{2\pi}\sqrt{\frac{k}{m}}$

Pendulum: only simple harmonic for small angles, $f = \frac{1}{2\pi}\sqrt{\frac{g}{L}}$

WAVES

Wavelength: λ is the distance between corresponding points on consecutive pulses.

$v = f\lambda$: (1) v is the same for all waves in the same medium; (2) f is constant when a wave passes into a new medium.

Waves in a string: $v = \sqrt{\dfrac{tension}{mass/length}}$

STANDING WAVES

String attached at each end: $\lambda_n = \frac{2L}{n}$ $(n = 1, 2, \ldots)$

Open pipe: $\lambda_n = \frac{2L}{n}$ $(n = 1, 2, \ldots)$ **Closed pipe:** $\lambda_n = \frac{4L}{n}$ $(1, 3, 5 \ldots)$

SOUND

Sound propagates through a deformable medium by the oscillation of particles along the direction of the wave's motion; this longitudinal pressure wave travels slowest in gases, fastest in solids.

Intensity (I) = P/A [SI units: W/m^2]

Sound level = $10 \log \left(\frac{I}{I_0}\right)$ [unit = decibel = (dB)] I_0 (threshold of hearing) = 10^{-12} W/m^2

Adding 10 dB corresponds to multiplying the intensity by 10. Subtracting 10 dB corresponds to dividing the intensity by 10.

Beats occur when two waves that have slightly different frequencies are superimposed: $f_{beat} = |f_1 - f_2|$

Doppler effect: When a source and a detector move relative to one another, the detected frequency of the sound received differs from the frequency emitted by the source.

$$f' = f \frac{(v \pm v_D)}{(v \mp v_S)}$$

LIGHT AND OPTICS

Light is an Electromagnetic (EM) Wave. EM Waves do not need a medium.

Speed of light in a vacuum: $c = 3 \times 10^8$ m/s

Energy of a photon (light particle): $E = hf$

Refraction:

$$n = \frac{c}{v} \quad (\text{speed of light} = 3 \times 10^8 \text{ m/s})$$

Snell's Law: $n_1 \sin\theta_1 = n_2 \sin\theta_2$ when $n_2 > n_1$, light bends toward normal, when $n_2 < n_1$, light bends away from normal.

Spherical Mirrors and Lenses

Mirror / lens equation: $\frac{1}{o} + \frac{1}{i} = \frac{1}{i}$

- o is always positive.
- i is positive for real images and negative for virtual images.

Magnification equation: $m = \frac{-i}{o}$

- m is positive for upright images and negative for inverted images.
- All real images are inverted; all virtual images are upright.

Spherical mirrors

- Real images are formed on the same side of the object.
- Virtual images are formed on the side opposite the object.

Thin spherical lenses

- Real images are formed on the side opposite the object.
- Virtual images are formed on the same side as the object.

CRITICAL ANALYSIS AND REASONING SKILLS

WORKING THE PASSAGE: ACTIVE READING BASICS

- Preview and highlight the question stems for references to passage content.
- Highlight the passage with a purpose: limit largely to question topics and words indicating tone and logical structure.
- Read for the major claims made by the author; skim over the evidence supporting those claims.
- Don't try to memorize the passage: treat it like an open book test.
- Don't get bogged down in the details or in rereading large sections: keep moving!
- Define the main point of each chunk or paragraph
- Think about how the chunks relate to each other as you read.
- Define the Bottom Line of the passage, including the author's tone/attitude.
- Pacing goal: 3–5 minutes for your first reading of the passage text.

QUESTION TYPES AND STRATEGIES

Question Type	Sample Wording	Strategy Tips	Common Types of Wrong Answers
1. Specific: Retrieval	"According to the passage, what is true of 'X'?" "The author states that 'X' is:"	• Go back to the passage first: find and paraphrase the relevant information.	• uses similar language as passage but changes meaning • supported by passage but doesn't answer question • too strong to be supported by passage • relies too much on speculation or outside knowledge
2. Specific: Inference	"The passage implies/suggests/ assumes that…" "Based on the passage, it is reasonable to conclude/infer that…" "With which of the following statements would the author be most likely to agree?"	• Go back to passage as soon as possible to find and paraphrase relevant information. • Answer in your own words.	
3. General: Main Point/Primary Purpose	"Which of the following best expresses the main point of the passage?" "The author's primary purpose in the passage is to:"	• Use your Bottom Line, including author's tone.	• too narrow • too broad • wrong tone
4. General: Overall Tone/ Attitude	"The author's apparent attitude towards 'X' can best be described as…"	• Use your Bottom Line. • Look for tone indicators you have highlighted in passage.	• positive or negative tone for a neutral passage • opposite tone (e.g., negative instead of positive) • too strong/extreme
5. Reasoning: Structure	"The author of the passage states 'X' in order to…" "The author's claim 'X' is based on evidence that:"	• Go back to the passage before POE. • Determine if the statement is a conclusion or evidence for a conclusion. • Pay attention to context of the cited statement.	• references wrong part of the author's argument • can be inferred from the passage, but doesn't describe logical structure
6. Reasoning: Evaluate	"How well supported is the author's claim that 'X'?"	• Go back to the passage and find the cited claim (or, if the question asks about the passage as a whole, remind yourself of the Bottom Line). • Use your highlighting to help locate the support, if any, given for claim.	• incorrectly describes logical structure of argument • opposite evaluation (e.g., strongly rather than weakly supported)
7. Application: Strengthen	"Which of the following, if true, most strengthens the passage author's argument?"	• Go back to the passage; find and paraphrase the relevant claim. • Define the necessary issue and direction (consistent or inconsistent with passage) of the correct choice.	• opposite • not relevant to cited claim • not strong enough to have a significant impact
8. Application: Weaken	"Which of the following statements, if true, most *weakens/ undermines/calls into question* the author's argument in the passage?"		
9. Application: New Information	"Elsewhere, the author of the passage states 'X.' Given the information in the passage, this is most likely due to:"	• Summarize theme of new info. • Define the relationship of new info to relevant parts of the passage/ Bottom Line.	• not relevant to new info and/or the passage • relevant only to wrong part of passage • incorrectly describes the impact or relevance of the new information on or to passage
10. Application: Analogy	"Which of the following relationships is most similar to 'X' as it is described in the passage?"	• Go back to passage; define the theme or logic of the relevant part of the passage.	• similar content but different logic • incomplete match • reverses/opposite of passage logic